PATHOLOGY

SECOND EDITION

Alan Stevens

MBBS FRCPath

Senior Lecturer in Histopathology,
University of Nottingham Medical School

Honorary Consultant Histopathologist
to Queen's Medical Centre,

University Hospital NHS Trust, Nottingham, UK

James Lowe

BMedSci, BMBS, DM, FRCPath

Professor of Neuropathology,
University of Nottingham Medical School

Honorary Consultant Histopathologist
to Queen's Medical Centre,

University Hospital NHS Trust, Nottingham, UK

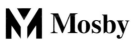 Mosby

EDINBURGH LONDON NEW YORK PHILADELPHIA ST LOUIS SYDNEY TORONTO 2000

MOSBY
An imprint of Harcourt Publishers Limited

© Harcourt Publishers Limited 2000

M is a registered trademark of Harcourt Publishers Limited

The rights of Alan Stevens and James Lowe to be identified as authors
of this work have been asserted by them in accordance with the
Copyright, Designs and Patents Act 1988

First edition published 1995
Second edition published 2000

ISBN 0 7234 3160 4
INTERNATIONAL EDITION 0 7534 32015
US edition ISBN 0 7234 3200 7

British Library Cataloguing in Publication Data
A catalogue record for this book is available from the British Library

Library of Congress Cataloging in Publication Data
A catalog record for this book is available from the Library of Congress

Note
Medical knowledge is constantly changing. As new information becomes
available, changes in treatment, procedures, equipment and the use
of drugs become necessary. The authors and the publishers have, as far
as it is possible, taken care to ensure that the information given in this
text is accurate and up-to-date. However, readers are strongly advised
to confirm that the information, especially with regard to drug usage,
complies with the latest legislation and standards of practice.

The
publisher's
policy is to use
paper manufactured
from sustainable forests

Printed in Grafos, arte sobre papel.

PATHOLOGY

SECOND EDITION

St James's

Commissioning Editor: Louise Crowe
Project Development Manager: Sarah Keer-Keer
Project Controller: Nancy Arnott
Page makeup: Kate Walshaw
Designer: Judith Wright
Indexer: Nina Boyd

Cover illustration by Lynda Payne:
Structure of the mesangium and its relationship
to the glomerular basement membrane.

Dedication

This edition we dedicate to the makers of the following wines:

BOTTACCIO – Rodolfo Cosimi 1993[*]

AMARONE – Capital de Roari 1993[*]

and **various BAROLOS** (none younger than 1993)[*]

(we are going through an Italian phase)

and to the staff of the University Club, University of Nottingham (particularly Liz, Kirby and Jane) who have kept us supplied with them all.

We would also like to dedicate it to the staff of the fabulous Capital Hotel, Basil Street, London, where much of the critical work on this second edition was carried out in a period of frenzied activity, with particular thanks to the chef and sommelier who did their excellent best to undermine our work ethic.

[*] but see pages 146, 181, 251, 291, 293 and 301 (MODERATION IN ALL THINGS!)

Credo – first edition

When we sat down to write *Pathology*, it was with several strongly held beliefs that were based on our combined experience of over thirty years of teaching pathology to medical students and post-graduates:

- The burden of knowledge required for clinical medical courses has become almost intolerable for students, and is increasing year by year; it is time to redefine a 'core curriculum'.

- Although education in the basic mechanisms of pathological processes is important in understanding disease, medical students do not need exposure to detailed pathology early in their training. For most medical students, the most important component of pathology will be a knowledge of which diseases exist, how they arise, their effects, and their usual (and sometimes unusual) outcomes. Thus an understanding of molecular pathology, although important and fashionable, should not be taught at the expense of clinically relevant pathology; the same applies to microscopical histopathology.

- It is the duty of the teacher/author to smooth the path of student learning by emphasizing the difference between the real and the speculative, the important and the trivial, and the central and the peripheral.

- A compartmentalized systems-based presentation of disease is out-dated and takes little account of the likely clinical exposure students will receive in hospital and community practice. A clinical grouping of pathology emphasizes the close links between pathology and clinical practice.

- Too many textbooks are biased towards hospital practice, with insufficient acknowledgement that most medical students will eventually work in community practice. As a result, inadequate coverage is given to conditions that are common and important in community practice but rarely seen in hospitals.

- Diseases that affect children are often very different from those that are common in adults, a fact rarely emphasized in non-specialized textbooks for medical students.

- The main desire of medical students is to pass their professional examinations with ease, using personal teaching and textbooks that are clear, concise, easy to use, and not overloaded with unnecessary detail that is not relevant to their stage of training.

- Seeing is often the key to understanding. Color photographs and graphics are essential to illuminate the more difficult concepts and to enhance learning.

Against this background, we have written a book with the needs of both teachers and students in mind. *Pathology* is not intended to be a reference book for all disciplines, it aims to present clinically relevant pathology in a compact and easily assimilated format, using an abundance of pictures to enhance understanding.

AS, JSL Nottingham 1994

Credamus – second edition

The second edition not only gives us a chance to correct our inaccurate Latin, but also allows us to reiterate our beliefs about the teaching of pathology to medical students, as outlined above. Our views about the inappropriate size of the curriculum remain unchanged, and have become reinforced in the years since the first edition; there is a limit to the neuronal storage capacity of medical students. Our expectation that students would not need microbiology, hematology and immunology in this book proved ill-founded, and we have expanded these areas where they are clinicopathologically relevant. Students will still need to read dedicated texts to learn more details, particularly the laboratory-based aspects of the subjects. We are grateful to the many students and teachers who contacted us with comments about the first edition and suggestions for additions to the second edition; unfortunately, if we had acted on them all, this edition would have run to three volumes.

AS, JSL Nottingham 1999

Acknowledgements – first edition

The authors wish to thank many people who have helped in the preparation of this book. Many of our professional colleagues and friends in Nottingham, including Dr Nick Griffin, Dr Peter James, Dr Peter Smith, Dr Margaret Balsitis, Dr Malcolm Anderson, Dr Iain Leach, Dr Keith Robson, Prof. David Turner, Dr Ian Ellis, Dr Sarah Pinder, Dr Richard Allibone and Dr David Ansell, passed on to us microscope slides for photomicrography and were very supportive and helpful in supplying suitable material for photomacrography. Many colleagues were generous with slides from their own collections, and these are acknowledged separately below; if there are any whom we have over-looked we apologize. The following people gave valuable assistance by reading and commenting on individual chapters, and making suggestions:

Chapter 5	Dr Jane Zuccollo
Chapter 10	Dr Iain Leach
Chapter 12	Jocelyn Germaine and Prof. D. Williams, Department of Oral Pathology; and Dr M. Thornhill, Department of Oral Medicine, London Hospital Medical College, Mr K. Gibbin and Mr P. Bradley, Queen's Medical Centre, Nottingham.
Chapter 17	Prof. David Turner
Chapter 20	Dr Sarah Pinder, Department of Histopathology, City Hospital, Nottingham.

We are grateful to all the laboratory staff in the Department of Histopathology, University Hospital, Nottingham for the sectioning and staining of paraffin and frozen sections for photomicrography, particularly Janet Palmer, Dave McQuire, Lianne Ward, Kath Fowkes, Kate Barker and Denise McLean, Ian and Anne Wilson, Angela Crossman and the staff in the Surgical Histopathology Laboratory. Trevor Gray and Kevin Randall prepared the electron micrographs, Ken Morrell and Richard Church the immunocytochemical preparations, and Neil Hand the undecalcified resin sections of bone. We would like to thank Isabella Streeter, Linda Dewdney and Gina Goode for the secretarial and word processing work, and John Ben, John Mulligan, Philip Dawes, Lynette Newbery and Kerry Wilkinson for their help with provision of macroscopic specimens for photography. The color photographs of gross specimens are largely the work of Bill Brackenbury of the Department of Histopathology at University Hospital, Nottingham, but some are the work of Sue Hirst at the City Hospital, Nottingham.

Finally we would like to thank all the staff at Mosby who have been involved in the book, particularly Harvey Shoolman, Rachael Miller and Jonathan Brenchley who have been our very patient and tolerant editors, Claire Hooper, Michele Campbell and Jennifer Prast who were involved in the early stages, and Richard Prime and Lynda Payne who converted our often rough illustrations into genuine artworks. Ian Spick and Anne-Marie Woodruff were responsible for design. Fiona Foley played her usual valuable role of emotional nursing, encouraging, gently bullying, buying lunch, and just generally being there (or in America).

Acknowledgements – second edition

We remain indebted to all those people named above who were involved in the production of the first edition of this book, particularly Fiona Foley, Lynda Payne and Richard Prime who taught us the importance of visual appeal in medical publishing.

We would like to thank our colleagues in Nottingham and from the nearby hospitals in Derby and Mansfield who regularly sent us slides of good examples for photomicrography and possible inclusion in the book. For this second edition, Dr David Clark kindly read and criticized chapter 15, and Dr Linda Morgan provided us with the laboratory diagnosis data sets; we are very grateful to them both.

We would like to thank the staff of Harcourt Publishers in Edinburgh and London who were involved in the production of this second edition, particularly Judith Wright (designer), Kate Walshaw (layout artist), Ailsa Laing (copy editor), Nicky Haig (proofreader) and Nancy Arnott (production manager). The excellent new illustrations are the work of Lynda Payne and MTG Design & Illustration. We are very grateful to Sarah Keer-Keer who was the project development manager who kept us pretty much up to the mark with charm and grace, to Alistair Christie who took over from Sarah near the end, and to Louise Crowe who was commissioning editor and the source of much fun, many good ideas and great lunches.

Picture acknowledgements

Dr R. Allibone
Department of Histopathology
University Hospital
Nottingham

Figs 11.10, 13.24, 17.24, 17.28b, 17.35 and 19.20

Dr M. Anderson
Department of Histopathology
University Hospital
Nottingham

Figs 19.13, 19.22, 19.23a and b, 19.24a and c, 19.25, 19.28 and 19.29

Dr I. G. Barrison
(taken from *Gastroenterology in Practice*,
Gower Medical Publishing, London, 1992)

Fig. 14.28a

Mr P. Bradley
ENT Department
University Hospital
Nottingham

Figs 12.36, 12.37 and 12.39

Dr K. Dalziel
Department of Dermatology
University Hospital
Nottingham

Figs 19.2–19.3 and 19.5

Mr R. Downes
Department of Ophthalmology
Queen's Medical Centre
Nottingham

Figs 22.6a–c

Dr R. Emerson
Department of Dermatology
Queen's Medical Centre
Nottingham

Fig. 23.24e

Mr I. Foster
Department of Trauma and Orthopaedics
Queen's Medical Centre
Nottingham

Figs 24.17 and 24.18

Mr K. Gibbin
ENT Department
University of Nottingham

Figs 5.28, 12.8, 12.9, 12.10a, 12.28–12.32, 12.42 and 12.43

Dr W. F. Jackson
(taken from *Color Atlas and Text of Clinical Medicine*,
Mosby–Wolfe, London, 1992)

Fig. 16.8

Dr P. D. James
Department of Histopathology
University Hospital
Nottingham

Fig. 11.5

Dr T. Jaspan
Department of Radiology
University Hospital
Nottingham

Fig. 16.2a

Dr I. Leach
Department of Histopathology
University of Nottingham

Figs 10.6b, 10.8, 10.37, 10.38, 10.40a, 10.41–10.43, 10.45–10.48, 10.50, 10.51 and 18.6

Dr Rita Mirakian
(taken from *Clinical Immunology*,
Gower Medical Publishing, London, 1991)

Fig. 7.8

Dr S. Pinder
Department of Histopathology
University of Nottingham

Fig. 20.14

Dr A. P. Read
(taken from *Medical Genetics: an Illustrated Outline*,
Gower Medical Publishing, London, 1989)

Fig. 5.8

Dr P. Small
Department of Radiology
University of Nottingham

Figs 4.9, 5.7 and 12.23

Dr P. G. Smith
Department of Histopathology
University Hospital
Nottingham
Figs 14.5, 14.33a and b, 16.13, 16.15 and 16.17

Dr M. Thornhill
Department of Oral Medicine
London Hospital Medical College
Figs 12.1a, 12.2–12.6 and 12.18

Dr J. Zuccollo
formerly Department of Histopathology
University of Nottingham
Figs 5.2, 5.3, 5.5 and 5.6

The authors are also grateful for permission to reuse the
following pictures from the textbook *Neuropathology*,
Ellison D, Love S (eds), Times Mirror Mosby, 1998:
Figs 21.1, 21.2b and c, 21.13, 21.14, 21.16, 21.29 and 21.35.

How to use this book

This book has been written with four main aims:

- To introduce students early in their studies to the basic pathological processes that underlie all diseases.

- To relate the disease processes to the clinical symptoms and signs that are manifest to the patients, and are noted and interpreted by the clinician.

- To provide sufficient factual detail about the common and important diseases so that students are aware of the predisposing factors, local and distant effects, and the natural outcome in each case.

- To indicate the relevant ways in which laboratory investigation can establish the true nature of the illness and monitor its progress and response to therapy.

After a brief introduction to the place of pathology in modern medicine, the book is divided into two parts: Basic Pathology (Chapters 2–9) and Systems Pathology (Chapters 10–25).

Chapters 2–9 are mainly designed for students before they begin their clinical studies, but contain material useful to more advanced students who wish to revise any aspects of basic disease processes. They cover the essential principles of disease processes including the mechanisms and, where known, the causative and predisposing factors. In most modern medical schools, students are now taught immunology, microbiology, hematology and clinical chemistry in dedicated courses. It is no longer appropriate for a general pathology text to attempt comprehensive coverage of these areas. We have therefore presented overviews of these areas relevant to histopathology, in the knowledge that students should own specialized texts in these subjects.

Chapters 10–25 cover the pathology of the systems, and are mainly aimed at students undertaking clinical studies, as well as postgraduate students who are specializing in, for example, obstetrics and gynecology, neurology, etc. The diseases that affect each system are sometimes presented in a way which relates to the clinical attachments the student will embark upon, rather than keeping strictly to the traditional 'system'. For example, diseases of the ears (special senses system), nose (respiratory and special senses systems), and throat (respiratory and alimentary systems) are normally encountered in an attachment to an otorhinolaryngology specialist, and it seems sensible to

deal with the pathology of the area under that heading, rather than fragmenting the pathological content into the separate systems.

Students need textbooks that are easy to read and contain sufficient factual detail to satisfy examination requirements, and the facts should be presented in such a way that they are easy to assimilate and remember. We have therefore organized the content so that it has a user-friendly layout, presented in a variety of visually attractive ways, using the best of contemporary design skills.

Telegraph headings help students learn facts

For rapid and easy assimilation of basic statements of pathological truth, we have used 'telegraph style' headings for many of the sections.

Blue boxes

Material in blue boxes deals with the more clinical aspects of disease, particularly the laboratory (and other) investigation of disease processes.

Some blue boxes are used to present details of laboratory medicine, for example different techniques used to perform biopsies, and how the laboratory assists in patient management. In the early chapters, blue boxes are also used to provide clinical examples which illustrate

Pink boxes

Material in pink boxes gives details of mechanisms, and up-to-date knowledge of the molecular biological or genetic basis of some diseases.

In many places these are used as the vehicle to illustrate how cell biology and molecular genetics are revolutionizing understanding of disease.

KEY FACTS

Key facts boxes

¥ Are planned to summarize material spanning several sections.

¥ Are used to present a brief overview of a subject.

In all sections of the book the basic information is on a white background, with occasional Key Facts entries, which summarize the major points and are to be used as an *aide mémoire* and for revision purposes.

DATA SETS

Data set boxes contain typical clinical chemical results, obtained in the laboratory investigation of diseases in which abnormal biochemical parameters are a vital component of the diagnostic armamentarium. There are many such, but we have selected those which illuminate, or correlate with, the structural and histological abnormalities of the disorder.

In the Data Sets, the actual numerical values are not as important as the general features (e.g. normal, slightly raised, greatly raised, slightly reduced, greatly reduced) and the combination of biochemical findings.

The authors welcome comments from teachers and students who have used this book for their courses and personal study; feedback is particularly welcome as to whether the content satisfies their requirements, and especially if there are any significant omissions that should be corrected in subsequent editions.

ERRATA
Please note that some text is omitted in Chapter 17.
The complete sentences are printed below.

Yellow box — Renal failure, page 353
Acute renal failure sometimes recovers when the damaging stimulus resolves.

Pink Box — Immune mechanisms in glomerular disease, page 358-359
The different patterns point to different diagnoses, discussed in descriptions of the main types of glomerulonephritis.

Pink box — Pathogenesis of membranous nephropathy, page 362
In cases with a drug related, neoplastic or infective cause, treatment of the underlying condition removes the source of circulating antigen and may cause remission of renal disease.

Pink box — Pathogenesis of MPGN, page 363-364
The complement activation may cause consumption of serum complement and serum levels of C3 are markedly reduced in most cases. There is a familial predisposition to development of this condition in some cases.

Yellow box — Membranoproliferative glomerulonephritis, page 364
Results in progression to renal failure over many years and tends to recur in transplants.

Contents

Contents

1 Pathology at the core of medicine

PATHOLOGY IS THE STUDY OF THE PATTERNS, CAUSES, MECHANISMS AND EFFECTS OF ILLNESS (DISEASE)

A thorough understanding of disease processes is essential if physicians and surgeons are to recognize, diagnose and treat all diseases with accuracy and competence. Pathology is therefore a vital component of medical education for all doctors, nurses and other health-care practitioners, greatly improving the skill and efficiency of all concerned.

For a doctor to be able to interpret the complaints of a patient (the **symptoms** of disease) and understand the abnormalities found on examination (the **signs** of disease), it is important to be familiar with the range of abnormalities possible in an organ or tissue. If such knowledge is supported by that of the potential **causes** of abnormality, it is possible to arrange investigations and, ultimately, to **treat** disease. Pathology is the bedrock of clinical medicine, and its study continues throughout clinical practice.

A knowledge of disease patterns forms the basis of a doctor's skill in diagnosis, which is rooted in listening to the patient's account of the features of the illness (the **clinical history**), and in simple **physical examination**.

Clinical symptoms

A man complains to his doctor of the sudden onset of severe, crushing, continuous central chest pain, radiating into the left side of the neck and down the left arm. The patient also mentions that he had previously transiently experienced similar, less severe, pain in his chest on physical exertion, but that the pain had gone away on resting. The latest episode is associated with severe breathlessness, and the patient feels very unwell. He has cold, clammy skin and low blood pressure.

Even without physical examination, the doctor can build up a picture of the most likely pathological processes at work, and will know what mechanisms are operating and what the causative factors and likely effects are. Thus, immediate, possibly life-saving, treatment can be instituted. From a knowledge of the range of diseases that can affect the heart, and their causes, the doctor deduces that the patient probably has severe disease affecting his coronary arteries, which have become partially blocked by a disease process called **atheroma** (see Chapter 10), and that this partial blockage has resulted in the heart muscle occasionally being short of oxygenated arterial blood in periods of strenuous physical activity, leading to heart muscle pain (**angina**) in the past.

The conclusion is that the most recent episode may have resulted from complete blockage of the artery, which has been made total by development of a blood clot (**thrombus**). This has caused complete cessation of arterial blood supply to part of the muscular wall of the heart, and consequent death of the heart muscle cells due to loss of oxygen supply. The doctor will make a working diagnosis of **myocardial infarction**. Knowing the likely etiology of a disease allows rational planning of investigations to confirm the clinical diagnosis. In this instance an electrocardiogram (ECG) will show diagnostic changes, and levels of enzymes liberated from dead heart muscle will be elevated in the blood.

A knowledge of the mechanisms involved (**pathogenesis**) also allows implementation of treatment; in this instance administration of an agent to promote lysis of thrombus allows reperfusion of heart muscle and may limit the extent of damage.

The thoughts in the doctor's mind will be as illustrated in *Fig. 1.1.*

▶

The history of chest pain which improved on rest must mean that the coronary arteries are severely narrowed by atheroma, causing partial blockage of the lumen.

presentation B

The constant chest pain must mean that the patient now has a true **myocardial infarct**, and that the coronary artery is completely blocked, perhaps by a thrombus.

presentation C

This patient's immediate complications are failure of the left ventricle, leading to reduced cardiac output (responsible for his cold, clammy skin and his low blood pressure). Also, his damaged left ventricle is unable to empty completely at systole, so there will be increased back pressure in the left atrium and pulmonary veins and capillaries. Water will pass from the pulmonary capillary blood into his alveoli, making him very breathless (**pulmonary edema**).

relevant pathology A

areas of narrowing of coronary arteries

relevant pathology B

complete occlusion of coronary artery

area of dead cardiac muscle (infarct)

relevant pathology C

reduced cardiac output

increased back pressure to pulmonary veins

cardiac chambers dilate as heart fails

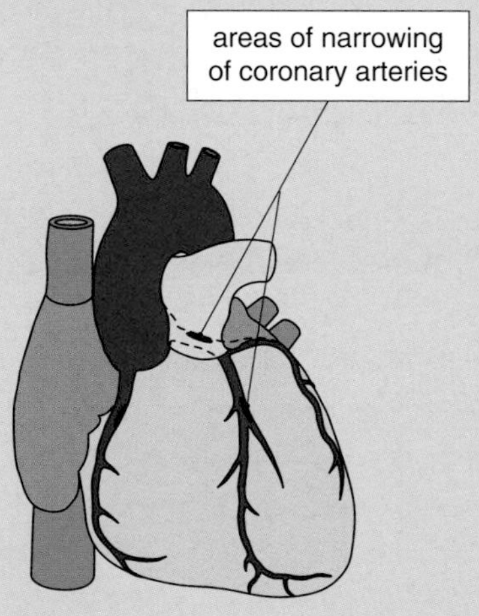

diagnosis A

Reduction in blood supply to the heart muscle will have produced symptoms of chest pain only on exertion, when the heart is working hard and has high blood and oxygen requirements. It is characteristic that this type of pain (**angina of effort**) disappears on resting.

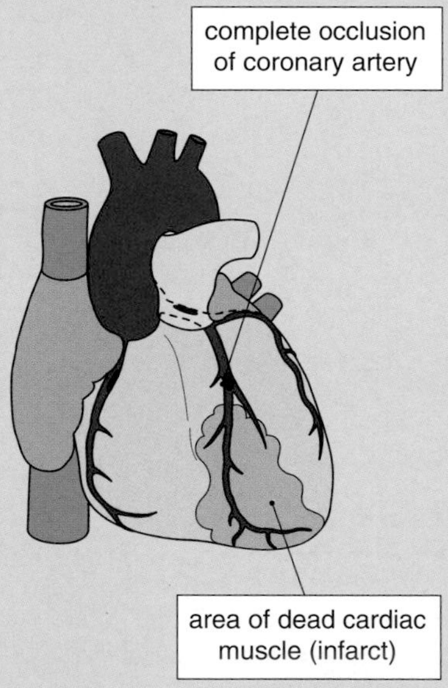

diagnosis B

There will now be an area of dead heart muscle in the wall of the left ventricle, and the patient's life is at risk. I must look out for symptoms and signs of the immediate complications of myocardial infarction. It will take about 8 weeks for the infarcted heart muscle to heal by scarring; until then he is at risk.

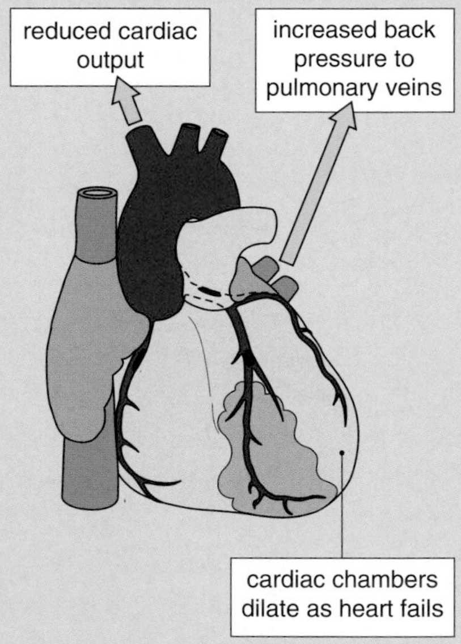

diagnosis C

The breathlessness and shock must mean that the patient has a failing left ventricle. I had better begin treatment immediately to improve the output and strength of the damaged left ventricular muscle.

Fig. 1.1 The diagnostic process requires an understanding of pathology.

Fig. 1.2
Common terms used in pathology

English	Pathology jargon	Explanations
Patterns of disease	Natural history	The natural history of a disease comprises many aspects including its origins, initial effects, progress, late effects and outcome (**prognosis**). Many diseases can be diagnosed at an early stage by a doctor's awareness of their origins and initial effects.
Causative factor or factors	Etiology or etiological factors	Some diseases have a single, clearly defined cause, e.g. an infection. In others, many different etiological factors operate to induce disease, and there is no single cause.
Mechanisms of disease	Pathogenesis	The mechanisms whereby the initial disease process produces structural and functional abnormalities and, hence, symptoms and signs.
Effects of disease	Sequelae	The sequelae (or complications) of a disease are the secondary 'knock-on' effects.

Pathology encompasses all aspects of disease

Special terms are used to refer to patterns, causes, mechanisms and effects of disease. These are given and explained in *Fig. 1.2*. Diseases can result from primary abnormalities at three levels:

- Genetic function.
- Physiological/biochemical function.
- Gross structural arrangement of cells, tissues and organs.

Many diseases reflect abnormalities at all three levels, since a genetic abnormality will induce a biochemical abnormality, and this can be manifest as a structural abnormality. An adequate understanding of pathology is therefore based on a sound grounding in normal cell biology, structure (histology and anatomy) and physiology. As most of this information is avaliable in specialized texts relating to other aspects of human biology, extensive presentations of normal material are avoided here.

A limited number of tissue responses underlie all diseases

Cells and tissues respond to disease processes in a limited number of ways, which can be considered as **basic pathological responses**. The first part of this book is devoted to the principles of these responses. These include:

- Adaptation of cells to changes in their environment (Chapter 2).
- What happens to cells when they cannot adapt, and how cells die (Chapter 3).
- Disorders due to abnormal cell growth, for example cancer (Chapter 6).
- Tissue responses to injury, and how tissues heal (Chapter 4).

- Genetic and immune factors in disease (Chapters 5 and 7).
- Adverse environmental factors that cause disease (Chapter 9).

These basic pathological processes are illustrated by examples from medical practice.

A single disease process has different effects in different systems

As well as understanding the basic types of pathological process in themselves, it is necessary to know how they affect various tissues and organs. For example, although Chapter 6 covers the basic pathology of benign tumors and cancers, you will also need to know which tumors occur in which tissues and organs, and their natural history, particularly in terms of progress and final outcome. For example, one common form of cancer called squamous cell carcinoma can occur in many organs and tissues, including the skin, mouth, esophagus, anus, uterine cervix, and in the bronchial tree. Although the tumor retains the same name wherever it arises, it behaves very differently in each different site. For example, a squamous cell carcinoma in the skin is slowly progressive, easily cured, and has a good outcome, rarely being life-threatening. Conversely, a squamous cell carcinoma in the esophagus or bronchial tree is more rapidly progressive, difficult to cure, and has a poor outcome, being life-threatening.

There is no short cut to this kind of knowledge, and it is necessary to be familiar with the details of the common pathology of the various organ systems. This approach is termed **systemic pathology** and is presented in Chapters 10 to 25. Full accounts of the pathology of each organ system are given, centered around the common and important diseases which, in our experience, it is essential to understand in some detail. For other less common or less important diseases, only the most significant facts are presented, often in an easily assimilable form such as a list or a table.

Pathology covers five main disciplines

Traditionally pathology has been subdivided into five main disciplines, reflecting the way in which clinical pathology is practiced in hospital centers.

Histopathology: the study of diseases from the perspective of structural, particularly histological, abnormalities of cells and tissues. Most of this book is about histopathology.

Hematology: the study of primary diseases of the blood, as well as the effects of other diseases on the blood.

Chemical pathology: the study of diseases from the perspective of biochemical abnormalities, both as primary disorders and as the effects of other diseases on biochemical parameters in the blood, urine and other tissues.

Microbiology: the study of diseases from the perspective of isolating, identifying and treating infections by bacteria, fungi, viruses and parasites. Microbiology is often further divided into virology and bacteriology.

Immunopathology: The study of diseases through analysis of immune function, particularly identifying primary diseases of the immune system, as well as the effects of other diseases on the immune system.

A reflection of modern developments in cell biology, the new discipline of **molecular pathology** is now emerging. Many diseases can now be defined by detection of molecular, rather than structural, abnormalities.

As specialist books now deal with hematology, chemical pathology, microbiology and immunopathology in great detail, this text presents only relevant aspects of these subjects, integrated into other chapters.

PATHOLOGY IS THE BASIS OF CLINICAL LABORATORY MEDICINE

Disease processes can have many effects, some of which are manifest as alterations in the cellular and biochemical composition of the blood. Frequently, the first manifestation of a disease process is not at its primary site, but takes the form of secondary effects. For example, in diabetes mellitus, although there is a primary abnormality in the pancreas, the diagnosis can be made by analysis of blood and urine glucose levels. Detection and analysis of similar secondary effects are of immense value in deducing the nature and site of underlying disease processes, and make a vital contribution to patient care. This is the basis of **diagnostic pathology**, increasingly being termed **laboratory medicine**.

To confirm or screen for disease the physician or surgeon sends samples from the patient to the pathology laboratory and asks for an appropriate analysis. The results, taken in conjunction with other investigations such as radiological examination, can pinpoint the site and likely nature of the disease process. If necessary, a tissue sample can be obtained from a diseased organ, and an accurate diagnosis established by histological examination. Two illustrative examples are shown in *Figs 1.3* and *1.4*.

Laboratory medicine is vital in medical and surgical practice

An early responsibility in medical and surgical training is to request relevant laboratory investigations to clarify the nature of disease in patients under your care. These laboratory investigations cover the whole range of laboratory medicine disciplines, the most common sample required being blood.

The development of techniques whereby small tissue samples (**biopsies**) can be obtained easily and painlessly from almost all areas of the body has had a huge impact on clinical medicine. There is now increasing reliance upon direct histological examination of abnormal cells, tissues and organs in establishing a diagnosis. For many diseases, current medical practice now revolves around accurate localization of an abnormality, using modern imaging methods (computerized tomography, magnetic resonance imaging and ultrasound scans), followed by direct sampling of the abnormal tissue by a guided biopsy method; the sampled tissue can then be examined by microbiological, histological, immunological, or biochemical techniques.

Good clinical practice requires:

- A knowledge of the systems pathology of each organ so that the range of disease processes likely to be causing an abnormality can be considered.
- A knowledge of the underlying basic pathology of each disease process, so that appropriate samples can be taken and relevant tests requested.
- An understanding of investigative techniques so that laboratory medicine results can be interpreted and a diagnosis established.

Pathology and laboratory medicine underpin much of clinical medical practice. This text is an introduction to pathology and laboratory medicine from a histopathological perspective. It offers an insight into the underlying basic pathology of the main disease processes and, through discussion of the systems pathology of each organ, provides a sound basis for clinical practice.

Pathological investigation in diagnosis – Case 1

HEMATOLOGY DEPARTMENT, UNIVERSITY HOSPITAL

Consultant/General Practitioner and patient location	Surname		Report no.
Clinical details Weakness,lethargy and pallor ?anemic ?type	Forename		Date received
	Age 63	Sex M	Hospital no.
Specimen Blood - full blood count please			

HEMOGLOBIN	W.B.C.	PLATELETS	M.C.V.	M.C.H.	R.B.C.	P.C.V.		
7.0	5.6	650.0	57	16.5	4.24	0.242		
M 13.0-18.0 F 11.5-16.5 g/dl	4.0-11.0×10⁹/1	150-400×10⁹/1	76.99 fl	27-32 pg	M 4.5-6.5 F 3.8-5.8 ×10¹²/1	M 0.40-0.54 F 0.37-0.47		

	NEUTROPHILS	LYMPHOCYTES	MONOCYTES	EOSINOPHILS	BASOPHILS	METAM'S BANDS	MYELOCYTES	PROM'CYTES	BLASTS	NUCLEATED RBC
×10⁹/1	2.11	2.99	0.31	0.13	0.06	<-(Cell counter estimates)				
%	37.7	53.4	5.5	2.3	1.1					
×10⁹/1	2.0-7.5	1.5-4.0	0.2-0.8	0.04-0.4	0.01-0.1	RETICULOCYTES (25-85)		E.S.R. mm/1hr		

Marked hypochromia & microcytosis 'Pencil cells' present
Iron deficiency anemia

(a) SNOP: **HEMATOLOGY**   Date of report

Fig. 1.3 (a) A 63-year-old man complains of increasing weakness and lethargy. On examination he appears very pale, suggesting that he is anemic. The physician takes a blood sample for hematological analysis. The hemoglobin level is low, the cells are small (low MCV) and each red cell contains reduced amount of hemoglobin (low MCH). Red cell numbers are also reduced (low RBC). The low packed cell volume (PCV) reflects the reduced number of small red cells. These are the typical features of an iron deficiency anemia which could be due to either inadequate iron intake or excessive blood loss. The high platelet count suggests that there has been recent blood loss. An increased number of reticulocytes would have supported this diagnosis but the estimation was not performed.

CHEMICAL PATHOLOGY DEPARTMENT, UNIVERSITY HOSPITAL

Consultant/GP and patient location	Surname		Report no.
Clinical details Anemic, iron deficiency & blood loss ?bleeding from GI tract	Forename		Date received
	Age 63	Sex M	Hospital no.
Specimen Feces - for occult blood			

Occult blood - positive

(b) SNOP: **CHEMICAL PATHOLOGY**   Date of report

Fig. 1.3 (b) On further questioning the patient admits that he occasionally passes very dark feces. A fecal sample is sent to the Chemical Pathology laboratory for analysis.

Fig. 1.3 (c & d) The patient is bleeding into his bowel, but where? Radiological examination by barium enema suggests an abnormality in the cecum. Using a colonoscope, the surgeon examines the full length of the colon and finds an ulcer with raised edges at the site of radiological abnormality in the cecum. Some samples of tissue are taken from the edges and floor of the ulcer, and sent to the Histopathology laboratory for histological examination.

HISTOPATHOLOGY DEPARTMENT, UNIVERSITY HOSPITAL

Consultant/GP and patient location	Surname		Report no.
Clinical details Iron deficiency anemia bleeding from gut. Colonoscopy - ulcer in gut. Biopsied	Forename		Date received
	Age 63	Sex M	Hospital no.
Specimen Fragments of cecal ulcer			

Histology - Biopsy of cecal ulcer shows invasive, poorly
differentiated adenocarcinoma

(c) SNOP: **HISTOPATHOLOGY**   Date of report

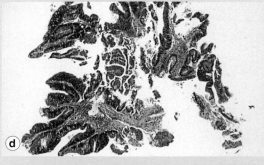

(d)

The underlying disease has been traced, and treatment can begin immediately. At the time of presentation the patient had no major complaints about his bowel, and the diagnosis was established by thorough investigation of a secondary effect.

Pathological investigation in diagnosis – Case 2

CHEMICAL PATHOLOGY DEPARTMENT, UNIVERSITY HOSPITAL

Consultant/General Practitioner and patient location	Surname		Report no.
Clinical details Urine thick & frothy ?proteinuria Edema - ?low serum albumin	Forename		Date received
	Age 47	Sex F	Hospital no.

Specimen (A) Urine - for protein (B) Blood - for albumin

(A) Urine - protein - 14.70g/save. Volume 1.5 litre/save

(B) Blood - albumin - 18g/litre (N=24-48)

(a) SNOP: CHEMICAL PATHOLOGY   Date of report

Fig. 1.4 (a) A 47-year-old woman is admitted because of weakness, lethargy and swelling of fingers and feet. She mentions that her urine has been unusually 'thick' and very frothy. Her physician sends samples of urine and blood to the Chemical Pathology laboratory for analysis.

HISTOPATHOLOGY DEPARTMENT, UNIVERSITY HOSPITAL

Consultant/GP and patient location	Surname		Report no. •
Clinical details Edema, proteinuria & hypoalbuminemia Nephrotic syndrome ?cause	Forename		Date received
	Age 47	Sex F	Hospital no.

Specimen Needle biopsy of kidney

Paraffin sections	- 5 glomeruli, all showing diffuse basement membrane thickening and mesangial increase
Electron microscopy	- immune complex deposition in subepithelial, subendothelial, intramembranous and mesangial locations
Immunofluorescence	- granular deposition of IgG, IgM, IgA, C_3 and C1q
Conclusion	- Lupus glomerulonephritis, with a membranous pattern

(b) SNOP: HISTOPATHOLOGY   Date of report

Fig. 1.4 (b) Armed with this evidence of severe protein loss in the urine, and a low serum albumin level, taken in conjunction with the clinical features, the physician knows that the patient suffers from the **nephrotic syndrome** (see page 351). The primary lesion will be in the kidney, and its true nature requires further investigation. Needle biopsy of the kidney is performed, and the small kidney samples are sent to the Histopathology laboratory for histological and electron microscopical examination. The locations of the immune complexes, and the pattern of immunofluorescence (demonstrating three types of immunoglobulin and two types of complement) are typical of glomerular involvement in systemic lupus erythematosus.

IMMUNOPATHOLOGY DEPARTMENT, UNIVERSITY HOSPITAL

Consultant/GP and patient location	Surname		Report no.
Clinical details Nephrotic syndrome Renal biopsy histology suggests SLE nephritis	Forename		Date received
	Age 47	Sex F	Hospital no.

Specimen Blood

```
C3 - 0.40g/l (N=0.63-1.19)
C4 - 0.07g/l (N=0.11-0.43)
C3dg   - 25units/ml (n=5-12)-grossly elevated
ANA    - 1:1600 (IgG class)
ENA    - Sm-positive
         Ro-negative
         La-negative
ds DNA - Crythidia Lucilliae-positive 1:80
         ELISA 1048iu/L-strong positive
```

The autoantibody profile is highly suggestive of SLE, and the hypocomplementemia indicates active disease.

(c) SNOP: IMMUNOPATHOLOGY   Date of report

Fig. 1.4 (c) The report suggests that the kidney disease is secondary to a widespread immunological disease, **systemic lupus erythematosus** (see Chapter 25). The physician therefore sends a further blood sample to the Immunopathology laboratory for confirmation of the diagnosis. The positive titer for double-stranded DNA is strongly suggestive of the diagnosis.

Et voila! The diagnosis is established, and treatment of this life-threatening disease can begin.

Cellular adaptations to disease

CELLS AS ADAPTABLE UNITS

Cells are constantly exposed to changes in their environment

The conditions to which cells are exposed are subject to constant change as a result of normal physiological processes, and also because of changes in the external environment, including the effects of medical treatment. For example, an individual's pattern of food intake may be modified, or the levels of circulating hormones may rise or fall. Alternatively, the individual may be exposed to drug therapy or to extremes of temperature.

If cells were static and rigid systems, these changes in the cellular environment would profoundly affect function of tissues, but there are homeostatic mechanisms which allow cells and tissues to cope with such stresses. Importantly, these mechanisms are brought into play not only in physiological situations but also to limit damage in response to disease processes.

Cells adapt to acceptable changes in their environment by modifying metabolism or growth pattern

To maintain normal function, cells have a physiological ability to adapt to acceptable environmental changes. Many of these modifications are **physiological metabolic adaptations**, and represent fine regulation of metabolic function at a biochemical level, not reflected in easily detectable changes in structure. For example:

- During periods of fasting, fatty acids are mobilized from adipose tissue to supply energy.
- During periods of relative calcium lack, calcium is mobilized from bone matrix by activity of osteoclasts under the influence of parahormone.
- Following administration of certain drugs (e.g. rifampin, an antimicrobial agent), hepatic microsomal enzymes are induced in cells to facilitate drug metabolism.

Other cell adaptations to environmental change are **physiological structural adaptations** caused by a change in the normal pattern of growth and accompanied by easily detectable structural changes. These normal adaptive structural changes can be divided into three broad types:

- **Increased cellular activity** (increase in size or number of cells) usually results from increased functional demands on a tissue or from an increase in hormonal stimulation.
- **Decreased cellular activity** (reduction in size or number of cells) usually results from reduction in hormonal stimulation of a tissue or from a decrease in functional demands.
- **Alteration of cell morphology** (change in cell differentiation) occurs when changes in the cellular environment cause an alteration in cell structure.

Severe changes in the cellular environment are termed pathological stimuli

Certain environmental changes lie outside an acceptable range of normality. Often the result of disease, these changes are then termed **pathological stimuli**. It must be emphasized that the boundary between pathological and physiological changes in the cellular environment is not rigid, nor is the definition of what is a significant injury to a cell or tissue. For example, exposure to UV radiation in sunbathing causes responses in the skin which vary from induction of melanin production (physiological) to severe blistering and loss of the epidermis (pathological).

The main causes of disease that lead to changes in the environment of cells are listed in *Fig. 2.1*.

THE CELL STRESS RESPONSE TO INJURY

Damaged cells produce proteins which protect them from damage

In response to some pathological stimuli, cells exhibit a series of metabolic changes known as the **cell stress response**, which is an important basic cellular mechanism that enables cells to survive environmental insults. Stressed cells turn down the genes coding for normal structural proteins (**housekeeping genes**) and show high levels of expression of genes coding for a set of proteins which have cell-organizing and protective functions (**cell stress genes**). Many of the cell stress proteins were originally described in response to experimental heat shock, hence a major group is termed the heat shock proteins (HSPs). The general terms 'heat shock protein' and 'cell stress protein' are synonymous.

Cell stress proteins are vital for cell viability

The stress proteins are expressed at low levels in normal cells, where they have important roles, but levels increase following exposure to damaging stimuli. Experimentally, a cell stress response can be induced in response to stimuli as diverse as heat, hypoxia, heavy metals, irradiation and viral infection. An indication of the fundamental biological importance of this cellular response is that the stress proteins exhibit a very high degree of inter-species conservation, with many of the stress proteins among the most conserved gene products in evolution. This evolutionary conservation suggest that the cell stress proteins are essential to cell survival, and their increased production in a cell stress response provides the extra stress proteins needed in pathological conditions.

Cell stress proteins are cytoprotective

The members of the HSP group of cell stress proteins are named according to size.

- The small heat shock proteins act as molecular chaperones, transiently associating with normal or damaged proteins to protect them from damage.
- **Ubiquitin** is an abundant protein in normal cells and has a role in removing old or damaged proteins by acting as a co-factor for proteolysis. Once ubiquitinated, such damaged proteins are recognized and degraded by specific proteases (*Fig. 2.2*).

In certain cells which undergo chronic stress, permanent aggregates of abnormal cell constituents and ubiquitin form visible masses known as **inclusion bodies** within the cytoplasm. One example of this phenomenon is when liver cells are chronically exposed to alcohol and form masses of the intermediate filament cytokeratin and ubiquitin, visible as pink-stained inclusion bodies. These are eponymously termed **Mallory's hyaline**. Another example is the **Lewy body** in nerve cells (see page 452).

Production of the cell stress proteins following exposure to a damaging stimulus is a rapid response that minimizes

Fig. 2.1
Causes of pathological stimuli

Type	Examples
Genetic	Gene defects, chromosomal defects
Nutritional	Deficiency or excess of dietary substances, e.g. iron, vitamins
Immune	Damage caused by the immune system, e.g. autoimmunity
Endocrine	Deficient or excessive hormone activity
Physical agents	Mechanical trauma, thermal damage, irradiation
Chemical agents	Toxicity due to many agents, e.g. heavy metals, solvents, drugs
Infective	Infection by viruses, bacteria, parasites, fungi and other organisms
Anoxia	Most commonly due to abnormal respiratory or circulatory function

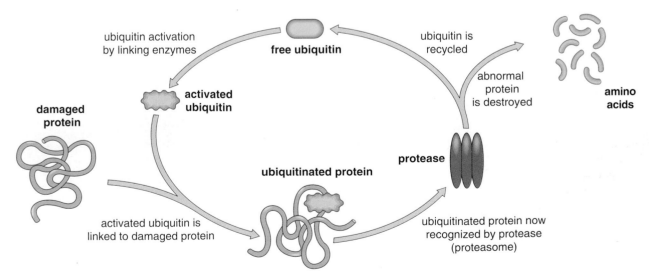

Fig. 2.2 The function of ubiquitin in cell stress.
Damaged proteins are recognized by a series of enzymes which covalently link the damaged protein to ubiquitin to form a ubiquitinated protein. Ubiquitination marks the protein for degradation by a cytosolic protease. As a result, ubiquitin is released and returns to form a pool of free ubiquitin in the cell cytoplasm while the damaged protein is eliminated.

cell damage and ensures cell viability. Cell stress proteins can only protect against certain levels of damage, more severe stimuli leading to cell degeneration or death (see Chapter 3).

ADAPTIVE RESPONSE IN DISEASE

Cells respond to damaging stimuli by extending adaptive processes

As well as mounting an immediate cell stress response, cells can adapt to damaging stimuli, becoming modified to achieve a new, steady state of metabolism and structure that better equips them for survival in the abnormal environment. Cells may adapt to a pathological (disease) stimulus by extending the three normal physiological adaptive responses:

- Increased cellular activity.
- Decreased cellular activity.
- Alteration of cell morphology.

Inability to adapt successfully to an environmental change leads to failure of cellular function and may result in sublethal cellular damage or cell death, as discussed in Chapter 3. This may be because the cell involved is particularly susceptible to the pathological stimulus or because the stimulus is so severe that it overwhelms the cell stress response and other adaptive reactions.

Different cell types show different degrees of susceptibility to environmental changes. Some cells, such as cerebral neurons, are highly sensitive to changes in their environment and die rapidly when conditions are outside the physiological norm. Other cells, such as fibroblasts, are extremely resistant to damage and can survive severe metabolic change, for example complete deprivation of oxygen, for relatively long periods of time without apparent harm.

Change in cellular growth pattern is an adaptive response in disease

Cells can adapt to certain pathological stimuli by altering their pattern of growth. This may be reflected in changes in the size, number or differentiation of cells in affected tissue. The terms used to describe such changes are outlined in *Fig. 2.3*.

Increased functional demand on a tissue can be met by increase in cell number (hyperplasia) as well as by increase in cell size (hypertrophy)

Certain organs or tissues may adapt to a disease process by increasing functional cell mass. There are two mechanisms of increase (*Fig. 2.4*).

Hyperplasia is an increase in the number of cells in a tissue caused by increased cell division. As this type of change can occur only in tissues that have the capacity for cell division, hyperplasia is not an adaptive response seen in skeletal muscle, cardiac muscle or nerve cells, which are non-dividing cell populations. Hormonal influences are important in this growth response.

Hypertrophy is an increase in the size of existing cells, accompanied by increase in their functional capacity. Cell enlargement is brought about by increased synthesis of structural components, associated with accelerated activity of cellular metabolism and rises in levels of RNA and organelles required for protein synthesis. Hypertrophy is particularly seen as a response to increased demand in tissues composed of cells which are unable to divide (skeletal and cardiac muscle).

Hypertrophy and hyperplasia may occur independently of each other or together, to meet a demand for increased function, and are usually associated with an increase in the size and weight of the organ or tissue concerned.

Increased cell mass in a tissue can result from physiological stimuli

An increase in functional cell mass through hypertrophy and hyperplasia may be physiological.

- The thyroid gland enlarges in pregnancy owing to the stimulus of pregnancy-associated high levels of TSH on thyroid epithelial cells (*hyperplasia*).
- In athletes, skeletal muscle fibers increase in size (*hypertrophy*) in response to exercise and increased metabolic demands (*Fig. 2.5*).
- Under the influence of endocrine stimulation in pregnancy, breast epithelial cells and myometrial smooth muscle cells both increase in size and number (*hypertrophy and hyperplasia*) (*Fig. 2.6*).
- Under the influence of ovarian endocrine stimulation in the menstrual cycle, endometrial glands increase in size as a result of proliferation of cells (*hyperplasia*) (*Fig. 2.7*).

Fig. 2.3 Changes in growth pattern of cells	
Change in size of cells	
Atrophy	Reduction in the size of cells
Hypertrophy	Increase in the size of cells
Change in number of cells	
Involution	Decrease in the number of cells
Hyperplasia	Increase in the number of cells
Change in differentiation of cells	
Metaplasia	Stable change to another cell type

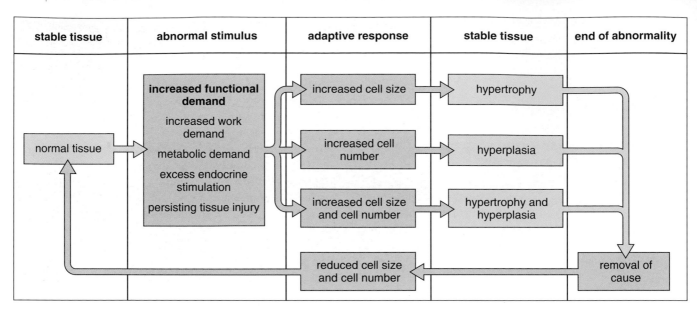

stable tissue	abnormal stimulus	adaptive response	stable tissue	end of abnormality
normal tissue	**increased functional demand** increased work demand metabolic demand excess endocrine stimulation persisting tissue injury	increased cell size	hypertrophy	removal of cause
		increased cell number	hyperplasia	
		increased cell size and cell number	hypertrophy and hyperplasia	
		reduced cell size and cell number		

Fig. 2.4 Adaptive responses resulting in increased tissue mass.
Increased functional demand or endocrine stimulation are what usually cause hypertrophy and hyperplasia. These new patterns of growth are stable while the causative stimulus persists, but once it is removed the tissue returns to a normal pattern of growth.

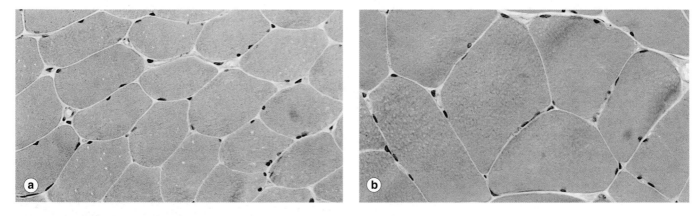

Fig. 2.5 Hypertrophy of skeletal muscle in response to exercise.
Hypertrophy in the absence of hyperplasia is typically seen in muscle where the stimulus is an increased demand for work. Taken at the same magnification, (a) shows muscle fibers in transverse section from the soleus muscle of a normal 50-year-old male and (b) shows fibers from the same muscle in a veteran marathon runner. Note the dramatic increase in the size of the fibers in response to the demands of marathon running.

Increased cell mass in a tissue can result from pathological stimuli. Increased functional cell mass also occurs as a response in disease states.

- If the serum calcium is abnormally low, the parathyroid glands increase the number of parahormone-secreting cells (*hyperplasia*).
- If the aortic valve outflow is severely narrowed by disease (see page 185), the muscle of the left ventricle of the heart responds with an increase in the size of cardiac muscle cells (*hypertrophy*) to overcome the resistance to flow and to ensure an adequate blood pressure (*Fig. 2.8*). This is also seen in myocardial muscle when systemic hypertension

causes an increased demand on cardiac function (see page 166).
- Obstruction of the colon by a tumor causes an increase in size (*hypertrophy*) of the smooth muscle cells of the bowel wall proximal to the obstruction.
- Estrogen produced by certain ovarian tumors causes abnormal proliferation of the endometrium (*hyperplasia*), which increases in bulk, and leads to an abnormal pattern of menstrual bleeding.
- If a kidney is removed or ceases to function, the remaining healthy kidney increases in size and weight to compensate for the loss. The process of hyperplasia leads to enlargement of structures such as glomeruli, and is often termed **compensatory hyperplasia**.

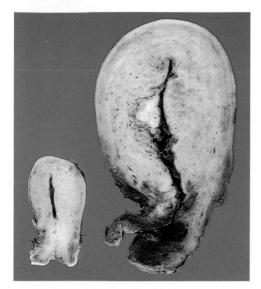

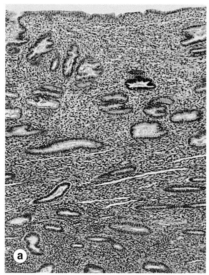

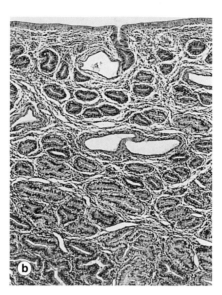

Fig. 2.6 Hyperplasia and hypertrophy of myometrium in pregnancy.
On the left is a normal uterus showing the normal mass of smooth muscle in its wall. On the right is a uterus from a recently pregnant woman, in which the striking increase in mass of smooth muscle is evident. At a cellular level, this is due to both hyperplasia and hypertrophy of uterine smooth muscle.

Fig. 2.7 Hyperplasia of endometrium in response to estrogen. (a) Inactive endometrium. (b) Proliferated endometrium.
Micrograph (a) shows glands in a state of absent stimulation by estrogen. Micrograph (b) shows that in response to secreted estrogen as part of the normal menstrual cycle there has been an increase in the number of cells in each gland, which are hyperplastic. This is an example of physiological hyperplasia.

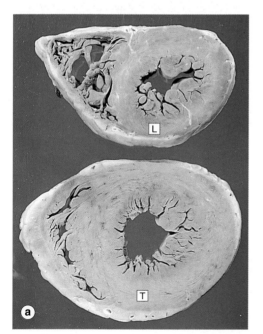

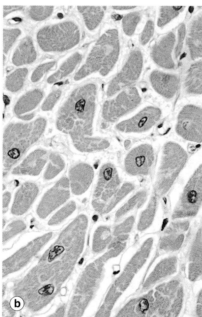

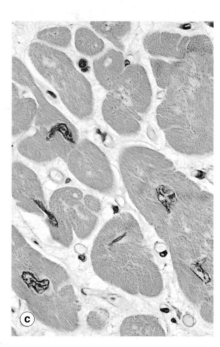

Fig. 2.8 Hypertrophy of cardiac muscle in response to valve disease. (a) Transverse slices of a normal heart and a heart with hypertrophy of the left ventricle. (b) Histology of cardiac muscle from a normal heart. (c) Histology of cardiac muscle from a hypertrophied heart.
The upper macroscopic specimen (a) demonstrates the normal thickness of the left ventricular wall (**L**) for comparison with the greatly thickened wall (**T**) in the lower specimen, taken from a heart in which severe narrowing of the aortic valve caused resistance to systolic ventricular emptying. The increased mass of the left ventricle is due to enlargement of cardiac muscle cells as a result of hypertrophy. This can be seen by comparing the diameter of fibers from the normal heart (b) with those from the diseased heart (c). Note that the size of nuclei in the hypertrophied cardiac muscle is also increased; it has been found that such nuclei are frequently polyploid (i.e. contain several times the normal quantity of DNA).

Hyperplasia may not be uniform and sometimes occurs as nodules

Hyperplasia may not occur uniformly throughout a tissue; instead, nodules of excessive cell growth (hyperplastic nodules) develop between areas of normal tissue, giving rise to the term nodular hyperplasia. Most examples of nodular hyperplasia occur in tissues in which cells are responding to a trophic hormone. It is likely that the hyperplasia seen in these conditions is a result of a disturbance in the hormone responsiveness of the target tissue. Nodular hyperplasia is seen most commonly in the prostate gland (*Fig. 2.9*), thyroid gland, adrenal gland and the breast.

Following removal of the stimulus causing hyperplasia or hypertrophy, tissue reverts to normal

A key feature of hyperplasia is that the altered pattern of growth ceases following removal of the causative environmental stimulus, and the tissue reverts to its normal state. For example, in cases of endometrial hyperplasia, removal of the cause of the abnormal levels of estrogen would trigger the endometrium to return to normal.

This feature distinguishes hyperplasia from neoplasia (the formation of tumors such as cancer – discussed in Chapter 6), in which there is excessive cell growth that does not regress on removal of the causal environmental stimulus.

Reduced functional demand leads to reduction in cell number or cell size

When the mass of functioning cells in a tissue becomes reduced, the tissue is said to have undergone **atrophy**. There are two mechanisms of reduction (*Fig. 2.10*).

- **Decrease in the size and volume of individual cells,** associated with reduction in cellular metabolism and reduced synthesis of structural proteins. Physical

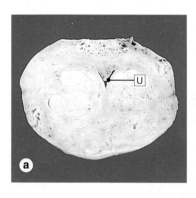
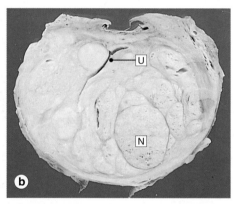

Fig. 2.9 Nodular hyperplasia of the prostate gland. (a) Normal prostate gland. (b) Nodular hyperplasia of prostate gland. These macroscopic specimens are transverse slices through the prostate gland. Note the nodules (**N**) in (b), which are the result of nodular hyperplasia. This is an extremely common condition in elderly men, resulting in compression of the prostatic urethra (**U**) and difficulty with micturition.

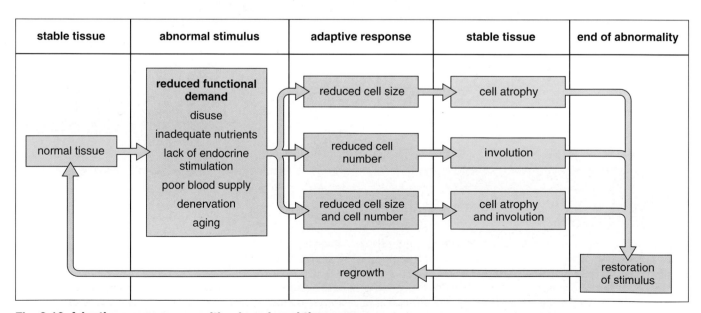

Fig. 2.10 Adaptive responses resulting in reduced tissue mass.
Reduced functional demand, reduction in trophic stimuli, or reduction in nutrients are the usual stimuli which cause involution or cell atrophy. Atrophic or involuted tissues are stable patterns of growth that persist while the lack of stimulation or demand causing them remains. However, once appropriate stimulation or demand returns, the tissue reverts to a normal pattern of growth.

reduction in the size of established cells is achieved through an increase in the catabolism of cytosolic structural proteins by the ubiquitin–proteosome system and by removal of organelles by autophagy, channelling redundant structural elements into the lysosomal system (*Fig. 2.11*).

- **Death of established cells** in an organ or tissue, causing a reduction in the number of functioning cells. This is brought about by the activation of specific cell systems which act to bring about cellular dissolution and elimination from tissues, sometimes called programmed cell death. The best studied example of this type of cell death is termed apoptosis (*Fig. 2.21* and pages 18–22). Involution is a form of physiological organ atrophy involving apoptosis of cells.

In many tissues that have undergone cellular atrophy, a brown pigment called lipofuscin accumulates within the shrunken cells. This pigment, composed of degenerate lipid material in secondary lysosomes, is produced by breakdown of the cell membranes and organelles through autophagy (*Fig. 2.12*). Lipofuscin builds up, particularly in the atrophic myocardial fibers of elderly people, giving rise to macroscopically evident brown coloration of the myocardium (**brown atrophy**).

Atrophy is usually associated with reduction in the size and weight of an organ or tissue. In some instances cell mass lost through cellular atrophy or involution is replaced either by adipose or by fibrous tissue, thus maintaining the overall size of an organ. This replacement tissue frequently appears as brightly eosinophilic material called **hyaline**.

Autophagy and cell atrophy

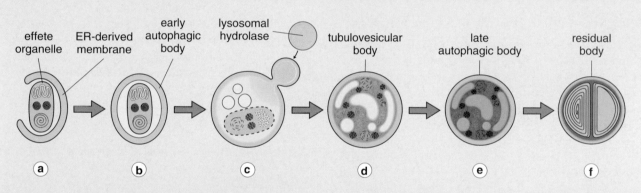

Fig. 2.11 In cellular atrophy, structural proteins and organelles of a cell are destroyed, with a parallel reduction in the size and functional capacity of the cell. This is an adaptive response as it allows the cell to survive in adverse conditions by reducing its metabolic overheads. Cell constituents are eliminated by a process of autophagy: unwanted cell organelles become enwrapped by membrane derived from the endoplasmic reticulum (ER) (a), forming an autophagic body (b) which subsequently fuses with vesicles containing lysosomal acid hydrolases (c). The action of the hydrolases brings about degradation of the organelles. Cells which are actively undergoing atrophy can be seen ultrastructurally to contain numerous autophagic vacuoles. These bodies become electron dense, but have internal tubular or vesicular profiles (derived from membrane-fusion events) that have earned them the alternative name of tubulovesicular bodies (d). Late autophagic bodies (e) become more electron dense and may form residual bodies (f) containing lamellar undigested lipid-rich cell material called lipofuscin (see *Fig. 2.13*).

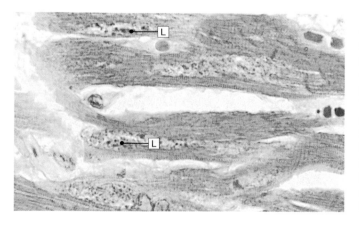

Fig. 2.12 Lipofuscin in cellular atrophy, seen in the cardiac muscle of an elderly patient.
Cellular atrophy is associated with autophagy of cellular structural elements and consequent reduction in size of the cell. One effect of this is that indigestible material, principally phospholipids, accumulates in lysosomal-derived bodies. This material can be seen on light microscopy as yellow-brown granules (**L**) called lipofuscin, here shown in the myocardium of a 90-year-old female. Ultrastructural examination of lipofuscin reveals it to consist of electron dense material within membrane-bound granules of varying size, which often have myelin-like figures. Lipofuscin commonly accompanies the cellular atrophy that occurs in many tissues with aging, and thus is often called **wear and tear pigment**.

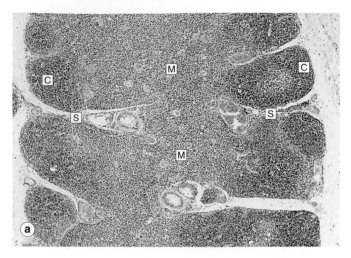

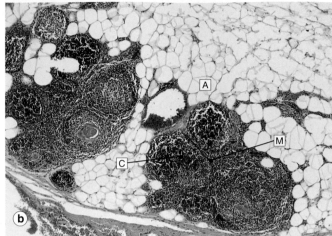

Fig. 2.13 Involution of the thymus. (a) Thymus in a child. (b) Thymus in an adult.
Micrograph (a) shows the dense cellularity of a child's thymus gland, heavily populated by lymphoid cells forming thymic cortex (**C**) and medulla (**M**) with dividing septa (**S**). In contrast, in the adult (b) the gland undergoes involution associated with dramatic reduction in size and, as with many examples of involution, becomes replaced by adipose tissue (**A**).

Reduction in cell mass may be physiological

Many physiological processes require that a tissue response is switched off as part of a reduction in functional demand. This is seen particularly when the mass of a target organ is maintained by endocrine stimulation which becomes reduced, for example when the thyroid gland returns to normal size after the physiological hyperplasia induced by puberty or pregnancy. In old age, a combination of factors such as reduced physical activity and changes in the pattern of endocrine secretion leads to reduced size (atrophy) of many organs and tissues. Examples of physiological atrophy or involution are:

- The thymus gland involutes during adolescence (*Fig. 2.13*).
- The myometrium involutes *post partum*.
- With reduced activity in old age, skeletal muscle fibers decrease in size (*aging atrophy*).
- In the aging parathyroid gland, hormone-secreting cells diminish in number and are replaced by fat cells.
- The testis undergoes atrophy as a result of reduced gonadotrophic stimulation in old age.

Reduction in cell mass occurs in some pathological states

Many disease processes lead to a reduction in functional demand, hormonal or nervous stimulation, or nutrition of tissues; atrophy or involution occurs as an adaptive response.

- Skeletal muscle fibers in the leg undergo cellular atrophy if the leg is immobilized, for example when splinting is used in the treatment of a fracture (*disuse atrophy*).
- Gradual reduction in blood supply to a tissue results in loss of functional cells through involution, as well as through cellular atrophy (*ischemic atrophy*).

- Damage to axons supplying muscle causes atrophy of affected muscle fibers (*denervation atrophy*) (*Fig. 2.14*).
- Following ablation of the pituitary gland by surgery, the cells of the adrenal cortex decrease in size and number owing to lack of ACTH stimulation (*Fig. 2.15*).
- After trauma to the spinal cord, skeletal muscle fibers supplied by affected spinal nerve roots undergo atrophy.

Developmental causes of reduced cell mass are termed 'agenesis', 'aplasia' and 'hypoplasia'

Certain developmental defects result in abnormally small organs or complete failure in development of organs or tissues. Such examples must be distinguished from atrophy and involution, in which the tissue or organ had originally developed in a normal fashion (*Fig. 2.16*).

- Complete failure to produce the embryonic cell mass destined to form an organ is termed **agenesis**.
- Failure of a correctly formed embryonic cell mass to differentiate into a developed organ is termed **aplasia**.
- If organ-specific structures develop correctly but are abnormally small the organ is termed **hypoplastic**.
- If organ-specific structures develop correctly but are histoanatomically abnormally configured the organ is termed **dysgenetic**.

Tissues may adapt to environmental stimuli by a change in cell differentiation termed 'metaplasia'

Certain long-standing environmental stimuli render the environment unsuitable for some specialized cell types and, as an adaptive response, the proliferating cells change their pattern of differentiation. These cells can adapt to a change in environment by differentiating to a new, mature,

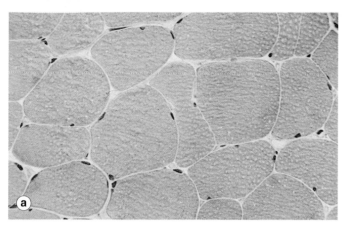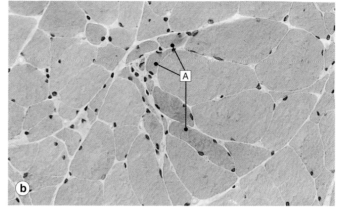

Fig. 2.14 Atrophy of skeletal muscle with denervation. (a) Normal muscle. (b) Denervated muscle.
Micrograph (a) shows normal skeletal muscle fibers. In micrograph (b) damage to many of the axons in the main nerve supplying the muscle has caused atrophy of fibers (**A**), which had been innervated by now-damaged axons. Fibers are small and angulated. With time, axon sprouting may reconnect some denervated fibers, which then return to normal size.

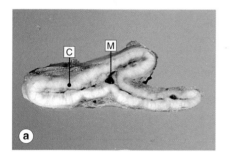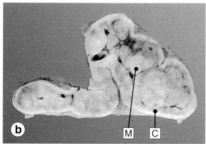

Fig. 2.15 Atrophy of the adrenal gland. (a) Atrophic adrenal. (b) Normal adrenal. Specimen (b) is a slice of normal gland, in which yellow cortex (**C**) can be distinguished from the small amount of grey medulla (**M**). The slice in (a) is from a patient who had surgical ablation of the pituitary gland, leading to lack of ACTH. This has resulted in reduction in the size of the adrenal gland, specifically affecting the cortex.

stable type of cell, which better equips them to withstand an environmental stress. This process is termed **metaplasia**, and examples are summarized in *Fig. 2.17*.

- In the bronchi, under the influence of chronic irritation by cigarette smoke, the normal ciliated columnar mucus-secreting respiratory epithelium is replaced by squamous epithelium (*squamous metaplasia*).
- In the cervix the normal columnar epithelium of the lower endocervix changes to squamous epithelium in response to exposure to the acid vaginal environment (*squamous metaplasia*).
- In the urinary bladder the normal transitional epithelium may be replaced by squamous epithelium in response to chronic irritation by bladder calculi or infection (*squamous metaplasia*) (*Fig. 2.18*).
- The esophageal squamous epithelium is replaced by columnar epithelium in response to exposure to gastric acid in cases of gastric reflux (see page 248).

Metaplasia most commonly occurs in epithelial tisuses, but may also be seen elsewhere. For example, areas of fibrous tissue exposed to chronic trauma may form bone (*osseous metaplasia*). In many settings, metaplasia co-exists with hyperplasia; for example, the squamous epithelium that arises by metaplasia in response to calculi in the bladder may also be hyperplastic.

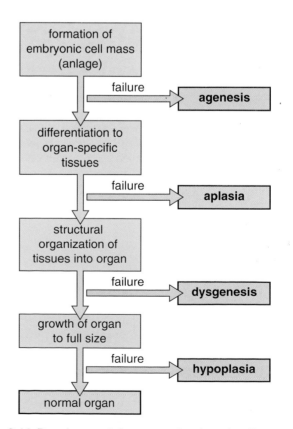

Fig. 2.16 Developmental causes of reduced cell mass.

Fig. 2.17
Examples of metaplasia

Original tissue	Stimulus	Metaplastic tissue
Ciliated columnar epithelium of bronchial tree	Cigarette smoke	Squamous epithelium
Transitional epithelium of bladder	Trauma of bladder calculus	Squamous epithelium
Columnar epithelium in gland ducts	Trauma of calculus	Squamous epithelium
Fibrocollagenous tissue	Chronic trauma	Bone (osseous) tissue
Esophageal squamous epithelium	Gastric acid	Columnar epithelium
Columnar glandular epithelium	Vitamin A deficiency	Squamous epithelium

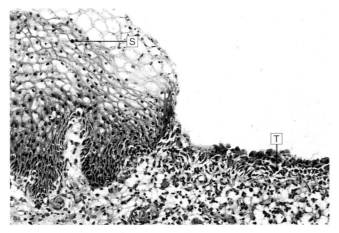

Fig. 2.18 Squamous metaplasia in urinary bladder.
The transitional epithelium of the urinary bladder (**T**) has become severely traumatized by a bladder stone (calculus), not seen in this micrograph. In response, squamous metaplasia has occurred, with replacement of the normal transitional epithelium by stratified squamous epithelium (**S**). Squamous metaplasia also occurs in the bladder when there is chronic irritation by the parasitic infection, schistosomiasis. In such cases the squamous epithelium is better suited to withstand the new environment than is the native transitional urothelial epithelium.

CELL BIOLOGY OF GROWTH ADAPTATION

Cell adaptation is influenced by growth factors accompanied by altered gene expression

The molecular signalling pathways that are involved in the adaptive responses of hyperplasia, hypertrophy and metaplasia are gradually being understood, but this is as yet an incomplete understanding. There is increasing recognition that cell growth is under the control of various **growth factors** (*Fig. 2.19*) which act upon specific cell-surface receptors that are then linked to internal cell signalling pathways.

Fig. 2.19
Growth factors

Epidermal growth factor family
Colony stimulating factors
Interferon family
Platelet-derived growth factor
Insulin-like growth factors
Fibroblast growth factors
TGFß family
Interleukin family
Erythropoietin
Nerve growth factor
Ciliary neuronotrophic growth factor

Growth factor receptors, many of which trigger secondary messenger systems through having tyrosine kinase activity, modulate transcription regulation and thereby directly affect the processes of gene regulation. Alterations in the relative concentrations of growth factors, in the expression of growth-factor receptors, in the activity of cell signalling pathways or transcription regulatory systems can result in altered cell growth.

For example, hyperplasia may be caused by a local increase in the concentration of a growth factor, or by an increase in expression of growth-factor receptors on cells, or by upregulation of a cell signalling system. It is clear that these factors have synergistic actions in promoting or regulating growth. Factors which inhibit cell growth have also been recognized in animal models, but are less well characterized in humans.

Increasingly, such growth factors are being manufactured by recombinant genetic techniques, and attempts are being made to administer them therapeutically. The finding that ciliary neuronotropic growth factor can prevent death of nerve cells in animal models of neurodegenerative

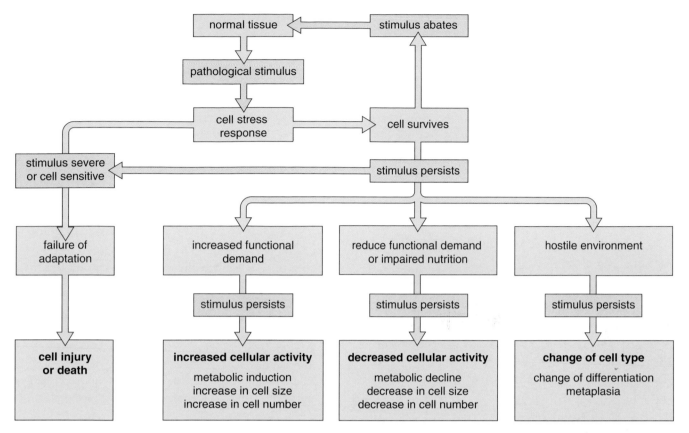

Fig. 2.20 Summary of tissue response to environmental change. Adaptive responses allow cells to survive in the face of a change in the cellular environment. Failure to adapt is associated with cell damage or cell death.

disease offers the exciting prospect of preventing certain neurodegenerative diseases in man. In cases in which the bone marrow has been suppressed or deprived of normal levels of growth factor, the use of recombinant erythropoietin to induce hyperplasia of the red cell compartment of bone marrow has also achieved encouraging results, e.g. preventing anemia in chronic renal failure.

Colony stimulating factors, involved in the control of cell growth of blood cells, are being used to help recovery of bone marrow function in patients who have received chemotherapy.

Unfortunately, important side-effects of systemic administration of some growth factors have included fever, loss of weight, loss of appetite, and hypotension – a reflection of the diverse effects of these factors, not limited to regulation of growth. It is likely that such systemic side-effects will limit many of the hoped-for therapeutic applications for these factors. A list of the most common factors is shown in *Fig. 2.19*.

The result of cellular activation by growth factors is the alteration of gene expression in cells. Many of the genes that are involved in control of cell growth and activated in cellular adaptive changes are also **proto-oncogenes**, implicated in the disorganization of cell growth that is the hallmark of neoplasia (development of cancer), discussed in Chapter 6.

Adaptive responses in disease occur only with tolerable environmental changes

The adaptive responses of hyperplasia, hypertrophy, atrophy, involution and metaplasia occur only if the damaging stimulus is tolerable to the affected cells. Failure to adapt leads to cell damage and, if the stimulus is severe or prolonged, may result in cell death, as summarized in *Fig. 2.20*.

KEY FACTS
Cell adaptation

- Cells are adaptable within physiological limits.
- Cells can respond to injury by producing cell stress proteins, which protect from damage and help in recovery.
- Increased demands are met by hypertrophy and hyperplasia.
- Reduced demand is met by atrophy.
- Cell loss from tissues can be achieved by programed cell death (apoptosis).
- Tissues can adapt to demand by a change in differentiation known as metaplasia.

Apoptosis is a fundamental cell process which serves several vital functions

Investigating the process of programed cell death leading to apoptosis has become one of the big growth areas in cell biology over the last few years. It has become apparent that this process of cell elimination is one of the most fundamental processes in cell biology and that it is the main mechanism of cell death in several important processes or diseases:

- Removal of excess cells in embryogenesis, for example in separating digits or in creation of the gut lumen.
- Elimination of cells after withdrawal of a hormonal growth stimulus, for example the estrogen-sensitive tissues in the female reproductive system.
- Clonal selection of lymphocytes in the induction of self-tolerance in development.
- Elimination of cells in tissues that require a high cell turnover, for example the lining epithelial cells of the gut.
- Killing of viral infected cells by cytotoxic T-cells.
- Elimination of cells with acquired DNA damage through viral infection, irradiation, or cytotoxic agents.
- Elimination of neoplastic cells in tumors.
- Death of nerve cells in neurodegenerative diseases such as Alzheimer's disease.

The structural changes in apoptosis are summarized in *Fig. 2.21*.

Apoptosis has four phases: induction, effector, degradation and phagocytosis

The terminology used in the biology of apoptosis is rich in analogies more usually heard in sword-and-sorcery games, such as executioner, executioner's sword, death domain and genes called 'Reaper' and 'Grim'. So far, the key players in cell death seem to be a group of proteases with defined specificities, termed the **caspases**, and factors which are either associated with or released from the mitochondria.

Apoptosis can be divided into four phases:

- **Induction/signalling phase:** death-inducing signals and cell-survival signals impinging on a cell are integrated and, if death signals are dominant, molecular systems that trigger apoptosis are activated. Importantly, cell survival is possible even in the face of signals which would normally cause death, provided that cell-survival signals have induced proteins that have anti-apoptotic effects. The most studied of this class of anti-apoptotic proteins is termed Bcl-2 which, if present in high quantities, prevents a cell from committing itself to apoptotic death.
- **Effector phase:** a cell becomes committed to die through the activity of what has been termed a cell executioner pathway. This is the point of no return for the cell, after which it is irreversibly committed to die. Increasing evidence suggests that it is mitochondrial membrane permeability that acts as the decision-making factor in

commitment to cell death. If mitochondrial membrane becomes permeable, factors that cause apoptosis enter the cytosol from mitochondria.

- **Degradation phase:** enzyme systems are activated which bring about the biochemical and structural features of apoptosis. The main enzymes involved are proteases called the caspases. The term caspase refers to the specificity of the proteases: 'c' refers to cyseine protease, 'asp' refers to cleavage after an aspartate residue in the target protein. The enzyme systems which are activated cleave or cross-link proteins, degrade DNA, expose phosphatidylserine on the outer cell membrane and bring about morphological changes in the cell which are now regarded as classical for apoptotic cell death.
- **Phagocytic phase:** cell fragments produced by the apoptotic process are recognized by macrophagic and other phagocytic cells and are engulfed. The expression of phosphatidylserine on the outer cell membrane and the binding of thrombospondin on the cell surface both facilitate specific phagocytic recognition by other cells. This aspect of apoptosis allows removal of dead cells without promoting an inflammatory response: dead cells are removed cleanly and with minimal disruption to adjacent cells.

Apoptosis may be started by activation of a surface receptor, cell membrane damage, direct mitochondrial damage, or unrepairable DNA damage

There are four main systems which are believed to be specially relevant to the triggering of apoptotic cell death in human pathology (*Fig. 2.22*).

1. Signal transduction pathway: binding of specific ligands at cell surface receptors triggers a signal transduction cascade that activates initiating caspases. The receptors have cytoplasmic 'death recognition domains' that interact with homologous death domains on so-called adaptor proteins, carrying that signal to the initiating parts of the apoptotic pathway. Examples include:

- Fas-Fas ligand-mediated apoptosis responsible for eliminating certain classes of lymphocyte from the immune system, as well as target-cell killing by cytotoxic T-cells.
- Cytokine-induced apoptosis of cells, as seen with tumor necrosis factor receptor (TNFR)-mediated apoptosis.

2. Cell damage pathway: cell damage initiates apoptosis by causing changes in mitochondrial membrane permeability – activating caspases and causing apoptosis. Examples include:

- Free radical-mediated damage.
- Cell anoxia.
- High intracellular free calcium levels.
- Perforin/granzyme-B-mediated cell death caused by cytotoxic T-lymphocyte-mediated cell death.

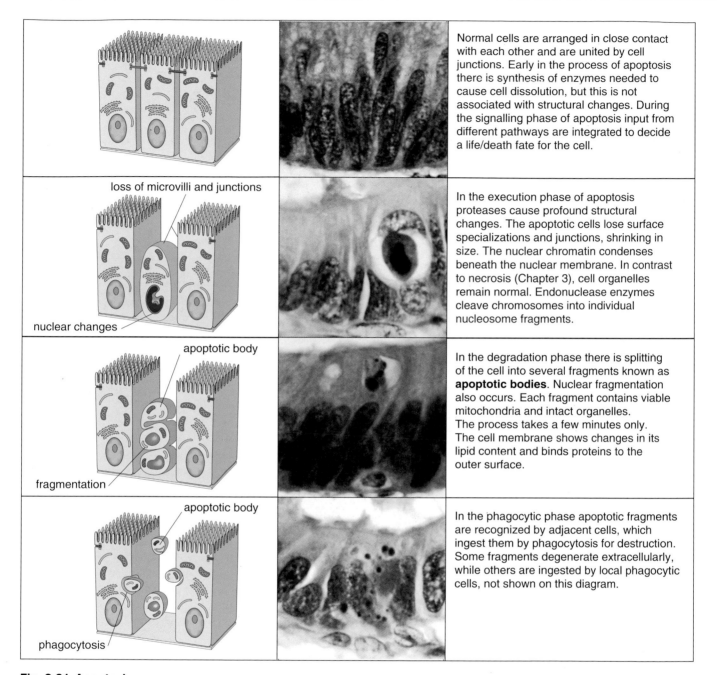

Normal cells are arranged in close contact with each other and are united by cell junctions. Early in the process of apoptosis there is synthesis of enzymes needed to cause cell dissolution, but this is not associated with structural changes. During the signalling phase of apoptosis input from different pathways are integrated to decide a life/death fate for the cell.

In the execution phase of apoptosis proteases cause profound structural changes. The apoptotic cells lose surface specializations and junctions, shrinking in size. The nuclear chromatin condenses beneath the nuclear membrane. In contrast to necrosis (Chapter 3), cell organelles remain normal. Endonuclease enzymes cleave chromosomes into individual nucleosome fragments.

In the degradation phase there is splitting of the cell into several fragments known as **apoptotic bodies**. Nuclear fragmentation also occurs. Each fragment contains viable mitochondria and intact organelles. The process takes a few minutes only. The cell membrane shows changes in its lipid content and binds proteins to the outer surface.

In the phagocytic phase apoptotic fragments are recognized by adjacent cells, which ingest them by phagocytosis for destruction. Some fragments degenerate extracellularly, while others are ingested by local phagocytic cells, not shown on this diagram.

Fig. 2.21 Apoptosis.
Apoptosis of cells is a programed and energy-dependent process designed specifically to switch cells off and eliminate them. This controlled pattern of cell death, termed programed cell death, is very different from that which occurs as a direct result of a severe, damaging stimulus to cells (discussed in Chapter 3).

3. DNA-damage/p53–p73 pathway: damage to DNA results in accumulation of p53 protein in the cell and this facilitates DNA repair. If this is not successful the p53 system modulates transcription of factors that favor apoptosis. Examples include:

- Apoptotic cell death after irradiation-induced DNA damage.
- Apoptotic cell death induced by anti-tumor chemotherapeutic drugs.

4. Cell membrane damage pathway: damage to the cell membrane results in activation of the enzyme sphingomyelinase, generating ceramide.

Ceramide then signals other intracellular events leading to apoptosis. Examples include:

- Apoptotic cell death due to irradiation-induced cell damage.
- Apoptotic cell death after free-radical-induced membrane damage.

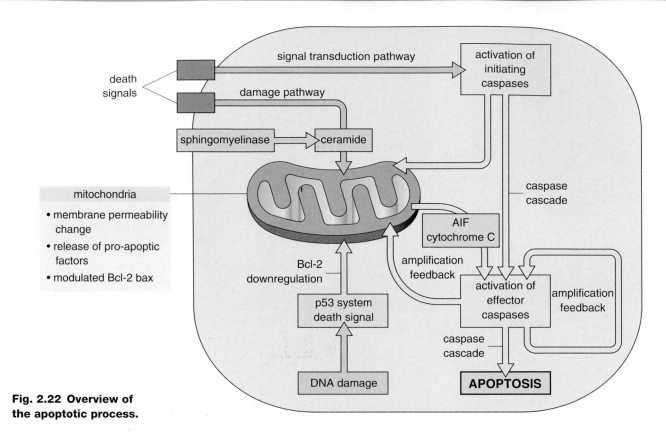

Fig. 2.22 Overview of the apoptotic process.

The caspase enzymes involved in apoptosis can be divided into two groups: initiating and effector, analogous to executioner and executioner's sword

Caspases exist in an inactive form in the cytosol of most cells as procaspases and require cleavage for activation. Caspases may cause activation of other caspases leading to the idea of a cascade of activation, analogous to that encountered in the blood coagulation cascade. The role of caspases is believed to be two-fold:

- In certain situations, specific caspase activation is the signal that commits a cell to apoptotic cell death (acting as the executioner signal). These are called initiating or 'upstream' caspases (mainly caspases 2, 8, 9 and 10).
- In all cases of apoptosis, specific caspases are the proteases which bring about structural degradation of the cell to give the classical morphological and biochemical features of apoptosis (acting as the executioner's sword). These are termed effector or 'downstream' caspases (caspases 3, 6 and 7).

Some caspases may be initiating proteases in some cell types, but effector proteases in other cell types.

In some systems some death-regulatory signals seem to act independently of caspase cascade activation, committing cells to die in the absence of 'upstream' caspase activation. While the executional 'upstream' signal is not caspase-related, the executioner's sword is still enacted via 'downstream' effector caspase activation.

Mitochondrial damage may trigger the point of no return for apoptosis in many cell systems

It is now realised that proteins released from mitochondria are vital players in the initiation of apoptosis. The integrity of the mitochondrial membrane systems has been proposed as the deciding factor in the fate of a cell: survival or death. In study of apoptosis it has been found that the ability of mitochondria to maintain a trans-membrane potential across their membrane systems becomes impaired before downstream, effector caspases are activated (*Fig. 2.23*).

The loss of mitochondrial potential is related to the opening of a huge composite ion channel that spans both inner and outer mitochondrial membranes, termed the **permeability transition pore complex** (PTPC) also referred to as the mitochondrial '*megachannel*'. This opening leads to release of material from mitochondria into the cytosol.

Important molecules released include cytochrome C (activates downstream caspases by forming an apoptosome) and apoptosis initiating factor (AIF) (a caspase activating factor) (*Fig. 2.23*).

Importantly, certain proteins associated with mitochondria can regulate the process of apoptosis. Bcl-2 and Bcl-XL are proteins which prevent opening of the megachannel and hence are protective against apoptosis. In contrast, mitochondrial-related proteins Bax and Bad serve to promote apoptotic opening of the megachannel.

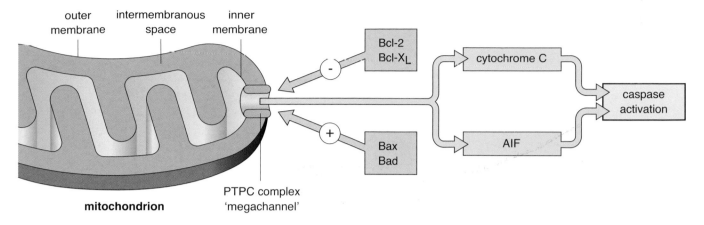

Fig. 2.23 Mitochondrial integrity is a key factor in apoptosis.

There is the suggestion that some activated caspases may act to cause mitochondrial damage, therefore amplifying a cell-death cascade involving both signal-tranduced caspase activation and mitochondrial-apoptosome caspase activation.

Direct mitochondrial damage, for example by toxins, free radicals or anoxia, can result in direct opening of the megachannel, releasing mitochondrial factors that activate apoptotic cell death. In this process, although effector (downstream) caspases are activated, the input of initiating (upstream) caspases is not required to trigger apoptotic cell death.

It therefore seems that factors which influence mitochondrial membrane permeability are the important players in regulating apoptosis in the cell. Pro-apoptotic factors increase permeability and allow release of cytochrome C and apoptosis initiating factor, while anti-apoptotic factors sequester vital proteins and preserve mitochondrial membrane integrity.

The executioner's sword of apoptosis can be activated by protein derived from disrupted mitochondria

Cytochrome C, and a protein called apoptosis initiating factor (AIF), both derived from mitochondria, are powerful activators of the effector or 'downstream' caspases. Cytochrome C forms a complex with other proteins to form an important caspase cascade activator which has been called an **apoptosome**.

It seems that a crucial event in activating downstream caspases via formation of the apoptosome is the availability of cytochrome C in the cytosol. The Bcl-2 protein (an anti-apoptotic factor) sequesters cytochrome C and prevents it activating apoptosis via the apoptosome. This partly explains why high levels of expression of Bcl-2 protect cells from apoptotic cell death. Bcl-w probably also has anti-apoptotic effects by sequestering the pro-apoptotic protease activating factor (Apaf-1), stabilizing mitochondrial membrane, and also by antagonizing opening of the mitochondrial megachannel.

Laboratory recognition of apoptosis is important in biological research

With a central role of apoptosis being found in so many disease processes, identifying apoptotic cells has become an important aspect in the investigation of the pathogenesis of disease. The recognition of apoptosis can be achieved by several techniques:

- Conventional morphology using light microscopy, or more specifically electron microscopy, will reveal characteristic structural features of apoptosis.
- If DNA is extracted from tissues and agarose gel electrophoresis performed, then a ladder pattern is seen corresponding to cleavage of DNA at nucleosomes by apoptosis-related endonucleases.
- Endonuclease activity results in breaks in double-stranded DNA. This can be detected in tissue sections by the tunel technique.
- Immunohistochemistry for transglutaminase can be used to identify cells in the effector stage of apoptosis.
- Immunohistochemistry for annexin-V on the cell surface can be used to identify cells that are in suspension, for example cells in culture using flow cytometry.

Apoptotic fragments are recognized by receptors on phagocytic cells

The cell fragments generated by the apoptotic processes are characterized by a change in the lipid composition of the outer cell membrane with flipping of phosphatidylserine from the inner leaflet to the outer surface.

Vitronectin and thrombospondin bind to the surface of apoptotic cells and these proteins are recognized by phagocytic cells such as macrophages and lead to engulfment and elimination of apoptotic remnants.

The apoptosis signalling pathways are characterized by several branching and convergence points

Fig. 2.24 summarizes the events in apoptosis. It can be seen that there are several branching and convergence points in the four main pathways involved in this process. Importantly, mitochondrial factors, caspases, ceramide, and free radicals are involved at several points.

- The signal transduction pathway, activated by binding a ligand at a cell surface receptor, induces apoptosis by direct activation of initiating caspases and also acts by modulating pro-apoptotic and anti-apoptotic factors of the Bcl-2 family.

- DNA damage activates the p53 system and this regulates the balance between pro-apoptotic and anti-apoptotic factors to cause cell death. This system is important as it eliminates cells that have irreparable DNA damage. Failure of this system leads to the generation of tumors (Chapter 6).

- Direct damage to cells via a variety of mechanisms, especially related to generation of free radicals, induces apoptosis by increasing the permeability of mitochondria and liberating pro-apoptotic factors into the cell that activate the effector arm of the apoptotic caspase enzyme system.

- Plasma membrane damage from a variety of stimuli, including irradiation, activates sphingomyelinase to generate ceramide from membrane lipids. Ceramide is then capable of initiating apoptosis.

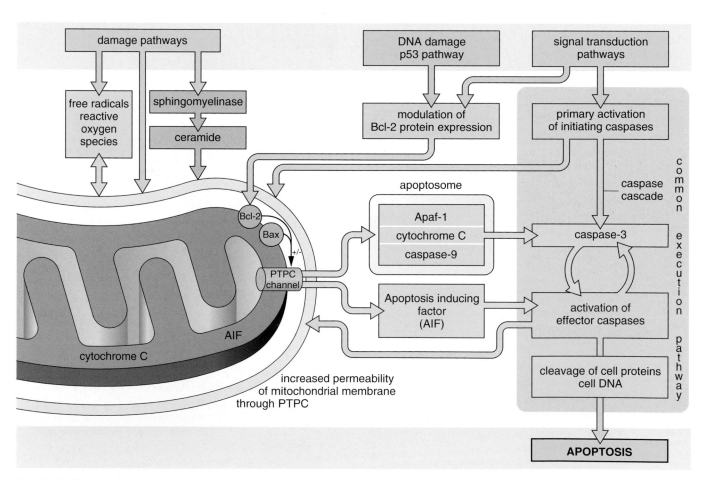

Fig. 2.24 Summary overview of the apoptotic process.

3 Cell injury and death

Pathological cell death is due to irreversible cell injury

Exposure of cells to damaging stimuli results in pathological cell death. This may occur via two fundamentally different processes:

- Certain damaging stimuli, particularly those mediated by the immune system and cytokines, cause cell death by switching on **apoptosis** (*Fig. 2.12*), a form of **programed cell death**. This type of response has been discussed in detail in Chapter 2, and is of great importance in disease.
- Other types of damaging stimuli impair key cellular systems, causing dysfunction outside an adaptable range, after which cell death occurs by a process termed **necrosis**.

Severe cell injury damages key cellular functions

Several interdependent cell components are primary targets for damaging stimuli:

- Cell membranes.
- Mitochondria.
- Cytoskeleton.
- Cellular DNA.

Because of interdependence, damage to one system leads to secondary damage to others and, ultimately, cell death occurs when a threshold of accumulated damage is passed. One example, which illustrates the concept of a cascade of accumulated damage, is seen in cells that are subject to lack of oxygen and nutrients owing to failure of blood supply (ischemia) (*Fig. 3.1*).

- Primary impairment of mitochondrial energy production is due mainly to lack of oxygen (hypoxia) and glucose (hypoglycemia), but may also be caused by toxins, for example cyanide, which directly inhibit cytochrome oxidase.
- Primary cell membrane injury is due mainly to free radical-mediated damage, immune-mediated damage (particularly via the complement system), and direct actions of bacterial toxins.

Molecular mechanisms that are considered important in cell death are discussed in more detail in the pink box on page 24.

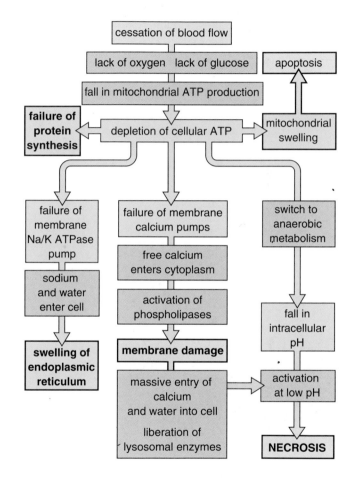

Fig. 3.1 Cellular response to ischemia.
ATP production by mitochondria relies on an adequate supply of oxygen and of energy substrates such as glucose. Mitochondrial function is therefore compromised soon after failure of blood supply, resulting in failure of production of ATP. One consequence of lack of ATP is failure of ATP-dependent membrane pumps, which normally pump sodium (and with it water) out of cells. Failure of membrane ion pumps leads to accumulation of sodium and water in the cell cytoplasm, with disruption of internal membrane systems. Failure of internal membrane pumps also allows free calcium to enter the cytosol, where it activates many destructive enzyme systems. Structural damage to internal membranes and the cytoskeleton, coupled with lack of ATP, leads to impairment of key synthetic pathways including those of protein synthesis. Rupture of lysosomes and intracellular liberation of powerful hydrolytic enzymes, active at a low pH, brings about further cellular dissolution.

Molecular mechanisms in damaged cells

ATP loss causes failure of biosynthesis and ion pumps

If cells become hypoxic or mitochondria are directly damaged, they cannot produce adequate ATP. The capacity that cells have for anaerobic production of ATP is limited by accumulation of lactate and is usually soon exhausted. Lack of ATP causes failure of membrane pumps, probably contributing to swelling of internal membrane systems in cells, seen as so-called 'cloudy swelling'. There is also failure of many biosynthetic processes, most of which require ATP.

Cytosolic free calcium is a potent destructive agent

The normal concentration of calcium in the cytosol is very low and there are finely tuned regulatory systems to ensure that this is not disturbed. Free calcium is used by secondary messenger systems to activate a variety of cytosolic enzymes:

- Protein kinases which bring about phosphorylation of other proteins.
- Phospholipases, which can attack membrane lipids.
- Calpain, a protease which can cause disassembly of cytoskeletal proteins in cells.

Calcium is usually rapidly removed from the cytosol by ATP-dependent calcium pumps. In normal cells, calcium is bound to buffering proteins, such as calbindin or parvalbumin, and is contained in the endoplasmic reticulum (ER), as well as in mitochondria. If there is abnormal permeability of calcium-ion channels, direct damage to membranes, depletion of ATP, or damage to mitochondria, calcium increases in concentration in the cytosol. If this cannot be buffered or pumped out of cells, uncontrolled enzyme activation takes place with further damaging consequences. It has become evident that uncontrolled entry of calcium into the cytosol (*Fig. 3.2*) is an important final common pathway in many causes of cell death.

Reactive oxygen metabolites damage cells

In all cells, highly reactive oxygen metabolites are constantly generated. Because they are potentially damaging to cells, they are constantly scavenged by protective systems, the integrity of which, in turn, is dependent upon an adequate nutrient supply (*Fig. 3.3*).

```
          calcium stores
    sequestered in mitochondria
    sequestered in ER lumen
    pumped to extracellular space
    bound to calcium-binding proteins
                  │
                  ▼
     release following cell damage
                  │
                  ▼
             free Ca++
         ┌────────┼────────┐
         ▼        ▼        ▼
   activation  activation activation
   of protein  of         of
   kinases     phospholipases proteases
         │        │        │
         ▼        ▼        ▼
  phosphorylation membrane cytoskeletal
  of protein     damage   disassembly
```

Fig. 3.2 Cytosolic free calcium is a potent destructive agent.

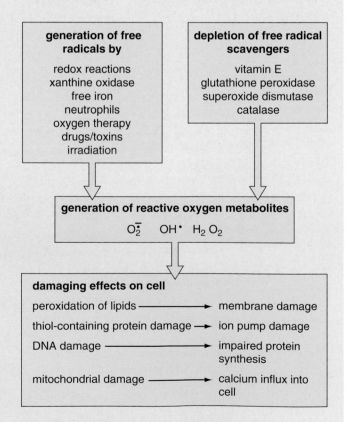

Fig. 3.3 Reactive oxygen metabolites damage cells.

▶ The main scavenging systems are:

- Antioxidants such as vitamin E.
- Glutathione peroxidase.
- Superoxide dismutase.
- Catalase.

The most important of the reactive oxygen species are generated when oxygen is reduced to water, and most are created by systems involved in electron and oxygen transport:

- Superoxide anion (O_2).
- Hydroxyl radical (OH).
- Hydrogen peroxide (H_2O_2).

Certain generative reactions are catalyzed by the presence of free iron in cells, which is therefore potentially damaging.

Another important source of reactive oxygen species is xanthine, which accumulates in hypoxic tissues as a metabolite of ATP. In hypoxic conditions, accumulated xanthine can be oxidized by the enzyme xanthine oxidase to generate reactive oxygen species.

Reactive free radicals can also be produced as intermediates in the metabolism of certain toxins (e.g. carbon tetrachloride) and drugs (e.g. paracetamol/acetaminophen), by irradiation, and by neutrophil leukocytes as part of the mechanism for bacterial killing. These reactive species have several damaging effects:

- Peroxidation of lipids in cell membranes takes place, causing membrane permeability.
- Thiol groups in proteins are attacked. Certain critical proteins are then damaged, for example membrane Na/K ATPase pumps.
- DNA strands become fragmented.

- Mitochondria become depleted of NADPH and liberate free calcium into the cytosol.

Following ischemia, cells become depleted of energy, but reactive oxygen species do not develop as there is no oxygen in the tissues. If, as a consequence of re-establishing a blood supply, tissues are reperfused, huge amounts of reactive oxygen species are generated, both by mitochondria and by xanthine oxidase. Depleted energy-dependent scavenging mechanisms are overwhelmed, and extensive cell damage and death ensue.

This is the basis of so-called **reperfusion necrosis**: tissue necrosis takes place, not on cessation of blood supply, but on re-establishment. For this reason the xanthine oxidase inhibitor drug allopurinol has been used clinically in attempts to limit the extent of cardiac muscle necrosis following myocardial infarction, thought to be mediated by reactive oxygen species on reperfusion.

Membrane and cytoskeletal damage

The integrity of the cell membrane is essential for cell survival following damage. Direct damage to cell membranes is a primary event in immune-mediated injury, for example when complement activation causes C9 to form transmembrane pores, allowing influx of calcium into the target cell. In energy-depleted cells there is failure of biosynthesis of new membrane phospholipids; depletion of phospholipids also takes place when phospholipases are activated by free calcium, and membrane damage is inevitable. In addition, calcium-activated proteases destroy the cytoskeletal bracing of cell membranes by demolishing cytoskeletal link proteins, rendering cells abnormally fragile under contractile or osmotic stresses.

KEY FACTS
Cell injury

- The main targets for cell injury are cell membranes, mitochondria, cytoskeleton and cellular DNA.
- Because of interdependence, damage to one cellular system leads to secondary damage to others.
- Reactive oxygen metabolites are extremely harmful to cells and are produced on reperfusion after ischemia.

- ATP loss causes failure of biosynthesis and membrane pumps.
- Free calcium in the cytosol activates intracellular enzymes and causes cell death.

Cell response ranges from recoverable damage to instant death

If damage to a cell is minimal, the cell can recover following removal of the damaging stimulus. Damaged proteins and organelles are removed by a cell stress response and autophagy (*Fig. 2.11*), with new structural components being synthesized. This is termed sublethal cell damage and is associated with recognizable structural changes.

In other situations a damaging stimulus may first cause sublethal damage and then, because the cell cannot recover, progress to cell death. There are two main structural routes of cell death that may occur after a lethal damaging stimulus: apoptosis (page 18) and necrosis. It is becoming apparent that the magnitude and type of injurious stimuli can determine whether a cell undergoes death through apoptosis or necrosis: severe damaging stimuli tending to result in necrosis, and lower grade damaging stimuli and stimuli from immune-mediated damage tending to cause apoptosis. A critical factor in determination of whether a cell follows an apoptotic or necrotic path to death seems to be how much cellular ATP is available after cell damage. In conditions where there is severe depletion of ATP, the necrotic pathway is followed.

In unusual circumstances, if the damaging stimulus to a cell is massive, the cell is killed immediately without passing through the stages of apoptosis or necrosis. This occurs most commonly with overwhelming physical agents such as severe heat or strong acids, both of which coagulate cell proteins. These relationships are summarized in *Figs 3.4* and *3.5*.

Sublethal damage is associated with reversible structural abnormalities

Sublethal damage can be identified from microscopic changes in affected cells. The first evidence of such damage is seen ultrastructurally as swelling of membrane-bound organelles, particularly endoplasmic reticulum and mitochondria.

- Mitochondrial swelling can be seen as an early event after cell damage. At first, spaces or vacuoles develop within the mitochondrion, distorting and separating the normally regular stacks of cristae. This change, termed **low-amplitude swelling**, is potentially reversible if the noxious stimulus is insufficient to cause cell death. Persisting insult leads to actual destruction of the cristae, the development of electron dense aggregates in the mitochondrial stroma, and more severe swelling. At this stage, termed **high-amplitude swelling**, the changes are irreversible and the mitochondrion is permanently damaged. Proteins leak from mitochondria, leading to generation of apoptosis. Depletion of cellular ATP develops (*Fig. 3.6*).

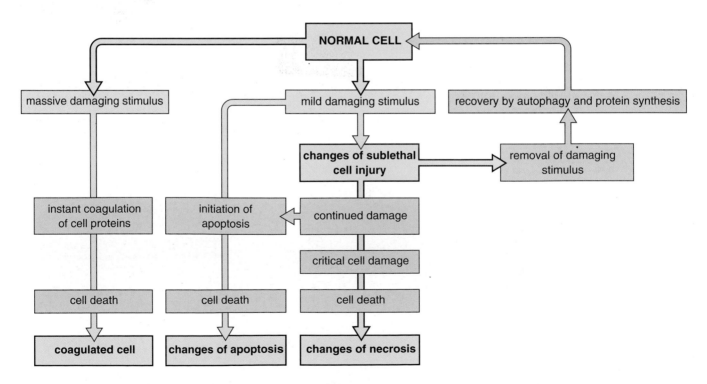

Fig. 3.4 Relationships between sublethal and lethal cell damage.
Normal cells that are subject to a damaging stimulus may initiate apoptosis or may become sublethally damaged. If the stimulus abates cells may recover by resynthesis of proteins and elimination of damaged components. If a damaging stimulus continues cells die either through apoptosis or, when critical cell damage takes place mainly through critical lack of ATP, cells die and undergo necrosis. Massively damaging stimuli, e.g. great heat or strong acids, cause immediate coagulation of proteins and death of cells (see *Fig. 2.12*).

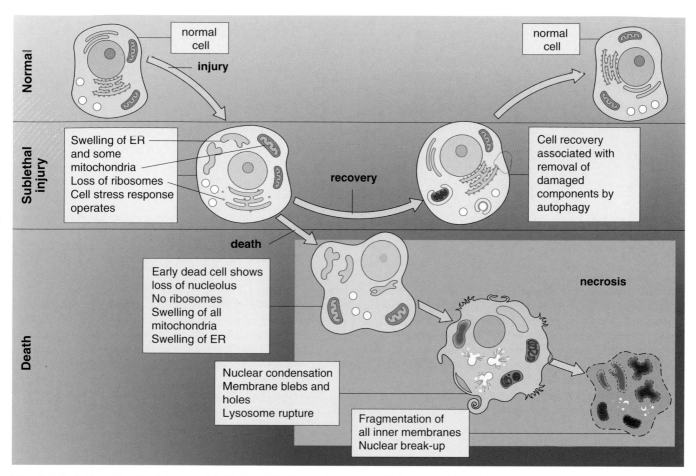

Fig. 3.5 Relationships between sublethal and lethal cell damage. Following sublethal damage a cell may recover or, with persistence of the damaging stimulus, cell death may result. The sequential structural changes of cell death are termed 'necrosis'.

Mitochondrial damage can cause apoptosis

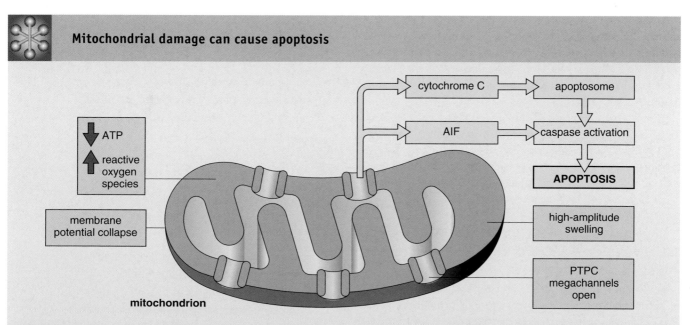

Fig. 3.6 After damage to mitochondrial membranes there is failure of ATP production and loss of the normal membrane potential of the mitochondrion. The mitochondrial membrane pores (PTPC *megachannels*) open and release proteins into the cytosol, which can cause apoptosis, as described in Chapter 2. If many mitochondria in a cell fail, causing a catastrophic reduction in ATP production, the cell will die by a non-apoptic route.

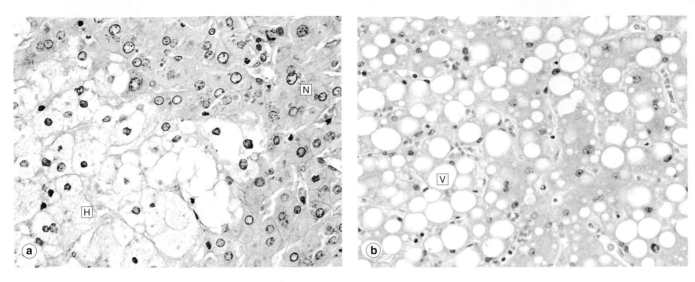

Fig. 3.7 Sublethal cell damage. (a) Hydropic degeneration. (b) Fatty change.
Micrograph (a) shows a section of liver damaged by the poison paraquat. Normal liver cells (**N**) contrast with injured cells, which are swollen, pale and vacuolated (**H**). The normal cell cytoplasm is pink with a faint hint of purple, the purple coloration (basophilia) being due to ribosomes, mainly on the RER. With swelling of ER, ribosomes become detached and reduced in number, so the normal purple cytoplasmic tint is reduced. Further cytoplasmic pallor is due to progressive swelling of ER and mitochondria that is known as **cloudy swelling** when mild, and **hydropic degeneration** when small, discrete vacuoles develop in the cytoplasm. Another example of sublethal damage is seen in micrograph (b), taken from the liver of an alcoholic patient. This shows extensive **fatty change** with large vacuoles (**V**) of fat within hepatocytes. As solvents used in conventional histological preparations dissolve out the fat to leave a clear space, lipid can be positively demonstrated only by using frozen sections.

- Swelling of endoplasmic reticulum (ER) is also seen early in the course of cell injury and is associated with loss of ribosomes attached to the rough endoplasmic reticulum (RER).

At the light microscopic level these reversible changes caused by organelle swelling are reflected in cellular swelling, paleness of cell cytoplasm, and development of small intracellular vacuoles, giving rise to the widely used descriptive terms **cloudy swelling** and **hydropic degeneration** (*Fig. 3.7*).

Another manifestation of sublethal cell damage is impairment of fatty acid metabolism. Affected cells accumulate lipid within cytoplasmic vacuoles, giving rise to the term **fatty change**. This is seen particularly in cells that have central roles in fatty acid metabolism, especially hepatocytes (*Fig. 3.7*). Mechanisms involved in fatty change are presented in *Fig. 3.8*.

Dead cells go through a series of structural changes termed necrosis

Lethal injury is followed by distinct structural changes in cells, which reflect disintegration of cellular structure due to activation of intracellular lysosomal enzymes. The dissolution of cells through the activity of intrinsic hydrolytic enzymes is termed **autolysis**. Autolysis brings about changes in both cytoplasm and nucleus during the evolution of a necrotic cell, as summarized in *Fig. 3.9*.

KEY FACTS
Sublethal damage

- Sublethal damage is recoverable, necrosis is not.
- The earliest visible sign of sublethal damage is ultrastructural damage to mitochondria.
- Later sublethal damage can be seen as swelling of cellular organelles (hydropic degeneration).
- Fatty change is a manifestation of sublethal impairment of metabolism and is common in the liver.

KEY FACTS
Necrosis

- Intense eosinophilia of the dead cell is due to loss of RNA and coagulation of proteins.
- Nuclei undergo phases of pyknosis, karyorrhexis, and karyolysis, leaving a shrunken cell devoid of nucleus.
- Proteins may be liberated from the dead cells and be detected in the blood in diagnosis.

Fatty change

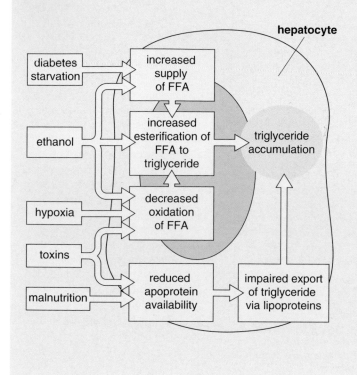

hepatocyte

Fig. 3.8 Fatty change. This is a manifestation of sublethal metabolic derangement, seen in certain cells which have a high throughput of lipid as part of normal metabolic requirements. Such change is usually seen in the liver, but it also occurs less commonly in the myocardium and the kidney. Common causes of fatty change are toxins (particularly alcohol and halogenated hydrocarbons such as chloroform), chronic hypoxia and diabetes mellitus. Impaired metabolism of fatty acids leads to accumulation of triglycerides (fat), which form vacuoles in cells.

There are four main metabolic reasons for the accumulation of triglyceride in cells:

- Increased peripheral mobilization of free fatty acids (FFA) and uptake into cells (diabetes mellitus and nutritional deprivation).
- Increased conversion of fatty acids to triglycerides (alcohol).
- Reduced oxidation of triglycerides to acetyl-CoA (hypoxia and toxins including ethanol).
- Deficiency of lipid acceptor proteins, preventing export of formed triglycerides (carbon tetrachloride and protein malnutrition). Fatty change is reversible if the abnormality responsible is removed. It may be associated with other types of sublethal injury in cells.

Several different patterns of necrosis are described

Several patterns of tissue necrosis have been traditionally described, reflecting the varying macroscopic appearances of the necrotic tissue.

- **Coagulative necrosis** describes dead tissue that appears firm and pale, as if cooked. In areas of coagulative necrosis, much of the cellular outline and tissue architecture can still be discerned histologically, even though the cells are dead. It is likely that this type of response takes place because affected cells have relatively few lysosomes to bring about complete breakdown of cellular proteins. The most common cause of this pattern of necrosis is occlusion of the arterial supply to a tissue (*Fig. 3.10a*). Proteins liberated from dead cells can enter the blood (*Fig. 3.11*).
- **Liquefactive** or **colliquative necrosis** describes dead tissue that appears semi-liquid as a result of dissolution of tissue by the action of hydrolytic enzymes. The most common types of damage leading to the liquefactive pattern are necrosis in the brain owing to arterial occlusion (cerebral infarction, *Fig. 3.10b*), and necrosis caused by bacterial infections.

In the brain, the huge lysosomal content in neurons, together with the relative lack of extracellular structural proteins (reticulin and collagen), leads to rapid loss of tissue architecture and liquefaction when lysosomal enzyme release takes place. In bacterial infection, microorganisms attract neutrophils into the area, which then release neutrophil hydrolases and cause liquefaction.

- **Caseous necrosis** describes dead tissue that is soft and white, resembling cream cheese. With this type of necrosis, dead cells form an amorphous proteinaceous mass but, in contrast to coagulative necrosis, no original architecture can be seen histologically. This pattern is invariably associated with tuberculosis (see *Fig. 3.10c*).
- **Gummatous necrosis** describes dead tissue when it is firm and rubbery. As in caseous necrosis the dead cells form an amorphous proteinaceous mass in which no original architecture can be seen histologically. However, the gummatous pattern is restricted to describing necrosis in the spirochetal infection syphilis (*Fig. 3.10d*).
- **Hemorrhagic necrosis** describes dead tissues that are suffused with extravasated red cells. This pattern is seen particularly when cell death is due to blockage

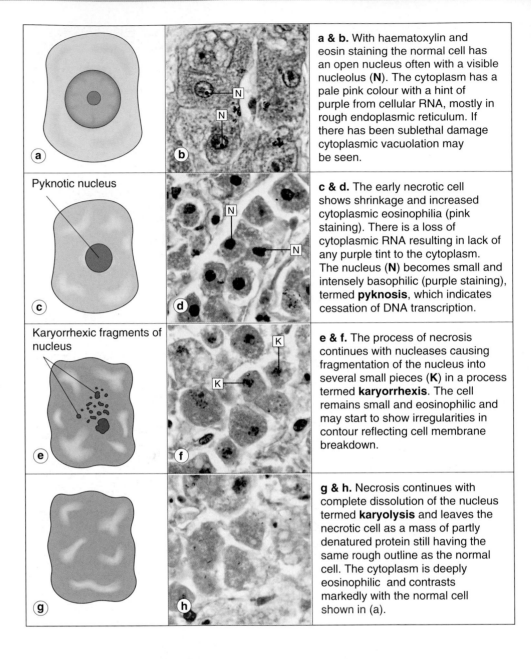

Pyknotic nucleus

Karyorrhexic fragments of nucleus

a & b. With haematoxylin and eosin staining the normal cell has an open nucleus often with a visible nucleolus (**N**). The cytoplasm has a pale pink colour with a hint of purple from cellular RNA, mostly in rough endoplasmic reticulum. If there has been sublethal damage cytoplasmic vacuolation may be seen.

c & d. The early necrotic cell shows shrinkage and increased cytoplasmic eosinophilia (pink staining). There is a loss of cytoplasmic RNA resulting in lack of any purple tint to the cytoplasm. The nucleus (**N**) becomes small and intensely basophilic (purple staining), termed **pyknosis**, which indicates cessation of DNA transcription.

e & f. The process of necrosis continues with nucleases causing fragmentation of the nucleus into several small pieces (**K**) in a process termed **karyorrhexis**. The cell remains small and eosinophilic and may start to show irregularities in contour reflecting cell membrane breakdown.

g & h. Necrosis continues with complete dissolution of the nucleus termed **karyolysis** and leaves the necrotic cell as a mass of partly denatured protein still having the same rough outline as the normal cell. The cytoplasm is deeply eosinophilic and contrasts markedly with the normal cell shown in (a).

Fig. 3.9 Cellular events in necrosis.
These sections are from the liver of a person poisoned by paracetamol (acetamenophen), a hepatic toxin. Many of the changes seen in necrosis are caused by the action of lysosomal hydrolases, which are released into the cell when cell membrane integrity is lost.

The nucleus of a necrotic cell first becomes small, condensed, and intensely stained with hematoxylin (basophilic). This appearance is termed pyknosis. Next, pyknotic nuclei become fragmented into several particles, a change known as karyorrhexis. Complete breakdown of karyolysis of the nucleus then takes place.

When tissue is damaged in this way, tissue defences are activated to limit the damage and restore tissue function (see Chapter 4).

of the venous drainage of a tissue, leading to massive congestion by blood and to subsequent arterial failure of perfusion (*Fig. 3.10e*).

- **Fat necrosis** describes foci of hard, yellow material seen in dead adipose tissue. This reaction can occur after liberation of pancreatic enzymes into the peritoneal cavity, following inflammation of the pancreas (see page 300). It may also be seen after trauma to fat, for example in the breast (see page 421).

- **Fibrinoid necrosis** is a term used to describe the histological appearance of arteries in cases of vasculitis (primary inflammation of vessels) and hypertension, when fibrin is deposited in the damaged necrotic vessel wall (see *Fig. 3.10f*).

KEY FACTS
Patterns of necrosis

Several tissue patterns of necrosis are identifiable:

- The most common pattern is coagulative necrosis caused by occlusion of vascular supply.
- Liquefactive necrosis is seen in the brain and in infections.
- Caseous necrosis is seen in tuberculosis.
- Gummatous necrosis is seen in syphilis.
- Fibrinoid necrosis is seen in vessel walls in hypertension and vasculitis.

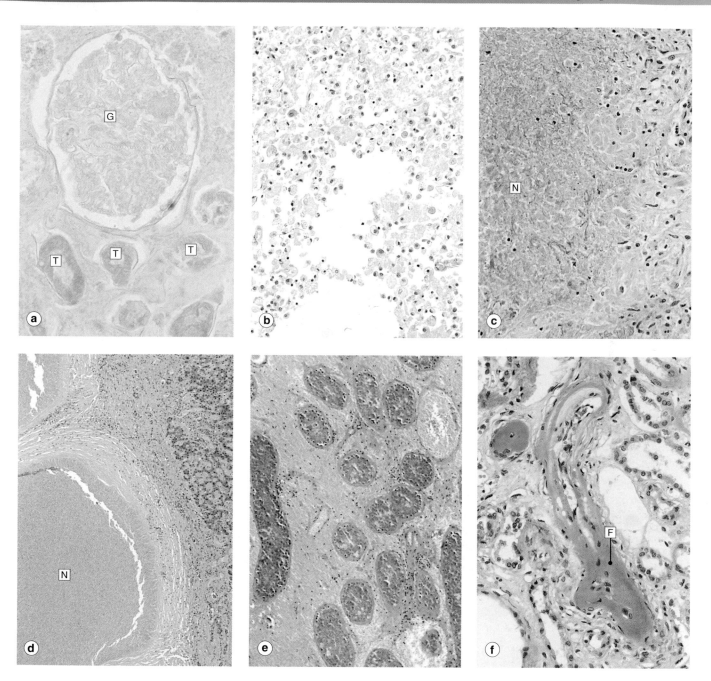

Fig. 3.10 Patterns of tissue necrosis. (a) Coagulative necrosis: kidney. (b) Liquefactive necrosis: brain. (c) Caseous necrosis: kidney. (d) Gummatous necrosis: liver. (e) Hemorrhagic necrosis: testis. (f) Fibrinoid necrosis: artery.
Micrograph (a) is an example of coagulative necrosis in an area of kidney which has been killed by interruption of its blood supply (infarction). The outlines of a glomerulus (**G**) and surrounding tubules (**T**) are recognizable, despite the fact that all the cells are dead. Micrograph (b) shows liquefaction in a cerebral infarct. In contrast to (a), no residual tissue architecture has been preserved. The necrotic brain area has been transformed into a semi-fluid mass of protein with phagocytic macrophages. Micrograph (c) shows an area of caseous necrosis from a kidney infected by *Mycobacterium tuberculosis*. The necrotic area (**N**) is homogeneously pink and, compared to (a), has no semblance of underlying renal architecture. This pattern is also illustrated in Chapter 4.

Micrograph (d) shows an area of gummatous necrosis (**N**) in the liver of a patient with syphilis caused by long-standing infection by the spirochete *Treponema pallidum*. Micrograph (e) demonstrates an area of testicular hemorrhagic necrosis caused by torsion (twisting) of the testis on the end of the spermatic cord, such that the venous return is cut off. This leads to ischemia of the testis, as it becomes massively suffused with blood that cannot escape. Micrograph (f) shows a vessel that has undergone fibrinoid necrosis. The wall of the affected vessel is replaced by bright pink staining material (**F**). In this instance, damage to the vessels was due to severe hypertension.

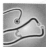

Laboratory medicine

Proteins liberated into the blood following necrosis are used in diagnosis

When cells die some of their proteins and enzymes are liberated and may be detected in the blood. Their presence can thus be used in clinical practice to establish whether a tissue or cell type has been damaged by disease. For the purposes of diagnosis the protein must be relatively restricted to one cell type and must normally be present in the blood in relatively low concentration, so that an elevation following cell damage can be detected. Several clinical chemistry tests rely on this general principle.

Fig. 3.11
Enzymes used in diagnosis of tissue damage by blood testing

Cell damaged	Enzyme elevated in blood
Cardiac muscle	Creatine kinase (MB isoform) Aspartate transaminase (AST) Lactate dehydrogenase (LDH-1)
Hepatocyte	Alanine transaminase (ALT)
Striated muscle	Creatine kinase (MM isoform)
Exocrine pancreas	Amylase

Damage to DNA causes sublethal damage long after the event

Certain damaging agents, most notably irradiation, injure the genetic apparatus of cells, resulting in abnormal genetic functioning. This may not be manifest as immediate cellular dysfunction, but may predispose affected cells to later problems.

- Cell division to repair damage may not be effective, leading to poor healing in damaged tissues (see Chapter 4).
- Mutations in DNA may predipose to development of tumors such as cancers (see Chapter 6).
- Cells with irradiation-induced DNA damage may be triggered to enter the apoptotic pathway of cell death.

Some cells are sensitive to damage while others are robust

Not all cells are equally susceptible to damaging agents. This is illustrated by the range of sensitivity exhibited by cells following cessation of oxygenation (hypoxia) to the whole body, as might happen after a cardiac arrest.

- The most sensitive cells are the large neurons of the hippocampus and cerebellum, which die after only 2–5 minutes without oxygen. More prolonged hypoxia causes damage to the majority of pyramidal cells in the cerebral cortex.
- The most robust cells are fibroblasts. They remain in an area of tissue damage even after all specialized parenchymal cells have been destroyed. It is possible to culture fibroblasts from the tissues of a person who has been declared somatically dead for many hours.

The reason why some cells are more sensitive to hypoxia than others lies in the varying metabolic capacities of the different cell types to survive ATP depletion and calcium influx, and to buffer free radical-induced damage. Differing metabolic capability of apparently similar cells also occurs. For example, hepatocytes in the periportal region of the liver have low levels of enzymes which generate toxic metabolites from paracetamol (acetamenophen), while centrilobular hepatocytes have high levels. This explains why liver necrosis following paracetamol toxicity is limited to centrilobular hepatocytes.

Aging is a form of cell degeneration that is not understood

Aging is associated with degeneration and loss of function of many cellular systems. With increasing age the incidence of many important diseases increases, some of which are probably due to a cumulative environmental exposure to a causative agent. However, others are due to the process of biological aging itself. Several theories seek to explain aging at a molecular level, but none entirely explains aging as a single biological phenomenon.

KEY FACTS
Aging

There are several theories of aging:

- Programed aging proposes that cells have a limited number of divisions.
- Other proposals suggest inefficient DNA repair, free radical damage, or failure of protein catabolism as the root cause of aging.
- Cumulative injury theories propose that damage to any systems sustained through life summate and are manifest as aging.

Somatic death is followed by autolysis and putrefaction

Death of cells and tissues does not result in the inevitable death of the individual. However, if physiological functions are critically impaired through tissue damage, for example respiration or cardiac output, death of the individual (known as **somatic death**) occurs. Following somatic death there is death of all cells in the body, and release of lysosomal enzymes causes decomposition of tissues through **autolysis**, being similar to the events of necrosis. Microorganisms, for example from the gut, also invade tissues and cause further putrefaction.

The processes of autolysis and bacterial decomposition can be slowed by refrigeration or by preservation in preservative solutions. This is the main reason for fixation of surgically resected organs and tissues in preservatives such as formaldehyde solution (formalin); morphology is thus preserved and autolysis is prevented.

 Cell biology of aging

- **Programed aging.** It has been proposed that cells have a programed capacity for a limited number of cell divisions, after which cells are not replaced and atrophy ensues with loss of function. Alternative theories suggest that essential neuroendocrine stimuli from brain or endocrine glands are programed to stop at a certain biological age, resulting in lack of essential trophic factors to maintain cell growth.
- **DNA repair defects.** It has been suggested that aging is merely the result of the known inefficiencies in repair of DNA, which occur at a low level in normal people. With time the proportion of cells carrying abnormal DNA increases and tissue function is impaired. This applies not only to nuclear DNA but also to mitochondrial DNA, which has much less effective systems for repairing damage.
- **Degeneration in extracellular matrix materials**, through protein cross-linking, modification such as glycosylation, and oxidation, has been proposed as a mechanism that impairs function of the specialized parenchymal cells, leading to cell dysfunction with age.
- **Free radical damage.** Decrease in the availability of free radical scavenging systems has been proposed as the mechanism whereby free radical-mediated damage becomes more significant with age and begins to cause cellular dysfunction and death. This would also cause damage to DNA, as well as to proteins.
- **Protein catabolic inefficiency.** All cells depend for survival on efficient systems for eliminating damaged or effete cell constituents. It has been suggested that a major contributor to aging is inefficiency in such systems, leading to cellular dysfunction and death.
- **Cumulative injury theories** propose that aging is the result of all cellular impairments sustained throughout life, whether through DNA damage, protein modification, free radical damage, or disease.

Tissue responses to damage

OVERVIEW OF TISSUE RESPONSES TO INJURY

When tissue is damaged and cells die, more than one outcome is possible, as summarized in *Fig. 4.1*.

The damaged area may be replaced by organized tissue identical in structure and function to that originally present.

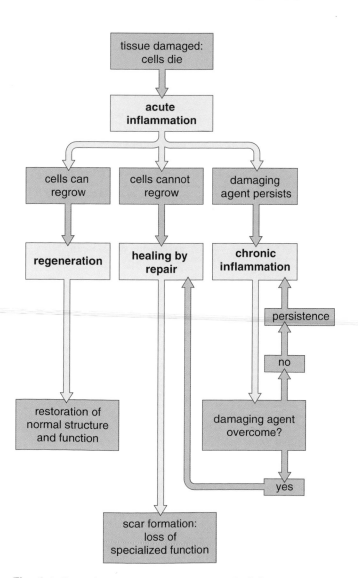

Fig. 4.1 Overview of tissue responses to injury.

Termed restitution, this is the ideal outcome. It can take place only if the damaging agent is removed, the cell debris is cleared from the site, and the specialized cells which have been destroyed have the capacity to regrow or **regenerate**.

If damaged cells cannot regrow, or local damage is so severe that tissue architecture is entirely destroyed, complete restitution of a damaged area is not always possible. In this case, the tissue response is to heal the damaged area by replacing it by non-specialized **scar tissue**, a process termed **fibrous repair**. This is the most frequent outcome of substantial tissue damage.

If the damaging agent persists (particularly if it involves infection), continuing tissue destruction, attempts to heal by fibrous repair, and immune responses occur concurrently, a process known as **chronic inflammation**.

Irrespective of the ultimate outcome of tissue damage, the initial response of the tissue is termed **acute inflammation** or the **acute inflammatory reaction**. This response is relatively non-specific, its main roles being to clear away dead tissues, protect against local infection, and allow the immune system access to the damaged area.

Acute inflammation is the most common early tissue response to tissue damage and destruction

The acute inflammatory response has three main functions:

1 The affected area is occupied by a transient material called the **acute inflammatory exudate**. The exudate carries proteins, fluid, and cells from local blood vessels into the damaged area to mediate local defences.
2 If an infective causative agent (e.g. bacteria) is present in the damaged area, it can be destroyed and eliminated by components of the exudate.
3 The damaged tissue can be broken down and partly liquefied, and the debris removed from the site of damage.

The acute inflammatory response is controlled by the production and diffusion of chemical messengers derived both from damaged tissues and from the acute inflammatory exudate. These **mediators of acute inflammation** are discussed in a later section (see pages 42–45), after the features of acute inflammation have been presented.

The acute inflammatory exudate is derived from local vessels

The acute inflammatory exudate is composed of:

- **Fluid** containing salts and a high concentration of proteins including immunoglobulins.
- **Fibrin**, a high molecular weight, filamentous, insoluble protein.
- Many **neutrophil polymorphs**, from the blood white cell population.
- A few **macrophages**, phagocytic cells derived from blood monocytes.
- A few **lymphocytes**.

All of these components are derived from the blood as a result of changes that occur in blood vessels in the surviving tissue around the area of damage. These changes, the vascular and cellular responses of acute inflammation, are illustrated diagrammatically in *Fig. 4.2*. Briefly, the steps are:

1 Small blood vessels adjacent to the area of tissue damage initially become dilated with increased blood flow, then flow along them slows down.
2 Endothelial cells swell and partially retract so that they no longer form a completely intact internal lining.
3 The vessels become leaky, permitting the passage of water, salts, and some small proteins from the plasma into the damaged area (**exudation**). One of the main proteins to leak out is the small soluble molecule, fibrinogen.
4 Circulating neutrophil polymorphs initially adhere to the swollen endothelial cells (**margination**), then actively migrate through the vessel basement membrane (**emigration**), passing into the area of tissue damage.

Clinical effects of acute inflammation

The four cardinal effects of acute inflammation were described nearly 2000 years ago by Celsus:

Rubor (redness)   **Dolor (pain)**
Calor (heat)   **Tumor (swelling)**

The redness and heat of acute inflammation are the result of vessel dilatation and increased blood flow to the inflamed part, and the swelling is caused by accumulation of exudate, particularly the fluid component. The pain is due to a combination of factors including pressure on nerve endings from swelling, and a direct effect of certain chemical factors which are released to mediate the response.

When swelling and pain are marked, there is loss of function, partial or complete, of the inflamed structure.

5 Later, small numbers of blood monocytes (macrophages) migrate in a similar way, as do lymphocytes.

Local vascular flow and permeability alter in acute inflammation

The main vascular changes that arise in acute inflammation are slowing of flow and dilatation of vessels, and increase in

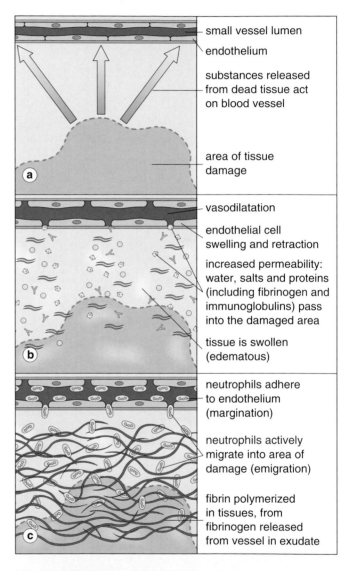

Fig. 4.2 Formation of acute inflammatory exudate.
(a) Death of tissue leads to release of substances (chemical mediators) which act on nearby blood vessels. (b) Mediators produce: (i) persistent vasodilatation and loss of axial flow; (ii) endothelial cell swelling and separation; (iii) increased permeability, with exudation of water, salts and small proteins, including fibrinogen. Fibrinogen is converted to fibrin. (c) Mediators cause neutrophils to adhere to endothelium (margination), and move through vessel walls into damaged tissue (emigration). Blood monocytes/macrophages also emigrate by a similar mechanism slightly later. The damaged area becomes progressively replaced by the components of the exudate.

the permeability of their walls, allowing diffusion of large proteins and fluid. The main structural changes in the vessel walls, and the factors that mediate increased permeability, are described in the later section on chemical mediators of acute inflammation (see pages 42–45).

Fibrin in the acute inflammatory exudate may have roles in allowing cell movement

Fibrin is a long, insoluble, filamentous protein, formed by the polymerization of numerous molecules of the smaller, soluble, precursor plasma protein **fibrinogen**. The fibrinogen passes out from vessels with the fluid and salts, polymerizing into insoluble fibrin threads once outside the vessel lumen, by activation of the blood coagulation cascade.

It is widely speculated that the network of fibrin threads prevents migration of microorganisms and produces a scaffold which might assist the migration of neutrophils and macrophages through the damaged area. However, there is no real proof that these are the precise functions of the network.

Fluid in the acute inflammatory exudate carries nutrients, mediators and immunoglobulins

It is logical to assume that the presence of fluids and salts may dilute or buffer any locally produced toxins in an area of tissue damage, but little more is known about their precise functions in the acute inflammatory reaction. Glucose and oxygen can diffuse into the area of inflammation to support macrophages. Fluid also allows diffusion of mediators of the inflammatory process, particularly plasma-derived precursors (see pages 42–43).

If immunity to an invading organism already exists, immunoglobulins in the exudate act as opsonins for neutrophil phagocytosis (see below).

The fluid in the exudate is not static but is constantly circulating from local vessels, through the extracellular space of the damaged tissue, to be re-absorbed by lymphatics. This increased flow of lymph takes antigens to the local nodes and assists in later development of a specific immune response.

Cellular reactions are also needed in acute inflammation

The main cellular events in acute inflammation, all of which are caused by chemical mediators, are as follows:

- The normally inactive endothelium has to be activated to allow adhesion of neutrophils.
- Normally inactive neutrophils have to be activated to enhance their capacity for phagocytosis, bacterial killing, and generation of inflammatory mediators.
- Neutrophils have to develop the ability to move actively, in a directional fashion, from vessels towards the area of tissue damage.

Neutrophils are the main effector cells in acute inflammation

The neutrophil is the main cell to mediate the effects of acute inflammation. If tissue damage is slight, an adequate supply is derived from normal numbers circulating in blood. If tissue damage is extensive, stores of neutrophils, including some immature forms, are released from bone marrow to increase the absolute count of neutrophils in the blood. To maintain the supply of neutrophils, growth factors derived from the inflammatory process stimulate division of myeloid precursors in the bone marrow, thereby increasing the number of developing neutrophils.

Neutrophils adhere to endothelial cells prior to emigration

The adhesion of neutrophils to endothelium causes them to aggregate along the vessel walls in a process termed **margination**. There are three stages to this process (see *Fig. 4.3*) mediated by different cell adhesion mechanisms:

- **Rolling** – neutrophils roll along the endothelium in close contact.
- **Adhesion** – neutrophils firmly adhere to the endothelium.
- **Aggregation** – adjacent neutrophils adhere to each other and undergo shape changes.

Neutrophils actively emigrate from vessels into tissues down a concentration gradient of chemotactic factors (see *Fig. 4.4a*)

KEY FACTS
Neutrophils

- Produced by maturation of precursor cells in bone marrow.
- Most numerous white cell in blood, increasing in number in acute inflammation.
- Short life-span once activated in tissues.
- Motile (ameboid) and able to move from vessels into tissues.
- Movement can be directional, attracted by chemotaxins (see *Fig. 4.4*).
- Actively phagocytic (see *Fig. 4.6*).
- Contain granules rich in a variety of proteases.
- Generated free radicals kill phagocytosed bacteria.
- Are a source of arachidonic acid to facilitate prostaglandin production.
- Increased neutrophil production by bone marrow is caused by cytokines generated in the inflammatory response.

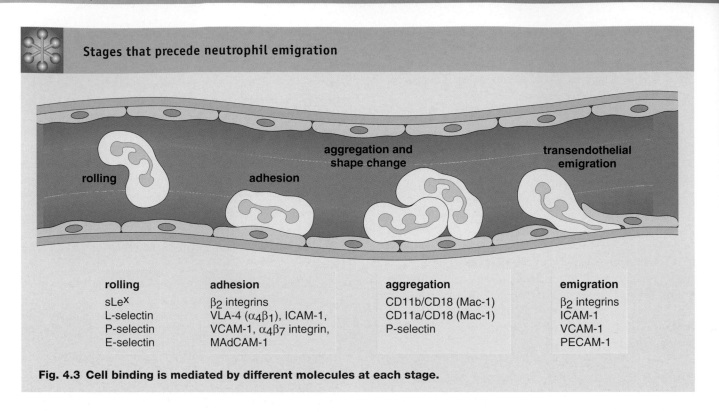

Stages that precede neutrophil emigration

rolling	adhesion	aggregation	emigration
sLe^X	β_2 integrins	CD11b/CD18 (Mac-1)	β_2 integrins
L-selectin	VLA-4 ($\alpha_4\beta_1$), ICAM-1,	CD11a/CD18 (Mac-1)	ICAM-1
P-selectin	VCAM-1, $\alpha_4\beta_7$ integrin,	P-selectin	VCAM-1
E-selectin	MAdCAM-1		PECAM-1

Fig. 4.3 Cell binding is mediated by different molecules at each stage.

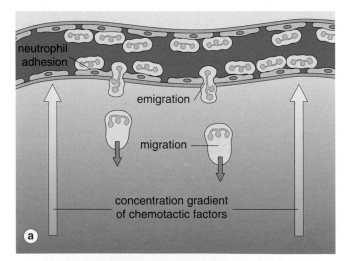

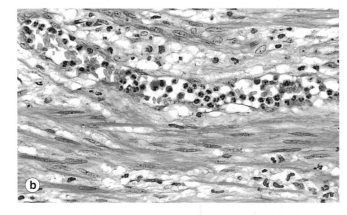

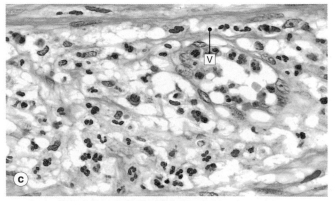

Fig. 4.4 Neutrophil emigration in acute inflammation.
(a) Margination, emigration and migration of neutrophils.
(b) Neutrophils marginated along vessel wall.
(c) Neutrophils emigrating into damaged tissue from vessel (V).

Activation of endothelium is a key process in acute inflammation

Endothelium in local vessels is activated both by products of tissue damage and by cytokines. This induces the expression of surface cell adhesion molecules, which interact with complementary molecules in the neutrophil cell membrane.

Some of the factors involved in the activation of endothelial cells, together with its role in neutrophil rolling and adhesion, are summarized in the pink box. The endothelium is modified to become sticky for neutrophils, to secrete factors mediating vasodilatation and to promote platelet adhesion and aggregation.

Endothelial activation in acute inflammation

The endothelium plays a vital role as a physical barrier against diffusion of plasma outside vessels, as well as being the source of many regulatory molecules. Because of its extent and its constant secretion of messenger substances, the endothelium has been called the largest endocrine organ in the body.

The main factors secreted by the endothelium are:

- Nitric oxide and prostacyclin, which induce vascular relaxation and inhibit platelet aggregation.
- Endothelin, thromboxane A2, and angiotensin II, which cause vascular constriction.
- Growth factor PDGF, which promotes inhibitors, e.g. heparin-like substances.
- Chemokines.

In the normal state the endothelium provides a surface that prevents platelet aggregation and degranulation. The balance of secreted factors is a major determinant in control of regional blood flow. In acute inflammation this balance is changed and there is increased synthesis of a lipid-derived molecule known as platelet activating factor (PAF), which increases vascular permeability; increased synthesis of nitric oxide, which promotes vascular

dilatation; and more cell adhesion molecules are expressed, which allows neutrophil adhesion. In addition to modulation of secreted factors, the surface properties of the endothelium are altered in acute inflammation (*Fig. 4.5*).

- IL-1 TNF and chemokines increase the expression of adhesion molecules on the endothelium, especially selectins which cause rolling of neutrophils.
- Chemokines on the endothelial surface bind to receptors on neutrophils and signal expression of leukocyte integrins.
- Intercellular adhesion molecule 1 (ICAM-1) promotes adhesion of neutrophils and lymphoid cells.
- Vascular cell adhesion molecule 1 (VCAM-1) promotes adhesion of lymphoid and monocyte cells.

At the same time, other mediators of inflammation, particularly the C5a fragment of complement, induce increased expression of complementary cell adhesion molecules on neutrophils (Beta-2 integrins). The endothelium in acute inflammation is therefore metabolically altered to produce vasoactive factors (particularly PAF and nitric oxide) as well as to be sticky for neutrophils.

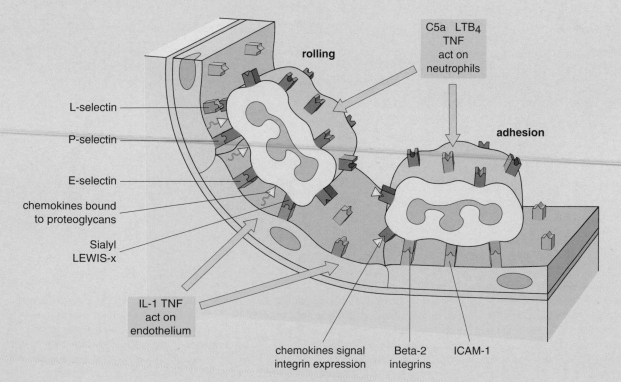

Fig. 4.5 Cell adhesion molecules involved in neutrophil adhesion.
IL-1 interleukin-1, **TNF** tumor necrosis factor, **LTB$_4$** leukotriene B$_4$

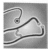

Systemic inflammatory response syndrome

This is an acute illness, the main features of which are caused by systemic activation of endothelium. This leads to generalized vasodilatation, platelet aggregation and widespread secondary organ dysfunction, particularly in the kidneys, liver, lungs, and heart.

The main clinical situation in which this syndrome occurs is septicemia from Gram-negative bacteria. The pathogenesis is due to inappropriate endothelial activation mediated by cytokines.

As more is understood about the pathogenesis of this syndrome, treatment by attempted blockade of IL-1 receptors or by administration of TNF neutralizing antibodies is under trial.

Neutrophils are attracted to the area of tissue damage by chemical mediators

The movement of neutrophils from the vessel lumen into a damaged area is mediated by substances known as chemotactic factors, which diffuse from the area of tissue damage. The main neutrophil chemotactic factors are listed in the Key Facts on mediators (see page 45). These factors bind to receptors on the surface of neutrophils and activate secondary messenger systems, stimulating increased cytosolic calcium, with resulting assembly of cytoskeletal specializations involved in motility.

Neutrophils kill microorganisms and break down damaged tissue

The neutrophil polymorph is packed with large numbers of lysosomal cytoplasmic granules that are rich in proteolytic enzymes capable of breaking down both cells and extracellular matrix materials. Neutrophils also have great phagocytic potential and can actively ingest pathogens, which are then destroyed both by lysosomal enzymes and by mechanisms that generate toxic free radicals. Neutrophil phagocytosis is illustrated in *Fig. 4.6*.

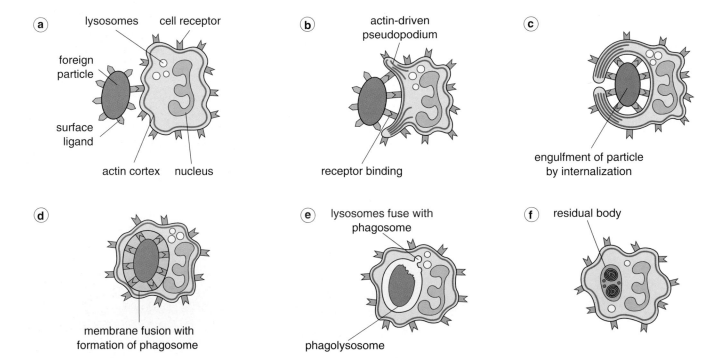

Fig. 4.6 Neutrophil phagocytosis.
(a) Neutrophils have membrane receptors (mainly for the Fc portion of antibodies), complement factors bound to foreign particles, and bacterial polysaccharides. Neutrophils do not phagocytose material to which they do not bind. (b) As the first step in phagocytosis, the neutrophil binds to the abnormal particle by its specific receptors. The cell pushes out pseudopodia to surround the particle, driven by assembly and disassembly of actin filaments. (c) The pseudopodia fuse to enclose the abnormal particle completely, forming an endocytic vesicle. Special proteins probably allow final sealing of the membrane. (d) The internalized particle in the endocytic vesicle is called a phagosome. (e) The phagosome fuses with neutrophil granules, particularly primary granules, which discharge their contents, exposing the particle to a potent mixture of lysosomal enzymes. If the particle is a bacterium, killing is enhanced by hydrogen peroxide and superoxide, which are generated by the enzymatic reduction of oxygen by respiratory burst oxidases (RBOs) (membrane enzymes). (f) Foreign particle destruction is associated with formation of a residual body containing degraded material.

Neutrophils are short-lived phagocytic cells

The disadvantage of neutrophils is that they are short-lived, surviving only a few hours once in the tissues. Consequently, the supply of neutrophils to a damaged area needs to be constantly replenished.

Any area of tissue damage will contain large numbers of viable, actively phagocytosing neutrophils, which are mixed with the remnants of dead neutrophils. As neutrophils die, they release some of their lysosomal enzymes into the surrounding tissue, and these enzymes may continue to act outside the cell, breaking down structural proteins and partly liquefying the tissue.

Neutrophils are stimulated to emigrate in their greatest numbers where the tissue damage is caused by bacterial invasion, as many bacterial products are potent chemoattractants. This large-scale emigration is particularly beneficial because neutrophils not only break down and eradicate the damaged tissue, but also phagocytose and kill the causative bacteria. Where there has been massive emigration associated with tissue breakdown, a thick, liquid substance called pus is formed, containing necrotic cell debris, live and dead neutrophils and, sometimes, microorganisms.

Macrophages play a small part in acute inflammation

A minor component of the acute inflammatory exudate is formed by macrophages derived from monocytes in the circulating blood, which migrate into the damaged area later than neutrophils. They are present in very small numbers early in the course of acute inflammation but, with time, increase in numbers to facilitate elimination of dead material. They are actively phagocytic and have powerful systems for bacterial killing. Because of a capacity for oxidative metabolism, they survive very much longer than neutrophils.

In addition to their phagocytic function, macrophages have secretory roles, producing growth factors and cytokines, which mediate some of the events in the inflammatory response. They also assist in repair following tissue

KEY FACTS
Acute inflammatory exudate

- Derived from local blood vessels.
- Contains fluid and electrolytes.
- Contains proteins, particularly fibrinogen/fibrin and immunoglobulins.
- Brings chemical mediators of inflammation into site of damage.
- Contains neutrophils, which are the main cells involved in acute inflammation.

damage. Macrophages have more important roles in chronic inflammation (see page 53).

The acute inflammatory exudate varies in its composition

The components of the acute inflammatory response may vary in their relative proportions depending on the site and cause of the inflammatory response.

- When neutrophils dominate the composition, and material is liquefied to form pus, the exudate is termed **purulent**.
- If fibrin is abundant, as often seen in relation to serosal surfaces (e.g. surface of the pericardium, lung or peritoneum), the exudate is termed **fibrinous**.
- When fluid is the major component the exudate is termed **serous**.

Examples of purulent, fibrinous, and serous exudates are illustrated in *Figs 4.7, 4.8* and *4.9.*

Acute inflammation may be harmful

It is paradoxical that the acute inflammatory process, which is meant to be protective and reparative, often produces severe illness and even death. To illustrate, in the two examples of common conditions given below, the symptoms and complications of the disease are the result of the acute inflammatory process.

- In **acute epiglottitis**, infection of the upper airway by Haemophilus bacteria causes acute inflammation. The extensive outpouring of exudate into the soft tissues of the laryngeal submucosa can lead to such severe narrowing of the airway that respiration is compromised. Ultimately, the acute inflammatory response to infection can result in death through asphyxia.
- In acute meningitis (*Fig. 4.7*), infection of the leptomeninges by bacteria induces an acute inflammatory response. Although the bacteria may be of low pathogenicity and, in themselves, cause little tissue damage, the acute inflammatory response causes thrombosis of local blood vessels and prevents perfusion to the cerebral cortex, leading to severe brain damage. In this way, the acute inflammatory response to the infection produces more damage than the infective organism it is attempting to combat. Many other examples, and their clinical implications, are presented later in this book.

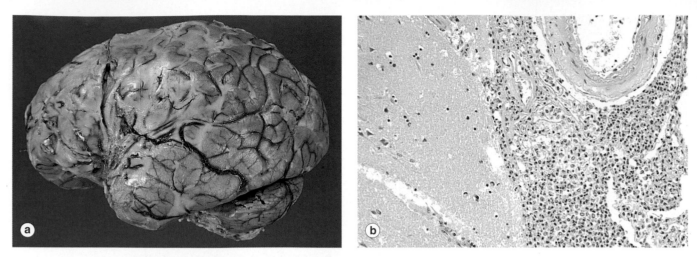

Fig. 4.7 Purulent exudate in the brain in meningitis. (a) Macroscopic specimen. (b) Histological section.
In (a), which shows a child's brain, a thick, creamy exudate is visible beneath the arachnoid, most prominent in the frontal and temporal areas. This creamy appearance is due to the predominance of neutrophil polymorphs in the exudate, as illustrated in (b). The diagnosis of purulent meningitis can be made by the identification of large numbers of neutrophils in a sample of cerebrospinal fluid removed by lumbar puncture; the causative bacterium can sometimes be seen in such samples, and the specimen should be sent for microbiological culture to identify the specific organism.

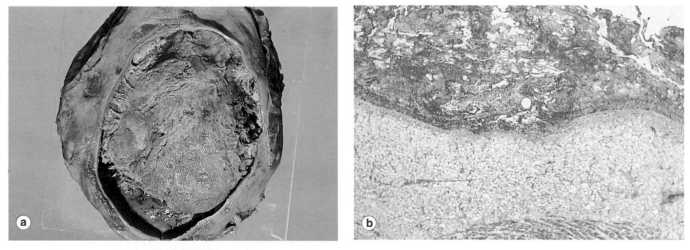

Fig. 4.8 Fibrinous exudate in the pericardium. (a) Macroscopic specimen. (b) Histological section.
In (a) a 'shaggy' exudate covers the entire surface of both the visceral and the parietal pericardium, seen through a window cut in the parietal pericardium. This shaggy appearance is due to the predominance of fibrin in the exudate, as seen in (b). The exudate destroys the normal, smooth surfaces of the pericardial cavity, and its presence can be detected clinically on auscultation, when a scratching noise can be heard with every heartbeat (pericardial friction rub).

An abscess results from local tissue breakdown

If an area of tissue necrosis is extensive, and the cause is a pus-forming (pyogenic) bacterium, an acute abscess may form. An abscess is a mass of necrotic tissue, with dead and viable neutrophils, suspended in the fluid products of tissue breakdown by neutrophil enzymes. In its early stages it is surrounded by a layer of acute inflammatory exudate, and is called an **acute abscess** (see *Fig. 4.10*). At this stage it may continue to enlarge if the bacteria are able to survive, proliferate and cause necrosis.

If the acute abscess enlarges only slowly or not at all, the acute inflammatory exudate forming the wall of the abscess is gradually replaced by scar tissue. The central area of damaged tissue is not eradicated, and the central debris still contains viable proliferating bacteria, which remain capable of causing tissue damage; this is a **chronic abscess**.

Acute inflammation is orchestrated by chemical mediators

Many factors which mediate and orchestrate the events of acute inflammation have been documented. These chemical

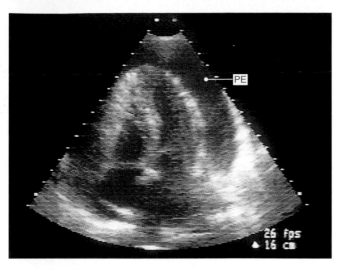

Fig. 4.9 Serous pericardial effusion.
Serous effusions are important only when they occur within a confined space, e.g. in the pericardial cavity. This echocardiogram shows a typical pericardial effusion greatly distending the pericardial sac (**PE**). The clinical problems arise because the substantially increased pressure in the pericardial cavity interferes with atrial filling.

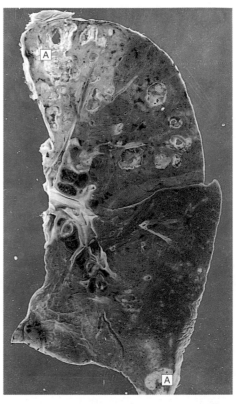

Fig. 4.10 Acute abscess. Lung showing multiple acute abscesses (**A**) due to staphylococcal infection.

Fig. 4.11	
Main groups of mediators involved in acute inflammation	

Cellular mediators of acute inflammation

Stored	*Active synthesis*
Histamine	Prostaglandins
	Leukotrienes
	Platelet activating factor
	Cytokines
	Nitric oxide
	Chemokines

Plasma-derived mediators of acute inflammation

Kinin system	– Bradykinin
Clotting pathway	– Activated Hageman factor
Thrombolytic system	– Plasmin
Complement pathway	– C3a, C3b and C5a

mediators of inflammation are important, since the process can be modified by drug therapy to minimize unwanted and potentially damaging effects. The mediators either come from cells or are plasma-derived (*Fig. 4.11*). Plasma-derived mediators gain entry to the damaged area via the inflammatory exudate. They are mostly precursor proteins, which are activated by proteolytic enzymes and, once activated, generally have short half-lives. Once in tissues, they are rapidly inactivated by a variety of enzymatic or scavenging systems.

Histamine is the main pre-formed mediator of inflammation. Released from mast cells, basophils and platelets, it causes transient dilatation of arterioles, increases permeability in venules, and is the primary cause of increased vascular permeability in the first hour after injury.

Both prostaglandins and leukotrienes are derived by local synthesis from arachidonic acid. This long-chain fatty acid is liberated from cell membranes by activation of the enzyme, phospholipase A_2. There are two main pathways in arachidonic acid metabolism:

1 The cyclo-oxygenase pathway produces: thromboxane A_2 (TXA_2), which aggregates platelets and causes vascular constriction; prostacyclin (PGI_2), which inhibits platelet aggregation and dilates vessels; and stable prostaglandins (PGE_2, $PGF_{2\alpha}$, PGD_2), which cause vasodilatation and increase vascular permeability. PGE_2 also causes pain. There are two forms of cyclo-oxygenase termed COX-1 and COX-2. COX-1 is normally present in cells as a constitutively expressed enzyme, whereas COX-2 is specially induced in cells where it plays a role in inflammation.
2 The lipoxygenase pathway produces leukotrienes (LTC_4, LTD_4, LTE_4), which cause vasoconstriction and increase permeability in venules. Leukotriene LTB_4 stimulates leukocyte adhesion to endothelium.

Platelet activating factor (PAF) is synthesized by mast cells/basophils and can be stimulated by IgE-mediated release. Also synthesized by platelets, neutrophils, mono-cytes, and endothelium, it is a specialized phospholipid compound, which causes vasoconstriction, increased vascular permeability, and platelet aggregation, and is at least a thousand times more potent than histamine. It also stimulates the synthesis of arachidonic acid metabolites.

Cytokines are polypeptide products of activated lymphocytes and monocytes. The main cytokines participating in acute inflammation are interleukin-1(IL-1) interleukin 8 (IL-8) and tumour necrosis factor alpha (TNFα). These are responsible for:

- Induction of cell adhesion molecules on endothelium.
- Induction of PGI_2 (prostacyclin) synthesis.
- Induction of PAF synthesis.
- Fever, anorexia, and stimulation of acute-phase protein synthesis by the liver.
- Stimulation of fibroblast proliferation and secretory activity.
- Attraction of neutrophils into damaged area (IL-8).

The chemokines are a family of factors secreted by leukocytes and endothelial cells in response to tissue damage and in response to other inflammatory mediators. They are locally bound to the extracellular matrix and heparin-sulphate proteoglycans of cells, and establish a concentration gradient away from the focus of inflammation. Neutrophil rolling causes neutrophils to encounter chemokines bound to proteoglycans on endothelial cells. Specific chemokine receptors are activated and this signals for activation of leukocyte integrins, mediating adhesion and emigration (see pages 37–38). Chemokines are removed from the circulation by the Duffy antigen receptor for chemokines (DARC) expressed on red cells.

Nitric oxide is a small molecule that is locally synthesized by endothelium and macrophages through the activity of the enzyme, nitric oxide synthase. It is a powerful cause of vascular dilatation, and increases vascular permeability. As an important reactive oxygen intermediary, it can also mediate cell and bacterial killing.

The complement system comprises a set of plasma proteins with important roles in immunity and inflammation. There is a cascade of activation, with production of numerous intermediary activated peptides. The main products with roles in acute inflammation are as follows:

- C3a increases vascular permeability by liberating histamine from mast cells/platelets.
- C5a increases vascular permeability by liberating histamine from mast cells/platelets, is chemotactic to neutrophils, and induces endothelial cell adhesion molecules.
- C$\overline{345}$ is chemoattractive to neutrophils.
- C3b opsonizes bacteria and facilitates neutrophil phagocytosis.

The kinins are small peptides derived from plasma precursors by proteolytic cleavage. The system is activated by one of the coagulation proteins, activated **Hageman factor** (**Factor XII**); this cleaves the peptide prekallikrein to kallikrein. Kallikrein stimulates a high molecular weight kininogen to form bradykinin, which is a powerful mediator of increased vascular permeability, causes pain, and activates the complement system.

The clotting pathway is responsible for coagulation of blood by formation of fibrin from fibrinogen. Factor XII (Hageman factor) is activated in the inflammatory exudate when it comes into contact with collagen outside the vessel. It then stimulates deposition of fibrin, activates the kinin system, and also stimulates the thrombolytic system. When fibrinogen is converted to fibrin, fibrinopeptides are formed. These cause increased vascular permeability, as well as being chemotactic for neutrophils.

The thrombolytic pathway. The enzyme plasmin (generated by plasminogen activator derived from endothelium by the action of bradykinin) is a proteolytic enzyme with several roles in inflammation. It:

- Activates the complement system.
- Activates Hageman factor.
- Lyses fibrin to form fibrin degradation products, which increase permeability of vessels.

In acute inflammation, these factors act in concert to bring about the structural and functional changes.

Laboratory medicine

Clinical indications of an acute inflammatory process include:

- General malaise.
- Fever.
- Pain, often localized to the inflamed area, e.g. the right iliac fossa in acute appendicitis.
- Rapid pulse rate.

Laboratory investigations usually reveal:

- A raised neutrophil count in the peripheral blood.
- An increased erythrocyte sedimentation rate (ESR).
- An increase in the concentration of **acute-phase proteins** in the blood. These are normally present in small concentrations, but increase dramatically in response to acute inflammation. Produced by the liver, they are induced by circulating IL-1. Specific examples, the most common being **C-reactive protein**, may be measured in blood to monitor inflammatory processes.

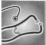

Drug therapy of acute inflammation

The acute inflammatory response can be treated with anti-inflammatory drugs, which prevent production of key mediators of inflammation.

- Phospholipase A_2 activity is inhibited by steroids, limiting the production of arachidonic acid and, therefore, the formation of arachidonic acid metabolites.
- Aspirin and indomethacin inhibit the cyclo-oxygenase pathway and prevent production of prostaglandins and thromboxane A_2.

KEY FACTS
Mediators in acute inflammation

Vasodilatation	Histamine, prostaglandins, nitric oxide, bradykinin, PAF
Increased permeability	Histamine, C3a, C5a, bradykinin, leukotrienes, PAF, nitric oxide
Neutrophil adhesion	IL-1, TNFα, PAF, LTB_4, C5a, chemokines
Neutrophil chemotaxis	C5a, LTB_4, bacterial components, chemokines
Fever	IL-1, TNF, prostaglandins
Pain	Prostaglandins, bradykinin
Tissue necrosis	Neutrophil lysosomal granule contents. Free radicals generated by neutrophils

Factors involved in vascular permeability in acute inflammation

There are two mechanisms for increased permeability of small vessels following tissue damage (*Fig. 4.12*).

- Toxins and physical agents may cause necrosis of vascular endothelium, leading to abnormal leakage (non-mediated vascular leakage).
- Chemical mediators of acute inflammation may cause retraction of endothelial cells, leaving intercellular gaps (mediated vascular leakage).

Experimental work has isolated three patterns of increased leakage of fluid from vessels, which occur at different times following injury.

1 An immediate response that is transient, lasts for 30–60 minutes, and is mediated by histamine acting on endothelium.
2 A delayed response that starts 2–3 hours after injury and lasts for up to 8 hours. This is mediated by factors synthesized by local cells, e.g. bradykinin, factors derived from complement, and factors released from dead neutrophils in the exudate.
3 An immediate response that is prolonged for over 24 hours and is seen if there has been direct necrosis of endothelium, e.g. in a burn or by a chemical toxin.

In disease it is likely that all three responses are activated, with an immediate prolonged response close to the centre of damage, and mediated responses at the interface between the damaged and healthy tissues.

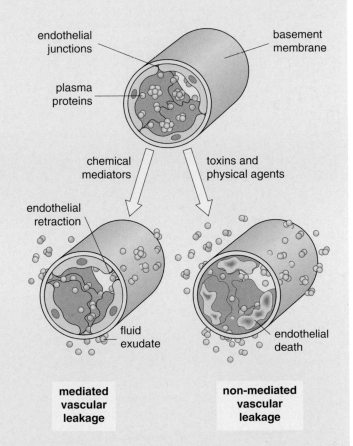

Fig. 4.12 The two main mechanisms for increase in vascular permeability.

OUTCOME OF THE ACUTE INFLAMMATORY REACTION

Under favorable circumstances the acute inflammatory reaction is adequate to deal with a damaging event and to prepare the ground for healing. The outcome of the reaction depends upon the removal of the inflammatory exudate, and its replacement either by regenerated cells of the original type (restitution) or by scar tissue (fibrous repair). The possible end-results are summarized in *Fig. 4.13*.

Resolution occurs where there has been minimal damage to the tissue architecture and cells can regrow

In some circumstances, although there may be extensive destruction of cells, damage to the support tissues is minimal. An acute inflammatory exudate forms which, on resolution, leaves the supporting stroma undamaged, and the only deficiency is in epithelial cells. The exudate can be removed from the inflamed area by a combination of liquefaction by neutrophil enzymes (with re-absorption of the fluid into lymphatics), and phagocytosis of particulate debris by macrophages.

Damaged cells regenerate, leaving the structure virtually as before, and normal function can be regained. This process, termed **resolution**, is obviously the best possible outcome but, unfortunately, it is not common. In most instances the support stroma is damaged and healing is by scar formation.

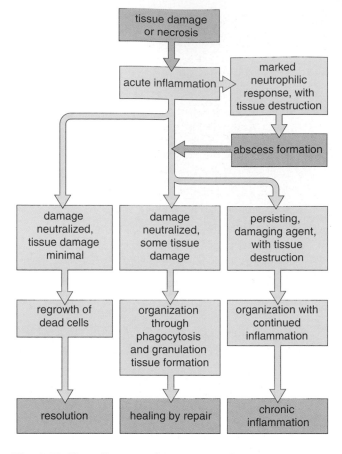

Fig. 4.13 Flow diagram of outcomes of acute inflammation.

Lobar pneumonia as an example of resolution of an exudate

Lobar pneumonia is a type of acute inflammation of the lung. It results from damage caused by certain types of pathogenic bacteria within the alveolar air sacs. The presence of the bacteria and their excreted toxins causes the death of epithelial cells (Type 1 and Type 2 pneumocytes) lining the alveolar spaces. The body's response is to produce an acute inflammatory exudate, the components of which (fluids, salts, fibrinogen/fibrin, other proteins, neutrophils and macrophages) pass out from the network of capillaries lining the alveolar sacs into the alveolar lumen.

As the infection develops, the air in a large number of alveoli is replaced by exudate (see *Fig. 4.14a*). This change tends to spread rapidly throughout all of the air sacs of a particular lobe of the lung (hence 'lobar' pneumonia), and a considerable proportion of the patient's gaseous exchange capacity is lost. Importantly, although cells lining alveoli die, the support stroma and vascular structure of the lung remain intact. Under favorable conditions, especially if the patient is treated with antibiotics, the neutrophils in the exudate phagocytose and destroy all of the causative bacteria, at which point the process of resolution can begin.

Enzymes released by neutrophils break up structural proteins (e.g. the fibrin) and remnants of dead cells, rendering the exudate highly liquid. Some of it is coughed up in sputum, but much of it can be re-absorbed into the alveolar capillary network or into the pulmonary lymphatic system. Macrophages phagocytose any residual undigested debris, pass into the lymphatic system, and are transmitted to regional lymph nodes.

At the same time, remnant epithelial stem cells divide to re-line the alveolar air spaces, differentiating into new Type 1 and Type 2 alveolar lining cells.

▶ Resolution can take place only if the damaged cells can divide and repopulate the injured area. Once the exudate is removed from the alveolar air spaces and epithelial cells are regenerated, gaseous exchange can begin again.

If this process of resolution of an inflammatory exudate (see *Fig. 4.14b*) does not take place, usually because of more severe structural damage to the supporting stroma, an area of scar tissue will eventually form in the lung.

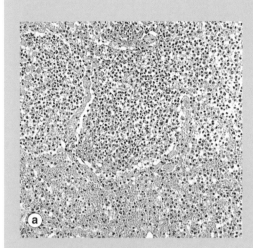 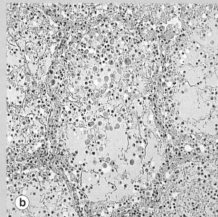

Fig. 4.14 Resolution of acute inflammatory exudate in lobar pneumonia.
In (a) the photomicrograph shows the fully formed exudate, rich in neutrophils and fibrin, filling all the alveolar spaces between alveolar walls.
In (b) the exudate is in the process of resolution. The alveolar spaces largely contain fluid (which will be re-absorbed) and some residual macrophages (which will re-enter the blood or lymphatic circulations).

KEY FACTS
Resolution

- End-result is restoration of normal structure and function without scarring.
- Acute inflammatory exudates removed by liquefaction and phagocytosis.
- Support stroma must be intact.
- Damaged cells must be able to regenerate.

Regeneration of cells is limited to certain types. Nerve cells and cardiac muscle cells cannot divide, so any loss is permanent. Cells of liver and kidney do not normally divide but, following damage, can divide to replace cells that have been lost. Other cells, such as surface epithelia, are constantly dividing and have a large capacity for regeneration following damage.

Organization and repair of acute inflammation lead to healing by collagenous scar

When there has been substantial structural damage to the tissue stroma, healing occurs not through resolution of the exudate, but by a process known as organization and repair, which eventually leads to the formation of a scar. The sequence of changes, shown diagrammatically and histologically in *Fig. 4.15*, is as follows:

- Pre-existing capillaries in the undamaged tissue form new capillaries by budding into the damaged area,

which is also infiltrated by macrophages, fibroblasts, and myofibroblasts. Macrophages phagocytose inflammatory exudate and dead tissue. Vascular granulation tissue, a fragile complex of interconnecting capillaries, macrophages and support cells, replaces the area of tissue damage (*Figs 4.15b* and *c*).

- There is progressive growth of fibroblasts and myofibroblasts, and the tissue defect is filled with the complex capillary network, proliferating fibroblasts, and a few residual macrophages (fibrovascular granulation tissue) (*Figs 4.15d* and *e*). With continued proliferation of the fibroblasts, and active collagen synthesis, many of the newly formed capillaries regress until a comparatively small number of vascular channels remain, connecting the damaged area of tissue to the normal undamaged area around it, and providing nutrients for the fibroblasts. Some of the persisting vessels acquire smooth muscle in their walls, and remain as functioning venules and arterioles.

- The intervening spaces between the vessels become progressively filled with fibroblasts synthesizing collagen (fibrous granulation tissue). The fibroblasts align themselves so that they deposit collagen in a mainly uniform pattern, running in a direction that provides maximum strength in the face of the physical stresses encountered. Contraction of the area of granulation tissue frequently occurs, partly through the contractile effects of the myofibroblasts. The size of the damaged area is thus reduced.

- Production of dense collagen by the fibroblasts forms a collagenous scar.

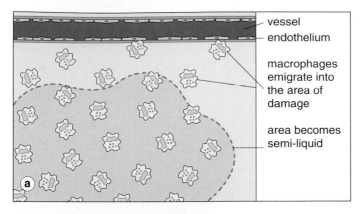

vessel
endothelium

macrophages emigrate into the area of damage

area becomes semi-liquid

Fig. 4.15 Organization and repair.
(a) Removal of debris by macrophages. (b) Vascular granulation tissue. (c) Vascular granulation tissue. This photomicrograph shows the abundant thin-walled vessels of vascular granulation tissue. The intervening tissue contains residual macrophages. (d) Fibrovascular granulation tissue. (e) Fibrovascular granulation tissue. This photomicrograph shows the tissue between the vascular network becoming filled with proliferating fibroblasts, which are already tending to align themselves in the direction of tensile stress. (f) Collagenous scar formation. (g) Early collagenous scar. This photomicrograph shows the nuclei of the fibroblasts becoming compressed. The formerly active fibroblasts have become inactive resting fibrocytes.

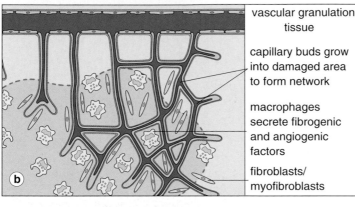

vascular granulation tissue

capillary buds grow into damaged area to form network

macrophages secrete fibrogenic and angiogenic factors

fibroblasts/ myofibroblasts

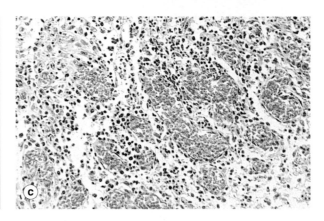

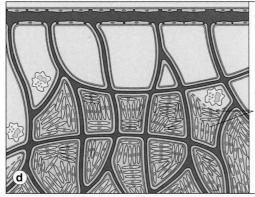

fibrovascular granulation tissue

fibroblasts proliferate and begin to deposit collagen

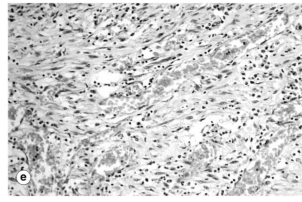

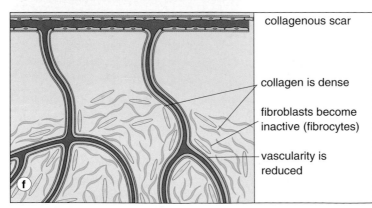

collagenous scar

collagen is dense

fibroblasts become inactive (fibrocytes)

vascularity is reduced

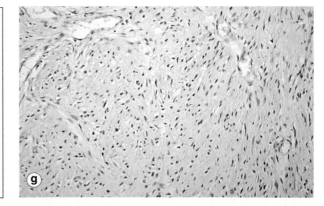

- Once the fibroblasts have synthesized sufficient collagen to fill the defect, they assume a resting status, in which they exhibit scanty cytoplasm and an elongated spindle-shaped nucleus (*Figs 4.15f* and *g*). These inactive fibroblasts are known as fibrocytes.

The process whereby the inflammatory exudate is replaced by granulation tissue is called **organization of the exudate**; that by which the granulation tissue is subsequently replaced by fibrous scar is called **fibrous repair**.

Healing of wounds is also achieved by organization, repair and scar formation

The healing of tissue wounds, including those caused by surgical procedures, also occurs through the processes of organization and formation of granulation and scar tissue.

The ideal situation for healing is of a surgical wound in which adjacent surfaces are closely apposed and held together by suture material. The classic example of a sutured skin wound is given in *Fig. 4.16*. The key feature of this type of healing is that there is only a narrow space between the adjacent tissues, with a minimal amount of dead tissue limited to the very edges of the wound.

Where there has been extensive loss of cells, a large tissue defect results, which has to be filled by granulation tissue. Examples include large surface ulcers or open wounds that cannot be sutured. Because the damage is extensive, the inflammatory response at the edges of the wound is usually intense, and the large amount of granulation tissue required means that healing takes a long time. However, the ultimate size of the collagenous scar is reduced by shrinkage of the healing wound. Myofibroblasts contract at the stage of granulation tissue formation, and this process, termed **wound contraction**, can reduce the surface area of an open wound to 10% of its original size.

Healing of closely apposed surfaces has been termed healing by **primary intention**; the healing of open wounds is sometimes termed healing by **secondary intention**. The differences between the two relate to the amount of in-fill required to bridge the tissue defect, rather than any special mechanistic differences.

Fig. 4.16
Stages in the healing of a sutured skin wound

Day 1	Neutrophils appear at margins of incision and there is an acute inflammatory response on each side of the narrow incisional space, leading to swelling, redness, and pain at the wound site. Epithelial cells at edge of wound undergo mitosis and begin to migrate across wound.
Day 2	Macrophages begin to infiltrate the incisional space and to demolish fibrin. Surface epithelial continuity is re-established in the form of a thin surface layer.
Day 3	Granulation tissue begins to invade tissue space. Surface epithelial continuity is reinforced by thickening of epithelial layer.
Day 5	Incisional space is filled with vascular granulation tissue: collagen is progressively deposited. Surface epithelium achieves normal thickness. Acute inflammatory response at wound margins begins to subside, and swelling and redness of adjacent tissues is reduced.
Day 7	Sutures commonly removed from skin wounds. Wound has approximately 10% of tensile strength of normal skin.
Day 10	Further fibroblast proliferation and collagen deposition occur in granulation tissue in the incisional space, adding to strength of wound.
Day 15	Collagen deposition follows the lines of tissue stress. Granulation tissue loses some of its vascularity, but still appears pinker than adjacent tissues.
Day 30	Wound now has 50% of tensile strength of normal skin.
3 months	Wound achieves maximal 80% of tensile strength of normal skin. It now appears only marginally more vascular than adjacent skin. Complete blanching of scar takes several more months.

Local and systemic factors influence healing

Many factors, whether encountered in the course of inflammation or during wound healing, impair organization and repair processes:

- Inadequate nutrition impairs repair. Protein is required for collagen synthesis, as are vitamin C and zinc.
- Ischemia to tissues markedly impairs repair.
- Infection of tissues causes continued tissue damage, promoting a continued acute inflammatory response.
- Foreign material (including large areas of dead tissue) retained in an area of tissue damage acts as a nidus for infection, promoting inflammation. This is the rationale behind surgical debridement of necrotic material from large wounds.
- Steroids hinder the formation of granulation tissue, and their immunosuppressive effects may predispose to local infection.
- Radiation exposure reduces a damaged area's capacity for repair, e.g. a wound in an area of previous radiotherapy will heal poorly.
- Diabetes is associated with poor wound healing for several reasons, including susceptibility to vascular disease and ischemia, and increased susceptibility to infection.
- Denervation of an area impairs healing.

Healing is promoted by:

- Removal of dead tissues to allow apposition of healthy tissues.
- Administration of appropriate antibiotics in cases of infection.

Damaged brain heals by growth of astrocytes rather than by formation of collagenous scars

Brain damage is generally not repaired through proliferation of fibroblasts, but through proliferation of the support cells of the brain, the astrocytes. The necrotic tissue is removed and replaced by fluid, which forms a cystic lesion. Surrounded by compacted glial fibers produced by astrocytes, this is termed a glial scar or astrocytic gliosis. The changes that follow damage to brain tissue are described in more detail in Chapter 21.

A fibrous scar is an inadequate end-result in bone healing

When bone is damaged, most commonly in fracture, collagenous scarring alone is insufficiently strong to repair the bone. Although bone fracture undergoes the same processes of organization, granulation tissue formation and fibroblast in-growth, an additional proliferation of osteoblasts produces the highly specialized collagen extracellular matrix known as osteoid, which is then mineralized to form bone. The mixture of fibrous granulation tissue and developing new bone, which is called callus, bridges the defect between the broken bone ends. At a later stage, the callus is refashioned to re-establish the normal structure of the bone prior to fracture. The details of fracture healing are given in Chapter 24.

Cellular events in wound healing

There are five key events in healing by organization and repair.

Local vessels:

1 Are stimulated to form outgrowths (**angiogenesis**).

Local support cells:

2 Divide to form fibroblasts and myofibroblasts (**mitogenesis**).
3 Migrate towards the area of tissue damage (**chemotaxis** and **motility**).
4 Secrete collagen (**fibrogenesis**).
5 Produce collagen-degrading enzymes (**remodelling**).

Peptide growth factors stimulate angiogenesis, promote cell division and migration, and stimulate collagen secretion. The main examples are platelet-derived growth factor (mitogenesis and chemotaxis), basic fibroblast growth factor (angiogenesis, mitogenesis, chemotaxis), transforming growth factor (fibrogenesis), IL-1 and tumor necrosis factor (fibrogenesis).

Molecules in the extracellular matrix facilitate adhesion of cells and act as signals, affecting differentiation and growth, e.g. fibronectin increases in tissues during healing, and mediates adhesion of growing capillaries and fibroblasts, as well as enhancing their response to basic fibroblast growth factor.

As part of the increase in the strength of a wound, the secreted collagen undergoes maturation. The molecular basis of this involves degradation as well as increased cross-linking. Degradation involves secretion of metalloproteinases by support cells that degrade collagen. The molecular type of collagen secreted early in granulation tissue formation is Type III, which is later replaced by degradation and secretion of Type I collagen.

CHRONIC INFLAMMATION

When a damaging stimulus persists, complete healing cannot occur, and chronic inflammation ensues

The sequence of **tissue damage → acute inflammation → exudate → organization of exudate → granulation tissue → fibrous scar** occurs only when the damaging stimulus is of short duration and does not persist. In such cases the changes leading to scar formation are consecutive.

If the damaging stimulus persists, the processes of continuing tissue necrosis, organization and repair all occur **concurrently**. In addition to acute inflammation, the specific defences of the **immune system** are activated around the area of damage, and tissues are infiltrated by activated lymphoid cells. Histological examination of an affected area will show necrotic cell debris, acute inflammatory exudate, vascular and fibrous granulation tissue, lymphoid cells, macrophages and collagenous scar. This state, termed **chronic inflammation**, will persist until the damaging stimulus is removed or neutralized.

Chronic inflammation is a balance between repair and continued tissue damage

Chronic inflammation is the result of a balance between continuing tissue damage on the one hand, and eradication of the damaging stimulus, followed by healing and scar formation, on the other (*Fig. 4.17*).

- If the damaging stimulus is neutralized or eradicated, further tissue necrosis does not occur and the repair response progresses to complete scarring.
- If the damaging stimulus cannot be eradicated or neutralized, the balance between tissue damage and

tissue repair is maintained in a kind of stalemate, and a state of chronic inflammation will persist, often for many years. During this time, the balance may alter, often because of changing local or systemic factors in the patient.

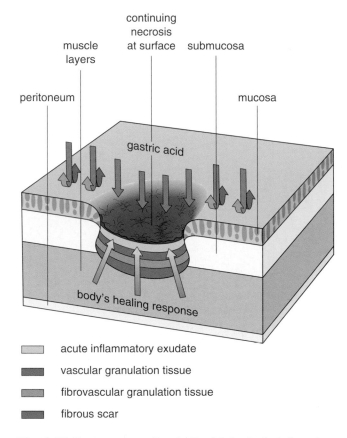

acute inflammatory exudate

vascular granulation tissue

fibrovascular granulation tissue

fibrous scar

Fig. 4.17 Factors operating in the biological stalemate of an active chronic peptic ulcer.

 Chronic peptic ulcer illustrates the basic principles of chronic inflammation

The lining of the upper alimentary tract is normally protected from the adverse effects of the dilute hydrochloric acid and proteolytic enzymes produced in the stomach mucosa for food digestion. If the protective mechanisms break down, the acid and enzymes destroy the epithelium and supporting stroma (cause ulceration) of the wall of the alimentary tract, usually affecting the stomach or duodenum. This damaging stimulus is persistent, since the stomach is always producing acid and enzymes. Tissue damage stimulates an acute inflammatory reaction, with the formation of exudate close to the damaging acid in the stomach lumen. In the depths of the ulcer, furthest away from the acid, attempts are made

to organize the exudate, and granulation tissue forms, which then progresses to collagenous scar.

In an established ulcer, all of these processes are occurring at the same time. A chronic peptic ulcer is therefore an example of chronic inflammation caused by the persistence of the damaging stimulus.

Fig. 4.17 shows diagrammatically the factors operating in a chronic peptic ulcer. *Fig. 4.18* shows the possible outcomes of such an ulcer, which depend on whether reparative responses are vigorous, or whether destructive responses cause progressive damage. The aim of treatment in peptic ulcer is to facilitate healing by removing or greatly reducing the damaging stimulus, i.e. the acid and enzymes secreted.

Outcomes of peptic ulcer

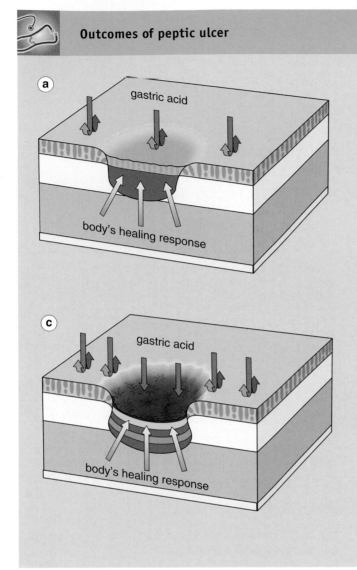

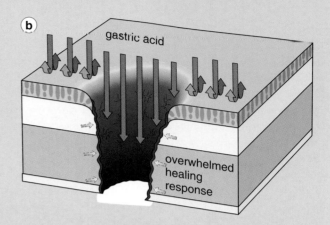

Fig. 4.18 Possible outcomes of peptic ulcer.
(a) **Healing**. The damaging stimulus is overcome by the healing process, usually because gastric acid secretion is reduced or neutralized. The defect becomes filled with fibrous scar and is re-covered with gastric mucosa. **The ulcer heals completely**.

(b) **Perforation**. The healing and repair process is overwhelmed by continuing damage caused by increased levels of gastric acid. The process of ulceration continues, penetrating the full thickness of the wall leading to **perforation**.

(c) **Chronicity**. The damage caused by acid is counterbalanced, but not overcome, by the body's healing response. This stalemate situation leads to chronic gastric ulcer, that may persist for many years. Any change in the balance of the conflicting factors may lead to (a) or (b) above.

Some of the possible outcomes are presented in relation to the example of chronic acid-induced ulceration of the stomach and duodenum (chronic peptic ulcer), illustrated in *Fig. 4.18*.

Immune mechanisms dominate the cellular responses in chronic inflammation

Although neutrophils are the key effector cells in acute inflammation, those in chronic inflammation are lymphoid cells and macrophages, a reflection of a tissue-based immune response to the damaging agent.

In chronic inflammation, macrophages not only act as phagocytic cells (removing and destroying cell debris), but they become activated to fulfil other immunological and secretory functions.

Because lymphocytes, plasma cells and macrophages are invariably present in chronic inflammatory reactions, they are sometimes referred to as chronic inflammatory cells (*Fig. 4.19*).

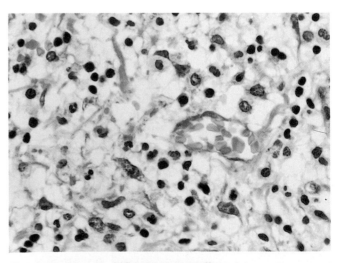

Fig. 4.19 Chronic inflammatory cells.
Photomicrograph showing the lymphocytes, macrophages and plasma cells commonly found in areas of chronic inflammation, mainly the result of the immune responses involved in chronicity.

KEY FACTS
Chronic inflammation

- Predisposed by factors that prevent elimination of a damaging stimulus.
- Tissue damage, acute inflammation, granulation tissue, repair, and immune response all take place concurrently.
- Associated with an immune response in tissues, visible as infiltration by lymphocytes.
- Chronic inflammation eventually heals by scarring.
- May develop after acute inflammation, or may be a primary response to certain stimuli, e.g. in tuberculosis.
- Predisposing factors include: persistent damaging stimulus, e.g. gastric acid in peptic ulcer; inadequate host response to infection; and persistent autoimmune disease, e.g. rheumatoid disease, chronic ulcerative colitis.

The macrophage is a main effector cell in chronic inflammation

Macrophages are among the main effector cells in chronic inflammation, and have several roles. They are converted from inactive monocytes to functioning macrophages by trophic signals, the best characterized being γ-interferon.

The morphology of activated macrophages changes, particularly as the subcellular apparatus for protein synthesis develops. Such cells develop voluminous cytoplasm, at which stage they are known as epithelioid cells. In addition, fusion of activated macrophages is a common event, whereby multinucleate histiocytic giant cells are formed.

Once activated, macrophages have both a phagocytic and a major secretory role in defence against injurious agents, and are important in cell-mediated immunity, e.g. antigen presentation. They secrete:

- Mediators of acute inflammation, particularly platelet-activating factor and arachidonic acid metabolites.
- Highly reactive oxygen metabolites, which participate in bacterial and cell killing.
- Proteases and hydrolytic enzymes, which cause dissolution of extracellular material. This is particularly relevant to macrophages' role in removing damaged material from areas of injury.
- Cytokines, IL-1, and TNFα. These stimulate fibroblast proliferation and collagen synthesis, which are important in any reparative response.
- Growth factors (PDGF, EGF, FGF). These stimulate growth of blood vessels, and division and migration of fibroblasts.

Granulomatous inflammatory reactions occur when neutrophil phagocytosis is inadequate to neutralize the causative agent

In certain diseases the acute inflammatory response, dominated by neutrophils, is transient and quickly replaced by an immune-based cellular reaction, which is characterized by aggregations of macrophages and lymphocytes. The macrophages often form discrete clusters called **granulomas**. A pattern of this kind is therefore frequently called **granulomatous inflammation**. It is an example of a chronic inflammatory response, as persistence of the damaging agent leads to concurrent tissue damage, inflammation and repair.

Damaging stimuli which provoke a granulomatous inflammatory response include:

- **Microorganisms which are of low inherent pathogenicity but which excite an immune response.** The most important group are the mycobacteria, which are intracellular pathogens with a resistant lipoprotein coating to the cell membrane. The most important mycobacteria in human disease are *Mycobacterium tuberculosis* (responsible for tuberculosis) and *M. leprae* (responsible for leprosy).
- **Non-living foreign material deposited in tissues.** As the material is non-viable, neutrophil enzymes are powerless to destroy it, and the material remains as a constant irritant within the tissues. Examples include both exogenous materials, which gain access to the tissues (e.g. inhaled inorganic dust in the lungs), and endogenous materials, which become misplaced or deposited in large quantities (e.g. precipitated urate crystals in gout (see page 526), and keratin that has escaped from traumatized epidermoid cysts).
- Certain fungi cannot be dealt with adequately by neutrophils, and thus excite macrophage granulomatous reactions.
- Unknown factors, e.g. in the disease 'sarcoid' (see page 539).

Tuberculosis is an example of granulomatous inflammation

The most common pattern of human tuberculosis (TB) is pulmonary. The *M. tuberculosis* organism is inhaled into the alveolar spaces of the lung, but other tissues are also affected, as described in the systems pathology later in the book.

Once in the lung the mycobacteria excite a transient but marked immune-mediated response, manifest by sensitization of T-cells to produce cytokines. Neutrophils are inadequate to deal with the organisms, the cell walls of which are resistant to degradation and, after 3 weeks or so, once bacteria have been presented to the immune system, the initial acute inflammatory response is replaced by a chronic inflammatory pattern. This is dominated by aggregates of macrophages, recruited by the cytokines. The type of immune response caused by TB is termed Type IV hypersensitivity.

A granuloma in TB is termed a 'tubercle'

In the context of TB, aggregates of macrophages, i.e. the granulomas, are often called **tubercles**.

Each tubercle has an area of caseous tissue necrosis at its centre. This is characterized by its homogeneity, and no ghost pattern of the original tissue structure remains. Viable mycobacteria are present within the necrotic debris. To the naked eye, this necrotic tissue resembles cream cheese, hence its descriptive name **caseous necrosis**. The reason for the necrosis at the centre of tubercles is uncertain, as it is not seen in the centre of granulomas caused by other agents.

A tubercle is composed of activated macrophages with surrounding lymphoid cells and fibroblasts

The structure of a typical tuberculous granuloma is shown in *Fig. 4.20*. Around the central area of caseous necrosis lies a collection of large, activated macrophages. Histologically, this functional activation is manifest by the presence of bulky pale-staining granular cytoplasm, which is rich in endoplasmic reticulum, with a prominent Golgi. Because

of a minimal resemblance to some epithelial cells, the term **epithelioid** cells was originally coined for these macrophages.

Some of the activated macrophages cells fuse to form large multinucleate cells (macrophage polykaryons) with many nuclei arranged around the periphery, and a large central cytoplasmic mass. In TB these giant macrophages are called **Langhans' cells**.

Around the zone of macrophages bordering the central caseous necrosis lies a collar of lymphocytes, reflecting the immunological response to the presence of mycobacteria.

As the tubercle persists, some fibroblasts appear within the lymphocyte collar and outside it. These are recruited by secretion of cytokines from the activated macrophages.

The outcome of tubercle formation depends on the adequacy of the host immune response

Because *M. tuberculosis* is resistant to destruction, infections tend to be chronic and persistent, being difficult to eradicate by natural defence mechanisms. The outcome of tubercle formation depends on the balance between two

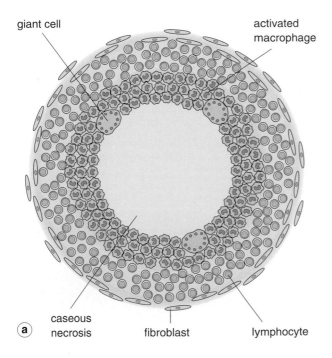
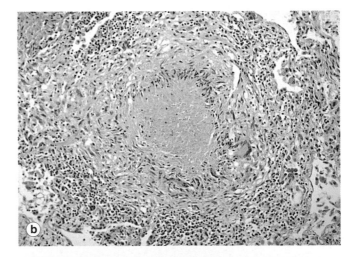
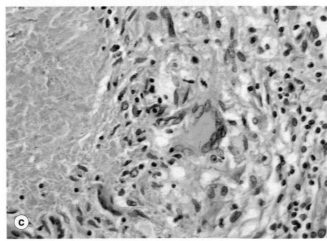

Fig. 4.20 A tuberculous granuloma.
In (a) the typical structure of a tubercle is shown diagrammatically. A central area of amorphous caseous necrosis is surrounded by a zone of activated macrophages, in which multinucleate macrophages (Langhan's giant cells) are present. There are outer layers of lymphocytes and fibroblasts. The low-power photomicrograph (b) shows a tubercle in the lung, demonstrating the features illustrated in (a). The medium-power photomicrograph (c) shows greater detail of the edge of the tubercle.

conflicting sets of factors: those predisposing to extension of infection, and those predisposing to containment, or healing and eradication of infection.

Factors predisposing to extension of the infection include:

- Ingestion of large numbers of highly virulent organisms.
- Poor immune response, e.g. due to malnutrition, extreme youth, old age, intercurrent disease or immunosuppressive therapy.

Factors predisposing to containment or eradication include:

- Ingestion of small numbers of poorly virulent organisms.
- Good immune response, e.g. robust health, heightened immune status due to immunization.
- Administration of appropriate antibiotics.

TB is most severe in patients with poor natural immunity, such as the malnourished, the poor and, increasingly, the underprivileged in the western world. Those immuno-suppressed by AIDS or treatment for organ transplantation are also greatly at risk. Worryingly, new strains of *M. tuberculosis*, resistant to formerly successful antituberculous chemotherapy, are now emerging, so the disease is becoming important once again.

Pulmonary tuberculosis exhibits different tissue patterns according to the level of host immunity.

- If there has been no previous exposure to the organism, a pattern of disease termed **primary tuberculosis** develops.

- If a person has previously been exposed and is sensitized to the organism, a pattern called **secondary tuberculosis** develops.
- If exposure has occurred, but immune responses become abnormal (e.g. by immunosuppression), the pattern of primary TB develops.

In primary TB the initial lung lesion remains small, but infection spreads to peribronchial lymph nodes

When infection with TB first occurs (e.g. in childhood), the organisms are inhaled and come to proliferate in alveoli at the periphery of the lung, often just beneath the pleura (a **Ghon focus**, *Fig. 4.21*). Although organisms are of low intrinsic pathogenicity, they cause cell death in adjacent lung. An ineffective acute inflammatory response occurs, which fails to destroy bacteria. Bacteria are then conveyed to local nodes at the lung hilum, where they also proliferate. After about 3 weeks, an immune response develops, and activated T-cells recruit macrophages to the lung and nodes, with resulting granulomatous inflammation and caseation. These early changes may produce no significant symptoms, and the outcome of the infection will depend on the balance between the host response to disease, and the virulence and number of organisms.

The primary complex will heal in most cases, with development of immunity to TB

In the vast majority of cases the Ghon focus and caseating granulomas in the lymph nodes heal by the deposition of collagen around the tubercles. The healed lesion comprises an area of central caseation surrounded by a wall of dense collagen (see *Fig. 4.22*). Calcium salts are frequently deposited in the collagen and are sometimes found in the caseous material.

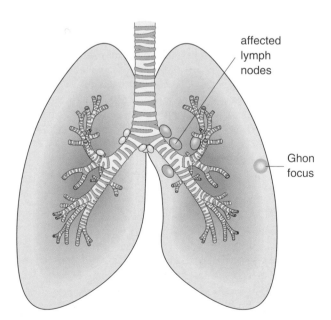

Fig. 4.21 The primary pattern in pulmonary TB.
The peripheral Ghon focus and enlarged peribronchial lymph nodes constitute the **primary complex**. The usual outcome is healing by progressive fibrosis surrounding the caseous necrosis.

affected lymph nodes

Ghon focus

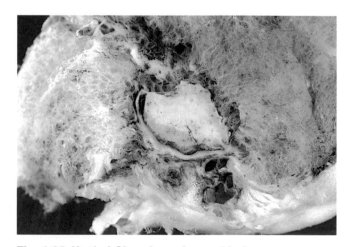

Fig. 4.22 Healed Ghon focus in an elderly man.
This close-up photograph shows an old, healed Ghon focus at the periphery of the lung. An incidental finding at autopsy, the lesion is a mass of yellowish caseous necrosis surrounded, in this case, by only a thin fibrous capsule.

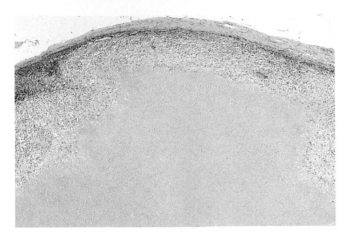

Fig. 4.23 Caseating TB in peribronchial lymph node.
This photomicrograph shows part of a lymph node which has been virtually replaced by pink-staining caseating tuberculous necrosis; only a thin rim of the original lymph node remains. Nodes such as this can rupture into the airways or bloodstream to initiate spread of tuberculosis.

Once the immune system has been exposed to *M. tuberculosis* the patient is sensitized to the organism. The disease does not progress, because the organisms are confined within the shell of collagen. Importantly, viable bacteria may remain walled off within the healed primary complex (latent tuberculosis).

Rarely, the primary complex will progress in patients with poor natural immunity

In patients who are unable to mount a vigorous immune and reparative response, further spread of mycobacteria occurs, with continuing enlargement of the caseating granulomas in the lymph nodes (*Fig. 4.23*). Known as progressive primary tuberculosis, spread occurs by the enlarging nodes eroding either through the wall of a bronchus or into a thin-walled blood vessel.

The Ghon focus usually remains small although, rarely, it may rupture through the visceral pleura, discharging organisms into the pleural cavity to produce tuberculous pleurisy.

Bronchial spread of organisms produces tuberculous bronchopneumonia

If an infected lymph node erodes into a bronchus, tuberculous caseous material containing living tubercle bacilli passes down bronchi and bronchioles under the influence of gravity, spreading the infection to the furthest reaches of the lungs (see *Fig. 4.24*), where extensive, confluent caseating granulomatous lesions develop. Known as 'galloping consumption', this is usually rapidly fatal.

Bloodstream spread of organisms produces miliary TB

If the enlarging caseating infected lymph node erodes a vessel wall, tubercle bacilli are carried in the bloodstream to

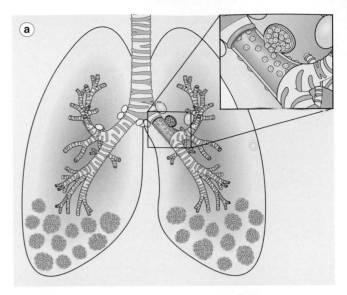

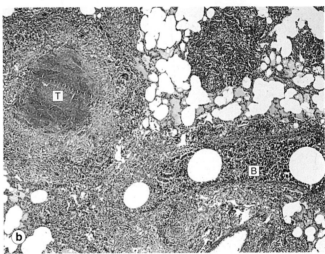

Fig. 4.24 Tuberculous bronchopneumonia.
As shown in the diagram (a), if the enlarged caseous nodes erode the bronchial wall, tubercle bacilli can enter into the lower portions of both the same and the opposite lung. New enlarging caseating granulomas form, often in the lower lobes. This is shown in the photomicrograph (b), where a caseating tubercle (**T**) is situated close to an infected bronchiole (**B**), down which the tubercle bacilli have passed.

many parts of the body, including the remainder of the lung, causing miliary tuberculosis (*Fig. 4.25*).

In secondary TB initial tuberculous infection is at the apex of the upper lobe of a lung, with little lymph node involvement

In secondary TB, organisms may be acquired exogenously or from healed primary complexes.

An apical lesion (often called an **Assmann focus**) begins as a small caseating tuberculous granuloma. Histologically similar to the Ghon focus, it has a central area of caseous necrosis that is surrounded by a granulomatous inflammatory

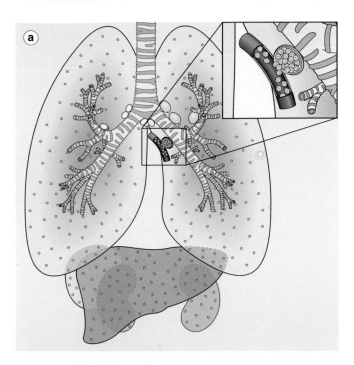

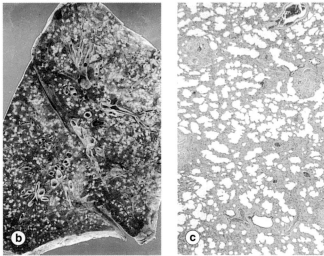

Fig. 4.25 Miliary tuberculosis of lung.
If an enlarged caseous node drains into a pulmonary vein (a), there is systemic dissemination of organisms (kidneys, liver, spleen). If drainage is into a pulmonary artery, miliary dissemination into the lung occurs (b). This slice of the lung of a child shows numerous tiny yellow-white dots. Each of these is a small caseating tuberculous granuloma caused by bloodstream spread. In (c) the photomicrograph shows the histological appearances of miliary TB in the lung; there are many small early tubercles, most of which have giant cells at their centre. There is, as yet, little caseation.

response. In most cases, destruction of lung leads to cavitation. There is little involvement of lymph nodes, as spread of organisms to regional nodes is prevented by a vigorous tissue-based hypersensitivity response. The outcome of the infection depends entirely on what happens to the Assmann focus.

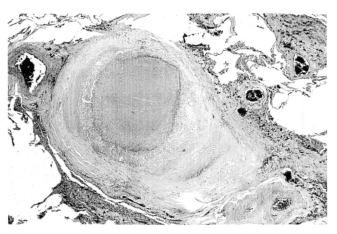

Fig. 4.26 Healed fibrocaseous TB.
This photomicrograph shows the histology of a small nodule from the apex of an adult who had no history of TB. There is a central area of pink-staining caseous material surrounded by a thick, pale-pink collagenous shell, representing healing of a small Assmann focus.

In adults secondary TB heals by fibrosis around the caseating granulomatous mass

In adults, with vigorous immune responses, healing of the apical lesion occurs through precisely the same process as that for the Ghon focus (*Fig. 4.26*). Thus, the lesion contains a central area of caseous necrotic material, surrounded by a thick dense collagenous wall in which calcium salts are frequently deposited. This achieves containment of the infection and there is no further spread of the organism. Nevertheless, if the fibrous wall breaks down, this latent tuberculosis can lead to spreading infection at a much later stage (reactivated fibrocaseous tuberculosis).

In adults with poor immune responses, secondary TB progresses locally, with risk of spread to other sites

In adults with poor immune responses, progressive enlargement of the apical lesion occurs, with caseous necrosis destroying lung tissue. A large caseous mass is formed as a result, which is surrounded by a thin cellular reaction, inducing little collagen to wall off the lesion (progressive pulmonary tuberculosis). As the lesion grows, so too does the risk of erosion into blood vessels or airways.

The release of tubercle bacilli into the main bronchi allows them to be coughed into the atmosphere in droplets, transmitting the infection to other people (so-called open tuberculosis), as well as producing TB bronchopneumonia by passage down bronchi to lower lobes.

Bloodstream spread of organisms can lead to single-organ infections

Sometimes only small numbers of tubercle bacilli escape into the blood and, if host defences are effective, most of the organisms die. However, for reasons that are not yet certain, some bacilli settle in specific organs and may remain dormant for many years, only proliferating and producing overt disease at a later date, often after the initial lung and lymph node lesions have healed. Known as metastatic tuberculosis or isolated organ tuberculosis, those organs particularly involved in this pattern of disease include: adrenal glands, kidney (see page 371), fallopian tube (see page 410), epididymis (see page 384), brain and meninges (see page 445), and bones and joints.

Tuberculous lesions may become reactivated long after apparent healing

In some patients, after collagenous walling-off of a primary or secondary focus, immune defences wane (often due to immunosuppression or malnutrition), and mycobacteria escape into adjacent lung. There the mycobacteria are able to proliferate rapidly, producing tissue necrosis, with new caseation and granulomatous inflammatory reaction. In the patient's debilitated state, the infection may progress rapidly, and is commonly fatal. Called reactivated pulmonary TB, it may, like other types, progress to miliary TB or tuberculous bronchopneumonia.

This illustrates that maintenance of adequate immune and reparative processes is needed to suppress a persisting damaging stimulus, in this instance a latent mycobacterial infection.

Mycobacteria of other types cause different patterns of infection

Like pulmonary TB, other mycobacterial diseases are characterized by a chronic inflammatory granulomatous response, with little induction of acute inflammatory response (see Chapter 4). These include:

- **Leprosy** (*M. leprae*), a chronic indolent lesion, mainly of skin. If immunity is high, it may cause a reaction similar to granulomas in TB. If immunity is low, generalized intracellular proliferation of organisms in phagocytic cells results.
- **Bovine TB** (*M. bovis*) is manifest as tuberculous infection of cervical lymph nodes, due to drinking infected cows' milk.
- *M. marinum* causes **chronic skin lesions**, usually on the hands ('fish tank granuloma' or 'swimming pool granuloma').
- *M. scrofulaceum* produces **enlarged lymph nodes** in the neck similar to those in bovine TB, particularly in children.

M. avium-intracellulare is increasingly being seen in AIDS patients, in whom it is characterized not so much by a granulomatous reaction (as the immune system is inactivated), but by vast numbers of organisms proliferating within macrophages in many organs, resembling lepromatous leprosy. This organism may also produce a classic caseating granulomatous disease of the lung, similar to that seen in pulmonary TB due to *M. tuberculosis*.

KEY FACTS

Tuberculosis

- Caused by *Mycobacterium tuberculosis*.
- Organism induces Type IV hypersensitivity response.
- Histological hallmark is caseating granulomatous inflammation.
- Main site of infection is in lungs.
- Lung infection in childhood comprises Ghon focus and nodal disease (primary complex).
- Infection in adult life causes Assmann focus.
- Blood-borne spread leads to miliary tuberculosis.
- Bronchial spread leads to tuberculous bronchopneumonia.
- Reactivation of disease may take place in later life if host response is weakened, e.g. due to immunosuppression.

OTHER CAUSES OF GRANULOMATOUS INFLAMMATION

Granulomatous inflammation can be a tissue response to some foreign materials

Foreign material (inorganic or organic) introduced into tissues commonly excites a predominantly macrophagic reaction, since neutrophils are unable to phagocytose and destroy the material. Clearly defined granulomatous aggregates with giant cells sometimes form around the material, but more often the aggregation of macrophages is irregular and ill-defined.

Foreign material may be either endogenous or exogenous. Commonly found endogenous materials include:

- Keratin – from traumatized epidermal cysts.
- Urate crystals in patients with soft-tissue deposits of urates in gout.
- Degenerate altered collagen – in the skin condition 'necrobiosis lipoidica', and rheumatoid nodules.
- Degenerate and altered elastin – in the walls of arteries affected by giant cell arteritis.

Exogenous materials usually gain access to tissues as a result of trauma, although some particles may be inhaled, producing a granulomatous reaction in the lungs (e.g. beryllium). The materials seen most frequently clinically are:

- Non-lysable suture material used in surgery.
- Talcum powder (used on surgeons' gloves during surgical operations) has occasionally induced numerous 'talc granulomas', with a particle of silicaceous talc at the centre of each.
- Fragments of vegetable material, e.g. thorn fragments.

Sarcoidosis is a granulomatous disease of unknown cause

In sarcoidosis, discrete granulomas with histiocytic giant cells form, mainly in lymph nodes, lungs, liver, spleen and skin, although other organs (e.g. brain and bone) are occasionally affected. Histologically, the granulomas resemble those of TB, although there is never any true caseation. The granulomas are multiple, and slowly increase in size, often becoming confluent. The cause of the disease is unknown. Affected patients most commonly present with clinical disease related to lung involvement, or with evidence of lymph node enlargement. The multinucleate giant cells in sarcoidosis occasionally contain laminated calcific spherical concretions (**Schaumann bodies** or **asteroid bodies**).

The disease is slowly progressive, but frequently burns itself out, the formerly cellular granulomas becoming progressively smaller and more collagenized. Where there has been significant lung involvement, this healing phase may produce widespread pulmonary fibrosis. This is discussed in Chapter 25.

5

Developmental and genetic factors in disease

Clinical Overview

This chapter presents a brief outline of developmental abnormalities and genetic factors in disease.

DEVELOPMENTAL DISORDERS

Factors that induce abnormal embryological development are known as 'teratogens'

Most teratogens induce abnormal development only if the mother and embryo are exposed to them at a particular stage of embryological development, often during the first 3 months (trimester) of fetal development, which is the period when there is most active embryological change. The likelihood of abnormality depends on:

- Dose and duration of exposure.
- Time of exposure.
- Individual susceptibility.

Many factors have been shown to be teratogenic in experimental animals, but largely harmless in humans. However, because for some factors the reverse is true, species specificity renders testing for drug teratogenicity using experimental animals something of a lottery.

The most important teratogenic factors recognized in man are:

- Drugs and chemicals, e.g. thalidomide, alcohol.
- Ionizing radiations, e.g. X-rays.
- Maternal infections, e.g. toxoplasmosis, rubella, herpes simplex, syphilis.
- Genetic/chromosomal abnormalities, e.g. Down's syndrome, Turner's syndrome.

Failure of normal embryological development is usually evident at birth

In many cases, the embryological error is so great that the embryo cannot survive and dies soon after fertilization.

Less severe abnormalities permit the embryo to develop to a later stage, but the fetus dies late in the pregnancy or shortly after birth; an example is bilateral renal dysplasia.

Some embryological abnormalities are not immediately lethal but produce disease in later life. For example, there are many embryological disorders that affect the final proper development of the heart; in some, the abnormality is not immediately fatal but produces severe illness (e.g. Fallot's tetralogy), whereas others are so mild that they are compatible with a normal existence (e.g. a small atrial or ventricular septal defect). Some of the more common and important congenital diseases of the heart are discussed in Chapter 10.

Examples of abnormal embryological development affecting the various systems are examined in the relevant chapters later in the book. The most important patterns of embryological maldevelopment are detailed in *Fig. 5.1*.

GENETIC FACTORS IN DISEASE

The use of new molecular genetic techniques has revolutionized the whole of medical practice. Three levels in the development of human genetics are now recognized: classic genetics, cytogenetics, and molecular genetics.

A full description of basic genetics, together with the detailed mechanisms of genetic and chromosomal disorders, is beyond the scope of this book. Readers are referred to one of the excellent student texts on clinical genetics.

Classic genetics is based on analysis of pedigrees and patterns of inheritance

Clinical analysis of diseases that run in families has allowed the delineation of distinct patterns of inheritance. Although many diseases follow Mendelian genetic principles of dominant, recessive, and sex-linked patterns, others reveal a pattern of inheritance suggestive of a polygenic or multi-factorial pattern. Increasingly, forms of maternal inheritance are seen, explicable by inheritance through mitochondrial, rather than nuclear, DNA.

The importance of classic genetics is that it allows counseling of families, based on the statistical chances of inheriting a disease. The recent developments in molecular genetic techniques can frequently reinforce such analysis by enabling precise diagnosis of disease, based on identification of abnormal genes. Prenatal diagnosis and confident prediction of whether a fetus has inherited abnormal genes from the parents are now possible. Until all genes related to disease are identified, classic genetics, and counseling based on statistical risk, remain important parts of clinical practice.

Fig. 5.1
Patterns of embryological maldevelopment

Pattern	Mechanism	Common examples
Complete failure of organ development (agenesis)	Early failure of development of all or part of organ primordium	Renal agenesis (see *Fig. 5.2*)
Incomplete organ development (hypoplasia)	Probably due to influence of external teratogen during organ growth phase	Microcephaly (e.g. alcohol teratogenicity) Phocomelia (e.g. thalidomide teratogenicity, see *Fig. 5.3*)
Abnormal tissue organization (dysplasia)	Failure of organized tissue differentiation and maturation	Renal dysplasia (see *Fig. 5.4*)
Failure of embryological fusion (dysraphism)	Defects arise by failure of complete fusion of embryological primordia	Myelomeningocele (see *Fig. 5.5*) 'Ectopia vesicae'
Failure of involution	Temporary embryological structures that normally involute fail to do so	Persistent urachus Persistent thyroglossal duct Syndactyly (see *Fig 5.6*)
Failure of lumen formation (atresia)	Solid cylinders of cells fail to undergo central programed cell death to create a lumen	Esophageal atresia (see *Fig 5.7*) Biliary atresia
Organ or tissue displacement (ectopia)	Failure of normal migration of cells during embryological development	Maldescent of testes

Examples of common patterns of embryological maldevelopment

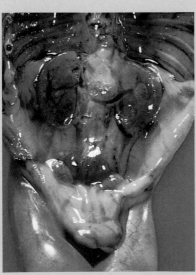
Fig. 5.2 Renal agenesis: an example of complete failure of organ development. This fetus shows total failure of kidney development. The masses located at the site normally occupied by the kidneys are large fetal adrenals.

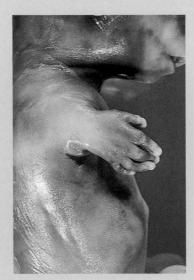
Fig. 5.3 Phocomelia: an example of incomplete organ development. This fetus shows incomplete development of the arm (phocornelia). This congenital malformation may occur spontaneously, but is particularly associated with the chemical teratogen, thalidomide.

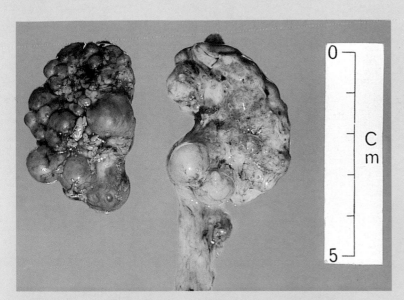

Fig. 5.4 Renal dysplasia: an example of abnormal tissue organization. This child died shortly after birth, without passing urine. The kidneys show dysplasia, and are being converted into a connected mass of cysts.

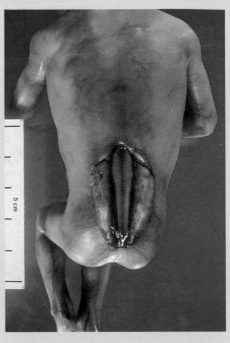

Fig. 5.5 Myelomeningocele: an example of failure of embryological fusion. This common congenital malformation is known as 'spina bifida'.

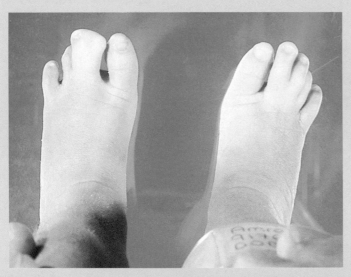

Fig. 5.6 Syndactyly: an example of failure of involution. Fusion of digits is a common congenital malformation, and is the result of failure of the tissues between the digits to involute during development.

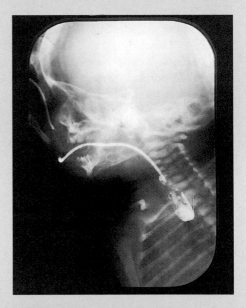

Fig. 5.7 Esophageal atresia: an example of failure of lumen formation. In this radiograph injection of radio-opaque medium into the upper esophagus of a new-born infant demonstrates the failure of the lumen to develop.

Cytogenetics is based on analysis of chromosomal abnormalities

The production of chromosomal spreads and the staining of chromosomes to show bands have allowed direct observation of abnormalities of chromosomes (*Fig. 5.8*). The two principal types of abnormality apparent using these techniques are:

- Abnormalities in the number of individual chromosomes.
- Structural abnormalities in individual chromosomes.

Such cytogenetic analyses are an important aspect of medical investigation (see page 69), and identification of carrier states allows genetic counselling to be given to at-risk families. Moreover, identification of specific forms of chromosomal abnormality provides an insight into prognosis of certain types of tumor, particularly leukemias.

Knowledge of how gross changes of chromosomal material lead to abnormal phenotypes is growing through the application of molecular genetic techniques. Until the molecular nature of all such disorders is defined, cytogenetic methods remain important clinical and research tools.

Certain genetic disorders can be identified by detection of abnormal gene products

For many years, several genetic abnormalities have been confidently diagnosed by identification of abnormal gene products. Some of these conditions have been diagnosed *in utero*, using prenatal tests based on identification of the abnormal product or the lack of a specific enzyme activity. Examples include identification of abnormal hemoglobins in the hemoglobinopathies (e.g. sickle-cell disease), identification of children affected by phenylketonuria (PKU), and demonstration of the loss of specific enzyme activities in many of the metabolic diseases leading to storage of abnormal metabolites (e.g. the glycogenoses).

Interestingly, molecular genetic techniques have shown several types of genetic abnormality to underlie single apparently well-defined conditions (molecular genetic heterogeneity), which goes some way to explaining the variation seen in clinical expression of disease.

Genetic disorders are now identifiable by molecular genetic techniques

Recombinant DNA technology has revolutionized the diagnosis and investigation of genetic diseases. The main techniques enable individual genes to be identified and sequenced, and probes can be created for use in molecular genetic diagnosis of disease. The use of specific restriction enzymes, together with Southern blotting to separate DNA fragments, allows the identification of the linkage between specific chromosomal areas and disease, so that such regions may be searched to locate specific genes. The technique of DNA amplification using the polymerase chain reaction means that DNA diagnostic tests can be performed rapidly and on very small amounts of material.

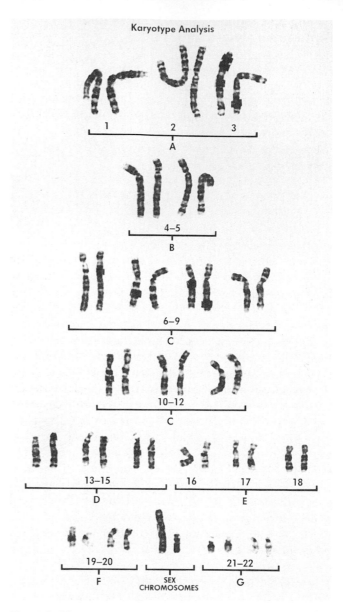

Karyotype Analysis

Fig. 5.8 Chromosome spread.

CYTOGENETIC ABNORMALITIES AND DISEASE

A normal haploid gamete has 22 autosomes and 1 sex chromosome

The normal (diploid) chromosome complement of the human somatic cell consists of 46 paired chromosomes, with 44 autosomes and 2 sex chromosomes (XX in females and XY in males); one half is contributed by the haploid maternal ovum, the other by the haploid paternal spermatozoon. Thus, after meiosis, the haploid maternal ovum will contain 22 autosomes and an X chromosome.

Similarly, the fertilizing paternal spermatozoon will contain either 22 autosomes and an X chromosome, or 22 autosomes and a Y chromosome, the sex of the embryo

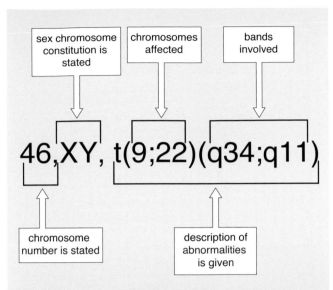

$$46,XY, t(9;22)(q34;q11)$$

- sex chromosome constitution is stated
- chromosomes affected
- bands involved
- chromosome number is stated
- description of abnormalities is given

Additional whole chromosomes are listed as '+' followed by the number, e.g. +21 for trisomy 21.

Abnormalities such as deletions, inversions, translocations (t) and fragile sites are denoted by an abbreviation (see *Fig. 5.11*), located to specific chromosome areas according to the following scheme:

- The short arm of a chromosome is termed 'p'.

- The long arm of a chromosome is termed 'q'.

- Chromosome regions are defined as numbered regions from the centromere outwards.

- Within each region, individual bands are given a number.

Fig. 5.9 Nomenclature and notation of karyotype analysis. The above example is a male with a translocation between chromosomes 9 and 22, both involving the long arm. This is the Philadelphia chromosome, seen in certain forms of leukemia (Chapter 15).

depending on which type of spermatozoon fertilizes the ovum. For successful blending of chromosomes, it is vital that the meiotic division in both ova and spermatozoa be faultless. However, abnormal chromosome separation during meiosis may result in deletion, non-disjunction or translocation of chromosomal material in either autosomes or sex chromosomes.

The convention used for describing the chromosomal complement of a cell on karyotype analysis is given in *Fig. 5.9*.

Abnormalities of chromosomes are a common cause of congenital abnormality

Abnormal chromosome numbers usually result from non-disjunction (i.e. failure of paired chromosomes to separate properly during cell division), and can occur in meiotic or mitotic divisions.

Gametes with only one of a pair of autosomes (monosomy) do not usually survive, and the majority of autosomal number disorders are due to extra chromosomal material, particularly trisomies (three copies).

Breaking and rejoining leads to structural chromosomal abnormalities

If there is a break in chromosomal material, the break can be rejoined. If a segment is involved, material may be lost (deletion), transposed into another chromosome (translocation), or abnormally inserted (inversion), as illustrated diagrammatically in *Fig. 5.10*.

The symbols used to describe the main structural abnormalities of chromosomes are listed in *Fig. 5.11*.

Translocation of one part of a chromosome to another is caused by breaking and rejoining (*Fig. 5.10a*). Translocation of chromosomal material is frequently reciprocal, thus there is no overall loss or gain of genetic material in the carrier, who is phenotypically normal. The problem with this type of abnormality is that when segregation takes place, two sets of material from one chromosome may end up in one gamete. For example, a translocation of chromosome 21 onto chromosome 14 may be present in the mother. An ovum may be then be produced with the normal chromosome 21, together with the abnormal chromosome 14 carrying the additional chromosome 21 material. If the gamete is then fertilized by a normal haploid sperm, three copies of chromosome 21 material are contained in the gamete.

Robertsonian translocation describes a special situation in which chromosome breaks occur close to the centromere of two chromosomes, resulting in one very large chromosome and one very small chromosome, which is frequently lost (*Fig. 5.10b*). Affected individuals appear to have 45 chromosomes on karyotype analysis. As with other forms of translocation, problems arise in gametogenesis, with the formation of unbalanced gametes containing both copies of the chromosomal material.

Ring chromosomes are associated with loss of genetic material. They are a special form of deletion in which a chromosome, having lost material from both ends, rejoins in a closed circle (*Fig. 5.10c*).

Inversions occur when two breaks in a chromosome take place. The resulting fragment is turned 180° and is re-united in the same chromosome.

The most common **deletion** syndrome is the *cri du chat* syndrome, caused by deletion of part of chromosome 5 (*Fig. 5.10d*). Microcephaly, muscular hypotonia and mental retardation are associated, and the affected infant has a characteristic shrill cry (hence *cri du chat*), arising from maldevelopment of the posterior part of the true vocal cords.

Abnormal chromosomes resulting from various types of translocation are rare. They cause 'functional' trisomy syndromes, the most common being those which produce the features of Down's, Edwards' and Patau's syndromes.

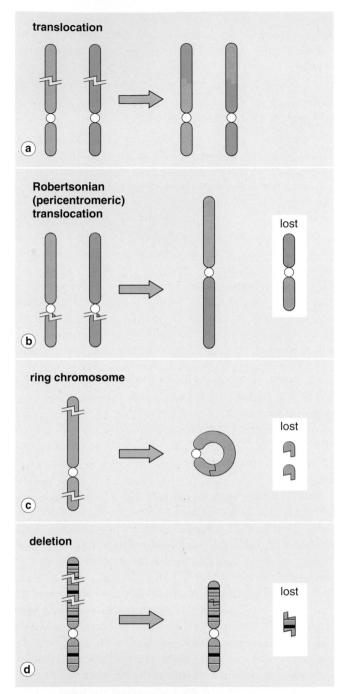

translocation

(a)

Robertsonian (pericentromeric) translocation

lost

(b)

ring chromosome

lost

(c)

deletion

lost

(d)

Fig. 5.10 Structural abnormalities of chromosomes. (a) Translocation. (b) Robertsonian translocation. (c) Ring chromosome. (d) Deletion.

Fig. 5.11
Main structural changes of chromosomes

Type	Symbol	Nature
Translocation	t	Two chromosomes break, rejoin, and exchange segments
Deletion	del	A segment of chromosome is lost
Inversion	inv	Two breaks occur; the middle piece is rotated and rejoins
Fragile site	fra	A chromosomal site with a tendency to break
Heterochromic site	h	Chromosomal region that stains differently from the rest, often of variable size in the normal population
Duplication	dup	Duplication of a segment of chromosome
Ring	r	Arises from breaks in both arms, with loss of both ends to form a ring

From observations after the nuclear explosions in Hiroshima and Nagasaki, exposure to ionizing radiations is known to be a causative factor in spontaneous mutations. Chemical agents and some viruses induce genetic abnormalities in cells in tissue culture, but there is no incontrovertible evidence that they have this effect in humans *in vivo*, although they can induce congenital malformations through interfering with embryological development .

It is known that some fetal chromosomal abnormalities, particularly those of chromosome number, become more common with increasing maternal age.

An abnormality in a haploid gamete is transmitted to all its daughter cells

An abnormality of chromosome segregation during meiosis gives rise to haploid gametes containing an abnormal chromosome complement. If the gamete goes on to form a cell by fertilization, all daughter cells will be affected.

Fortunately, many such abnormal gametes are probably incapable of participating in fertilization and, if fertilization does occur, the fetus usually dies *in utero*. (A high proportion of fetuses that spontaneously abort in early pregnancy have chromosomal abnormalities.)

However, a few fetuses with an abnormal chromosome complement survive *in utero*, growing to reproductive

Translocations may be associated with abnormal gene expression, resulting in tumor formation (see Chapter 6).

Most new genetic and chromosomal abnormalities have no identifiable cause

As the reason for the development of most new genetic aberrations is unknown, they are referred to as being 'spontaneous'.

maturity. As all of their cells have the chromosomal abnormality, the gametes will be abnormal, and the chromosomal disorder is thus passed on to the next generation. The various patterns of inheritance are discussed below.

MOSAICISM is caused by a chromosomal abnormality that develops during mitotic division AFTER fertilization

A problem in chromosome separation that originates in the embryo after fertilization is transmitted only to daughter cells formed after the defect has occurred. Non-disjunction is the most important chromosomal abnormality, producing the most common mosaic syndromes. The resulting embryo therefore contains at least two cell lines and is described as a **mosaic**.

Mosaicism may involve abnormalities in the autosomes, e.g. Down's syndrome (see below), or the sex chromosomes, e.g. Turner's syndrome (see page 69).

Genomic imprinting is the differential expression in a child of a gene, depending on whether it is inherited from the mother or the father

In normal Mendelian inheritance, genes inherited from either parent would be expected to have an identical and equal effect. Genomic imprinting describes the situation where certain genes function differently depending on whether they are derived from the mother or the father. The best known example of diseases resulting from genomic imprinting is in the two quite distinct diseases, Prader–Willi syndrome and Angelman syndrome. Both are due to a deletion of certain genes in the q11–13 region of chromosome 15.

If the deletion is on the chromosome derived from the father, then the Prader–Willi syndrome results, whereas if the deletion is on the chromosome 15 from the mother, the child will suffer from Angelman's syndrome. Brief details of these rare but important syndromes are outlined in *Fig. 5.12*. Genomic imprinting has also been implicated in some cases of nephroblastoma (see page 376).

Uniparental disomy is a rare cause of non-Mendelian inheritance

In uniparental disomy both chromosomes in the child are inherited from the same parent. For example, a percentage of cases of Prader–Willi syndrome do not show genomic imprinting with the deletion described above on the paternal chromosome 15, but both chromosomes 15 are derived entirely from the mother, without deletion. This seems to have the same effect as a deletion on the paternal chromosome.

The cause of uniparental trisomy is not known but it may follow a trisomy in which one of the three chromosomes is lost. As well as Prader–Willi syndrome, uniparental disomy

Fig. 5.12
Summary of clinical features of Prader–Willi and Angelman's syndromes

Prader–Willi syndrome	Angelman's syndrome
Neonatal hypotonia ('floppy baby')	Microcephaly
Mental retardation and learning difficulties	Severe mental retardation
Initial failure to thrive	Ataxic gait
Uncontrollable appetite → obesity	Epilepsy
Hypogonadism, small hands and feet	Absent speech
Characteristic facies	Characteristic 'happy face'

is rarely the cause of anomolous inheritance patterns, for example, a hemophiliac father having an affected son.

The most important abnormalities of autosomal numbers are the TRISOMIES

A trisomy describes the situation in which there are three chromosomes of a particular type, rather than the normal pair. The most common example is trisomy 21, which produces Down's syndrome (*Fig. 5.13*).

In Down's syndrome, the additional chromosome 21 is usually the result of non-disjunction (failure of separation during meiosis) of chromosome 21 during formation of the haploid maternal ovum. The incidence of this disorder rises with increasing maternal age (1 in 3000 when the maternal age is below 30, 1 in about 300 in women aged 35 to 40, and about 1 in 30 in women over 45). In a small percentage of cases, Down's syndrome is due either to translocation or to mosaicism. The likelihood of Down's syndrome occurring in a subsequent pregnancy depends on whether the abnormality has arisen by meiotic non-disjunction (relatively low), maternal translocation (high) or mitotic mosaicism (relatively low); this is important in genetic counselling.

Non-disjunction is responsible for 95% of cases, which have a recurrence risk of approximately 1%.

About 4% of cases are due to translocations:

- Robertsonian translocation 14;21. Recurrence is 15% if mother is carrier, and 1% if father is carrier.
- Translocation 21;22. Recurrence is 10% if mother is carrier, and 5% if father is carrier.

Other autosomal trisomies are much rarer (*Fig. 5.14*), accounting for 1% of cases.

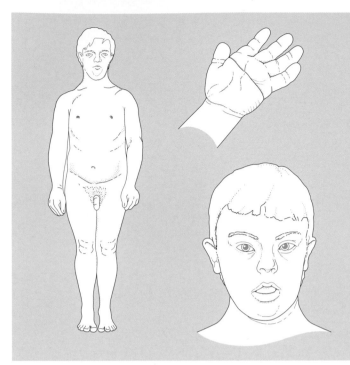

- Characteristic facies (flat facial profile, oblique palpebral fissures, low-bridged nose, epicanthal fold, open mouth, enlarged protruding tongue).

- Short stature (long bones of limbs are short).

- Short middle phalanx of little fingers.

- Horizontal palmar crease in short, broad hands.

- Hyperflexibility of joints.

- Poor muscle tone.

- Pelvic abnormalities.

- Congenital heart disease.

- Mental retardation.

- Alzheimer's disease beyond age of 40.

Fig. 5.13 Features of Down's syndrome.

Fig. 5.14
Rarer autosomal trisomies

Name	Chromosomal abnormality	Features
Patau's syndrome	Trisomy 13	Mental retardation Microcephaly and microphthalmos Hair lip and cleft palate Cardiac abnormalities, e.g. venticular septal defect (VSD) Abnormal feet ('rocker bottom') Polydactyly Mental retardation
Edwards' syndrome	Trisomy 18	Hypotonia/hypertonia Flexion deformities of fingers Cardiac abnormalities, e.g. VSD Abnormal feet ('rocker bottom') Abnormal head shape (prominent occiput) Low-set abnormal ears

Disorders of sex chromosome number arise by non-disjunction

The most important abnormalities of sex chromosome number arise from non-disjunction of chromosomes during meiotic division of male and female gametes.

- Meiotic division in female gametogenesis should produce two cells (ova), each with a single X chromosome. Non-disjunction may produce one cell with two X chromosomes (XX), and one with no sex chromosome at all (−).

- Meiotic division in male gametogenesis should produce two cells (spermatozoa), one with a single X chromosome, the other with a single Y chromosome. Non-disjunction may provide one with both X and Y chromosomes, and one with no sex chromosomes (−).

The most important syndromes produced by non-disjunction affecting sex chromosomes are:

- Turner's syndrome (mainly X−) (*Fig. 5.15*).
- Klinefelter's syndrome (mainly XXY) (*Fig. 5.16*).

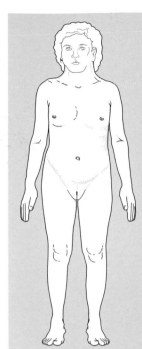

- Infantile genitalia (even when adult).

- Widely spaced nipples.

- Micrognathia and prominent ears.

- Short stature.

- Redundant skin of neck (webbing).

- Primary amenorrhea.

- Cubitus valgus (wide carrying angle).

- Short fourth metacarpal bone.

- Congenital renal and aortic abnormalities.

Fig. 5.15 Turner's syndrome.
Turner's syndrome is mainly due to non-disjunction in the meiotic division of gamete formation, but non-disjunction in mitotic division in the early embryo may produce Turner mosaics. About 20% of spontaneously aborted fetuses show the Turner chromosome pattern (X–).

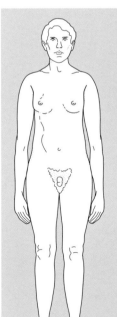

- Tall stature with long arms and legs.

- Testes and penis small.

- Gynecomastia.*

- Female pubic hair profile.*

- High pitched voice.*

- Reduced facial and body hair.*

*feminization features

Fig. 5.16 Klinefelter's syndrome.
Men with XXY Klinefelter's syndrome have greatly reduced fertility, but patients with mosaic types may be fertile. Other Klinefelter patterns include XXXY and XXXXY, with which mental retardation may be associated.

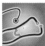

Laboratory medicine

Karyotype analysis of chromosomes is usually performed for prenatal diagnosis, or for investigation of conditions in postnatal life.

In postnatal diagnosis, cells are derived from blood lymphocytes, or from biopsy of skin to obtain fibroblasts. In prenatal diagnosis, cells are derived from amniocentesis or chorionic villus biopsy.

Cells are cultured and a chromosome preparation is made. Chromosomes can be specially stained by a variety of methods which produce a banding pattern, the most common being Giemsa staining (G-banding). Increasingly, specific DNA probes are being used to analyse the presence of specific chromosomes or chromosome regions.

The main clinical situations in which it is useful to examine for chromosomal abnormalities are:

- **Pediatric practice**
  Congenital abnormalities or dysmorphic state.
  Mental handicap or learning difficulty.
  Growth retardation.
  Failure of sexual development at puberty.

- **Obstetric practice**
  Infertility.
  Recurrent spontaneous abortions.
  Pregnancies in older females.

- **Oncology**
  Malignancies, particularly leukemias.

GENE DEFECTS AND DISEASE

Many important diseases are due to abnormalities in single genes or small gene clusters, the chromosome numbers being normal. Such defects either may be expressed as dominant or recessive disorders with a Mendelian inheritance pattern, or may require the co-existence of environmental factors before producing the disease (polygenic or multifactorial inheritance, see page 76).

Single gene defects are of varied Mendelian pattern

Single gene defect diseases can be classified according to two criteria:

- Whether the abnormal gene is located on one of the 22 autosome pairs (autosomal) or on the sex chromosomes (sex-linked).

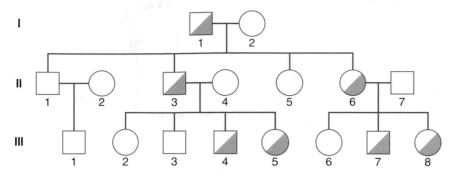

Fig. 5.17 A typical pedigree in autosomal dominant inheritance.

Fig. 5.18 Punnett square for autosomal dominant inheritance.

- Whether the disease is produced only when the abnormal gene is present on both members of the chromosome pair (homozygote), or can occur when the abnormal gene is present on only one member of the chromosome pair (heterozygote).

The following Mendelian patterns of inheritance of single gene defects occur:

- **Autosomal dominant inheritance** (expressed in heterozygotes).
- **Autosomal recessive inheritance** (expressed in homozygotes).
- **Sex-linked recessive inheritance**. Virtually all sex-linked abnormalities are associated with genes on the X chromosome, and are therefore expressed mainly in males who only have one copy and cannot compensate with a normal X chromosome as in females. They are not usually expressed in heterozygous females, who have one normal and one abnormal X chromosome, but 'manifesting carriers' can occur in some X-linked disorders, e.g. Duchenne's muscular dystrophy (see page 469).

Sex-linked dominant inheritance is very rare.

In autosomal dominant inheritance the abnormal gene produces disease in heterozygotes, where a normal allele is also present

Theoretically, in autosomal dominant inheritance the gene can produce disease either in homozygotes, i.e. when the abnormal gene is present in both members of a chromosome pair, or in heterozygotes, when only one member of the chromosome pair has the abnormal gene. Since homozygous affected individuals are very rare, the usual mating is between a homozygous normal individual and a heterozygous affected individual.

Each affected individual is a heterozygote for the disease and will have a genotype **Aa** for the relevant gene (**A** is the abnormal gene, **a** its normal allele); unaffected individuals will have the genotype **aa**. The gametes produced by the

KEY FACTS
Autosomal dominant inheritance

- Homozygotes and heterozygotes manifest the disease, but the great majority are heterozygotes (i.e. all affected individuals in *Fig. 5.17*).
- Both males and females are affected, e.g. **III**, 4 and 5.
- Only affected individuals can pass on the disease to their children; clinically unaffected individuals do not pass on the disease (e.g. **II**, 1).
- The disease is therefore passed on (on average) to only half of their children.
- The disease appears in every generation.

affected male in the first generation (**I**) will be **A** and **a**, and the non-affected female will produce **a** and **a** gametes. Thus, the possible combinations after fertilization are as shown in *Fig. 5.18*.

The affected progeny (approximately 50%) are heterozygotes (**Aa**) like the affected parent. Affected homozygotes (in this case, **AA**) are rare, since they can only arise from matings between two affected heterozygotes. This is unlikely where the gene abnormality is rare, but the chances are greater when parents are related. The common autosomal dominant disorders are listed in *Fig. 5.19*.

As a result of a new mutation or non-penetrance, autosomal dominant disease may affect offspring of clinically unaffected parents

Spontaneous mutation is a common event in certain diseases that subsequently show an autosomal dominant inheritance, although the rate varies greatly from disease to disease. It is believed that new mutations are responsible for approximately 50% of cases of neurofibromatosis, and 80% of cases of achondroplasia.

Fig. 5.19
Common and important autosomal dominant diseases

Achondroplasia	Dwarfism due to short limb bones	
Adult polycystic disease	Enlarging cysts replacing kidney	see page 381
Neurofibromatosis 1 Neurofibromatosis 2	Multiple nerve sheath tumors Acoustic neuromas	see page 459
Familial polyposis coli	Multiple colonic adenomata and carcinomas	see page 261
Hereditary spherocytosis	Spherical red cells with short life-span	see page 320
Huntington's disease**	Progressive neuronal degeneration	see page 452
Myotonic dystrophy**	Muscle weakness and wasting	see page 470
Familial hypercholesterolemia	Increased cholesterol levels	
Osteogenesis imperfecta	Brittle bones, fracturing with minimal trauma	see page 522
Marfan's syndromes	Abnormal elastic tissues – skeletal, cardiovascular and ocular disease	
Some Ehlers–Danlos syndromes*	Abnormal collagen – skin, joint and vascular effects	
Retinoblastoma	Malignant tumor of eye	see page 480

*Other Ehlers–Danlos syndromes show autosomal or sex-linked recessive inheritance.
** These neurological disorders are known to be the result of inserts of multiple triplet repeats.

Non-penetrance is where the abnormal genotype is not manifest in the form of disease. The phenotype appears normal, and there is no clinical expression of the disease (*Fig. 5.20b*).

The identification of specific gene abnormalities for several of the autosomal dominant conditions now allows molecular diagnostic evaluation using specific gene probes.

Unstable tandem trinucleotide repeat sequences underlie several major diseases

Molecular genetic analysis of several dominant heritable diseases has revealed a common factor in the underlying genetic abnormality.

Myotonic dystrophy, Huntington's disease, X-linked bulbospinal neuronopathy, fragile-X syndrome, and several spinocerebellar ataxias have all been shown to have expansion of tandem repeats of three nucleotides. In the Huntington's disease gene on chromosome 4, there are as many as 100 trinucleotides, whereas in normal subjects these areas are 9–34 trinucleotides long. In Huntington's disease and myotonic dystrophy there is an inverse correlation between the length of the repeat sequence and the age of onset of disease.

This finding provides an explanation for the clinical phenomenon of 'anticipation', whereby a dominantly inherited disease becomes more severe with each generation. As the repeat enlarges, the disease worsens clinically and has an earlier onset. Recent findings have also suggested that apparently unaffected parents may have repeats at the upper limit of normal, suggesting that the mutational event is amplification of the gene.

Fragile-X syndrome, the most common cause of mental retardation (1 in 2000 births), is also due to an expanded trinucleotide repeat at the fragile site on the X chromosome. This abnormality can be demonstrated in karyotype analysis as a discontinuity of staining at the end of the long arm of the X chromosome.

Autosomal recessive disorders produce clinical disease in homozygotes

In autosomal recessive inheritance, the disease is manifest only by homozygotes who have received one abnormal gene from each unaffected parent, the parents being heterozygotes for the abnormal gene. A typical pedigree is shown in *Fig. 5.21*. The incidence of the autosomal recessive disease state will depend on the number of heterozygotes in

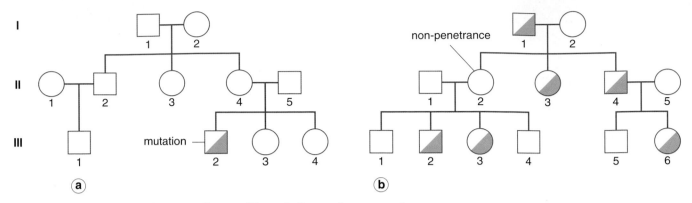

Fig. 5.20 Autosomal dominant pedigree with mutation and non-penetrance.

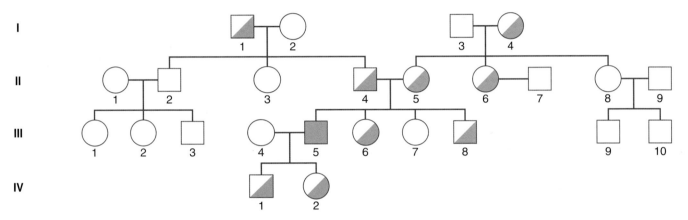

Fig. 5.21 Typical pedigree in autosomal recessive inheritance (see *Fig. 5.22* for Punnett squares).

the general population, i.e. the gene frequency. If the abnormal gene is rare in the general population, the chances of a mating between two non-affected heterozygotes are low. If the gene is common, the chances are accordingly greater, and the disease incidence will be high. Thus, mating between close relatives will increase the incidence of disease. Some autosomal recessive genes have a high frequency in certain races, e.g. the gene frequency for cystic fibrosis is high in Caucasians (approximately 1 in 25 are heterozygotes), and the gene for sickle-cell disease (*Fig. 5.23*) is common in Afro-Caribbeans (approximately 1 in 12).

Note that, with small average family sizes in western society, the incidence of most clinically apparent autosomal recessive diseases is low; it is therefore tempting to consider each new case as a new spontaneous mutation, since any heterozygote carriers are usually asymptomatic (see *Fig. 5.22*). However, for genetic counselling purposes, it is vital to try to identify all related non-affected heterozygotes. Fortunately, in many of the diseases it is possible to identify heterozygotes. For example, where the homozygous state is associated with complete absence of a particular enzyme, the heterozygotes have a reduced level of the enzyme, lying somewhere between normal levels and complete absence. Similarly, heterozygotes for the

hemoglobinopathies have a mixture of normal and abnormal hemoglobins.

The identification of specific gene abnormalities for several of these conditions now allows molecular diagnostic evaluation using specific gene probes. This has opened the way both for population screening for carrier states in heterozygotes, and for confident genetic counseling in cases of prenatal diagnosis.

Cystic fibrosis is a very common autosomal recessive disorder with a frequency of 0.5–0.6 per 1000 live births.

Disease is caused by mutations in the gene coding for a chloride transporter called the cystic fibrosis transmembrane conductance regulator (CFTR). A genetic test is available to detect individuals who carry a mutant gene (heterozygotes) and there is debate on the ethical and cost–benefit issues related to implementing any screening program.

It has been advised that genetic testing for CF should be offered to adults with a positive family history of CF, to partners of people with CF, to couples currently planning a pregnancy, and to couples seeking prenatal care. It is presently not advocated that CF genetic testing be offered to the general population or newborns. The ability to detect carriers of genetic traits raises issues of potential discrimination and stigmatization.

	B	b
B	**BB** (homozygote affected)	**Bb** (heterozygote carrier)
b	**Bb** (heterozygote carrier)	**bb** (homozygote normal)

e.g. **II**, 4 and 5

	B	b
b	**Bb** (heterozygote carrier)	**bb** (homozygote normal)
b	**Bb** (heterozygote carrier)	**bb** (homozygote normal)

e.g. **I**, 1 and 2; **I**, 3 and 4

	B	B
b	**Bb**	**Bb**
b	**Bb**	**Bb**

(all heterozygote carriers)

e.g. **III**, 4 and 5

	B	B
B	**BB** (homozygote affected)	**BB** (homozygote affected)
b	**Bb** (heterozygote carrier)	**Bb** (heterozygote carrier)

Not shown in *Fig. 5.21*.

Fig. 5.22 Punnett squares for autosomal recessive inheritance (see also *Fig. 5.21*).

Fig. 5.23
Common and important autosomal recessive diseases

Cystic fibrosis	Abnormal ion-transport protein	see page 221
Sickle-cell anemia	Abnormal hemoglobin	see page 321
Thalassemias	Abnormal hemoglobin	see page 320
Glycogenoses	Enzyme deficiency	see Chapter 25
Mucopolysaccharidoses	Enzyme deficiency	
Lipidoses	Enzyme deficiency	
Phenylketonuria	Enzyme deficiency	
Albinism	Enzyme deficiency	
Wilson's disease	Copper accumulation	see page 292

KEY FACTS
Autosomal recessive inheritance

From the typical pedigree shown in *Fig. 5.21*, it can be seen that autosomal recessive diseases show the following characteristics:

- Affected individuals are homozygotes (see **III**, 5).
- Inheritance of clinical disease is from two unaffected heterozygous parents (see **II**, 4 and 5).
- Both males and females are affected.
- There is a 25% chance of two unaffected heterozygous ('carrier') parents producing an affected homozygous child (see **III**, 5).
- There is a 50% chance of two unaffected heterozygous parents producing an unaffected heterozygous child (carrier) (see **III**, 6 and 8).
- There is a 25% chance of two unaffected heterozygous (carrier) parents producing an unaffected non-carrier child with normal genes (see **III**, 7).
- All offspring of an affected homozygote and a normal non-affected homozygous individual will be unaffected heterozygous (carrier) children (see **IV**, 1 and 2).
- The disease is not manifest in every generation. In the pedigree shown, the disease is manifest only in generation **III**, although there are non-affected (carrier) heterozygotes in generations **I**, **II**, **III** and **IV**.

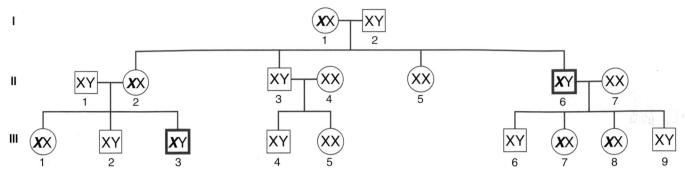

Fig. 5.24 Typical pedigree for X-linked recessive inheritance.

	X	Y
X	**X**X (carrier female)	**X**Y (affected male)
X	XX (normal female)	XY (normal male)

	X	Y
X	**X**X (carrier female)	XY (normal male)
X	**X**X (carrier female)	XY (normal male)

*	**X**	Y
X	**XX** (affected homo- zygous female)	**X**Y (affected male)
X	**X**X (carrier female)	XY (normal male)

Fig. 5.25 Inheritance possibilities in X-linked recessive inheritance (Punnett squares).

Sex-linked disorders are almost entirely due to abnormalities of the X chromosome

Most diseases associated with abnormal genes on the sex chromosomes are due to mutant genes on the X chromosome and show recessive inheritance (X-linked or sex-linked recessive, *Fig. 5.26*).

In the female, the abnormal gene on one X chromosome is balanced by the possession of a normal allele on the other X chromosome, so the abnormal gene is not manifest. The

KEY FACTS
X-linked recessive inheritance

From the pedigree shown in *Fig. 5.24* it can be seen that X-linked recessive disorders show the following characteristics:

- The abnormal gene is on an X chromosome (**X**).
- The disease affects males (**II**, 6 and **III**, 3).
- The disease is transmitted by heterozygous females who are unaffected (**I**, 1 and **II**, 2).
- Unaffected males do not carry or transmit the gene (e.g. **II**, 3).
- Each male offspring of a heterozygous female carrier has a 50% chance of being affected (e.g. **II**, 3 and **II**, 6; **III**, 2 and **III**, 3).
- Both affected males and unaffected heterozygous females can transmit to produce unaffected heterozygous female carriers (e.g. **III**, 1, **III**, 7 and **III**, 8).

female manifests no features of the disease, but is a carrier. In the male, the abnormal gene on the sole X chromosome is not balanced, for there is no normal allele on the Y chromosome; the abnormal gene is therefore expressed, and males carrying the abnormal gene will display the disease.

Fig. 5.24 shows a typical pedigree for an X-linked recessive disorder. The mating combination shown in the third example in *Fig. 5.25* is extremely unlikely in most X-linked recessive disorders, but may occur where the gene frequency of the abnormal X-linked gene is fairly high. For example, in some Afro-Caribbean communities the X-linked gene that produces one type of glucose-6-phosphate dehydrogenase deficiency is fairly common (about 1 in 10 male homozygotes), and there is a relatively high percentage of heterozygous females. In these circumstances it is not rare to find a homozygous (XX) female with clinical manifestations of the enzyme defect (see third Punnett pattern in *Fig. 5.25* (*)).

Fig. 5.26
Common and important X-linked recessive diseases

Hemophilia A	Bleeding tendency due to clotting factor VIII deficiency
Hemophilia B	Bleeding tendency due to clotting factor X deficiency
G-6-PD deficiency	Attacks of hemolytic anemia after certain drugs
Duchenne muscular dystrophy	Progressive muscle weakness due to dystrophin deficiency — see page 469
Becker muscular dystrophy	Relative dystrophin deficiency — see page 469
X-linked (Bruton) agammaglobulinemia	Decreased gamma globulins due to B-cell maturation failure — see page 105
X-linked ichthyosis	Permanently thick, scaly skin due to steroid sulphatase deficiency

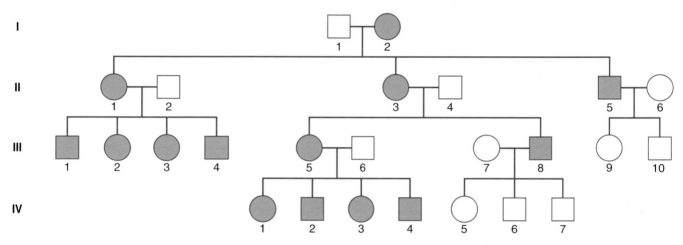

Fig. 5.27 Typical pedigree of mitochondrial inheritance.

X-linked dominant inheritance diseases are very rare

One example of an X-linked dominant inheritance disease is hypophosphatemic osteomalacia (vitamin D-resistant rickets), in which failure of proper mineralization of bone results from excessive phosphate loss in the urine and low blood phosphate levels. The abnormal dominant gene is on the X chromosome, and is expressed in both males (XY) and females (XX) who have received an abnormal X chromosome from an affected heterozygous mother (XX). Affected fathers (XY) transmit the gene only to their daughters.

Several mitochondrial proteins are encoded by mitochondrial DNA rather than by genes in the nucleus

Although most genetic material is located in the cell nucleus, DNA is also found in mitochondria. This type of DNA is transmitted to offspring by maternal inheritance to both male and female, and thus defects can be passed on to the offspring (**mitochondrial inheritance**). A typical pedigree is shown in *Fig. 5.27*.

KEY FACTS
Mitochondrial inheritance

See *Fig. 5.27*.

- Inheritance is only through maternal lines, as mitochondria in the embryo are derived from the ovum.
- All children of an affected mother receive a dose of abnormal mitochondria in the ovum (e.g. **II**, 1, 3 and 5; **III**, 1–5 and 8; **IV**, 1–4).
- If an affected male has children, his progeny are unaffected (e.g. **II**, 5, **III**, 8).
- The severity of disease may vary, as the dose of abnormal mitochondria may vary in different tissues. A mixture of genetically normal and abnormal mitochondria in tissues is termed **heteroplasmy.**

Although both males and females are affected, only affected females can transmit to offspring. The most important group of diseases inherited in this way are the mitochondrial cytopathies, which commonly manifest as progressive disease involving skeletal and cardiac muscle or brain in adult life. Associated with deficiencies in a number of mitochondrial respiratory enzymes, they are characterized by the presence of large abnormal mitochondria, often containing large inclusions, beneath the sarcolemma.

There are many disorders in which genetic factors play only a partial role

The terms **polygenic** and **multifactorial** are often used synonymously when describing inheritance. However:

- Polygenic diseases result from the interaction of a number of scattered genes, each of which has a slight effect on the phenotype. The final clinical picture is a summation of each of the individual gene effects.
- Multifactorial diseases result from a combination of genetic (often polygenic) and environmental factors. Genetic make-up is believed to produce predisposition to a disease, environmental factors acting as the trigger.

Many diseases observed to have a high incidence within families but with no evidence of a recognizable inheritance pattern (**familial tendency**) are diseases with polygenic or multifactorial inheritance. Such diseases are common, and include congenital malformations present at birth (e.g. hare lip, cleft palate, *Fig. 5.28*), some congenital heart malformations, and diseases which manifest themselves in childhood, adolescence and adult life (e.g. psoriasis, see page 489), diabetes mellitus (see page 540), hypertension (see page 166), atopic diseases, schizophrenia, manic depressive psychosis, rheumatoid arthritis (see page 524), gout (see page 526). In most cases the nature and location of the abnormal genes are not known.

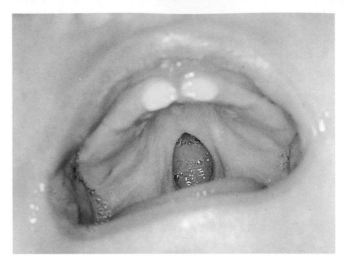

Fig. 5.28 Cleft palate.

MOLECULAR GENETICS AND DISEASE

Molecular biology techniques have made investigative genetics possible

Modern molecular genetics, using DNA isolation, fragmentation with restriction enzymes, and probes to specific genes, have a wide application to clinical medicine. If the gene for a disease is known, abnormalities in gene structure can be determined in individuals and the presence of a mutation established. In cases of familial disease in which the genetic abnormality is not known, linkage analysis of the disease to specific chromosome regions is possible, with ultimate isolation of the gene responsible.

The ultimate aim of molecular genetic approaches to disease is to develop techniques of gene therapy to repair or complement the defective gene, thereby preventing disease.

Molecular genetic investigation techniques

Restriction analysis and Southern blotting

DNA, usually taken from white blood cells, is digested with a restriction endonuclease. The resulting fragments are separated on an agarose gel by electrophoresis, the smaller fragments migrating furthest down the gel. The fragments are transferred to a nylon membrane after denaturing in alkali by capillary blotting (Southern blotting). A gene probe to a known gene sequence is applied to the nylon membrane, and the resulting pattern of hybridization compared to normals.

Two main methods are used to analyze DNA in the search for an abnormal gene.

1 A change in a gene may introduce or remove a restriction site, thereby changing the size of DNA fragments hybridizing to a specific probe.

Such analysis can be performed only for genetic abnormalities for which the base change causing a mutation that alters a restriction site for a particular restriction enzyme is known. This technique is used to look for the mutation in the β-globin gene causing sickle-cell disease. This mutation removes a site for the restriction enzyme, MstII. Instead of being cut into three small fragments, as in the normal gene, the β-globin gene is cut into only two pieces. Probing the ▶

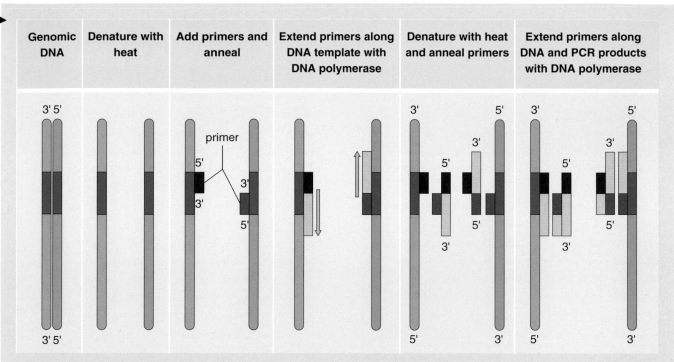

| Genomic DNA | Denature with heat | Add primers and anneal | Extend primers along DNA template with DNA polymerase | Denature with heat and anneal primers | Extend primers along DNA and PCR products with DNA polymerase |

Fig. 5.29 Polymerase chain reaction.

resulting digested DNA with a cDNA probe to the β-globin gene shows that, compared to normals, loss of the cutting site leads to an abnormal, large fragment of DNA hybridizing to the probe.

2 A synthetic DNA probe, typically 15–20 base pairs in length (oligonucleotides), can be made to complement the normal gene, with a second probe to complement the point mutation gene.

Under stringent conditions, the point mutation is sufficient to impair hybridization with the normal probe, allowing hybridization with the probe to the mutant gene. Unfortunately, such techniques are technically difficult and the exact mutation must be known. In practice, it is common for a genetic abnormality to be heterogeneous in terms of mutation, which severely limits the usefulness of the technique.

The polymerase chain reaction

The polymerase chain reaction (*Fig. 5.29*), which is used to amplify the gene sequence in which a mutation is being sought, is a more rapid technique than Southern blotting.

The sequence of the normal gene must be known so that primers that bind at one end of the gene can be made. DNA polymerase is used to extend the primer along the normal DNA template. Unlike analysis with a specific oligonucleotide probe, where the specific mutation being sought must be known, with the PCR technique the gene

sequence between the primers will be amplified irrespective of the mutation involved. Repeated cycles of amplification produce millions of copies of the gene region between the primers.

If a restriction site is affected by the mutation, the PCR products can be digested and probed as for whole-cell DNA, above. Alternatively, the PCR fragments, representing huge numbers of copies of the original cellular gene, can be sequenced and compared with the known normal gene sequence. In comparison with the technical problems involved in sequencing native DNA, those involved in sequencing the PCR products are not arduous.

Linkage analysis

When a disease is known to be familial but the gene product and pathogenesis of the disease are unknown, linkage analysis can be used to find which part of a specific chromosome is associated with disease. Once identified, the chromosomal region of interest can be cloned from affected individuals and sequenced to find the specific gene responsible.

This approach has been spectacularly successful in finding the genes for disorders such as cystic fibrosis, adult polycystic kidney disease, Duchenne's muscular dystrophy, neurofibromatosis, familial Alzheimer's disease, Huntington's disease, myotonic dystrophy, and familial motor-neuron disease. Once the gene is identified, its

▶ protein product can be predicted and identified. This technique of going from disease to chromosome to gene to protein has been termed 'reverse genetics' as, previously, it was usual to look for genes only after a protein product was known and characterized.

Linkage analysis depends on knowing which chromosome has been inherited in affected and non-affected individuals in a family. The identification of large pedigrees by classic genetics is a vital start point in such a study.

Between 1 in 250 and 1 in 500 bases in the human genome is polymorphic, i.e. alternative versions are present in the normal population. These variations are mostly in non-coding regions, but serve to create or remove restriction sites for one of the many specific restriction enzymes that cut DNA into fragments depending on specific bases on each side of the cut site. Fragments of DNA generated from different individuals by a restriction enzyme therefore differ in size, and this is the basis of detecting restriction fragment length polymorphisms (RFLPs).

Probes that detect RFLPs spaced over all of the chromosomes have been derived from DNA sequence libraries screened by Southern blotting. These are applied to restriction DNA fragments from the pedigree under investigation, and segregation of the disease, together with segregation of an RFLP, is sought. Once linkage with a particular probe is found, further study in pedigrees can show how tightly the probe is linked with the disease. Once an area of a chromosome has been located, other markers that are closer to the gene can be isolated and used, until it becomes feasible to clone the chromosome region involved and laboriously to sequence the region until the actual gene is found. Such studies are not easy. Even tightly linked markers are frequently more than a million bases away from the actual gene.

Neoplasia

INTRODUCTION

A key characteristic of the adaptive responses of cells, as discussed in Chapter 2, is that if the stimulus is removed, any alteration in cell growth reverts to normal. In contrast to these reversible adaptive responses, certain stimuli cause changes in genetic material that result in permanent alteration of the normal cellular growth pattern. Such altered cells, which are termed neoplastic, fail to respond normally to signals controlling cell growth. They proliferate excessively in a poorly regulated manner, forming a lump or tissue mass called a neoplasm (literally, new growth).

This chapter considers the nature of neoplasia, the clinical study of which is termed oncology, and the classification and diagnosis of tumors. Causes of neoplasia are discussed, and the basic science relating to properties of neoplastic cells reviewed.

CHARACTERISTICS AND TERMINOLOGY OF NEOPLASTIC DISEASES

Terms used to describe neoplastic diseases

By convention, a neoplastic mass of cells is known as a tumor. The Latin derivation was originally used to refer to any tissue swelling, although this literal use has largely gone out of fashion. The term **cancer** is frequently in lay use and is equated with any malignant neoplasm. The name is derived from the Latin word for a crab, as such tumors were perceived to seize upon adjacent tissues with pincer-like outgrowths. Study of different tumors reveals that cancers originating from different tissues display varying degrees of aggressiveness: some are slow-growing and indolent, others spread rapidly to many parts of the body and rapidly cause death. The generic term cancer is, therefore, not always suitable for professional use, as it conveys no information about the likely biological behaviour of a tumor.

A neoplasm is composed of cells that grow in a poorly regulated manner

In a neoplastic state, cellular proliferation and growth occur in the absence of any continuing external stimulus. The term neoplasia therefore describes a state of poorly regulated cell growth, in which the neoplastic cells are said to be transformed. In neoplastic cells and tissues, there is a failure of the normal mechanisms that control cellular proliferation and maturation. The molecular nature of these events is part of the study of carcinogenesis, reviewed towards the end of this chapter.

Each neoplastic cell has an alteration in its genome, responsible for abnormal growth

The state of neoplasia arises out of changes in genetic material, which are then transmitted to each new generation of cells within the neoplasm. Neoplastic growth contrasts with hyperplasia (discussed in Chapter 3) in that although there is abnormal proliferation of cells in the latter, this ceases with removal of the causative stimulus. Recent molecular genetic study has shown that alteration in key genes controlling growth of cells underlies the majority of tumors (*Fig. 6.1*). Such genes are termed oncogenes, and examples are discussed in the later section on carcinogenesis (see page 94).

There are two main types of neoplasm: benign and malignant

Early in the study of tumors, clinical observation identified two main patterns of neoplastic growth:

- If the margins of the tumor were well defined and the tumor grew only locally, the neoplasm was termed benign.
- If the margins of the tumor were poorly defined and the neoplastic cells were growing into and destroying the surrounding tissues, the neoplasm was termed malignant.

Benign tumors generally have a very good prognosis and lead only rarely to death. In contrast, malignant tumors are a major cause of mortality.

FAILURE TO ACHIEVE CELLULAR DIFFERENTIATION IS A PARTICULAR FEATURE OF MALIGNANT NEOPLASMS

Following cell division from a precursor or stem cell, normal cells assume a specific function, which involves development of specialized structures such as mucin vacuoles, microvilli or cilia, known as differentiation. Whereas stem cells can be said to be relatively undifferentiated, the fully

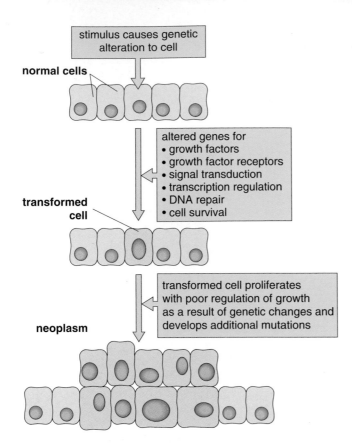

Fig. 6.1 Events in neoplastic transformation.
Normal cells develop abnormalities in key genes regulating growth and are transformed into neoplastic cells.

mature cell of any particular cell line is said to be highly differentiated. In association with loss of regulation of cell growth, neoplastic cells commonly fail to achieve a highly differentiated state. Histological features associated with this are shown in *Fig. 6.2*.

In general the cells of benign neoplasms are differentiated to a degree which fairly closely corresponds to that of the cells from which they were derived (*Fig. 6.2b*). This differentiation frequently extends to the retention of the functional attributes of the tissue of origin. For example, benign tumors of endocrine tissues frequently secrete hormones and may have endocrinological effects.

In the case of malignant neoplasms, variable degrees of differentiation may be seen.

- When the constituent cells closely resemble the tissue of origin the tumor is termed a well differentiated malignant neoplasm (*Fig. 6.2c*).
- When tumor cells show only a passing resemblance to the tissue of origin the neoplasm is termed a poorly differentiated malignant neoplasm (*Fig. 6.2d*).
- When, because of failure of differentiation, it is not possible to identify the cell of origin on morphological observation, the growth is termed an anaplastic malignant neoplasm (*Fig. 6.2e*).

The degree of differentiation of a neoplasm is generally related to its behaviour. A poorly differentiated neoplasm tends to be more aggressive than a well differentiated neoplasm.

Along with failure of differentiation in neoplasia, cells are said to show atypical cytology. The associated features are:

- Increased variation in the shape and size of cells (cellular pleomorphism).
- Increased variation in the shape and size of nuclei (nuclear pleomorphism).
- Increase in the density of staining of nuclei (nuclear hyperchromatism).
- Disproportionately large increase in the size of nuclei, relative to the size of the cell cytoplasm (increased nuclear:cytoplasmic ratio).

Fig. 6.2e shows how the cytological features of neoplasia become more marked with loss of differentiation.

Benign tumors grow locally, are generally slow growing, and compress adjacent tissues

Benign tumors, the cells of which closely resemble the tissue of origin, generally do not have highly abnormal dysregulation of growth. Such tumors grow locally, and generally have a very slow pace of growth. Two main factors influence the effects of such tumors:

- As a benign tumor grows, it causes compression of adjacent tissues. This may have adverse effects if the resulting mass causes blockage of a lumen, e.g. gut or airway.
- If a benign tumor has an endocrine function, it may cause disease due to uncontrolled secretion of hormone.

An example of a benign tumor of the thyroid gland is illustrated in *Fig. 6.3*.

Malignant tumors grow into adjacent tissues and can spread to other parts of the body

The most significant property of malignant neoplasms is that growth is not confined to the site of origin of the tumor, i.e. the primary tumor. Control of cell growth becomes so abnormal that cells can grow into adjacent local tissues, in a process termed invasion (*Fig. 6.4*). As neoplastic cells invade they usually do so at the expense of the local tissues, causing damage and destruction.

The most sinister property of malignant neoplasms is that cells from the primary tumor can become detached, move to a different part of the body, and grow as a separate mass of tumor. This process is known as metastasis, and the resulting detached masses of cells are termed metastases or secondary tumors. As with the malignant primary tumor, metastases grow at the expense of local tissues and usually result in tissue destruction.

The ways in which benign and malignant tumors differ are shown in *Fig. 6.5*.

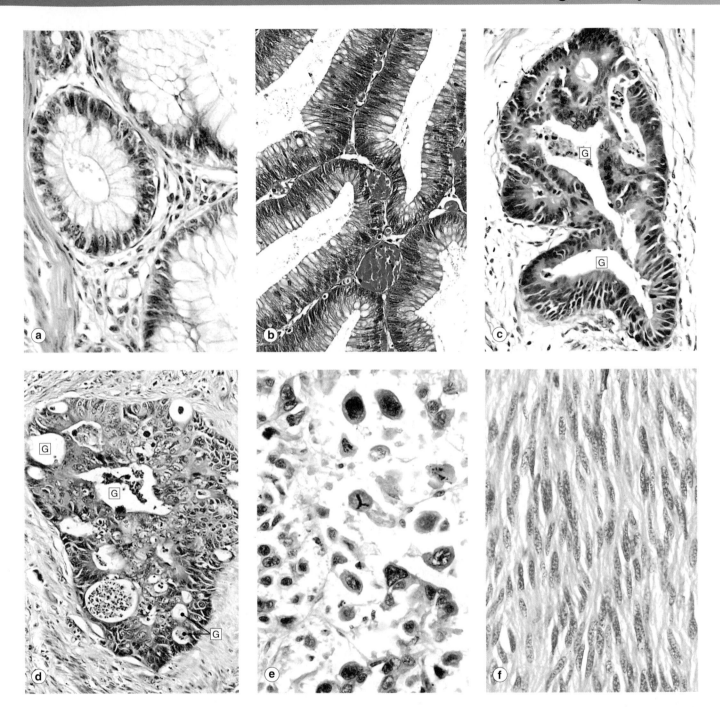

Fig. 6.2 Histological features of loss of differentiation. (a) Normal colonic epithelium. (b) Benign neoplasm of colon. (c) Well differentiated malignant neoplasm of colon. (d) Poorly differentiated malignant neoplasm of colon. (e) Anaplastic malignant neoplasm of colon. (f) Benign neoplasm of smooth muscle.

The cells of a benign neoplasm (b) resemble those of the normal epithelium (a), in that they are columnar and have an orderly arrangement. Loss of some degree of differentiation is evident in that the neoplastic cells do not show mucin vacuolation. The cells of the benign neoplasm of smooth muscle (f) closely resemble normal muscle cells. Cells of the well differentiated malignant neoplasm (c) have a haphazard arrangement and, although gland lumina (**G**) are formed, they are architecturally abnormal and irregular. Nuclei vary in shape and size. Cells in the poorly differentiated malignant neoplasm (d) have an even more haphazard arrangement, with very poor formation of gland lumina (**G**). Nuclei show greater variation in shape and size compared to (c).

Cells in anaplastic malignant neoplasm (e) bear no relation to the normal, with no attempt at gland formation. There is tremendous variation in the size of cells and of nuclei, with very intense staining (nuclear hyperchromatism) of the latter. Without knowing the site of origin it would be impossible to tell what sort of tumor this was by histology. Well differentiated tumors of support cells resemble their cell of origin, as shown in this example of a benign tumor of smooth muscle (f). In a poorly differentiated malignant neoplasm of smooth muscle, cells show marked variation in size and shape of nuclei, with hyperchromatism and numerous mitoses. A smooth muscle origin can then be established only by the use of electron microscopy or immunohistochemistry.

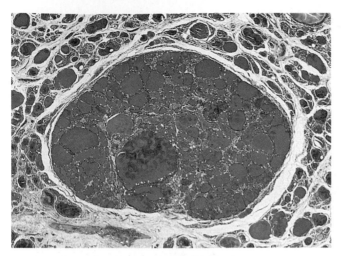

Fig. 6.3 Benign neoplasm of thyroid gland.
This low-power micrograph shows the features of a benign epithelial neoplasm. The tumor is very well circumscribed, and although it compresses adjacent tissue, it does not grow into it.

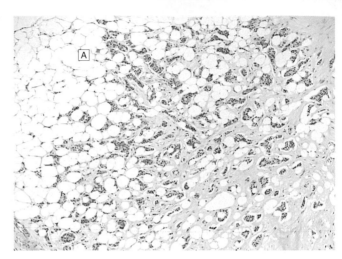

Fig. 6.4 Edge of malignant tumor of breast showing invasion. Islands of neoplastic cells can be seen extending into adjacent adipose tissue (**A**) by invasion. The edge of the tumor is therefore not well circumscribed, in contrast to a benign lesion.

Fig. 6.5
Histological features of neoplasms

	Benign	Malignant
Behavior	Expansile growth only; grows locally	Expansile and invasive growth; may metastasize
Histology	Resembles cell of origin (well differentiated)	Shows failure of cellular differentiation
	Few mitoses	Many mitoses, some of which are abnormal forms
	Normal or slight increase in ratio of nucleus:cytoplasm	High nuclear:cytoplasmic ratio
	Cells are uniform throughout the tumor	Cells vary in shape and size (cellular pleomorphism) and/or nuclei vary in shape and size (nuclear pleomorphism)

A neoplasm must develop stromal support components if it is to grow

If neoplastic cells are to grow, they must obtain adequate nutrients by developing an appropriate set of support tissues, particularly an adequate vascular supply. Just as normal cells interact with support tissues and induce stroma formation, neoplastic cells also retain this ability. Tumors develop a vascular stroma by secretion of **angiogenesis factors**. The ability of a tumor to induce and maintain a vascular supply is a key factor in its growth (see pink box, right). A tumor mass therefore contains the genetically abnormal neoplastic cells and a component of normal support tissues.

In well differentiated lesions, induction of stroma is usually well developed and the neoplastic cells grow without problems. In less well differentiated neoplasms, induction of stroma may be poor and outstripped by proliferation of neoplastic cells. This may limit the speed of growth of a tumor and frequently leads to death of cells in the centre of a tumor mass. Certain tumors induce a stromal response that is disproportionate to the number of tumor cells. Such tumors are often termed desmoplastic.

The growth rate of a neoplasm is determined by several factors

Different tumors grow at different rates. In general terms, benign tumors and well differentiated malignant tumors grow more slowly than poorly differentiated lesions, although there are many exceptions.

The rate of growth of a tumor depends on many factors:

- The proportion of cells which are in the cell cycle as opposed to cells which have differentiated and entered the G0 (non-proliferating) part of the cell cycle.

Tumor angiogenesis is controlled by positive and negative regulatory factors

If tumor cells fail to recruit an adequate blood supply then they will not grow. Additionally, a vascular network is required by tumors for spread by metastasis: studies have shown a good correlation between the density of vessels in certain tumors and the probability of spread by metastasis.

The two most important angiogenesis factors secreted by cells, including tumor cells are:

- Vascular endothelial growth factor (VEGF): secreted by many cell types and acts on receptors expressed on endothelial cells to induce endothelial cell growth, migration, and vessel formation (see *Fig. 6.6*).
- Basic fibroblast growth factor (bFGF): inducing endothelial cell growth and migration.

Angiogenesis is also modulated by proteins termed angiopoietins which interact with endothelial cell receptors:

- Ang1 promotes stabilization and growth of vessels from capillary types to larger types by recruiting peri-endothelial cells.
- Ang2 promotes remodeling and maturation of developing vascular networks.

Anti-angiogenesis factors are normally produced by cells to prevent angiogenesis and include:

- Thrombospondin (platelet factor 4).
- Angiostatin: cleavage product of plasminogen.
- Endostatin: cleavage product of collagen type XVIII.
- Vasostatin: cleavage product of calreticulin.

A key molecular event in some tumors may be failure of production of anti-angiogenic factors. Therapeutic trials are presently underway to see if endostatin can inhibit tumor growth, already suggested in some experimental tumors in mice. The drug thalidomide has anti-angiogenic effects and this is being used in clinical trials for some tumors.

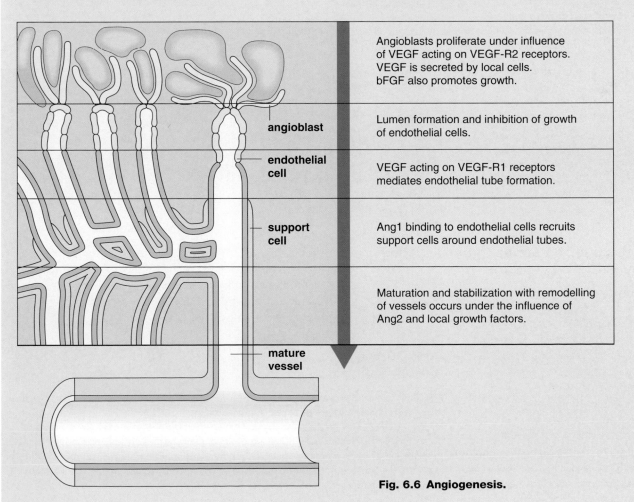

angioblast	Angioblasts proliferate under influence of VEGF acting on VEGF-R2 receptors. VEGF is secreted by local cells. bFGF also promotes growth.
endothelial cell	Lumen formation and inhibition of growth of endothelial cells.
	VEGF acting on VEGF-R1 receptors mediates endothelial tube formation.
support cell	Ang1 binding to endothelial cells recruits support cells around endothelial tubes.
	Maturation and stabilization with remodelling of vessels occurs under the influence of Ang2 and local growth factors.
mature vessel	

Fig. 6.6 Angiogenesis.

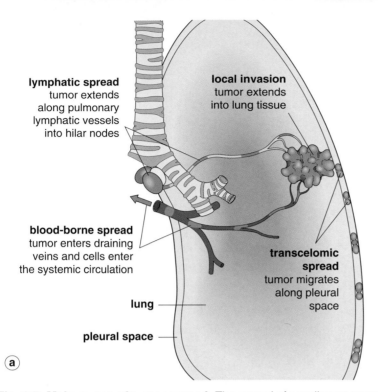

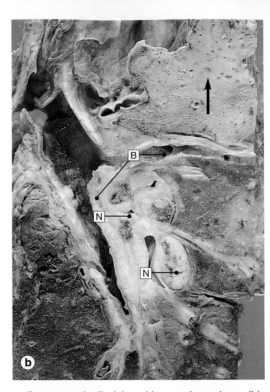

Fig. 6.7 Main routes of tumor spread. The spread of a malignant tumor is shown diagrammatically (a) and in a real specimen (b) for a carcinoma of the lung. The four main routes, i.e. local, lymphatic, blood-borne and transcelomic, are shown. In (b) the malignant neoplasm originated in a bronchus (**B**) and spread locally into adjacent lung (arrow). Tumor has also spread via lymphatics and is evident as white deposits in hilar lymph nodes (**N**), which also contain carbon pigment.

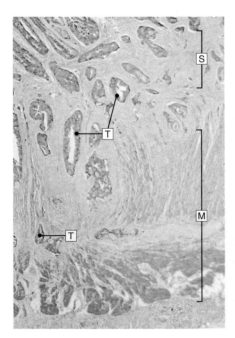

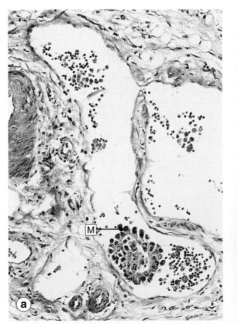

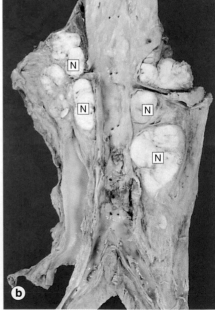

Fig. 6.8 Local invasion in malignant neoplasm of colon. This low-power micrograph shows purple-stained malignant tumor (**T**) extending through submucosa (**S**) and muscle (**M**) of the colon wall by local invasion. Via this route, neoplastic cells may invade adjacent organs such as the bladder.

Fig. 6.9 Lymphatic invasion by tumor. (a) Histology of invasion of lymphatic vessel. (b) Tumor in para-aortic lymph nodes.
Micrograph (a) shows malignant cells (**M**) in a small lymphatic vessel. Cells break off from the primary tumor, enter small lymphatics, and are carried to lymph nodes, where they frequently grow as metastases. The macroscopic appearance of tumor in nodes is shown in (b); the nodes (**N**) are enlarged and replaced by tumor which, in this instance, originated from the testis.

- The death rate of cells in the tumor. Tumor cells are particularly prone to programed cell death by the process of apoptosis (see *Fig. 2.21*). Tumors which develop genetic changes that allow them to escape from growth control by apoptosis tend to become rapidly growing.
- The adequacy of supply of nutrients to the tumor, derived from induction of a stroma by the neoplastic cells.

If cell proliferation greatly exceeds cell death in the tumor, it will grow in size rapidly.

Malignant neoplasms spread to other sites by four main routes

Spread of a malignant tumor from its primary site (metastasis) is by four main routes (*Fig. 6.7*):

- **Local invasion**. The most common pattern of spread of malignant tumors is by direct growth into adjacent tissues (*Fig. 6.8*). Tumors may also spread along natural tissue planes, e.g. along nerves.
- **Lymphatic spread**. Tumor cells frequently spread via draining lymphatic vessels and are conducted to local lymph nodes, where they grow as secondary tumors (*Fig. 6.9*).
- **Vascular spread**. Tumor cells can spread via the veins draining the primary lesion. Gastrointestinal tumors are frequently conducted via the portal vein giving rise to metastases in the liver. Tumor cells that enter systemic veins most frequently form metastases in the lung, bone marrow, brain and adrenal glands (*Fig. 6.10*).
- **Transcoelomic spread**. Primary tumors in the abdominal cavity or the thorax can spread directly across coelomic spaces, e.g. the peritoneal or pleural cavities, by seeding cells which then migrate to the surface of other organs.

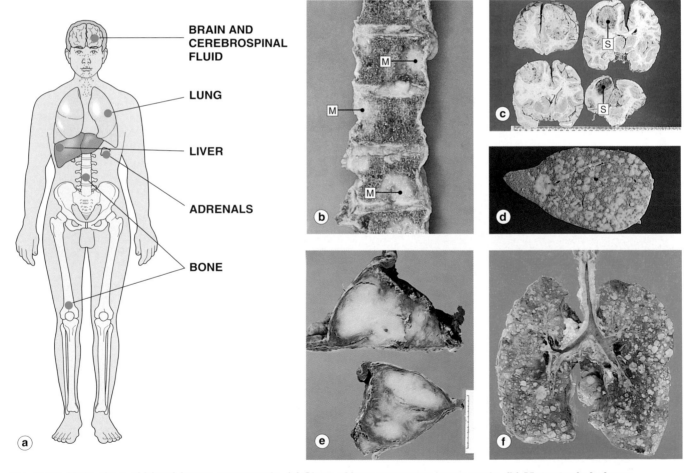

Fig. 6.10 Main sites of blood-borne metastasis. (a) Sites of hematogenous metastasis. (b) Metastasis in bone. (c) Metastasis in brain. (d) Metastasis in liver. (e) Metastasis in adrenals. (f) Metastasis in lungs.
Blood-borne tumor metastasis leads to growth of secondary tumors in several main sites. The macroscopic appearances of bone metastasis are shown in (b), where lesions are seen in vertebrae (**M**). Numerous metastases from a neoplasm of the stomach (**S**) are seen in the brain in (c). The liver is the most common site for metastases from tumors in the gastrointestinal tract, as seen in (d), which arose from a colonic neoplasm. In (e) metastatic tumor has replaced both adrenal glands, as is commonly seen with spread from lung and breast tumors. The lung (f) is the most common site for blood-borne metastases from tumors outside the gastrointestinal tract, particularly mesenchymal tumors.

For invasion and metastasis to occur, neoplastic cells have to acquire special attributes

Neoplastic cells have to develop several attributes in order to metastasize, as summarized in *Fig. 6.11*. Within any primary tumor it is likely that only a proportion of cells acquire these attributes by developing additional genetic mutations as part of further abnormalities in cell growth.

To grow through basement membrane into the extracellular matrix and then enter a vessel, neoplastic cells must express surface molecules for adhesion (particularly specific integrins that bind to laminin and fibronectin). To grow into adjacent tissues or vessels, cells must also be motile and capable of migration.

The production of enzymes that degrade extracellular matrix appears to be an important factor in metastasis, one of the most studied being the matrix metalloproteinases, which degrades the Type IV collagen in basement membranes.

Whether, once in the circulation, a cell establishes a metastasis in a particular organ is probably determined by many factors. It is likely that both tumor cell and host organ tissues must express complementary cell adhesion molecules. The host organ should also have an appropriate environment including the absence of protease inhibitors and the presence of appropriate growth factors.

The specific requirements for individual tumors and target organs are, as yet, poorly understood. However, they continue to represent an important research area, as understanding why tumors metastasize opens the way for direct therapeutic intervention.

Despite the uncertainties surrounding metastatic potential of tumors, there are recognizable patterns or 'fingerprints' of metastasis, which relate to the site and histological type of tumors. For example, certain tumors frequently spread to bone (kidney, lung, thyroid, prostate, breast), whereas other types, such as melanoma, have a much greater latitude and can invade and grow in a wide range of foreign tissues.

Lysis of basement membrane takes place by secretion of proteases, as well as inhibition of protease inhibitors

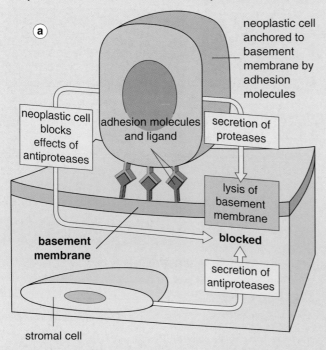

Migration of cell is stimulated by self-secreted motility factor and anchorage of cell to molecules in extracellular matrix

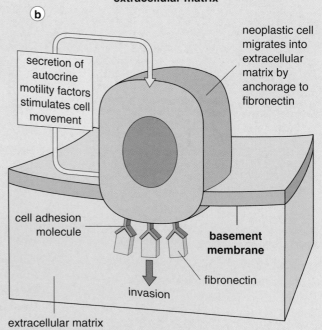

Fig. 6.11 Cellular events needed for metastasis.
Neoplastic cells have to develop special attributes of altered growth in order to metastasize. In order to escape the confines of the basement membrane (a), cells secrete proteases. As these can normally be inactivated by inhibitors secreted by stromal cells, inhibition of this process is required to allow disruption of basement membrane. Once the basement membrane is breached, cells have to acquire receptors that can anchor them to the extracellular matrix (b) and must develop motility.

Neoplasms are frequently associated with systemic effects

Patients with a neoplasm frequently have systemic symptoms, the most frequent being:

- Weight loss.
- Loss of appetite.
- Fever.
- General malaise.
- Anemia.

In many cases the cause of these constitutional symptoms is uncertain, but they are most probably due to effects of secreted cytokines such as tumor necrosis factor and IL-1. These are released from inflammatory cells present in areas of tumor.

Some tumors, benign or malignant, retain the function of their organ of origin; if this happens to be an endocrine function, the tumor may exert harmful effects by secretion of excess hormone.

Paraneoplastic syndromes are also frequently recognized in association with tumors. These are syndromes that are not the result of direct effects of the tumor or metastases. For instance, certain tumors derived from non-endocrine cells can secrete hormones (ectopic hormone secretion); lung tumors derived from squamous epithelium can secrete a parathormone-related product, resulting in hypercalcemia. Other tumors are associated with weakness of muscle (myopathy), malfunction of peripheral nerves (neuropathy), or cerebellar ataxia.

Increasingly, it is being shown that these syndromes are due to autoantibodies generated to tumor cells, which cross-react with normal tissues and cause immune-mediated damage.

Both benign and malignant neoplasms can cause death

Malignant tumors, once disseminated, often lead to the death of a patient, the main reasons being:

- Cachexia and development of poor nutrition from the effects of widespread tumor metastases. Progressive weakness and death result, often from a secondary infection such as a pneumonia. Tumor cachexia is believed to be mediated by activation of cytokines from tumor and inflammatory cells responding to the tumor.
- Obliteration of a vital organ or system by either primary or metastatic tumor.

Most benign tumors will behave in a relatively innocuous manner and, for the most part, are not life-threatening. However, although the main problems caused by the presence of a mass lesion are amenable to surgical resection, the location of a benign tumor may be important in influencing the outcome; for example, a benign tumor of the brain stem may lead to rapid death because of its critical site.

Histological assessment of neoplasms allows prediction of likely tumor behavior

Examination of the pathological features of a neoplasm provides a useful guide to its likely behavior. Two main assessments are made: analysis of the degree of differentiation and growth pattern of the tumor, and evaluation of how far a tumor has spread. In addition, special techniques may be used to obtain further prognostic information. These are listed towards the end of the chapter, where diagnosis of neoplasia is discussed.

Grading of tumors is performed by looking at cellular cytology

To allocate a grade to a tumor the following cellular features are assessed:

- The degree of differentiation of tumor cells, with reference to the tissue of origin.
- Variation in size and shape of constituent cells of the tumor. The degree of variation (**pleomorphism**) increases with failure of differentiation, and a high degree of variability is seen in malignant tumors (*Fig. 6.2d*).
- The number of cells containing mitotic figures. Known as the mitotic index, this provides a crude indication of the rate of cell proliferation. The index is generally high in more malignant tumors and low in benign tumors.

As an example, a well differentiated malignant tumor of the breast epithelium (carcinoma of the breast) would be expected to show structures that resemble small ducts or gland-like spaces while a poorly differentiated malignant tumor of the breast epithelium would not show any attempt to form a glandular pattern. Similarly, mitoses would be expected to be in small number in the well differentiated tumor but in high density in a poorly differentiated tumor (*Fig 6.12*).

Staging of a tumor offers an indication of how far it has spread

The size of a primary tumor, the degree to which it has locally invaded, and the extent to which it has spread, ultimately determine the chances of survival once a neoplasm has been diagnosed. Assessment of such factors is termed tumor staging. There are several schemes for standardized staging of individual tumors, one of the most frequently applied being the Dukes' staging for neoplasms of the rectum (page 263). The TNM system is based upon extent of local tumor spread, regional lymph node involvement and the presence of distant metastases (*Fig. 6.13*). It can

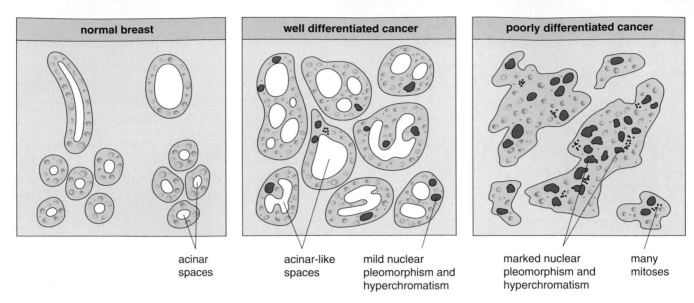

normal breast	well differentiated cancer	poorly differentiated cancer

acinar spaces — acinar-like spaces — mild nuclear pleomorphism and hyperchromatism — marked nuclear pleomorphism and hyperchromatism — many mitoses

Fig 6.12 Grading of tumors. Distinction between a well differentiated and a poorly differentiated tumor is assessed by grading. In this example the well differentiated tumor resembles its normal counterpart but shows some architectural and cytological abnormality. In a poorly differentiated tumor there is little architectural resemblence to the tissue of origin and cells show more pronounced cytological abnormalities.

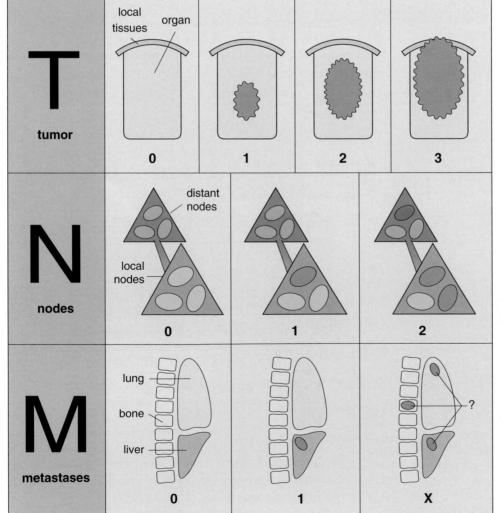

Fig. 6.13 Staging of carcinoma by TNM system.

The general principles of TNM staging are as follows:

T refers to primary tumor. The accompanying number denotes the size of tumor and its local extent. The number varies according to site.

N refers to lymph node involvement, and a high number denotes increasing extent of involvement.

M refers to the extent of distant metastases.

As an example, the TNM system for staging malignant neoplasms of the breast is:

T0 = breast free of tumor
T1 = lesion <2 cm in size
T2 = lesion 2–5 cm
T3 = skin and/or chest wall involved by invasion

N0 = no axillary nodes involved
N1 = mobile nodes involved
N2 = fixed nodes involved

M0 = no metastases
M1 = demonstrable metastases
MX = suspected metastases

be applied to many different types of tumor, although the criteria are different for each tumor site.

The stage of a tumor is generally the most important indicator of likely prognosis and of appropriate therapy; tumors at an advanced stage (extensive spread) may require aggressive treatment, while early stage tumors (localized) may be treatable by relatively conservative measures.

In situ neoplasia is a stage of neoplasia prior to development of invasion

Although an epithelial neoplasm may show the cytological features of malignancy, i.e. cellular pleomorphism and increased mitotic activity, it may not be invasive on histological examination. This phenomenon, termed carcinoma *in situ*, represents a very early stage of neoplasia. In molecular terms it is probable that the genetic abnormalities allowing metastasis (*Fig. 6.11*) have not yet developed.

Neoplasms of this type are most commonly encountered in epithelial tissues, for example, squamous epithelium of the cervix (see page 401), skin, and breast, where cytologically malignant cells may be confined within ducts (intraduct carcinoma) or within lobules (intralobular carcinoma, see pages 425 and 426).

The diagnosis of tumors at the stage of *in situ* neoplasia is clearly important as, if left, such lesions would progress to become invasive, whereas early detection and treatment at this pre-invasive stage is often completely curative.

Dysplasia is a histological term applied to cells that have some of the cytological features of neoplasia

The term dysplasia is used to describe the histological appearance of cells that show an increased rate of cell division, coupled with incomplete maturation. Like neoplastic cells, dysplastic cells tend to exhibit a high nuclear to cytoplasmic ratio and there is an increased number of mitoses. Dysplastic tissues may also show loss of the normal architectural relationships between cells.

Dysplasia most frequently arises in epithelial tissues that have been subject to chronic irritation. In these instances there is usually evidence of an associated inflammatory response. However, dysplasia can occur in the absence of obvious tissue damage or repair, and in such cases the cytological features of the dysplastic tissue may merge with those described in early neoplasia. It is important to identify dysplasia as, in some circumstances, true neoplastic change follows after a period of time, and can develop over many years. A sequence from dysplasia through *in situ* neoplasia to invasive neoplasia is now well recognized in several tissues (*Fig. 6.14*).

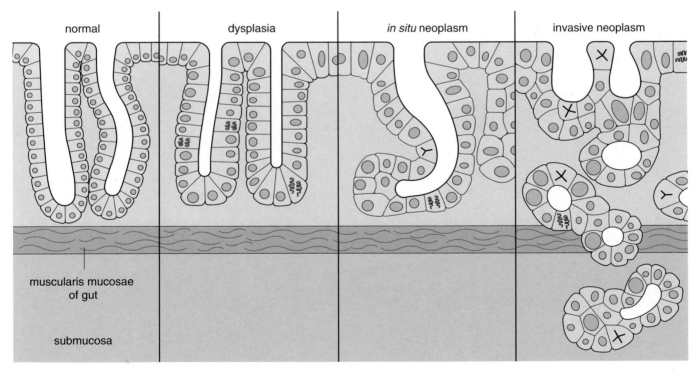

Fig. 6.14 Progression of dysplasia to neoplasia.
A sequence of progression from dysplasia through *in situ* neoplasia to invasive neoplasia is often seen in several tissues. In the diagram, as in real life, the distinction between dysplasia and *in situ* neoplasia is difficult and emphasis is placed on loss of normal tissue architecture to signify development of neoplasia. The main areas in which this situation develops are: squamous epithelium at the squamocolumnar junction of the uterine cervix; epidermis of sun-exposed skin; colonic mucosa after long-standing chronic colitis, and gastric mucosa after long-standing chronic gastritis. The altered cell turnover in dysplasia probably allows local environmental factors to cause genetic abnormalities leading to neoplasia.

Pre-malignant lesions can be treated to prevent later development of invasive neoplasia

Certain lesions, including some benign neoplasms, are known to progress, with time, to invasive neoplasia. The recognized progression from dysplasia through carcinoma *in situ* to invasive neoplasia has already been mentioned. Important conditions which can be treated in their pre-malignant stage are:

- Adenomatous polyps of the colon (see page 260).
- Cervical epithelial *in situ* neoplasia (see page 401).
- Dysplasia of the colon in long-standing ulcerative colitis.
- Dysplasia of the stomach epithelium.

Fig. 6.15
Nomenclature of tumors of support cells and muscle

Tissue of origin	Benign	Malignant
Fibrous	Fibroma	Fibrosarcoma
Bone	Osteoma	Osteosarcoma
Cartilage	Chondroma	Chondrosarcoma
Adipose	Lipoma	Liposarcoma
Smooth muscle	Leiomyoma	Leiomyosarcoma
Skeletal muscle	Rhabdomyoma	Rhabdomyosarcoma

The dysplasia is not, in itself, a neoplastic condition, and removal of the adverse environmental stimulus responsible often allows restoration of the normal cell growth pattern.

Treatment of dysplastic conditions by surgical removal or ablation of affected tissue is often undertaken to minimize the risk of subsequent malignancy.

TUMOR NOMENCLATURE AND CLASSIFICATION

The name given to a tumor should provide information about its cell of origin and its likely behavior (benign or malignant). Unfortunately, as with many areas of medicine, the classification and nomenclature of tumors has evolved over many years and is full of inconsistencies. Some tumors are named on the basis of a macroscopic feature, or histological and behavioral observation. Others are given eponymous or semi-descriptive names, which were coined when there was poor understanding of histogenesis but have been retained because they have been in use for so long. It is not unusual for a single tumor to have many synonyms.

Nomenclature of tumors of epithelial origin

Some benign neoplasms of surface epithelia, e.g. skin, are known as **papillomata** (singular: **papilloma**) because they form frond-like growths. This is prefixed by the cell of origin, e.g. squamous cell papilloma of skin.

Benign neoplasms, of both solid and surface epithelium, are termed **adenomata** (singular: **adenoma**), and are also prefixed by the tissue of origin, e.g. thyroid adenoma, renal adenoma, adrenal adenoma, colonic adenoma.

A malignant tumor of any epithelial origin is termed a **carcinoma**. Tumors of glandular epithelium (including that lining the gut) are termed **adenocarcinomas**. Tumors of other epithelia are prefixed by the cell type of origin, e.g. squamous cell carcinoma, transitional cell carcinoma, hepatocellular carcinoma. To classify a carcinoma further, the tissue of origin is added, e.g. adenocarcinoma of prostate, adenocarcinoma of breast, squamous carcinoma of larynx.

Nomenclature of tumors of mesenchymal tissues

For tumors composed of mesenchymal tissues (support cells or muscle) the nomenclature is more consistent than that for epithelial types. The tissue of origin takes the suffix **-oma** if the tumor is benign, or **-sarcoma** if it is malignant. For example, a benign tumor of cartilage is termed a chondroma, and a malignant tumor is termed a chondrosarcoma. A summary of nomenclature of other tumors of support cells is shown in *Fig. 6.15*.

Nomenclature of other tumors

Neoplasms that do not fit into either the epithelial or the support cell categories are named according to their tissue of origin (histogenetic nomenclature). The main categories are:

Lymphomas. These tumors of the lymphoid system are composed of neoplastic lymphocytes, and vary in grade of malignancy from slow-growing to highly aggressive (see Chapter 15).

Malignant melanoma. Highly malignant tumors derived from melanocytes, usually identifiable by their melanin content.

Leukemias. Malignant tumors derived from hemopoietic elements in bone marrow which circulate in the blood (see Chapter 15).

Embryonal tumors. A group of malignant tumors seen mainly in childhood, derived from primitive embryonal blastic tissue; the most common types are nephroblastoma of the kidney (*Fig. 17.26*) and neuroblastoma of the adrenal medulla (*Fig. 16.23*).

Gliomas. Tumors derived from the non-neural support tissues of the brain. They may be benign or malignant and are named according to the cell of origin, e.g. astrocytoma, oligodendroglioma (see Chapter 21).

Germ cell tumors. Tumors derived from germ cells in the gonads, but also rarely arising in non-gonadal sites (Chapters 18 and 19).

Teratomas. A type of germ cell tumor which differentiates to form elements of all three embryological germ cell layers: ectoderm, endoderm, and mesoderm. Teratomas may be benign or malignant and, as well as arising in the gonads, they also occur in non-gonadal sites in young people, particularly in the sacrum and mediastinum.

Neuroendocrine tumors. Tumors of neuroendocrine cells, which secrete polypeptide hormones or active amines. Examples include pheochromocytoma of the adrenal medulla (see page 343), carcinoid tumor of the appendix (page 264) and medullary carcinoma of the thyroid (page 338). Some of these growths are grouped under the term APUD tumors, in recognition of the role of functional amine precursor uptake and decarboxylation. Others are also given functional names, e.g. insulinoma, prolactinoma.

Hamartomas. Non-neoplastic overgrowths of tissues, which would normally occur in the site in question. Although they are developmental abnormalities rather than true neoplasms, they are often grouped with neoplasms because they appear as localized tissue masses. Common examples are hemangiomas (see page 172), and melanocytic nevi (moles).

Choristomas. Non-neoplastic overgrowths of tissues which would not normally occur in that site. Although developmental, like hamartomas, they are considered alongside tumors because they present as a mass of tissue.

Tumors with eponymous names

Many tumors continue to be named after the person who recognized or popularized them. The most common examples are:

Ewing's sarcoma. A malignant tumor of bone seen in young people, probably derived from primitive neuro-endocrine cells.

Hodgkin's disease. A malignant proliferation of lymphoid tissues, classified as a sub-group of the lymphomas.

Kaposi's sarcoma. A malignant tumor thought to be derived from endothelium, now commonly seen in association with AIDS.

Burkitt's lymphoma. A form of lymphoma derived from B-cells, in which Epstein–Barr virus has a causative role.

BIOLOGY OF NEOPLASIA

Carcinogenesis is the train of biological events that underlies the development of neoplasia. At the cellular level, neoplasms are ultimately caused by genetic mutations, resulting in abnormal control of growth. There is now much evidence to suggest that this genetic damage is a multi-step development, requiring the interaction of several processes, often over a period of many years.

Abnormalities in genes regulating cell proliferation underlie neoplastic transformation

Four main genetic mechanisms are thought to have a role in the development of most human neoplasms:

- Expression of genes resulting in inappropriate activity of products which, under normal circumstances, stimulate growth. Such genes are termed oncogenes and act in a dominant fashion. (Phenotype is affected even if one allele is present, which abnormally stimulates growth.)

- Loss of activity of genes which, under normal circumstances, produce products that inhibit cell growth. Such genes are termed **tumor suppressor genes** or **anti-oncogenes**. They can rarely act in a dominant manner to cause benign tumors (heterozygotes with one abnormal gene), but generally act in a recessive manner to produce malignant tumors. (Malignant phenotype only develops if both alleles fail to suppress growth.)

- Over-expression of genes which, under normal circumstances, produce products that prevent normal cell death. Failure to eliminate genetically damaged cells allows continued growth of tumors.

- Loss of activity of gene products which, under normal circumstances, would repair damaged DNA. Loss of activity leads to a state of DNA instability with the development of somatic mutations in oncogenes or tumor suppressor genes.

The genetic reason for neoplastic transformation is variable:

- Point mutations in oncogene causing production of abnormally functioning product or loss of a suppressor.
- Gene amplification causing excessive production of oncoprotein product.
- Chromosomal rearrangements whereby an oncogene is activated inappropriately by another promoter region.

It is now recognized that tumors normally have several genetic aberrations, the sum of which results in neoplastic transformation of cells. A tumor may develop additional oncogene abnormalities with time, resulting in a more aggressive growth pattern. The mechanisms by which oncogenes act are summarized in *Fig. 6.16*.

Growth factors regulate cell division

Cells are induced to proliferate by specific growth signals from a variety of growth factors which include hormones, cytokines and classical growth factors. These bind to cell surface receptors which are virtually all transmembrane proteins having a cytosolic domain with tyrosine kinase activity. In response to a positive growth signal cells undergo internal reorganization of actin-dependent adhesion mechanisms, show an increase in intracellular calcium, and following activation and nuclear translocation of transcription factors, the cell cycle is entered.

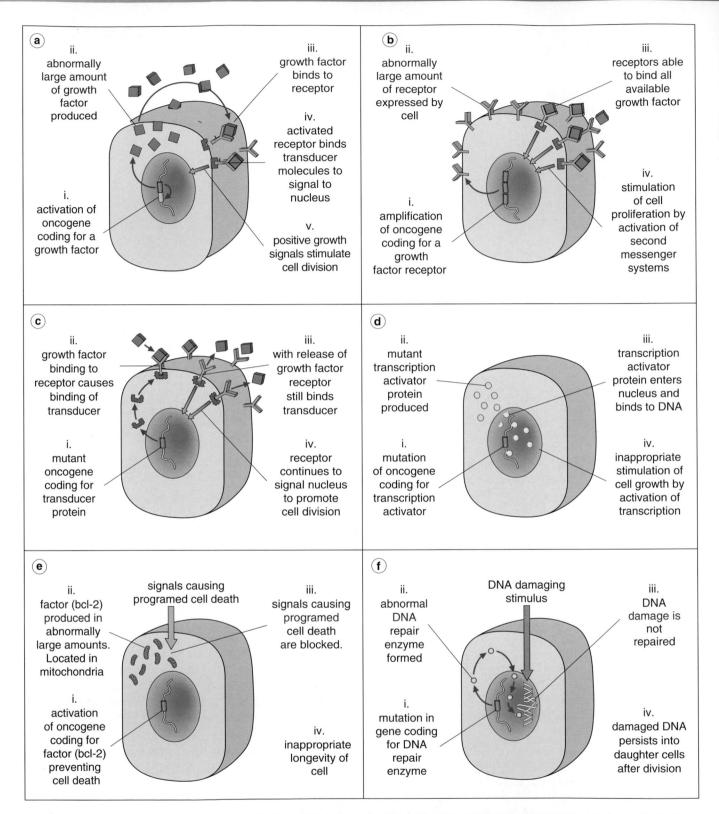

Fig. 6.16 Action of oncogenes in neoplastic transformation of cells. (a) Increased production of secreted growth factor. (b) Increased expression of growth factor receptors. (c) Mutation in transducer protein gene. (d) Mutant transcription factor production. (e) Over-production of factor that prevents cell death. (f) Loss of activity in DNA repair systems.

The cell cycle is controlled at several points

The cell cycle is controlled by complexes of cyclins and cyclin-dependent kinases

Cells which are in an active state of proliferation are said to be in the cell cycle (*Fig. 6.17*).

Progression of a cell through this cycle is controlled by the synthesis, degradation and state of phosphorylation of proteins called cyclins (cyclins A, B, E). The cyclins form complexes with cyclin-dependent kinases (CDKs) and these complexes control progress through the cell cycle by activating a variety of proteins by phosphorylation. A variety of cyclin-dependent kinase inhibitors (CDKIs) are also present which modulate the activity of the cell cycle.

- p21, p27 and p57 have broad activity as inhibitors of CDK activity.
- p15, p16, p18 and p19 (INK4 proteins) inhibit CDK4 and CDK6.

Cell cycle check points make sure that only normal cells complete replication

There are important check points in the cell cycle which are policed by surveillance systems in the cell nucleus which are designed to prevent cells replicating if they become damaged, especially is there is existing DNA damage. A cell which has been halted in its progresson through the cell cycle can either activate DNA repair mechanisms or, if these fail, switch on apoptosis to eliminate itself.

- The transition from the G1 to the S phase of the cell cycle can only happen when a transcription factor factor called E2F is free in the nucleus. During G1, E2F is normally bound to Rb protein and must be released to allow movement through G1 to S phase, past a point late in G1 called the restriction point. This is achieved by the phosphorylation of Rb, releasing E2F. Phosphorylation of Rb is achieved by synthesis of D cyclin, which forms a complex with CDK4 and 6, and then formation of a cyclin E–CDK2 complex. If a cell has an abnormal Rb protein then it will not be checked in its passage through this important cell cycle checkpoint. Cells which overexpress CDK4 or cyclin D will also functionally fail to prevent check point arrest after G1, as Rb will tend to be phosphorylated.

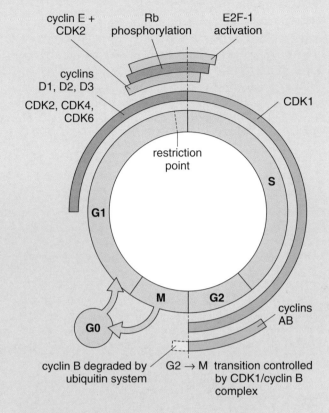

Fig. 6.17 Cell cycle.
Following the M (mitosis) phase cells can either enter a non-dividing state, termed G0, or continue through the cell cycle. Phases G1, S and G2 constitute so-called interphase cells. During the S phase, cells replicate DNA. Two of the important cell cycle check points are shown: the G1–S transition regulated by the state of phosphorylation of Rb, releasing the E2F transcription factor and the G2–M transition regulated by the CDK1–cyclin B complex.

- The transition between the G2 and the M phases is regulated by the formation of the CDK1–cyclin B complex. After entry to M phase, cyclin B is rapidly destroyed by the ubiquitin–proteasome system.
- The gene coding for p53 protein is activated in the presence of DNA damage and causes increase in the cyclin-dependent kinase inhibitor (CDKI) p21 protein termed WAF1. This inhibitor prevents phosphorylation of cyclins and hence arrests the cell in its progression through the cycle. If a cell has an abnormal form of p53 protein then this regulatory function will be impaired and so cells with damaged DNA may complete mitosis, thereby propagating a mutation.

Oncogenes are central to the development of tumors

Oncogenes were originally isolated from tumor-forming RNA retroviruses (v-onc).

Viral concogenes (v-oncs): genes within a virus that code for a protein involved in the development of neoplasia.

Proto-oncogenes (p-oncs): genes that code for proteins involved in the control of cell growth.

Cellular oncogenes (c-oncs): genes that code for proteins in the development of neoplasia A proto-oncogene can lead to the development of a tumor by three main mechanisms:

- Mutation – leading to a mutant protein product.
- Gene amplification – leading to excess protein product.
- Abnormal gene promotion – the oncogene is driven by an abnormal promotor:
  —Host-derived: usually in association with a chromosome translocation.
  —Viral-derived: in the setting of a retroviral infection.

Oncogene products, all key molecules in signal transduction and control of normal cell growth, are referred to by the abbreviated name of the tumor virus or system in which they were discovered. For example, *ras*, found in rat sarcoma virus, is a protein that acts on the GTP intracellular secondary messenger system.

In humans, abnormalities of oncogenes are found in tumors, and are thought to be primary events in malignant transformation. Usually, multiple oncogene abnormalities are seen in a single tumor.

Fig. 6.18 summarizes the important oncoproteins, giving examples of associated tumors and the respective reasons for their activation.

Absence of tumor suppressor genes promotes neoplasia

The first suppressor gene to be discovered was found in a malignant tumor of the retina in childhood, known as a retinoblastoma. The gene is located on chromosome 13 and is termed Rb. Familial forms of disease are inherited as an autosomal dominant trait, in which affected children have one mutant gene (inactive) and one normal gene (active). To develop a retinoblastoma, the second gene must undergo a somatic mutation in the child. In sporadic retinoblastoma both genes must undergo mutation, a chance event which means that sporadic tumors are rare. Since the discovery of the Rb gene's absence in retinoblastoma, its absence has been established in many other tumors.

Located on chromosome 17, another suppressor gene, p53, has been found to be lost in so many types of tumor that it has been proposed as the most common genetic abnormality in neoplasia. In a normal cell p53 is activated in response to DNA damage, activating systems that bring about DNA repair and arresting the cell cycle. In cells where repair is not achieved p53 can cause the cell to enter the apoptotic pathway of cell death, eliminating the

---

Fig. 6.18
Main oncogene products and mechanisms of abnormal regulation

Proto-oncogene	Function	Oncogene type	Reason for activation
ras	GTP binding	Signal transduction	Point mutation
myc	Transcription activator	Nuclear regulator	Translocation
n-*myc*	Transcription activator	Nuclear regulator	Translocation
erb-B1	EGF receptor	Growth factor receptor	Amplification
erb-B2 (new)	EGF-like receptor	Growth factor receptor	Amplification
Bcl-2	Mitochondrial protein	Inhibit apoptosis	Translocation
abl	Tyrosine kinase	Signal transduction	Translocation
sis	PDGF β chain	Growth factor	Over-expression
hst-1	FGF	Growth factor Follicular lymphoma	Over-expression

EGF - epidermal growth factor   FGF - fibroblast growth factor
PGDF - platelet derived growth factor   GTP - guanosine triphosphate

possibility of division of a cell with damaged DNA. Loss of activity of p53 in a cell allows the proliferation of cells with DNA damage.

The absence of APC, another tumor suppressor gene, is responsible for the development of familial adenomatous polyposis coli. People who inherit a single inactive copy of the gene develop multiple benign adenomata of the large bowel (see page 261). If cells develop a second mutation of the normal inherited gene on the other allele, it leads to development of carcinoma of the colon. The molecular basis of defective APC function has been determined. In normal cells, APC protein binds another protein termed alpha-catenin and brings about its degradation. Alpha-catenin is a transcription factor and if APC function is defective through mutation, raised levels of alpha-catenin occur in the cell, driving cell proliferation.

Many of the tumor suppressor genes have been called 'gatekeeper' genes, in that they normally directly control the proliferation of cells, and a loss of function allows a cell to enter a state that leads to fully developed neoplasia.

Damage to genes that regulate DNA repair predispose to neoplasia

Cells are constantly exposed to stimuli that cause damage to DNA and there is a well developed system for detection and repair of DNA, including the action of p53 discussed above.

Mutation in DNA repair genes allows the proliferation of cells with DNA mutations, so-called replication error positive phenotype (RER+). This state can be assessed by looking at microsatellite sequences (tandem repeated DNA sequences) in cells, which normally remain constant. With DNA repair errors, cells develop changes in the repeat length of microsatellite DNA, a condition termed microsatellite instability.

Several genes have been characterized which code for DNA repair elements (hMSH2, hMLH1, hPMS1, hPMS2).

Mutations in such genes are found in those patients who have an inherited predisposition to colonic carcinoma not linked to the APC gene. Development of a replication error positive phenotype is also encountered in many sporadic tumors as a result of a somatic mutation in DNA repair genes. The genes coding for DNA repair systems are sometimes called 'caretaker' genes, in that they look after the DNA, defective function leading to genetic instability in which there is an overall increased risk of a cell developing a mutation in any gene, including a proto-oncogene.

Tumors are composed of several genetic clones derived by acquired mutations

It is widely recognized that tumors become less well differentiated and more aggressive with time. This property, termed progression, is due to the emergence of subpopulations of cells with new genetic abnormalities that make growth control more abnormal and facilitate metastasis. Any large tumor is therefore composed of a whole set of slightly different cells (tumor heterogeneity) as a result of further acquired somatic mutations (*Fig. 6.19*). Any mutations that favour tumor survival or spread are chosen by a form of natural selection.

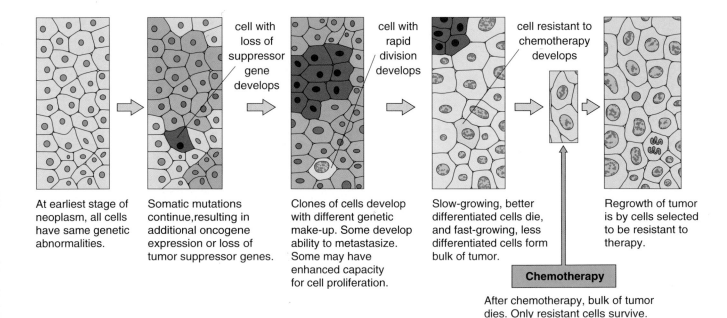

At earliest stage of neoplasm, all cells have same genetic abnormalities.

Somatic mutations continue,resulting in additional oncogene expression or loss of tumor suppressor genes.

cell with loss of suppressor gene develops

Clones of cells develop with different genetic make-up. Some develop ability to metastasize. Some may have enhanced capacity for cell proliferation.

cell with rapid division develops

Slow-growing, better differentiated cells die, and fast-growing, less differentiated cells form bulk of tumor.

cell resistant to chemotherapy develops

Regrowth of tumor is by cells selected to be resistant to therapy.

Chemotherapy

After chemotherapy, bulk of tumor dies. Only resistant cells survive.

Fig. 6.19 Tumor progression and genetic heterogeneity.
As tumors develop they undergo further somatic mutation, which causes abnormalities in other oncogenes. Mutations may also lead to cell death. A mutation which puts a cell at a survival disadvantage will cause that clone to be eliminated. A tumor will ultimately consist of many different sub-clones of cells, those with greater growth potential gradually coming to dominate the lesion.

This is an important concept as it explains how a primary tumor may respond to therapy, and yet metastatic lesions do not, as they are composed of cells with properties allowing invasion, motility, and growth in another site. It also explains how, after apparent clinical response, tumor may re-emerge as lesions resistant to chemotherapeutic drugs: resistant cells are selected and eventually come to dominate the tumor.

Cytogenetic studies have documented a mixture of molecular genetic and cytogenetic features which accompany clinical and histological evidence of tumor progression. As research continues, it is hoped that the precise gene abnormalities underlying the cytogenetic abnormalities will be identified, allowing a molecular assessment of the likely biological behaviour of a neoplasm.

Recurring cytogenetic abnormalities are seen in some tumors

Cytogenetic examination of the chromosomal complement of cells has identified several recurring chromosomal abnormalities in specific tumors.

More recent molecular biological investigation has demonstrated some of the genetic effects of these structural abnormalities. In most instances this takes the form of over-expression of an oncogene or deletion of a suppressor gene. The most important abnormalities are listed in *Fig. 6.20*. Detection of these cytogenetic abnormalities in tumor samples is not only useful in determining either

Techniques for detecting cytogenetic changes in tumors

Traditional karyotypic analysis is performed on metaphase spreads and requires viable tumor maintained in culture for a short time. Technical limitations mean that it only works for solid tumors in about 40% of cases and can only detect relatively large changes.

Structural changes for which sequence data is available, for example certain translocations producing fusion oncogenes, can be detected by FISH (fluorescent *in situ* hybridization) or RT-PCR (reverse transcriptase polymerase chain reaction). Spectral karyotyping (SKY) allows simultaneous labeling of all chromosomes by fluorescent probes and allows detection of complex and small chromosomal abnormalities.

diagnosis or prognosis, but also important because they are ultimately related to abnormal gene expression.

Chemical carcinogens have a role in several human tumors

Many chemical carcinogens have been identified, and their effects documented in experiments in which animals

Fig. 6.20
Cytogenetic abnormalities in human neoplasms

Tumor	Cytogenetic abnormality	Effects
Chronic myeloid leukemia	T(9;22)(q34;q11) (Philadelphia chromosome)	Fusion oncogene bcr-abl leads to protein with tyrosine kinase activity
Follicular lymphoma	T(14;18)(q32;q21)	IgH gene from chr14 fused to Bcl-2 gene on chr21 leading to prevention of apoptosis
Ewing's sarcoma	T(11;22)(q24;q12)	Fusion of the FLT-1 gene from chr11 with the EWS gene on chr22 leading to a fusion protein with high transcription activator activity
Alveolar rhabdomyosarcoma	T(2;13)(q35;q14)	PAX3 gene from chr2 is fused with the FKHR gene on chr13 leading to a fusion protein with transcription factor activity
Synovial sarcoma	T(X;18) (p11;q11)	SYT gene from chr18 is fused to SSX1 SSX2 gene on X chromosome. Possible ectopic expression of SSX1/2 products
Neuroblastoma	Homogeneous staining regions and double minute chromosomes	Amplification of n-myc
Burkitt's lymphoma	T(8;14)(q24;q32)	Fusion of c-myc on chr8 with IgH from chr14 leading to c-myc expression

exposed to the agents develop neoplasia. The main groups of relevance to human disease are as follows:

- Polycyclic hydrocarbons, found in tars, are among the potent agents in cigarette smoke that cause lung cancer.

- Aromatic amines are mainly encountered through industrial exposure (e.g. rubber or dye industry) and are converted to active agents in the liver. They become concentrated by excretion in the urine, and so have their main effect on the urothelium, where cancers develop.

- Nitrosamines have been shown to be potent carcinogens in animals, and in humans there is a pathway for conversion of dietary nitrites and nitrates to nitrosamines by gut bacteria. These agents are thought to cause cancer in the stomach and gastrointestinal tract.

- Alkylating agents can bind directly to DNA and are directly mutagenic. They are rare in the environment, but examples are used in cancer chemotherapy (e.g. cyclophosphamide), raising the possibility that the use of such agents to treat one tumor may predispose a patient to development of another.

There are three main groups of chemical carcinogens

Chemical carcinogens may cause development of neoplasia either directly or indirectly. They can be grouped into three classes according to the mechanism by which they stimulate development of neoplasia:

Genotoxic: cause direct damage to DNA by forming chemical DNA adducts. The abnormal areas of DNA are prone to damage in replication and some adducts are resistant to normal DNA repair mechanisms.

Mitogenic: bind to receptors on or in cells and stimulate cell division without causing direct DNA damage. In experimental skin carcinogenesis such agents have been shown to bind to and activate protein kinase C, causing sustained epidermal hyperplasia.

Cytotoxic: produce tissue damage and lead to hyperplasia with cycles of tissue regeneration and damage. In some cases it is believed that cytokines generated in response to tissue damage act as mitogenic factors.

Chemical carcinogens can be further divided into two groups:

Direct acting: the agent is capable of directly causing neoplasia.

Procarcinogens: the agent requires conversion to an active carcinogen. This conversion takes place by normal metabolic pathways.

In procarcinogens the cytochrome P450 oxygenase system plays an important role in conversion in many instances. Detoxifaction reactions also occur, the accumulation of carcinogen being determined by a balance between:

- Dose of procarcinogen.
- Rate of detoxification and elimination.
- Rate of conversion to the active form.

Chemical carcinogens can be divided into initiating and promoting agents

The original concepts of chemical carcinogenesis were largely derived from work on experimental induction of malignant skin tumors in mice. It was found that some agents, such as polycyclic aromatic hydrocarbons, could cause cancer of the skin if they were painted onto mice in high doses. In low dosage they would not cause cancer but would render the skin susceptible to developing cancer on exposure to another agent which, on its own, would not induce cancer. From this work it was possible to define two types of chemical carcinogen (*Fig 6.21*).

Initiating agents:

- Exposure of cells to an initiating agent does not directly cause neoplasia but renders cells susceptible to developing neoplasia if they are later exposed to certain other agents.

- The initiating agent causes genetic abnormality of exposed cells. The genetic damage will cause an abnormality which is not in itself enough to result in abnormal cell growth.

- Most initiating agents are examples of mutagenic carcinogens.

Promoting agents:

- Exposure of normal cells to a promoting agent causes no abnormality.

- Prolonged exposure of initiated cells to a promoting agent causes development of neoplasia.

- Transient exposure of initiated cells to a promoting agent will also not result in development of neoplasia.

- The promoting agent causes increased cell turnover (inducing cell proliferation). With continued exposure to the promoting agent cells which have a genetic abnormality (caused by the initiating agent) develop

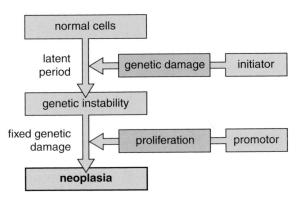

Fig. 6.21 Action of initiating and promoting carcinogens.

Predicting carcinogenicity of chemical agents

Important emphasis has been placed on the determination of whether an agent is a carcinogen. Two types of test can be used.

- **Mutagenicity studies**
Strains of *Salmonella typhimurium* which are unable to synthesize histidine are mixed with a microsomal fraction from rodent liver and a test chemical. The microsomes enable conversion of a procarcinogen to an active form. If the chemical is a mutagen then some bacteria undergo mutation and acquire the ability to make histidine. This is detected by plating out the test bacteria on a medium which is deficient in histidine.

This type of test (**the Ames test**) will detect genotoxic chemical carcinogens but is insensitive to cytotoxic or mitogenic types.

- **Carcinogenicity studies**
Chemical agents are administered to rodents at high-dose exposures and the incidence of tumors evaluated on pathological and histological examination after near life-long exposure. This approach appears valid for genotoxic carcinogens but may not be appropriate for non-genotoxic agents because of dose considerations and species specificities.

secondary genetic abnormalities in key genes regulating cell growth (oncogenes).
- With increased cell proliferation clones of cells develop which have loss of growth control and characteristics of a neoplasm.
- Many promoting agents are examples of mitogenic carcinogens.

Three stages have been defined in chemical carcinogenesis

From experimental work three stages of chemical carcinogenesis have been defined as:

Initiation: induction of genetic changes in cells. The nature of the initial changes in cells is still uncertain. In experimental chemical carcinogenesis in skin, the Harvey *ras* gene has been identified as being frequently mutated. This gene is involved in epidermal proliferation and when it becomes abnormal epidermal cells are less responsive to signals that normally cause terminal differentiation. Only relatively few genes have been identified as being mutated in other animal models of chemical carcinogenesis.

Promotion: induction of cell proliferation. In this phase of carcinogenesis a promoting agent, either a mitogen or a cytotoxic agent, brings about increased cell proliferation. Promotion is initially reversible if the promoting agent is withdrawn.

Progression: If there is persistent cell proliferation then initiated cells acquire secondary genetic abnormalities in oncogenes which first lead to dysregulation and eventually to autonomous cell growth. The ultimate end-point of progression is development of an invasive neoplasm.

While many environmental agents fit into the categories of initiating and promoting agents, some factors can act as both initiator and promotor (complete carcinogens).

Study of chemical carcinogenesis is relevant to the treatment of human disease

The understanding of molecular aspects of chemical carcinogenesis have lead to development of the concept of chemoprevention. This proposes strategies for intervention at the phase of pre-malignancy using drugs to reverse or halt the process of carcinogenesis. Drugs that are under investigation include:

- Tamoxifen in breast carcinoma.
- Retinoids and beta-carotene in head, neck and lung tumors.

KEY FACTS
Chemical carcinogenesis

- Most work on chemical carcinogensis has been developed in experimental animal studies.
- Following exposure to a carcinogenic agent there is a long latent period before a neoplasm develops. It is thought that altered cells are primed but require a second change to bring about molecular genetic changes expressed as neoplasia.
- From the evidence supplied by animal models, carcinogenesis is a multi-stage process:
Initiation: an event that alters the genome occurs.
Promotion: an event that causes proliferation of the transformed cell takes place, giving rise to a neoplasm.
Progression: new genetic mutations occur, with development of sub-clones of neoplastic cells.

Only a few infections are implicated in human neoplasia

Based on the fact that viruses are known to be directly responsible for some neoplasms in animals, it is not unreasonable to assume that similar viruses cause certain human neoplasias; relatively few viruses have been implicated, as summarized in *Fig. 6.22*.

Two types of viral carcinogenesis have been described related to activation of oncogenes:

- Slow-transforming viruses insert viral-derived DNA into the genome randomly. If chance dictates that the viral DNA is integrated next to a proto-oncogene, then the viral DNA causes abnormal promotion of the proto-oncogene, leading to neoplasia.
- Acute-transforming viruses contain a viral oncogene and when viral-derived DNA is inserted into the host genome the transcribed viral oncogene is expressed leading to neoplasia.

The precise molecular mechanisms whereby viruses cause neoplastic transformation are beginning to be determined, e.g. papillomaviruses produce proteins that inactivate certain products made by tumor suppressor genes (see page 94), thereby allowing cells to escape normal regulation of growth. Bacteria have been implicated in neoplasia. The development of gastric lymphoma has been directly related to infection by *Helicobacter pylori*.

Irradiation is a potent cause of neoplastic transformation

An increased incidence of neoplasia following exposure to ionizing radiation has long been documented and is due to direct increase in DNA damage. There are two main effects of DNA damage through irradiation:

- Formation of DNA breaks.
- Development of DNA instability.

Direct exposure to ionizing radiation, for example repeated exposure to X-rays, increases the risk of tumors in bone marrow and in the skin of exposed areas. Exposure to radioactive material in the environment is a more complex issue as the type of tumor is related to the type of exposure and to possible incorporation of radioactive material in body tissues. For example:

- Inhalation of radioactive dust or gas (e.g. radon) increases the risk of carcinoma of the lung.
- Ingestion of radioactive iodine increases the risk of carcinoma of the thyroid.
- Incorporation of radioactive metals into bone increases the risk of tumors of bone marrow and bone.

A frequently overlooked source of radiation, which is a major cause of neoplasia, is UV light in sunlight (see Chapter 9). This is known to increase the risk of development of many types of malignant skin tumor (see page 143).

Fig. 6.22
Viruses implicated in human neoplasia

Virus	Neoplasm
Epstein–Barr virus	Burkitt's lymphoma Nasopharyngeal carcinoma Other B-cell lymphomas and some cases of Hodgkin's disease
Hepatitis B virus	Hepatocellular carcinoma
Human papillomavirus	Cervical carcinoma Some forms of carcinoma of the skin
HTLV-1	T-cell leukemia/lymphoma
HSV-8	Kaposi sarcoma

Biological agents such as hormones play a role in tumor growth

In some circumstances hormones are thought to contribute to the etiology or growth of neoplasia:

- Hormones may be required to promote growth of tumors. Estrogens stimulate proliferation of breast and endometrial tissue and can predispose to the development of carcinoma of the breast and endometrium in animal models. Certain tumors depend on hormones for continued growth.
- Carcinomas of the breast that express estrogen receptors can be treated by anti-estrogen drugs and this often causes regression of tumor.
- Carcinoma of the prostate can be treated by removal of testosterone stimulation by orchidectomy or administration of estrogenic drugs.
- In a unique situation, children of women treated during pregnancy with the synthetic estrogen diethylstilboestrol develop carcinoma of the vagina. This is an example of an agent acting *in utero* causing neoplasia in later life.

Cytokines may also be involved in control of growth of neoplastic cells. For example, one form of tumor of white blood cells, termed hairy-cell leukemia, can be treated with interferon.

Asbestos is an example of a physical agent that causes neoplasia

Asbestos fibers (see page 210) which are inhaled are a potent cause of neoplasia in the lung and pleura. This is often after a long latent period following exposure. The association with primary malignant tumors arising in the pleura is particularly strong as, in the absence of previous asbestos exposure, they are extremely rare (see page 220). The precise mechanism whereby asbestos fibers cause neoplasia is unresolved.

Many dietary factors are implicated in neoplasia but their role is uncertain

A variety of dietary substances have been implicated in the cause of neoplasia, particularly related to neoplasia in the gut. A diet high in fat is associated with a higher risk of development of carcinoma of the breast and colon compared to populations with a low-fat diet. A diet low in fiber is associated with an increased incidence of carcinoma of the colon compared to populations with a high-fiber diet. High levels of nitrates or nitrites in the diet are associated with an increased risk of development of carcinoma of the stomach.

Preneoplastic conditions are diseases associated with an increased risk of developing tumors

Certain non-neoplastic diseases are known to carry an increased risk of later development of neoplasia and are termed preneoplastic conditions.

Hyperplasia is one such condition; endometrial hyperplasia and hyperplasia of the epithelium of breast lobules and ducts both predispose to development of carcinoma.

In some instances a chronic increased proliferation of cells results in **dysplasia**, which then progresses to carcinoma. For example:

- Chronic gastritis predisposes to the development of carcinoma of the stomach.
- Chronic colitis predisposes to the development of carcinoma of the colon.
- Hepatic cirrhosis predisposes to development of liver cell carcinoma.

Chronic autoimmune diseases are associated with the development of localized neoplastic transformation of lymphoid cells to form a lymphoma. For example:

- Celiac disease predisposes to later development of gut lymphoma.
- Autoimmune thyroiditis predisposes to development of thyroid lymphoma.

Immune responses are being explored to combat established human tumors

Neoplastic transformation results in an abnormal phenotype of cells and may be associated with development of abnormal antigens. Although immune responses to tumors are evident, they seem weak and, in human disease, do not normally appear to contribute significantly to the response to an established tumor.

There are two main classes of tumor-related antigens:

- Tumor-specific antigens are present only on tumor cells. These are well established in animal models, but their role in human tumors is, at present, uncertain. The presence of a significant lymphoid infiltrate, including cytotoxic lymphocytes in certain tumors, suggests that an immune response to tumor-specific antigens may be taking place. Clinical observations have indicated that patients with tumors that have a lymphoid infiltrate have a better prognosis than those without an infiltrate. This has prompted treatment protocols whereby lymphocytes are harvested from surgically excised tumors, cloned in culture to produce killer cells, and transfused back to the patient in an attempt to enhance any tumor-related immune response. Great interest is being shown in developing tumor vaccines against tumor-specific antigens. For example, MAGE proteins are normally expressed in germ cells in the absence of class II antigen and hence cannot be recognized by the immune system. MAGE proteins are also expressed on several tumors with class II antigens so it is possible that vaccination against MAGE proteins could be used to combat certain tumors. The identification of similar novel tumor antigens with a view to developing a vaccine is an active research area.
- Tumor-associated antigens are present on both tumor cells and some normal cells. Included in this group are the oncofetal antigens, which are normally expressed in development but become re-expressed in the neoplastic cells. For example, alpha fetoprotein (AFP) is expressed in hepatocellular cancer, and carcinoembryonic antigen (CEA) is expressed in cancers of the gastrointestinal tract.

EPIDEMIOLOGY OF NEOPLASTIC DISEASE

In humans there is an association between the incidence and types of cancer encountered and age, as summarized in *Fig. 6.23*.

There is a small number of tumors of childhood. These are distinct from those that occur in adult life, being mainly tumors recapitulating embryonal tissues ('blastomas') and leukemias.

Tumors in early adult life are uncommon, being mainly tumors of bone, lymphomas, and germ cell tumors. These lesions may well be precipitated by an abnormal response to normal growth and endocrine stimuli.

An increasing incidence of a wide range of epithelial neoplasms is seen with age in later adult life. This is probably the result of an accumulation of events required for a multi-step causation of neoplasia. The incidence of the most common neoplasms is shown in *Fig. 6.24*.

Epidemiological studies are important in the search for etiological factors in the development of a wide range of neoplastic diseases. The observation of 'clustering' of cases of a certain type of cancer in a particular geographical location may provide a pointer to an environmental etiological factor.

- Cancer is the second most common cause of death (after ischemic heart disease) in most developed countries, accounting for about 23% of all mortality.
- The incidence of the different histological types of cancer varies greatly between different populations, and is attributable to occupational, social and geographic factors.
- The incidence of lung cancer is increasing rapidly in women as a result of cigarette smoking. It now exceeds breast cancer as the leading cause of cancer death (as opposed to incidence).
- The incidence of malignant melanoma of the skin is increasing among Caucasians in many countries. This is the result of exposure to UV radiation because of the fashion for sun-tanning.

- There is a high incidence of stomach cancer in Japan compared to other countries, which has been attributed to dietary factors (particularly smoked, raw fish).
- The survival rate for many tumors has been greatly increased over the past two decades as a result of advances in, and greater availability of, treatment.
- Cancer prevention strategies depend, for the most part, on elimination of causative factors, largely identified through epidemiology.
- Cancer detection strategies depend on screening populations for early forms of neoplasia at an early stage of development, e.g. cervical carcinoma and breast carcinoma.

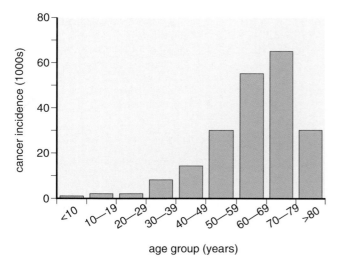

Fig. 6.23 Annual number of registered cases of malignant neoplasia, by age group, in the UK.
The number of reported cases of malignancy increases markedly after the age of 50. The reduction in cases after the age of 79 is because there are few individuals alive and at risk in this age range. In addition, case ascertainment is probably less robust in this age group.

Heritable neoplastic conditions have revealed genetic abnormalities important in neoplasia

Several neoplastic conditions are heritable, and genetic analysis has led to the identification of several of the molecular genetic abnormalities underlying neoplasia discussed earlier in this chapter. The most important heritable neoplastic syndromes are given in *Fig. 6.25.*

Detailed studies of family groups in which there has been a high incidence of either a single type of cancer, or a particular group of cancers, has led to the understanding that certain families have a genetic predisposition to develop cancers of a particular type. Often, in these 'familial tendency' cancers, the tumors which occur tend to be atypical in some way. Most commonly, the tumors present at an earlier age than is usual for that specific tumor, and it may be of an unusual histological type.

The best-known example is in colorectal carcinoma. The role of the autosomal dominant disorder, familial plyposis coli, in the development of colorectal carcinoma has long been known, but recent studies in families with a high incidence of colorectal carcinoma have pointed to another, much larger, group in which a gene disorder predisposes to the development of colorectal carcinoma. The tumors typically occur a decade or two before the usual age for development of colorectal carcinoma. This is dealt with in more detail in Chapter 13, page 260.

A similar genetic basis for malignant tumor has been found in families with a high incidence of adenocarcinoma of the breast (see Chapter 20, page 429).

The importance of these findings is twofold. First, it enables the gene defect specific to the affected family members to be identified, with the eventual potential for more widespread screening tests applied to the population as a whole, but particularly in the members of the affected family. Secondly, it allows early screening of family members with the gene defect before the tumor has developed; for example, in the colorectal cancer group, regular colonoscopies are performed to detect and treat the developing tumors at an early stage when there is every chance of successful surgical treatment.

(a) Estimated 10 leading sites of new cancer cases grouped by sex, as a percentage of all new cancer cases (United States 1999)*

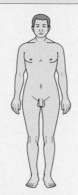
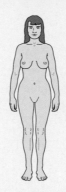

prostate	29
lung and bronchus	15
colon and rectum	10
urinary bladder	6
non-Hodgkin's lymphoma	5
melanoma of skin	4
oral cavity and pharynx	3
kidney and renal pelvis	3
leukemia	3
pancreas	2
all other sites	20

29	breast
13	lung and bronchus
11	colon and rectum
6	uterus
4	ovary
4	non-Hodgkin's lymphoma
3	melanoma of skin
3	urinary bladder
2	pancreas
2	thyroid
23	all other sites

(b) Estimated 10 leading sites of cancer leading to death, grouped by sex, as a percentage of all cancer death (United States 1999)*

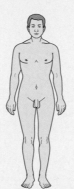
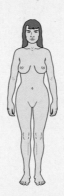

lung and bronchus	31
prostate	13
colon and rectum	10
pancreas	5
non-Hodgkin's lymphoma	5
leukemia	4
esophagus	3
liver and intrahepatic bile duct	3
urinary bladder	3
stomach	3
all other sites	20

25	lung and bronchus
16	breast
11	colon and rectum
5	pancreas
5	ovary
3	non-Hodgkin's lymphoma
4	leukemia
2	uterus
2	brain and other nervous system
2	stomach**
2	multiple myeloma**
21	all other sites

* excludes basal and squamous cell skin cancers and *in situ* carcinomas except urinary bladder.

** these two cancers both received a ranking of 10: they have caused the same number of deaths and contribute the same percentage.

Fig. 6.24 (a) Estimated new cancer cases for the ten leading sites by sex, USA, 1999. (b) Estimated cancer death cases for the ten leading sites by sex, USA, 1999. Data derived from: Landis SH, Murray T, Bolgen S, Wingo PA 1999 Cancer Statistics. CA: A cancer journal for clinicians. 49: 8–31.

Fig. 6.25
Characterized heritable neoplasia syndromes

Syndrome	Tumor caused	Defect
MEN syndromes	Multiple tumors in endocrine organs	Mutations on chromosomes 10 and 11
Polyposis coli	Adenomata and carcinomas of the colon	Absent tumor suppressor gene APC
Li–Fraumeni	Breast cancer and sarcomas	Mutated tumor suppressor gene P53
Xeroderma pigmentosum	Skin cancer	Abnormal DNA repair
Familial retinoblastoma	Malignant tumor of the retina	Absent tumor suppressor gene rb
Neurofibromatosis Type 1	Benign and malignant tumors of peripheral nerves	Abnormal tumor suppressor gene NFI

DIAGNOSIS OF NEOPLASIA

The diagnosis of neoplasia is based on clinical investigation, imaging, and laboratory testing which, ultimately, will involve histological examination of suspect tissue. It is now common for oncology services to work as a team, the pathological diagnosis being made only after detailed consultation over clinical features and imaging. Precision in diagnosis is particularly important as chemotherapy regimes are now closely matched to specific tumor types.

There are several techniques for obtaining tissue from a suspected neoplastic lesion.

Biopsy of tissues can be performed by several techniques (*Fig. 6.26*), and material processed for histology. Samples can also be assessed by electron microscopy.

Cytology can be performed on many types of tissue sample to look for neoplastic cells (*Fig. 6.27*). Increasingly, diagnoses of deep-seated solid tumors are being made by aspiration of cells, using a fine needle placed in the tumor under radiological control.

Cytological sampling of cells from some epithelial surfaces can be done without radiological control, and in some cases can be carried out in family practices without hospital admission. For example, cells from the surfaces of the cervix can be obtained easily by family practitioners, smeared onto microscopic slides, placed in fixative, and transported to a local laboratory for staining and microscopical examination. This technique not only identifies established malignant change in the epithelia, it also detects early dysplastic abnormalities in the epithelial cells which might indicate a pre-malignant change, so that full investigation can be performed, and the abnormal area treated or removed before full malignant change supervenes (see page 402).

Fig. 6.27
Methods of obtaining cells for cytological examination

Cells shed naturally into body fluids

Sputum, urine, CSF, fluid in pleural or peritoneal cavities

Cells obtained by exfoliation

Scrape smear of cervix
Brush cytology of lesions in gastrointestinal tract by endoscopy

Cells aspirated by needle

Blood and bone marrow
Needle aspiration of solid tumors (breast, thyroid, pancreas)

Fig. 6.26
Techniques for obtaining tissue samples by biopsy

Needle biopsy

Uses cutting needle to sample tumor
Sample is a core of tissue 1–2 mm wide and 2 cm long
Small size can make histological interpretation difficult
Can be applied to any lesion, including those in brain

Endoscopic biopsy

Uses small forceps to sample lesions seen at endoscopy
Samples are fragments 2–3 mm in size
Small size can make histological interpretation difficult
Applied to lesions in GI, respiratory, genital and urinary tracts

Incision biopsy

Scalpel used to remove sample of lesion
Sample is variable in size depending on nature of lesion
Applied to surgically accessible lesions only

Excision biopsy

Whole abnormal lesion surgically removed
Sample is variable in size depending on nature of lesion
Applied to surgically accessible lesions only

 Tumor markers

Certain tumors liberate products that can be detected in blood samples, thereby acting as tumor markers. These may aid diagnosis but may also be used to follow up therapy when blood levels become increased, often before imaging can detect tumor recurrence (*Fig. 6.28*).

Fig. 6.28
Examples of tumor markers

Tumor marker	Tumor
Alpha fetoprotein (AFP)	Hepatocellular carcinoma Germ cell tumors
Human chorionic gonadotrophin (HCG)	Trophoblastic tumors
Acid phosphatase	Prostatic carcinoma
Carcinoembryonic antigen (CEA)	Gastrointestinal tract neoplasia
Hormone products	Endocrine tumors

Special techniques for analysis of tumors

Once a tissue sample has been removed, special histological techniques can be used to assist diagnosis. To facilitate this the clinician must preserve the biopsy in an appropriate fashion, and it is usual to consult the laboratory over tissue handling in difficult cases.

Formaldehyde solution: routine histology.

Glutaraldehyde solution: electron microscopy.

Fresh-frozen: tumor marker or molecular genetic studies.

Cell culture medium: cytogenetic analysis.

Electron microscopy: used to look for ultrastructural evidence of cell differentiation that may not be evident on light microscopy, e.g. epithelial junctions, neurosecretory granules.

Immunohistochemistry: now frequently applied in the diagnosis of tumors, particularly when small samples of tissue are submitted for diagnosis.

Antisera to specific cell proteins can be used to stain slides, aiding identification of the cell of origin of a lesion. The most useful antibodies in general use are:

- Leukocyte common antigen and other lymphoid markers, which detect and type lymphoid tumors.
- Cytokeratin and polymorphic epithelial mucin, seen in epithelial tissues.
- Desmin and myoglobin, seen in muscle tumors.
- Prostate specific antigen, seen in carcinoma of the prostate.
- Alpha fetoprotein, seen in germ cell tumors.
- HCG, seen in trophoblastic tumors.
- Glial fibrillary acidic protein, seen in astroglial tumors.

Tumor markers, cytogenetic and molecular genetic studies are increasingly being used in diagnosis as well as in prognostic assessment of tumors. Examples are given, where relevant, with specific tumors discussed in the systems pathology section of the book.

Survival rates for tumors vary greatly between the different types

The length of survival following a diagnosis of neoplasia varies according to the biological nature of the tumor, how far it has spread, and whether any effective therapy can

be given. One of the most useful facts to remember for each of the tumor types is the average 5-year survival rate, as this allows the disease to be put into perspective during discussion with a patient. *Fig. 6.29* shows the current 5-year survival for a range of common tumors.

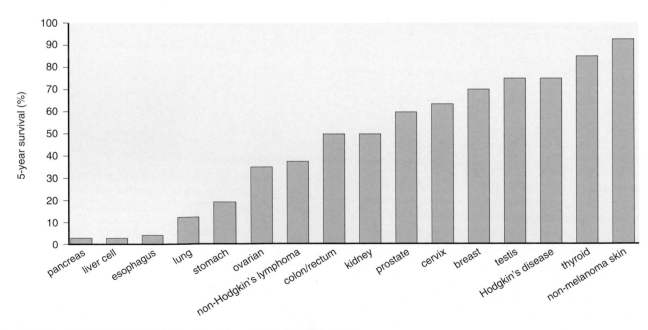

Fig. 6.29 Average 5-year survival rates for common neoplasms.
The chances of surviving for 5 years after diagnosis vary greatly according to the type of neoplasm.

IMMUNOLOGICAL FACTORS IN DISEASE

Designed to combat the effects of invasion by adverse environmental factors such as microorganisms and toxic chemical agents, the immune response is a normal defence mechanism. It usually works effectively, but illness may result from:

- Inadequate immune response.
- Excessive immune response.
- Unwanted or inappropriate immune response.

It is not our intention to present the various components and mechanisms of immune responses in disease, as these are covered in standard immunology texts, but rather to give a succinct outline of clinically relevant immunopathology.

INADEQUATE IMMUNE RESPONSES

Inadequate immune responses can result from immuno-deficiency states. There are two classes of immunodeficiency syndrome:

- Primary immunodeficiency, which is present at birth and often the result of a genetic disorder (*Fig. 7.1*).
- Secondary immunodeficiency, which is acquired secondary to drug treatment or disease process (*Fig. 7.2*).

X-linked agammaglobulinemia (Bruton's) is associated with low or absent B-cells and low levels of IgG

This occurs in male infants and is a panhypoglobulinemia. The levels of IgG are greatly reduced and other immuno-globulin levels are very low or absent. Although B-lymphocytes are greatly reduced or almost absent, cellular immunity is intact since T-cells are not involved. The infants present with recurrent pyogenic infections which characteristically begin sometime after about 6 months of age when all the maternal transplacental antibodies have disappeared. Common sites for infection are the lungs and bones and the commonest infecting bacteria are streptococci, pneumococci and *Haemophilus influenzi*. Normal mature B-cells do not form and therefore the lymph nodes lack lymphoid follicles and germinal centres, and no plasma cells are found in peripheral tissues. Failure of mature B-cells to form occurs at the pre-B-cell stage and

Fig. 7.1
Primary immunodeficiency states

Abnormal component of immune system	Example
Antibodies	X-linked hypogammaglobulinemia (Bruton's disease: X-linked recessive) Isolated IgA deficiency
T-cells	Thymic aplasia (DiGeorge's syndrome)
B-cells and T-cells	Severe combined immunodeficiency • Swiss type (autosomal recessive) • Adenosine deaminase deficiency (autosomal recessive) • X-linked recessive
Phagocytes	Chronic granulomatous disease
Complement	C2, C4 deficiency

Fig. 7.2
Main causes of secondary immunodeficiency

Old age
Chronic malnutrition
Widespread malignancy
Metabolic diseases (diabetes, chronic liver failure, chronic renal failure)
Drug therapy (cytotoxic therapy, steroid therapy)
Splenectomy (pneumococcal septicemia)
AIDS (acquired immune deficiency syndrome)

is associated with an abnormal gene on the X-chromosome responsible for the production of a tyrosine kinase.

Isolated IgA deficiency is a very common primary immunodeficiency but it is usually asymptomatic

In this condition there is a marked reduction in the level of serum IgA but other immunoglobulins are normal.

Lymphocytes responsible for producing IgA fail to mature into secreting IgA plasma cells. In most cases this isolated IgA deficiency is detected by accident, but some patients have an increased tendency to respiratory and other infections. Occasionally the isolated IgA deficiency is associated with a partial deficiency of other immunoglobulins, particularly IgG, and these patients have a greater incidence of recurrent infections.

Common variable immunodeficiency is a bit of a mixed bag

Patients with this disorder are predisposed to the development of recurrent infections. It occurs equally in men and women and the onset of the recurrent infections usually begins in the second or third decade of life. They are found to have markedly low immunoglobulin and antibody levels. It can be distinguished from X-linked Bruton's agammaglobulinemia by the fact that normal numbers of B-cells are present, although their function appears disordered, in some cases associated with impaired T-cell signalling. Sometimes there is an excess of T-suppressor cell activity or inadequate T-helper cell activity. Some cases are associated with intrinsic failure of pre-B-cells to mature. Patients with this condition have a high associated incidence of the common autoimmune disorders including Hashimoto's disease and rheumatoid arthritis.

The most important failure of T-cells is DiGeorge's syndrome

In these infants there is partial or complete failure of T-cells to form, associated with hypoplasia of the thymus gland. This failure is the result of failure of development of the third and fourth pharyngeal pouches and therefore the parathyroid glands are also absent. The affected infants have a characteristic facial appearance with midline facial clefts, mainly cleft palate, a small receding mandible and low-set ears. There is a high incidence of congenital cardiac malformations and the absence of the parathyroid glands leads to hypocalcemia.

Onset of recurrent infections begins soon after birth and the infants are particularly vulnerable to infections by viruses and intracellular bacteria. If a child has some thymic remnant and survives the early years, then T-cells may increase in number and efficiency of cell-mediated immunity may be almost normal by the age of 5 years. The prognosis is often associated more with the severity of the cardiac defect than the immunological defect.

The most common combined primary immunodeficiency of B- and T-cell function is called 'severe combined immune deficiency'

This condition may be inherited in either an autosomal recessive (Swiss type) pattern, or an X-linked recessive disorder. Some of the autosomal recessive types are associated with adenosine diaminase deficiency. The condition is due

to a failure of the development of both B-cell and T-cell precursors from the primitive stem cell. As a result of B- and T-cell failure the thymus is small or absent and lymphoid tissue in lymph nodes and the gut is also greatly reduced.

Children present early in life with recurrent infections including Candidal thrush, pneumonia and diarrhea. There is a very low blood lymphocyte count and low blood immunoglobulin levels. Without treatment (usually bone marrow transplantation), death occurs within the first 2 or 3 years of life. One of the most common fatal infections is *Pneumocystis pneumonia*, see page 199).

Ataxia–telangiectasia and the Wiskott–Aldrich syndrome are very rare forms of combined immune deficiency

Ataxia–telangiectasia is inherited as an autosomal recessive disorder and the syndrome comprises predisposition to infection associated with low IgE and IgA levels and depressed cell-mediated immunity, cerebellar degeneration and atrophy of the spinocerebellar tracts and peculiar areas of telangectatic blood vessels in the conjunctiva and on the flexor aspects of the forearm. The commonest site for recurrent infections is the upper respiratory tract including the nasal sinuses, and severe bronchiectasis is a long-term complication. The neurological manifestations become apparent when the child begins to walk and progressive mental retardation may occur. There may also be associated endocrine abnormalities including gonadal dysgenesis. There is an increased incidence in chromosome breaks, possibly suggesting a defect in repair of DNA. There is a high incidence of malignancy, particularly lymphoma, leukemia and brain tumors.

Wiskott–Aldrich syndrome presents clinically with eczema, recurrent infections and a low platelet count, and is an X-linked recessive disease affecting male infants. The earliest manifestations are usually due to the low platelet count and include hemorrhagic episodes, often from the alimentary tract. Recurrent respiratory infections develop later and children who survive to the age of 8 or more have a very high incidence of malignant lymphoma and acute lymphoblastic leukemia. Immunologically there is a low IgM level but the IgA and IgE levels are usually raised. Hematologically these children have small platelets and at least part of the reduction in number is due to increased destruction of circulating platelets by the spleen. Splenectomy may lead to a rise in platelet numbers. Bone marrow transplantation is the treatment of choice.

The most important primary abnormality of phagocytic cells is called 'chronic granulomatous disease'

This disease mainly occurs in boys and is due to an X-linked recessive inheritance pattern; a small proportion of cases show an autosomal recessive pattern. Blood and marrow neutrophils are deficient in the nicotinamide adenine dinucleotide phosphate (NADPH) oxidase system and are unable to produce hydrogen peroxide and superoxide, which destroys their bactericidal killing ability, leading to foci of persisting infection, particularly in the skin, bones, lung and lymph nodes. The infecting bacteria are often unusual organisms which are not usually severely pathogenic. The neutrophils are able to respond to infection by migration to the site and are able to phagocytose the bacteria. However once phagocytosed, the neutrophils are unable to kill the bacteria. As a result there is often a secondary macrophagic response in the area of infection producing histiocytic granulomas.

Secondary immunodeficiency is much more common than primary immunodeficiency

In general the immune system does not work well in early infancy and in old age, although infants are partly protected by the presence of maternal antibodies which have crossed the placenta. On a worldwide scale severe malnutrition is an important cause of an impaired immune response. An increasingly common and important cause of secondary immunodeficiency is as the result of drug therapy, either corticosteroid therapy for a wide range of diseases, or the specific immunosuppressive therapy given in transplantation to prevent rejection and as part of a cytotoxic chemotherapy regime for the treatment of malignant disease.

AIDS is an important cause of secondary immunodeficiency

AIDS (acquired immune deficiency syndrome) leads to severe impairment of the cell-mediated immunity system. In brief, infection by the human immunodeficiency virus (HIV-1) leads to destruction of CD4 lymphocytes and a decreased helper/suppressor T-cell ratio in the blood. The virus gains entry to T-cells by attaching to surface CD4 molecules in concert with one of the chemokine receptors, taking over cellular metabolism to synthesize new virus. The virus has several key protein components that can be used in diagnosis.

An immune response to virally infected cells develops, with both humoral and cell-mediated components. This initially contains the infection but, importantly, does not eliminate it. After several years, this immune response fails to control infection due to antigenic variation in virus proteins. (The median time from infection with HIV to development of clinical AIDS in transfusion cases is 4.5 years. For other groups the time-scale is unknown.) As the virus proliferates, there is depletion of CD4 cells, leading to severe immunosuppression.

Most disease is caused by RNA retrovirus HIV-1, but HIV-2, originally identified in Senegal, also causes AIDS and is most common in West Africa. Transmission is by sexual contact, blood transfusion, intravenous drug abuse,

---

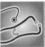

There are four clinical phases of HIV infection

Following infection with HIV, changes are seen in the number of circulatory T-lymphocytes and the presence of HIV antigen and antibody (*Fig. 7.3*), relating to four phases of infection.

1. Primary infection (seroconversion). After infection, a median time of 2 months elapses before antibodies to

HIV are detected in the blood. Rapid viral replication occurs in all organs (p24 antigen from the virus is detectable in blood), and an immune response develops, with increased numbers of CD8 cells in blood directed against viral antigen. About 50% of patients develop an influenza-like illness, rashes or lymphadenopathy at this

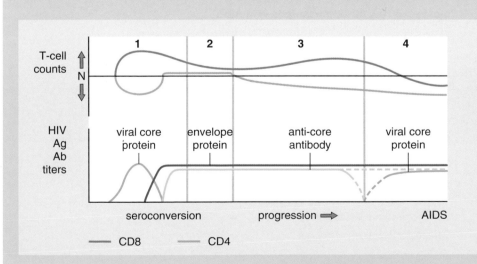

Fig. 7.3 Serological and cellular markers during HIV infection.
Chart showing relation of T-cell numbers to phase of infection with HIV.

1 = seroconversion
2 = asymptomatic
3 = AIDS-related complex
4 = AIDS

A fall in core antibody, with a subsequent rise in core antigen, is seen in some but not all patients progressing to HIV disease.

▶ time, associated with transient fall in CD4 lymphocytes. Antibody tests for HIV become positive around 6 weeks after infection.

2. Asymptomatic phase (incubation period). Individuals have antibodies to HIV in blood, but are otherwise asymptomatic. They are infective and can transmit the disease. The length of this phase is uncertain. There is a polyclonal hypergammaglobulinemia, and CD8 cells directed against viral antigens are increased in number in blood; numbers of CD4 cells remain within the normal range.

Symptoms relating to loss of immune regulation may become evident, such as worsening of pre-existing psoriasis, folliculitis or eczema, or development of immune thrombocytopenia.

3. AIDS-related complex. In this phase of HIV infection, as the proportion of CD4 infected cells increases, function of T-cells is partially impaired and their numbers in blood fall to around 400 cells/µliter. It is associated with non-specific general malaise, fever lasting longer than 3 months, night sweats, weight loss and diarrhea. Generalized lymphadenopathy is common (persistent generalized lymphadenopathy), with hematological and serological evidence of impaired cell-mediated immunity and reduced T-cell numbers.

Superficial fungal infections are frequent and infections with pathogens such as *Salmonella* and *Haemophilus* are severe. Similarly, gynecological infections such as candidiasis and pelvic inflammatory disease are increased.

The incidence of cervical intraepithelial neoplasia (see page 401) is increased because of greater susceptibility to genital human papilloma virus infection.

4. AIDS. In the late phase of HIV infection there is fully developed immunodeficiency, with complications of opportunistic infection, development of HIV infection of the central nervous system and development of neoplastic disease. In addition, infections with non-opportunistic organisms occur more frequently and with greater clinical severity. CD8-positive cells reacting against HIV become virtually undetectable in blood. The type of opportunistic infections that develop can be related to the degree of loss of CD4 cells, as summarized in *Fig. 7.4*.

Infection of the central nervous system by HIV produces an encephalitis that leads to a syndrome of motor slowing, cognitive decline and spinal cord disease in the late stages of HIV infection (see page 447).

Development of neoplastic disease is a common feature of late HIV infection.

- Kaposi's sarcoma produces purple-coloured tumors in any organ, but most typically in the skin. It is thought to be derived from an endothelial-like cell (see page 173).

- High-grade lymphomas of B-cell type are common, including primary lymphomas of the nervous system (see page 464).

- Invasive carcinomas of the cervix may develop as a result of human papillomavirus infection (see page 403).

Fig. 7.4
Opportunistic infections in AIDS

CD4 positive cells in blood (normal lower limit 450–500 cells/µliter)	Increased risk for opportunistic infection
Fewer than 300 cells/µliter	Tuberculosis and syphilis may become reactivated
Fewer than 200 cells/µliter	*Pneumocystis carinii* pneumonia Cerebral toxoplasmosis Systemic fungal infections including cryptococcal meningitis and histoplasmosis Progressive multifocal leukoencephalopathy due to papovavirus infection of CNS
Fewer than 150 cells/µliter	*Mycobacterium avium* infections
Fewer than 50 cells/µliter	Cytomegalovirus infection Parasitic infestations of the gut

and vertically from mother to child. High-risk groups are male homosexuals and bisexuals, IV drug abusers, Central Africans and their sexual partners, and hemophiliacs transfused with infected material.

Children with AIDS show clinical differences from adults

Children with vertical transmission of HIV show certain clinical differences from adult cases. About 25% of affected children die in the first year of life, with rapid development of immunosuppression, usually through development of *Pneumocystis* pneumonia. The 75% with a longer course of disease develop severe bacterial infections, with both routine pathogens and a range of opportunistic infections similar to those seen in adults.

Lymphocytic interstitial pneumonia occurs in 50% of affected children, but is rare in adult cases. CNS infection is manifest by developmental delay and progressive motor abnormalities.

EXCESSIVE IMMUNE RESPONSES

Excessive immune responses can cause 'hypersensitivity' reactions

Although immune mechanisms have a protective role in eliminating damaging agents, they may be abnormally amplified so that the response is damaging rather than beneficial. Such excessive immune responses can produce a severe and damaging reaction in a person exposed to a 'routine' antigen and are termed **hypersensitivity reactions**.

Hypersensitivity reactions have been divided into four types, known as Type I, Type II, Type III and Type IV responses. It is important to realize that more than one immunological mechanism may be involved in a single disease. Although it is possible to identify a predominant hypersensitivity response underlying an immune-related disease, other aspects of the immune response network are nearly always operating. Examples of diseases caused by hypersensitivity responses are presented in the systems chapters in this book (Chaps 10–25).

Type I hypersensitivity reactions are due to an excessive response of IgE to the presence of an allergen (antigen)

In this type of response (also known as immediate hypersensitivity or anaphylactic sensitivity) an often harmless antigen reacts with specific IgE antibodies located on membrane receptors on mast cells and blood basophils. The reaction between the antigen and the antibody causes rapid release of pre-formed potent chemicals from the mast cell into the surrounding tissue. The substances released include potent vaso-active and inflammatory mediators such as histamine and triptase. The reaction also causes the rapid production of leukotrienes and prostaglandins from

the precursor substance arachidonic acid within the mast cell, and these are also released in large quantities into adjacent tissues. These chemicals produce marked vasodilatation, smooth muscle spasm, increased permeability of small blood vessels, and excessive secretion by epithelial glandular tissue. The affected tissue also becomes heavily infiltrated by eosinophils and some other inflammatory cells. A group of patients who are particularly prone to develop Type I hypersensitivity reactions are those who produce excessive amounts of IgE which is specific as an antibody to normally innocuous protein antigens in the environment; these people are said to have an **atopic** tendency and can suffer from a wide range of the various clinical manifestations of Type I hypersensitivity. Many of these conditions are discussed elsewhere in this book. The commonest and most important are:

- Atopic dermatitis (acute eczema).
- Allergic rhinitis (hay fever), often associated with…
- Atopic conjunctivitis.
- Extrinsic allergic asthma.
- Food allergies.

A severe form of Type I hypersensitivity reaction is **anaphylaxis**. This is a severe acute IgE-mediated systemic reaction occurring in a person who is exposed to an antigen to which they have previously been sensitized. Important causative antigens include insect stings, drugs (particularly antibiotics), transfused blood products, and some food items, for example peanuts. The onset of symptoms is rapid. Within a short time after exposure to the sensitizing antigen, the patient becomes flushed and fretful and may complain of palpitations, odd tingling sensations, itching of the skin and difficulty breathing. They develop urticaria in the skin and in the larynx and often develop bronchospasm. If untreated they may develop shock, with cardiovascular collapse leading to death. These acute widespread systemic reactions are due to the antigen reaching the blood circulation. The potent mediators released by the mast cells when the antigen–antibody reaction occurs flood the circulation and produce widespread smooth muscle contraction and vascular dilatation. The fluid component of the blood passes quickly from the dilated, highly permeable blood vessels, leading to urticaria and angio-edema. This massive movement of fluid from the vascular compartment into the tissues is a major cause of shock, and similar movement of fluid from pulmonary wall capillaries into the alveoli produces pulmonary edema which may be fatal.

Type II hypersensitivity reactions result from circulating antibodies attaching to specific body antigens leading to death of the cells and tissues bearing the specific antigen

The circulating antibody binds specifically to some antigen as part of a tissue component, and this is followed by damage or death to the cells bearing the antigenic epitope.

The antibody-coated cells may be killed either as a result of lysis of the cell membrane following activation of the complement system or by killer cells directed against the antibody-coated cell. The target cells may also be phago-cytosed by macrophages. Important clinical examples include:

- Immune hemolytic anemia. Common and important examples include hemolytic disease of the newborn, autoimmune hemolytic anemia and incompatible blood transfusion.
- Antibody-induced thrombocytopenic purpura and neutropenia.
- Pemphigus and pemphigoid. In pemphigus there is an antibody to an antigen in the intracellular cement of the keratinocytes in the epidermis, mainly in the prickle cell layer. In pemphigoid the antibody is to an antigen situated in the epidermo-dermal basement membrane (see page 496).
- Goodpasture syndrome. This is due to a reaction between an antibody and the endothelium and basement membrane of glomerular capillaries in the kidney and the alveolar capillaries in the lung (page 364).
- Hyper-acute graft rejection of a renal transplant (see page 373).

Type III hypersensitivity reactions are due to the deposition in vessel walls or other tissues of soluble circulating antigen–antibody complexes

The immune complexes, after deposition, activate complement, leading to the attraction of neutrophil polymorphs and platelets to the site. Release of lysosomal enzymes from the attracted neutrophils and factors released from the attracted platelets initiate the tissue damage. This may be augmented by the formation of occlusive platelet aggregates within the lumen of very small blood vessels. Not all immune complexes lead to this type of damage; very small complexes may pass through the glomerular tuft and be excreted in the urine without causing any damage. Type III hypersensitivity reactions are characterized by the occurrence of a vasculitis in which there is fibrinoid necrosis of small blood vessel walls. Because complement is activated and consumed there is also usually a low blood level of some complement components.

Type IV hypersensitivity reactions do not involve antibodies but are cell-mediated and caused by sensitized T-lymphocytes

In Type IV reactions sensitized T-lymphocytes contact with a specific antigen and may cause damage by a direct toxic effect involving cytokine release which influences the activity of neutrophils, macrophages and lymphocyte killer cells. Some Type IV reactions are characterized by the presence of large numbers of lymphocytes and macrophages,

KEY FACTS
Hypersensitivity reactions

- Type I: IgE/mast cell-mediated liberation of histamine. Local and systemic anaphylaxis.
- Type II: antibodies bind to cell surface. Damage by complement activation or cellular cytotoxicity, or may stimulate/block a receptor.
- Type III: antigen–antibody complexes, either local or circulating types. Cause damage by activating complement in tissues at site of trapping of complexes.
- Type IV: T-cell-mediated: CD4 cells recruit macrophages; CD8 cells cause cytotoxicity.

sometimes with macrophage accumulation to produce granulomas. There are three main patterns of Type IV hypersensitivity:

- Reactions stimulated by microorganisms, particularly certain bacteria (tuberculosis and leprosy), some fungi (histoplasmosis, chronic candidiasis) and some viruses (see page 53).
- Contact dermatitis due to a reaction between sensitized T-lymphocytes and a complex antigen produced by a foreign substance and a carrier protein in the skin.
- Rejection of tissue or organ grafts.

INAPPROPRIATE IMMUNE RESPONSES

The most important inappropriate immune responses produce autoimmune diseases

Autoimmune diseases are the result of the body producing an immune response against its own tissues or individual tissue components. Sometimes the immune response is an antibody response (autoantibodies), sometimes it is a cell-mediated immune response. In many instances cell damage is by a cell-mediated cytotoxic response, and abnormal antibodies are generated to internal cell constituents, which are not, in themselves, damaging to cells. Such auto-antibodies are useful in diagnosis and typing of certain immune-mediated disease.

In autoimmune diseases it is recognized that the normal mechanisms ensuring tolerance for self-antigens have broken down. It is known that some autoimmune diseases have a genetic component, e.g. certain diseases are associated with particular HLA histocompatibility types. In other situations, an autoimmune disease can be triggered by a microbial infection, although the mechanisms underlying this are uncertain.

Fig. 7.5
Organ-specific autoimmune disease

Organ	Disease	Associated autoantibody	Comment
Skin	Vitiligo	Antityrosinase antibodies	Hypopigmentation
Thyroid	Graves' disease	Thyroid-stimulating antibodies Thyroid growth-stimulating antibodies	Hyperthyroidism caused by Type III stimulatory hypersensitivity response
Thyroid	Hashimoto's disease	Anti-thyroid specific antibodies	Hypothyroidism
Adrenal cortex	Addison's disease	Anti-adrenal antibodies	Hypoadrenocorticalism
Stomach	Autoimmune (Type A) gastritis	Anti-intrinsic factor and parietal cell antibodies	Pernicious anemia
Pancreatic islet cells (insulin-producing)	Type I diabetes mellitus	Anti-islet β-cell (insulin) antibody	Diabetes mellitus due to cell-mediated cytotoxicity to pancreatic β-cells
Skeletal muscle	Myasthenia gravis	Antibody to acetylcholine receptors	Muscle fatigue due to Type III inhibitory hypersensitivity response

Autoimmune diseases may either be organ-specific or affect many tissues

In some cases an autoimmune response is directed against a single component of a single tissue (**organ-specific autoimmune disease**) but, more often, it is against a tissue component present in many tissues and organs throughout the body (**non-organ-specific autoimmune disease**).

The organ-specific autoimmune diseases are listed in *Fig. 7.5*, each being discussed in more detail in the relevant later chapters. There is a tendency for several organs to be involved in affected individuals, suggesting that there is a general autoimmune predisposition for this group of diseases.

Autoantibodies directed against the diseased tissue are often found in the blood. In many cases it is uncertain whether the antibodies are pathogenic. It is known that healthy individuals produce small amounts of antibody against certain tissue components, but no harm ensues. For example, many people may have small titers of antibodies against nuclear DNA, but this is not associated with tissue damage. High titers of autoantibodies are nearly always associated with disease.

The most important **non-organ-specific autoimmune diseases** are summarized in *Fig. 7.6*, and each is discussed in greater detail in other chapters. Multiorgan involvement is frequently caused by secondary damage due to circulating immune complexes. For example, in systemic lupus erythematosus (SLE), there are autoantibodies against components of cell nuclei, particularly double-stranded DNA, which are not, in themselves, damaging to cells. Immune complexes form and are deposited in blood vessels, glomerular capillaries, skin, joints, skeletal muscle and brain, leading to tissue damage. This group of disorders is often

Fig. 7.6
Non-organ-specific autoimmune disease

Disease	Main organs involved	Page reference
Systemic lupus erythematosus	Skin, kidney, joints, heart, lung	see page 533
Progressive systemic sclerosis and variants	Skin, gut, lung	see page 536
Polymyositis and dermatomyositis	Skeletal muscle, skin	see page 470
Rheumatoid disease	Joints, lungs, systemic vessels	see page 537

collectively called the 'connective tissue diseases' as they have a major impact on blood vessels and support tissues throughout the body.

Immune responses prevent transplantation of organs from one individual to another

Organ transplantation is increasingly being used to treat irreversible diseases of the kidney, liver, heart, lung, and bone marrow. Unfortunately, the action of the immune system can lead to the transplanted tissue being destroyed, a process termed **transplant rejection**. For the best chance of survival, antigens in the graft and recipient must be alike.

After blood group identity, the most important set of antigens in transplantation immunology are the histocompatibility antigens, human leukocyte associated antigens (**HLA antigens**). The endothelial cells that line the blood vessels of the graft are particularly rich in both HLA antigens and blood group antigens, thus blood vessels are an important target of the host's immune response to a transplanted allograft. The effects of transplant rejection are discussed in relation to the transplanted kidney (see page 373), heart (see page 186) and bone marrow (see page 327).

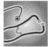

Laboratory medicine

Fig. 7.7
Autoantibodies used in the diagnosis of disease

Disease	Autoantibody correlating with disease diagnosis
Hashimoto's disease	Anti-microsomal, anti-thyroglobulin
Graves' disease	Anti-TSH receptor
Diabetes mellitus Type I	Anti-islet cell
Pernicious anemia	Anti-parietal cell, anti-intrinsic factor
Chronic active hepatitis	Anti-smooth muscle
Primary biliary cirrhosis	Anti-mitochondrial
Autoimmune thrombocytopenia	Anti-platelet
SLE	Anti-double-stranded DNA
Sjögren's syndrome	Anti-ribonucleoprotein
Scleroderma	Anti-centromeric
Rheumatoid disease	Rheumatoid factor (Anti-IgG)

Autoantibodies can be detected in the blood in many diseases (*Fig. 7.7*). Although it is not always certain that they are responsible for initiating the tissue damage, their detection in high titers provides a useful pointer to the diagnosis of some of these diseases (*Fig. 7.8*). The autoantibodies listed in the right hand column of *Fig. 7.7* have a high correlation for the diseases indicated. However, it is not uncommon to have several positive autoantibodies and, for some diseases, to have clinical and pathological overlap.

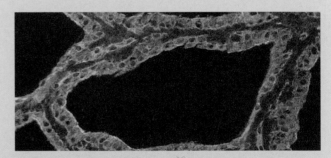

Fig. 7.8 Hashimoto's thyroiditis.
Unfixed cryostat section of human thyroid stained with labelled serum from a Hashimoto's patient.

8

Introduction to infectious diseases

Clinical Overview

In this section we present an overview of the body's response to infection. It is beyond the scope of this book to describe fully the many types of microorganisms and parasites that can produce disease in humans. Readers are referred to textbooks of microbiology and parasitology for the details of taxonomy and cultural characteristics. Examples of important specific infectious diseases are given in the relevant systems chapters of the book.

Infection is prevented by both specific and non-specific defence mechanisms

The body has non-specific and specific defence mechanisms, both of which serve to prevent organisms gaining access to tissues and causing infection.

Non-specific defence mechanisms play an important role in preventing infection, and the main ways in which these are breached are summarized in *Fig. 8.1*.

The acute inflammatory response (see Chapter 4) is able to immobilize and kill many types of infective organism in a non-specific manner. The immune system is able to mount a response against infections by both humoral and cell-mediated mechanisms, different organisms being neutralized by different mechanisms.

Spread of infection can be by several routes

Once an infective organism has gained entry to the body, it seldom remains localized but spreads to other tissues via several possible routes:

- **Local spread**. This route is facilitated by destruction of local tissues, especially if exotoxins are produced by the organism.
- **Lymphatic spread**. Organisms may be taken in macrophages to lymph nodes, or may gain access to lymphatic fluid. Enlargement of lymph nodes may be due to generation of an immune response, but may also be as a result of infection by the organism.
- **Hematogenous spread**. Organisms may travel freely in plasma (e.g. many bacteria and hepatitis B virus) or within cells such as monocytes (herpes, cytomegalovirus, HIV, mycobacteria). There are several terms used to

Fig. 8.1
Barriers to bacterial invasion

Barriers to invasion	Predisposition to infection
Keratin of skin	Wounds, insect bites
Glandular secretions and IgA e.g. in gut and lungs	Reduced in isolated IgA deficiency (*Fig. 7.1*)
Secretion currents e.g. in respiratory tract	Reduced by cigarette smoking Reduced in cystic fibrosis (see page 221) Reduced in immotile cilia syndromes (see page 221)
Bacterial commensals e.g. in vagina and gut	Changed by antibiotic therapy

describe blood spread of an infecting agent. Viremia and bacteremia are used to describe passive carriage of viruses and bacteria respectively, without growth in the bloodstream. The term 'septicemia' is used when there is severe systemic manifestation of bacteremia, with growth of bacteria in the bloodstream. This commonly leads to toxic shock syndrome.
- **Spread in tissue fluids**. This takes place in pleural and abdominal cavities, and is an important feature of peritonitis and pleural infections.
- **Neural spread**. The rabies virus and the varicella zoster virus produce infection by travelling along nerves.

BACTERIAL INFECTIONS

Bacterial pathogenicity is due to factors in the organisms as well as the host response

Pathogenicity describes the capacity of an organism to cause disease. Pathogenic bacteria can cause damage in several main ways:

- Bacteria can produce **exotoxins** that directly lead to cell and tissue damage.
- Bacteria can liberate **endotoxins** that cause systemic disease.

- Bacteria can produce toxins that functionally impair cells without cell death.
- Bacterial products may directly excite an acute inflammatory reaction.
- Antigens from the bacteria stimulate a Type III hypersensitivity reaction by the host.
- Bacterial antigens excite a chronic inflammatory response by stimulating a Type IV hypersensitivity reaction.

There is frequently overlap between these factors, and one organism may cause damage via several mechanisms.

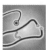

Endotoxic shock syndrome

Bacterial endotoxins are derived from the lipopolysaccharide (LPS) component of the outer bacterial cell wall. The most important endotoxins are those produced by Gram-negative organisms such as *Escherichia coli*, *Proteus* and *Pseudomonas aeruginosa*. They produce local effects, but the most important disorders are those associated with a Gram-negative septicemia in which the release of large amounts of endotoxin in the bloodstream produces **endotoxic shock syndrome**. The consequences are summarized in *Fig. 8.2*.

- Macrophages are stimulated to produce TNF-α.
- Neutrophils become activated and adhere to endothelium.
- The endothelium is activated, and releases nitric oxide, producing vasodilatation.
- Factor XII is activated by LPS and causes secondary activation of the coagulation/fibrinolytic system, kinin system, and complement system.

The major clinical features are profound hypotension, respiratory difficulty, tissue hypoxia, and systemic acidosis. The syndrome may cause death within hours of onset and is complicated by secondary changes in the lungs, termed 'adult respiratory distress syndrome' (ARDS) (see pages 205–207). If the patient survives, renal and liver failure commonly develop. The generalized activation of mediators of inflammation throughout the circulatory system has led to coinage of the term 'systemic inflammatory response syndrome' (SIRS).

Recently, monoclonal antibodies directed against LPS have been used therapeutically to block its effects in septicemic states. Additionally, monoclonal antibodies have been used to neutralize circulating IL-1 and TNF, thus preventing secondary damaging effects.

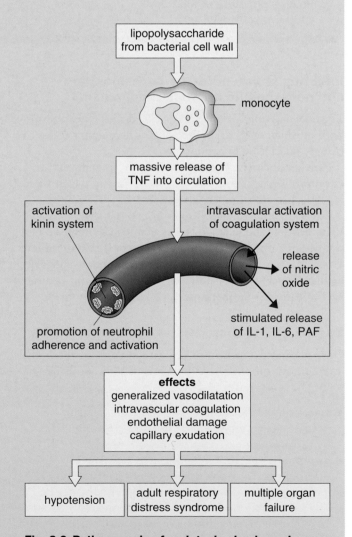

Fig. 8.2 Pathogenesis of endotoxic shock syndrome.

Some bacteria have a propensity to produce pus and are termed 'pyogenic'

Some bacteria produce a particularly vigorous acute inflammatory reaction, leading to local tissue necrosis. The reason for this is the presence of chemical factors in the bacterial walls which are chemoattractants for neutrophils. The infected necrotic area is liquefied by the effects of enzymes released by dying neutrophils, and is converted to a homogeneous semi-liquid material composed of dead host tissue, live and dead neutrophils, and live and dead bacteria, all suspended in the fluid component of the exudate.

The combination of necrotic tissue, acute inflammatory exudate and bacteria produces a semi-liquid material known as **pus**. For this reason, causative organisms are termed **pyogenic bacteria**.

Some bacteria produce a chronic granulomatous inflammatory response

Some organisms fail to excite an acute inflammatory response. Instead, the body mounts a Type IV hypersensitivity reaction, and the resulting tissue response is in the form of granulomatous inflammation (see page 53), as exemplified by pulmonary TB (see page 55).

The main organisms that excite a granulomatous response to infection are:

- TB, caused by *Mycobacterium tuberculosis*.
- Leprosy, caused by *Mycobacterium leprae*.
- Other mycobacterial infections.
- Syphilis (*Fig. 8.3*) and other spirochetal infections.
- *Yersinia enterocolitica* infection.
- Organism of cat-scratch disease (see page 307).

Syphilis causes chronic inflammation with Type IV hypersensitivity

Syphilis is caused by a spirochete, *Treponema pallidum*, which is mainly transmitted through sexual contact. The organisms gain access at the site of inoculation, usually the genitalia, and produce the primary lesion, known as a **chancre**. The organism is then disseminated throughout many organs from the site of inoculation. An immune response develops and the primary infection heals but, thereafter, the disease becomes a chronic inflammatory condition, affecting many organs. Serological tests can be performed to detect infection.

The pattern of disease is usually divided into four stages:

1 **Primary syphilis**. A chronic inflammatory nodule (chancre) forms in the skin or mucosa at the site of entry of the organism (typically penis, vulva or cervix). There is a heavy infiltrate of chronic inflammatory cells, particularly lymphocytes and plasma cells, which develops 1–12 weeks after exposure. The chancre ulcerates and there may be painless enlargement of local lymph nodes. Many spirochetes are present in the chancre, which is highly infectious. Long before the primary lesion develops, organisms have migrated to regional lymph nodes and throughout the body via the bloodstream. Frequently, the primary lesion is not noticed by the patient.

2 **Secondary syphilis**. This stage typically occurs 1–3 months after onset of the infection, resulting from spread of the organism to many sites in the body.

The most obvious manifestations are: any of a number of **skin rashes** (most frequently a coppery brown, diffuse, macular rash); mucosal involvement, with the formation of ulceration in the buccal mucosa (**snail-track ulcers**); shallow ulcers in the genital mucosa; and, often, the formation of warty growths around the genitalia (**condylomata lata**). Not only is this secondary stage the most infective, with large numbers of organisms in the ulcerated and warty mucosal lesions, the organism is also most likely to be transmitted to another person at this point. Generalized enlargement of the lymph nodes may also occur, and organisms are numerous in the lymph nodes. This stage typically lasts 4–12 weeks.

3 **Latent syphilis**. This is a stage in which an infected person is asymptomatic but still harbours the infection. There may be recurrence of secondary syphilis during this period.

4 **Tertiary syphilis**. This occurs after a period of latency, typically after 3–30 years. It affects about one-third of patients who have untreated syphilis. There are two main histological patterns of disease:
- Small vessels develop proliferation of their intimal lining, with surrounding plasma cell infiltration (endarteritis obliterans). This leads to tissue damage because of poor blood supply. The main consequence is development of **thoracic aortic aneurysm** (*Fig. 8.3*).

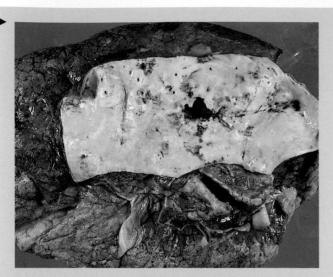

Fig. 8.3 Syphilitic aortitis and atheroma.
Inflammation of the aorta causes wall destruction and dilatation in the thoracic region.

- A Type IV cell-mediated immune response causes areas of necrosis to develop in several tissues. These areas of necrosis, known as 'gummas', are surrounded by activated macrophages, fibroblasts, and lymphoid cells including plasma cells.

The main effects of tertiary syphilis are summarized in *Fig. 8.4*.

Congenital syphilis is the result of transmission of the organism from an affected pregnant mother to the fetus, and many fetuses are stillborn as a result.

Active multiplication of the organisms in the fetus produces a characteristic pattern of syphilitic hepatitis, syphilitic pneumonia, and desquamation of skin, leading to early death.

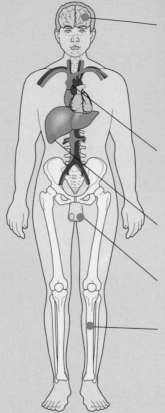

CEREBRAL DISEASE
Meningovascular disease: ischemic lesions, cranial nerve damage, strokes, sensory abnormalities
Parenchymal disease: infection by spirochetes causes dementia
Tabes dorsalis: Loss of spinal posterior columns

CARDIOVASCULAR SYSTEM
Aortic aneurysm formation (*Fig. 8.3*), widening of aortic valve ring, producing incompetence

LIVER
Gummas (pale areas of liver necrosis) resolve to scars (hepar lobatum appearance)

TESTIS
Gummas produce firm swelling simulating tumor

BONE
Gummas produce areas of bone necrosis – hard palate may be perforated

Fig. 8.4 Systemic involvement in tertiary syphilis.
Syphilis has its main effects on blood vessels, and the nervous system.

Osteochondritis and perichondritis cause bone deformities, e.g. malformation of tibiae (sabre shins) and inadequate development of the bones of the nose, which produces a flattened bridge (saddle nose). There may also be malformation of the teeth.

BRIEF REVIEW OF COMMON BACTERIA AND THEIR DISEASES

In this section we give a brief summary of the more frequently encountered bacteria and the important diseases they cause. For fuller details of taxonomy, cultural characteristics and laboratory investigation, students should consult a medical microbiology textbook.

Staphylococci are pyogenic (pus-forming) bacteria which can also cause disease by the exotoxins they secrete

These are Gram-positive cocci which normally colonize human skin. There are three common species, *S. aureus*, *S. epidermidis* and *S. saprophyticus*, of which *S. aureus* is most commonly responsible for pyogenic infection and the enterotoxin-associated syndromes.

S. aureus is an important cause of common bacterial skin infections such as superficial folliculitis, boils, and particularly wound infections. It may also cause pneumonia and lung abscess (particularly in children), lactational breast abscess and osteomyelitis (children), all characterized by the production of tissue necrosis and pus-formation. Exotoxins secreted by *S. aureus* can produce a range of disorders, including an acute gastroenteritis (see *Fig. 8.5*)

An important group of *S. aureus* are those which have developed resistance to the potent antibiotic methicillin (**methicillin resistant staphyloccus aureus – MRSA**). This is an important cause of hospital-acquired infections.

Fig. 8.5
Important diseases due to *S. aureus* exotoxins

Toxin	Disease	Clinical features
Enterotoxins A and D	Acute gastroenteritis	Food poisoning, usually vomiting only, 3–6 hrs after ingestion Processed meats, dairy products
Toxic shock syndrome toxin	Toxic shock syndrome	Septicemia and toxemia, exfoliating rash on palms and soles *S. aureus*-colonized tampons a cause in women
Epidermolytic toxin ('exfoliatin')	Staphylococcal scalded skin syndrome	Usually infants Toxin destroys intercellular connections between keratinocytes → blistering → desquamation/exfoliation

Fig. 8.6
Important diseases caused by *Streptococcus pyogenes*

Direct infection

Skin	Impetigo	Pustular infection of epidermis
Skin	Erysipelas	Spreading infection of dermis (see page 492 and *Fig. 8.7*)
Soft tissues	Cellulitis and necrotizing fasciitis	Severe spreading infection of subcutis and deeper tissues (see page 492)
Upper respiratory tract	Pharyngitis and tonsillitis	Bacterial sore throat
Uterus	Puerperal sepsis	From skin, nose or throat of medical attendants – now rare

Toxin/immunologic infection

Skin	Scarlet fever	Red rash due to erythrogenic toxins
Kidney	Acute glomerulonephritis	Immune reaction of streptococcal pharyngitis (see page 360)
Heart and other organs	Rheumatic fever	Immune reaction to cell wall component of *Streptococcus pyogenes* (see page 189)

S. epidermidis is less pathogenic than *S. aureus*, but is a particularly important infecting organism of prostheses, such as prosthetic heart valves, ventriculo-peritoneal shunts, and other long-term catheters including indwelling urinary catheters. *S. saprophyticus* rarely causes post-coital urinary tract infection in women.

Streptococci of medical importance can be divided into β hemolytic and α hemolytic types

The pathogenic β hemolytic streptococci can be divided into two groups, A and B. Group A (*Streptococcus pyogenes*) is the most important and produces a wide range of diseases (see *Figs 8.6* and *8.7*). Group B (*Streptococcus agalactiae*) is a much less important pathogen, but can cause neonatal meningitis and septicemia. The organism is a commensal in the vagina and infection may occur at birth during passage through a colonized birth canal.

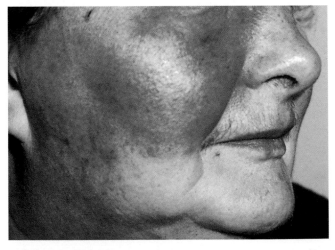

Fig. 8.7 Erysipelas of the face.
Spreading acute inflammation of the dermis and subcutis due to infection by *Streptococcus pyogenes*.

The most important α hemolytic streptococcus is *Streptococcus pneumoniae*

This organism (also called the pneumococcus) colonizes the human respiratory tract in up to 5% of the normal population, rising particularly in winter and early spring to 40–50%. Spread is by droplet cross-infection. The most common infections are:

- Acute otitis media, particularly in infants and children (see page 238).
- Pneumonia, particularly of lobar pattern (see page 196).
- Acute purulent meningitis, particularly after otitis media, infection of paranasal sinuses, and pneumonia (see page 445).

In the early stages of acute pneumococcal infections, there is frequently a transient bacteremia, and blood culture can be a useful investigation.

Other streptococci are important causes of bacterial endocarditis

The *Streptococcus viridans* group includes members which are important infectors of previously damaged heart valves (subacute bacterial endocarditis – see page 183) and *Streptococcus bovis* also causes bacterial endocarditis. The organisms formerly grouped as *Streptococcus faecalis* are now reclassified as enterococci. Their normal habitat is the gut of humans and animals. They cause urinary tract and wound infections, and occasionally infect heart valves.

Neisseria are Gram-negative cocci which can produce gonorrhea or meningitis, and a particularly virulent form of septicemia

Neisseria gonorrhoeae ('gonococcus') is the bacterium responsible for the sexually transmitted disease gonorrhea, which infects urethra, prostate, epididymis and testis in men, and vagina, cervix, uterus and fallopian tubes in women (see pages 384 and 410). It can also produce a gonococcal bacteremia with pustular skin lesions and arthritis. In women, the infection may lead to a salpingitis which, if severe, may proceed to pelvic inflammatory disease and infertility.

Neisseria meningitidis ('meningococcus') is carried in the pharynx of 5% of people and is an important cause of acute bacterial meningitis (see page 445), particularly in young children. It tends to occur in minor epidemics, mainly in closed or semi-closed institutions such as schools and colleges. Acute meningococcal septicemia (which may occur without evidence of meningitis) is one of the septic shock syndromes. It is clinically characterized by rapid onset, circulatory collapse, multiorgan failure and widespread disseminated intravascular coagulation, with a high fatality rate. A rapidly spreading petechial rash in the skin (see page 497) and bilateral hemorrhagic necrosis of the adrenals (see page 343) are characteristic.

Corynebacteria are mainly commensal, but one species causes diptheria

Corynebacteria are widely distributed in nature and are mostly harmless. Diphtheria, however, is caused by certain toxigenic strains of *Corynebacterium diphtheriae*, normally located in the pharynx, nasopharynx or tonsils. Occasionally the primary focus is in the skin, usually an infected abrasion, cut, ulcer or burn. Local production of exotoxin produces necrosis and acute inflammation in adjacent cells and tissues, in the pharynx and tonsil producing the so-called 'diphtheric membrane' composed of necrotic mucosal cells, submucosa, and the associated acute inflammatory exudate.

Systemic distribution of the toxin may produce degeneration and necrosis of myocardial fibres, and cranial and peripheral nerves, and impaired kidney function due to interstitial nephritis. There is also generalized toxemia and prostration.

The genus *Bacillus* are soil organisms: one type produces food poisoning and the other causes anthrax

Bacillus cereus is an important cause of food poisoning with two different patterns, each due to different bacterial toxins. One toxin produces vomiting 1–4 hours after ingestion, and the other causes diarrhea about 12 hours after ingestion. The toxins are food-borne, and are common on rice and other pulses. This form of food poisoning is most common after eating previously cooked rice which is reheated.

Bacillus anthracis causes anthrax, a potentially fatal disease which is now rare. Anthrax is primarily a disease of herbivorous farm and domestic animals, and human disease is acquired by contact with feces, urine or saliva of affected animals. The anthrax spores can enter through human skin, and produce swelling and ulceration, with the ulcer being covered by a characteristic black necrotic scab. In most cases the lesion and infection remain localized to the area of primary penetration, but in a small percentage of cases a severe septicemia develops, which is usually fatal.

Inhalation of spores leads to the site of primary penetration being in the lung alveoli ('pulmonary anthrax') with pulmonary edema and hemorrhage. Direct infection from infected animals is now very rare except in the developing world, and occasional cases are still attributed to contact with animal products such as hides, skins, wool, etc. It is known that anthrax spores are very long-lived.

Clostridial diseases are mainly due to the effects of potent toxins

Clostridia are anaerobic bacilli which produce long-lived spores, which may be found in the soil and in the gut of humans and animals. There are four main types, each producing a different toxin-mediated disease (see *Fig. 8.8*).

Fig. 8.8
Diseases due to clostridial toxins

Clostridium difficile	Pseudomembranous colitis	See page 255
Clostridium perfringens	Gas gangrene	Infection of dirty (e.g. soil-containing) wounds Toxins lead to spreading destruction of tissue
Clostridium tetani	Tetanus (lockjaw)	Neurotoxin (tetanospasmin) causes muscle spasms and convulsions Frequently fatal Soil contamination of penetrating wound
Clostridium botulinum	Botulism	Ingestion of pre-formed neurotoxin in inadequately sterilized or processed food Muscle paralysis and death

Listeria monocytogenes causes meningitis in the newborn and elderly, and abortions in pregnant women

The organism *Listeria monocytogenes* is excreted in large amounts in cows' milk, and may therefore be present in unpasteurized dairy products. However, it is also an occasional component of the normal gut flora. Infection of neonates usually results from trans-placental infection from an infected mother, and adults acquire the infection by ingestion of contaminated food. Significant clinical infection is associated with some element of immune incompetence in many cases.

Escherichia coli is responsible for a wide range of diseases according to the type of virulence factors possessed by the particular pathogenic strain

E. coli is a normal commensal in the human gut, and all strains produce an endotoxin. Pathogenic varieties have additional virulence factors which produce different patterns of disease. One of the most important virulence factors is a group of enterotoxins which produce diarrheal disease, some varieties of which also induce the hemolytic uremic syndrome, leading to acute renal failure and death. The important pathogenic elements of *E. coli* infection are:

- urinary tract infection – local spread from anus.
- neonatal meningitis – the virulence factor is the presence of a capsule (K1 capsular type) around the bacterium.
- diarrheal diseases – often severe, watery and hemorrhagic, associated with strains which produce strong enterotoxins. The strain known as *E. coli* 0157:H7 (enterohemorrhagic *E. coli*) has a high mortality rate because it is complicated by hemolytic–uremic syndrome. Spread is by the feco-oral route, and from contaminated foods such as undercooked beef.

Proteus species are gut commensals which can also cause urinary tract infection

Like *E. coli*, this Gram-negative bacillus normally colonizes the colon, but can spread locally from the anus to produce urethritis, cystitis and pyelonephritis.

They may also produce wound infections, particularly hospital-acquired, and rarely produces an atypical pneumonia, otitis media or suppurative mastoiditis.

Enterobacter, *Serratia* and *Klebsiella* are also Gram-negative rods commensal in the gut, and may cause lower urinary tract infections: The infections usually occur in the elderly or immune-suppressed who are in hospital. *Klebsiella* can produce a severe atypical hemorrhagic pneumonia, often with lung abscess, in vulnerable individuals such as the immunosuppressed, malnourished and diabetic.

Salmonella and Shigella species are not normally present as commensals in the gut, and cause diarrheal disease

The Salmonella group contains many members (belonging to *S. enteritidis* group), most of which cause diarrheal disease which remains confined to the bowel with no spread of bacteria beyond. *Salmonella typhi* and *paratyphi* produce systemic diseases ('typhoid fever' and 'paratyphoid fever') in which bowel involvement is only part of a widespread symptomatic bacteremia. The organisms are ingested in contamined water (in underdeveloped countries) or in food which has been contaminated during handling by someone who is a carrier of the organism. Asymptomatic carriers excrete *Salmonella typhi* in feces and urine. The onset is gradual with non-specific malaise, fever and headache, sometimes with myalgia and arthralgia. This represents the stage when the organisms have entered via the gut and are being disseminated by lymphatics and thence to the bloodstream. The mucosa-associated lymphoid tissue in the gut, particularly the Peyer's patches in the small intestine, become enlarged, and larger lymphoid aggregations become ulcerated, often manifest as diarrhea which is sometimes bloody. Perforation through the necrotic Peyer's patches in terminal ileum may occur. Recovery and relapse are frequent, and after recovery the patient may become a chronic carrier, and a potential source of infection to others.

The Shigella group comprises four important organisms responsible for bacillary dysentery: **Shigella dysenteriae** causes the most severe symptoms. There is sudden onset of watery and bloody diarrhea often with abundant mucus, with severe dehydration (which may be fatal in children without proper medical care). The symptoms and outlook are generally most severe in children; adults may have a more gradual onset and milder symptoms. Infection is by the feco-oral route from the feces of carriers or convalescents, and flies and food may be intermediate stepping stones. Pathologically, the bowel mucosa is hyperemic, acutely inflamed and focally ulcerated.

Vibrio cholerae produces severe watery diarrhea, and leads to dehydration and electrolyte imbalance

The organism *Vibrio cholerae* is usually spread by the ingestion of water contaminated by the feces of an infected person, and is endemic in the summer months in areas of the world where public and personal sanitation is poor. In addition, small or large epidemics may occur at any time when there is a major breakdown in public sanitation, for example after severe flooding destroys sewage systems and fresh water supplies.

The symptoms are due to an enterotoxin and the organism has to be ingested in very large numbers to produce disease, since gastric acid destroys most of them. Any surviving bacteria pass into the small intestine which, if conditions are suitable for the organism, rapidly becomes colonized by adherence of the bacterium to the mucosal surface. The enterotoxin is produced in large quantities and leads to profuse outpouring of large quantities (up to 1 L every hour) of fluid, passed as a clear watery stool ('rice water stool'). Loss of water and electrolytes leads to severe dehydration and metabolic disturbance (mainly hypokalemia and metabolic acidosis due to loss of bicarbonate). Unless the fluid and electrolyte imbalance is restored by intravenous fluid and electrolyte therapy, hypovolemic shock, cardiac irregularities and death will occur.

Yersinia enterocolitica produces an enterocolitis which can be clinically similar to acute appendicitis

Infection results from eating contaminated food of many types. During a sub-clinical incubation period of about a week, it is believed that the organism invades the epithelium of the small intestine and finds its way into the mucosa-associated lymphoid tissue, particularly the Peyer's patches, where they cause necrosis. Histologically, the foci of necrosis are surrounded by macrophages and giant cells to form granulomas, and may sometimes be difficult to distinguish from tuberculous infection and Crohn's disease. Mesenteric lymph nodes are enlarged and may contain granulomas. These developments are clinically matched by abdominal pain, diarrhea and fever. The pain is often in the right iliac fossa, similar to acute appendicitis. The symptoms may last for some weeks.

Another Yersinia, *Y. parahaemolyticus*, causes a more acute diarrheal illness, sometimes with vomiting and fever, following the ingestion of contaminated fish and shellfish. Symptoms begin any time from 12 to 48 hours after ingestion, and last for 24–48 hours.

Another Yersinia (*Y. pestis*) causes the historically famous disease called 'the plague'

Now rare, the plague was a common epidemic illness in Europe, the Middle East and the Far East for hundreds of years. Major epidemics in Europe in the 14th century (the 'Black Death') and in England in 1665 caused a significant reduction in population (estimated to be as high as 25% in some areas). Some small towns and villages, such as Eyam in Derbyshire, England, were almost completely wiped out in a matter of months. The organism causes mild infection in a variety of rodents, which form its natural reservoir. The major human epidemics are caused by transmission from rats to humans via bites from the rat flea, which become heavily infected by feeding on the blood of rats.

The bacteria proliferate and pass in lymphatics to lymph nodes which enlarge and become necrotic and hemorrhagic ('buboes') within a few days. From these the bacteria may pass in the bloodstream to the lungs to cause pneumonic plague, which is almost invariably fatal. Acute septicemia is associated with disseminated intravascular coagulation which produces extensive internal hemorrhage and a confluent petechial and blue-black ecchymotic rash in the skin, the reason for the ancient name 'the Black Death'.

Campylobacter species are a common and important cause of diarrhea

The most common Campylobacter is *C. jejuni* which is responsible for most cases of Campylobacter diarrhea. Clinically, the illness resembles Salmonella enteritis (see page 119) but may persist for longer, up to 3–4 weeks. In persistent disease the symptoms and signs may be difficult to distinguish from an attack of ulcerative colitis. Endoscopic examination of the colon may show inflamed and reddened mucosa, with focal superficial hemorrhage and ulceration; however, similar changes are also seen in the ileum and jejunum, not a feature of ulcerative colitis.

The organisms are widespread in many domestic animals, including cattle, sheep and poultry, and human infection is thought to be acquired through ingestion of contaminated food, particularly milk and poultry.

The organism formerly known as *Campylobacter pylori* associated with gastritis and duodenal ulcer has been re-classified and renamed *Helicobacter pylori* (see page 251).

Actinomyces israelii causes chronic suppurating abscesses in the neck, and less commonly in the appendix region

Actinomyces are common commensals in the mouth, particularly in the crypts of the tonsils and around the necks of the teeth. Occasionally, the organism becomes pathogenic, with spread into the soft tissues of the neck to produce a lumpy swelling (see *Figs 8.9* and *8.10*) which can discharge onto the surface through numerous sinuses. A thin watery fluid discharges, within which can be seen small yellow fragments ('sulphur granules') which are large aggregated colonies of the organism. The original source of the infection may be an infected tooth.

Actinomycosis may also occur in the abdomen, particularly in the right iliac fossa after appendix surgery.

Haemophilus influenzae causes a range of infections, including meningitis in children

Haemophilus species are common commensals in the upper respiratory tract, but only *Haemophilus influenzae* produces disease. It is responsible for acute exacerbations of chronic bronchitis in adults, but is mainly a disease of young children, causing acute tracheobronchitis and pneumonia, sinusitis, otitis media and epiglottitis. It was formerly an important cause of acute purulent meningitis in young children, but is becoming less so as a result of vaccination.

One of the most important virulence factors for *Haemophilus influenzae* is the possession of a capsule; non-capsulated forms are rarely pathogenic except as secondary invaders of the respiratory tract.

Haemophilus ducreyi causes the mainly tropical disease called chancroid, in which painful ulcers develop on the genitalia, often associated with inguinal lymph node enlargement.

Mycobacteria are the causative organism of tuberculosis and leprosy

Mycobacteria are characterized by the possession of a resistant cell wall containing mycolic acids which are long-chain fatty acids, and are able to resist dehydration and destruction both in the environment and in the animals which they infect, e.g. humans, cows, fish, birds. Two varieties produce the most important diseases. *M. tuberculosis* (see *Fig. 8.11*) produces tuberculosis in man and other

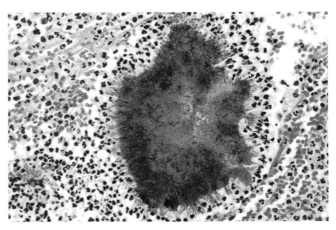

Fig. 8.10 Actinomycosis.
A colony of *Actinomyces israelii* in a jaw abscess. The colony is surrounded by neutrophils. These colonies form the so-called 'sulphur granules' which are extruded when the abscess discharges.

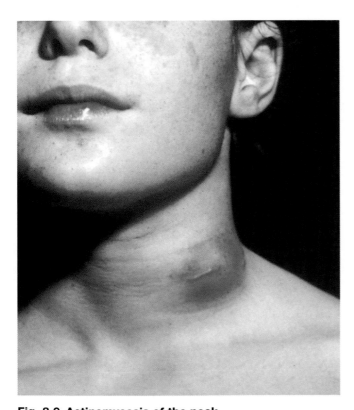

Fig. 8.9 Actinomycosis of the neck.
Actinomycotic abscess oozing clear fluid at its center, which will soon discharge to produce yellow 'sulphur' granules.

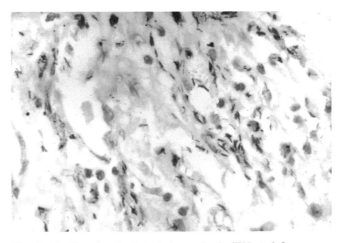

Fig. 8.11 *Mycobacterium tuberculosis* (ZN stain).
The acid-fast mycobacteria are stained a reddish color, other cell components being blue.

animals, and *M. leprae* causes leprosy. These conditions are discussed elsewhere in this book. *Fig. 8.12* shows brief details of other mycobacterial diseases.

Treponema pallidum is a spiral bacterium which causes syphilis

The organism *Treponema pallidum* is very sensitive, and is easily destroyed by heat and drying, so successful transmission is largely confined to intimate sexual contact between mucosal surfaces. The pathology of syphilis is illustrated and discussed on pages 115–116.

Other treponemes cause diseases which are not sexually transmitted, summarized in *Fig. 8.13*.

The Treponema species cannot be grown successfully in artificial culture media, so diagnosis is made on clinical features, microscopic examination of infected tissue and serology.

Leptospirosis is contracted by contact with rat urine in water

Leptospira are spiral bacteria which cause kidney infection in small mammals, particularly rats, which then pass the organism into rivers in their urine. Human infection can be by ingestion or penetration (e.g. through broken skin) of the organism, which passes into the bloodstream, the bacteremia being associated with a mild febrile illness which usually resolves with no further symptoms. In a small percentage of such cases, rapid proliferation of the organism

in the blood leads to septicemia with kidney failure, jaundice, hemorrhage and liver failure due to leptospiral hepatitis (Weil's disease).

Lyme disease is caused by a spirochete transmitted to humans through tick bites

The causative organism is *Borrelia burgdorferi*, a spirochetal bacterium which occurs in a wide range of mammals, but most human infections come from sheep, deer or dogs. The bacterium is transmitted to man through tick bites, the ticks jumping from the host mammal directly onto human skin, or more commonly from the grass on which the animals graze. The ticks are normally small and difficult to see until they have been attached to human skin for sufficient time to become distended with human blood; the bacterium is transmitted to humans during this blood-sucking phase.

The usual first symptom of the disease is a red spot or patch of erythema at the site of the bite, the characteristic pattern of progression being the pattern known as **erythema migrans**, in which the red patch enlarges peripherally and shows central clearing. This is accompanied by systemic symptoms such as fever, lethargy and muscle and joint pains. Later on most patients develop flitting and intermittent arthritis, particularly involving the knees, and these arthritic symptoms may occur on and off for months or even years. A few patients develop CNS symptoms, particularly meningoencephalitis and cranial nerve lesions.

Fig. 8.12
Mycobacterial diseases other than tuberculosis and leprosy

Mycobacterium ulcerans	Chronic skin ulcerated nodule (Buruli ulcer)	Africa and Australia
Mycobacterium marinum	Chronic skin ulcerated nodules	From contaminated water, e.g. aquaria, swimming pools
Mycobacterium avium (intracellulare)	TB-like cervical lymphadenopathy or lung lesions. Disseminated colonization of macrophages throughout body (AIDS-related)	Opportunistic infection in AIDS patients

Fig. 8.13
Other treponemal diseases

Endemic syphilis ('bejel')	West Africa Eastern Mediterranean	Nodular skin lesions Gummatous lesions later	*Treponema pallidum endemicum*
Yaws	Tropical equatorial	Nodule in skin at inoculation site, widespread skin granulomas, gummas, periostitis	*Treponema pallidum pertenue*
Pinta	Central and South America	Nodule at inoculation site becoming indurated plaques with depigmentation	*Treponema carateum*

Brucellosis is contracted by contact with infected animals or their products

The Brucella group are primary animal pathogens, and human infection is acquired by direct contact, ingestion (e.g. in infected milk) or inhalation. Organisms gain access to the bloodstream via lymphatics, and produce an illness characterized by malaise and fever with no localizing signs other than occasional lymphadenopathy. Histologically, the lymph nodes, liver, spleen and bone marrow may contain foci of granulomatous inflammation with central necrosis in some granulomas. The ill-defined symptoms may persist for weeks or months, and a few cases go on to chronic brucellosis, with the relapsing illness lasting for more than a year. There are three main pathogenic species, each with a different animal host:

- *Brucella abortus* (cow): worldwide, but most commercial herds are now Brucella-free.
- *Brucella melitensis* (sheep and goats): countries around the Mediterranean Sea, South America and Mexico.
- *Brucella suis* (pigs): southeast Asia, South America and the USA.

Legionella causes a severe atypical pneumonia known as Legionnaire's disease

Legionella is a recently discovered organism (Gram-negative rod) which is usually contracted by inhaling water droplets from contaminated water supplies such as cooling towers, domestic and institutional shower systems and air-conditioning devices. There are about 20–30 species, but *Legionella pneumophila* is responsible for most cases. Inhalation may lead to:

- Development of anti-Legionella antibodies, but without the development of symptoms.
- A mild transient flu-like illness, called Pontiac fever.
- Full-blown Legionnaire's disease.

In Legionnaire's disease, an incubation period of 2–10 days, during which the patient may develop fever, malaise and flu-like symptoms, is followed by evidence of lung infection. This is signified by cough with mucoid sputum, high fever, and X-ray changes of patchy lung consolidation. There may also be diarrhea and mental confusion. The patchy lung consolidation spreads to become confluent and often bilateral, with rapidly deteriorating lung function. Even with early diagnosis and appropriate antibiotic therapy, the overall mortality rate is as high as 10–20%. In severe infections, investigations show evidence of impaired liver and kidney function. Legionella pneumonia is an important community- and institution-acquired lung infection (see page 198).

Chlamydia are increasingly becoming recognized as associated with a wide range of diseases

Chlamydia are intracellular organisms, formerly thought to be viruses, but now classified as bacteria. There are three main groups. The commonest, *Chlamydia trachomatosis*, has many sub-types which give rise to a wide range of diseases:

C. trachomatosis sub-types D–K are the organisms responsible for a large number of sexually transmitted diseases the most frequest of which are cervicitis, urethritis, salpingitis and pelvic inflammatory disease in women, and urethritis and epididymo-orchitis in men. It is a cause of Reiter's syndrome (see page 528). Members of this group may infect newborn infants on their passage through an infected maternal birth canal, particularly producing conjunctivitis.

C. trachomatosis subtype L produces the sexually transmitted disease, lymphogranuloma venereum.

The other two main groups are *C. psittaci* which causes the human pneumonitis, psittacosis (see page 198) transmitted from birds, and *C. pneumoniae* which causes atypical pneumonia, particularly in the young. This last organism has been postulated to play a role in the development of atheroma.

The most common disease caused by Bartonella is cat-scratch fever

Bartonella are small Gram-negative bacilli which are passed to humans by an insect vector from an animal reservoir. The most widespread organism is *Bartonella henselae* (formerly *Rochalimaea henselae*) which exists as a commensal in the tissues and blood of up to 50% of domestic cats.

The human illness cat-scratch disease is thought to result from the organism gaining access to the human skin by way of a scratch from the cat's claws, but many patients give no history of a scratch and have no evidence of a primary inflammatory skin lesion, so it is possible that in some cases the organism is transmitted via the cat flea. The main abnormality in the patient with cat-scratch disease is regional lymphadenopathy (see page 306), in which the histological features are characteristic, and almost diagnostic.

In AIDS patients, severe systemic infections may cause a severe feverish illness, often associated with raised red polypoid lesions in the skin ('bacillary angiomatosis') which may be clinically confused with the early lesions of Kaposi's sarcoma.

Other varieties of Bartonella cause 'trench fever', a feverish condition common in foot soldiers in both World Wars, and a disease in the Andes ('Oroya fever').

Rickettsial diseases are transmitted by insect vectors (usually ticks) and cause a range of febrile illnesses with headaches, rash and malaise

Rickettsiae are intracellular cocco-bacilli, usually transmitted to humans by tick bites from an animal reservoir which consists mainly of rodents of various types. There is significant geographical localization in most cases (see *Fig. 8.14*).

Fig. 8.14
Diseases due to rickettsial infection

Disease	Location	Organism	Host(s)	Transmitted by	Usual symptoms	Severe complications
Rocky Mountain spotted fever	USA	*Rickettsia rickettsii*	Small mammals, e.g. dog, rabbit	Ixodid ticks	Fever, headache, myalgia Hemorrhagic rash	Encephalitis, pneumonia, circulatory collapse
Epidemic typhus	Worldwide	*Rickettsia prowazekii*	Humans	Human body louse	Prolonged fever, headache, rash (often hemorrhagic)	Encephalitis, pneumonia, hypotension and renal failure
Endemic (murine) typhus	Worldwide (sporadic)	*Rickettsia typhi*	Rodents	Cat and rat fleas	Similar to epidemic typhus	Rare
Q fever	Worldwide	*Rickettsia burnetii*	Goats, sheep, cattle, rodents	In humans by inhalation or ingestion	Fever, headache, myalgia, pneumonia	Aortic valve endocarditis, granulomatous hepatitis Atypical lobar pneumonia
Scrub typhus (Tsutsugamushi disease)	Far East	*Rickettsia tsutsugamushi*	Rodents	Mite	Fever, headache, rash, ulcer at site of bite, lymphadenopathy	Severe pneumonitis Myocarditis

FUNGAL INFECTIONS

Fungi are ubiquitous in the environment. Many reside innocuously on the skin surface, some are commensals on the mucosal surfaces (e.g. the mouth and vagina), but very few are pathogenic. Pathogenic fungal infections can be divided according to the pattern of involvement:

- Superficial and deep fungal infections of the skin (see page 491).
- Infections of mucosal surfaces.
- Lung infections due to inhaled fungi (see page 198).
- Systemic blood-borne infections.

Immunosuppression is an important predisposing factor for fungal infections.

The main fungal infections of clinical significance are: dermatophytic fungi (skin), *Candida albicans* or thrush (mucosal and systemic), Aspergillus spp. (lung and systemic), zygomycoses (nasal sinuses), Cryptococcus (lung and brain), and Histoplasma (lung).

The reaction of tissues to fungi depends on the infection and site involved

The reactions seen to fungal infection are:

- **Minimal tissue reaction**. This is a particular feature of superficial skin infections by dermatophytic fungi. Histologically the tissue response is very low-key, with dilatation of dermal vessels and very minor neutrophil accumulation in the epidermis. *Cryptococcus neoformans* often shows minimal tissue reaction in the lungs and meninges, but this may be a manifestation of the patient's depressed immune-suppressed state.
- **Acute inflammatory reaction**. This is seen mainly in primary mucosal fungal infections, such as oral, esophageal and vaginal Candida infections. There is vascular dilatation and a heavy neutrophil infiltration in the epithelium, often with ulceration. In the early stages of systemic blood-borne infection, there is an acute inflammatory reaction, often followed by microabscess formation.
- **Granulomatous inflammatory reaction**. One of the characteristic tissue responses to fungi, particularly seen in deep subcutaneous and some systemic infection is the so-called 'suppurating granuloma'. There is a central purulent neutrophil reaction, surrounded by a granulomatous histiocytic and giant-cell reaction. The fungi can usually be found within the purulent neutrophilic material. Some fungi, particularly yeasts (e.g. chromoblastomycosis), excite a purely histiocytic and giant-cell granulomatous reaction, without suppuration.

Dermatophytic fungi are common and cause a range of skin diseases

These fungi are mainly located on the skin surface but hyphae insert themselves between epidermal keratinocytes. Both surface epidermis and the keratinocytes of hair follicles may be involved, as may finger and toe nails. Details of the common organisms and their clinical effects are given on page 491 of Chapter 23. The effect in most cases is to disorder normal keratinocyte maturation so that

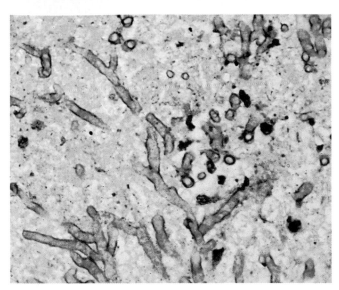

Fig. 8.15 Aspergillosis in the lung.
Photomicrograph showing the branching system of *Aspergillus fumigatus* at the edge of an area of lung necrosis.

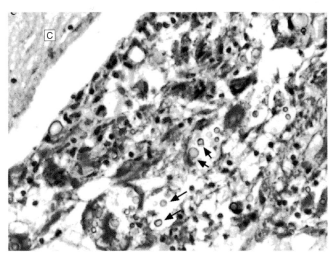

Fig. 8.16 Meningitis due to cryptococci.
High-powered photomicrograph showing a granulomatous inflammatory exudate in the meninges, with a piece of cerebral cortex (**C**). The cryptococcal yeast forms (arrowed) are present in the exudate, along with a few poorly formed giant cells.

parakeratotic scale is formed instead of normal stratum corneum, and inflammatory changes in the dermis, often due to localized immune-based hypersensitivity reactions.

Candida albicans is a normal commensal of skin and alimentary tract, and superficial pathogenic infections are particularly common in orificial mucosa

This organism occurs in both a yeast and a hyphal form. The commonest sites for infection are the mouth (oral thrush – see page 224) and at the vulvo-vaginal orifice (see page 397). In immunosuppressed individuals, systemic blood-borne infection can occur with small candidal abscesses in many organs. Intravenous drug abusers, and patients with long-standing intravenous lines are particularly at risk; sometimes candidal endocarditis, with large mitral and aortic valve vegetations, is the basis of the widespread blood dissemination. In surface skin/mucosal lesions the hyphal forms predominate, with scanty yeast forms, whereas in endocarditis and the systemic micro-abscesses the yeast forms predominate.

Aspergillus fumigatus is an important opportunistic fungus in immunocompromised individuals

This fungus is widely distributed in the environment and is usually non-pathogenic. In severely immunocompromised patients it may gain access to the lung periphery and proliferate rapidly (see. *Fig. 8.15*). An important feature of the organism is its ability to penetrate the walls of blood vessels, leading to thrombosis, vessel occlusion and tissue necrosis, particularly in the lung. Aspergillus lung disease is discussed and illustrated on page 198. Although the main lesions are in the lung, Aspergillus can become systematized through the bloodstream to produce small Aspergillus lesions which are often necrotic or semi-cystic due to the vessel occlusion by masses of hyphae and thrombus.

Aspergillus niger is a cause of otitis externa; the black fungus can be easily seen clinically in the external auditory canal.

Cryptococcus neoformans can cause pneumonia and meningitis

This fungus exists only in the form of a spherical yeast, and has a thick capsule. It is common in bird droppings. Human infection occurs by inhalation of the yeast, particularly when it is air-borne in dry dusty soils. In an immune-competent individual, the presence of Cryptococci inhaled into lung alveoli may be asymptomatic or associated with only a mild flu-like illness. The disease is at its worst in the immune-compromised individual in whom the Cryptococci proliferate within the lung to produce pneumonic consolidation. The yeasts can spread to the meninges to give a meningitis (see *Fig. 8.16*) and sometimes intracerebral accumulations of the capsulated yeast. There is often little or no inflammatory response of any type to the presence of the yeasts in either lungs or meninges, particularly in immunosuppressed patients, but a low-grade granulomatous reaction sometimes occurs.

Histoplasma capsulatum produces cavitating lung lesions, and can become disseminated in immunosuppressed individuals

Like Cryptococcus, Histoplasma occurs in soil which is extensively contaminated by infected bird droppings. Human infection is by inhalation of dust containing the spores of the fungus. In healthy immune-competent individuals, symptoms are usually mild, with slight cough, malaise and occasionally fever ('acute primary histoplasmosis'); rarely, an acute pneumonia develops. Some patients, possibly slightly or moderately immune-impaired, or repeatedly exposed to large quantities of spores, develop a chronic cavitating lung disease ('chronic cavitating histoplasmosis') which affects the apices of the upper lobes, and therefore resembles adult-pattern tuberculosis (see page 55).

Disseminated systemic infection occurs in partly immunocompromised individuals, the fungus spreading from a lung lesion via the bloodstream to colonize lymph nodes, spleen, liver and bone marrow. The illness is chronic, with surprisingly mild non-specific symptoms. Severe symptoms may occur in patients with AIDS (for which it is one of the defining opportunistic infections), the disseminated systemic infection sometimes occurring many years after the initial exposure in an endemic area.

Histoplasmosis is uncommon in Europe, but endemic in parts of the central USA, mainly the Ohio and Mississippi river valleys.

Coccidioidomycosis and blastomycosis show similar clinical and pathological features to histoplasmosis

Coccidioidomycosis is endemic in the south western USA. Like histoplasmosis, human infection is acquired by inhalation of dusty soil containing fungal spores, and a mild respiratory illness follows which resembles acute bronchitis. The tissue response in the lungs is the formation of a giant cell granulomatous reaction, which may enlarge and cavitate to produce radiologically obvious lesions. Healing is by fibrosis. In some cases the lung lesions fail to heal, and organisms persist, occasionally becoming systematized. This may occur in individuals who are mildly or transiently immunocompromised, e.g. the elderly, malnourished or on immunosuppressive therapy. AIDS patients may have particularly severe systemic lesions, involving brain, bones, soft tissues and visceral organs. In this group the original pulmonary lesions frequently enlarge rapidly, with progressive respiratory impairment.

Blastomycosis is very similar in clinical and pathological features to coccidioidomycosis, with inhalation of soil dust-borne spores causing lung lesions characterized by a giant cell granulomatous reaction to the organism in the lungs, associated with trivial symptoms. Some patients have more severe pulmonary involvement with respiratory failure. It differs from coccidioidomycosis in that the main manifestation of systemic spread is the development of numerous enlarging and spreading skin lesions which undergo pustulation.

Pneumocystis carinii is an important cause of disease and death in immunosuppressed patients

This organism was regarded until recently as a protozoan but has now, by some taxonomic sleight-of-hand, emerged center-stage as a fungus. It is widespread and innocuous except in patients who have inadequate cellular immune mechanisms, and is particularly common in patients with AIDS and heavily immunosuppressed patients such as transplant recipients. It causes progressive pulmonary consolidation, leading to respiratory failure and death, unless successfully treated. *Pneumocystis pneumonia* is illustrated and discussed on page 199 (Chapter 11).

VIRAL INFECTIONS

Three main outcomes of viral infection are cell death, cell proliferation, and latent infection

The most commonly seen viral diseases are manifest either by producing cell death or by stimulating cell proliferation.

Cell necrosis is the most common manifestation of viral infections. It may be due to direct cytopathic effect of the virus or may be the result of host immune defences recognizing viral proteins in contact with class I antigen expression. For example, herpes and chickenpox produce skin blistering and mucosal lesions as a result of necrosis of epithelial cells, and influenza produces necrosis of the epithelial cells of the respiratory mucosa. With proliferation of poliovirus and rabies, neurons are killed, and liver cells are killed when infected with yellow fever virus.

Cell proliferation is stimulated by infections caused by variants of the human papillomavirus (HPV), responsible for warty overgrowth of the epidermal cells of the skin in viral warts, and overgrowth of the cervical epithelium in wart-virus infection of cervical epithelium. This group is important because of the increasingly recognized link between HPV infection and the subsequent development of epithelial malignant tumors. HPV inactivates the product of p53 gene, which normally prevents cell division.

Latent infection is seen in several diseases when virus becomes integrated into the host genome. Reactivation of virus may then occur at a later date, causing episodes of cell necrosis. For example, herpes zoster may be latent in dorsal root ganglia, reactivating to cause shingles. Virus travels down axons to reach the skin, where productive infection leads to epithelial cell death and a painful blistering rash. Similarly, herpes simplex may be latent in epithelial cells, reactivating to cause cold sores, as well as active genital herpes.

Slow replication of virus inside the host cells may lead to persistent infection

In some situations virus may continue to replicate in host cells, evading immune responses, and thereby causing persistent infections. Such infections may be clinically asymptomatic and, because the individual is infective, are an important reservoir for disease spread. For example, human immunodeficiency virus (HIV) is present at low levels as persistent infection in asymptomatic individuals, and hepatitis B virus can remain as a persistent active infection in certain cases.

Parvoviruses cause two important conditions, both in children

Parvoviruses are single-stranded DNA viruses which cause:

- 'Slapped cheek syndrome', a febrile illness in children associated with a red maculo-papular rash on the cheeks, due to Parvovirus B19.
- Aplastic crises in children with sickle-cell anaemia.

Parvovirus may also cause arthritis in adults, and a form of summer diarrhea.

Papovaviruses include papilloma virus, polyomaviruses and simian vacuolating viruses

These are double-stranded DNA viruses, with many sub-types, particularly in the papillomavirus group.

Papilloma viruses stimulate the proliferation of squamous epithelial cells to produce proliferating lesions called warts (hence often called 'wart virus'). They are transmitted from person to person by direct or indirect contact, and the virus persists in basal epithelial cells long after the original wart has clinically resolved, with potential for reactivation. Different sub-types of the virus are responsible for warts in different sites. Human papilloma virus (HPV) causes warts in:

- Skin – due to HPV1 and 2, with plantar warts mainly due to HPV1 (see *Fig. 8.17*), and the rarer flat 'plane' wart due to HPV3. Warts in the skin around penis, vulva and anus may be due to HPV6, the genital wart virus.
- Anogenital skin – most are due to HPV6 and HPV11.
- Uterine cervix – mainly HPV16 and HPV18. These two sub-types are oncogenic, and infection is a factor

predisposing to cervical intraepithelial neoplasia (CIN) and invasive malignancy.

- Larynx – 'juvenile papillomatosis' in young children. Where HPV is identified it is usually HPV6 and HPV11, the viruses responsible for anogenital warts. It is thought that infection is acquired during birth.

These conditions are discussed and illustrated in more detail on pages 243, 397, 401 and 490.

The polyoma viruses are two in number, called JC and BK. Although both are frequently present in the urinary tract and kidneys, they very rarely produce infective symptoms. In severely immunosuppressed patients JC virus causes progressive multifocal leukoencephalopathy (see page 448).

Adenoviruses cause epidemics of acute respiratory disease with pneumonia, conjunctivitis and infantile gastroenteritis

Adenoviruses are double-stranded DNA viruses, and there are over 40 types. Common conditions due to this group are:

- A range of upper and lower respiratory tract infections, particularly in children, including pharyngitis (sore throat) and non-specific 'colds'. Atypical adenovirus pneumonia due to Types 3, 4 and 7 can occur in young adults.
- Conjunctivitis associated with Types 3, 7, 8 and 19.
- Acute diarrhea in children associated with Types 40 and 41.

Hepadnaviruses cause hepatitis B

Hepadnaviruses are double-stranded DNA viruses with a circular shape. The only recognized pathogenic member is the hepatitis B virus, causing hepatitis. This is discussed in detail on page 282, Chapter 14.

Herpes viruses are a large and important group, responsible for a wide range of diseases

Herpes viruses are double-stranded DNA viruses which cause many important acute and chronic human diseases. There are eight important types, numbered 1–8 (HHV1–8), but many have synonyms:

- HHV1 is also known as herpes simplex virus 1 (HSV1). It is the cause of cold sores around the mouth and gingivostomatitis (see *Fig. 8.18*). Also can cause encephalitis (see page 447).
- HHV2 is also known as HSV2. It causes genital herpes and cutaneous herpes (see pages 397 and 490). This virus may rarely cause meningoencephalitis in the newborn and infants, possibly contracted during passage down the birth canal.
- HHV3 is also known as the varicella-zoster virus. This causes varicella (chicken-pox) and zoster (shingles) – see page 490.

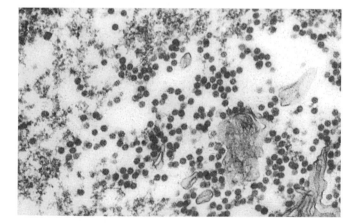

Fig. 8.17 HPV in a plantar wart.
Numerous HPV1 particles in a keratinocyte from an active plantar wart (verruca).

- HHV4 is also known as the Epstein–Barr virus (EBV). This causes infectious mononucleosis (glandular fever), but is also involved in Burkitt's lymphoma and nasopharyngeal carcinoma.
- HHV5 is also known as cytomegalovirus (CMV). It causes a wide range of diseases, including a mononucleosis syndrome resembling that due to HHV4, congenital infection, CMV pneumonitis and hepatitis. It is an important pathogen in the immunosuppressed, particularly AIDS patients.
- HHV6 and 7 have no synonyms. Both cause roseola infantum, a mild feverish illness in infants and young children, followed by a red maculo-papular rash.
- HHV8 was recently shown to be present in Kaposi's sarcoma.

The poxvirus group cause a wide variety of skin lesions

The poxviruses are double-stranded DNA viruses and are the largest viruses. The most frequently occurring is *Molluscum contagiosum* which is transmitted from human to human (see *Fig. 8.19*). The others pass from animals to humans and include:

- Orf contracted from sheep (blistering skin lesions).
- Cowpox contracted from cows (blistering skin lesions on the hands of those milking infected cows).

The orthomyxoviruses cause influenza

These are single-stranded RNA viruses, and there are three types named influenza A, influenza B and influenza C. The A and B types are the cause of influenza, and the emergence of new strains is fairly frequent, leading to epidemics and pandemics.

The new strains emerge as a result of either small mutations (antigenic drift) affecting the H (hemagglutinin) and N (neuraminidase) type-specific antigens in the viral envelope, or to a major change in the same antigens (antigenic shift). People with established immunity to previous strains of the virus have no resistance to the new strains. Influenza A also affects other animals, particularly birds, and new strains can develop in these animal reservoirs before infecting humans.

The paramyxoviruses cause mumps and measles, and the common cold

These are single-stranded RNA viruses, and there are four clinically important types:

- Mumps virus causes mumps (parotitis, encephalitis, orchitis).
- Measles virus (morbillivirus) causes measles (see *Fig. 8.20*).
- Respiratory syncytial virus causes the common cold in adults and occasionally acute bronchitis and pneumonia in infants.
- Parainfluenza viruses cause the common cold and pneumonia.

The picornaviruses are a large group causing a variety of different diseases including poliomyelitis

There are two main sub-groups, the enteroviruses and the rhinoviruses. The latter are responsible for some cases of the common cold, whereas the former (poliovirus, coxsackievirus and echoviruses) are mainly important for producing aseptic meningitis including poliomyelitis. One of the enteroviruses (enterovirus 72) is the causative organism in hepatitis A (see page 281).

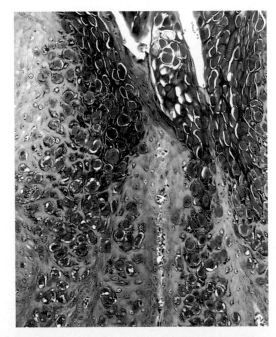

Fig. 8.19 Poxvirus inclusions in *Molluscum contagiosum*. Showing the keratinocytes of the skin in a lesion. Infected squamous cells show very large intranuclear inclusions composed of vast number of poxvirus particles. Originally red-staining with H&E, the inclusions become blue-staining when they are shed on the surface of the keratin mass.

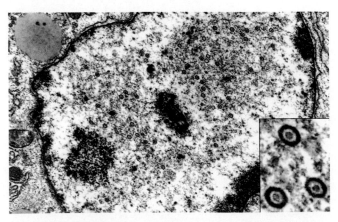

Fig. 8.18 HHV1 (herpes simplex virus) in the nucleus of a keratinocyte from an active cold sore in the mouth.

The only rhabdovirus of clinical significance is the rabies virus

The virus can infect all types of mammals, and human infection is usually acquired by a bite from an infected animal, most frequently a diseased dog.

The togaviruses cause rubella, hepatitis C and a variety of severe feverish illnesses, including yellow fever

The following groups produce important diseases:

- Rubivirus causes rubella (German measles).
- Arbovirus is *arthropod-borne* and causes a variety of serious encephalitic diseases such as Eastern equine encephalitis and St. Louis encephalitis, and diseases characterized by liver involvement and jaundice (yellow fever, dengue).
- Hepatitis C virus (see page 284).

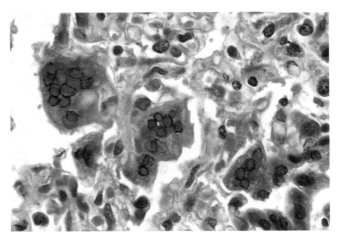

Fig. 8.20 Measles inclusion bodies.
Giant cells from a case of fatal measles pneumonia in an immunosuppressed child. The giant cells contain intranuclear and cytoplasmic eosinophilic inclusions of the virus.

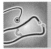

Histological diagnosis of viral infection

In addition to using microbiological techniques, it is possible, to diagnose viral infection on histological examination of biopsy tissue. This is increasing in importance because severe viral infections become manifest as a result of immunosuppression states.

Intracellular inclusion bodies are produced in many infections, e.g. cytomegalovirus (*Fig. 8.21*), and can be recognized by light microscopy. The main inclusions of diagnostic use are given in *Fig. 8.22*.

Immunohistochemistry to detect specific viral proteins is now an important aid to diagnosis, e.g. detection of herpes simplex in biopsy of necrotic tissue from brain can confirm a diagnosis of herpes encephalitis (see page 447).

***In situ* hybridization** to detect viral genome is increasingly being used as an aid to diagnosis. Detection of different sub-types of HPV in skin and cervical lesions can be achieved in some cases.

Polymerase chain reaction (PCR) techniques, as with many areas of pathology, can also be used to detect small numbers of virus in biopsy material.

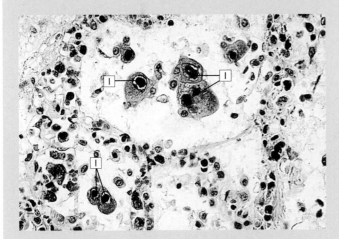

Fig. 8.21 Inclusion bodies in viral infection.
These cells in the lung of a patient with immunosuppression show large intranuclear inclusions (**I**) caused by cytomegalovirus.

Fig. 8.22
Inclusion bodies of diagnostic use in viral infection

Virus	Inclusion body
Cytomegalovirus	Intranuclear inclusion surrounded by a halo
Rabies	Eosinophilic rounded cytoplasmic inclusions (Negri bodies)
Hepatitis B	Ground-glass cytoplasm in hepatocytes
Molluscum contagiosum	Eosinophilic cytoplasmic inclusions
Herpes simplex	Eosinophilic intranuclear inclusions
Papovavirus	Basophilic intranuclear inclusions

The arenaviruses mainly affect rodents, from whom humans become infected, usually via rodent urine or feces

Infection is followed by a febrile illness. In some cases the illness progresses to lymphocytic choriomeningitis (LCM) or one of the severe, often fatal, hemorrhagic fevers such as Lassa fever.

The retroviruses are an important group because they include the AIDS virus and the oncoviruses HTLV1 and HTLV2

The HIV virus is the cause of AIDS (see page 107). HTLV1 is associated with T-cell leukemia, and HTLV2 with hairy cell leukemia (see page 325).

Finally, **coronaviruses** cause the common cold, and the **rotaviruses** (types A–D) produce acute onset of vomiting and diarrhea, particularly in young children.

Prion diseases are caused by an infectious protein

In a unique biological situation, certain diseases of man and animals appear to be due to an infective protein-only agent. These include: diseases of the nervous system, Creutzfeldt–Jakob disease and kuru in humans (see page 448), scrapie in sheep, and bovine spongiform encephalopathy in cattle. These diseases were formerly called slow-virus diseases.

The infective agent is a normal host protein, termed **prion protein**. Found in many tissues, it is a membrane-associated protein of unknown function. The structural change responsible for making it infective is, at present, unknown. It is thought that the protein undergoes a conformational change and, once inoculated into a normal host, is able to catalyze a chain reaction in which host proteins are also conformationally changed.

PROTOZOAN AND HELMINTHIC PARASITES

Protozoa are unicellular eukaryotic organisms. Helminths are multicellular worms, which are divided into roundworms (nematodes), flatworms (cestodes) and flukes (trematodes).

Diseases associated with protozoan and helminthic parasites are common in tropical countries and in underdeveloped areas where public hygiene standards are poor. However, with the increasing frequency and speed of international travel, many diseases that were rarely seen in Britain, Europe and the USA are now becoming more common.

Significantly, formerly clinically mild and transient diseases caused by protozoa are now becoming more important, occurring more frequently and with greater severity in the immune-suppressed population, e.g. transplant recipients, patients receiving immunosuppressive therapy, and AIDS patients.

The main protozoan and helminthic infections of clinical relevance are presented according to organ involvement in *Figs 8.23* and *8.24*. The most important life-threatening protozoal infections worldwide are:

- Malaria caused by several types of Plasmodium. Parasites in red cells cause hemolysis associated with splenomegaly.
- Schistosomiasis is caused by several types of worm. The main pathology is caused by inflammatory and fibrotic reactions to eggs, which are laid in tissues, especially bladder, gut and liver.

The most important protozoal disease worldwide is malaria caused by the Plasmodium species

There are four species of Plasmodium involved (*P. vivax, P. falciparum, P. ovale* and *P. malariae*), but the complicated life-cycle of the parasite is much the same in all (see *Fig. 8.25*).

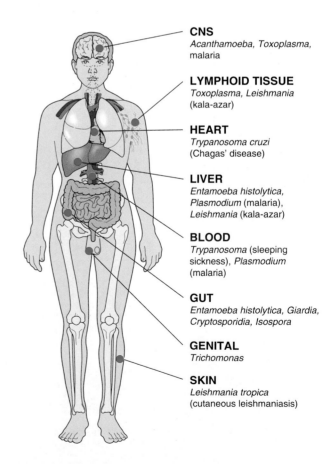

CNS
Acanthamoeba, Toxoplasma, malaria

LYMPHOID TISSUE
Toxoplasma, Leishmania (kala-azar)

HEART
Trypanosoma cruzi (Chagas' disease)

LIVER
Entamoeba histolytica, Plasmodium (malaria), Leishmania (kala-azar)

BLOOD
Trypanosoma (sleeping sickness), Plasmodium (malaria)

GUT
Entamoeba histolytica, Giardia, Cryptosporidia, Isospora

GENITAL
Trichomonas

SKIN
Leishmania tropica (cutaneous leishmaniasis)

Fig. 8.23 Protozoan infections.

The symptoms, signs and pathological changes in malaria are related to the sequelae of various aspects of the parasite's life-cycle in man:

- Cyclical fever with rigors and sweats coincides with red cell rupture cycles at the release of merozoites. In *P. falciparum* the fever cycle is not always regular due to non-synchronous cycles, but occurs more frequently, usually daily.
- Severe anemia mainly due to excessive red cell destruction, but marrow suppression may play a part.
- Hepatosplenomegaly due to excessive sequestration of red cells and red cell debris in spleen and hepatic Kupffer cells.
- Cerebral malaria, only in *P. falciparum*. Coma, often of rapid onset, following convulsions and severe headache.

CNS
Taenia solium (pork tapeworm),
Echinococcus granulosus
(hydatid cyst), *Trichinella spiralis*

EYE
*Onchocerca volvulus, Loa-loa,
Toxocara*

LUNG
Paragonimus westermani (liver fluke),
*Strongyloides stercoralis,
Wuchereria bancrofti* (filariasis),
Ascaris lumbricoides (roundworm),
Echinococcus granulosus (hydatid cyst)

LYMPHOID TISSUE
Wuchereria bancrofti (filariasis)

HEART
Trichinella spiralis

LIVER
Clonorchis sinensis, Fasciola hepatica
(liver fluke), *Schistosoma,
Echinococcus granulosus* (hydatid cyst)

LARGE INTESTINE
Enterobius vermicularis (pinworm),
Trichuris trichiura (whipworm)

SMALL INTESTINE
Ascaris lumbricoides (roundworm),
Necator americanis (hookworm),
Ancylostoma duodenale (hookworm),
Taenia solium (pork tapeworm),
Taenia saginata (beef tapeworm)

BLADDER
Schistosoma

SKELETAL MUSCLE
Trichinella spiralis, Taenia solium
(pork tapeworm)

SKIN
*Onchocerca volvulus, Loa-loa,
Toxocara*

Fig. 8.24 Helminthic infestations.

Usually rapidly fatal. Brain shows petechial hemorrhages associated with occlusion of capillaries by infected red cells (see *Fig. 8.26*), often bound up in fibrin/platelet thrombi. Similar capillary occlusion in the myocardium can produce acute cardiac failure, with fatal acute pulmonary edema.

Entameba histolytica is an important gastrointestinal parasite

This organism is confined to humans, and is transmitted by the feco-oral route by ingesting food or water contaminated by amebic cysts passed in human feces. In brief, the life-cycle is:

- Ingestion of food or water containing encysted ameba from human feces.
- Cyst wall breaks down in small intestine to release ameba trophozoites.
- Ameba trophozoites penetrate mucosa of colon to produce shallow flask-shaped ulcers.
- Ameba trophozoites may gain access to submucosal blood vessels, with potential for extra-colonic spread (see below).
- Some trophozoites in the colon become encysted and are passed out in the feces.

Sometimes the ameba trophozoites feed harmlessly on colonic bacteria without significantly damaging the mucosal cells, and the infection is asymptomatic. When significant ulceration occurs (see *Fig. 8.27*), amebic dysentery ensues, with abdominal pain and profuse diarrhea (which is often

**KEY FACTS
Tissue reaction to protozoan
and helminthic infection**

The tissue response to protozoan and metazoan infections varies greatly between different organisms. Some common factors are evident:

- The immune response is operative in most infections with Type I and Type IV hypersensitivity responses. Immunosuppression is an important reason for fatal parasitic infection.
- Eosinophils play an important role in defence against parasitic infestation. Tissue and blood eosinophilia are frequently seen in such infections.
- Certain organisms induce tissue necrosis and acute inflammation, e.g. amebas.
- Certain organisms induce hypersensitivity responses and tissue damage is the result of the host immune response, e.g. fibrosis caused by Schistosoma.

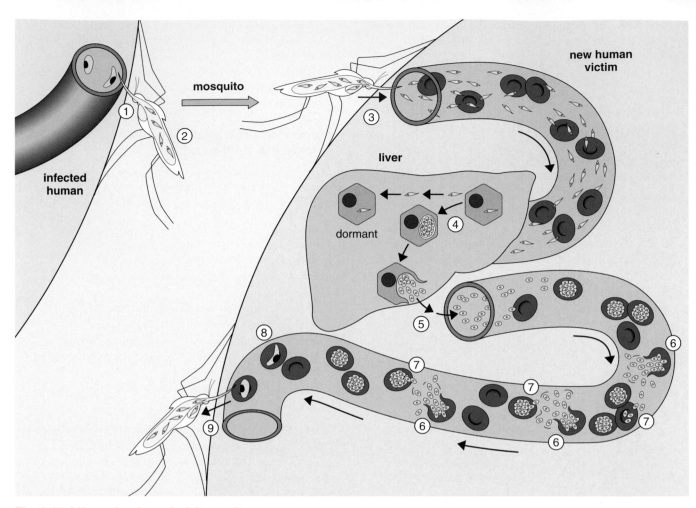

Fig. 8.25 Life-cycle of a malarial parasite.
A female Anopheles mosquito feeds on the blood of a human suffering from malaria and ingests red blood cells containing male and female Plasmodium gametocytes (1). In the gut of the mosquito, the gametocytes reproduce sexually to produce infective sporozoites (2), some of which enter the mosquito salivary glands to be injected into the next human victim the mosquito bites (3). In the human, the parasites pass in the bloodstream to the liver where they mature and reproduce asexually within hepatocytes to produce many thousands of merozoites (4), which are released into the bloodstream when the affected hepatocytes rupture and die (5). The merozoites invade human red cells and transform into trophozoites, which grow in size and then divide asexually to produce even more merozoites, which are released when the affected red cell ruptures (6). These merozoites invade other red cells and initiate another cycle of asexual reproduction in red cells → red cell rupture → merozoite release → re-invasion of red cells, etc (7). This cyclical asexual reproductive phase continues for months, even years, occurring every 48 or 72 hours (72 hours for *P. malariae*, 48 hours for the others). Some merozoites in red cells produce male and female gametocytes instead of entering the asexual reproductive cycle (8), and it is these which infect the next female mosquito to feed on the victim's blood (9). Some parasites (at stage 4) can remain sequestered and dormant in liver cells instead of maturing and dividing into merozoites; these dormant parasites are responsible for late relapses.

blood-stained) during acute exacerbations, with intermittent cramping abdominal pain and mild diarrhea between major attacks. The disease has a tendency to become chronic without treatment, and involvement of the appendix and cecal regions may lead to a large chronic inflammatory mass ('ameboma') in the right iliac fossa. Chronicity, with repeated acute exacerbations, over a period of months or years leads to chronic anemia (due to intermittent blood loss), and emaciation.

Extra-colonic amebiasis results from invasion of colonic submucosal vessels by amebic trophozoites in the ulcers.

They pass in the portal venous system to the liver where amebic abscesses may form. Enlargement of a liver abscess may lead to local sub-diaphragmatic abscess and an abscess in adjacent lung tissue. Blood-borne spread from a lung or liver abscess, or from a large ameboma, may rarely produce a brain abscess.

Amebiasis is most common in tropical and subtropical countries, and cases in more temperate climes are usually acquired while living or working abroad. However, it can be a sexually transmitted disease in male homosexuals, due to anal sexual activity.

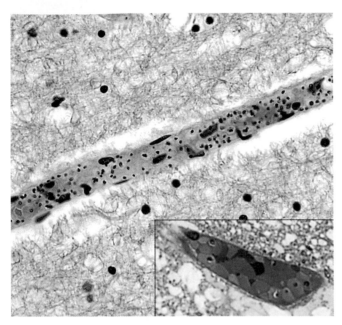

Fig. 8.26 Cerebral malaria.
Main picture shows a tiny capillary with numerous black dots apparently within it. This is 'malarial' pigment, a fixation artefact occurring in association with red cells which contain malarial parasites. The inset is an epoxy resin thin section stained with Toluidine blue showing the parasites within some of the tightly packed red cells.

The Trypanosoma group of protozoa contains three distinct species which cause disease via insect vectors

Two of the species (*T. brucei gambiense* and *T. brucei rhodesiense*) are transmitted by tsetse flies and cause sleeping sickness in different parts of sub-Saharan central Africa ('African trypanosomiasis'). After inoculation by a tsetse fly bite, a small inflammatory skin nodule forms at the site but later heals. The parasites disseminate in lymphatics and bloodstream to produce fever, headaches and malaise, often with generalized lymphadenopathy. After a few months (in *T. brucei rhodesiense*) or months to years (in *T. brucei gambiense*), brain involvement becomes manifest as trypanosomes eventually reach the brain in significant numbers. Mixed cerebral symptoms include persistent headache, personality changes, lassitude and somnolence, tremor and ataxia, but progression is towards coma and death, within a year in *T. brucei rhodesiense* and 3 years in *T. brucei gambiense*.

The third species is *Trypanosoma cruzi* which is responsible for 'American trypanosomiasis' or **Chagas' disease**. It is largely confined to Central and South America but is seen in the USA in immigrants from these areas. Although most cases are transmitted to humans by an insect vector (reduviid bugs) from a large range of mammalian hosts (dogs, opossums, rats, etc), human-to-human transmission via blood transfusion is possible.

There is an **acute phase** during which organisms spread through the tissues via bloodstream and lymphatics to

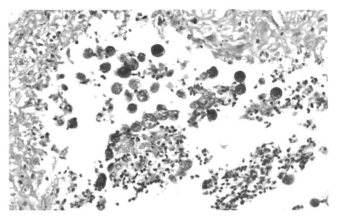

Fig. 8.27 Amebas in a colonic mucosal ulcer.
In this photomicrograph the amebas are stained magenta by the PAS stain.

infect many tissues, but particularly the nervous system, skeletal and myocardial muscle and tissues and organs of the immune system. This phase may be asymptomatic, or marked by fever, malaise and lymphadenopathy. In a small percentage of patients there are severe symptoms with acute myocarditis or acute meningoencephalitis, often fatal ('acute Chagas' disease').

The patient enters a **chronic phase** lasting many years in which there may be very gradual tissue destruction, with immune damage playing an important part. The main features of this chronic Chagas' disease are:

- Slowly progressive cardiomyopathy (see page 182) leading to a dilated, chronically failing heart, ventricular aneurysms and dysrhythmias.
- Chronic dilatation of the esophagus and colon due to destruction of myenteric nerve plexuses, to produce changes similar to achalasia of the cardia (see page 249) and Hirschsprung's disease (see page 270).
- Potential for cross-placental transmission from infected mother, with high incidence of stillbirth or early abortion.
- Potential for reactivation to produce severe acute Chagas' disease if patient becomes severely immunosuppressed.

Leishmaniasis is transmitted by sandfly bites from a wide range of animal reservoirs, and produces three patterns of disease

The most common animal reservoirs in the West are dogs and rodents. The three patterns are cutaneous, mucocutaneous and systemic (visceral) leishmaniasis.

Cutaneous leishmaniasis is usually due to *Leishmania tropica* in Europe, and comprises a chronic ulcerating papule, usually in the skin of the face or arms following a sandfly bite, usually acquired in Southern Europe and the Mediterranean coastline or islands. The lesion is indolent, and takes many months to heal, with scarring. The organisms are easily seen within dermal macrophages in early lesions (see *Fig. 8.28*) but can be difficult to find in

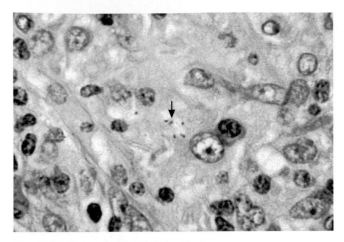

Fig. 8.28 Cutaneous leishmaniasis.
Taken from a skin lesion which had been present for
14 days following a sandfly bite while on holiday in Cyprus.
The organisms (arrowed) can be seen within the macrophages
in the early dermal inflammatory infiltrate.

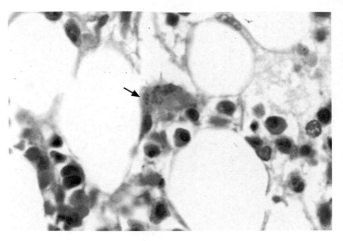

Fig. 8.29 Systemic leishmaniasis.
From the bone marrow of a patient with systemic leishmaniasis.
The parasites (*Leishmania donovani* – arrowed) are present in
swollen macrophages in the hemopoietic bone marrow.

long-standing lesions. Different species in Asia, Africa, and
Central/South America cause similar skin lesions. One of
the American species (*L. braziliensis*) occasionally produces:

Mucocutaneous leishmaniasis, in which a lesion of
cutaneous leishmaniasis is followed, usually within months,
by involvement of the nasal and nasopharyngeal mucosa
resulting in destructive chronic inflammatory masses.

Systemic (visceral) leishmaniasis is also known as kala-
azar, and is due to *L. donovani*. It occurs in para-equatorial
areas such as Central/South America, India and the
Mediterranean coastline. Following a sandfly bite, the
parasites are distributed in the bloodstream, particularly to
organs of the immune defence system such as the spleen,
lymph nodes, bone marrow (see *Fig. 8.29*) and liver. There
is lymphadenopathy, hepatosplenomegaly, and evidence of
marrow abnormality in the form of pancytopenia. Up to
80% of patients die if untreated.

Toxoplasmosis commonly produces benign reactive lymph node enlargement, but can be a fatal infection in the immunosuppressed patient

The usual animal reservoir for *Toxoplasma gondii* is the
domestic or feral cat, and most human disease is thought to
be acquired by feco-oral contact with Toxoplasma oocysts
in cat feces, either directly or indirectly, via contaminated
soil. In pregnant women the infection can be passed trans-
placentally to the fetus. There are the three main clinical
patterns.

Acute lymphadenopathic toxoplasmosis is by far the
most common. The main clinical feature is benign reactive
enlargement of lymph nodes, particularly in the neck.
This may be accompanied by an illness with many of
the clinical features of infectious mononucleosis, including
fever, malaise, sore throat and muscle discomfort. The

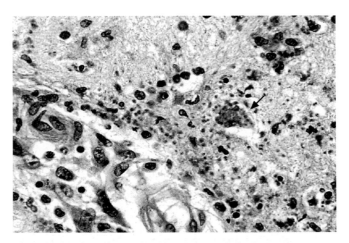

Fig. 8.30 Acute encephalitis due to toxoplasmosis.
In a portion of the brain alongside a small blood vessel, a
toxoplasma cyst has ruptured to release large numbers of
minute organisms (arrow).

blood picture shows similar features, with anemia and the
presence of atypical mononuclear cells (atypical lymphocytes) in the blood smear. These symptoms may persist for
weeks, and the lymphadenopathy may not return to normal
for months.

Acute toxoplasma encephalitis is almost confined to
immunosuppressed patients, and is now an important
infective complication of AIDS. Most cases are probably
the result of reactivation of quiescent or latent infection
in patients who have previously had, and overcome, lymphadenopathic toxoplasmosis. The brain shows focal areas
of necrosis and microvascular thrombosis associated with
the presence of intact and ruptured toxoplasmal cysts, the
ruptured cyst releasing large numbers of tachyzoites (see
Fig. 8.30). The CNS symptoms relate to the area of the
brain involved, but in most cases there is raised intracranial
pressure, altered mental state, fits and coma.

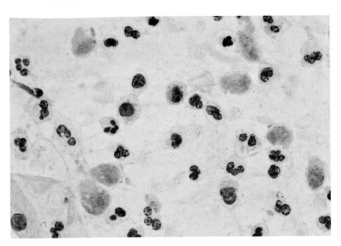

Fig. 8.31 *Trichomonas vaginalis* **in a vaginal smear.**
Taken from a young woman with vaginal soreness and discharge, showing the greyish protozoan and some darker staining neutrophil polymorphs.

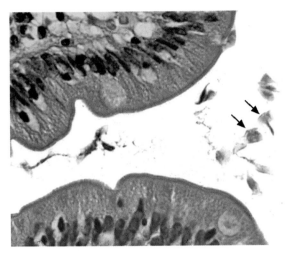

Fig. 8.32 *Giardia lamblia* **near duodenal mucosa.**
The ill-defined slightly purplish-stained organisms lie mainly free above the surface of the mucosa.

Congenital toxoplasmosis is due to transplacental spread from the infected mother. Severe infection early in pregnancy usually leads to spontaneous abortion or stillbirth. If the child survives *in utero*, it may be born with a structural brain disorder such as microcephaly or hydrocephaly, usually with foci of calcification in the brain, and choroidoretinitis. At birth, such neonates may have persisting jaundice, with a palpably enlarged liver. Less severe infections acquired when the mother contracts toxoplasmosis late in pregnancy may lead to an apparently normal infant, but symptoms due to toxoplasmosis may present later in childhood, particularly in the form of a choroidoretinitis (ocular toxoplasmosis).

Trichomonas vaginalis most commonly causes vaginitis in women, and occasionally mild urethritis in men

This protozoan parasite is flagellated and highly motile, and can be easily identified under the microscope in a wet preparation of vaginal fluid in cases of infection. They are also frequently seen in cytological smear preparations taken for the diagnosis of cervical dysplasia (see *Fig. 8.31*). The organism is transmitted by sexual intercourse, and in women produces a heavy vaginal discharge with an offensive smell, with secondary inflammation of the vaginal mucosa and often the vulval skin. Men are usually asymptomatic or, at the most, have a mild urethritis. Because of sexual transmission, both partners should be treated whether symptomatic or not.

Giardia lamblia is a common intestinal parasite and may cause malabsorption syndrome

Giardia cysts occur in water, and infection is particularly likely to occur in areas of the world where sanitation is poor and water supplies are contaminated by human feces. The cysts are passed in the feces by infected humans and some other mammals, and there is potential for direct feco-oral transmission. The organism is flagellated and attaches to the surface enterocytes of the duodenum and proximal jejunum (see *Fig. 8.32*), and may interfere with the absorption of sugars and fats, leading to chronic malabsorption syndrome with the frequent passage of offensive soft or semi-liquid feces. Even without malabsorption, the patient suffers from abdominal cramps and flatulence, although many patients remain asymptomatic carriers, passing both the sensitive trophozoites and the resistant cysts (which are the important source of reinfection and spread) in their feces.

Cryptosporidiosis is an important cause of infective diarrhea and is highly contagious

Infection can be spread from humans or animals by the feco-oral route, but most outbreaks are the result of water supplies contaminated by human or animal feces.

The parasites live and replicate within the brush border of the absorptive enterocytes of the small intestine (see *Fig. 8.33*), eventually producing oocysts which pass to the external environment in the feces. The infection produces profuse diarrhea and abdominal cramps, often lasting 2–3 weeks, being most severe and prolonged in patients with AIDS. Even after the patient has recovered from the acute illness, infective occysts continue to be excreted in the feces.

FLUKE (TREMATODE) INFECTIONS

There are many types of fluke infection worldwide, but the most important is schistosomiasis (bilharziasis) in which the water snail is the intermediate host. Different schistosoma species affect different areas of the human body, and have different geographic distributions.

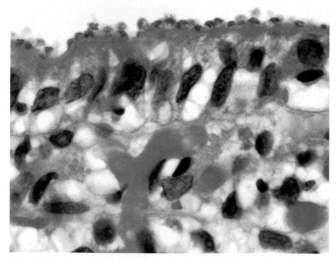

Fig. 8.33 Cryptosporidiosis in the small intestine.
Showing the purple-staining Cryptosporidia colonizing the surface of the enterocytes.

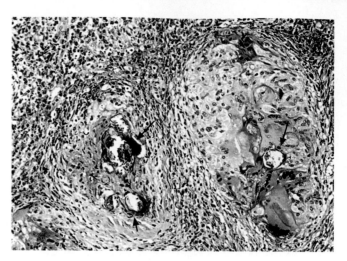

Fig. 8.34 Schistosoma in the bladder.
There is a florid foreign body giant cell reaction and severe chronic inflammation in response to the presence of partly calcified schistosome eggs (arrows).

Schistosomiasis due to *Schistosoma haematobium* predominantly affects the human bladder

Schistosoma haematobium is widespread throughout Africa, including some tourist resorts on the North African coast. In simple terms, the organism's eggs pass in the urine of an infected human to contaminate fresh water where they hatch and infect a fresh-water snail, within the body of which they multiply to produce large numbers of infective cercariae which swim freely in the water. These can penetrate the skin of humans walking in the water and eventually migrate to the veins in the wall of the bladder, where they develop into sexually active adult worms which reproduce to form eggs. In the early stages there may be a localized itchy rash or lump at the site or sites of human skin (usually feet and lower legs), where the cercariae have penetrated. In the late stages (chronic schistosomiasis) the symptoms are due to the chronic inflammatory reaction in the bladder wall to the presence of schistosome eggs (see *Fig. 8.34*). There is initially a florid chronic inflammatory and granulomatous reaction, followed by fibrosis. This leads to ulceration of bladder mucosa which becomes chronic and is often attended by repeated attempts at re-epithelialization, which produces papillomatous masses of transitional epithelium, some of which may become malignant. The chronic inflammation affecting the urothelium frequently leads to **squamous metaplasia**, and this may also be followed by the development of malignancy in the form of squamous carcinoma of the bladder.

Schistosomiasis due to *S. mansoni* and *S. japonicum* affects the alimentary tract and the liver

S. mansoni occurs in Africa and Central and South America, and *S. japonicum* occurs in the Far East. They gain access

to humans in the same way as *S. haematobium* but the organisms migrate not to the bladder but to the intestinal wall, where they produce ulceration, strictures and chronic fibrosis by chronic inflammatory, granulomatous and fibrous reaction to the presence of eggs. From the intestine some organisms migrate via the portal venous system to the liver, where they can produce a periportal fibrosis, sometimes leading to a pseudo-cirrhosis pattern. Because the damage is particularly marked in the portal triads, portal hypertension and hematemesis is an important complication. Occasionally the eggs can be transferred to the lungs where a foreign body granulomatous and fibrotic reaction can occur.

TAPEWORM (CESTODE) INFESTATIONS

Adult tapeworms are flat segmented worms (see *Fig. 8.35*), each comprising:

- Head (or 'scolex') which bears hooklets with which it attaches to the small intestinal mucosa of the host.
- Neck, from which the linked segments arise.
- Segments (proglottides) which are very small when they are formed in the neck region, but become larger and more mature as they are pushed distally by new small segment formation.

The larger distal segments are sexually mature, and contain a uterus within which eggs are formed (the worms are hermaphroditic). In most types (*Taenia saginata*, *Diphyllobothrium latum* and usually *Taenia solium*), the eggs pass out in the human host feces, to be ingested by a variety of other animals (according to tapeworm species) within which the eggs hatch into 'oncospheres' which

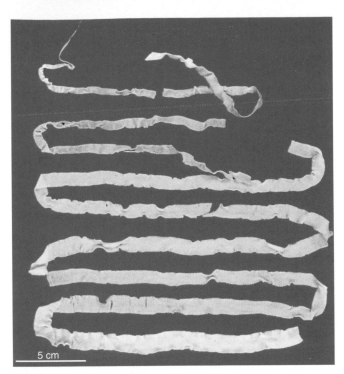

Fig. 8.35 A tapeworm (*Taenia saginata*).
Mounted museum specimen of an almost entire tapeworm. From the scale, it is easy to calculate its full length. At the top the worm is extremely small, with progressively enlarging segments distally.

5 cm

penetrate the blood vessels in the animal's intestinal wall and are carried around the body, often lodging in skeletal muscle where they become encysted and develop to contain a scolex or head.

Human infection is acquired by eating the affected animal's meat. In this pattern, the main effects on the human host are usually mild, often without significant symptoms. There may be mild abdominal pain and diarrhea, but sometimes large tapeworms may produce weight loss, malnutrition and vitamin deficiencies. This is because tapeworms have no alimentary tract, and nourish themselves by direct absorption of food and vitamins from the human small bowel lumen.

An important exception to this life-cycle pattern is hydatid disease and one variant of *Taenia solium* infestation (see below).

Taenia saginata infestation is acquired by eating raw or undercooked infected beef

This disease has been largely eradicated in affluent nations due to strict herd control, abattoir inspection, and examination of the butchered beast. It still occurs in poor countries, for example in parts of Africa, South America, Eastern Europe and the Middle East. In these areas, the use of human feces as a soil fertilizer, and inadequate treatment and disposal of sewage, play a part in the perpetuation of the cyclical infestation.

Diphyllobothrium latum infestation is acquired by eating raw or undercooked infected freshwater fish

The worm gets into fish after a fresh-water environment, particularly a lake, is contaminated by human feces due to inadequate sewage treatment and disposal. The eggs hatch into minute larvae in the water and are consumed by small crustaceans which, in turn, are eaten by fish, some of which are caught and eaten by humans. It occurs worldwide, particularly in cold or temperate zones with abundant lakes. In the human small intestine, the mature worms absorb food and vitamins, particularly Vitamin B_{12}, and may cause megaloblastic anemia (see page 318).

Taenia solium infestation is usually acquired by eating undercooked infected pork, but humans can also act as intermediate hosts by direct feco-oral infection

Taenia solium can behave exactly like *T. saginata*, the ingestion of undercooked infected pork leading to the development of a mature worm in the small intestine. Like *T. saginata*, this infestation is usually asymptomatic or, at the worst, responsible for mild abdominal discomfort and intermittent diarrhea. However, there is a much more serious pattern of illness when humans act as the intermediate host, in which the oncospheres hatch and spread. This may occur by direct human-to-human feco-oral spread, the eggs hatching into oncospheres in the human stomach, then spreading in the bloodstream in the pattern normally seen in the cow (*T. saginata*) and pig. The oncospheres may spread to many sites (skin, muscle, internal organs, etc) where they encyst and form scolices, but the main target organ is the brain and spinal cord. The enlarging cysts may produce symptoms of a brain or spinal cord tumor. The symptoms are particularly severe when the cyst dies, since a vigorous inflammatory reaction results. Dead cysts are usually calcified and can be identified by brain imaging.

Echinococcus granulosus produces 'hydatid disease', characterized by the formation of cysts, mainly in the liver

In this pattern, like the severe systemic variant of *T. solium* infection described above, humans act as the intermediate host, ingesting the eggs and developing migrating oncospheres, most of which pass to the liver (occasionally lungs) to produce slowly enlarging cysts containing daughter cysts within each of which is a scolex (see *Fig. 8.36*). Rupture of a liver or lung cyst can lead to wide dissemination of scolices.

The main host is the dog, and the main alternative intermediate host is the sheep. Dogs acquire the infection by eating infected sheep, and humans become infected through contact with dog feces containing the eggs, probably by hand-to-mouth contamination. The disease is particularly important in sheep farming areas such as Australia, New Zealand, the Mediterranean, South America, etc.

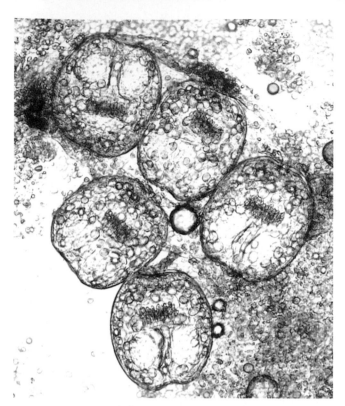

Fig. 8.36 *Echinococcus granulosus*.
A collection of scolices of *Echinococcus granulosus* found on microscopy of the fluid contents of a hydatid cyst of the liver.

In the United Kingdom, Wales is the most common area for the disease to originate. The disease is also seen in some areas of North America, particularly Canada and Alaska; in these areas the moose is the main host rather than sheep.

ROUNDWORMS (NEMATODES)

Unlike tapeworms (cestodes) and flukes (trematodes), roundworms have a body cavity. They can affect humans in various ways, a few of which are briefly outlined below.

- Occupation of human alimentary tract. Heavy infestations may produce abdominal pain and malnutrition, e.g. *Ascaris lumbricoides*, **trichuriasis**, or anemia due to the worm sucking blood from the intestinal mucosa, e.g. **Ancylostoma species**.
- Larval migration through the lungs may cause Löffler's syndrome (eosinophilic pneumonia), e.g. *Toxocara canis, Toxocara catis, Ascaris lumbricoides*.
- Multiple cysts containing larvae in tissues, particularly skeletal muscle, e.g. *Trichinella spirosis*.
- Obstruction of lymphatics, e.g. **filariasis**, often leading to marked lymphedema.
- Acute and chronic dermatitis, chronic skin ulcers and nodules, e.g. **Guinea worm**, **strongyloidiasis**, **Ancylostoma, Onchocerca, Loa-loa**.

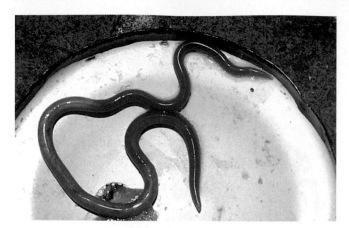

Fig. 8.37 *Ascaris lumbricoides*.
A freshly passed Ascaris roundworm in an enamel toilet bowl.

- Eye lesions, e.g. **Toxocara** (ocular larva migrans), **Onchocerca** (river blindness), **Loa-loa** (migrating larva in conjunctiva).

The majority of the above are mainly tropical and subtropical diseases. Students are advised to read a microbiology or tropical medicine text for details of life-cycles and variety of clinical manifestations. A few of the more important are detailed below.

Ascaris lumbricoides eventually occupy the gut as mature roundworms but the larval stage passes through the lungs

Ingested eggs hatch into larvae in the duodenum, the larvae passing into the bloodstream and reaching the lungs, where they may produce a transient Loffler's syndrome (eosinophilic pneumonitis). The larvae climb up the bronchi into the pharynx and are then swallowed to pass into the small intestine where the larvae develop into mature roundworms (see *Fig. 8.37*). Unless there are large numbers of worms in the intestine, the infestation may be asymptomatic, except in children where there may be abdominal pain and failure to thrive. Heavy infestations in adults may produce similar symptoms. Mature worms produce eggs which are excreted in the feces. The disease is most common in tropical and subtropical areas, but may occur in rural areas in Europe and the USA, wherever sanitation facilities are poor.

Ancylostoma species are hookworms which attach to the small intestinal mucosa and feed on the host's blood

Eggs in moist soil hatch into larvae which penetrate human skin and pass in the bloodstream to the lungs, from where they gain access to the small intestine in a similar manner to Ascaris larvae, as described above. On the way in, the penetrating larvae may cause a localized itchy rash, and blood eosinophilia and Löffler's syndrome may occur as the larvae pass through the bloodstream and lungs. When the worms are attached in the small intestine there may be only mild abdominal symptoms, but persistence leads to a chronic iron deficiency anemia due to the constant removal of blood from the small intestinal mucosa by the hookworm.

Toxocariasis is a potentially important infection contractable by contact with dog and cat feces

This condition is particularly important in children who play in an environment where they may come into contact with dog and cat feces, and employees such as kennel maids. There are two main varieties, *Toxocara canis* and *Toxocara cati*, affecting dogs and cats respectively. Eggs are passed from the animal's alimentary tract in the feces and may be ingested by humans by feco-oral contamination. The eggs hatch in the human small intestine, and penetrate into intestinal blood vessels and are carried to the liver, brain, eyes, lungs and many other tissues where they excite a florid chronic inflammatory granulomatous response, in which eosinophils are very numerous. There are two important clinical syndromes, one associated with the larvae locating the eye ('ocular larva migrans' or 'ocular toxocariasis') and the other with widespread larval dissemination to other internal organs ('visceral larva migrans').

Ocular larva migrans is due to the florid granulomatous reaction in the eye, particularly in the retina where it may lead to severe visual impairment. This pattern is mainly confined to children.

Visceral larva migrans is accompanied by severe systemic manifestations such as fever, raised white cell count with greatly increased numbers of eosinophils, with asthmatic symptoms and pneumonitis (if the larvae are numerous in the lungs) and hepatosplenomegaly (if the liver and spleen are involved). This mainly occurs in young children under the age of 6. The larvae in the skin may produce an itchy rash, and severe cerebral symptoms may occur if the larvae reach the brain, although this is uncommon.

Pinworm infestation is very common in young children and usually presents clinically with perianal itching or soreness

The small pinworm (*Enterobius vermicularis*) is a very common parasite in children in temperate zones and of all social classes. The worm is small and difficult to see unless special methods are used to trap and identify it. The female worm is about 1 cm long, and is 2–3 times as big as the male. Infection is by direct or indirect feco-oral transmission, directly from finger to mouth in young children who have scratched an itchy ova-laden perineum, or indirectly by contact with clothing or bedding in which the ova have come to rest. The ova hatch and mature into worms in the colon and rectum. The mature female migrates to the anus and perianal skin to deposit its ova, and the worms can sometimes be identified and trapped in the child's perianal skin at night when the child is complaining particularly of itching. Sometimes the placement of a strip of transparent sticky tape over the anus may pick up eggs and even trap the female worms when they emerge to lay eggs at night. Once the eggs have been laid successfully, there is a very high chance of repeated reinfection by the feco-oral route. However, the eggs can survive in clothing and bedding, etc, for some days or even weeks.

9

Environmental and nutritional factors in disease

ENVIRONMENTAL FACTORS IN DISEASE

Although an interplay between genetic and environmental factors often modifies the host response, many diseases are predominantly due to adverse environmental factors, the most important of which are mechanical trauma, extremes of temperature, exposure to radiation, electricity and chemicals, environmental pollution, and nutritional factors.

MECHANICAL TRAUMA

Mechanical trauma is responsible for a considerable proportion of emergency hospital admissions. The effects of the trauma will be dependent on:

- The nature of the trauma.
- The force of impact.
- The site or sites traumatized.

A special type of mechanical injury occurs with sudden changes in pressure, exemplified by blast injuries due to proximity to explosions. In such cases, pressure waves may enter the body through air passages, causing traumatic rupture of lungs and intestines.

Skin and soft tissue injuries are common in trauma

The most frequent types of mechanical trauma are skin and soft tissues injuries. These may be divided into:

- **Abrasion.** Removal of surface layers by friction.
- **Contusion**. Rupture of small blood vessels, leading to extravasation of blood into tissues (bruising).
- **Laceration**. Ragged tear in tissue.
- **Incision and puncture wounds**. These are caused by penetrating sharp objects, e.g. a knife, wooden stake, or broken glass.

Injuries to bone and tendon may be acute or chronic

Certain types of trauma lead to acute injuries. The most common type of acute bony injury after trauma is partial or complete fracture of the bone. Fracture is associated with pain centered on the site of injury, and there is

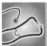
Motor vehicle accidents

Trauma from motor vehicle accidents is of major clinical and social importance. Damage inflicted is related to several factors, the most important of which are speed of travel, restraint, and protection from impact. There are three main types of injury:

1 **Injuries caused by sudden deceleration.** When a body is accelerated and then suddenly brought to a stop, the resulting internal stresses may cause severe damage.
  - The aorta may be transected, leading to severe internal bleeding
  - The brain may sustain internal tearing of white matter tracts.

2 **Injuries caused by direct trauma.** These occur when a body impacts with parts of a vehicle or with road surfaces. There may be:
  - Lacerations to face and hands from windshield glass.
  - Fracture of sternum and ribs from impact with steering column.
  - Fracture of legs from collapse of car frame, or from impact of car on a pedestrian.
  - Contusional damage and laceration of liver, spleen and lungs.
  - Contusions of brain, and fracture of neck from impact damage to head.

3 **Injury secondary to impaired cardiorespiratory function.** Blood loss, unconsciousness, and interruption of the airway are common in victims of trauma and lead to secondary damage.
  - Brain is extremely vulnerable to hypoxia, developing neuronal death (see page 441).
  - Kidneys may develop tubular necrosis (see page 372).

often considerable bleeding into the muscles and other tissues around the bone. Bone fracture is discussed in Chapter 24.

Acute musculotendinous injuries, such as torn muscle fibers, partially or completely ruptured tendons, and dislocated joints (particularly of the fingers and shoulder), are common sporting injuries.

More insidious is chronic trauma resulting in chronic musculoskeletal injuries, particularly osteoarthritis of joints (see page 523). Thickening of tendon sheaths may result from repetitive minor trauma over a long period. It is particularly common in certain occupations, e.g. those that involve typing, and is a major contributor to so-called 'repetitive strain injury' (RSI).

Musculotendinous and joint injuries are discussed in Chapter 24.

DAMAGE FROM EXTREMES OF TEMPERATURE

Burns are caused by local heat injury

Direct exposure of the skin to severe heat produces burns, the severity of the burn being related to the degree of heat and the length of exposure.

The two factors that influence the outcome of burn injury are the depth of burn (*Fig. 9.1*), and the surface area of skin affected.

Burns may be classified as major or minor, according to extent and depth. First-degree burns, although painful, are classed as minor and have little systemic impact. The immediate systemic consequence of a second-degree burn to more than 20% of the body is extravasation of fluid, including high protein exudate, from the burn site. This loss causes hypovolemic shock, manifest by low blood pressure and failure to perfuse tissues. There is a hypermetabolic state, frequently requiring special nutritional support.

Victims involved in a fire frequently have other injuries which influence outcome, e.g. airways injury by heat of carbon monoxide inhalation, and chemical inflammation of lung caused by inhalation of toxic smoke.

In the period following a major burn, there are several further potential complications. There may be secondary infection of the burn, particularly by *Pseudomonas aeruginosa*, *Staphylococcus aureus*, streptococci and *Candida*, and lung damage due to shock (ARDS, see page 205) can develop.

First-degree burns heal rapidly without scarring. Keratinocytes migrate from skin appendages such as hair follicles and eccrine ducts to form a new layer over the intact dermis and dermoepidermal basement membrane.

Full-thickness burns heal with dermal scarring. The only natural way to re-epithelialize is by migration of keratinocytes from the edges of the wound. This is assisted by skin-grafting from an intact area of skin elsewhere.

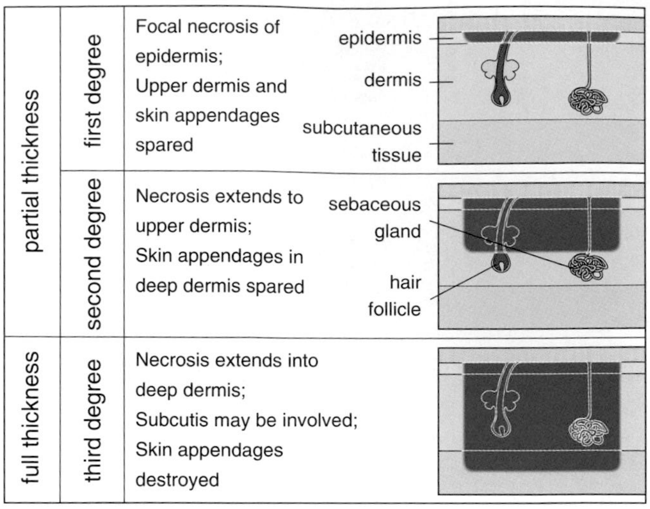

Fig. 9.1 Depth of burns.

Despite grafting, excessive tissue scarring with contractures is a frequent complication.

Generalized heat injury can lead to death if untreated

Generalized heat injury (hyperthermia) is common and may be seen in those exposed to a hot environment for a prolonged period.

Heat cramps are due to disturbance of electrolytes, which are lost in sweat. Treatment is by salt replacement.

Heat exhaustion occurs when hemoconcentration due to fluid loss has occurred. Hypotension develops and the patient feels weak and nauseous. Treatment involves oral rehydration and removal to a cool environment.

Heat stroke is a life-threatening condition associated with delirium and loss of consciousness. Hypotension develops and body temperature rises to 41–44°C. Treatment is by fluid replacement and rapid lowering of body temperature.

Localized cold injury leads to frostbite

The main syndrome caused by localized injury due to cold is frostbite, which occurs when part of the body is exposed to temperatures below freezing point. There is vasoconstriction and thrombosis in arteries, leading to tissue necrosis within a few hours (*Fig. 9.2*).

Hypothermia can cause death due to failure of cellular metabolism

Hypothermia is a generalized reduction in body temperature, usually due to prolonged exposure to low temperatures. It is most common in the elderly, in whom thermoregulatory mechanisms may be inefficient, and is particularly likely to occur if the person is immobile. It is not uncommon for hypothermia to complicate collapse from another disease process. For example, elderly patients

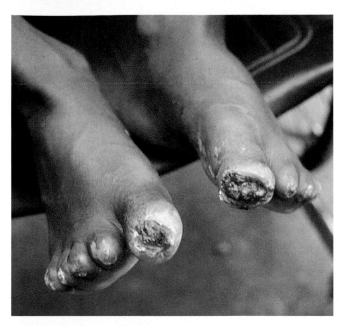

Fig. 9.2 Frostbite of toes.
Localized cold injury has caused necrosis of the toes in this person, exposed to the extreme cold while on a climbing expedition in the Himalayas. Similar changes may also occur in the fingers.

are often found unconscious or semi-comatose in their poorly heated houses in winter. As well as an initial cause for collapse, such as a stroke, they are also found to have a low body temperature. Patients with hypothyroidism (myxedema) are particularly prone to developing hypothermia.

If the patient is warmed, recovery is possible. In severe cases patients die from cardiac failure or secondary bronchopneumonia. Acute pancreatitis is another complication.

DAMAGE FROM IRRADIATION

Ultraviolet radiation causes acute and chronic forms of skin damage

Melanin pigment in the keratinocyte cell layers of the skin has a protective function against the effects of ultraviolet (UV) radiation. As a result, Caucasians are particularly vulnerable to skin damage.

The most frequent type of damage is sunburn, in which dermal capillaries dilate and the epidermis undergoes necrosis, with blistering and eventual shedding. Healing occurs by reformation of the epidermis from keratinocytes that migrate from undamaged basal cells.

Several skin rashes occur largely in areas exposed to light, and exposure to UV radiation is thought to be one of the factors involved in producing the skin damage (**photodermatitis**). However, there are other contributory factors, e.g. exposure to plant-derived allergens or an underlying intrinsic disease such as systemic lupus erythematosus.

Testing may demonstrate skin sensitivity to UV radiation of a particularly narrow wavelength, and the application of a topical UV-blocking cream cures the rash.

UV radiation is a predisposing factor for development of neoplasia in skin

UV radiation is known to damage DNA in epidermal cells, and several malignant tumors of skin in Caucasians are believed to be caused by exposure to this type of radiation, particularly **malignant melanoma** and **basal cell carcinoma** (see Chapter 23).

In the rare autosomal recessive disease, **xeroderma pigmentosum**, there is an inherited deficiency of endonuclease, the enzyme partly responsible for the repair of DNA damaged, for example, by UV radiation. Children with this disorder develop severe abnormalities in the epidermis, followed by development of multiple squamous cell carcinomas. Protection of the skin from sunlight prevents or greatly delays the development of malignant skin tumors in such cases.

Ionizing radiation causes damage to DNA

In terms of tissue damage, the main impact of ionizing radiation is on cell DNA. Ionizing radiation is normally present in the environment, and individuals may also be exposed to artificial sources, e.g. radiation used in diagnostic imaging.

The ionizing radiations of medical importance are:

- X-rays and gamma rays.
- Alpha particles, beta particles and neutrons.

To cause damage, ionizing radiation has to be absorbed by tissues. It removes electrons from atoms of the tissue through which it passes, generating free radicals. These interact with DNA and cause strand breaks, base alterations and abnormal cross-linking. The DNA damage can either lead to immediate cell death or cell death at next division, or may cause alteration in the genome, rendering a cell susceptible to neoplasia (see page 99).

The extent and severity of radiation damage depends on dose, duration of exposure, and sensitivity of individual cell types to the radiation.

The dose of radiation absorbed is expressed in grays (Gy). (1 Gy is equivalent to 100 rads, the previous dose unit.) Because different types of ionizing radiation penetrate tissues to varying degrees, and different tissues vary in their sensitivity to radiation, doses are corrected mathematically as dose equivalents expressed in sieverts (Sv). (1 Sv is equivalent to 100 rems, the previous dose unit.)

In general, cell types with a high turnover (frequent mitoses) are the most sensitive, those with a low turnover being the least sensitive. This differential sensitivity of cells with a rapid mitotic and replication rate is the basis of the treatment of malignant tumors (composed of rapidly replicating cells) by ionizing radiation (radiotherapy).

There are three main types of exposure to ionizing radiation

The body is exposed to harmful amounts of ionizing radiation in three main ways:

1 Slow, cumulative, whole-body exposure. This is usually due to natural or low output industrial and medical sources. An important source of natural radiation is radon, a radioactive gas which naturally diffuses from hard rocks such as granite and may reach high concentrations in some buildings.

2 Sudden, whole-body exposure. This is usually due to industrial or military sources.

3 High-dose, localized exposure. This is mainly a result of therapeutic ionizing radiation used to treat tumors.

In the UK the annual average exposure to radiation is 2.5 mSv. Just over 10% of this is from medical usage of radiation. The clinical response to total body irradiation ranges from none to rapid death depending on the dose (*Fig. 9.3*).

Long-term effects of irradiation are related to chronic vascular damage

In addition to the acute effects of irradiation, tissues frequently show long-term or delayed effects of exposure. A common factor in such delayed effects is damage to blood vessels, which show intimal proliferation, hyalinization, and occasionally fibrinoid necrosis, long after exposure (*Fig. 9.4*). These changes cause secondary ischemic changes

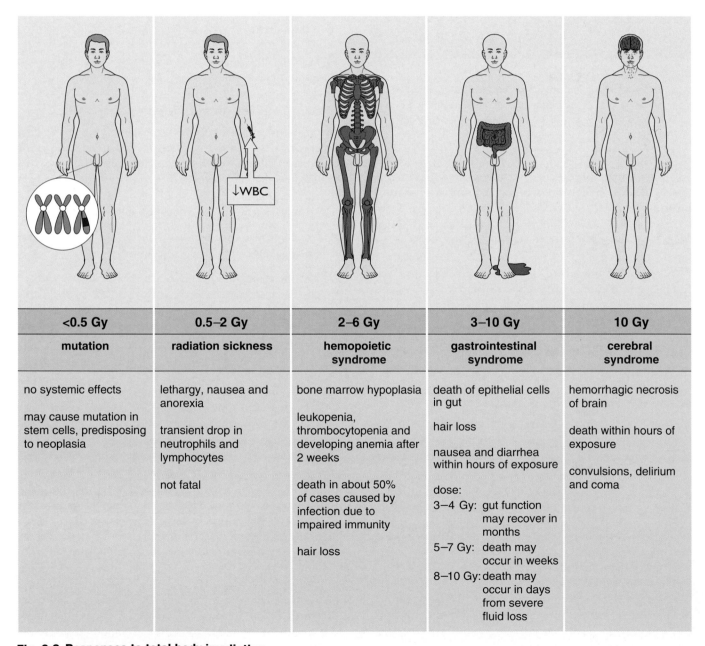

<0.5 Gy	0.5–2 Gy	2–6 Gy	3–10 Gy	10 Gy
mutation	**radiation sickness**	**hemopoietic syndrome**	**gastrointestinal syndrome**	**cerebral syndrome**
no systemic effects may cause mutation in stem cells, predisposing to neoplasia	lethargy, nausea and anorexia transient drop in neutrophils and lymphocytes not fatal	bone marrow hypoplasia leukopenia, thrombocytopenia and developing anemia after 2 weeks death in about 50% of cases caused by infection due to impaired immunity hair loss	death of epithelial cells in gut hair loss nausea and diarrhea within hours of exposure dose: 3–4 Gy: gut function may recover in months 5–7 Gy: death may occur in weeks 8–10 Gy: death may occur in days from severe fluid loss	hemorrhagic necrosis of brain death within hours of exposure convulsions, delirium and coma

Fig. 9.3 Responses to total body irradiation.

in tissue, with fibroblast proliferation and scarring. A summary of acute and delayed effects of radiation exposure is shown in *Fig. 9.5*.

ELECTRICAL INJURY

Electrical energy can cause tissue damage proportional to the amount of current flowing. Factors that maximize current flow, e.g. high voltage and low resistance of contact such as wet skin, predispose to more severe damage. There are two main effects of electrical injury:

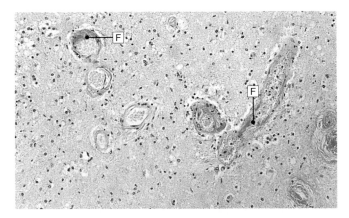

Fig. 9.4 Photomicrograph of irradiation vascular damage. After irradiation, vessels develop fibrinoid necrosis in walls (**F**) and hyalinization. Fibroblasts develop large hyperchromatic nuclei. The vascular changes lead to secondary ischemic damage to tissue.

- **Interference with normal body electrical activity.** Passage of current through the brain causes cessation of activity in cardiorespiratory centers. Passage of current through the heart causes cardiac arrhythmia, particularly ventricular fibrillation. Spasms of skeletal muscles may cause bone fractures.
- **Generation of heat, causing burns.** If there is prolonged contact with the electrical source, local generation of heat will cause burns. Prolonged exposure is frequently seen with AC sources as they cause tetanic spasm of muscles, preventing escape. Burns occur at entry and exit points of the electrical current and are useful in forensic practice, aiding reconstruction of the scene of a fatality from electrocution.

CHEMICAL DAMAGE

Toxic chemicals can gain access to the body by many routes including skin contact, inhalation, ingestion, and injection.

Exposure may be accidental (due to environmental or industrial exposure) or deliberate (the result of therapeutic or addictive or suicidal self-administration). Some chemicals

Fig. 9.5
Summary of effects of irradiation on various tissues

Tissue	Acute effect	Chronic effect
Skin	Desquamation and edema	Pigmentation and thinning Carcinoma
Bone		Bone necrosis Premature closure of epiphyses in children
Bone marrow	Marrow hypoplasia	Risk of leukemia
Ovary/testis	Destruction of germ cells	Atrophy and fibrosis
Lungs	Acute radiation pneumonitis	Alveolar wall fibrosis
Gut	Mucosal necrosis	Submucosal fibrosis and stricture
Kidney	Acute radiation nephritis with acute renal failure	Gradual loss of renal parenchyma, with chronic renal failure
Brain	Transient somnolence	Developmental delay in young children
Eye		Cataracts
Ear		Deafness
Thyroid		Hypothyroidism Risk of thyroid carcinoma

have a direct toxic effect on cells, whereas others produce damage indirectly by acting as antigens and initiating a damaging immune response.

Ethyl alcohol is a potent toxin that affects many major organs

Ethyl alcohol consumption in alcoholic beverages is common in most societies. The pathopharmacology of ethanol and its psychological effects are important aspects of social medicine. In terms of structural pathology, ethanol has several main effects.

Acute intoxication. Ethanol is a depressant, leading to impaired consciousness and, ultimately, to respiratory depression at high levels. A frequent complication of excessive consumption is coma, during which aspiration of vomit into the lungs leads to death. Other acute effects of very high concentrations are acute gastritis (see page 251) and acute alcoholic hepatitis (see page 291).

Chronic ethanol abuse. This is frequently part of physical and psychological dependence on alcohol. The main pathological effects are:

- Chronic liver disease, leading to liver failure.
- Cardiomyopathy, leading to cardiac failure (see page 181).
- Pancreatitis, causing severe, intractable abdominal pain (see page 301).
- Peripheral neuropathy, often caused by associated vitamin deficiency.
- Brain damage, leading to cognitive decline and ataxia due to neuronal death.
- Fetal alcohol syndrome, seen in the offspring of mothers who are dependent on alcohol.

Substances of abuse cause disease by both direct and indirect effects

Substances of abuse taken for recreational purposes are a major social problem. Drugs abused are commonly stimulants, depressants, or hallucinogenics. They are taken by injection into skin (skin popping), intravenous injection (mainlining), smoking, sniffing (snorting) or orally. Solvents are abused by inhalation (glue sniffing) and butane gas is inhaled. Associated pathology can be attributed to both direct and indirect effects.

Addiction to heroin and other opiates can lead to a wide range of pathologies

The pathological sequelae of opiate addiction can be divided into those due to the drug itself, those due to the presence of a contaminant in the injected drug (e.g. powdered talc, quinine, etc), those due to unsterile administration, and those due to social pathology (risk of violence, etc).

- **Direct opiate effect** – usually due to overdose, leading to depression of the cardiorespiratory center in the brain. Progressively slowing heart and breathing rates, with hypotension, eventually lead to coma, cardiorespiratory arrest and death due to acute pulmonary edema. Regurgitation of gastric contents whilst semi-comatose, with inhalation into the respiratory tract, is also a common cause of death.

- **Effects due to drug contaminants** – occur only with illegally purchased opiates which have been diluted ('cut') from the pure form with white powdery or crystalline substances such as talc or quinine. If talc has been used, there is a risk of multiple talc granulomas forming in the lung after intravenous drug injection, leading to progressive pulmonary fibrosis. Chronic quinine intoxication can lead to amblyopia. When the drugs are injected into the subcutaneous tissue (usually early in the addictive process), the contaminants may play a role in the frequent occurrence of skin ulcers.

- **Effects due to unsterile administration** – are extremely important and common, and are due to a combination of injecting through dirty skin, use of dirty needles, and the sharing of needles and syringes between addicts. Bacterial infection (often staphylococcal) leads to bacteremia, septicemia and bacterial endocarditis, from which septic emboli can spread to anywhere in the body. Fungal infection (usually due to *Candida albicans*, another skin commensal – see page 186) has a similar pattern. Both candidal and staphylococcal endocarditis produce bulky vegetations on the heart valves (see *Fig. 10.47*). The most important viral infections, usually acquired through the sharing of needles and syringes with previously infected addicts, are hepatitis B and C (see pages 282 and 284) and HIV, leading to AIDS (see page 107).

- **Social pathology** is beyond the scope of this book, but it is worth noting that opiate addicts are very prone to accidental injury when under the influence of drugs and to criminal violence from fellow addicts and dealers. Addicts who turn to prostitution to fund their drug habit also have a high incidence of sexually transmitted disease.

Cocaine addiction produces little structural pathology, but significant social pathology

Although an overdose of cocaine can produce severe cerebral over-stimulation leading to fitting and death, this is rare. Probably the commonest cause of death in habitual cocaine users is due to involvement in road traffic and other accidents as a result of the inappropriate feelings of confidence and impregnability which the drug gives.

Persistent heavy nasal inhalation of cocaine can rarely lead to necrosis of the nasal septum due to intense persistent vasoconstriction of the small blood vessels in the septal mucosa and submucosa.

The social pathology of heavy cocaine abuse is immense, but beyond the scope of this book.

MDMA (also known as Ecstasy or 'E') can lead to death by a combination of hyperpyrexia and dehydration or by disseminated intravascular coagulation

MDMA is 3.4 methylenedioxymethylamphetamine, and is now widely available on the illegal drugs market. It is commonly used by young people attending dance events. Under the influence of this stimulant and euphoriant drug, and the stimulating environment, they dance beyond exhaustion, and may suffer severe dehydration and hyperpyrexia. A few individuals react inappropriately to the drug and develop a rapidly fatal disseminated intravascular coagulation state, with widespread rash, cerebral petechial hemorrhages, coma and death. The mechanism of this is not known.

Solvent abuse is an important drug-related cause of death in young teenagers

The most commonly used solvents currently inhaled by teenagers are the solvents used in various glues ('glue sniffing'), and butane aerosols (e.g. cigarette lighter fuel). Inhalation leads to intoxication due to transient cerebral stimulation. Excessive dosage can lead to profound CNS depression and sudden death from cardiorespiratory arrest or inhalation of vomit.

Metals cause disease as a result of environmental, occupational and therapeutic exposure

Many metals have adverse effects if present in high levels. In most instances it is possible to distinguish acute toxic effects (often the result of suicidal or homicidal administration) from chronic toxic effects (usually environmental and occupational exposure). Complete lists of metals and their toxicity are presented in specialist texts. Some of the more common agents are listed in the blue box below.

Iron and copper accumulate in tissues as a result of inborn errors of metabolism

Iron can accumulate in tissues as a result of an inborn error of metabolism that leads to a disease termed **hemochromatosis**, in which cells contain vast excess of iron as ferritin. The defect causes excessive iron absorption from the gut, which comes to light because the accumulated iron causes cell death and dysfunction in several tissues. There may be:

- Cardiomyopathy leading to heart failure (see page 181).
- Diabetes because of iron in islet cells of pancreas (see page 540).
- Chronic liver disease due to cirrhosis (see page 292).
- Female infertility due to pituitary involvement.

Excessive iron can also accumulate in tissues in diseases associated with excessive breakdown of red cells,

---

Metals and toxicity

Lead toxicity
Exposure: gasoline, earth, paints, water, car battery burning, foundries.
At risk: workers in industry, children in poor socioeconomic circumstances.
Effects: anemia with basophilic stippling of red cells (lead interferes with normal heme formation), motor neuropathy, contractions of intestinal smooth muscle and colic, deposition in growth lines in bones (visible in epiphyses on X-ray), encephalopathy in children.

Mercury toxicity
Exposure: common industrial waste product.
Acute toxicity: suicidal ingestion, gastrointestinal ulceration, and acute tubular necrosis.
Chronic toxicity: (Minimata disease) cerebral and cerebellar atrophy with loss of neurons, dementia and ataxia; nephrotic syndrome.

Aluminium toxicity
Exposure: ubiquitous in environment, but poorly absorbed.
At risk: renal dialysis patients and some patients on total parenteral nutrition (TPN).
Effects: osteomalacia-like syndrome, dementia with cerebral atrophy.

Arsenic toxicity
Exposure: agricultural chemicals, particularly pesticides.
Acute toxicity: suicidal or homicidal ingestion results in abdominal pain and collapse.
Chronic toxicity: arsenical keratoses, skin cancer, peripheral neuropathy with myelin loss, angiosarcoma of liver.

Gold toxicity
Exposure: therapeutic administration in arthritis.
Effects: glomerulonephritis, skin rash.

Fig. 9.6
Common chemical toxins available in domestic settings

Agent	Effects
Methyl alcohol	Metabolic acidosis, neurological damage
Ethylene glycol	Metabolic acidosis, oxalate deposition in kidneys, acute tubular necrosis
Carbon tetrachloride	Centrilobular necrosis in liver, tubular necrosis in kidneys
Carbon monoxide	Tissue hypoxia by forming carboxyhemoglobin
	Headache, dizziness and confusion (early features)
	Delayed damage to basal ganglia and white matter
	Coma and death with high saturation
Strong alkalis	Ulceration of oropharynx and esophagus

Agrochemicals and disease

- **Organophosphates** are pesticides that work as acetylcholinesterase inhibitors. Chronic exposure causes muscle paralysis, autonomic dysfunction, and abdominal pain.
- **Paraquat** is a herbicide that causes massive free-radical generation. Accidental or suicidal ingestion leads to diffuse alveolar damage, renal necrosis, and hepatic necrosis.
- **Dioxin** causes chloracne in humans and has been shown to be embryotoxic in animals. It has been a contaminant in several processes producing other herbicides.

necessitating repeated blood transfusion. This is termed **secondary hemosiderosis** and mainly affects the liver (see page 292).

Copper toxicity is seen in an inborn error of metabolism termed **Wilson's disease**. Excessive copper is absorbed and accumulates in liver and brain due to mutation in a gene coding for a copper transport protein. If untreated, there is death of neurons and hepatocytes, leading to permanent damage. The main effects are abnormal movement disorders, psychiatric disease, and chronic liver disease.

Insecticides and herbicides are frequently implicated in disease

Environmental awareness has led to increasing scrutiny of the potential role of agrochemicals in disease. Several compounds have been found to accumulate in the food chain but, as yet, their significance in causing disease in man is uncertain. For example, chlorinated hydrocarbons (DDT, dieldrin) are insecticides, chronic exposure leading to accumulation in the liver. Although toxicity to certain birds and carcinogenicity in rats is established, there is little evidence of toxicity in man, despite extensive epidemiological surveys and evidence of massive exposure. However, recent concerns have been expressed that some compounds accumulating in the environment have estrogenic effects.

Importantly, the presence of agrochemicals must be weighed against the presence of highly toxic natural agents that are produced in plants as a result of infection by insects and fungi. Many of the toxins produced by nature are proven carcinogens, e.g. aflatoxins are highly carcinogenic substances produced by fungi in stored crops such as nuts.

Domestically available toxins are commonly used in suicides

There is ready access to chemicals in the domestic setting. Toxicity is mostly related to accidental or suicidal ingestion. The common agents are listed in *Fig. 9.6*.

Take a drug history: therapeutic agents are a frequent cause of disease

Therapeutic agents are a frequent cause of disease, and adverse drug reactions are responsible for many episodes requiring medical care, particularly skin rashes. Some reactions are dose related and may be attributable to pharmacokinetic variation between individuals. Others are idiosyncratic, often related to allergic and hypersensitive responses. Importantly, certain adverse reactions are delayed, e.g. drugs which are carcinogenic, impair fertility, or induce congenital malformations.

In addition to adverse effects of prescribed drugs taken in the correct dosage, therapeutic drugs are frequently used in suicide attempts.

NUTRITIONAL FACTORS IN DISEASE

Worldwide, nutritional factors are a very important cause of morbidity and mortality. In the developing world the major problem is under-nutrition; in the developed world, over-nutrition is a greater problem, in the form of obesity. A normal diet should provide energy, proteins, fatty acids, vitamins and minerals.

Under-nutrition can be caused by many factors, with a marked geographical variation

The causes of under-nutrition (starvation) in the developing world are usually:

Protein energy malnutrition

Protein energy malnutrition (PEM) is particularly seen in children in the developing world during periods of famine. When body weight falls to 60% of normal, a child is considered to have **marasmus**. Metabolic changes of starvation lead to loss of subcutaneous adipose tissue and loss of skeletal muscle bulk. In addition, the hair is lost, the skin becomes thin and atrophic, and there is predisposition to develop severe bacterial and viral infections, particularly TB and gastroenteritis, due to the effects of malnutrition on the immune system. There is also vitamin deficiency.

When protein deprivation is greater than deprivation of energy (carbohydrates still being available in the diet), the condition of **kwashiorkor** develops, in which affected children are 60–80% of normal weight. However, the marked protein lack leads to severe hypoalbuminemia and generalized edema. A scaly skin rash develops and the liver is enlarged and shows fatty change because lipid carrier proteins cannot be made. As with marasmus, there is immune deficiency and vitamin deficiency.

- Insufficient food available.
- Severe infection, particularly gastroenteritis.

Elsewhere, the main causes are:

- Malabsorption, due to intestinal disease.
- Anorexia nervosa and related psychological disorders.

In starvation there is inadequate intake of protein and carbohydrates. Hepatic stores of glycogen are rapidly depleted and the liver then breaks down amino acids and fatty acids to convert to glucose. The amino acids are derived from the breakdown of muscle protein, and the fatty acids from the breakdown of the fat stores, leading to loss of muscle bulk and subcutaneous fat. Lastly, serum proteins are catabolized to generate energy, resulting in abnormally low levels of albumin. These metabolic disturbances can be reversed if a normal dietary intake of food can be resumed.

Many factors play a role in the etiology of obesity

Obesity can be regarded as a form of chronic calorie overdose, due to a combination of excessive calorie intake and inadequate calorie breakdown. The surplus calories are stored in the body's fat deposits as fat within adipocytes; the most obvious externally visible fat depot is the subcutaneous adipose tissue, leading to the appearance of obesity, but the surplus is also stored internally, for example in omental, mesenteric, perinephric and epicardial adipose tissue.

Briefly, the factors involved in obesity are:

- **Excessive food intake** (particularly of fats) – excessive or gluttonous eating habits are often imposed by parents in infancy and early childhood. Such strongly imprinted patterns are difficult to break. It is the calorie content, not the physical bulk, of the food which is important, though most obese persons consume large quantities of high-calorie food and drink.
- **Inadequate calorie breakdown** – due to insufficient physical activity. The largely sedentary, car-dependent lifestyle in the developed world is a particularly important factor.

Genetic factors have been claimed to play a role following the discovery of leptin, a protein made in the adipocytes which controls body fat levels, probably through an influence on those parts of the brain which regulate energy utilization. Mutations in the gene which codes for leptin may play a role in the predisposition to obesity.

Obesity predisposes to many diseases, serious and mild

Obesity has been linked to many diseases that are common in the developed world, the most serious and important of which are:

- Systemic hypertension.
- Type 2 diabetes mellitus.
- Hyperlipidemia and increased severity of atherosclerosis.
- Increased predisposition to heart disease.
- Osteoarthritis and other degenerative joint diseases.
- Gallstones and obstructive biliary disease.
- Increased predisposition to leg vein thrombosis and pulmonary embolus.

In addition, obese people frequently suffer from a wide range of mild disorders, including breathing disorders on exertion, fungal infections in skin creases, and the tendency to lower-leg ulcers which heal slowly and poorly.

Vitamin deficiencies produce distinct clinical syndromes

In people with a well-balanced diet, vitamin deficiency is extremely rare. In most cases the manifestations of vitamin deficiencies are combined with some elements of protein–calorie malnutrition when the cause is starvation. However, individual vitamin deficiency syndromes can result from a number of factors including impaired absorption due to bowel disease, impaired synthesis, and specific absence from diet. The most important features of single vitamin deficiencies are given in *Fig. 9.7.*

Fig. 9.7
Vitamin deficiency syndromes

Vitamin	Function	Consequences of deficiency
A	Retinal function, epithelial growth control	Night blindness, keratomalacia, xerophthalmia
B_1 (thiamine)	Co-enzyme	Beriberi, Wernicke's encephalopathy
B_2 (riboflavine)	Co-enzyme	Dermatitis, glossitis, keratitis, neuropathy, confusion
B_6 (pyridoxine)	Co-enzyme	Neuropathy
B_{12} (cobalamin)	Nucleic acid synthesis	Megaloblastic anemia Subacute combined degeneration of spinal cord
Niacin	Co-enzyme NAD, NADP	Pellagra (diarrhea, dermatitis and dementia)
Folate	Co-enzyme in nucleic acid synthesis	Megaloblastic anemia, villous atrophy of gut
Vitamin C	Co-factor in hydroxylation	Scurvy
Vitamin D	Calcium and phosphate absorption	Rickets (childhood) Osteomalacia (adults)
Vitamin E	Antioxidant	Spinocerebellar degeneration
Vitamin K	Co-factor for coagulation factor synthesis	Bleeding due to coagulation defects

10 Blood circulatory system

Clinical Overview

Diseases of the blood circulatory system are the commonest cause of death in the western world. An adequate blood supply is vital for the functioning of every organ and tissue in the body, and anything which interferes with the adequacy of the arterial supply of oxygenated blood and the removal of relatively deoxygenated venous blood will have significant impact on the functioning of cells and tissues.

In the well-nourished (not to say frequently obese) western society, the disease process known as **atheroma** is virtually ubiquitous and is the basis of many diseases causing severe morbidity and death, such as **myocardial infarcts**, **gangrene**, **cerebral infarcts**, **aneurysms of large arteries**, and many others. Atheroma is a degenerative disease of large and medium-sized arteries which produces many complications including the important lesion called **thrombosis**, in which the solid cellular components of the circulating blood cluster together to form a solid mass which may lead to blockage of the vessel. Veins do not suffer from atheroma but under certain circumstances may also become blocked by thrombosis. In both the arterial and venous systems the solid masses of thrombotic material may pass in the circulation until they reach a vessel which is too small to allow further passage, when they become impacted leading to acute blockage of the vessel. This is called **thromboembolism**.

Another important disorder of the blood circulatory system is when the blood within the vascular channels is at a much higher pressure than it should be. In the systemic arterial system this is called **systemic hypertension**, and in the pulmonary arterial system, **pulmonary hypertension**. Systemic hypertension is much the most common and is responsible for a wide range of disorders including heart failure, brain hemorrhage, renal failure, worsening of atheroma, and predisposition to aneurysms of the aorta.

Tumors of the cardiovascular system are extremely rare, with the exception of small tumor-like masses composed of capillaries and similar small vessels. These are called '**hemangiomas**' and are common in the skin, particularly in infants and children. They are probably hemartomatous malformations rather than true tumors. The only significant malignant tumors of the blood vascular system are **angiosarcomas** which occur in the skin of elderly people, and **Kaposi's sarcoma** which occurs in patients with AIDS.

Congenital malformations of the arterial system are uncommon, but congenital malformations of the heart are a very important cause of morbidity and death in infants and children.

GENERAL PATHOLOGY OF THE CIRCULATORY SYSTEM

Accumulation of excess fluid in tissues is termed 'edema'

One of the important consequences of disease of the blood circulatory system is development of excess fluid in tissues, termed **edema**. Under normal circumstances, only a little fluid leaks from vessels to form interstitial fluid, which is removed by lymphatic vessels. Excess fluid leaks from capillaries into tissues in three main circumstances:

1   More fluid leaves capillaries if the hydrostatic pressure in vessels is increased (interference with venous drainage, heart failure).
2   More fluid leaves capillaries with reduced plasma oncotic pressure (hypoproteinemia).
3   More fluid leaves capillaries if vascular permeability is altered (allergic responses liberating histamine, acute inflammation).

The two most important types of edema are seen as a consequence of cardiac failure:

Pulmonary edema is the accumulation of fluid in the alveoli of the lung. It is caused by increased hydrostatic pressure in the pulmonary vascular bed, resulting from failure of the left side of the heart (see page 174).

Subcutaneous edema is the accumulation of fluid in subcutaneous tissues. It is caused by increased hydrostatic pressure in the systemic venous system, resulting from failure of the right side of the heart (see page 174).

Hemorrhage is caused by rupture of blood vessels

Hemorrhage is caused by rupture of blood vessels. Massive exsanguination is usually caused by trauma to a major artery or vein, but may also result from bursting of a vessel weakened by disease. Bleeding into tissues or body cavities results in several types of hemorrhage.

- **Hematoma** is an accumulation of blood within soft tissues. It is usually due to traumatic damage to vessels, but occasionally follows spontaneous rupture of diseased vessels.
- **Hemopericardium** is a collection of blood in the pericardial cavity, usually due to rupture of the heart or the aorta.
- **Hemothorax** is a collection of blood in the pleural cavities, usually due to trauma or rupture of the aorta.
- **Hemoperitoneum** is a collection of blood in the peritoneal cavity, usually due to rupture of an aortic aneurysm or traumatic damage to liver, spleen or aorta.
- **Hemarthrosis** is a collection of blood in a joint space. It is usually due to either direct trauma, or a bleeding disorder such as hemophilia (see page 75).

- **Petechiae** (1–2 mm diameter) and purpura (2–10 mm diameter) are small tissue hemorrhages, often seen in the skin (see *Fig. 10.25*), due to either abnormal small vessel fragility, abnormal blood clotting or abrupt increase in pressure within small venules and capillaries.

A clotted mass of blood forming in the circulation is called a 'thrombus'

A thrombus is a structured, solid mass composed of blood constituents that forms in the cardiovascular system. This distinguishes it from a coagulum, which is unstructured and forms when blood clots outside the circulatory system.

The process of thrombus formation, termed **thrombosis**, is due to activation of the normal blood coagulation system (*Fig. 10.3*). Aggregation of platelets, held together with a meshwork of fibrin, is a normal hemostatic mechanism, occurring constantly to plug small defects in blood vessel walls. Once the defect is plugged effectively, and the vessel wall is repaired, the small platelet/fibrin thrombus is normally removed by **fibrinolysis**, a multienzyme process that breaks down the supporting mesh of fibrin filaments, allowing dissolution of the thrombus (see *Fig. 10.4*).

In normal vessels, excessive thrombosis is prevented by several physiological mechanisms (see pink box). In **pathological thrombosis** the process of thrombus formation proceeds beyond the capacity of the endogenous fibrinolysins to eradicate the thrombus. Thrombus continues to enlarge by deposition of fresh layers of platelets and fibrin until a substantial mass is formed, which may reduce the lumen of the vessel. The morphology of a thrombus is shown in *Fig. 10.1*.

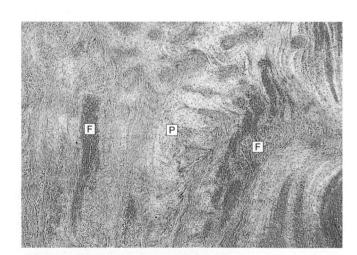

Fig. 10.1 Thrombus morphology.
A thrombus is composed of elements derived from activation of the coagulation cascade, i.e. aggregated platelets, insoluble fibrin derived from soluble plasma fibrinogen, and entrapped red cells. These elements are usually arranged in a laminated pattern, layers of platelets alternating with layers of fibrin and entrapped red cells. This is shown in the photomicrograph of a thrombus, in which pale layers of platelets (**P**) are separated by pink-stained layers of fibrin and red cells (**F**).

Events in thrombus formation

Endothelial damage results in exposure of collagen and von Willebrand factor, which mediate adhesion of platelets. Platelets express surface glycoprotein receptor which bind to these ligands.

- Glycoprotein Ia (GPIa) binds directly to collagen
- Glycoprotein Ib (GPIb-IX) binds to von Willebrand factor (VIII:vWF) and this in turn binds to collagen. (Inherited deficiency of GPIb-IX results in a bleeding disorder termed Bernard-Soulier syndrome. Deficiency of VIII:vWF is termed von Willebrand's disease.)

Adherent platelets undergo a shape change and aggregate.

- ADP is released from granules which stimulates further aggregation of platelets (as well as adhesion of further platelets), forming a platelet plug.
- Prostaglandin thromboxane A2 (TXA2) is synthesized by platelets and causes platelet aggregation and vasoconstriction.
- Receptors are expressed on the platelet surface which interact with coagulation factors collectively referred to as Platelet Factor 3 (PF3). The coagulation system generates the insoluble protein fibrin, discussed below.
- Platelets express glycoprotein complex IIb-IIIa on their surface (GPIIb-IIIa), which act as receptors for fibrinogen and vWF helping formation of a firm hemostatic plug. (Inherited deficiency of GPIIb-IIIa results in a bleeding disorder termed Glanzmann's thrombasthenia.)

NORMAL

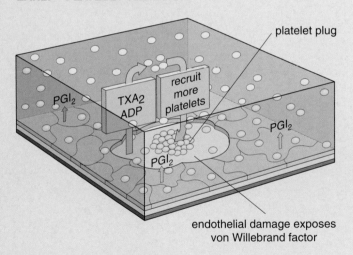

EARLY – PLATELET ADHESION

LATE – FIBRIN DEPOSITION

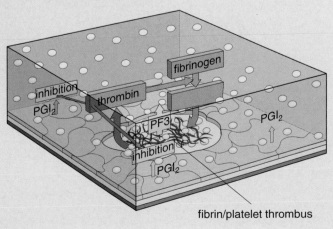

Fig. 10.2 Events in thrombus formation.

The coagulation cascade is activated to produce fibrin at the site of damage

The ultimate aim of the coagulation cascade is to generate a solid plug of cross linked protein that seals a defect in a blood vessel wall. The protein which is deposited is fibrin, generated from its circulating precursor protein, fibrinogen. To achieve this end point a large number of different proteins interact in a cascade, illustrated in *Fig 10.3*. The coagulation factors have been given numbers (I–XIII). Functionally nearly all these factors are proteases with the exception of factors V and VIII which act as co-factors.

Traditionally the coagulation cascade has been divided into three compartments

Common pathway: a series of steps that leads to the generation of cross-linked fibrin. A key protease generated in this part of the pathway is thrombin. This is an important factor as it feeds back to activate co-factors and other proteases early in the system, providing feedback amplification of the cascade.

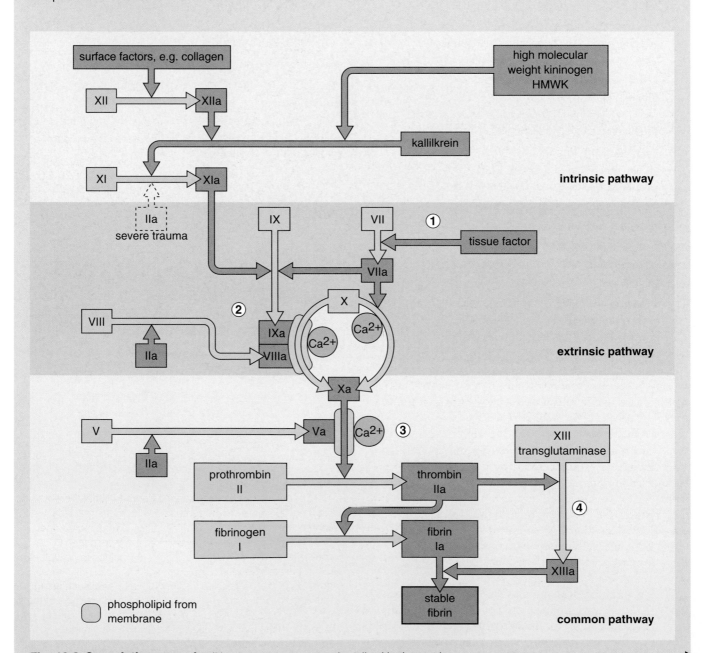

Fig. 10.3 Coagulation cascade. (Numbers refer to steps described in the text.)

▶ **Extrinsic pathway:** coagulation is initiated by a substance generated from damaged tissues called Tissue Factor by interaction with factor VII

Intrinsic pathway: coagulation is initiated by contact with surface agents such as collagen or by proteases such as kallikrein, acting through factor XII (Hageman factor). It is now believed that the intrinsic pathway is of little relevance for coagulation in-vivo and that the activities described mainly pertain to in-vivo systems. Activation of factor XI and stimulation of coagulation is seen mainly after severe injury such as severe trauma.

1 Coagulation is initiated by tissue factor, generated on the surface of cells adjacent to vessels and exposed following injury to the vessel wall. Tissue factor and activated factor VII activate factor IX and can also directly activate factor X.

2 Activated factor IX with activated factor VIII and calcium ions act at the phospholipid surface of platelets to convert factor X to its active form (Xa). Factor VIII consists of two parts: a large component with activity in the coagulation pathwas (VIII-C) and a component which is involved in platelet adhesion (VIII:vWF). This acts as a co-factor by being activated by thrombin.

3 Activated factor X forms a complex on platelet phospholipid surfaces with activated factor V and calcium ions to convert prothrombin to thrombin. Thrombin has several vital activities as a protease in the coagulation cascade:

- cleavage, if fibrinogen, to form fibrin and fibrinopeptides A and B
- activation of factor XIII (transglutaminase) which cross links fibrin to form a stable thrombus
- activation of factors XI, VIII, and V in the coagulation cascade.

In addition thrombin acts through thrombin receptors to activate endothelial cells and promote expression of vasoconstrictive factors and plasminogen activator (see later).

4 Fibrin initially formed by the action of thrombin is unstable and need to be cross-linked by the action of a transglutaminase, factor XIII.

Full details of the coagulation cascade are available in standard hematology texts.

Fibrinolytic systems are activated to remove thrombus once formed

The products of the coagulation cascade are usually restricted to the immediate site of vessel wall damage.

Plasma inhibitors of coagulation act to limit the coagulation cascade. The most potent inhibitor of coagulation is antithrombin III, the action of which is potentiated by the action of heparin. Protein C is a vitamin-k-dependent factor which is activated by thrombin in the presence of thrombomodulin and in concert with protein S works by destroying activated co-factors V and VIII. Protein C also inactivates something which normally prevents fibrinolysis (PAI-1).

Fibrinolysis is brought about by formation of the protease plasmin (*Fig. 10.4*). This is formed by activation of its precursor, plasminogen and acts to degrade fibrin into fibrinopeptides collective termed fibrin degradation products (FDPs), together with fragments of cross-linked fibrin termed D-dimer. Plasminogen is converted into plasmin by the activity of plasminogen activators. The most important are tissue plasminogen activator, derived from endothelial cells (tPA) and urinary-type plasminogen activator (uPA). Under normal circumstances uPA and tPA are inhibited by plasminogen activator inhibitor 1 (PAI-1). However activated protein C prevents this, thereby facilitating local fibrinolysis. Circulating alpha2-antiplasmin is a potent inhibitor of formed plasmin.

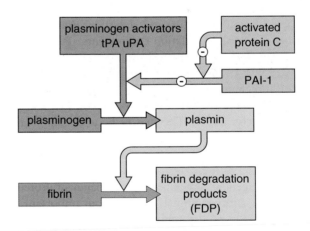

Fig. 10.4 Fibrinolysis.
The fibrinolytic system functions to degrade fibrin, thereby allowing lysis of formed thrombus. The enzyme that cleaves fibrin is termed plasmin and this is formed from a precursor protein in plasma, termed plasminogen. Plasminogen is converted to plasmin by the aciton of plasminogen activators. Other factors, grouped as plasminogen activator inhibitors, antagonize the process of forming plasmin. One such being PAI-1, which interacts with protein C. The end products of the fibrinolytic process are fibrin degradation products. These products also have anticoagulant activity. Plasminogen activators have been considered for therapeutic administration to promote lysis of thrombus, for example in the immediate management of coronary artery thrombosis.

The endothelium normally prevents thrombosis in vessels

Normal endothelial cells act to prevent activation of the coagulation cascade, generating factors that bring about thrombus lysis.

- Intact endothelium prevents platelets from coming into contact with collagen and von Willebrand factor (which cause platelet aggregation and degranulation).
- Prostacyclin (PGI2) and nitric oxide prevent adhesion and aggregation of platelets to endothelium.
- Thrombomodulin, on the endothelial surface, binds to any locally formed thrombin generated as part of the activation of the coagulation cascade. The thrombomodulin/thrombin complex can then initiate the anticoagulant effects of the vitamin-k-dependent factor protein C and its co-factor protein S. Active protein C destroys factor V and factor VIII

- Endothelium produces heparin-like molecules, which inhibit elements of the normal coagulation cascade.
- Endothelium synthesizes plasminogen activators, which produce plasmin, a proteolytic enzyme that lyses fibrin and inactivates parts of the coagulation cascade.
- Antithrombin III (AT-III) is a potent inhibitor of coagulation and works by inactivating proteases operating in the coagulation cascade. Heparin potentiates the activity of this system.

Three main factors predispose to thrombus formation

Among the main predisposing factors to thrombus formation is **endothelial dysfunction**. Direct injury to endothelium, as seen in trauma and inflammation, may lead to thrombosis. Damage to endothelium occurs in association with atheroma (see page 162).

Change in the flow pattern of blood is a major factor in causing thrombus. Stasis allows platelets to come into contact with endothelium, and slow flow prevents blood diluting activated coagulation components. Turbulence of blood flow may cause physical trauma to endothelial cells and, with loss of laminar flow, bring platelets into contact with endothelium.

Changes in potential blood coagulability predispose to thrombus formation. This may be because of an increase in the concentration of fibrinogen in acute phase responses. Increase in concentration of prothrombin and fibrinogen can also occur with estrogen-containing oral contraceptive therapy. Congenital lack of natural anticoagulant protein C, protein S or antithrombin III are rare but important predisposing factors to thrombosis. Abnormal autoantibodies directed against platelet phospholipids (**antiphospholipid** antibodies) are an increasingly recognized cause of arterial and venous thrombosis.

A mutation in the coagulation factor V, so called Leiden mutation, renders this factor resistant to inactivation and is a predisposing factor to abnormal arterial or venous thrombosis in 2–10% of the Caucasian population.

Thrombosis can occur at any place in the circulatory system

Thrombi that occur in different parts of the circulation have different causative factors and different macroscopic appearances. Those formed in fast-moving blood in arteries and cardiac chambers have a relatively high platelet/fibrin content and are very firm and pale, with prominent laminations. Thrombi that form in slow-moving blood, such as that in veins, have a high proportion of trapped red cells relative to fibrin/platelets, and are typically red, soft and gelatinous in texture, with poor laminations.

As most thrombi that form in small- or medium-sized vessels occlude the lumen and prevent blood flow, they are termed **occlusive thrombi**. However, thrombi that form in the heart or aorta generally do not cause complete occlusion, appearing as raised plaques applied to the wall (**mural thrombi**). Thrombi that occur on heart valves appear as polypoid masses and are termed **vegetations**. The main predisposing factors to thrombosis at different sites are shown in *Fig. 10.5*.

Fig. 10.5
Predisposing factors to thrombus at different sites

Site	Predisposition to thrombosis
Artery	Atheroma, aneurysms
Heart valve	Inflammation caused by infection
Ventricle	Inflammation following infarction Ventricular aneurysm
Atrium	Atrial fibrillation (→ stasis) Mitral valve stenosis
Vein	Slow flow Changes in coagulability of blood
Cerebral venous sinus	Inflammation following infection Change in coagulability of blood

There are four main outcomes following vascular occlusion by a thrombus

Once a thrombus develops in a vessel there are several possible outcomes. The thrombus may enlarge along the vessel (a process termed **propagation**) or it may undergo lysis by the fibrinolytic system. The latter process may, in certain circumstances, be assisted by therapeutic administration of a fibrinolytic agent such as streptokinase.

There may be **organization** of the thrombus by ingrowth of granulation tissue from the vessel wall. Gradually the thrombus is replaced by granulation tissue, and new vascular channels develop, bridging the site of occlusion and re-establishing flow. This is termed **recanalization** (*Fig. 10.6*).

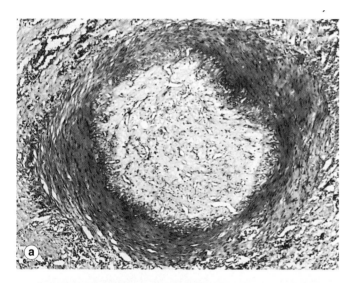

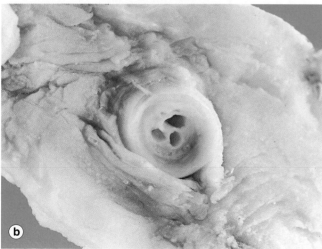

Fig. 10.6 Organization and recanalization of thrombus. (a) Histology. (b) Macroscopic.
Granulation tissue containing many small blood vessels has completely replaced the thrombus that was occluding this vessel (a). Eventually, some of these vessels enlarge and flow is re-established. Such a recanalized artery is shown in (b), in which a coronary artery lumen has been replaced by three small lumina having been previously blocked by thrombus.

Alternatively, fragments may break off the thrombus and be carried by the circulation to impact in other vessels, a process termed **thromboembolism**.

EMBOLISM

Occlusion of a vessel by material travelling in the circulation is termed 'embolism'

Embolism can be defined as 'occlusion of a vessel by a mass of material that is transported in the bloodstream'. The mass of material is termed an **embolus**, and the most common type is due to fragments of circulating thrombus, termed **thromboemboli**.

Thromboembolism occurs when a mass of thrombus breaks off from its site of formation to enter the blood circulation, where it travels until it meets a blood vessel with a lumen too small to permit further passage. At this site it impacts, usually occluding the lumen of the vessel.

- Thromboemboli originating in systemic veins travel round to the heart to impact in the pulmonary arterial system, causing **pulmonary thromboembolism**.
- Thromboemboli originating in the heart (mural thrombus or vegetations) travel via the aorta to the systemic arterial circulation. There they commonly impact in arteries leading to brain, kidneys, spleen, gut and lower limbs.
- Thromboemboli originating from mural thrombus in the common carotid arteries impact in the cerebral arterial system.
- Thromboemboli originating from mural thrombus in the abdominal aorta commonly impact in the renal arteries and arteries of the lower limbs.

Pulmonary thromboembolism is an extremely common preventable condition

The most common preventable cause of death in hospital patients is pulmonary thromboembolism (*Fig. 10.7*). The vast majority of cases are caused by emboli arising from thrombosis of deep leg veins (calf, popliteal, femoral and iliac veins). Diagnosis of leg vein thrombosis is notoriously difficult as symptoms and signs are non-specific; most cases are silent, resolving without detection.

The two main consequences of embolization to the pulmonary arterial tree are an increase in pulmonary arterial pressure (which puts a strain on the right side of the heart) and ischemia of the lung, with ventilated areas not being perfused by blood. The clinical consequences of pulmonary embolism depend on the extent of the pulmonary vasculature blockage and the time-scale involved.

If 60% of the pulmonary vasculature is suddenly blocked, the heart cannot pump blood through the lungs. There is cardiovascular collapse, with electromechanical dissociation of the heart as it continues to beat but develops no output. This pattern of blockage is known as **massive pulmonary**

embolism. Causing rapid death, it accounts for about 5% of all cases of pulmonary thromboembolism.

Accounting for about 10% of all cases of pulmonary thromboembolism, **major pulmonary embolism** occurs when there is blockage of middle-sized pulmonary arteries. Patients commonly experience breathlessness. Infarction of lung develops in only about 10% of such cases. It can lead to hemoptysis and, if adjacent to the pleura, pleuritic chest pain. It is not uncommon for patients to develop a subsequent massive thromboembolism if untreated.

In about 85% of all cases of pulmonary thromboembolism there is blockage of small peripheral vessels by small emboli (**minor pulmonary embolism**). Patients may be asymptomatic or may experience breathlessness and pleuritic chest pain as a result of small infarcts. As with major pulmonary embolism, it is not uncommon for patients to develop a subsequent massive thromboembolism if untreated.

A very small number of patients develop **recurrent minor pulmonary embolism**. There is blockage of many small peripheral arteries over a period of many months by recurrent small emboli. This leads to obliteration of the vascular bed and right heart strain, causing pulmonary hypertension (see page 169).

Not all pulmonary emboli originate from thrombosis in leg veins

Although thrombus formed in the deep veins of the calf is the commonest site of origin, in a few cases the primary thrombosis occurs in the peri-prostatic venous plexus of veins in men and (much less commonly) in the small pelvic veins in women. Usually the reason for thrombosis at these sites is not apparent since no predisposing pelvic disease is present.

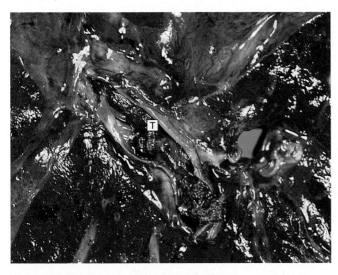

Fig. 10.7 Pulmonary thromboembolism.
The main pulmonary artery contains a mass of red thrombus (**T**), a thromboembolus. This originated by embolization from one of the femoral veins.

KEY FACTS
Pulmonary embolus

- Usually follows thrombosis in leg veins, often deep veins in calf.
- Small pulmonary emboli impact in peripheral branches of pulmonary artery and cause **pulmonary infarcts** (often with clinical pleurisy).
- Large pulmonary emboli may impact in, and obstruct, a major pulmonary artery to cause sudden death (**massive pulmonary embolus**).
- A small pulmonary embolus (with infarction) may be followed by a much larger, fatal, embolus ('**premonitary embolus**').
- Prevention of leg vein thrombosis is the best way of preventing pulmonary embolus.

Clinical conditions predisposing to leg vein thrombosis

Thrombosis arising in deep leg veins may be completely asymptomatic or may cause mild pain and tenderness in the muscles, sometimes with development of ankle edema.

Clinical situations predisposing to development of deep leg vein thrombosis are:

- Immobility and bed rest.
- Postoperative period.
- Pregnancy and *post partum* period.
- Oral contraceptive therapy with high-estrogen preparations.

- Nephrotic syndrome (see page 351).
- Severe burns.
- Trauma.
- Cardiac failure.
- Disseminated malignancy.

In many of these situations it is clinical practice to give prophylactic treatment with heparin to prevent development of thrombosis, combined with physiotherapy to the legs.

Embolism of material other than embolus is less common

The most common material to embolize in the blood stream is thrombus, but other types of embolus can occur. The most important and clinically significant is malignant tumor.

Tumor embolism is the way in which malignant tumors spread from the site of origin to distant metastatic sites using the blood stream route. The malignant tumor infiltrates through the wall of a blood vessel (usually a venule or vein) at the primary site to occupy the lumen, and clumps of tumor cells of various sizes break off and are carried in the venous system until they reach a vessel too small to permit further passage, then impact there and often grow to produce a distant metastasis. For this reason, histological evidence of vascular invasion at the primary site at the time of tumor excision is regarded as a poor prognostic feature in tumor grading (see page 85).

Fat and bone marrow embolus may occur following severe fracture trauma to bones. Fragments of fat released from traumatized adipocytes in the fatty bone marrow may enter the blood circulation through thin-walled veins torn by the fracture trauma. They pass through the venous system to the right side of the heart, and thence via pulmonary arteries to the lung capillaries where some are trapped. However, some small lipid droplets can pass completely through the pulmonary capillary bed to enter the pulmonary veins and thereby gain access to the systemic circulation. They are then distributed to the small capillaries throughout the body; if many such fat droplets enter the cerebral circulation, they can occlude many brain capillaries, leading to coma and death. Larger fragments of bone marrow (including hemopoietic tissue) are too large to pass through the pulmonary capillaries, so are usually trapped in the lung.

Air embolism is usually due to accidental pumping of air into the venous circulation during intravenous injection or transfusion. If large quantities of air mixed with blood enter the right atrium, a bloody froth is formed and the patient may suffer cardiac arrest. In deep-sea divers, inhaled air may dissolve into the plasma due to the increased pressure at great depths, only to reform into bubbles of gas within the circulation if the diver comes to the surface too quickly. This decompression sickness (known to divers as 'the bends') and the embolization of the bubbles of mainly nitrogen gas may occlude small vessels, leading to widespread anoxia of tissues, and even death.

Amniotic fluid embolism may occur rarely during childbirth; some of the amniotic fluid (containing fetal cells from the skin surface) may enter the maternal circulation through the exposed and bleeding placental bed in the uterus. The material passes in the venous circulation to the lung capillaries and may cause acute alveolar wall damage and disseminated intravascular coagulation (see pages 205 and 327).

Therapeutic embolization is being used increasingly to treat inoperable vascular malformations of the brain by interventional radiology. Wire, gelfoam, glue and balloons are all used to deliberately block vessels.

INFARCTION

Lack of perfusion of tissues by blood leads to infarction

Failure of adequate blood supply to a tissue causes cell damage through ischemia. Tissue necrosis due to interference with local blood flow is termed **infarction**. The vast majority of infarcts are due to obstruction of the arterial supply to a tissue, a minority being caused by interference to the venous drainage. The ischemic damage results in coagulative necrosis in tissues.

Infarction is a major cause of morbidity and mortality, the most important examples being myocardial infarction ('heart attack', see page 177), cerebral infarction ('stroke', see page 438) pulmonary infarction, gangrene of lower limb, and bowel infarction (see page 264).

Blockage of an artery generally causes coagulative necrosis in the target organ

Infarcts caused by blockage of an artery are shaped according to the territory of supply of the blocked vessel. Occlusion of small arteries in an organ such as the kidney or lung usually results in wedge-shaped infarcts, with the occluded vessel at the apex (*Fig. 10.8*).

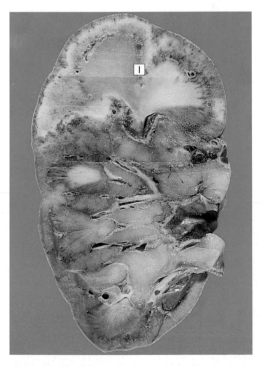

Fig. 10.8 Renal infarct. A recent infarct of the kidney shows a pale area of infarction (**I**), with an adjacent hyperemic border separating it from normal kidney.

Immediately following arterial occlusion, a damaged area is typically poorly defined, pale and swollen. Within about 48 hours the dead tissue becomes better demarcated and is pale and yellowed. As an acute inflammatory response develops in adjacent viable tissue, a red hyperemic border becomes visible, separating normal tissue from the area of infarction. After 10 days or so, ingrowth of granulation tissue and organization are advanced. The infarcted area is ultimately replaced by collagenous scarring.

Blockage of veins causes hemorrhagic necrosis (venous infarction)

Infarcts caused by blockage of venous drainage develop because tissue becomes massively suffused by blood. Blood is unable to drain from the tissue via the veins, but arterial blood continues to pump in, causing congestion and a rapid rise in pressure in small blood vessels, which lead to vessel wall rupture. Eventually, when the pressure is so high that arterial blood cannot enter, the tissue is deprived of oxygenated blood and undergoes anoxic necrosis.

Affected areas are deeply congested by deoxygenated blood and may appear almost black (hemorrhagic infarction). The usual cause of venous infarction is torsion of the vascular pedicle of an organ. Examples include torsion of the testis, bowel volvulus, and strangulated hernia. Venous infarction is also seen in the brain with venous sinus occlusion by thrombosis.

Slow occlusion of a vessel may cause ischemia and not infarction

Infarction usually occurs when vascular occlusion is abrupt; when the blood flow is reduced over a period of time there are two possibilities. Alternative vascular channels can open up to compensate for the obstruction in the diseased vessel (collateral circulation). Development of collateral vessels is possible in many tissues, but not when an area is supplied by a single artery (end artery).

Alternatively, the tissue undergoes ischemic atrophy. Specialized cells shrink and eventually die over a long period of time, and tissue is converted into hyaline, pink-staining amorphous support tissue. Robust support cells such as fibroblasts may survive in the face of ischemia.

KEY FACTS
Infarction

- **Infarction** is death of tissue due to anoxia following abrupt interference with the blood supply.
- **Arterial infarction** follows sudden obstruction to the arterial supply to a tissue or organ.
- **Venous infarction** follows sudden and persistent obstruction to venous drainage of an organ or tissue.

SHOCK

Shock is a clinical state associated with generalized failure of tissue perfusion

In contrast to local failure of vascular flow, a systemic reduction in tissue blood flow, manifest by profound low blood pressure (hypotension), is clinically termed **shock**.

Among the many causes of shock are severe failure of the pumping mechanism of the heart (**cardiogenic shock**), blockage of major arteries (**obstructive shock**), and lack of blood to pump (**hypovolemic shock**) due to hemorrhage or severe fluid loss. Abnormal dilatation of peripheral vessels causing lack of venous return of blood may also be responsible, arising in cases of septicemic shock/endotoxic shock, anaphylactic shock and neurogenic shock.

Events in the early and later stages of shock are summarized in *Fig. 10.9*. During the development of shock, protective mechanisms first operate to maintain perfusion of vital organs. The renin–angiotensin–aldosterone system causes retention of sodium and fluid, expanding blood volume. There is increased catecholamine production by the adrenals, and increased sympathetic activity, causing tachycardia and vasoconstriction in certain vascular beds (skin is cold and pale). ADH secretion is also increased, causing sodium and water retention.

With persistence of shock, systemic acidosis develops. This causes dilatation of previously constricted vessels, and blood pressure consequently falls. Blood is diverted from gut and kidneys to maintain perfusion of heart and brain. Output of urine falls and there is damage to renal epithelial cells. Gut stasis also develops, with necrosis of lining epithelial cells. In the late and irreversible stages of shock there is necrosis of cells in liver, heart and brain. Death is due to multiple organ failure.

Fig. 10.9
Early and late manifestations of shock

Tissue	Early shock	Late shock
Skin	Pale and cold	Cyanosed
Kidneys	Low urine production	Necrosis of tubular epithelium
Gut	Bowel stasis	Necrosis of lining epithelium
Lung	Tachypnea	Necrosis of alveolar epithelium
Liver	Fatty change	Necrosis of centrilobular cells
Brain	Reduced conscious level	Necrosis of neurons, coma
Heart	Tachycardia	Myocardial necrosis

ARTERIAL DISEASES

Arterial disease and its complications are important causes of morbidity and mortality in most western societies, the main disease being atherosclerosis.

Thickening and hardening of arterial walls is termed 'arteriosclerosis'

Arteriosclerosis is the term used to describe thickening and hardening of the walls of arteries, without implying any particular cause. The effect of arteriosclerosis on the functions of the artery are twofold:

- the internal diameter of the arterial lumen is almost invariably reduced, with consequent reduction in the amount of blood flowing through it
- the thickened and rigid artery wall loses some of its ability to contract and relax, and also loses some of its elasticity.

Arteriolosclerosis is the term used to describe thickening and hardening of the walls of the arterioles. In most cases the structure of the wall of the affected arteriole is completely effaced with destruction of the thin smooth muscle layer. Arteriolosclerosis is most frequently a consequence of systemic hypertension (see page 166) or diabetes mellitus (see page 540).

Atheroma is a specific degenerative disease affecting large and medium arteries in the systemic circulation. Although it begins as a disease affecting the tunica intima, eventual involvement of the tunica media leads to thickening and hardening of the artery wall. At this stage the disease is called atherosclerosis, and is the most common cause of arteriosclerosis affecting large and medium-sized arteries.

Arteriosclerosis affecting small arteries is usually due to the affects of prolonged systemic hypertension (see page 166).

The main consequence of these structural abnormalities affecting arteries and arterioles are due to a combination of factors:

- the **reduction of the size of the lumen** leads to poor perfusion of blood to the tissues supplied by the affected vessels, with the consequent tissue hypoxia which may be severe enough to cause cell death, particularly in cells which have a high oxygen requirement
- the changes in the structure in the tunica intima, particularly the potential for damage to the lining endothelium, predisposes to **thrombus** formation (see page 156)
- the changes in the structure of the media may result in loss of elasticity of the vessel wall. This is a major factor in the pathogenesis of **aneurysm** formation (see page 164), and mainly occurs in the large arteries affected by severe atherosclerosis, particularly the abdominal aorta below the origin of the renal arteries.

Atherosclerosis accounts for half of all deaths in the western world

Atheroma and its consequences constitute the most common and important cause of disease and death in the western world. Atheroma affects large- and medium-sized arteries, rarely involving arteries under 2 mm in diameter, and is confined to arteries exposed to the high pressures in the systemic circulation. The pulmonary arteries, which are accustomed to the low blood pressures of the pulmonary circulation, normally show no evidence of atheroma except when heart or lung disease leads to pulmonary hypertension. Similarly, atheroma does not affect veins, although atheroma-like lesions can be seen in veins exposed to systemic arterial pressures, e.g. when lengths of vein are used to bypass blocked coronary arteries.

The arteries most severely affected by atheroma are the aorta, coronary, carotid, mesenteric, iliac and femoral arteries, and the cerebral arteries derived from both the vertebrobasilar and internal carotid arteries.

Atheroma is a disease of the intima of arteries

Atheroma is the accumulation of lipid-rich material in the intima of arteries associated with cellular reactions. The lesions are termed **plaques**. Although atheroma is essentially a disease of the tunica intima, it has an impact on the structure and function of the media.

The macroscopic appearance of atheroma varies according to the stage of evolution of a plaque (*Fig. 10.10*). The sequence of changes that occurs in the development of a severe atheromatous lesion is summarized in *Fig. 10.11*.

Histologically, plaques show varying amounts of free lipid, collagen, and macrophages containing lipid (foam cells) (*Fig. 10.12*).

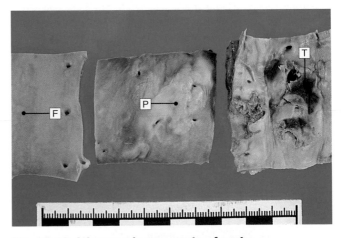

Fig. 10.10 Atheroma in segments of aorta.
The earliest changes are small fatty streaks (**F**), visible as pale areas beneath the endothelium in the aortic segment on the left. The central segment shows pearly white fibrolipid plaques (**P**), and the segment on the right shows ulcerated advanced plaques with adherent fibrin–platelet thrombus (**T**).

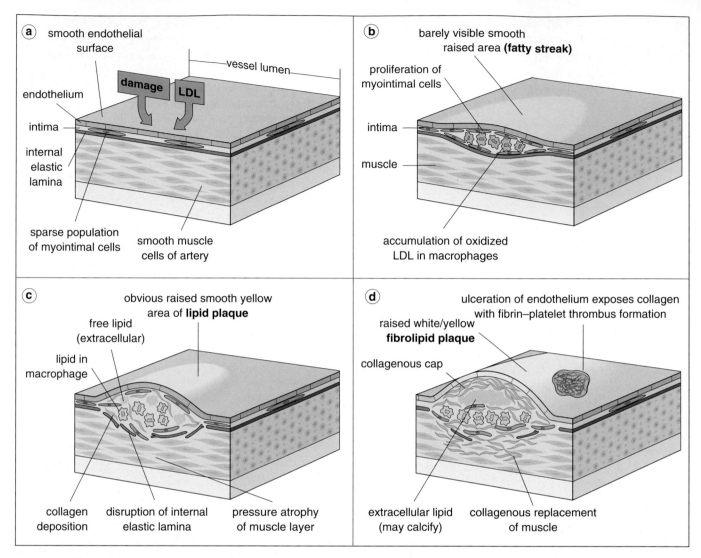

Fig. 10.11 Atheroma formation.

(a) The pathogenesis of atheroma is believed to be damage to the endothelium associated with a variety of risk factors discussed later. This allows entry of cholesterol-rich low-density lipoproteins (LDLs) into the intima. (b) The lipid is taken up by macrophages in the intima. Normal receptor-mediated uptake of lipid can be bypassed by oxidization of LDL, which is taken up by a receptor-independent pathway. In this way, excessive lipid accumulates in intimal macrophages to form a visible pale bulge termed a 'fatty streak'. (c) With development and increased accumulation of lipid, macrophages release lipid into the intima. Cytokines secreted by macrophages stimulate proliferation of intimal cells with features of myofibroblasts. These cells secrete collagen and the plaque starts to become fibrotic. At this stage lesions are raised and yellow (lipid plaques). As the lesion develops, there is pressure atrophy of the media and the elastic lamina is disrupted. (d) Increased secretion of collagen forms a dense fibrous cap to the plaque which is now hard and white (fibrolipid plaque). The advanced plaque shows free lipid as well as lipid in macrophages. Collagenization also affects the media, weakening the arterial wall. The endothelium is fragile and often ulcerates, allowing platelet aggregation and thrombosis. It is possible that platelet-derived growth factor causes further development of plaques by stimulating cell proliferation.

The pathogenesis of atheroma is still uncertain

There have been many hypotheses as to the pathogenesis of atheroma, which must explain the origin of the lipid seen in plaques, the reason for development of the cellular elements of plaques and the relation to known risk factors for atheroma development.

The thrombogenic hypothesis proposes that thrombus is incorporated into the intima of vessels, lipid being derived from platelet membranes and cells stimulated to proliferate by platelet-derived growth factors (PDGFs).

The clonal proliferation hypothesis is based on observations that smooth-muscle cells in plaques are derived from one clone of cells, raising the possibility that atheroma is caused by a primary abnormality in cell growth.

The lipid insudation hypothesis proposes that LDLs are taken up into the intima, where they become chemically oxidized to act as toxic, pro-inflammatory and chemotactic

Understanding of risk factors for atheroma is largely based on epidemiological studies

Atheroma is almost ubiquitous in the western world, virtually all adults developing the disease to some degree. Fatty streaks can be seen in childhood, small fibrofatty atheromatous plaques in teenagers and young adults, and complicated atheroma lesions in early middle age; atheromatous lesions increase in number with age.

Epidemiological studies have identified risk factors associated with atheroma development. These can be grouped into constitutional factors, hard risk factors, and soft risk factors.

Constitutional risks for atheroma

- **Age** – The number and severity of atheromatous lesions increases with age.
- **Sex** – Clinically significant atheroma is considerably more common in men than in women up to the age of 55 years; thereafter the incidence and severity increases rapidly in women, although men remain marginally more severely affected. It has been suggested that women are protected by estrogens before the menopause.
- **Familial traits** have an important bearing on atheroma in a small number of cases in which, independent of traits for hyperlipidemia, there is a familial increase in predisposition.

Hard risk factors for atheroma

- **Hyperlipidemia** – The severity of atherosclerosis has a direct correlation with serum levels of **cholesterol** or **LDL**. The risk increases in a linear fashion with serum

cholesterol levels above 3.9 mmol/L (150 mg/dL) There is a less significant association with increased levels of triglyceride and elevated very-low-density lipoprotein. There is a *reduced* risk of atherosclerosis with high levels of high-density lipoproteins, and this is favoured by modest ethanol consumption (less than 30 mg/day).

Atherosclerosis is much more common in patients with some forms of familial hyperlipidemia (Types II and III).

- **Hypertension** – There is a link between persistent high blood pressure and the severity of atheroma, most evident for raised diastolic blood pressure.
- **Diabetes mellitus** is a major risk factor for development of atheroma, and has been related to induced hypercholesterolemia in this disease.
- **Cigarette smoking** – There is a link between cigarette smoking and deaths from coronary artery disease, the most important clinical consequence of severe atheroma. The mechanism of the link is uncertain.

Soft risk factors for atherosclerosis

- **Exercise** reduces the incidence of sudden death from ischemic heart disease, one of the main effects of atherosclerosis, but it is uncertain whether it has an effect on the development of atheroma.
- **Overweight** individuals have an increased risk of death from ischemic heart disease, but this may be a reflection of diet and resultant hyperlipidemia.
- **Stress and personality** traits have been linked to death from ischemic heart disease in some studies.

factors. This is supported by the fact that antioxidant drugs can inhibit atherogenesis in animals.

The response to injury hypothesis (*Fig. 10.13*) proposes that the atheromatous plaque is a response to chronic low-grade injury to the endothelium. Metabolic disturbance to endothelial cells (as a result of hemodynamic stresses and toxic effects of LDL) allows platelet adhesion, diffusion of plasma proteins, and migration of monocytes into the intima of arteries. Platelets release PDGF and this stimulates proliferation of intimal smooth-muscle cells (myointimal cells). These, in turn, synthesize excess collagen and elastin in the intima. Oxidization of LDL facilitates its uptake into monocytes by non-receptor-mediated pathways.

Recently the organism *Chlamydia pneumoniae* has been found in atheromatous lesions, with antibodies to the organism detected in blood, consistent with infection. It has been proposed that *Chlamydia pneumoniae* may be

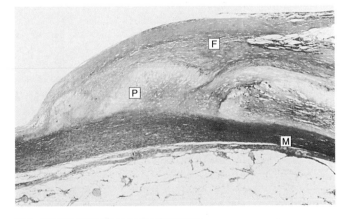

Fig. 10.12 Histology of atheroma.
The plaque shows pale lipid-rich areas (**P**) and pink-stained fibrous areas (**F**). Late in the fibrolipid stage the media (**M**) is thinned beneath the plaque.

either a causative or possibly potentiating agent in atheroma. Trials are being conducted to investigate if antibiotic therapy affects the natural history of atheromatous lesions.

Clinicopathological consequences of atheroma

Atheroma produces disease in several ways:

- **Reduction of blood flow through arteries.** When atheroma affects small arteries, the enlargement of an intimal atheromatous plaque may severely reduce the size of the lumen (*Fig. 10.14a*). The main clinical implications are ischemic heart disease (page 176), peripheral vascular disease (page 166), and cerebrovascular disease (page 437).

- **Predisposition to thrombosis.** If the fibrous cap over an atheromatous plaque breaks down, collagen fibres in the abnormal intima are exposed to the circulating blood, and this initiates the formation of thrombus (*Fig. 10.14b*). In small bore vessels, such as the coronary or cerebral arteries, this thrombus may suddenly complete the occlusion of an already narrowed artery. In larger vessels, such as the aorta, a plaque of mural thrombus is formed, which may embolize to distal vessels.

- **Bleeding into a plaque.** If there is breakdown of the fibrous cap of a plaque, blood may dissect into the centre of the plaque, causing it to balloon into the vessel lumen and reducing blood flow (*Fig. 10.14c*). This is occasionally seen in coronary arteries, leading to myocardial infarction.

- **Weakening of vessel wall and aneurysm formation.** Severe atheroma in the intima eventually leads to thinning of the media, loss of smooth-muscle cells and elastic fibers, and progressive replacement by non-contractile inelastic collagen. The media becomes

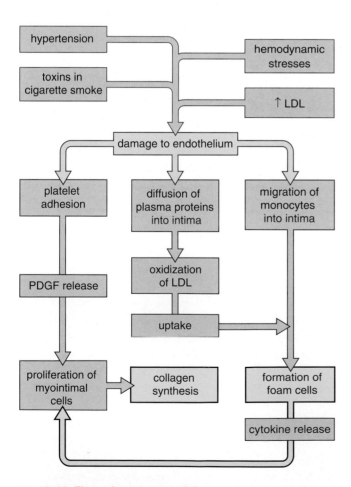

Fig.10.13 Flow-chart summarizing events involved in pathogenesis of atheroma.

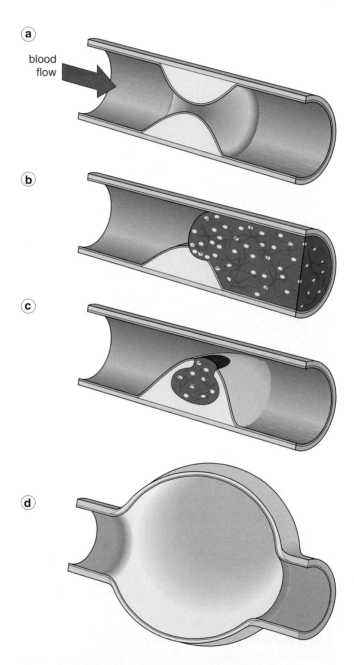

Fig. 10.14 Complications of arterial atheroma. (a) Narrowing of artery by atheroma. (b) Thrombus on plaque. (c) Bleed into a plaque. (d) Aneurysm.

functionally incompetent and this leads to generalized dilatation of the artery over a period of some years to form an aneurysm (*Fig. 10.14d*). The abdominal aorta is the most common site for aneurysms secondary to atherosclerosis.

KEY FACTS
Atheroma

- A disease of the intima of systemic arteries, NOT veins.
- Plaques composed of macrophages, muscle cells, lipid (cholesterol rich), and collagen.
- Main risk factors are hypertension, smoking, high cholesterol, and diabetes.
- Complications are reduction of flow, initiating thrombosis, and aneurysm formation.

ANEURYSMS

Diseases that damage the arterial media predispose to aneurysm formation

An aneurysm is an abnormal focal dilatation of an artery, the main complications being rupture and predisposition to thrombosis. Although it is the most frequent cause, atherosclerosis is not the only disease that produces aneurysms; any abnormality that weakens the media may produce an aneurysm, although permanent or transient hypertension is also an important factor in their enlargement and rupture. Other types and causes of aneurysm are given in *Fig. 10.15*.

'Dissecting aneurysm' is not a true aneurysm

In dissecting aneurysm, a tear in the intima leads to tracking of blood into the arterial media, which splits. The most common site for this is the aorta, where the split forms a false channel, usually between the inner two-thirds and outer third of the medial thickness. The possible outcomes are summarized in *Fig. 10.16*.

Fig. 10.15
Types of aneurysm

Type	Site	Cause	Incidence
Atherosclerotic	Abdominal aorta	Thinning and fibrous replacement of media	Common
Syphilitic	Ascending aorta and arch	Inflammatory destruction of media and fibrous replacement	Now rare
Berry	Cerebral arteries	Congenital defect(s) in elastic lamina/media	Common
Infective (mycotic)	Any	Destruction of wall by bacteria in infected thrombus	Rare

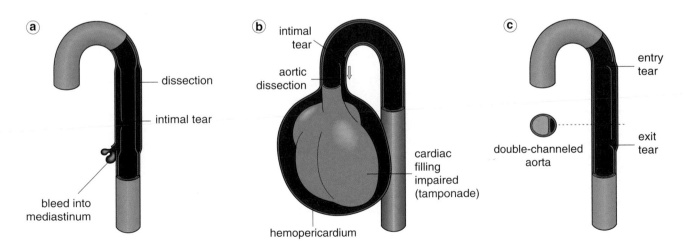

Fig. 10.16 Outcome following aortic dissection.
(a) External rupture, usually lower down the thoracic aorta, with massive fatal hemorrhage into the thoracic cavity. (b) Retrograde spread (back towards the heart) with rupture into the pericardial cavity, with fatal hemopericardium. (c) Internal rupture, with blood tracking back into the lumen by rupturing through the inner media and intima, to produce a double-channeled aorta. This is rare.

Atherosclerotic peripheral vascular disease causes gangrene

Atherosclerosis of arteries supplying the lower limbs is particularly common in diabetics, affecting them more than any other risk group. The iliofemoral and popliteal arteries are most commonly involved. Reduced flow leads to hypoxia of the calf muscles when their oxygen demands are high, e.g. while walking briskly or running. Patients complain of cramp-like pains in the calf muscles on exercise, which disappear after rest (**intermittent claudication**). More severe reduction in flow can produce similar changes at rest, and there are associated skin changes; there is hair loss, and the skin is smooth, shiny and slow to heal if traumatized.

Complete occlusion, usually by thrombus deposition on the atheroma, produces **gangrene** (ischemic necrosis of all tissues), manifest as blue-purple, painful discoloration of the skin, followed by progressive blackening of the tissues. Toes are involved first, but the changes progress proximally until a line becomes demarcated where oxygenation is just adequate.

Among the predisposing factors are hypertension, present in 70% of cases, and degenerative changes in the aortic media (medial mucoid degeneration), which sometimes arise as part of a recognized hereditary disorder of support tissues, e.g. Marfan's syndrome due to defective fibrillin, and Ehlers–Danlos syndrome.

Atherosclerosis is also a predisposing factor, the original intimal tear occasionally occurring at the edge of an atheromatous plaque. This pattern is particularly important in the distal aorta.

Dissection due to instrumentation of an artery wall is a rare complication of arterial puncture or cannulation. It often heals spontaneously without rupture, since the medial wall is usually healthy, limiting the extent of blood tracking.

HYPERTENSION

Hypertension may be classed as primary or may be secondary to a known cause

Elevated blood pressure (hypertension) is an important and treatable cause of disease, which is divided into primary or secondary groups. In the population, blood pressure is a continuous variable, with increasing risk of disease associated with increasing blood pressure. Hypertension can be arbitrarily defined as sustained diastolic pressure greater than 90 mmHg. However, there is no threshold below which a person has no risk of developing diseases in which blood pressure is a pathogenic factor.

Primary (essential) hypertension is elevation of blood pressure with age, but with no apparent cause. It accounts for over 90% of all cases and is usually seen after the age of 40 years. The phenotype of high blood pressure in essential hypertension is the result of interactions between genetic predisposition, obesity, alcohol consumption, physical activity and other, as yet unidentified, factors.

Accounting for about 10% of all cases, **secondary hypertension** is due to an identifiable cause, the most common of which is renovascular disease that elevates blood pressure by activation of the renin–angiotensin–aldosterone system.

Depending on the clinical course of disease, both primary and secondary hypertension can be classified into two types. With **benign hypertension** there is stable elevation of blood pressure over many years, and with **accelerated hypertension** blood pressure elevation is severe and becomes worse over a short period of time.

Artery wall thickening and hyaline arteriolosclerosis are features of benign hypertension

In benign hypertension, vessel changes develop gradually in response to a persistent stable elevated blood pressure. The changes in small arteries are shown in *Fig. 10.18*, and those in arterioles in *Fig. 10.19*.

These degenerative changes in the walls of small vessels such as arterioles lead to reduction in effective lumen, with consequent tissue ischemia, and to increased fragility of vessels in the brain, predisposing to hemorrhage.

Destruction of small vessel walls is seen in malignant hypertension

When the blood pressure rises suddenly and markedly, acute destructive changes occur in the walls of small blood vessels, together with proliferative reparative responses in the walls of small arteries (*Figs 10.20* and *10.21*).

These changes lead to cessation of blood flow through the small vessels, with multiple foci of tissue necrosis, e.g. in the glomeruli in the kidney.

Hypertension mainly affects the heart, brain, kidneys and aorta

The pathological consequences of hypertension are seen in four main tissues:

- **Heart.** With increasing pressure, the left ventricular myocardium undergoes hypertrophy. Since hypertension

Factors that regulate blood pressure

Blood pressure can be elevated by increasing cardiac output or by increasing peripheral vascular resistance. The former is raised by increasing the blood volume or by increasing cardiac contractility and rate, and the latter may be increased by humoral, neural and autoregulatory factors. These regulatory processes are summarized in *Fig. 10.17*.

Great interest is being taken in understanding genetic predispositions to hypertension. Very rare single-gene disorders have been identified that can cause hypertension:

- Mutations in genes coding for proteins involved in aldosterone metabolism.
- Mutations in genes coding for sodium ion handling.

The search is on to identify common polymorphisms in genes that will explain both population and individual predispositions to hypertension.

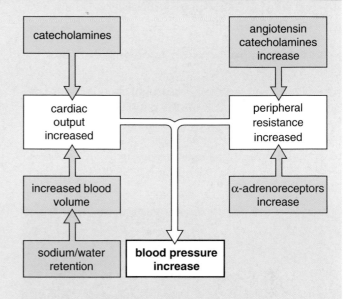

Fig. 10.17 Regulation of blood pressure.

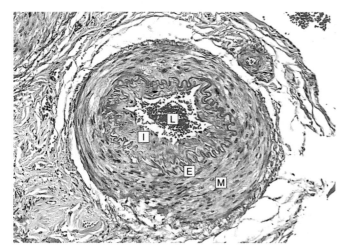

Fig. 10.18 Small arterial changes in benign hypertension. There is hypertrophy and thickening of muscular media (**M**), thickening of elastic lamina (**E**), fibroelastic thickening of the intima (**I**), and reduction in the size of the vessel lumen (**L**).

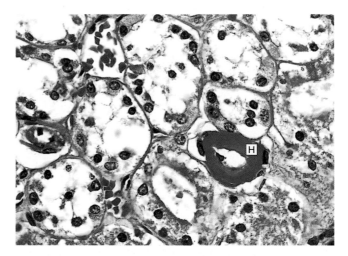

Fig. 10.19 Arteriole changes in benign hypertension. There is hyaline wall thickening (hyaline arteriolosclerosis) (**H**), increased rigidity (with limited capacity for expansion and constriction), and reduction of lumen size.

is usually associated with increased severity of atherosclerosis, coronary blood flow may be insufficient, leading to ischemic heart disease. **Left ventricular failure** is a common result of hypertensive heart disease.

- **Brain.** Hypertensives are particularly prone to developing massive **intracerebral hemorrhage** due to rupture of intracerebral blood vessels (see page 440). Small vessel damage within the cerebral hemispheres produces microinfarcts in the form of small areas of brain destruction filled with fluid (**hypertensive lacunae**).

- **Kidney.** Arteriolosclerosis leads to progressive ischemia of the nephron, with eventual destruction of glomeruli, and atrophy of the associated tubular system. This disease is slowly progressive, as individual nephrons are picked off one at a time. When sufficient nephrons have been rendered non-functional through ischemia, the patient develops slowly progressive **chronic renal failure**. When hypertension has produced significant nephron ischemia, the kidney is said to have developed **benign hypertensive nephrosclerosis**. It is a common and important cause of chronic renal failure in the middle-aged and elderly population.

- **Aorta.** Hypertension predisposes to development of severe atheroma, abdominal aortic aneurysms, and dissections (page 165).

Secondary hypertension accounts for less than 10% of cases

In a minority of cases, some structural abnormality is considered to be responsible for the development of systemic hypertension. For example, **stenosis of one renal artery** (usually at its origin) by atherosclerosis can produce hypertension, treatable by surgery. Associated with a rise in renin and angiotensin II levels in the circulation from the ischemic kidney, the hypertension can be cured in the early stages by removal of the affected kidney.

Hypertension is also a feature of **diffuse renal disease** such as glomerulonephritis and pyelonephritis. The hypertension is transient in the initial acute phase of glomerular diseases (e.g. acute nephritic syndrome), but is permanent in chronic diffuse renal disease.

Pheochromocytoma, an adrenaline–noradrenaline (epinephrine–norepinephrine)-secreting tumor, usually of the adrenal medulla produces hypertension that is initially paroxysmal (see page 343).

Coarctation of the aorta is a congenital malformation in which there is increased peripheral resistance due to a structural narrowing of the aorta. In such cases the hypertension is not truly systemic as it affects only the arterial system proximal to the coarctation and, thus, mainly the arms, head and neck (see page 188).

Hypertension is a feature of **adrenal cortical diseases**, conditions associated with excess production of

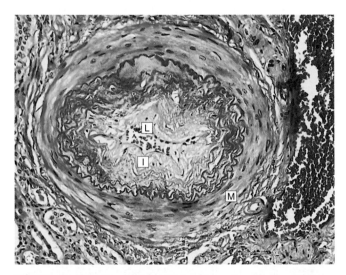

Fig. 10.20 Accelerated hypertension change in small arteries. Loose myxomatous fibrous intimal proliferation (**I**) can be seen, together with reduction of lumen (**L**) and normal media (**M**).

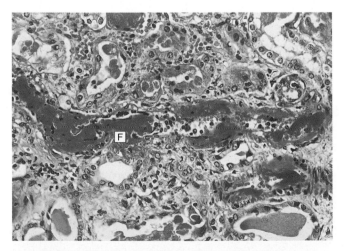

Fig. 10.21 Accelerated hypertension change in arterioles. Fibrinoid necrosis, visible as replacement of the wall by material stained bright red (**F**), is seen in the wall of a renal arteriole in malignant hypertension.

Fig. 10.22 Causes of pulmonary hypertension
Increased pulmonary blood flow
Cardiac shunts (ASD, VSD) (see page 187)
Pulmonary venous congestion
Mitral valve disease especially stenosis (see page 184)   Chronic left ventricular failure (see page 174)
Mechanical arterial occlusion
Multiple pulmonary thromboemboli (see page 158)   Foreign body emboli (drug addicts)
Alveolar hypoxia causing pulmonary vasoconstriction
High altitude   Obesity   Chronic obstructive airways disease
Destruction of lung capillary bed
Emphysema   Interstitial fibrosis of lungs
Idiopathic
Primary pulmonary hypertension: rare disease of young women due to increased tone in pulmonary vessels, leading to progressive vascular changes and death.
Pulmonary veno-occlusive disease: rare disease causing fibrous obliteration of pulmonary vessels. Some cases thought to be due to vascular thrombosis.

glucocorticoids and mineralocorticoids by the adrenal cortex (Cushing's syndrome and Conn's syndrome, see page 341).

It is also a feature of **preeclampsia** (see page 416), may be seen in association with endocrine disorders such as thyrotoxicosis, acromegaly and, occasionally, hypothyroidism, or there may be a **neurogenic cause** such as raised intracranial pressure.

Pulmonary arterial hypertension is usually due to disease in the lung or left side of the heart

Most pulmonary hypertension is 'secondary' in that it develops as a consequence of one of two types of raised pressure in the pulmonary capillary bed.

Pulmonary capillary pressure may be raised due to raised pressure in the left atrium and left ventricle. This back pressure is the result of inadequate emptying of the left heart chambers (left heart failure), the increased pressure in these chambers being reflected along the pulmonary veins and into the pulmonary capillary beds (pulmonary congestion). Important causes are left ventricular failure due to hypertensive or ischemic heart disease, aortic valve stenosis, and mitral valve stenosis (leading to left atrial failure).

Alternatively, pulmonary capillary pressure may be raised due to destruction of the pulmonary capillary bed as a result of primary lung diseases.

The classification and causes of pulmonary hypertension are shown in *Fig. 10.22*.

VASCULITIS

Vasculitis syndromes are a mixed group of diseases, affecting blood vessels of all types

Vasculitis implies inflammation and damage to the vessel wall. It can affect capillaries, venules, arterioles, arteries and, occasionally, large veins. In the most severe cases this leads to irreversible vessel wall destruction. In mild cases the damage is transient and may be marked only by cellular infiltration and vessel wall damage manifest by leakage of red blood cells.

There are three main groups of vasculitis syndromes:

- Hypersensitivity vasculitis is the most common pattern. It affects capillaries and venules, and is usually manifest as a skin rash. It is often a manifestation of allergy to a drug ('drug-induced vasculitis'), occasionally arising as an allergic rash in viremia or bacteremia. It also occurs in Henoch–Schönlein purpura, serum sickness, and cryoglobulinemia.
- Vasculitis can be a major element of multiorgan autoimmune diseases such as systemic lupus erythematosus (SLE) and rheumatoid disease.
- Systemic vasculitides are an important group of diseases, characterized by differing patterns of vessel-wall destruction, which is of unknown causation, e.g. polyarteritis.

Many diseases have a vasculitis as a main, possibly causative, feature. *Fig. 10.23* lists diseases that have vasculitis

Fig. 10.23
Vasculitis syndromes

Disease	Vasculitis	Clinical features
Hypersensitivity angiitis	Neutrophilic, fibrinoid necrosis	Skin, kidney
Polyarteritis nodosa	Neutrophilic, fibrinoid necrosis	Multiorgan
Wegener's granulomatosis	Neutrophilic and giant cell	Nasal, lung and renal involvement
Churg–Strauss syndrome	Histiocytic and eosinophils	Lung, kidney, heart, skin
Kawasaki arteritis	Lymphocytic; endothelial necrosis	Skin, heart, mouth, eyes
Takayasu's disease	Histiocytic; giant cell	Aorta and arch branches
Buerger's disease	Neutrophil; granulomatous	Leg arteries and veins; gangrene
Connective tissue diseases, e.g. SLE	Lymphocytic Occasional neutrophil	Skin, muscle, brain
Erythema nodosum	Venulitis and panniculitis	Deep tender lumps in legs
Pyoderma gangrenosum	Vasculitis and skin ulcers	Necrotizing ulcers of skin and subcutis

as a component, several of which are discussed in other systems chapters, according to the main organs involved.

Hypersensitivity vasculitis commonly presents with petechial hemorrhagic lesions in the skin

Hypersensitivity vasculitis mainly involves the post-capillary venules, with some capillary involvement (*Fig. 10.24*). The pathogenesis is due to immune complexes between an antigen and antibody becoming trapped in the walls

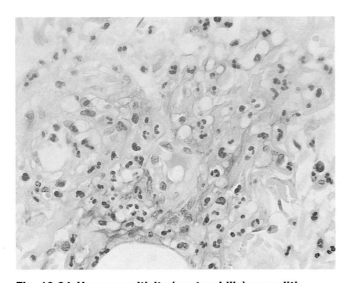

Fig. 10.24 Hypersensitivity (neutrophilic) vasculitis. Histologically the capillaries and venules in the upper dermis show destruction of small vessel walls by neutrophils, with adjacent dark-stained particles of neutrophil nuclear debris (neutrophilic vasculitis), and extravasated red cells in the area around the vessel. Occasionally the vessel walls show fibrinoid necrosis. This pattern of vasculitis mainly affects skin, but occasionally a similar small-vessel vasculitis occurs in the kidney, lining of the joints and alimentary tract mucosa in Henoch–Schönlein syndrome.

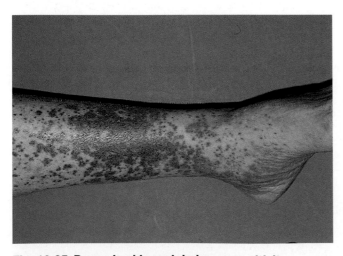

Fig. 10.25 Purpuric skin rash in hypersensitivity angiitis.

of venules. These activate complement, setting off a local acute inflammatory response, with neutrophil chemotaxis. Destruction of the vessel wall is mediated by release of neutrophil enzymes.

In many cases this pattern of vasculitis is associated with drug therapy or infection. The extravasation of red cells in the dermis is manifest as a transient palpable purpuric skin rash (*Fig. 10.25*), which disappears when the drug is stopped or the infection passes.

Polyarteritis nodosa (PAN) is a systemic disease that affects small- and medium-sized arteries

Polyarteritis nodosa is a systemic disease characterized by inflammatory necrosis of the walls of small- and medium-sized arteries (*Fig. 10.26*). Although the disease is systemic, it is patchy and focal, only parts of some arteries being involved. The clinical effects of the disease are the result of vessel occlusion leading to small areas of infarction, and the tissues most seriously affected are the kidneys, heart, alimentary tract, liver, central nervous system, peripheral nerves, skeletal muscle, and skin (*Fig. 10.27*).

The cause of the disease is unknown, but it is likely to be immune-complex-mediated. There is an association with chronic hepatitis B virus antigenemia.

Lymphocytic vasculitis is an important feature of the systemic connective tissue disorders, particularly SLE

Most of the severe vasculitides are characterized by the presence of neutrophils in the vessel wall (neutrophilic vasculitis). However, in some disorders the walls are disrupted

Laboratory medicine

In cases of neutrophilic vasculitis it is possible to detect auto-antibodies that react against neutrophils; one type reacts with neutrophil cytoplasm on immunofluorescence (c-ANCA) and is directed to proteinase-3; the other shows a pattern of perinuclear staining (p-ANCA) and is directed against myeloperoxidase.

c-ANCA, in the absence of p-ANCA, is present in the serum of 90% of patients with Wegener's granulomatosis and, rarely, in other types of vasculitis. p-ANCA is present in polyarteritis nodosa and other types of necrotizing vasculitis.

Identification of these antibodies in serum is used in diagnostic evaluation of patients with possible vasculitis.

by lymphocyte infiltration (lymphocytic vasculitis). This is particularly seen in SLE and mixed connective tissue disease, and is frequently observed during histological examination of skin and muscle biopsies. Similar lesions may be seen in the brain in SLE. Although lymphocytic vasculitis is seen in most cases of connective tissue disease, there may also be an acute neutrophilic vasculitis similar to that described on page 170 (hypersensitivity vasculitis).

Lymphocytic vasculitis may also be seen in some drug reactions, particularly in the skin.

Giant cell arteritis is common in the elderly

Giant cell arteritis is a systemic disease that mainly involves arteries in the head and neck region. It particularly affects the temporal arteries, hence the alternative name of **temporal arteritis**. Increasing in incidence with age, it is rare under the age of 50 years, and is more common in females.

Patients have ill-defined symptoms of malaise and tiredness with headaches. In many cases there is an associated disease of muscle, polymyalgia rheumatic. Investigations characteristically reveal a very high ESR. Diagnosis is by biopsy of the temporal artery, and histological findings are shown in *Fig. 10.28*.

As a frequent complication is sudden blindness from involvement of the ophthalmic artery, treatment with steroids is urgently indicated in this condition.

Buerger's disease is an inflammatory disease of vessels that is related to smoking

Buerger's disease causes inflammatory occlusion of peripheral arteries in the upper and lower limbs. It is related to heavy cigarette smoking and is mainly seen in males. Pathologically there is segmental chronic inflammatory infiltration of the walls of arteries and veins, with secondary thrombosis. Small foci of neutrophils may also be seen.

Patients develop peripheral vascular insufficiency, with eventual development of gangrene.

Fig. 10.27
Pathological effects of polyarteritis nodosa

Organ	Effects	Clinical features
Kidney	Microinfarcts	Acute renal failure
Gastrointestinal tract	Microinfarcts	Mucosal ulceration
Central nervous system	Infarction	Focal neurology
Nerves	Necrosis	Mononeuritis multiplex
Skeletal muscle	Fiber necrosis	Myalgia and weakness
Heart	Infarction	Cardiac failure

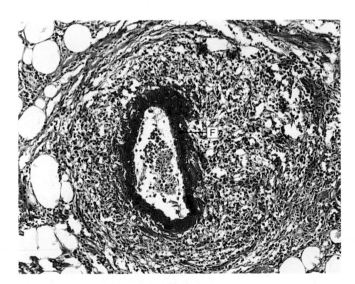

Fig. 10.26 Polyarteritis nodosa.
The artery wall shows infiltration by mixed inflammatory cells, in which neutrophils and eosinophils are most numerous. Fibrinoid necrosis (**F**) of a segment of the artery wall is very common. The inflammatory destruction leads to disruption of the normal architecture of the vessel wall, with necrosis of muscle cells and destruction of the elastic lamina; healing is followed by fibrous replacement of these specialized structures. During the acute inflammatory phase, the extensive damage to the intima predisposes to thrombosis, which is often followed by vessel occlusion and infarction of the target tissue.

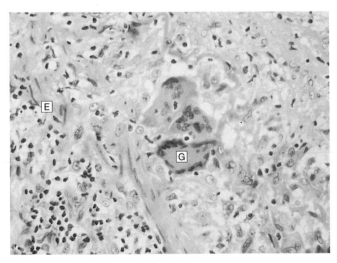

Fig. 10.28 Giant cell arteritis.
In giant cell arteritis the vessel wall is thickened and infiltrated by a mixture of inflammatory cells. This is largely composed of T-lymphocytes, but has foci of histiocytes and giant cells (**G**). The histiocytic giant cells are mainly related to fragments of the disrupted elastic lamina (**E**). Complication by thrombosis is common.

STRUCTURAL ABNORMALITIES OF VEINS

Dilatation and congestion of veins is common in many sites

The most common abnormality of veins is dilatation and congestion with blood. Such abnormal veins are given different names in different sites.

Varicose veins are persistently distended superficial veins in the lower limbs (long and short saphenous veins). They are the result of incompetence of the valves, which allows the veins to become engorged with blood under the influence of gravity. A saphenovarix is a localized distension of the superficial saphenous veins in the groin, producing a smooth rounded mass.

Hemorrhoids (or 'piles') are greatly distended veins of the internal hemorrhoid plexus of submucosal veins in the anal canal and at the anorectal junction. They present as prolapsed mucosa-covered masses, which often protrude through the anal orifice. Bleeding may follow trauma, and pain may follow from gross protrusion and anal sphincter spasm.

Varicocele is persistent distension of the veins of the pampiniform plexus of veins in the spermatic cord within the scrotum.

All of these conditions in the pelvis and lower limbs can be aggravated by any pelvic or abdominal condition that causes pressure on the veins preventing adequate venous return. For example, pregnancy is an important and common precipitating factor in the development of varicose veins and hemorrhoids.

Esophageal varices and prominent umbilical veins are distended venous channels that develop in portal hypertension secondary to cirrhosis of the liver (see page 280).

TUMORS AND MALFORMATIONS OF VESSELS

Angiomas are developmental malformations derived from blood vessels

Developmental malformations derived from blood vessels are very common and are termed **angiomas** or **hemangiomas**.

- Hemangiomas are composed of dilated vascular spaces.
- Capillary angiomas are composed of small capillary-like vessels.
- Cavernous angiomas are composed of wide, vein-like vessels (*Fig. 10.29*).
- Angiomas with mixed patterns are common.

Vascular tissues (usually abnormal) are an important, often predominant, component of mixed connective tissue hemartomatous malformations in the subcutaneous tissue of the neck and upper trunk in young people. In some cases lymphatic vessels are the predominant feature, and in

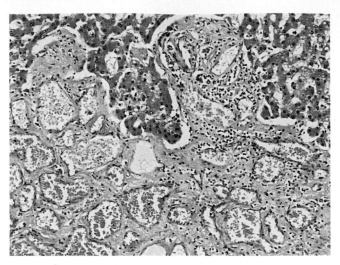

Fig. 10.29 Cavernous angioma.
Cavernous angioma is composed of vein-like vascular spaces filled with blood. In this example the lesion has arisen in the liver.

children such malformations may consist almost entirely of enormously dilated lymphatic vessels (**cystic hygroma**). Other connective tissues present include adipose tissue, abnormal nerves, and some smooth muscle.

Large vascular malformations are an important cause of intracerebral hemorrhage

The brain is an important site for vascular malformations. They are usually large and consist of both arterial- and venous-type vessels. These often communicate directly and are termed **arteriovenous malformations** (AVM). They may produce symptoms by local brain compression, resulting in focal neurological signs. The most serious complication is spontaneous bleeding leading to intracranial hemorrhage.

True vascular tumors are rare

True tumors of blood vessels are rare, but include Kaposi's sarcoma, which is becoming a more important and common tumor.

Numerically the most common tumor is the so-called **glomus tumor (glomangioma)**, which presents as a tender, painful nodule on the finger, often close to the nail. The tumor contains vascular channels surrounded by glomus cells.

Angiosarcoma (*Fig. 10.30*), a malignant tumor of blood vessel endothelium, most commonly occurs as a raised bluish red patch on the face or scalp of elderly people. It enlarges progressively, often ulcerating, and later metastasizes to regional lymph nodes. This tumor may also occur in limbs that have very long-standing chronic lymphedema but this is now very rare, and was most commonly seen in the arms of women who had had a total axillary clearance as part of radical surgery for breast cancer. Angiosarcomas in

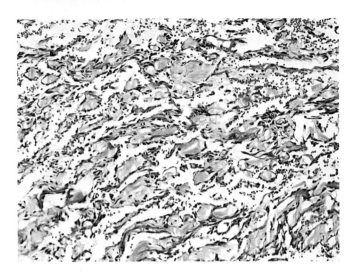

Fig. 10.30 Angiosarcoma.
An angiosarcoma is composed of neoplastic endothelial cells, which form vascular-like channels in tissues. This is a highly malignant tumor.

the liver have been associated with industrial exposure to vinyl chloride, which is used in various chemical industries (particularly plastic manufacturing).

Hemangioendotheliomas behave as low-grade malignant tumors and are derived from endothelial cells. **Hemangiopericytomas**, also of low-grade malignant potential, are derived from the pericytes surrounding blood vessels. Occurring mainly in the subcutaneous tissues of the limbs, they occasionally develop in other sites.

One form of Kaposi's sarcoma is seen with AIDS

Kaposi's sarcoma is believed to be derived from endothelial cells. However, evidence for this is controversial and there have been proposals that the tumor arises from multipotential mesenchymal cells. There is a strong and possible causative association with human herpesvirus Type 8 (HHV8). There are four patterns of disease, the natural histories of which seem to be related to the clinical setting in which the tumor develops. Only one form is seen in AIDS.

Endemic Kaposi's sarcoma is seen in Africa. In children it is a highly malignant condition based in lymph nodes, but in adults it runs a more indolent course, with hematogenous spread.

Classic Kaposi's sarcoma is a rare tumor that develops in the lower limbs of elderly males. It behaves as a low-grade malignant skin neoplasm, with hematogenous and lymph node metastasis.

Kaposi's sarcoma in therapeutic immunosuppression resembles classic Kaposi's sarcoma, behaving as a low-grade malignant neoplasm in the skin.

Epidemic Kaposi's sarcoma is seen in patients with AIDS, particularly in homosexual males. It is a highly

Fig. 10.31
Stages of Kaposi's sarcoma

Phase	Macroscopic appearance (skin and oral mucosa)
Patch phase	Flat, bruise-like, purple lesions
Plaque phase	Slightly raised, firm, purple lesions
Nodular phase	Dome-shaped, firm, purple lesions

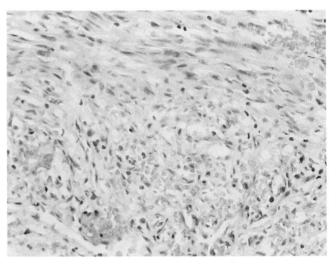

Fig. 10.32 Nodular phase of Kaposi's sarcoma.
Histology shows plump spindle cells with compressed, slit-shaped vascular channels containing red cells.

malignant tumor of skin with spread to lymph nodes and visceral organs.

Kaposi's sarcoma progresses through three phases, which are summarized in *Fig. 10.31*. The nodular phase is shown in *Fig. 10.32*.

DISEASES OF THE HEART

HEART FAILURE

Cardiac failure develops when the heart cannot maintain the circulation

When the pumping effort of the heart falls short of sustaining a circulation sufficient for metabolic needs, **cardiac failure** is said to have occurred. Conditions in which the circulation fails because of a low blood volume, e.g. bleeding or fluid loss, are excluded from this definition. The main broad groups of conditions causing cardiac failure are those demanding extra work of the heart (e.g. hypertension, valve diseases) and those that damage heart muscle (e.g. ischemia).

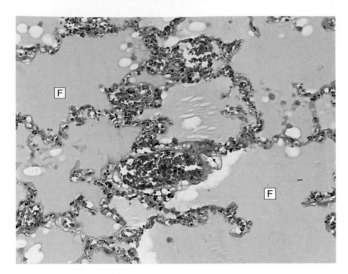

Fig. 10.33 Pulmonary oedema – left heart failure.
This histological section shows lung alveoli filled with pink-stained edema fluid (**F**).

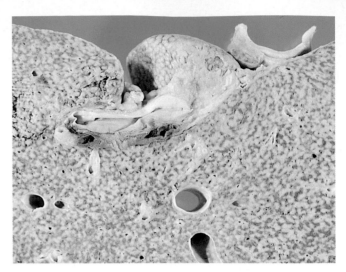

Fig. 10.34 Congested liver – right heart failure.
Chronic passive venous congestion of the liver causes dark areas where centrilobular zones are congested by blood, contrasting with pale periportal areas. This appearance is similar to that of the cut surface of a nutmeg, hence the term 'nutmeg liver'.

Cardiac failure can be either acute or chronic

Acute cardiac failure takes place when there is a sudden onset of pathology. There is abrupt failure of chamber emptying, the failing chambers dilate, and compensatory mechanisms cannot be brought into operation. Circulatory collapse with low blood pressure is termed 'cardiogenic shock' (see page 160).

Chronic cardiac failure takes place when there is gradual increase in severity of a disease. It has a major impact on organ systems other than the heart, and is manifest by tiredness, breathlessness and development of edema. In the face of inadequate circulation, several compensatory responses take place:

- The ventricles of the heart enlarge in size, and contract more effectively.
- Constriction of arterioles causes redistribution of blood flow.
- Activation of sympathetic and renin–angiotensin systems causes retention of salt and water, and changes in vascular tone.
- There is desensitization of cardiac muscle to sympathetic stimulation.

Acute or chronic cardiac failure may develop when compensatory mechanisms break down.

Failure of the left side of the heart leads to poor systemic arterial perfusion and increased pressure in the pulmonary venous and capillary system

When the left heart fails to pump efficiently, the chambers fail to empty completely at systole and they become dilated. A dilated chamber is a failing chamber. Incomplete emptying

leads to a progressive rise in pressure in one chamber, which is reflected back into the chamber or vessels preceding it in the circulation. In the left heart this leads to dilatation of the left atrium, dilatation and increased pressure in the pulmonary veins and, eventually, to increased pressure in the pulmonary capillaries. The high pressure in the pulmonary capillary system forces the fluid component of blood out into the alveolar air sacs, which become filled with low-protein fluid. This is manifest clinically as **pulmonary edema**, and presents with acute breathlessness due to fluid in the air sacs (*Fig. 10.33*).

Another consequence of left heart failure is that insufficient blood is pumped out into the aorta and arterial system, which leads to hypotension, poor perfusion of tissues, and poor tissue oxygenation.

Failure of the right side of the heart leads to poor perfusion of the lungs and increased pressure in the systemic venous system

As the right side of the heart fails, the chambers dilate and there is increased intrachamber pressure, preventing adequate emptying of the systemic venous blood from the superior vena cava and inferior vena cava into the right atrium. This rise in systemic venous pressure has a number of clinical manifestations:

- The raised pressure in the superior vena cava can be observed in the neck in the form of jugular vein engorgement (**raised jugular venous pressure**).
- The raised pressure in the inferior vena cava is reflected back into the venous system of the liver and other organs, and may manifest as a **tender,**

Molecular changes in the myocardium are important in the pathophysiology of cardiac failure

Increasing interest is being shown in the phenotype of cardiac myocytes in the failing heart.

In heart failure, compensatory mechanisms are brought into play at the level of changes in signalling pathways aimed to improve cardiac reserve and function. While beneficial, these augmentations have cumulative damaging effects.

- Cardiac muscle is extensively remodeled in the failing heart both in terms of contractile proteins and in the extracellular matrix.
- In the failing heart expression of the myosin isoforms involved in contraction are reduced, correlating with impaired systolic function.
- Uncoupling of adrenergic receptors to the G-protein cAMP pathway is seen in failing hearts due to abnormal receptor phosphorylation.

Signal	Benefit	Adverse effects
Adrenergic	Contractility Myocardial hypertrophy	Myocyte toxic effects Myocyte apoptosis
Angiotensin II	Myocardial hypertrophy	Change in gene expression of contractile proteins
Cytokine (TNFα)	Myocardial hypertrophy	Remodelling of extracellular matrix with dilatation

These insights into the molecular pathophysiology of cardiac failure are directing the search for new therapeutic agents.

KEY FACTS
Heart failure

- Left-sided failure causes pulmonary edema.
- Main causes of left-sided failure are myocardial infarction, hypertension, and valve disease.
- Right-sided failure causes venous congestion and peripheral edema.
- Main causes of right-sided failure are chronic lung disease and chronic left-sided failure.
- Congestive cardiac failure is failure of both sides of the heart.

enlarged, congested liver (*Fig. 10.34*), palpable beneath the right costal margin.
- The raised pressure in the small venules and capillaries of the lower limb, supplemented by the effect of gravity, leads to increased pressure in the lumen of these small vessels, with transudation of fluid into the interstitial tissues producing **subcutaneous edema**, particularly around the ankles.

Congestive cardiac failure is failure of both the right and the left side of the heart

Failure of both sides of the heart is termed 'congestive cardiac failure'. Biventricular failure most commonly arises when there is right heart failure secondary to pulmonary capillary congestion as a result of primary left heart failure.

When left heart failure is long-standing and severe, the back pressure effects cause permanent congestion and increased pressure in the pulmonary capillary system. This gives rise to increased back pressure in the pulmonary arterial system, which leads to right heart failure as a result of the right heart having to pump against an increased peripheral resistance.

Congestive cardiac failure may also be caused by unusual diseases that simultaneously affect the muscle of both ventricles.

ISCHAEMIC HEART DISEASE

The most common disease of the heart is caused by myocardial ischemia

Ischemic heart disease is the most common type of cardiac disease and the leading cause of death in the western world, accounting for about 30% of all male deaths and 23% of all female deaths.

The main cause of ischemic heart disease, also called **coronary heart disease**, is atheroma of coronary arteries. The risk factors predisposing to development of ischemic heart disease are similar to those predisposing to development of atheroma (see page 163).

Because of its greater bulk and work requirement, the myocardium of the left ventricle has the higher oxygen demand and is more prone to ischemia.

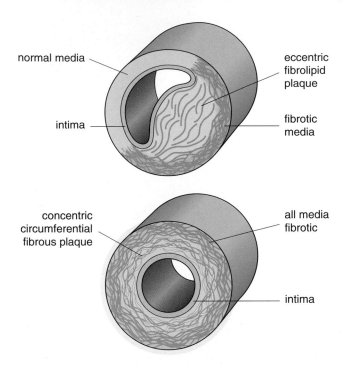

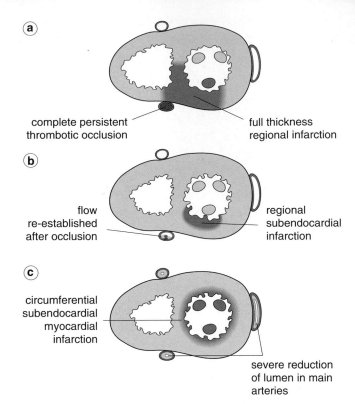

Fig. 10.35 Plaques in coronary arteries.
Eccentric plaques, often rich in lipid, affect only one segment of the wall of a coronary artery. Improvement of flow at the site of such plaques may be achieved by vasodilator drugs, which can cause relaxation of the normal (unaffected) part of the vessel wall. **Concentric plaques**, usually mostly collagenous, affect the whole of the arterial wall and, as the whole wall is abnormal, drug therapy cannot improve flow over a narrowed segment.

Fig. 10.36 Patterns of myocardial infarction.
The three main patterns of myocardial infarction are regional full-thickness (a), regional subendocardial (b), and circumferential subendocardial (c).

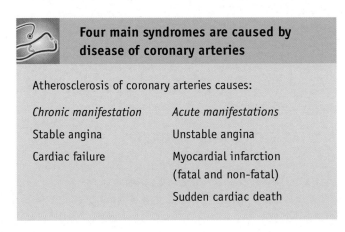

Four main syndromes are caused by disease of coronary arteries

Atherosclerosis of coronary arteries causes:

Chronic manifestation	*Acute manifestations*
Stable angina	Unstable angina
Cardiac failure	Myocardial infarction (fatal and non-fatal)
	Sudden cardiac death

depending on the nature of the plaque. Atheromatous plaques in coronary arteries may be one of two types (*Fig. 10.35*).

Over a long period, repeated episodes of impaired flow may lead to development of fine fibrosis in the myocardium, with death of individual cardiac muscle fibers. Anastomotic vessels frequently develop to compensate for areas of vascular stenosis.

Acute ischemic heart disease is largely caused by complications to atheromatous plaques

Thrombus formation, stimulated by the presence of an atheromatous plaque, is the main cause of episodes of acute ischemic heart disease. Thrombosis at this location is caused by two main processes:

- 25% of cases are due to superficial ulceration of endothelium over a plaque.
- 75% of cases are due to plaque fissuring, resulting in a deep cleft in a lipid-rich plaque that either precipitates thrombus development in the lumen or causes bleeding into the body of the plaque, with resultant ballooning into the lumen.

Importantly, such complications may be in low-grade stenoses, areas that will not have caused previous angina on

Stable angina is caused by low flow in atherosclerotic coronary arteries

Angina is episodic chest pain that takes place when there is a demand for increased myocardial work, usually through exercise, in the presence of impaired perfusion by blood. Pathological studies of patients with angina show that they have at least one stenosis over 50% of the lumen in a main coronary artery (high-grade stenosis). The high-grade stenosis limits flow, but this may be modifiable by drugs,

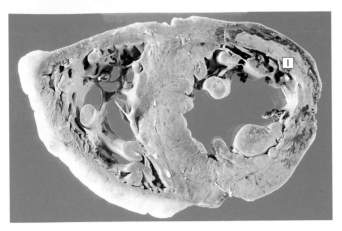

Fig. 10.37 Regional full-thickness myocardial infarction. The full thickness of the lateral wall of the left ventricle is infarcted (**I**).

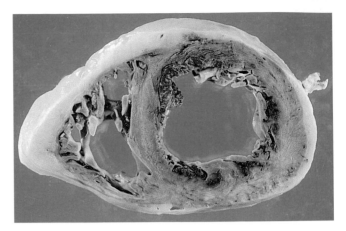

Fig. 10.38 Circumferential subendocardial infarction. The subendocardial zone around the whole circumference of the left ventricle is infarcted and dark in color.

exertion. The initial manifestation of coronary artery atherosclerosis may therefore be sudden cardiac death, with no history of previous chest pain on exertion.

Unstable angina is caused by fissuring of atherosclerotic plaques

Fissuring of plaques may cause a syndrome of sudden-onset angina that increases in frequency and severity, termed **crescendo angina** or **unstable angina**.

As there is a plaque fissure and thrombosis has been initiated, there is a risk of subsequent total thrombotic occlusion of the vessel. A proportion of patients with unstable angina will progress to myocardial infarction or may die from secondary development of a ventricular arrhythmia.

Acute myocardial infarction may be regional or subendocardial

There are two main patterns of myocardial infarction, each having a somewhat different pathogenesis (*Fig. 10.36*).

Regional myocardial infarction (90% of cases) involves one segment of the ventricular wall. The cause of this pattern of infarction is nearly always thrombus formation on a complicated atheromatous plaque. If there is complete persisting occlusion of the arterial branch supplying that area, the infarct is full thickness (*Fig. 10.37*). If there is lysis of the thrombus or a collateral supply to the myocardium, the infarct will be limited to the subendocardial zone (**regional subendocardial infarction**).

Circumferential subendocardial infarction (10% of cases) involves the subendocardial zone of the ventricle and is caused by a general hypoperfusion of the main coronary arteries. This is usually due to an episode of modest hypotension critically reducing flow in arteries already affected by high-grade atherosclerotic stenosis. The region at the end of the arterial perfusion zone, the subendocardial zone, fails to be perfused and undergoes necrosis (*Fig. 10.38*).

Thrombolytic therapy and infarction

The main cause of regional infarction is thrombus developing as a complication of an atheromatous plaque in a coronary artery. In cases of plaque fissure, the thrombus present in and overlying the fissure is platelet-rich, whereas the thrombus in the lumen of the vessel, often comprising the major obstructing element, is generally fibrin-rich.

Administration of fibrinolytic drugs such as streptokinase or tissue-plasminogen activator (TPA) can bring about clot lysis and reestablish flow in previously occluded vessels. Lysis is usually confined to the luminal, fibrin-rich thrombus but, occasionally, achieves lysis of thrombus in a plaque fissure.

If clot lysis is achieved shortly after onset of occlusion, it is possible to minimize the extent of ischemic damage to the subendocardial zone.

The site of regional myocardial infarction depends on which vessel is involved

The extent and distribution of the area of myocardial infarction depends upon which coronary artery branch is occluded (*Fig. 10.39*). The vast majority of infarcts affect the left ventricle and the septal region. Infarction of the right ventricle can occur but is very rare by comparison.

Myocardial infarction induces acute inflammation, followed by organization and scarring

The end result of myocardial infarction is replacement of the necrotic area by collagenous scar. The entire process, from fiber necrosis to scar formation, takes 6–8 weeks, the macroscopic and histological appearances of the infarct changing with time (*Fig. 10.40*).

Sudden cardiac death is due to either infarction or arrhythmias

Most deaths caused by ischemic heart disease do not occur in hospital. Patients either have no warning symptoms or die shortly after their onset. Death is usually due to ventricular fibrillation.

Patients who have had symptoms of previous ischemic heart disease, e.g. angina or previous infarction, tend to develop cardiac arrhythmias arising from muscle adjacent to an area of old scarring, and have not had a new thrombotic episode.

Those with no previous cardiac history have usually had a new thrombotic event arising from a complicated atheromatous plaque. This has given rise to acute myocardial ischemia, which precipitates the arrhythmia.

Sudden cardiac death is the most important immediate consequence of myocardial ischemia.

Many complications of myocardial infarction occur in the first 2 weeks

If the patient survives the immediate impact of acute myocardial infarction, or is successfully resuscitated from cardiac arrest or acute pulmonary edema, the next hurdle is the short-term complications. These include:

- **Further episodes of cardiac dysrhythmia**, particularly ventricular fibrillation. Bradyarrhythmias are particularly seen with posterior (inferior) infarcts, as the AV node is often involved.
- **Development of left ventricular failure** is most common with very large areas of infarction, which cause cardiac dilatation as the necrotic wall softens in organization.
- **Rupture of the ventricular wall** at any time, usually 2–10 days after the infarct, particularly during early organization and softening (*Fig. 10.41*). Blood bursts through the wall, instantly filling the pericardial cavity (hemopericardium). The sudden rise in intrapericardial cavity pressure prevents cardiac filling (**cardiac tamponade**), leading to rapid death. Rarely, intracardiac rupture may occur through the septum, causing a left-to-right shunt and development of severe left ventricular failure if large.
- **Papillary muscle dysfunction or infarction** leads to mitral valve incompetence, as one valve leaflet is no longer able to close during systole.
- **Mural thrombus formation** on the inflamed endocardium over the area of infarction (*Fig. 10.42*). Fragments can break off and embolize to various organs (particularly the brain, spleen, kidney, gut and lower limbs), producing infarction.

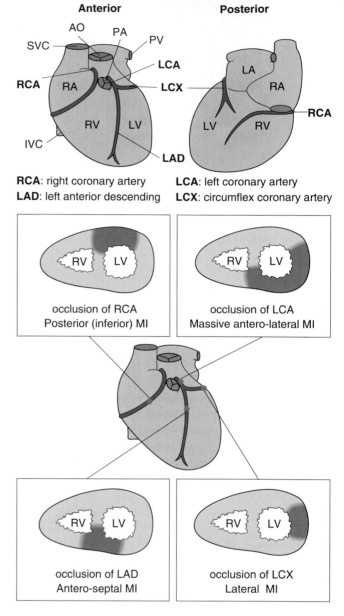

RCA: right coronary artery   **LCA**: left coronary artery
LAD: left anterior descending   **LCX**: circumflex coronary artery

occlusion of RCA
Posterior (inferior) MI

occlusion of LCA
Massive antero-lateral MI

occlusion of LAD
Antero-septal MI

occlusion of LCX
Lateral MI

Fig. 10.39 Site of myocardial infarction and vessel involvement.

- **Acute pericarditis** may occur due to inflammation over the infarct surface.

Because blood flow is slower, patients may be confined to bed, and there is a phase of hypercoagulability of blood, increasing the risk of leg-vein thrombosis.

Long-term complications of myocardial infarction

If patients survive the immediate and short-term effects of myocardial infarction, long-term complications may arise, among which is **chronic intractable left-heart failure** due to inadequate left ventricular pumping action. This is particularly common when the infarct has been extensive and full-thickness.

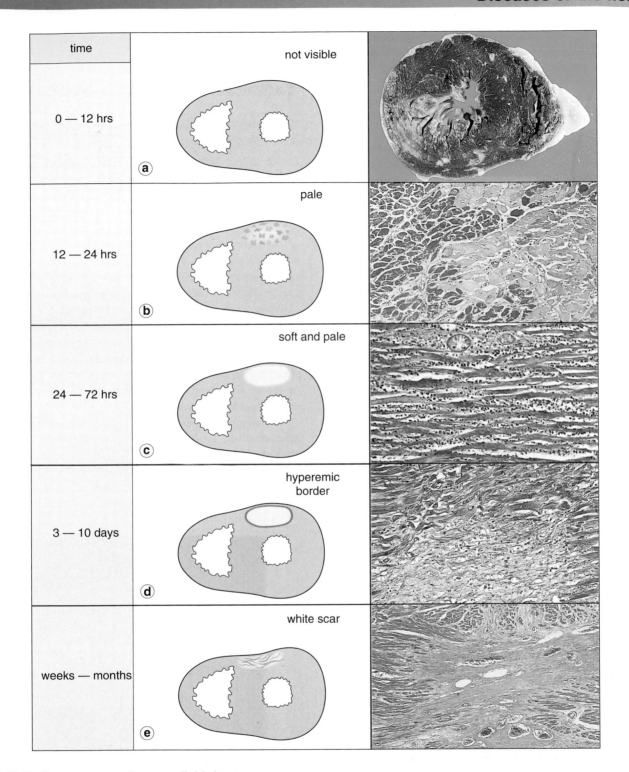

Fig. 10.40 Appearances of myocardial infarct.
Myocardial infarcts go through a series of changes with time. Between 0 and 12 hours an infarct is not macroscopically visible, however the ischemic muscle can be detected by showing loss of oxidative enzymes by nitro-blue-tetrazolium (NBT) when the infarcted area appears uncolored (a). Between 12 and 24 hours the infarcted area is macroscopically pale with blotchy discolouration. Histologically (b) infarcted muscle is brightly eosinophilic with intercellular edema. Between 24 and 72 hours the infarcted area excites an acute inflammatory response. Macroscopically the dead area appears soft and pale with a slight yellow colour. Histologically neutrophils infiltrate between dead cardiac muscle fibers (c). Organization of the infarcted area occurs between 3 and 10 days. Macroscopically a hyperemic border develops around the yellow dead muscle. Histologically there is replacement of the area by vascular granulation tissue (d). With time, progressive collagen deposition occurs and over a period of weeks to months the infarct is replaced by collagenous scar (e).

There may be **ventricular aneurysm formation** due to gradual distension of that part of the left ventricular wall where the muscle has been replaced by rigid but inelastic fibrous scar. Ventricular aneurysms frequently become filled with laminated thrombus, but embolic complications are uncommon (*Fig. 10.43*). This occurs in around 10% of long-term survivors.

Recurrent myocardial infarction is a risk because of the underlying coronary artery insufficiency; a patient who has had a myocardial infarct is always prone to develop a further episode.

Dressler's syndrome is a form of immune-mediated pericarditis associated with a high ESR. It develops in a very small number of cases after infarction (2–10 months after the acute event).

CARDIOMYOPATHY AND MYOCARDITIS

Cardiomyopathies are diseases primarily affecting heart muscle

Once cases of ischemic heart disease, valvular heart disease, and hypertensive heart disease have been excluded, there remains a group of patients who have presented with abnormal cardiac function due to primary disease of the myocardium.

These disorders, termed **cardiomyopathies**, can be considered together, as the diseases have a primary impact on cardiac muscle function. Many have a defined cause and can be classed as **secondary cardiomyopathies** (*Fig. 10.44*).

Other diseases have, as yet, no defined cause and are classed as **idiopathic primary cardiomyopathies**.

The cardiomyopathies usually cause progressive development of cardiac failure. The time-scale varies according to the cause of disease; development may occur over weeks or years. In some instances, sudden cardiac death is the first manifestation of disease.

The diagnosis of disease is based on clinical features supplemented by imaging (radiology and echocardiography) and cardiac catheter studies. These investigations allow cardiomyopathies to be grouped according to functional abnormalities of myocardium, and structural changes to the heart. To obtain a histological diagnosis of disease,

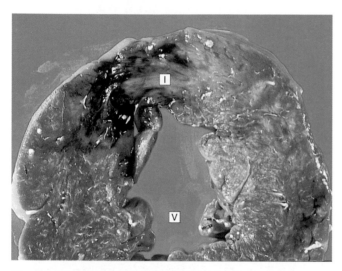

Fig. 10.41 Rupture of myocardial infarct.
The area of infarction (**I**) has ruptured and a track of blood runs from the ventricular chamber (**V**) to the epicardial surface. In this instance death was rapid after development of hemopericardium.

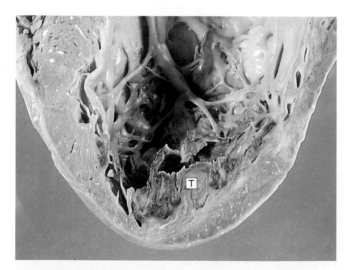

Fig. 10.42 Mural thrombus over myocardial infarct.
A plaque of mural thrombus (**T**) lies over an area of infarction at the apex of the left ventricle.

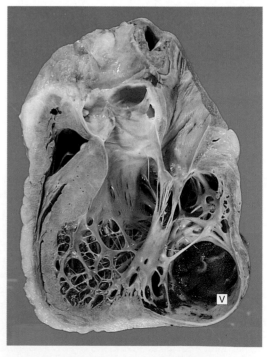

Fig. 10.43 Left ventricular aneurysm. After an infarct, stretching of collagenous scar causes aneurysmal bulging of the ventricular wall (**V**).

endomyocardial biopsy may be performed at the same time as cardiac catheterization.

Diseases that infiltrate the myocardium causing abnormal rigidity are termed **restrictive cardiomyopathies**, e.g. amyloid.

Primary cardiomyopathies are classified according to myocardial dysfunction

Primary cardiomyopathies follow two main patterns according to the dysfunction of the myocardium.

In **hypertrophic cardiomyopathy** the heart walls (especially the left ventricle) are enormously thickened and hypertrophied, often in an asymmetrical pattern, particularly affecting the interventricular septum (*Fig. 10.45*). Catheter studies show an abnormal pressure gradient along the left ventricular cavity. Histologically there is disorganized branching of hypertrophied muscle fibers, which show loss of the normal parallel orientation. In about 50% of cases, hypertrophic cardiomyopathy is inherited as an autosomal dominant disorder; it occurs most often in young adults and juveniles, and may present with sudden, unexplained death on exertion. Less dramatic presentations include angina and breathlessness on exertion in a young person, or repeated fainting attacks. There have been developments in the genetic understanding of this group of disorders (see pink box on page 182).

In **dilated (congestive) cardiomyopathy** the ventricles are dilated, the chamber walls stretched thin, and the muscle is poorly contractile (*Fig. 10.46*). Typically, there is an elevated ventricular end-diastolic pressure. The cause is not known, but some cases may follow viral myocarditis. It has been suggested that causative viruses produce proteolytic cleavage of cardiac myofibrillar proteins.

Arhythmogenic right ventricular dysplasia (ARVD) is a condition in which the wall of the right ventricle is extensively replaced by adipose tissue. This is a developmental problem and the condition is heritable (1 : 5000 population). An important aspect of this condition is that it is a cause of sudden cardiac death, accounting for 10–15% of cases of sudden death in childhood and adolescence. Patients known to have this condition have an annual death rate of 2.5% per year. A gene has been mapped to chromosome 3p23 in one affected family.

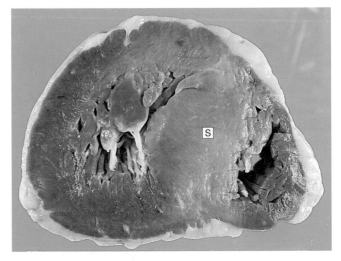

Fig. 10.45 Hypertrophic cardiomyopathy.
In hypertrophic cardiomyopathy there is marked left ventricular hypertrophy. This often preferentially affects the septum (**S**).

Fig. 10.44
Causes of secondary cardiomyopathies

Multisystem diseases

Diabetes
Amyloid
Thyroid disease
Hemochromatosis

Inflammatory and infective diseases

Myocarditis
Chagas' disease

Toxic and metabolic disturbances

Alcohol
Drugs (e.g. daunorubicin)

Primary muscle disorders

Muscular dystrophy
Mitochondrial cytopathy

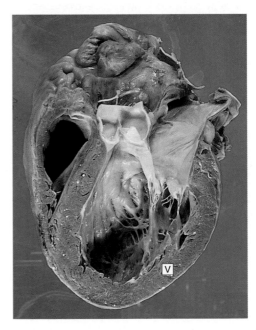

Fig. 10.46 Congestive cardiomyopathy. The dilated left ventricle (**V**) has a thin wall.

Genetic basis of hypertrophic cardiomyopathy

A genetic basis has now been identified in most cases of hypertrophic cardiomyopathy. It is thought that mutations result in varying degrees of abnormality of the myofibrillary proteins in the muscle cell, and that the abnormal myofibrils lie in disorganized patterns leading to misshapen cardiac muscle cells. The three main gene abnormalities are:

- About 50% of cases are due to an abnormality in the β-heavy chain myosin gene on chromosome 14 due to a replaced amino acid. The affected members are all heterozygous for the mutated gene.

- 15% of familial cases are associated with an abnormality of the Troponin T gene on chromosome 1. This genetic abnormality produces less severe disease than the myosin gene defect on chromosome 14.

- About 3–5% of familial cases are due to an abnormality in the α-tropomyosin gene on chromosome 15; this also produces a less severe form of disease.

- Very few cases of familial hypertrophic cardiomyopathy are associated with gene loci on chromosomes 7 and 11 but little is known of the function of these genes.

Myocarditis is a rare disease in which diffuse inflammation of the myocardium occurs

Inflammation of the myocardium, termed **myocarditis**, is generally rare. Although it is considered by many to be grouped best as a cardiomyopathy, others categorize this pattern of disease separately. The myocardium shows interstitial edema and infiltration with lymphocytes and macrophages.

The disease can be caused by **direct infection**, e.g. *Trypanosoma cruzi* (Chagas' disease), Coxsackie A and B viruses, HIV, influenza, Epstein–Barr virus, and fungi; **toxin-mediated damage**, e.g. diphtheria, typhoid and septicemic states; and **immune hypersensitivity**, e.g. acute rheumatic fever (see page 189). There are also idiopathic causes, such as giant-cell myocarditis. Diagnosis can be helped by endomyocardial biopsy.

CARDIAC TUMORS

Neoplasia affecting the heart is uncommon

The pericardium and heart may be involved by metastatic disease, the most common cause being local extension of a carcinoma of the lung.

Atrial myxoma is a tumor composed of stellate cells in a myxoid matrix, which arises from the atrial lining and may cause symptoms similar to infective endocarditis.

Cardiac rhabdomyomas are tumors of muscle seen in association with tuberose sclerosis.

DISEASES OF THE PERICARDIUM

The main disorder of the pericardium is pericarditis

The main disorder of the pericardium, pericarditis, is often complicated by development of an effusion.

In acute pericarditis there is acute inflammation of the pericardium, in which both pericardial surfaces are coated with a fibrin-rich acute inflammatory exudate. Loss of smoothness leads to the clinical sign of a friction rub.

The most common cause of acute pericarditis is myocardial infarction (see page 176). The next most common cause encountered in community practice is the transient pericarditis that can occur in some **viral disorders**; many are probably sub-clinical and most are clinically mild, presenting to the family practitioner and rarely requiring hospital treatment. Other causes of clinically significant pericarditis are:

- **Postoperative**, following open heart surgery. The pericarditis is diffuse, involving the entire pericardial surface, and heals by fibrosis, largely obliterating the pericardial cavity.

- **Bacterial pericarditis**, usually associated with severe bacterial infection of the lungs. An important cause in the past was pulmonary TB, producing tuberculous pericarditis. Healing by fibrosis became heavily calcified and rigid, often producing restriction to cardiac filling (constrictive pericarditis).

- **Malignant pericarditis**, usually due to infiltration of the pericardium by local spread from a primary bronchial tumor. Less commonly the cause is blood-borne metastases from a distant site, e.g. malignant melanomatosis.

- **Uremic pericarditis**, rarely seen now that chronic renal failure can be treated by dialysis and transplantation.

- **Immune pericarditis**, formerly an important component of the pancarditis associated with rheumatic fever, is now rare. Occasionally, patients with systemic autoimmune disease, such as SLE and rheumatoid disease, may develop pericarditis.

DISEASES OF ENDOCARDIUM AND VALVES

Primary diseases of the non-valvar endocardium are rare

As a long-term result of myocardial infarction that involves the endocardial surface, the endocardium is damaged and thickened, and may be a predisposing site for mural thrombosis, although this complication is more frequent in the immediate postinfarctive period.

Similar patchy areas of endocardial thickening can be seen (particularly in the left atrium) where the flow through the mitral valve has been modified by valve disease. A jet of blood squirting through the incompetent mitral valve during systole can produce a patch of endocardial thickening (jet lesion) where the jet hits the atrial wall.

Endocardial thickening in the right side of the heart is rare, but may occur in the carcinoid syndrome or in some congenital heart disease, where there is a left-to-right shunt.

Diffuse endocardial thickening in the left heart is seen in two diseases, both of which are rare in the UK, Europe and USA. In **endocardial fibroelastosis** the endocardium becomes greatly thickened and replaced by fibroelastic tissue, mainly in the left heart, often extending over the papillary muscles. This disease occurs in babies and young children, presenting with unexplained heart failure. Its cause is not known.

In **endomyocardial fibrosis** there is fibrous thickening of the endocardium and the inner myocardium, leading to limitation of cardiac contraction. Occurring particularly in Central Africa, this condition is often associated with peripheral blood eosinophilia; its cause is not known.

Both of the above conditions lead to cardiac failure by restricting contraction of the cardiac chambers during systole; they are sometimes classified as a form of cardiomyopathy (**restrictive cardiomyopathy**) by clinicians, despite the fact that the primary structural abnormality is endocardial.

Mechanical disturbance of heart valves results in cardiac disease

Mechanical disturbances of heart valves are an important cause of cardiac disease. The two main types of mechanical defect are narrowing or abnormal rigidity of a valve resulting in **stenosis**, and failure of the valve to close fully, resulting in **incompetence**.

The principal causes of valve disease are congenital abnormality, postinflammatory scarring, degeneration with ageing, dilatation of the valve ring, degeneration of collagenous support tissue of the valve, and acute destruction by necrotizing inflammation.

Any structurally abnormal valve is more liable than usual to develop colonization by microorganisms (infective valvulitis).

Inflammatory disorders of heart valves cause vegetations and late scarring

Inflammation of the endocardium of heart valves (valvulitis) is an important cause of valve disease, which results either from **immune-mediated damage** initiating inflammation in the valve cusps (seen in acute rheumatic fever, see page 189), or from **damage due to infection**, e.g. in bacterial and fungal endocarditis.

Inflammatory damage to heart valves has two important consequences:

- Valve collagen is exposed, causing **thrombus deposition**. The thrombus develops as exophytic nodules or irregular warty growths on the valve leaflets, called **vegetations** (*Fig. 10.47*).

- Inflammation and thrombus formation on the valve causes organization with collagenous scarring. This causes physical distortion to the valve cusps and renders them mechanically and functionally abnormal.

The valves on the left side of the heart (mitral and aortic) are much more frequently the site of endocarditis and thrombotic vegetation formation than the valves of the right side of the heart (tricuspid and pulmonary); thus, embolic material from valve thrombosis passes into the systemic circulation and produces infarcts in the systemic organs.

Some vegetations form on valves as a consequence of hypercoagulability of blood

In patients who are severely debilitated, for example with widespread metastatic carcinoma or severe chronic infections, small, non-infective, firm, platelet-rich vegetations (**marantic vegetations**) may form on the heart valves of the left side of the heart. The reason for this is hypercoagulability of blood caused by an acute phase response, manifest by a very high ESR.

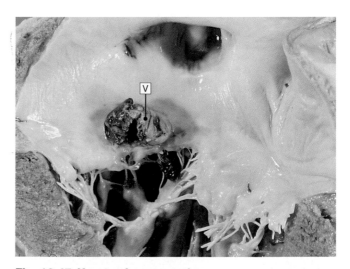

Fig. 10.47 Heart valve vegetations.
A thrombotic vegetation (**V**) on the mitral valve caused by inflammation of the valve.

Vegetations may form on the heart valves in SLE (Libman–Sacks endocarditis). This is related to the presence of high titers of anticardiolipin antibodies, which cause platelet aggregation.

Rheumatic fever is a major cause of chronic scarring of heart valves

The main cause of chronic scarring of valves is rheumatic fever, the incidence of which has decreased in many countries in recent years. Acute rheumatic fever is a disease of children, and is discussed on page 189.

The rheumatic pericarditis and myocarditis that arise in the acute phase usually resolve without long-term ill-effect. However, the damage to the valves heals by progressive fibrosis, with fibrous thickening of the valve leaflets and associated chordae tendineae. The valve leaflets become thickened, fibrotic and shrunken, often with fusion to their partners, and there is frequent secondary deposition of calcium.

Many patients with chronic scarring of valves give no history of having had rheumatic fever; the non-committal term 'postinflammatory scarring' is used in such cases.

Mitral stenosis causes left sided heart failure and predisposes to atrial thrombosis

Mitral stenosis is caused by postinflammatory scarring of the valve cusps. A history of rheumatic fever is obtained in only about half of the cases, and a chronic rheumatic etiology cannot be assumed in all instances.

Valve cusps are thickened and there is fusion of commissures. Chordae tendineae are thickened and fused, resulting in a funnel-shaped, narrowed valve orifice with a slit-like opening (*Fig. 10.48*).

Failure of the left atrium to empty through the stenosed valve leads to left atrial hypertrophy and dilatation. Back

pressure causes pulmonary hypertension and pulmonary vascular congestion, which commonly causes hemoptysis. Left-sided cardiac failure develops. Atrial fibrillation is a common complication, with resultant development of left atrial thrombosis. (*Fig. 10.49*).

Mitral incompetence leads to left-sided heart failure and has many causes

Regurgitation from the left ventricle back into the atrium is the result of mitral valve incompetence, the main causes of which are postinflammatory scarring (commonly rheumatic), papillary muscle dysfunction after infarct, left ventricular dilatation, cusp destruction by infection (infective endocarditis), and floppy mitral valve syndrome.

If the valve is suddenly rendered incompetent (papillary muscle rupture or infective perforation), severe acute pulmonary edema develops.

In most cases regurgitation develops slowly and results in left ventricular enlargement and a giant left atrium (caused by its filling with blood in systole). Progressive left-sided cardiac failure develops with time.

Mitral valve prolapse (floppy valve syndrome) is now much more common than rheumatic mitral valve disease. The valve leaflet becomes degenerate, with myxoid degeneration of the central zona fibrosa. The valve leaflet is soft and bulges upwards into the atrium during systole (*Fig. 10.50*). The posterior mitral leaflet is most commonly involved, and mild valve incompetence is the result of the

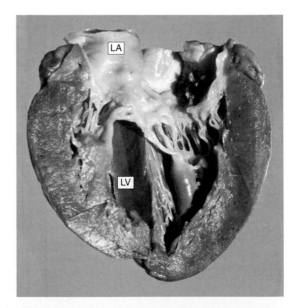

Fig. 10.49 Mitral stenosis with left atrial thrombosis. This heart has been opened to show the left atrium (**LA**) and left ventricle (**LV**), with the mitral valve between them. The valve and its chordae tendineae have been damaged by rheumatic endocarditis, leading to thickening and fusion of both, with functional stenosis. The combination of stenosis in the dilated left atrium and co-existing atrial fibrillation has led to thrombus formation (arrow).

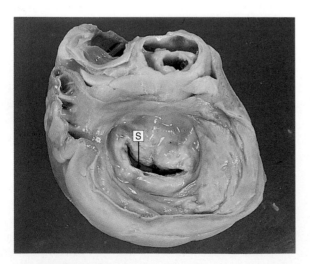

Fig. 10.48 Mitral stenosis. Looking down onto the valve from above, the mitral valve orifice is reduced to a narrow slit (**S**). This is caused by chronic rheumatic heart disease.

hypermobility of the leaflet. However, there is a danger of rupture of one of the chordae, leading to severe valve incompetence. It is most common in women and usually presents in young adulthood. In some cases there is a family history.

Aortic valve disease is a cause of sudden cardiac death

The aortic valve is frequently affected by disease resulting either in stenosis or in incompetence.

Aortic stenosis is most commonly due to calcification of a congenital bicuspid aortic valve (*Fig. 10.51*), post-inflammatory scarring after rheumatic fever, or senile

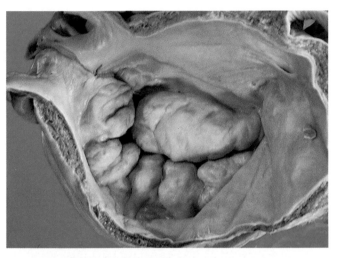

Fig. 10.50 Mitral valve prolapse. Looking down on the mitral valve, the ballooning of the leaflets due to mitral valve prolapse is seen.

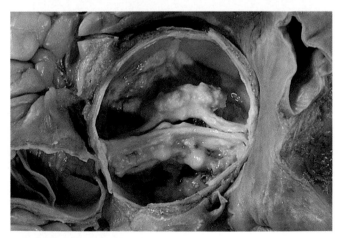

Fig. 10.51 Calcific aortic valve disease.
The valves become thick and fibrotic, with fusion of the commissures and heavy calcification. The thickening and fusion lead to reduction of the valve lumen, so that flow out of the valve is greatly reduced during systole (aortic stenosis). Furthermore, because the valve leaflets are rigid and fused, they are unable to close completely, and there is flow of blood back into the left ventricle during diastole (aortic regurgitation).

calcific degeneration. Isolated fibrosis and calcification of the aortic valve, with no evidence of mitral valve involvement or evidence of previous rheumatic fever, is the most common valve disease, although its cause is unknown. The disease is most commonly seen in bicuspid aortic valves, a common congenital malformation, but can also been seen in originally normal valves with three cusps.

Aortic regurgitation has four main causes:

- Retraction of cusps due to postinflammatory scarring.
- Erosion of cusps by inflammation in infective endocarditis.
- Retraction of cusps due to senile calcification.
- Dilatation of the aortic wall and valve ring caused by inflammatory diseases (e.g. syphilis, ankylosing spondylitis).

Mixed stenosis and regurgitation is common.

Progressive obstruction of the outflow of the left ventricle causes development of left ventricular hypertrophy. When stenosis is severe, patients may develop angina due to low flow in coronary arteries. They may also have episodes of syncope and are at risk of sudden cardiac death because of cardiac arrhythmias.

With aortic regurgitation, patients usually remain asymptomatic until the left ventricle, having undergone hypertrophy, fails acutely. Because of the serious nature of aortic valve disease surgical intervention is offered early in the course of disease.

Disease of the pulmonary and tricuspid valves is uncommon

The valves of the right side of the heart are infrequently involved in disease, but may be damaged by postinflammatory scarring in rheumatic heart disease. Endocarditis of the right side of the heart is seen in association with intravenous drug abuse.

For reasons that are as yet unclear, the carcinoid syndrome, caused by excess 5-hydroxytryptamine secretion by tumor, can result in endocardial fibrosis of the right side of the heart and pulmonary stenosis.

Infective endocarditis is caused by infection of heart valves or other areas of endocardium

Infection of the endocardium, whether on heart valves or elsewhere, is termed 'infective endocarditis'. There are two broad groups of cases.

In one group, patients are predisposed to infection by a **structural abnormality of heart valves** or by congenital cardiac defects. The incidence of this pattern has increased in western countries in recent years, mainly as a result of patients surviving with structurally abnormal hearts and heart valves. The infective organisms responsible are of low pathogenicity and are derived from normal commensal organisms of skin, mouth, urinary tract and gut. Organisms that enter the blood in trivial episodes of bacteremia become enmeshed in platelet aggregates on the surface of abnormal endocardium, growing to cause persistent infection. The main underlying abnormalities in this group are congenital bicuspid aortic valves, postinflammatory scarring, mitral valve prolapse syndrome, and prosthetic valves.

Infection of **normal valves** accounts for the remaining cases of infective endocarditis. In contrast to the first group, infection is with pathogenic organisms that directly invade the valve and cause rapid destruction. This pattern of disease is predisposed by conditions that promote entry of pathogenic organisms into the blood. It is seen in intravenous drug addicts, after open-heart surgery, and following septicemia from other causes.

Infective endocarditis occurs as two main clinical syndromes

Following on from the two main groups of cases of infective endocarditis described earlier, there are two main clinical disease patterns.

Acute infective endocarditis is usually due to a virulent organism, e.g. *Staphylococcus aureus*, and can occur on a previously normal heart valve. The bacteria proliferate in the valve, and cause necrosis, with generation of thrombotic vegetations. The pathogenic bacteria lead to destruction of the valve leaflets, with perforation and acute disturbance of valve function leading to acute cardiac failure. The disease is rapidly progressive and often fatal.

Subacute bacterial endocarditis generally occurs on structurally abnormal valves. The causative organisms are generally poorly virulent (e.g. *Streptococcus viridans*) and proliferate slowly in thrombotic vegetations on the damaged

valve surface. In most cases, they cause very gradual valve destruction, stimulating the formation of thrombus with potential for systemic embolization. Many of the effects of this pattern of infection are through immunological phenomena and generation of cytokines from persisting low-grade inflammation.

The main clinical effects of subacute infective endocarditis are:

- Small emboli of infected thrombotic material enter the systemic circulation, producing infarcts in many organs, particularly brain, spleen, and kidneys. These necrotic areas may, in turn, become infected by organisms in the occluding thrombus.
- Gradual destruction of valve cusps leads to features of valve incompetence with cardiac failure.
- Immune complexes against antigens in the infecting organism are trapped in small vessels. They cause skin petechiae and microhemorrhages seen in the retina and skin, particularly around the finger nails. They also cause a form of glomerulonephritis.

Cardiac transplantation is increasingly being performed for severe disease

Cardiac transplantation is now a technically straightforward surgical operation, and many of the problems of transplant rejection are being overcome; immunosuppression with cyclosporin has greatly improved the management of the almost inevitable rejection episodes.

Transplantation of the heart is mainly undertaken for advanced irreversible myocardial disease, particularly cardiomyopathy and severe ischemic disease, particularly in young people. Where the severe heart disease is associated with poor lung function, combined heart–lung transplants can be carried out. Since donor hearts are difficult to obtain, poor HLA matching is not usually a contraindication, although poor matches are usually associated with more severe rejection reactions.

Two patterns of rejection are seen:

- Acute cellular rejection, in which there is myocardial fiber necrosis, interstitial edema with lymphocytic infiltrate, and inflammation of the endocardial lining.
- Chronic rejection, in which there is ischemic damage in the myocardium, with interstitial fibrosis, associated with thickening of the intima in the coronary arteries.

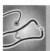

Diagnosis of infective endocarditis

The diagnosis of infective endocarditis is based on clinical suspicion, knowing the risk factors for development of disease. It should also be considered in patients with unexplained fever, septicemia, heart failure, or embolic infarct.

Investigations commonly reveal a raised ESR, raised white cell count, and a normochromic normocytic anemia.

The most important diagnostic procedure is **blood culture** to isolate an organism. A negative blood culture may be caused by prior administration of an antibiotic (which will not have cured the infection) or may be due to a special organism such as a fungus, *Coxiella* or *Chlamydia*.

Echocardiograms can be used for detection, if vegetations on valves are large.

- Cytokine generation from low-grade infection leads to systemic features of fever, weight loss and malaise. There may be anemia and splenomegaly.

HEART DISEASE IN CHILDREN

The most important heart disease in children are congenital cardiac malformations

Most cardiac malformations are manifest at or shortly after birth, usually by some manifestation of cardiac failure such as cyanosis, breathlessness, feeding difficulties, and failure to thrive. Certain maternal factors are known to increase the incidence of congenital cardiac malformations, particularly maternal rubella infections and chronic alcohol abuse, but in the majority of cases no teratogenic factors can be identified.

Congenital cardiac defects may be divided into two main groups: lesions that cause **obstruction to blood flow**, and those that cause **abnormal shunting** of blood between the two sides of the heart.

The latter group normally cause a left-to-right shunt because of the higher pressure in the left side of the heart. This is not associated with clinical cyanosis.

If there is an increase in resistance to blood moving on from the right side of the heart (either from obstruction of the right ventricular outflow or from pulmonary hypertension), there is a right-to-left shunt; with blood bypassing the lungs to enter the systemic circulation, cyanosis develops.

The most common congenital heart defects cause left-to-right shunts

The most common group of malformations result in a shunt of blood from the left side of the heart to the right.

Atrial septal defects (ASDs) are due to a defect in the interatrial septum. The lesion is usually located at the level of the fossa ovalis, which is incompletely closed (ostium secundum defect) (*Fig. 10.52*).

Ventricular septal defects (VSDs) are due to a defect in the interventricular septum. The larger defects involve the muscular wall of the septum, but small defects are often confined to the tiny membranous area (*maladie de Roger*) (*Fig. 10.53*).

Patent ductus arteriosus is due to persistent patency in the ductus arteriosus, an embryological connection between the aorta and the pulmonary trunk or left main pulmonary artery. In intrauterine life the ductus is an important channel, allowing blood oxygenated in the placenta to bypass the lungs, but it closes at or shortly after birth, when the lungs become aerated and expand. Persistence of the duct is most common in females, and there is a recognized association with maternal rubella (*Fig. 10.54*).

The severity of the symptoms depends on the size of the shunt between the left and right sides of the heart or main vessels. In the case of small ASDs or VSDs the flow can be minor and largely asymptomatic, sometimes presenting in mid-adult life with unexplained right heart failure. Patent ductus usually requires treatment in childhood.

Defects leading to permanent right-to-left shunts are less common

The most important and common congenital abnormality of the heart to cause right-to-left shunting is **Fallot's tetralogy** (*Fig. 10.55*), which consists of:

- **VSD**.
- **An overriding aorta**, which sits astride the VSD, so that it receives blood from both right and left ventricles.

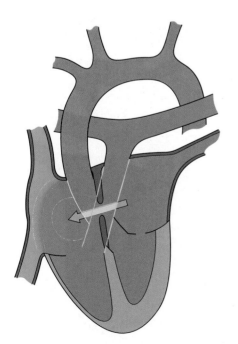

Fig. 10.52 Atrial septal defect.

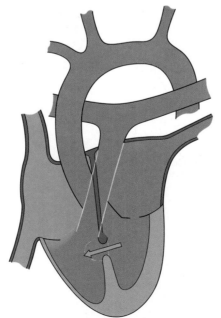

Fig. 10.53 Ventricular septal defect.

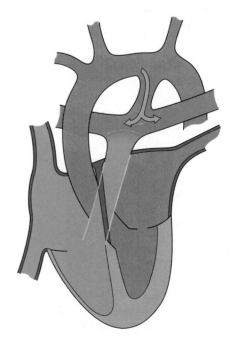

Fig. 10.54 Patent ductus arteriosus.

- **Pulmonary stenosis**, usually due to thickening of the subvalvar muscle in the pulmonary outflow tract, but sometimes associated with fused stenotic valve cusps.
- **Right ventricular hypertrophy**.

Because the abnormal aorta receives blood from the right ventricle as well as the left, the systemic circulation contains deoxygenated blood, and the patient has clinical **cyanosis**. The pulmonary stenosis leads to inadequate perfusion of the lungs. Affected individuals develop a right-to-left shunt and have cyanosis. With growth, the pulmonary stenosis remains fixed and eventually there is severe right ventricular outflow obstruction. Most cases are surgically corrected.

Surgical correction of this complex disorder is usually aimed at closing the VSD, rechannelling the flow into the aorta from the left ventricle only, and relieving the pulmonary stenosis. This technique has greatly increased survival. Complications include bacterial endocarditis (see page 186), and consequent cerebral infarction or brain abscess.

Some congenital malformations are not associated with significant shunting of blood

Of those congenital malformations not associated with significant shunting, the most common are aortic stenosis, coarctation of the aorta, and transposition of the great vessels.

With **aortic stenosis** there is stenosis of the valve, which is usually bicuspid. Symptoms tend to appear later in life, when fibrosis and calcification of the abnormal valve lead to functional stenosis and incompetence (*Fig. 10.51*). Less commonly the stenosis occurs in the muscular tissue below the aortic valve (**subvalvar stenosis**), or in the aortic wall above the valve (**supravalvar stenosis**). These two variants are present in infancy and may be associated with coarctation of the aorta.

In cases of **coarctation of the aorta**, there is a stenotic narrowing of the aorta, usually located at or just beyond the site of the ductus arteriosus, which appears closed (*Fig. 10.56*). The stricture produces hypertension proximal to the stenosis, and hypotension distal to it. The proximal hypertension can produce symptoms such as headache and dizziness, whereas the distal hypotension produces generalized weakness and poor peripheral circulation. Further symptoms may be due to the associated stenotic aortic valve that is present in about half of the cases. A rarer variant is the so-called infantile preductal coarctation, in which there is stenosis of a long segment of the aorta between the left subclavian artery origin and the ductus arteriosus, which remains patent.

Transposition of the great vessels is a complex malformation in which the connections between the right and left ventricle and aorta and pulmonary artery are disordered, the aorta emanating from the right ventricle and the pulmonary artery from the left. Survival is possible only if other shunts are present at either atrial (a), ventricular (b) or ductus (c) level (*Fig. 10.57*).

Cardiac disease is uncommon in children, with the exception of congenital malformations and rheumatic heart disease

Cardiomyopathy may occur in young children, but it is more common in juveniles. Some cardiomyopathies in young children are associated with abnormal storage in some of the autosomal recessive storage disorders, e.g. glycogen storage disease.

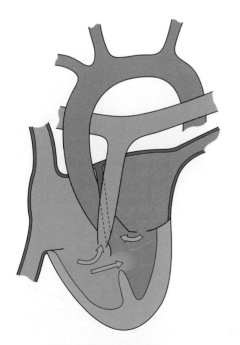

Fig. 10.55 Fallot's tetralogy.

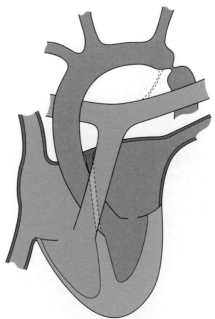

Fig. 10.56 Coarctation of the aorta.

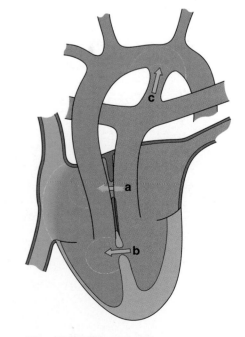

Fig. 10.57 Transposition.

The myocardium can be involved in some muscular dystrophies, but presentation in childhood is rare.

Acute rheumatic fever is still an important disease of children in certain developing countries

Rheumatic fever is an immune disorder that follows an infection in children, usually a streptococcal tonsillitis or pharyngitis. Certain strains of streptococci, especially group A β-hemolytic streptococci, produce particular antigens to which antibodies are developed by certain susceptible individuals; these antibodies may cross-react with host cardiac antigens.

The disease occurs mainly in children between the ages of 5 and 15 years, and was once prevalent in the UK, Europe and USA. It is now rare outside certain developing countries with low socioeconomic standards. The disease is a systemic disorder which, in the acute phase, presents with fever, malaise and, sometimes, synovitis and polyserositis. However, the most important target organ is the heart. Patients develop characteristic lesions (**Aschoff's nodules**) in various parts of the heart (*Fig. 10.58*). Diagnostic criteria have been established (*Fig. 10.59*).

Rheumatic fever causes a pancarditis in the acute phase

The components of the pancarditis are:

- **Rheumatic pericarditis**. Aschoff's nodules form in the pericardium, associated with an acute pericarditis. The acute inflammatory exudate is often predominantly of the serous type (mainly fluid with comparatively little fibrin or neutrophil components). The serous exudate can produce a pericardial effusion, which may distend the pericardial cavity.

- **Rheumatic myocarditis**. Aschoff's nodules developing in the myocardium are associated with interstitial edema and mild inflammation, sometimes with muscle-fiber necrosis. The myocarditis is usually clinically mild, but may produce left ventricular failure.

- **Rheumatic endocarditis**. Aschoff's nodules may form anywhere in the endocardium, producing slight irregularity of the endocardial surface. However, Aschoff's nodules in the valves lead to greater irregularity, and there may be erosion of the overlying endocardium, particularly at the points at which the valves contact each other at the line of closure. In these sites, small aggregations of fibrin and platelets accumulate to form small vegetations. The aortic and mitral valves are most prone to develop severe lesions, probably because of the higher pressures to which they are exposed and the more vigorous and traumatic valve closure.

In the acute phase of rheumatic fever the greatest dangers to the patient are the pericarditis and myocarditis; however, the main morbidity of rheumatic fever is the long-term effects of the immune damage causing chronic scarring of valves (page 184).

Clinical and laboratory diagnosis of acute rheumatic fever and investigation of chronic rheumatic endocarditis

Fig. 10.59
Jones' criteria for diagnosis of rheumatic fever

Major manifestations

Carditis
Polyarthritis
Skin rashes (erythema marginatum and
    subcutaneous nodules)
Neurological symptoms (Sydenham's chorea)
Fever

Minor manifestations

Polysynovitis (flitting arthropathy)
Arthralgia
Raised ESR or raised C-reactive protein
Prolonged PR-interval on ECG

Diagnosis requires two major features **or** one major and two minor features **plus** raised anti-streptococcal antibody levels (anti-streptolysin O titre) **or** positive throat culture for group A β-hemolytic streptococcus.

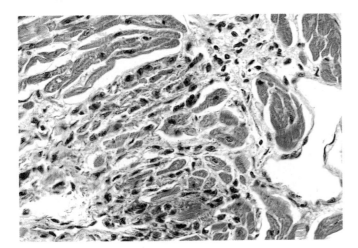

Fig. 10.58 Histology of the Aschoff's nodule.
The Aschoff's nodule is composed of an area of degenerate collagen, surrounded by activated histiocytic cells and lymphoid cells. These lesions stimulate fibroblast proliferation and lead to scarring.

11 Respiratory system

Clinical Overview

The most frequent diseases of the respiratory tract as a whole are bacterial and viral infections of the upper respiratory tract, mainly the nose, nasopharynx, pharynx and larynx (see Chapter 12). The trachea and large bronchi are frequently involved as well ('tracheobronchitis') and, in susceptible people such as the elderly or immunosuppressed, the infection may spread to distal small bronchioles and associated alveoli (bronchiolitis and bronchopneumonia). Other important lung infections such as lobar pneumonia, tuberculosis and opportunistic infection, originate in the alveolar air sacs, and are the result of the infecting organisms being inhaled directly into the lung.

Because of the enormous amount of air inhaled into the lungs every minute of every day, the lung tissues are exposed not only to air-borne microorganisms, but also to a wide range of toxic substances in the fumes from motor vehicles and industrial smoke, and various types of particulate matter. Chronic exposure to these plays a role in the development of various common chronic lung diseases such as asthma, chronic bronchitis, emphysema and pulmonary fibrosis. The risks to certain occupations such as coal miners and asbestos workers is well recognized.

Tumors of the bronchial tree and lung are common and important, and almost all are malignant; benign tumors are extremely rare. Most of the bronchial tumors originate in the main or large branch bronchi near the lung hilum. Surprisingly, the trachea which is only a few centimeters proximal, lined by the same type of epithelium, and exposed to exactly the same inhaled toxic influences, is almost never the site of either a primary benign or malignant tumor.

The lung is also important because it is frequently the secondary victim of malfunction elsewhere. Failure of the left side of the heart leads to back pressure, congestion in pulmonary capillaries, with constant transudation of fluid into pulmonary alveoli (pulmonary edema) seriously impairing air entry and gaseous exchange. Because the lung is at the end of the systemic venous drainage system, thromboses which form in systemic veins can embolize to the pulmonary arterial tree (pulmonary emboli), and malignant tumors which spread from their primary site by venous invasion will produce secondary tumors in the lung (pulmonary metastases).

Illness due to lung abnormalities is important in premature infants, since the lung is structurally and functionally immature. It is a common cause of death in this group.

THE RESPIRATORY SYSTEM COMPRISES THE UPPER RESPIRATORY TRACT, THE AIRWAYS AND THE LUNGS

The respiratory system consists of the upper respiratory tract, the airways and the lungs. Diseases of the nose and larynx are considered along with those of the ear in Chapter 12, as these conditions are clinically seen together.

The main diseases of the airways and lung are caused by infection and inflammation. Exposure to environmental agents has an important role in causing disease, especially smoking and occupational exposure to dusts. Carcinoma of the lung is particularly feared because of its aggressive nature.

One consequence of severe disease of the respiratory system is impairment of oxygenation of blood, resulting in respiratory failure.

RESPIRATORY FAILURE IS DEFINED BY THE PRESENCE OF A LOW LEVEL OF BLOOD OXYGEN

Normal respiratory function maintains blood gases within physiological limits. The normal PaO_2 varies between 10.7 kPa and 13.3 kPa (80–100 mmHg), and the normal $PaCO_2$ varies between 4.7 kPa and 6.0 kPa (35–45 mmHg). Respiratory failure is defined as when the PaO_2 falls below 8 kPa (60 mmHg)

There are two types of respiratory failure, which are defined according to whether blood carbon dioxide is also abnormal. In **Type I**, PaO_2 is low, but $PaCO_2$ is within normal range. In **Type II**, PaO_2 is low, and $PaCO_2$ is raised (above 6.7 kPa/50 mmHg).

There are several general causes of respiratory failure including failure of ventilatory drive, e.g. depression of respiratory center; upper airways obstruction; diseases of lung preventing normal gas exchange; and mechanical impairment of ventilation, e.g. massive rib fracture, diseases of muscle.

Chronic respiratory failure has major effects on the cardiovascular system

Chronic hypoxemia has two main consequences:

- **Pulmonary hypertension**. Due to pulmonary vasoconstriction leading to increased pulmonary artery pressure and increased work of the right ventricle, this occurs when the arterial PaO_2 falls below 8 kPa (60 mmHg). With chronicity, pulmonary arteries develop intimal proliferation and occlusion of lumina. Sustained demand on the right ventricle leads to right ventricular hypertrophy.

Blood gas analysis

Analysis of arterial blood gases is vital in distinguishing the severity and different types of respiratory failure. The only direct clinical sign of respiratory failure is central cyanosis, detected reliably when the PaO_2 is below 6.7 kPa (50 mmHg) in a person with a normal hemoglobin level. Loss of consciousness occurs when the PaO_2 is less than 4.0 kPa (30 mmHg).

Disorders of conduction of air and ventilation cause both hypoxia and CO_2 retention.

A low PaO_2 alone (breathing normal air) usually means that there is mismatch between ventilation and perfusion of lungs, but that alveolar ventilation is normal.

Hypoxia due to an increase in the proportion of blood passing through the lung without being oxygenated (increased shunt fraction) is seen in pulmonary collapse, and in situations in which the lung becomes consolidated.

Failure of diffusion of gas because of abnormal thickening in alveolar septa leads to hypoxemia, but hypercapnia does not develop.

- **Polycythemia** is due to stimulation of erythropoietin release from the kidney. This can lead to increased blood viscosity and predisposes to increased risk of thrombosis.

Hypercapnia, when severe, causes tremor of outstretched hands, bounding pulse, vasodilatation and increased cardiac output, and confusion leading to coma.

COLLAPSE OF THE LUNG IS TERMED 'ATELECTASIS'

Several conditions lead to atelectasis, which has important clinical consequences of disturbing respiratory function:

- Obstruction of an airway leads to resorption of air from the lung distal to the obstruction.
- Compression of the lung is most commonly seen when fluid or air accumulates in the pleural cavity (see page 218).
- Scarring in the lung may cause contraction of parenchyma and collapse.
- Loss of normal surfactant (developmental or acquired) from terminal air spaces leads to generalized failure of lung expansion, termed **microatelectasis**.

VASCULAR AND HEMODYNAMIC DISEASE OF THE LUNGS

The main cause of pulmonary edema is pulmonary capillary congestion due to left ventricular failure

Pulmonary edema is due to an increase of fluid in alveolar wall (pulmonary interstitium) which, if severe, subsequently affects alveolar spaces. The main cause of pulmonary edema is failure of the left ventricle, causing increased pressure in the alveolar capillaries.

Fluid leaks from capillaries into the pulmonary interstitium, and there is increase in flow of fluid into pulmonary lymphatics. This increases the stiffness of the lungs, giving rise to a subjective sensation of dyspnea. Such a condition may remain stable for a long period of time.

In severe left ventricular failure, fluid also leaks into alveolar spaces, resulting in severe acute impairment of respiratory function.

Capillary rupture leads to leakage of red cells into the interstitium, as well as into alveoli. Hemoglobin is phagocytosed by macrophages, which accumulate iron pigment and lie in alveoli and interstitium. They are often termed 'heart-failure cells' (*Fig. 11.1*).

Pulmonary hypertension results in structural damage to pulmonary vessels

Increased pulmonary arterial pressure is pulmonary hypertension, as discussed in Chapter 10. This causes irreversible structural changes in pulmonary arteries, and leads to increased demand for work on the right side of the heart and right heart failure (**cor pulmonale**). The main causes of pulmonary hypertension are listed in *Fig. 10.22*, the most important being:

- Chronic obstructive airways disease.
- Fibrosis of the lungs.
- Chronic pulmonary venous congestion.

In long-standing pulmonary hypertension, structural changes develop in the lung including medial hypertrophy in muscular arteries (with increase in amount of smooth muscle) and pulmonary veins (arterialization).

In severe long-standing cases, exposure of the pulmonary arterial wall to high pressures approaching or equalling those in the systemic circulation produces calcified atherosclerotic plaques in the main pulmonary arteries (see *Fig. 10.10*). This is most likely to occur when there is a long-standing shunt between systemic and pulmonary arterial systems, e.g. untreated patent ductus arteriosus.

There is occlusion of the lumen of pulmonary arteries by intimal proliferation, and alveolar macrophages containing hemosiderin are prominent (*Fig. 11.1*). Fibrosis in the interstitium of the lung develops in long-standing cases.

The clinical effects of pulmonary hypertension are breathlessness and development of right-sided cardiac failure.

Pulmonary emboli cause infarction of lung in a minority of cases

Occlusion of the pulmonary arteries by thromboemboli has been introduced on page 157. Most emboli arise in the deep leg veins and pass in the venous circulation, through the right side of the heart, to lodge in the pulmonary arteries.

Pulmonary infarction (*Fig. 11.2*) occurs in only about 10% of emboli because the normal dual circulation protects against ischemic necrosis. Recurrent thromboemboli may damage the pulmonary vasculature and cause pulmonary hypertension.

Massive coiled pulmonary emboli impacted in a main pulmonary artery lead to acute right heart failure and death (see pages 157 and 158).

Pulmonary vasculitis (angiitis) is caused by several disease processes

Several uncommon diseases are characterized by cellular infiltration of pulmonary blood vessels (**angiitis**), resulting in necrosis of pulmonary parenchyma.

The main forms of this process are caused by inflammatory destruction of vessels as part of a necrotizing vasculitis (see page 169).

In Wegener's granulomatosis, mainly the nose, lung and kidneys are affected: Churg–Strauss syndrome is caused by eosinophil infiltration of the lung.

Diagnosis is made on the basis of clinical features, in conjunction with lung biopsy.

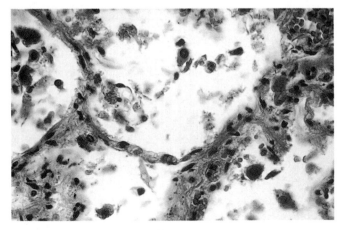

Fig. 11.1 Heart-failure cells.
The alveolar spaces contain macrophages which show brownish discoloration of their cytoplasm due to the hemosiderin content.

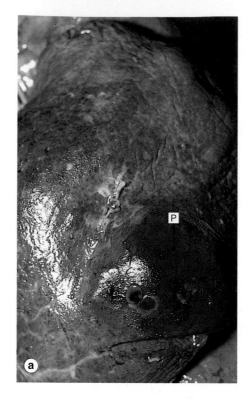

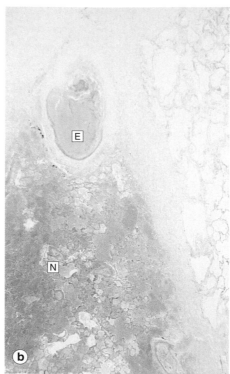

Fig. 11.2 Pulmonary infarction.
Macroscopically, pulmonary infarcts are typically hemorrhagic because of blood entering from the bronchial circulation. Infarcts are wedge-shaped and, as shown in (a), there is often an associated pleurisy (**P**), the cause of the chest pain experienced in such cases. With time, infarcts become organized to form a fibrous scar. Histologically (b), pulmonary infarction caused by thromboembolism (**E**) is characterized by extravasation of blood into the necrotic lung (**N**) (the cause of clinical hemoptysis).

KEY FACTS
Vascular and hemodynamic disease of the lungs

- Pulmonary edema is most commonly caused by left ventricular failure.
- Pulmonary hypertension causes right-sided cardiac failure.
- Pulmonary thromboembolism is most commonly from deep leg vein thrombosis.
- Large pulmonary emboli cause acute right heart failure and death.

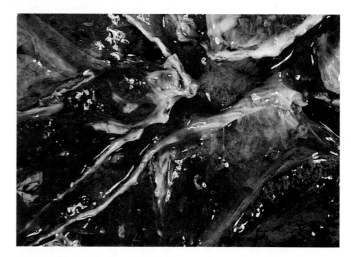

Fig. 11.3 Acute bronchitis.
In acute bronchitis the airway mucosa is red and edematous. There is often an overlying mucoid purulent exudate.

INFECTIVE DISEASE OF THE RESPIRATORY SYSTEM

Infective diseases of the upper respiratory tract (nose, pharynx, larynx, trachea and bronchi) are frequent in western countries, but most are minor and transient. Infections of the lower respiratory tract (bronchus to alveoli) are a serious cause of morbidity and mortality.

Infection of bronchi and bronchioles is most commonly due to viruses

Inflammation of bronchi and bronchioles is extremely common (*Fig. 11.3*). Most cases are due to self-limiting viral diseases. For example, influenza causes tracheobronchitis with necrosis of lining epithelium, and respiratory syncytial virus causes epidemics of bronchiolitis in very young children. In rare cases destruction and scarring of airways can occur.

Adenovirus and measles viruses can cause severe inflammation of bronchioles, which heals by fibrosis leading to permanent damage to lungs (obliterative bronchiolitis).

Bacterial infection of airways is common and precedes development of bronchopneumonia. *Bordetella pertussis* causes whooping cough and, in fatal cases, is associated with bronchial and bronchiolar inflammation.

Fig. 11.4
Classification of pneumonia

Pathological classification

How infection spreads within the lung
Bronchopneumonia
Lobar pneumonia

Microbiological classification

Causative organism determined by microbiology

Clinical classification

Circumstances surrounding development of disease
Community-acquired disease
Hospital-acquired disease (nosocomial)
Disease acquired in special environments
Disease in immunosuppressed patients
Aspiration pneumonia

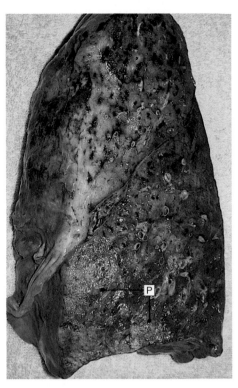

Fig. 11.5 Bronchopneumonia. The cut surface of the lung shows pale areas in the lower lobe (**P**), which are areas of consolidation.

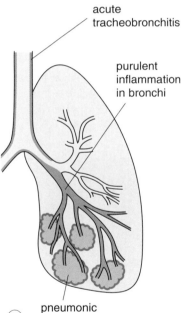

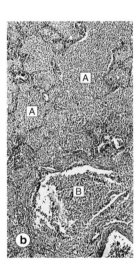

Fig. 11.6 Bronchopneumonia.
In bronchopneumonia, inflammation centered on bronchi (**B**) spreads out to cause inflammation in the alveoli (**A**), which contain acute inflammatory infiltrate. Consolidation is in the dependent parts of the lung.

Infective inflammation and consolidation of the lung is termed 'pneumonia'

Pneumonia is one of the most common infective conditions and is the fifth most common cause of death in the USA. There are three ways of classifying pneumonias, as shown in *Fig. 11.4.*

A clinical classification of pneumonia is best suited for planning investigation and initiating therapy. This is because knowledge of the circumstances in which a person develops a pneumonia is a strong clue as to the likely organism causing infection. Knowing the pathological pattern, be it bronchopneumonia or lobar pneumonia, gives little clue to the likely cause of infections.

Bronchopneumonia occurs when organisms colonize bronchi and extend into alveoli

In bronchopneumonia, primary infection centered on bronchi spreads to involve adjacent alveoli, which become filled with an acute inflammatory exudate, and affected areas of lung become consolidated. Initially, consolidation is patchy within the lung (involves lobules) but, if untreated, it becomes confluent (involving lobes).

This pattern of disease, which is most common in infancy and old age, is predisposed by the presence of debility and immobility. Patients who are immobile develop retention of secretions; these gravitate to the dependent parts of the lungs and become infected, hence bronchopneumonia most commonly involves the lower lobes.

Macroscopically, affected areas of lung are firm, airless and have a dark red or grey appearance (*Fig. 11.5*). Pus may be present in the peripheral bronchi. Histologically, there is acute inflammation of bronchi, and alveoli contain acute inflammatory exudate (*Fig. 11.6*). Involvement of the pleura is common and leads to pleurisy.

If treated, recovery usually involves focal organization of lung by fibrosis. Common complications include lung abscess, pleural infection (pleurisy, see page 218), and septicemia. The causative organisms for this pattern of pneumonia depend on the circumstances predisposing to infection.

Lobar pneumonia occurs when organisms widely colonize alveolar spaces

In lobar pneumonia, organisms gain entry to distal air spaces rather than colonizing bronchi (*Fig. 11.7*). Rapid spread through alveolar spaces and bronchioles causes acute inflammatory exudation into air spaces. Macroscopically, the whole of a lobe becomes consolidated and airless (*Fig. 11.8*).

This pattern of disease is seen in adults. Vagrants and alcoholics who have poor social and medical care are particularly prone to this pattern of pneumonia, which is often caused by *Pneumococcus* or *Klebsiella*.

Patients with lobar pneumonia are usually severely ill, and there is usually associated bacteremia. If treated promptly, many patients recover with the lungs returning to normal structure and function by resolution. In other cases the exudate in alveoli is organized, leading to lung scarring and permanent lung dysfunction. Common complications are development of pleurisy (*Fig. 11.9*), lung abscess, and septicemia.

Community-acquired pneumonia is usually caused by Gram-positive bacteria

No cause is identified by microbiology in about 30% of cases of community-acquired pneumonia, usually because of administration of antibiotics. The most common cause of community-acquired pneumonia is *Streptococcus pneumoniae*, accounting for about a third of all cases. In cases associated with bacteremia, there is a mortality rate of about 25%. In children, patients over the age of 60 years, and

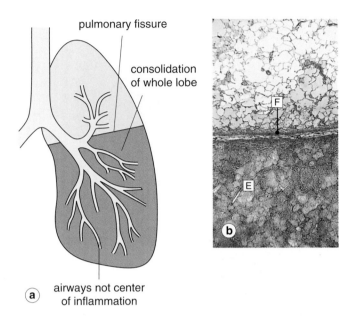

Fig. 11.7 Lobar pneumonia.
In lobar pneumonia, infection spreads rapidly through air spaces to consolidate a whole lobe (a). Histologically (b), alveoli are filled with acute inflammatory exudate (**E**), which is limited by the pulmonary fissures (**F**).

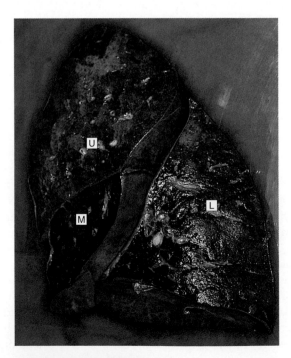

Fig. 11.8 Lobar pneumonia.
The upper (**U**) and lower (**L**) lobes are consolidated compared to the congested but uninvolved middle lobe (**M**).

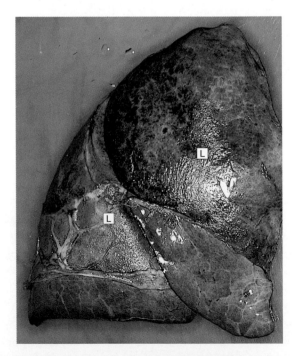

Fig. 11.9 Acute pleurisy in lobar pneumonia.
The pleural surfaces over consolidated lobes (**L**) are covered by a patchy, white, fibrinous exudate, causing acute pleurisy.

those with chronic obstructive airways disease, *Haemophilus influenzae* infection is common. *Legionella* causes disease particularly in mid-adult life, accounting for under 5% of cases (with a 10% mortality rate).

Atypical pneumonia caused by *Mycoplasma pneumoniae* accounts for about 10% of cases of community-acquired infection between the ages of 20 and 60 years. Increasingly, infection with *Chlamydia pneumoniae* is responsible for many cases of pneumonia in neonates and working adults.

Pneumonia due to *Mycobacterium tuberculosis* is particularly seen in socially deprived patients with poor medical care. It is common in developing countries and is once more an increasing cause of disease in developed countries.

Viral pneumonia probably accounts for 10–20% of cases, often complicated by development of superadded bacterial infection. *Staphylococcus aureus* may cause a very severe pneumonia following viral infection (especially influenza), and particularly causes development of lung abscesses (see *Fig. 11.13*).

In dramatic contrast to pneumonias acquired in hospital, Gram-negative bacteria account for under 1% of community-acquired pneumonias. The organism most commonly responsible is *Klebsiella pneumoniae*, which causes a lobar pattern of pneumonia in debilitated and poorly nourished patients such as alchoholics.

Hospital-acquired pneumonias are mainly due to Gram-negative bacteria

Hospital-acquired (nosocomial) infection is defined as 'that which occurs two days or more after admission to hospital'. This happens in up to 5% of all patients admitted to hospital and is predisposed by old age, serious illness, cigarette smoking, decreased lung defences (anesthetics, reduced consciousness), and mechanical ventilation in critical-care units.

Gram-negative bacteria (e.g. *Klebsiella*, *E. coli*, *Pseudomonas*, *Proteus*, *Serratia*) cause 60% of cases, and organisms responsible for community-acquired pneumonia also cause nosocomial disease, but with much reduced frequency. For example, *Pneumococcus* accounts for infection in about 5% of nosocomial cases. Importantly, certain institutions harbour *Legionella* (see pink box on page 198), which can be a cause of nosocomial pneumonia.

Microbiological diagnosis of nosocomial infection may be difficult because Gram-negative organisms frequently colonize the oropharynx following hospital admission, contaminating expectorated sputum. Specimens obtained by bronchial lavage are often more useful in establishing the cause of infection and the antimicrobial sensitivity.

Aspiration pneumonia is caused by chemical and infective damage to lungs

Aspiration into the airway is usually associated with regurgitation during episodes of unconsciousness, but is also seen in patients who have impaired swallowing due to neuromuscular disease, e.g. after a stroke, or with motor neuron disease.

Gastric acid causes chemical pneumonitis, which can lead to adult respiratory distress syndrome (see page 205). Patients develop increasing respiratory dysfunction, and chest radiography shows opacification of lungs. Food material excites a foreign body histiocytic response in the lung, and organisms from the oropharynx cause infection.

Organisms causing infection are usually mixed, but include anaerobes, e.g. *Fusobacterium* and *Bacteroides*. In cases of aspiration pneumonia in hospital patients, *Staphylococcus aureus* and oropharyngeal Gram-negative bacteria are common.

Development of lung abscess is a frequent complication of aspiration pneumonia.

Atypical pneumonia is characterized by inflammation in alveolar septa

In contrast with lobar pneumonia and bronchopneumonia, in which there is inflammatory exudation into air spaces, certain forms of infection of the lung are characterized by inflammation of alveolar septa by chronic inflammatory cells. This pattern of inflammation (acute interstitial pneumonitis), may be caused by several factors, including infection by some viruses, *Chlamydia* and *Rickettsia*.

Patients with this pattern of infection develop fever, dry cough and dyspnea, with little to find on clinical examination of the chest, e.g. absence of consolidation. This pattern of infection is therefore termed **atypical pneumonia**.

Virus infections of lung cause inflammation of lung interstitium

Most viral infections of the lung cause an interstitial inflammatory response by lymphoid cells (interstitial pneumonitis), which is self-limiting in most cases. In severe cases, damage to alveolar lining cells leads to alveolar exudation of fibrin similar to that seen in adult respiratory distress syndrome (see page 205).

Influenza causes rhinitis, pharyngitis, tracheobronchitis and interstitial pneumonitis. Lung infection may rarely cause a severe pneumonitis, leading to necrosis of alveolar lining cells and, ultimately, to death. More usual is superinfection with bacteria, especially *Staphylococcus aureus*.

Cytomegalovirus causes a self-limiting interstitial pneumonitis, commonly seen in small children. Severe infection may be seen in immunocompromised adults.

Measles may cause an interstitial pneumonitis characterized by formation of multinucleate giant cells. Inflammation of bronchioles with scarring can be a complication. In poorly nourished or immunocompromised individuals, measles infection of the lung can be fatal (see *Fig. 8.20*).

Varicella infection may cause an interstitial pneumonitis (chickenpox lung) and can lead to miliary small scars in the lung parenchyma, visible on chest radiography. This may be fatal in immunocompromised individuals.

Fungal infections of lung cause destructive inflammation

Fungal infections of the lung are seen in two populations: most are seen in immunosuppressed patients, but rare cases occur in otherwise healthy patients by exposure to a specific agent indigenous to a particular geographic area.

Aspergillus infection of the lung can cause several patterns of disease, including a pneumonia which leads to extensive necrosis and infarction of affected lung because of vessel wall invasion (*Fig. 11.10*) by the fungus.

Histoplasmosis, coccidioidomycosis and sporotrichosis all cause chronic granulomatous inflammation of the lung, with fibrosis in a pattern resembling TB (see page 54 *et seq.*).

Cryptococcal pneumonia is mainly seen in immuno-compromised patients. It causes granulomatous inflammation, with consolidation and cavitation of lung.

Pneumonia acquired in special environments is associated with unusual organisms

Certain pulmonary infections are associated with unusual environmental exposure to an organism.

- *Legionella* pneumonia is acquired from exposure to buildings with contaminated air-conditioning or water supplies.
- Psittacosis is caused by *Chlamydia psittaci*, usually acquired from avian excreta. It is therefore seen after exposure to pet birds, especially parrots.
- Histoplasmosis is a disease seen in the midwest and the south-eastern regions of the USA. Acquired from inhaling fungal spores in dust, the disease develops in a similar pattern to TB, with granulomatous inflammation and fibrosis (see page 54 *et seq.*).

Candida pneumonia is seen in severely debilitated patients and causes severe acute inflammation, leading to a bronchopneumonic pattern of disease.

Immunosuppressed patients develop opportunistic pneumonias

The diagnosis and treatment of pneumonia in immuno-suppressed patients is becoming increasingly important, particularly with the growing incidence of AIDS (see

KEY FACTS
Pneumonia

- Lobar pneumonia spreads through alveoli to involve whole lobes.
- Bronchopneumonia develops as spread from tracheobronchial infection.
- Atypical pneumonia causes predominantly interstitial inflammation in the lung (viruses, *Chlamydiae* and *Rickettsiae*).
- Different sets of organisms cause community-acquired (as opposed to hospital-acquired) infections.
- The most common community-acquired infections are due to *Streptococcus pneumoniae* and *Haemophilus influenzae*.
- The majority of hospital-acquired cases are due to Gram-negative organisms.
- Unusual environmental exposure is a factor in psittacosis, Legionnaires' disease, and fungal pneumonias.
- Aspiration pneumonia results in both chemical and mixed infective damage to lungs.
- Opportunistic infections affect patients with immunosuppression. The main groups include mycobacteria, viruses, fungi and protozoa.

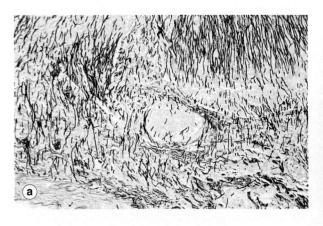

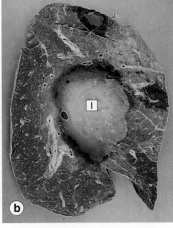

Fig. 11.10 *Aspergillus* pneumonia. *Aspergillus* invades widely in lung, frequently involving vessel walls. In (a) the section has been stained to show *Aspergillus* hyphae invading lung as well as vessel wall. This causes infarction of lung, seen on the cut surface (b) as large areas of organizing infarction (**I**).

page 107). Infection may be with several types of organism, many being opportunistic infections:

- Routine bacterial pathogens responsible for community pneumonias are generally more severe in immunosuppressed patients.
- Mycobacterial infection can be with *M. tuberculosis* or with atypical mycobacteria.
- Viruses, e.g. CMV and herpes simplex.
- Fungi, e.g. *Candida, Aspergillus* and *Pneumocystis carinii* (*Fig. 11.11*).

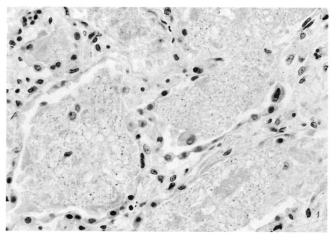

Fig. 11.11 *Pneumocystis carinii* pneumonia.
Infection of the lung by *Pneumocystis carinii* occurs as an opportunistic infection in immunocompromised patients. Histologically, alveoli are filled with a fine, foam-like material, in which the minute bodies of the organism can just be seen as a purple-stained stippling.

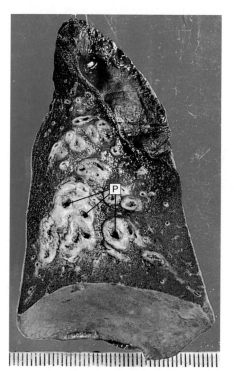

Fig. 11.12 Bronchiectasis. This is a lower lobe of lung surgically resected for bronchiectasis. Large dilated air passages (P) extend out to the lung periphery.

In some instances a diagnosis has to be made on the basis of the invasive techniques of bronchoscopy and analysis of washings, or percutaneous lung aspiration/biopsy.

Lymphocytic interstitial pneumonitis of unknown cause is seen in children with AIDS, but is unusual in adults.

Bronchiectasis is abnormal dilatation of the bronchial tree and predisposes to infection

Abnormal dilatation of main bronchi is termed **bronchiectasis** (*Fig. 11.12*). Patients have recurrent cough and hemoptysis, and expectorate copious quantities of infected sputum. Recurrent episodes of chest infection are common, with a mixed flora of organisms including anaerobes.

Although any bronchi may be involved, the most common site is at the base of the lungs. Airways are typically dilated to 5–6 times their normal diameter and may contain purulent secretions. Histological examination shows chronic inflammation in the wall of the abnormal bronchi, with replacement of the epithelium by inflammatory granulation tissue; it is this which bleeds, giving rise to the frequent clinical sign of recurrent hemoptysis. In less inflamed areas there is commonly squamous metaplasia of bronchial mucosa. With repeated episodes of infection extending into adjacent lung parenchyma, there may be fibrous scarring and obliteration of lung, leading to respiratory failure.

The pathogenesis of this condition is shown in the pink box below. Complications of bronchiectasis include chronic suppuration, formation of a lung abscess, hematogenous spread of infection (particularly predisposing to brain abscess), and development of serum amyloid A – derived systemic amyloidosis (see page 543).

Pathogenesis of bronchiectasis

Bronchiectasis is predisposed by two main factors:

Interference with drainage of bronchial secretions.

- Obstruction of proximal airway, e.g. tumor, foreign body.
- Abnormality in bronchial mucus viscosity, e.g. cystic fibrosis (see page 221).
- Immotile cilia syndrome in which cilia are abnormal, leading to stagnation of secretions (see page 221).

Recurrent and persistent infection weakening bronchial walls.

- Predisposed to by retention of secretions (as above).
- Immunodeficiency states, particularly hypogammaglobulinemia.

In many cases in adults, no cause can be found **(idiopathic bronchiectasis).**

Bacterial lung abscess is predisposed by several diseases

A bacterial lung abscess appears as a cavity, typically 1–3 cm in diameter, containing pus and surrounded by fibrosis and organizing lung (*Fig. 11.13*). There are many diseases that cause or predispose to development of a lung abscess including infection in a pulmonary infarct, unresolved acute pneumonia (particularly due to staphylococci), aspiration of gastric contents (see page 197), and bronchiectasis.

The main complications of an abscess are rupture into pleura, causing empyema and pneumothorax; hemorrhage from erosion into pulmonary vessel; and bacteremia causing cerebral abscess.

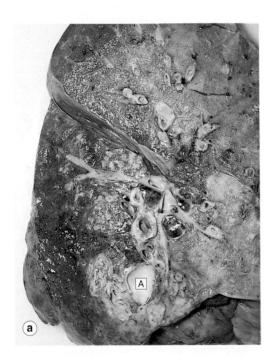

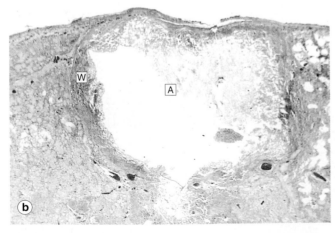

Fig. 11.13 Lung abscess.
(a) A lung abscess is seen as a cavity filled with green purulent material (**A**). The histological section (b) shows the cavity of a peripheral lung abscess (**A**) containing pus, with a wall (**W**) composed of acute inflammatory granulation tissue. This was derived from an infected area of infarction.

CHRONIC OBSTRUCTIVE AIRWAYS DISEASE

Chronic obstructive airways disease (COAD) is a term used to describe conditions in which there is chronic limitation to air flow in the lungs. Flow is reduced for one of two main reasons: either because **airways resistance is increased** (normally by narrowing of airways) or because the **outflow pressure is reduced** (elastic recoil of lungs is lost). The main diseases in this category are chronic bronchitis and asthma (narrowing of airways) and emphysema (loss of elastic recoil).

Asthma is characterized by reversible airways obstruction in small airways

Asthma is the most common cause of recurrent breathlessness, cough and wheeze. It is characterized by obstruction of small airways by a combination of bronchospasm and mucus plugging, which fluctuates with time and is frequently partially reversible with bronchodilator drugs. It is a common disorder, affecting around 10% of children and 5% of adults. There have been recent suggestions that the incidence of asthma is rising, with speculation that this increase might relate to environmental atmospheric pollution.

There are several known triggers for asthma:

- Allergy, e.g. to house dust mites.
- Infection. Viral infection triggers bronchoconstriction particularly in children.
- Occupational exposure. Some agents act as allergens, others by direct irritation of airway.
- Drug-induced, e.g. β-antagonists and aspirin.
- Irritant gases, e.g. sulphur dioxide, nitric oxide, ozone in smog.
- Psychological stress.
- Exertion.
- Cold air.

The concept that there are two types of asthma, extrinsic (due to allergy) and intrinsic (due to constitutional factors) is widely held; there is much overlap between asthma with different triggers.

Asthma is due to a complex chronic inflammatory response in bronchial mucosa

The main changes that take place in asthma are shown in *Fig. 11.14.*

This pattern of responses is seen in long-standing asthma, whatever the cause, and it has been difficult to separate distinct mechanisms in asthma triggered by different causes. The prevailing view is that asthma is a form of low-grade chronic inflammation of the airways, with a variety of triggers causing acute exacerbations. Some of the proposed mediators and mechanisms in the pathogenesis of asthma are described in the pink box on page 202).

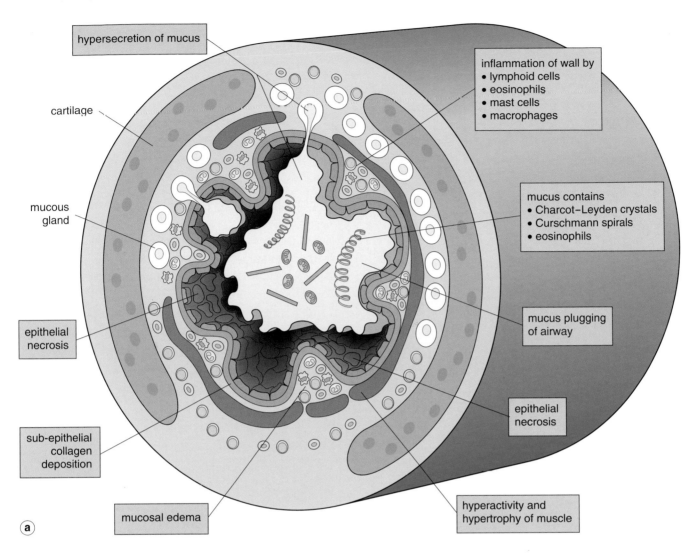

hypersecretion of mucus

cartilage

mucous gland

epithelial necrosis

sub-epithelial collagen deposition

mucosal edema

(a)

inflammation of wall by
• lymphoid cells
• eosinophils
• mast cells
• macrophages

mucus contains
• Charcot–Leyden crystals
• Curschmann spirals
• eosinophils

mucus plugging of airway

epithelial necrosis

hyperactivity and hypertrophy of muscle

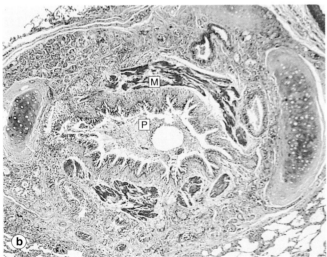

(b)

Fig. 11.14 Structural changes in asthma.
The main events that take place in the airways in asthma are shown diagrammatically (a) and histologically (b). There is:

- Bronchoconstriction due to increased responsiveness of bronchial smooth muscle (**M**).
- Hypersecretion of mucus leading to plugging of airways (**P**).
- Mucosal edema leading to narrowing of airways.
- Extravasation of plasma in submucosal tissues due to leakage from vessels.
- Infiltration of bronchial mucosa by eosinophils, mast cells, lymphoid cells and macrophages.
- Focal necrosis of airway epithelium.
- Deposition of collagen beneath bronchial epithelium in long-standing cases.
- Sputum contains Charcot–Leyden crystals (derived from eosinophil granules) and Curschmann spirals (composed of mucus plugs from small airways).

Most people with asthma have mild disease with acute episodes of bronchospasm that are triggered by well-recognized causes. Disease can be controlled by drug therapy with β_2-adrenoceptor agonists and corticosteroids.

In severe disease (chronic asthma), airway obstruction is persistent despite drug therapy; chronic alveolar hypo-ventilation may cause pulmonary vasoconstriction and pulmonary hypertension. **Status asthmaticus** refers to severe, acute disease that does not respond to drug therapy and may cause death from acute respiratory insufficiency.

Notes on cellular mechanisms of asthma

Immune mechanisms are dominant in many, but not all, cases of asthma (Type I hypersensitivity response); 80% of asthmatics show an atopic tendency.

Although **mast cells** are thought to be important in asthma, and they release histamine, antihistamines are not clinically useful in therapy. This suggests that there are not close parallels with some of the other Type I hypersensitivity responses in which antihistamines are effective.

T-cells are prominent in the mucosal cellular infiltrate. They can release IL-5 to recruit eosinophils.

Eosinophils are thought to be important in the pathogenesis of asthma. They migrate into mucosa in response to chemotactic factors, releasing many mediators of inflammation:

- Leukotrienes LTC_4 and LTD_4 constrict airways.
- Prostaglandins PGD_2, $PGF_{2\alpha}$ and thromboxane can constrict bronchial smooth muscle, but they probably

play little part, as treatment with aspirin does not benefit patients and may worsen or precipitate asthma in some people.

- PAF is probably an important mediator, as it causes long-lasting hyperresponsiveness of bronchial smooth muscle.

Stimulation of afferent nerves by inflammatory mediators can release local peptides, such as substance P, and cause edema and hypersecretion of mucus. Such neural mechanisms are believed to play an important role in pathogenesis and are beginning to be targeted by new therapies.

Inflammation of bronchial walls can give rise to airflow restriction by causing depletion of surfactant in small airways, making them open with difficulty. In long-standing cases, collagen is deposited beneath bronchial epithelium, and this may predispose to increased susceptibility to epithelial necrosis.

Generalized emphysema is characterized by dilatation of air spaces and destruction of alveolar walls without scarring

Emphysema can be defined as 'a permanent dilatation of any part of the respiratory acinus (air spaces distal to the terminal bronchiole), with destruction of tissue in the absence of scarring'.

In practical terms, there is loss of elastic recoil in lungs as respiratory tissue is destroyed and the area available for gas exchange is reduced. Individuals with severe emphysema have reduced oxygen uptake despite increase in ventilation. Although they manage to maintain blood oxygenation by a rapid respiratory rate, they feel breathless on the slightest exertion and become hypoxic (Type I respiratory failure). In pure emphysema, cyanosis, hypercapnia and cor pulmonale develop only late in the disease, after progressive decline in respiratory function.

The pathogenesis of emphysema is thought to be parenchymal destruction by secreted extracellular proteases, normal defensive protease inhibitors being either inactivated or absent (*Fig. 11.15*).

There are two main forms of generalized emphysema, defined by the location of damage in the respiratory acinus (*Fig. 11.16*). Macroscopically lungs are voluminous and, on cut surface, show large dilated air spaces. More than one pattern may exist in the same lung.

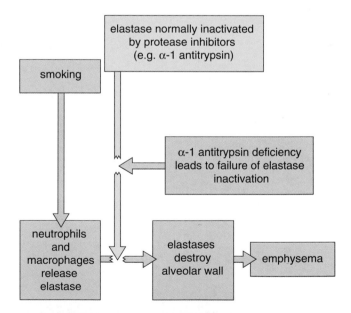

Fig. 11.15 Pathogenesis of emphysema.
Normally, proteases secreted by inflammatory cells are inactivated by extracellular proteases, particularly α-1 antitrypsin. If proteases are not inactivated they can destroy lung tissue. Emphysema is caused by imbalance in the activity of proteases and protease inhibitors. Smoking increases release of proteases. Congenital lack of protease inhibitors is an important cause of excess protease activity.

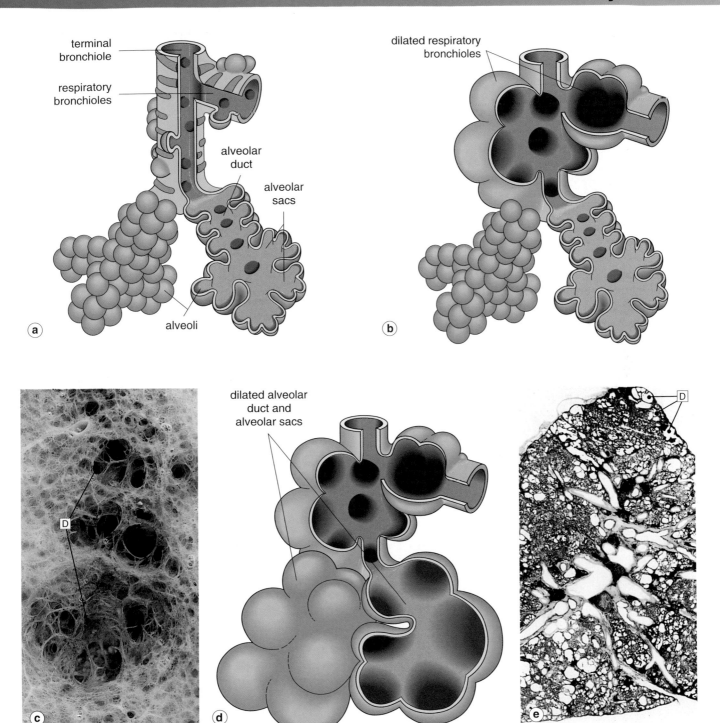

Fig. 11.16 Generalized emphysema. (a) Normal distal lung acinus. (b) Centriacinar emphysema. (c) Centriacinar emphysema. (d) Panacinar emphysema. (e) Panacinar emphysema (Gough–Wentworth section).
The normal lung acinus distal to the terminal bronchiole consists of respiratory bronchioles, alveolar ducts and terminal acini. In centriacinar emphysema, there is dilatation of the respiratory bronchioles at the center of the acinus (b). This is seen in a very high power macroscopic photograph (c) of a portion of affected lung, in which the dilated air spaces (**D**) are surrounded by normal-sized alveoli. In panacinar emphysema (d), there is dilatation of the terminal alveoli and alveolar ducts, which later affects respiratory bronchioles, thereby affecting the whole acinus. The extent of this process in a whole lung can be seen in (e), which is a Gough–Wentworth preparation made by taking a slice, 1 mm thick, through a whole lung and mounting it on paper. The dilated air spaces (**D**) caused by emphysema are evident in all lobes.

Centriacinar emphysema (centrilobular emphysema) is the most common form and is associated with cigarette smoking, chronic bronchitis and inflammation of distal airways (*Fig. 11.16b* and *c*). It is probable that chronic bronchiolitis seen in early cigarette smokers progresses to this form of emphysema. It is most often seen in the upper lobes.

It is likely that the pathogenesis of this type of emphysema is related to secretion of extracellular proteases by local inflammatory cells. Cigarette smoke may also inhibit the effect of protease inhibitor α-1 antitrypsin, thereby potentiating tissue destruction.

Panacinar emphysema involves the whole respiratory acinus and is commonly associated with smoking (*Fig. 11.16 d* and *e*). As with centriacinar emphysema, its pathogenesis is related to excessive activity of extracellular proteases secreted by inflammatory cells. Individuals with congenital deficiency in α-1 antitrypsin also develop this pattern of emphysema at an early age.

The term 'emphysema' is also used to describe other forms of dilated air space

Several conditions are traditionally called emphysema, but do not conform to the definition of the two generalized forms of emphysema, mainly because they are associated with scarring.

Localized emphysema (paraseptal emphysema), which is probably due to infection, is accompanied by inflammatory changes and fibrosis. Lesions are localized and are usually of little clinical significance. They are seen in the sub-pleural zones of the upper lobes, adjacent to lobular septa, around blood vessels and bronchi. When sub-pleural they may burst to cause pneumothorax (see page 218).

Scar emphysema is used to describe dilated air spaces that occur around scars in the lung, whatever the cause.

Focal dust emphysema describes a pattern of dilatation of centrilobular air spaces around aggregates of macrophages containing coal dust, leading to no functional disability.

Compensatory emphysema is used to describe the dilatation of air spaces that takes place in areas around collapsed lung or after surgical lung resection.

Chronic bronchitis causes increased airflow resistance in large airways

Chronic bronchitis is a functional disorder, defined clinically as 'cough productive of sputum on most days for 3 months of the year for at least 2 successive years'. The structural changes are shown in *Fig. 11.17*.

Airways obstruction in chronic bronchitis is due to luminal narrowing and mucus plugging. This leads to alveolar hypoventilation, hypoxemia and hypercapnia (Type II respiratory failure). Individuals with chronic bronchitis and Type II respiratory failure are typically cyanosed, but do not usually have distressing dyspnea. Hypoxic pulmonary

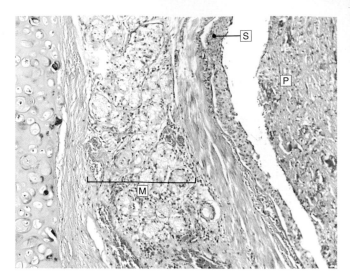

Fig. 11.17 Chronic bronchitis.
In chronic bronchitis the main abnormality is secretion of abnormal amounts of mucus, causing plugging of the airway lumen (**P**). Hypersecretion is associated with hypertrophy and hyperplasia of bronchial mucus-secreting glands (**M**). This can be appreciated by the **Reid index**, the ratio of gland : wall thickness in the bronchus, which is increased in cases of chronic bronchitis. Inflammation in chronic bronchitis is typically not present, although individuals with excessive mucus production frequently develop coincidental respiratory tract infections, leading to secondary inflammation. Squamous metaplasia (**S**) is common in patients who have persistent or recurrent superimposed infections.

vasoconstriction may cause secondary pulmonary hypertension and, with time, lead to right-heart failure (cor pulmonale).

Chronic bronchitis, emphysema and asthma are frequently seen together as a mixed disease

Chronic obstructive pulmonary disease (COPD) is a term commonly used to describe the lung disease commonly encountered in heavy smokers who have persistent cough with sputum, breathlessness on exertion, and airways obstruction. These patients have a mixture of the pathology of chronic bronchitis and emphysema, as described earlier. The situation is further clouded because such patients frequently have a reversible component to airways obstruction, as is typical of asthma.

The main risk factors for this type of disease are lifetime smoking exposure, and asthma in childhood. Acute episodes of infection superimposed on COPD cause acute decline in lung function and may precipitate acute deterioration of chronic cor pulmonale. For this reason, prophylaxis with pneumococcal and influenza vaccines is advisable in this group of patients. Although often suggested, there is no strong epidemiological evidence that such repeated infection is related to the long-term progression of airways obstruction seen in these cases.

KEY FACTS
Obstructive lung disease

- Chronic bronchitis and asthma cause airway narrowing; emphysema causes loss of recoil in lungs.
- Asthma is characterized by a chronic inflammatory response in airways, leading to reversible airways obstruction.
- Muscle spasm, mucus plugging and mucosal edema cause airway obstruction.
- Generalized emphysema is permanent dilatation of any part of the respiratory acinus, with destruction of tissue in the absence of scarring.
- Emphysema is caused by unregulated activity of extracellular proteases secreted from inflammatory cells.
- There are two patterns of generalized emphysema: centrilobular and panacinar.
- Chronic bronchitic airways show mucus hypersecretion with mucous gland hyperplasia.
- Many patients with chronic bronchitis have an asthmatic component to obstruction, as well as emphysema.
- Pulmonary hypertension and right-sided heart failure are common in long-standing obstructive pulmonary disease.

RESTRICTIVE LUNG DISEASES

Restrictive lung diseases cause reduced compliance of the lungs, i.e. they are difficult to expand with respiration. The main reason for this pattern of respiratory dysfunction is abnormality of alveolar walls that renders them rigid, usually by edema or fibrosis. Those affected complain of breathlessness (dyspnea), as they feel the greater effort needed to inflate the lungs. Fibrosis and edema of alveolar walls causes a diffusional defect so that hypoxia develops.

Diffuse alveolar wall damage is the main feature of restrictive lung diseases

The restrictive lung diseases are characterized by damage to alveolar walls. Injury to the alveolar walls leads to three main phases of reaction in lung:

- Hemorrhage and high protein exudation into alveoli (causes so-called **hyaline membranes**).
- Edema and inflammation of the interstitium.
- Fibrosis in the interstitium.

Two main clinical patterns of disease are recognized, depending on which phase of diffuse alveolar damage is most evident: **acute restrictive lung disease**, the main features of which are exudation and edema; and **chronic restrictive lung disease**, the main features of which are inflammation and fibrosis.

Adult respiratory distress syndrome (ARDS) is an acute restrictive lung disease caused by diffuse alveolar damage

The adult respiratory distress syndrome is a manifestation of diffuse alveolar damage leading to widespread systemic metabolic derangements. Many conditions predispose to this serious reaction in lung, most commonly systemic sepsis and severe trauma.

Systemic liberation of chemical mediators of inflammation, particularly cytokines, is important in progression of disease. The pathophysiology of this condition is presented in the pink box on page 206 (*Fig. 11.18*).

The clinical diagnosis of ARDS depends on:

- Presence of a condition known to precipitate ARDS (*Fig. 11.19*).
- Refractory hypoxemia ($PaO_2 < 8.0$ kPa on $> 40\%$ O_2).
- Radiographic evidence of evolving diffuse pulmonary shadowing.
- Clinical signs of lungs becoming abnormally rigid with low total compliance.

Treatment of ARDS is by continuous positive airway pressure ventilation, and intensive support of cardiac, circulatory and renal function. Patients with ARDS usually die from systemic inflammatory response syndrome (see page 40) with multiorgan failure, mortality being around 70%. Of those who survive ARDS, 20% have some permanent lung dysfunction due to organization of exudate and persisting restrictive defect.

Fig. 11.20 summarizes the main features and outcomes in ARDS.

Chronic interstitial lung diseases are characterized by inflammation and fibrosis in alveolar walls

Several conditions can be grouped together on the basis of a common process of inflammation in the walls of alveoli (chronic interstitial pneumonitis), leading to progressive diffuse fibrosis in the lung interstitium.

These are termed **interstitial lung diseases**, as the primary pathology is within walls rather than air spaces. Despite this grouping on the basis of a common lung response to damage, there are widely differing causes since the disease process can be initiated by a wide range of extrinsic factors, both inhaled (e.g. industrial dust disease) and non-inhaled (drugs, radiation), as well as intrinsic disease such as scleroderma and rheumatoid disease (*Fig. 11.21*).

It is notable that, as well as causing a chronic fibrosing syndrome, many of these conditions can also cause an acute exudative phase of diffuse alveolar damage and may present as ARDS.

Pathophysiology of ARDS

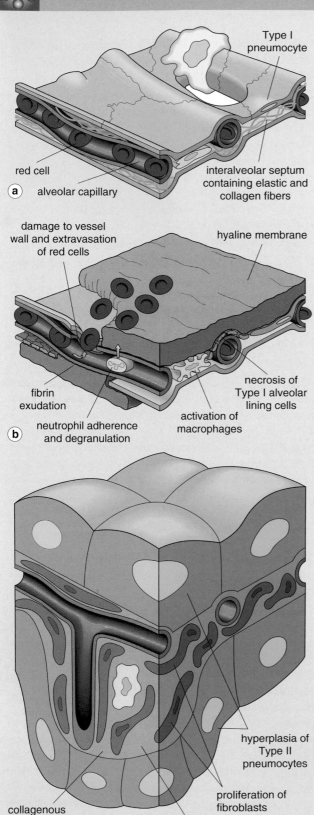

(a)
- Type I pneumocyte
- red cell
- alveolar capillary
- interalveolar septum containing elastic and collagen fibers

(b)
- damage to vessel wall and extravasation of red cells
- hyaline membrane
- fibrin exudation
- neutrophil adherence and degranulation
- activation of macrophages
- necrosis of Type I alveolar lining cells

(c)
- collagenous scarring
- fibrosis organizing alveolar exudate
- proliferation of fibroblasts
- hyperplasia of Type II pneumocytes

The normal alveolar wall is shown diagrammatically in *Fig. 11.18a*. The alveolar wall showing pathological charges centred on the same group of vessels can be seen in *Figs 11.18b* and *c*.

The events that take place in the lung in ARDS are termed **diffuse alveolar damage** (DAD) and occur in two phases:

1 Acute exudative phase, with destruction of alveolar lining cells.
2 Late organization phase, with cell proliferation and fibrosis.

Following the damaging stimulus, there is a latent period of 4–24 hours before symptoms develop. Dyspnea develops before changes are visible on chest radiographs. ARDS develops progressively over a period of 24–48 hours.

In the **acute phase** (*Fig. 11.18b*) there is:

- Necrosis of alveolar epithelium.
- Exudation of fibrin and fluid into alveolar spaces, forming hyaline membranes.
- Microthrombosis in alveolar capillaries.
- Adherence and activation of neutrophils, with release of neutrophil enzymes.
- Hemorrhage into alveoli.

In the **organization phase** the lungs are congested and ventilation is impaired by disturbance of alveolar walls with exudation into alveolar spaces (*Fig. 11.18c*). There is regeneration of Type II alveolar lining cells and organization of hyaline membranes with pulmonary fibrosis. Organization may result in interstitial fibrosis with thickening of alveolar walls, or may cause fibrous obliteration of alveolar spaces.

If ARDS has been caused by septicemia, endotoxin causes endothelial and neutrophil activation, with activation of complement. Treatment with high concentrations of oxygen may, paradoxically, increase damage by generation of oxygen-derived free radicals. ARDS is often complicated by secondary infection in the lungs.

In severe cases of ARDS from any cause, cytokines liberated from the lung vascular bed can enter the systemic circulation and may cause systemic endothelial activation with systemic neutrophil activation leading to multiorgan failure (**systemic inflammatory response syndrome**).

Fig. 11.18 Adult respiratory distress syndrome.
(a) Normal alveolar wall. (b) Acute phase of ARDS.
(c) Organization phase of ARDS.

The end-stage of chronic interstitial fibrosis is termed 'honeycomb lung'

The end-result of long-standing interstitial fibrosis, from whatever cause, is conversion of the lung into a mass of cystic air spaces separated by areas of dense collagenous scarring. This is termed 'honeycomb lung', as the cut surface has been thought to resemble a honeycomb (*Fig. 11.22*).

This is an end-stage process resulting from any of the causes of chronic interstitial lung disease given in *Fig. 11.21*, and is the result of the sequence of damaging stimuli and reparative changes summarized in *Fig. 11.20*. Honeycomb lung leads to chronic respiratory impairment because lung capacity and residual volume are decreased, and there is reduced compliance, with reduced diffusion capacity.

The alveolar wall fibrosis greatly reduces the pulmonary capillary network, leading to right ventricular hypertrophy and the development of pulmonary hypertension, with eventual right heart failure (cor pulmonale). Death results from a combination of respiratory and cardiac failure.

Fig. 11.19
Conditions causing ARDS

ARDS follows a wide variety of direct or indirect insults to the pulmonary vascular endothelium or the alveolar epithelium:

Major trauma, especially associated with raised intracranial pressure

Septicemia

Pulmonary aspiration of gastric contents

Inhalation of toxic fumes or smoke

Major burns

Near-drowning

Pneumonia from many causes requiring ventilation

Disseminated intravascular coagulation

Massive blood transfusion

Amniotic fluid embolism

Acute pancreatitis

Cardiac surgery with bypass

Radiation injury

Certain types of anti-tumor chemotherapy

Paraquat poisoning

Fig. 11.21
Causes of chronic interstitial lung disease

Idiopathic interstitial pneumonitis (also called 'usual interstitial pneumonia') (see page 208)

Connective tissue diseases (rheumatoid disease and scleroderma; see Chapter 25)

Drug-induced damage (particularly anti-tumor chemotherapeutic agents)

Atypical pneumonias (*Chlamydia*, *Mycoplasma*, some viruses)

Pneumoconiosis (diseases caused by inhaling mineral dusts)

Extrinsic allergic alveolitis (disease caused by immune reactions to inhaled organic dusts)

Sarcoidosis (see Chapter 25)

Radiation damage (see page 144)

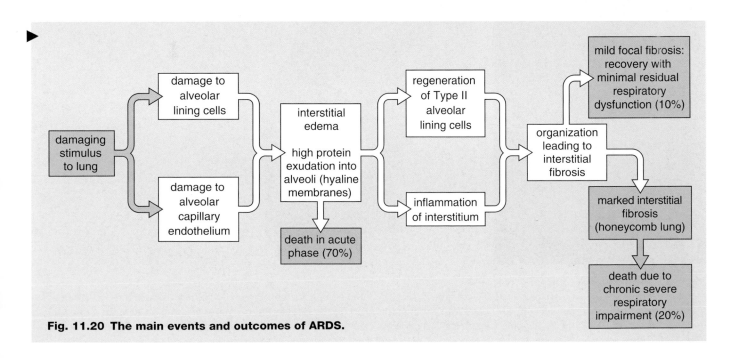

Fig. 11.20 The main events and outcomes of ARDS.

Idiopathic chronic interstitial pneumonitis leads to pulmonary fibrosis

Interstitial pneumonitis with no apparent cause on investigation is termed 'idiopathic'. The disease causes chronic fibrosis in the lung interstitium and is also termed **cryptogenic fibrosing alveolitis**. It presents with insidious onset of dyspnea and tachycardia, most commonly in the sixth decade. A restrictive pattern of respiratory disturbance develops, with impaired diffusion of gas across alveolar walls. These pathological findings are also referred to as **usual interstitial pneumonitis** (UIP). In patients whose disease progresses, honeycomb lung develops.

Desquamative interstitial pneumonitis (DIP) is a phase of UIP characterized by numerous macrophages in the alveoli. Some workers distinguish this as a separate entity, as it may respond to steroid therapy.

The pathogenesis of UIP is uncertain, although the finding of non-specific autoantibodies in serum points to some sort of autoimmune disease. There are also striking similarities between the pathology of UIP and that of lung disease associated with rheumatoid disease and scleroderma (see Chapter 25), suggesting a relationship with connective tissue disorders.

Extrinsic allergic pneumonitis is caused by immune reaction to inhaled allergens

Extrinsic allergic pneumonitis, also called **hypersensitivity pneumonitis**, is caused by immune reaction in the lung to inhaled antigens. There are two main groups of allergen: **animal proteins**, e.g. proteins in bird droppings, and **microbial agents** that contaminate vegetable-derived material. The latter are thermophilic actinomycetes and fungi that colonize rotting crops (e.g. hay, compost, sugar cane, maple bark).

Many clinical syndromes result from this process, their names reflecting the circumstances of allergen exposure, e.g. farmer's lung (*Actinomyces* in mouldy hay), bird fancier's lung (budgerigar and pigeon feces), bagassosis (*Actinomyces* in mouldy sugar cane, called 'bagasse').

There are two types of clinical problem caused by inhalation of allergens:

- Symptoms resulting from acute exposure to antigen. After inhalation, there is a Type III hypersensitivity response. Immune complexes generated at the site of allergen entry in the lung activate complement and there is inflammation. Those affected have dyspnea, fever and cough 4–8 hours after exposure to antigen, resolving after 12–24 hours.

- Symptoms resulting from chronic pulmonary fibrosis. Repeated exposure to antigen results in a Type IV cell-mediated hypersensitivity reaction, with small granulomas visible histologically. This causes interstitial fibrosis and insidious onset of cough and dyspnea, eventually leading to honeycomb lung in about 5% of cases.

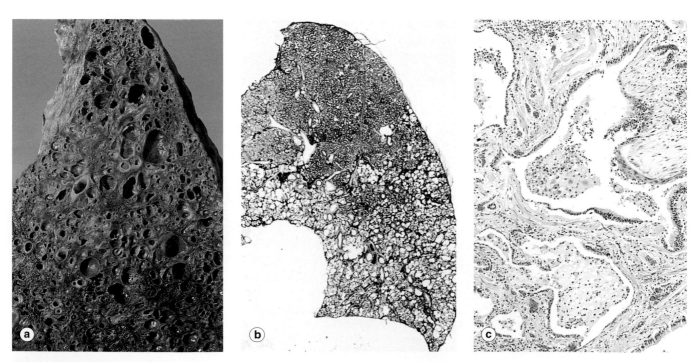

Fig. 11.22 Honeycomb lung.
Macroscopically (a) honeycomb lung appears as large, cystically dilated air spaces surrounded by fibrosis. The pleural surface has a bosselated, leathery appearance. In a Gough–Wentworth preparation (b) the extent of abnormality and interstitial fibrosis can be better appreciated. Histology (c) shows coalescence of air spaces, both alveoli and bronchioles, to form cysts lined with cuboidal epithelium. Focal squamous metaplasia is frequently seen, as well as proliferation of smooth muscle around terminal bronchioles.

Pneumoconiosis is respiratory disease caused by inhalation of dusts

Disease of the lungs caused by inhalation of dusts is termed 'pneumoconiosis', the majority of cases being caused by non-fibrous mineral dusts. Lung damage occurs when the dust interacts with defence mechanisms in the lung. The normal fate of inhaled dust is for it to be coughed out of the lung or ingested into macrophages. If a dust is toxic to macrophages, there is local inflammation, secretion of cytokines and stimulation of fibrosis. Fibrosis in the lung causes a restrictive pattern of respiratory dysfunction. The main dusts causing industrial pulmonary fibrosis are various forms of silicates, often mixed with other materials such as iron oxide or coal.

There are two types of coalworker's pneumoconiosis: one mild, one severe

The risk of developing coalworker's pneumoconiosis is related to degree of exposure to dust. There are two types of pathology.

Simple coalworker's pneumoconiosis (*Fig. 11.23*) is diagnosed by the presence of small nodules, 2–5 mm in diameter, in the lung fields on chest radiography. This pattern of disease is not associated with any clinically significant impairment of respiratory function.

Progressive massive fibrosis (PMF) is characterized by large nodules in the lungs, greater than 10 mm in diameter (*Fig. 11.24*). The disease progresses relentlessly and may present long after active exposure to coal dust. Patients have severe respiratory impairment, with a mixed restrictive and obstructive pattern.

Silicosis is caused by inhalation of quartz-containing dust

Silicosis is caused by inhalation of silicon dioxide (quartz). The main occupational exposure is from slate mining, metal foundaries, stone masonry, tunnelling, granite quarrying, and coal mining through granitic rocks. Changes are seen on chest radiograph as small nodules, 3–5 mm in diameter. There may also be calcification of the periphery of hilar lymph nodes. Disease may progress even after cessation of exposure.

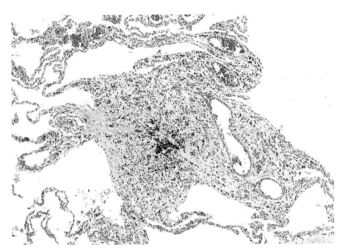

Fig. 11.23 Simple coalworker's pneumoconiosis. Histologically there is accumulation of anthrosilicotic dust in macrophages at the center of the acinus, with associated emphysema of focal dust type.

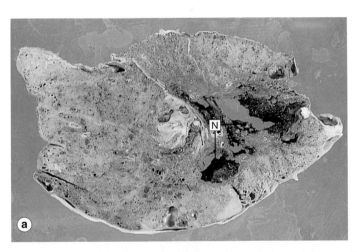

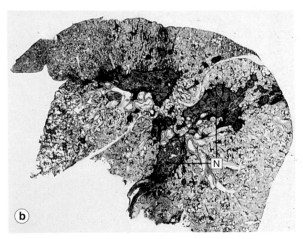

Fig. 11.24 Coalworker's pneumoconiosis: progressive massive fibrosis. (a) Cut surface (b) Gough–Wentworth thin section of whole lung. The nodules in progressive massive fibrosis (**N**) are most common in the upper lobes; they become so extensive as to occupy up to 30% of the lung fields. There is usually surrounding irregular emphysema. There are three main pathological types of nodule in PMF:
- Amorphous collection of acellular proteinaceous material containing little collagen and abundant carbon pigment, which frequently cavitates and liquefies. This type is seen in response to coal with a low silica content (a).
- Dense collagenous tissue and macrophages, heavily pigmented by carbon dust, seen in response to coal with high silica content (b).
- Caplan's syndrome occurs in miners with rheumatoid disease. The nodules have the appearance of large, carbon-pigmented rheumatoid nodules (see page 538).

Short heavy doses produce acute silicosis with pulmonary edema and alveolar exudation.

Prolonged exposure leads to formation of multiple fibrous nodules composed of collagen in the lungs (*Fig. 11.25*). These expand and cause extensive destruction of lung tissue. PMF may also develop. Histologically, silica particles can be seen in nodules, using polarized light.

The development of tuberculosis is a common complication of silicosis (silicotuberculosis). It is presumed to be due to impaired local defences, consequent on the accumulation of silica in macrophages.

The pathogenesis of silicosis is thought to be a toxic effect on macrophages, which stimulates cytokine generation, precipitating fibrogenesis.

Asbestos causes several major diseases of the lung and pleura

Now that its harmful effects have been realized, asbestos exposure has declined rapidly in most parts of the world. Patients who present with asbestos-related diseases are generally over the age of 40 years, and suffered exposure before legislation became effective in the late 1960s. An insidious feature of asbestos-related disease is that there is often a long latent period of up to 50 years between exposure and clinical onset of disease.

The diseases produced by asbestos are:

- Pleural plaques. Benign plaques of collagenous fibrosis in the pleural surfaces.
- Pleural effusions and pleural thickening. Spontaneous effusions in the absence of obvious other cause, and dense pleural thickening, which may compress the lungs.
- Asbestosis. Progressive chronic fibrosis of lungs.

- Malignant mesothelioma. A highly malignant tumor of the mesothelium (see page 220).
- Carcinoma of the lung (see page 212).

Occupational asbestos exposure has been extensive

Asbestos is a fibrous silicate mineral that was widely used between 1890 and 1970 as a building, insulating and fire-resistant material. As well as the hazards of mining and refining asbestos, exposure of individuals has occurred in the building industry, and in industries using asbestos for its insulating properties, e.g. affecting dockyard workers and spray-lagging operatives.

There are two main forms:

- Serpentine asbestos (including white asbestos) is the most common form, and fibers persist in lung for a limited time.
- Amphibole asbestos (including blue and brown asbestos), the fibers of which persist in lung for many years. This form is the main cause of malignant mesothelioma.

The risk of disease depends on duration of exposure (long exposure increases risk), intensity of exposure (heavy exposure to air-borne fibers increases risk), and the type of asbestos (short fibers are not very pathogenic; fibers over 8 μm long particularly cause disease).

Asbestosis causes pulmonary fibrosis, and fibers can be seen in lung

Asbestosis is caused by heavy exposure to asbestos, usually with a latent period of 25 years before clinical symptoms become evident.

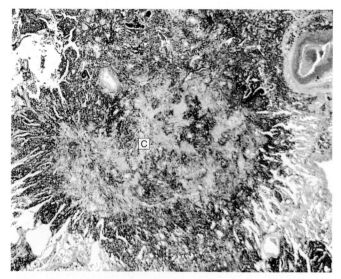

Fig. 11.25 Silicosis of lung.
In silicosis, nodules of collagen (**C**) contain silica particles. In this case, as is common when coal-mining exposure has occurred, there is additional carbon pigmentation, resulting in black peripheral staining.

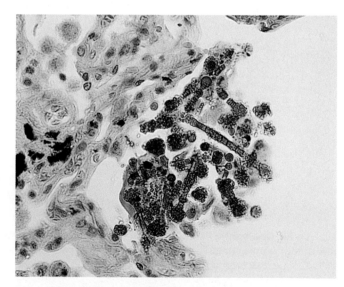

Fig. 11.26 Asbestos bodies.
Asbestos bodies are long, thin asbestos fibers coated with hemosiderin and protein to form brown filaments with a beaded or drumstick pattern.

Diagnosis is made on the basis of occupational exposure, changes on chest radiograph (linear shadows in lung bases), and a pattern of restrictive defects on lung-function testing.

Pathological findings are of interstitial fibrosis of the lungs which, in early stages, is maximal at the lung bases. Asbestos bodies may be seen histologically (*Fig. 11.26*).

The disease progresses with increasing restrictive defect, which is associated with interstitial fibrosis. Pulmonary hypertension and cor pulmonale develop in the late stages.

Lung involvement is common in non-organ-specific autoimmune diseases

Several of the non-organ-specific autoimmune diseases, such as rheumatoid disease, scleroderma and systemic lupus erythematosus (see Chapter 25), cause interstitial fibrosis in the lungs; restrictive lung disease develops, associated with marked diffusional defects as a result of alveolar wall fibrosis.

The histological features are very similar to those described for UIP. In severe cases there is progression of interstitial fibrosis to honeycomb lung.

Goodpasture's syndrome is caused by autoantibodies to the alveolar basement membrane

Diffuse damage to the interstitium of the lung is seen in Goodpasture's syndrome, which is caused by autoantibodies reactive to basement membrane in the lung and in renal glomeruli. The renal pathology of this syndrome is discussed on page 358. Patients develop intrapulmonary hemorrhage and hemoptysis.

Interstitial fibrosis and restrictive lung dysfunction can be caused by treatment for malignancy

Damage to the lung may be caused by radiotherapy, as well as by certain forms of chemotherapy used in treatment of tumors. Drug- or irradiation-induced damage causes diffuse alveolar damage and this may progress to interstitial fibrosis.

Drugs implicated in this type of damage are bleomycin, busulfan, chlorambucil, melphalan, and methotrexate. In some cases damage develops many years after therapy.

Radiation damage to the lung may be acute, causing dyspnea and cough with fever in up to 10% of patients within 6 months of being treated for thoracic or chest-wall diseases. If large volumes of lung have been irradiated, significant late pulmonary fibrosis may develop.

GRANULOMATOUS DISEASE IN LUNGS

Some progressive lung diseases are characterized by the presence of histiocytic and giant-cell granulomatous inflammatory responses. The most important are TB (caused by *M. tuberculosis*), sarcoidosis, granulomatous vasculitis, and fungal infections, e.g. histoplasmosis.

Granulomas also develop as a response to some foreign bodies in the lung, e.g. in some pneumoconioses such as chronic berylliosis, and in response to some inhaled allergens.

TB is discussed in Chapter 4.

Sarcoidosis causes granulomatous inflammation of the lung with interstitial fibrosis

A multisystem disease of unknown cause, sarcoidosis is characterized by the presence of non-caseating granulomas in tissues. From the histology it is evident that a Type IV immune response takes place, yet no allergen or infective organism has been conclusively demonstrated. In 90% of cases the main tissues involved are those of the lungs and draining hilar lymph nodes. Sarcoidosis is also discussed in Chapter 25.

Patients with lung involvement present with slowly progressive dyspnea and cough, and are found to have lung

KEY FACTS
Restrictive lung disease

- Caused by disease affecting the interstitium of lungs, resulting in fibrosis.
- Diffuse alveolar damage is the prototype pattern of initial response in lung.
- ARDS is an acute form of diffuse alveolar damage, mainly caused by severe sepsis and shock.
- Progressive pulmonary interstitial fibrosis leads to honeycomb lung.
- Idiopathic fibrosing alveolitis is a form of interstitial pneumonitis leading to progressive fibrosis of lung interstitium.
- Extrinsic allergic alveolitis is due to hypersensitivity to inhaled allergens, e.g. farmer's lung.
- Pneumoconioses are examples of interstitial fibrosis caused by reactions to inhaled mineral dusts.
- Coalworker's pneumoconiosis has two forms: simple and progressive massive fibrosis.
- Asbestos predisposes to interstitial fibrosis, lung cancer and mesothelioma of pleura.
- Sarcoidosis and connective tissue disease cause interstitial fibrosis of lung.

shadowing on chest radiography, with enlargement of hilar lymph nodes. Histology shows non-caseating histiocytic granulomas in the lung interstitium. Around 70% of patients recover with steroid therapy; 25% of patients show progression to interstitial fibrosis and development of honeycomb lung.

Pulmonary eosinophilia is caused by several diseases

Infiltration of the interstitium of the lungs with eosinophils is a feature of several diseases, and is often also associated with blood eosinophilia and elevated serum IgE. The clinical features of asthma with reversible airways obstruction are often present.

The main causes are:

- Allergic aspergillosis.
- Drug reactions (penicillin, nitrofurantoin, aspirin).
- Helminth infections (microfilariasis, schistosomiasis).
- Idiopathic (Churg–Strauss syndrome).

NEOPLASTIC DISEASE OF THE LUNGS

Carcinoma of the lung is the most common cause of death from neoplasia in industrialized nations. Once mainly a disease of males it is now increasingly common in females. The peak incidence is between the ages of 40 and 70 years, reflecting cumulative exposure to several potential causative carcinogens.

Incidence of lung cancer is related to the main causative factors of cigarette smoking and industrial carcinogens.

Cigarette smoking increases the risk of development of lung cancer, with precursor lesions of metaplasia and dysplasia occurring in the respiratory tract after exposure to cigarette smoke. The risk of cancer increases with the number of cigarettes smoked and with the age at which smoking was started.

Occupational and environmental factors are known to predispose to development of lung cancer, especially exposure to radioactive material, asbestos, nickel, chromium, iron oxides, and coal gas plants. Radon, the natural radioactive gas, is thought to contribute significantly to respiratory exposure to radiation in certain geographic areas.

There are four main histological types of lung cancer

The four main histological types of carcinoma of the lung are squamous cell carcinoma (50%), small-cell anaplastic carcinoma (oat-cell carcinoma) (20%), adenocarcinoma (including bronchoalveolar carcinoma) (20%), and large-cell anaplastic carcinoma (10%).

Because of differences in natural history and response to treatment, many clinicians group tumors into either small-cell lung carcinoma (SCLC) or non-small-cell lung

Smoking and lung cancer

- The increasing incidence of lung cancer in women reflects changes in smoking habits.
- Increase in smoking in developing countries is increasing incidence of lung cancer.
- If smokers who smoke fewer than 20 cigarettes a day stop, the increased risk of lung cancer decreases, reaching that of a non-smoker after 13 years.
- If smokers who smoke more than 20 cigarettes a day stop, they retain a small increased risk over non-smokers for life.
- For passive smokers the risk of developing lung cancer is twice as great as that for those not exposed to smoke.

cancers (NSCLC). A small proportion of tumors may show a mixed pattern of differentiation, particularly mixed adenocarcinoma/squamous carcinoma.

- 70% of all tumors arise in relation to the main bronchi (central or hilar tumors, *Fig. 11.27*).
- 30% of lung cancers arise from peripheral airways or alveoli (peripheral tumors, *Fig. 11.28*).

Lung cancers spread by four main routes

All types of carcinoma of the lung spread by the common routes of metastasis.

Local spread: a carcinoma that arises from a bronchus invades locally through the wall and into surrounding lung. Peribronchial spread, along the outside of bronchi to distant parts of the lung, is common. Direct extension into pleura and adjacent mediastinal structures is a feature of advanced disease.

Lymphatic spread: carcinomas spread to ipsilateral and contralateral peribronchial and hilar lymph nodes. Compression of adjacent tissues by infiltrated nodes may then cause symptoms.

Transcoelomic spread: tumor cells may seed within the pleural cavity, causing a malignant pleural effusion.

Hematogenous spread: the main sites of blood-borne spread are to brain, bone, liver and adrenal glands. Bone metastases are most common in the ribs, vertebrae, humeri, and femora, presenting with pain or pathological fracture.

Squamous cell carcinoma is the most common type of cancer of the bronchus

Squamous cell carcinomas are believed to be derived from metaplastic squamous epitheliums, which develops to line the main bronchi as the result of exposure to agents such as cigarette smoke (*Fig. 11.29*).

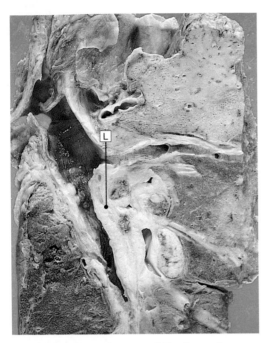

Fig. 11.27 Central carcinoma of the bronchus.
Central carcinomas of the lung (**L**) appear as friable white masses of tissue, which extend into the lumen of bronchi and invade into adjacent lung.

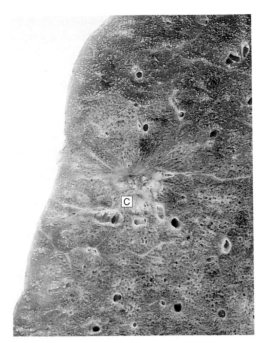

Fig. 11.28 Peripheral carcinoma of the lung.
Peripheral carcinomas of the lung (**C**) appear as ill-defined masses, often occurring in relation to scars, and frequently extend to the pleural surface.

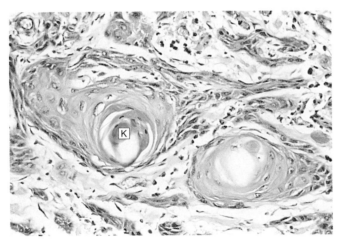

Fig. 11.29 Squamous cell carcinoma of the lung.
Squamous cell carcinoma of the lung shows a range of differentiation from well differentiated lesions producing lots of keratin (**K**), through to lesions with only a few keratin-producing cells.

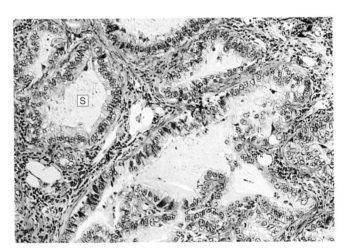

Fig. 11.30 Adenocarcinoma of the lung.
This micrograph shows an acinar pattern of adenocarcinoma of the lung, with prominent gland-like spaces (**S**) lined by a columnar epithelium.

Tumors, which are most common in males, are usually central and close to the carina, frequently presenting with features related to bronchial obstruction. Compared with other types, they are relatively slow-growing and may be resectable.

Adenocarcinoma of the lung is usually a peripheral tumor

Adenocarcinomas have an equal sex incidence and are not as closely linked with cigarette smoking as other types. They characteristically develop as a peripheral tumor, although they may also occur as a central lesion arising from a main bronchus. A proportion of adenocarcinomas are thought to originate in areas of pre-existing lung scarring (**scar cancers**).

There are four main histological patterns: **acinar** (gland-like spaces, *Fig. 11.30*), **papillary** (fronds of tumor on thin septa), **solid carcinoma with mucin production** (poorly differentiated lesions), and **bronchoalveolar carcinoma**.

Most tumors do not produce signs of airways obstruction because of their peripheral location. It is not unusual for extremely extensive systemic metastatic tumor to have originated from a very small peripheral adenocarcinoma of the lung.

Bronchoalveolar carcinoma is a special type of adenocarcinoma

Bronchoalveolar carcinoma of the lung is a special type of adenocarcinoma, accounting for about 5% of all cases and derived from alveolar or bronchial epithelial cells (Clara cells and Type II pneumocytes). A distinct histological feature is spread through lung along alveolar septa.

Half of all cases are multifocal diffuse infiltrative tumors, which replace areas of lung in a manner resembling pneumonic consolidation. Cells are tall, columnar and relatively uniform, have few mitoses and secrete mucin.

The remaining half are single, grey masses of tumor, up to 10 cm in diameter. Cells are cuboidal, with hyperchromatic nuclei and mitoses, and form papillary structures. There is often no mucin secretion. In the absence of metastasis, this sub-type has a better prognosis than other forms of lung cancer.

Small-cell anaplastic carcinoma is the most highly malignant of lung cancers

Small-cell anaplastic lung cancer (also called **oat-cell carcinoma** because the cell nuclei histologically resemble oat grains) is a highly malignant condition (*Fig. 11.31*). Tumors arise from bronchial epithelium, but exhibit differentiation into neuroendocrine cells containing neurosecretory granules.

Tumors are usually centrally located and are associated with a rapid rate of growth, relative to other forms of lung cancer. It is usual for metastases to be present at the time of diagnosis. Because of the neuroendocrine type, this form of cancer is often associated with ectopic hormone production (see page 215).

Large-cell anaplastic carcinoma lacks features of differentiation by light microscopy

Large-cell anaplastic carcinomas are insufficiently differentiated to permit further classification by light microscopy (*Fig. 11.32*). However, if electron microscopy is used, features that favor either squamous or adenocarcinomatous origin can be often seen. This is therefore a diagnostic grouping of convenience, as further histogenetic subdivision is of no clinical or biological importance. Lesions may be either central or peripheral, and are composed of large cells with nuclear pleomorphism and frequent giant cell forms. They have a poor prognosis and are frequently widely disseminated at the time of diagnosis.

The natural history of lung cancer allows no opportunity for screening

There are no early symptoms of lung cancer and it is usual for a lesion to have been growing for many years before

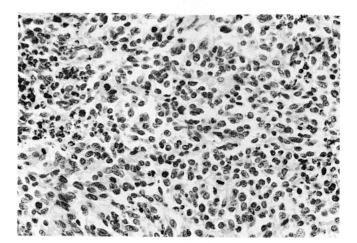

Fig. 11.31 Small-cell anaplastic carcinoma of the lung. This type of carcinoma shows neuroendocrine differentiation. Cells are round to oval and have little cytoplasm; in certain situations there can be diagnostic confusion with a tumor of lymphoid cells. Other types have elongated nuclei and more cytoplasm (intermediate cell variant).

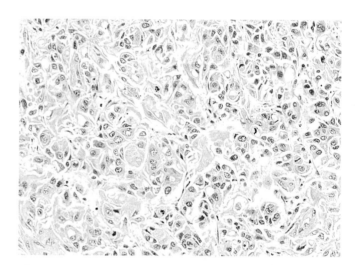

Fig. 11.32 Large-cell anaplastic carcinoma of the lung. These tumors are composed of pleomorphic large cells with no distinguishing differentiation features by light microscopy.

clinical presentation. Small-cell and large-cell anaplastic carcinomas have the fastest pace of growth, adenocarcinomas being the slowest. Symptoms at presentation are usually a manifestation of locally advanced disease.

- Cough (80% cases): infection distal to airway blocked by tumor.
- Hemoptysis (70% cases): ulceration of tumor in bronchus.
- Dyspnea (60% cases): local extension of tumor.
- Chest pain (40% cases): involvement of pleura and chest wall.
- Wheeze (15% cases): narrowing of airway.

Systemic features of malignancy, such as weight loss, anorexia and malaise, are also common at presentation.

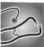

Tissue diagnosis of lung cancer

Diagnosis is made on the basis of clinical features, imaging and obtaining histological confirmation of the nature of the disease.

- Sputum cytology: examination of expectorated sputum by cytology
- Cytology of pleural effusion: examination of pleural fluid by cytology.
- Percutaneous needle aspiration under image guidance: cytological preparation obtained.
- Bronchoscopy and biopsy: small tumor biopsy obtained.

Molecular pathology of lung cancer

Lung cancer is characterized by multiple genetic alterations.

There is inactivation of tumor suppressor genes, e.g. RB tumor suppressor gene on the short arm of chromosome 3, and p53.

Dominant oncogenes are activated in particular; *ras* proteins are mutated in about 20% of NSCLC, but not in SCLC, and seem to be associated with a poorer prognosis.

Overexpression of epidermal growth factor receptor is commonly seen.

At present, such molecular information is used as a research tool. The expectation is that a temporal sequence of mutational events may be uncovered that gives insight into the behavior of these tumors.

Several initiatives to detect lung cancer by mass screening using chest radiography revealed that over half of the asymptomatic tumors detected at screening were inoperable and that there was no improvement in overall survival.

Metastatic spread is a frequent presenting feature of lung cancer

Metastatic spread is present in 70% of patients at presentation, 30% of patients presenting with symptoms caused by metastatic disease.

Bloodstream spread may present with pathological fracture (bone metastasis), leukoerythroblastic anemia (extensive marrow replacement), CNS symptoms (brain metastasis), or hepatomegaly and jaundice (liver metastasis).

Local spread and spread to intrathoracic nodes causes several important clinical syndromes. For example, Horner's syndrome (ptosis, enophthalmos, small pupil, lack of sweating on ipsilateral side of face) is caused by invasion of cervical sympathetic chain, and superior vein caval obstruction is caused by enlarged right paratracheal nodes compressing veins. Recurrent laryngeal nerve palsy results from spread to the left hilar region, and brachial neuritis is due to direct invasion of the plexus by apical tumors, leading to pain in T1 dermatome and wasting of intrinsic hand muscles. Pericarditis is due to direct tumor invasion.

Lung cancer frequently causes non-metastatic extrapulmonary syndromes

Systemic syndromes associated with non-metastatic effects are common in lung cancer and may be a presenting feature of disease.

Endocrine disturbances, seen in 12% of patients with lung cancer, are nearly all associated with small-cell lung cancer because it has a neuroendocrine phenotype with neurosecretory granules. Common syndromes include inappropriate ADH (low sodium and plasma osmolality with high urine osmolality) and ectopic ACTH secretion associated with a Cushing's syndrome (see page 341). Hypercalcemia, in contrast to other endocrinopathies, is most common with squamous cell carcinomas, and is due to secretion of parahormone-related peptide.

Several neurological syndromes can be caused by lung cancer including peripheral sensory/motor neuropathy, cerebellar degeneration causing ataxia, proximal myopathy, dermatomyositis, and Lambert–Eaton myasthenic syndrome, which is associated with small-cell tumors and may precede clinical detection of tumor.

Hypertrophic pulmonary osteoarthropathy (finger clubbing, swelling of wrists and ankles with periosteal new bone formation) is seen in 2–3% of squamous cell carcinomas and adenocarcinomas.

Staging and histological type determine outcome in lung cancer

The factors that determine the outcome of lung cancer, and its likely response to treatment, are histological type and stage. For example, squamous cell carcinomas grow slowly and carry a good prognosis if detected at an early stage and are operable, some forms of bronchoalveolar cell carcinoma have a better prognosis than other forms of lung cancer (see page 214), and small-cell tumors metastasize widely and have the poorest prognosis.

Survival is better for early stage disease, except for small-cell carcinoma. The TNM system and staging used for carcinoma of the lung is shown in *Fig. 11.33*.

Most lung cancers have a very poor 5-year survival with treatment

NSCLC: 75% of all cases are inoperable owing to age, poor lung function, or advanced stage on careful assessment (CT and MRI scanning or mediastinoscopy). If squamous carcinomas alone are considered, about 60% are resectable at presentation. Of patients who have a thoracotomy, about one-fifth will be found at surgery to have inoperable disease. Overall, of this group, only 20% of cases have successful resection of tumor. Longer follow-up reveals broncho-alveolar-cell carcinomas have a better prognosis than other types, with 20–50% 5-year survival rates. Overall, others show 5–30% of cases surviving for 5 years. Inoperable cases may be treated with radiotherapy depending on clinical circumstances. The role of chemotherapy is limited.

SCLC: cases with limited disease, in which tumor is confined to one side of the chest, are seen in only 30% of cases, the rest having extensive disease. SCLC is very sensitive to radiotherapy and chemotherapy, but the extent of disease means that survival is still poor despite local control of tumor. Treatment offers good palliation of pain, cough and dyspnea. Radiotherapy and combination chemotherapy cause complete local response in 30% of cases, with a median survival of 11 months, and a 1-year survival of 45%.

Carcinoid tumors of the lung have variable malignant potential

Carcinoid tumors of the lung are neuroendocrine tumors, representing about 5% of all pulmonary neoplasms. They grow either as bronchial lesions that protrude into the lumen, presenting early with airway obstruction, or as locally infiltrative lesions extending from the bronchus into adjacent lung.

Histological examination shows some lesions that have no atypical cytological features, and these behave in a benign fashion. Others lesions, particularly the infiltrative group, show mitoses and nuclear atypia. This group has

---

 Staging of carcinoma of the lung

Non-small cell lung cancer

For non-small cell lung cancer, tumor stage has an important bearing on prognosis. Tumours are evaluated using a lung cancer-specific TNM system and on this basis can be divided into stages I–IV.

For stages I and II the main form of therapy which will be considered is surgery. The key features which offer a reasonable prospect for surgery are listed in *Fig. 11.33*. For stages III–IV combinations of chemotherapy and radiation therapy offer the best option, mainly with an expectation for palliation of symptoms rather than cure.

Small cell lung cancer

For small cell lung cancer the detailed TNM staging system is not commonly used in clinical practice because metastatic disease is commonly present at diagnosis and survival is generally not affected by the local and regional extent of tumor. A 2-stage system has been devised which is of much more clinical relevance and is widely used in practice.

- **Limited stage**. Limited stage small cell lung cancer refers to tumor confined to one hemithorax, the mediastinum, and the supraclavicular nodes, and which can be encompassed within a clinically acceptable therapeutic irradiation field.
- **Extensive stage**. Extensive stage small cell lung cancer refers to any tumor that extends beyond the definition of limited stage disease.

Fig. 11.33
Features which go with a reasonable prospect for surgery in non-small cell lung cancer

- Tumors smaller than 3 cm in size.
- Tumors are in a lobar bronchus or at least 2 cm distal to the carina.
- No involvement of the chest wall, diaphragm, pericardium, trachea, great vessels, esophagus or vertebrae.
- No contralateral lymph node involvement.
- No distant metastases (including separate tumor nodules in same lobe).
- Absence of a malignant pleural effusion.
- Absence of associated atelectasis or obstructive pneumonitis in the adjacent lung.

For limited stage disease most patients will be offered treatment with combination chemotherapy and radiotherapy to the affected side of the chest. Those who respond may be offered prophylactic cranial irradiation in an attempt to minimize development of cerebral metastases.

For extensive stage disease most patients will be offered treatment with combination chemotherapy. Radiotherapy is generally used to treat sites of metastatic disease, especially in the brain, bone metastases, and for the relief of vena-caval obstruction.

the potential for local recurrence or metastasis in a small proportion of cases, being termed **atypical pulmonary neuroendocrine tumors**. The term 'pulmonary carcinoid' is perhaps inappropriate for such lesions, as a clinical carcinoid syndrome is unusual in most cases, and most lesions do not secrete 5-hydroxytryptamine.

There is about 80% 10-year survival for resected cases showing no atypical features, whereas atypical forms have about 50% 5-year survival.

Tumor permeation of pulmonary lymphatics leads to severe breathlessness

Metastatic tumor, whether from lung or extrapulmonary sites, may diffusely infiltrate pulmonary lymphatic vessels, producing the syndrome of **lymphangitis carcinomatosa** (*Fig. 11.34*).

This presents as severe breathlessness, as blockage of lymphatics causes failure of removal of interstitial fluid, which accumulates in lung parenchyma in much the same way as in early cardiogenic pulmonary edema. The chest radiograph shows diffuse shadowing, and dilated intrapulmonary lymphatic vessels may be visible as linear streaks.

This is a dire condition, which is rapidly fatal.

Metastases and hamartomas are common pulmonary mass lesions

After primary cancers, the two most common mass lesions in the lung are metastases and hamartomas.

Metastatic tumors are common by blood-borne spread, particularly from kidney, breast, testis, and gastrointestinal tract.

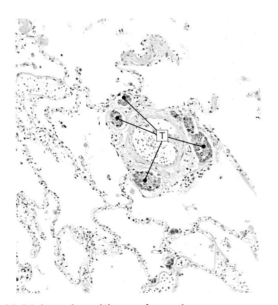

Fig. 11.34 Lymphangitis carcinomatosa.
Diffuse permeation of pulmonary lymphatics by malignancy may occur with lung tumors or from metastases. Macroscopically, surface lymphatics packed with tumor may be visible on the pleural surface. Histologically, tumor cell clumps (**T**) are evident in lymphatics throughout lung.

Bronchial hamartomas are common benign lesions composed of tissue normally encountered in the lung. Most are 1–3 cm in diameter and largely consist of cartilage, being firm and glistening white in appearance. Other elements are bronchial epithelium, fat, and muscle. They are asymptomatic and are mainly discovered at *post mortem* examination.

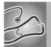

Coin lesions on chest radiograph

The discovery of a rounded solitary lesion on a chest radiograph is termed a 'coin lesion'. This appearance has several main causes.

If all age groups are considered, one-third of cases are caused by a carcinoma of the lung, increasing to a half of all cases in patients over the age of 50 years.

The common lesions are:

- Primary bronchial or lung carcinoma.
- Metastatic tumor (especially of the kidney).
- Bronchial hamartoma.
- Carcinoid tumor.
- Granulomatous inflammation (e.g. TB).
- Lung abscess.

The uncommon lesions are pulmonary cysts, pulmonary angiitis, fungal mycetoma, and vascular malformations.

KEY FACTS
Lung cancer

- Caused by inhaled environmental agents, particularly smoking and radon.
- Peak incidence 40–70 years, most common form of cancer.
- Four main types: squamous cell, small-cell anaplastic, adenocarcinoma and large-cell anaplastic.
- Tumors may be central (all types) or peripheral (mainly adenocarcinomas).
- Bronchoalveolar carcinoma is a special form of adenocarcinoma.
- Small-cell anaplastic tumors are neuroendocrine, highly malignant and frequently have ectopic endocrine syndromes.
- Overall survival 5–30% at 5 years, highly dependent on type and stage of disease.

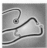

Mediastinal pathology

Mass lesions in the mediastinum can be caused by many different lesions arising from structures in its anterior, middle, posterior, inferior and superior parts (*Fig. 11.35*).

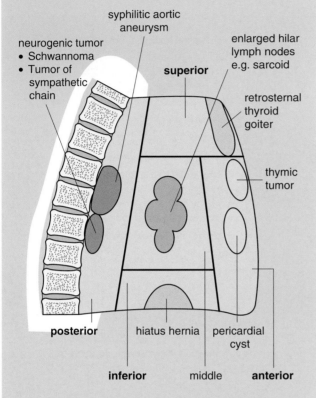

Fig. 11.35 Mass lesions in the mediastinum.

PATHOLOGY OF THE PLEURA

The pleura is lined by a sheet of mesothelial cells. There is constant generation of fluid from the parietal pleura and resorption of pleural fluid by the visceral pleural surface. The formation of fluid is influenced by hydrostatic and osmotic gradients, as well as by changes in the permeability of local vessels.

Several types of fluid may accumulate in the pleural space. If the accumulation is large, there may be compression of the lung.

- **Pus**: empyema due to infection.
- **Blood**: hemothorax due to trauma or surgery.
- **Chyle**: chylothorax due to leakage from the thoracic duct.
- **Fluid effusion** (either transudate or exudate): can be caused by several main diseases (*Fig. 11.36*).
- **Transudate**: low-protein fluid due to movement of excess fluid through normal vessel walls. Commonly due to high hydrostatic pressure in cardiac failure.

Laboratory medicine: diagnostic techniques for lung disease

Bronchoalveolar lavage (saline injected into a lung segment down a bronchoscope. Saline is aspirated and examined for cells and organisms):
- Atypical infections e.g. pneumocystis.
- Interstitial lung diseases.

Bronchial biopsy (biopsy down bronchoscope):
- Neoplasia.
- Sarcoid.
- Allergic aspergillosis.

Transbronchial biopsy (forceps advanced to lung periphery down bronchoscope and samples parenchyma):
- Diffuse lung disease.
- Transplant monitoring.
- Infection diagnosis.

Percutaneous lung biopsy by needle:
- Localized mass lesions.
- Atypical infections.

Open lung biopsy:
- Chronic diffuse lung shadowing of uncertain cause.

- **Exudate**: high-protein fluid (containing fibrinogen/fibrin) due to movement of fluid through damaged vessel walls. Commonly due to infection, infarction or tumor (see *Fig. 11.36*).
- **Air**: 'pneumothorax'.

Pneumothorax may be spontaneous, traumatic or iatrogenic

The presence of air in the pleural space is termed 'pneumothorax'. Spontaneous pneumothoraces can be divided into those that occur secondary to disease in the lungs, and those that occur in otherwise healthy individuals. Traumatic pneumothorax may be due to chest injury, or may be iatrogenic. The causes are summarized in *Fig. 11.37*.

Infection of the pleura is the most common cause of pleurisy

Acute inflammation of the pleura is termed **pleurisy**, the most common cause of which is infection. Macroscopically, fibrinous exudate is seen over the pleural surfaces (see *Fig. 11.9*), and there is variable exudation of fluid. Certain infections result in accumulation of pus in the pleural cavity (empyema). Aspiration of an infected pleural effusion reveals a high-protein exudate. Neutrophils predominate in

Fig. 11.36
Pleural effusion

Type of effusion	Pathogenesis	Causes
Transudate Less than 30 g protein/litre	Increased hydrostatic pressure	Cardiac failure
	Decreased oncotic pressure	Vena caval obstruction Hypoalbuminemia
Exudate More than 30 g protein/litre	Infections	Bacterial, including TB Other organisms
	Neoplasm	Metastatic carcinoma Primary carcinoma of lung Mesothelioma of pleura
	Pulmonary infarction	Thromboembolic disease
	Autoimmune disease	Rheumatoid disease Systemic lupus erythematosus
	Abdominal disease	Pancreatitis Subphrenic abscess Meigs' syndrome

Investigation of pleural effusion

The investigation of a pleural effusion involves aspirating a sample for laboratory investigation. It is also common for a biopsy sample of pleura to be taken, using a specialized needle.

- **Cytology**: this will detect neoplastic cells, and distinguish acute and chronic inflammatory conditions on the basis of the presence of appropriate inflammatory cells.
- **Biochemistry**: analysis of protein concentration helps in deciding whether an effusion is a transudate or exudate.
- **Microbiology**: if the aspirate is turbid, it is important to search for infective causes. TB is best cultured from a pleural biopsy rather than from fluid.
- **Histology**: biopsy of the pleura will assist in histological identification of neoplastic conditions and TB.

acute infections, whereas lymphoid cells predominate in TB. There is a wide range of causative organisms, mostly spreading from initial lung infection, including *Streptococcus pneumoniae*, *Haemophilus*, *Klebsiella*, *Pseudomonas*, and *Bacteroides*.

Fig. 11.37
Causes of pneumothorax

Spontaneous pneumothorax

Primary
Thin young men
Rupture of congenital subpleural apical bleb

Secondary
Rupture of emphysematous bulla
Asthmatics
Rupture of congenital cyst
Pleural malignancy
Cystic fibrosis
Pneumonia
Sarcoidosis
Whooping cough

Traumatic pneumothorax

Penetrating chest wounds
Rib fractures
Esophageal rupture

Iatrogenic pneumothorax

Subclavian cannulation
Positive pressure artificial ventilation
Pleural aspiration
Esophageal perforation during endoscopy
Lung biopsy

Viral infections of the pleura are most commonly due to Coxsackie viruses, echoviruses, and adenoviruses.

The fibrinous exudate of acute pleurisy may become organized to form fibrous pleural adhesions and can lead to fibrous pleural thickening. Calcification may also be seen in the pleura as a result of old tuberculous pleurisy.

The most common tumor of the pleura is metastatic carcinoma

Metastatic tumors are the most common cause of neoplasm in the pleura. The most frequent primary sites are lung and breast, causing pleural effusion.

Metastasis to the pleura is usually associated with a high-protein exudate. Diagnosis can be made by cytology of aspirated fluid or by needle biopsy of the pleura.

Malignant mesothelioma is caused by exposure to asbestos

Primary neoplasms of the pleura are rare except after exposure to asbestos, when tumors termed 'malignant mesotheliomas' develop. After exposure, there may be a latent period of up to 50 years before development of the tumor.

Patients have chest pain and breathlessness, and there is commonly a pleural effusion. Diagnosis is made on pleural biopsy. Histologically, mesotheliomas have spindle cells and glandular patterns.

These are highly malignant tumors that spread around the pleural cavity and pericardium, encasing the lung and mediastinal structures (*Fig. 11.38*). Death is usual within 10 months of diagnosis, and metastasis is rare.

Exposure to asbestos also causes development of benign collagenous thickenings of the pleura, termed **pleural plaques**.

LUNG DISEASE IN CHILDREN

Common developmental abnormalities of the lung

Bronchial atresia leads to severe narrowing of a bronchus supplying an area of lung. Overexpansion of the lung segment may occur from air trapping.

Pulmonary hypoplasia reflects incomplete development of the lung, which is smaller than normal. This is often seen with other congenital abnormalities and is associated with lung compression by other abnormal masses and oligohydramnios.

Bronchogenic cysts are usually attached to the trachea and represent accessory bronchial buds, which become sealed off from the rest of the main airways. They are lined by a respiratory epithelium and contain mucinous fluid.

Bronchopulmonary sequestration is due to development of a portion of lung that does not communicate with the normal bronchial tree. Patients develop an abnormal

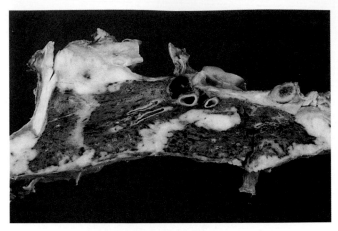

Fig. 11.38 Malignant mesothelioma.
Mesothelioma is seen as a thick sheet of white tumor, which encases the whole of the lung.

lung mass and the abnormal areas develop dilated airways. There are recurrent infections, with frequent development of an abscess.

Neonatal respiratory distress syndrome (hyaline membrane disease)

The neonatal respiratory distress syndrome (NRDS) is due to deficiency of surfactant in the lungs. It is primarily a disease affecting premature infants, but is also seen in infants born to diabetic mothers, as excess production of insulin by the fetus suppresses surfactant production.

A very common condition, the incidence of NRDS increases with increasing prematurity (20% incidence at 32–36 weeks' gestation; 60% incidence at < 28 weeks' gestation).

The pathogenesis of the disease is illustrated in *Fig. 11.39*. With development of disease, the chest radiograph shows a 'ground glass' opacity in the lung fields. The mortality from NRDS is 50% in infants weighing under 1000 g. The lungs from infants who die from the condition appear airless, dark red and dense. Depending on the stage of disease, atelectasis, epithelial necrosis, hyaline membranes, and organization may be seen histologically.

There are four main extrapulmonary complications of NRDS: hypoxic-related intracerebral hemorrhage; failure of closure of ductus arteriosus (normal closure stimulated by oxygenation); necrotizing enterocolitis caused by hypoxic/ischemic damage to gut; and bronchopulmonary dysplasia, which is caused by high-pressure ventilation and oxygen toxicity to alveolar lining cells. Lungs show fibrous obliteration of bronchioles, peribronchial fibrosis, and overdistended alveoli.

Administration of synthetic surfactant and respiratory support allows recovery in the majority of cases. Prevention can be assisted by administering corticosteroids to mothers about to deliver prematurely, as this stimulates surfactant production in the fetus.

Pathogenesis of NRDS

There are four main risk factors for development of NRDS. The immature or damaged lung is unable to make enough surfactant, the lecithin-rich surface-active lipid secreted by Type II pneumocytes. Normally this reduces surface tension in alveoli and keeps alveoli open. In NRDS, lack of surfactant means that alveoli collapse with microatelectasis.

Hypoxia leads to damage of alveolar lining cells, hypoxia and pulmonary arterial constriction. Endothelial damage causes plasma to leak into alveoli, being deposited as fibrin. The fibrin appears as bright, pink-stained membranes lining alveoli, hence the name **hyaline membrane disease.** The presence of fibrin further impairs gas exchange and makes hypoxia worse. The process is similar to that in diffuse alveolar damage, illustrated in *Fig. 11.20.*

Later, regenerative changes in the lung lead to organization of hyaline membranes and fibrosis.

Fig. 11.39 Pathogenesis of NRDS.

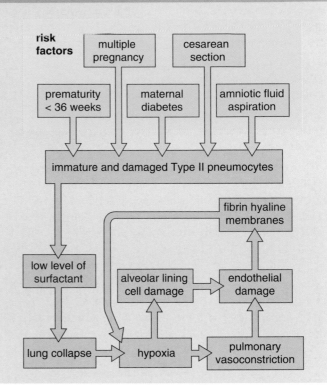

KEY FACTS
Neonatal respiratory distress syndrome

- Caused by deficiency of surfactant.
- Risk factors: prematurity, diabetic mother, neonatal aspiration, multiple birth.
- Lung collapse causes hypoxia, damage to endothelial and alveolar lining cells, and fibrin exudation.
- 50% mortality if weight < 1000 g.
- Complications: intracerebral bleed, patent ductus arteriosus, necrotizing enterocolitis, bronchopulmonary dysplasia.

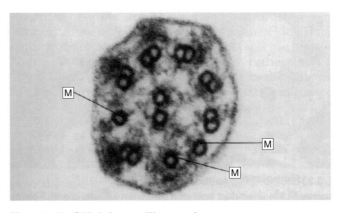

Fig. 11.40 Cilial dysmotility syndrome.
Electron micrograph of cilia from a person with recurrent chest infections since childhood. The outer dynein arms are absent and there are abnormal single microtubules (**M**), which prevent normal motility.

Immotile cilia syndrome leads to recurrent chest infections

Recurrent chest infections in childhood may be due to defective cilial function, the **immotile cilia syndrome.** Imaging studies show reduced clearance of tracer substances inhaled into the lungs, and biopsy of cilia-bearing nasal mucosa shows uncoordinated beating with time-lapse photography. In some individuals, cilia are seen to have an abnormal structure, with absence of structural components such as the dynein arms (*Fig. 11.40*).

A syndrome of absent frontal sinuses, bronchiectasis and situs inversus (organs on wrong side), termed **Kartagener's syndrome,** is due to defective cilial motility.

Cystic fibrosis is characterized by abnormally thick mucus

Cystsic fibrosis is the most common autosomal recessive disorder in the Caucasian population, with an incidence of 1 : 2500 newborns, 1 : 25 adults being a heterozygous carrier of the CF gene. It is a multisystem disease and, most importantly, causes recurrent chest infections in childhood, associated with pancreatic exocrine dysfunction. The disease is caused by the production of an abnormally viscid mucus that cannot be cleared from the lungs and causes blockage of the main pancreatic ducts.

- 40% of cases present with respiratory disease.
- 30% present as failure to thrive and malabsorption.
- 20% present at birth with meconium ileus (due to abnormally viscid intestinal mucus).
- 10% present with liver disease, recurrent nasal polyps or sinusitis.

Diseases of other organs are discussed in relevant chapters.

The molecular pathogenesis of the disorder is defective function in a membrane chloride channel of epithelial cells, which causes decreased release of sodium and water to liquefy mucus. This is shown in the pink box below (*Fig. 11.41*). In the respiratory tract, bronchi and bronchioles become obstructed by abnormally viscid mucus, which leads to four main problems.

- The obstruction and stagnation of secretions leads to repeated bouts of infection, particularly with *Staphylococcus aureus* and the mucoid form of *Pseudomonas.*
- Bronchiectasis is a frequent complication leading to hemoptysis (see page 199).
- Hyperinflation of lungs due to air trapping behind mucin plugs increases the risk of developing pneumothorax.
- Hypoxia, scarring and destruction of the pulmonary vascular bed lead to pulmonary hypertension and cor pulmonale (see page 193).

The median age of survival is just over 30 years.

Molecular pathogenesis of cystic fibrosis

The gene for cystic fibrosis (CF gene) is on the long arm of chromosome 7. It encodes a protein termed the **cystic fibrosis transmembrane conductance regulator** (CFTR).

In normal mucus-secreting epithelia (a) chloride channels open in response to increased concentration of cAMP (generated by stimulation of cell surface receptors), which activates a protein kinase (PKA). Phosphorylation of the CFTR protein opens the channels, and secretion of chloride, water and sodium is facilitated.

In the main mutation causing CF (b) (70% of cases), the protein is not present in the cell surface, stimulated chloride secretion cannot occur, cells do not secrete water and sodium, and mucus is extremely viscid. Such cases have severe clinical disease.

Over 100 other different mutations of the CF gene lead to expression of an abnormal CFTR in the cell membrane, with only partial activity in response to cAMP (c). Such cases have moderately viscid mucus and milder clinical disease.

The detection of the CF gene now allows for fetal diagnosis and carrier detection. Gene therapy to place a normal CF gene in respiratory tract epithelial cells is a real possibility, using an inhaled viral vector.

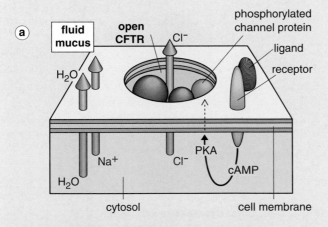

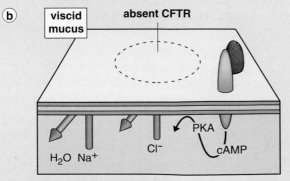

Fig. 11.41 Molecular pathogenesis of cystic fibrosis.

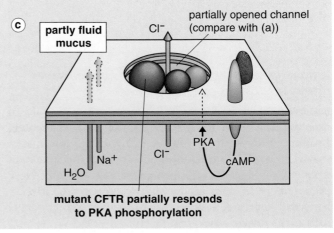

mutant CFTR partially responds to PKA phosphorylation

12 Oral and ENT pathology

Clinical Overview

In this chapter, we cover topics that cross many special disciplines of clinical practice. There is material here that students may encounter in their training in pediatrics, dermatology, dentistry, maxillofacial surgery, otorhinolaryngology, and general medicine and surgery. Most importantly, this chapter contains many diseases that are seen frequently in family practice clinics. Almost all of the topics in this chapter are either very common, or very important, or both. Dig in, and try to remember it all.

MOUTH AND OROPHARYNX

The mouth is largely lined by non-keratinizing squamous epithelium, but there is abundant scattered salivary tissue located in the submucosa, with ducts opening onto the surface. The mouth comprises the lips, the buccal cavity, the palate, the tongue, the alveolar ridges of the mandible and maxilla (in which the teeth are embedded), the teeth, and **Waldeyer's ring**, which is formed by the lymphoid tissue of the posterior tongue, the palatine tonsils, and the oropharynx.

Cleft palate and cleft lip are the most common major congenital malformations of the mouth

Cleft palate and cleft lip frequently occur together, as they arise as a result of the same process, i.e. a failure of fusion of embryological midline structures (see page 76) at about 8 weeks' gestation. A few cases are associated with a chromosomal abnormality (e.g. trisomies 13 and 18), but the teratogenic factors cannot usually be identified in individual cases. In minor degrees of cleft palate, only the soft palate is cleft, the most obvious feature on examination being a bifid uvula. Severe degrees also affect the bone of the hard palate, and the cleft may involve the alveolar ridge, in which case there is co-existent cleft lip.

A high, arched palate is a very frequent minor congenital abnormality. It is usually asymptomatic, although there may be a predisposition to middle ear infections and sinusitis.

Most infections of the lips and buccal cavity (infective stomatitis) are due to either viruses or fungi

Viral infections of the lips and mouth usually manifest as large blisters or crops of small, painful vesicles, which eventually erode to form shallow, tender ulcers.

Herpes virus Type 1 produces herpetic stomatitis. Blisters develop on the gingiva and palate in the early stages, leaving shallow ulcers after rupture. Severe herpetic stomatitis is important in immunosuppressed patients, particularly AIDS patients. Herpes labialis (coldsore) is the result of viral latency, with reactivation of previous virus infection producing vesicle formation at the mucocutaneous borders of the upper and lower lips.

Herpes zoster may affect the mouth when the disease involves the trigeminal nerve ('trigeminal shingles'), producing clusters of vesicles in the mouth, invariably unilaterally.

In infectious mononucleosis the **Epstein–Barr virus** (glandular fever) most commonly produces symptoms at the back of the mouth, particularly in the tonsils and pharynx. However, the anterior part of the oral cavity may show small petechial hemorrhages, usually on the palatal mucosa.

Coxsackie A virus produces tiny vesicles in the mouth, with small vesicles in the skin of the hands and, occasionally, that of the feet (hand, foot and mouth disease). This transient, mild infection is mainly seen in children, often in school-based epidemics.

Fungal infection of the mouth with *Candida albicans* is common

Candida albicans infection of the mouth is most frequently seen in infants in the form of 'thrush'. It is manifest as white patches on the palatal (*Fig. 12.1a*), buccal, and tongue surfaces; the white patches are composed of tangled fungal hyphae (*Fig. 12.1b*) mixed with acute inflammatory cells and some desquamated epithelium. The underlying epithelium is acutely inflamed and red, a feature that becomes apparent when the white patch is scraped away.

In adults, acute candidal infection of the mouth is less common unless there are predisposing factors such as diabetes mellitus, immunosuppressive therapy, or a natural immunosuppressed state, for example in advanced malignancy or with HIV infection. However, **denture stomatitis**, due to *Candida* lodging under the denture plate, is not uncommon in adults with no other predisposing factors.

Infective stomatitis due to bacteria is now rare

Bacterial infections are common and important at the back of the mouth and oropharynx. However, although dental caries and periodontal disease are a consequence of bacteria present on and around the teeth, bacterial infections of the front of the mouth are now uncommon.

Acute necrotizing ulcerative gingivitis occurs mainly in young males with poor dental hygiene (*Fig. 12.2*). There is acute sloughing ulceration of the interdental papillae, which rapidly spreads along the gingival margins, producing an expanding area of yellow slough surrounded by a narrow zone of hyperemic mucosa, which often bleeds heavily. The gingiva are very painful, and the breath smells foul. Extension of the necrosis and inflammation leads

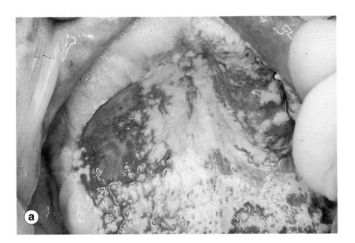

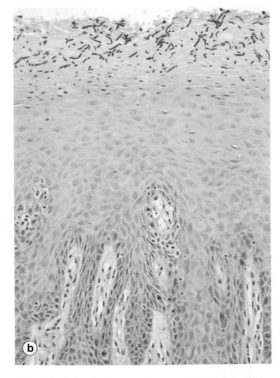

Fig. 12.1 *Candida albicans* infection of the palate.
In (a) the white sheets are fungal mycelium in a thickened horny layer. The underlying mucosa is red and inflamed. Palatal mucosa stained with PAS (b) shows masses of superficial fungal hyphae.

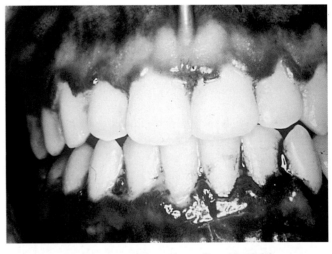

Fig. 12.2 Acute necrotizing ulcerative gingivitis.

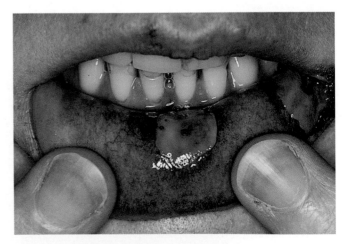

Fig. 12.3 Aphthous ulcer on lower lip.
This example is unusually large.

to destruction of the periodontal tissues. The necrotic areas are heavily populated by a mixture of fusiform and spirochetal organisms (*Fusobacterium* and *Borrelia* species), which are probably the causative organisms.

Secondary syphilis, which causes characteristic snail-track ulcers in the buccal mucosa, was formerly an important cause of mucosal ulceration, as was tertiary syphilis, in which the palate ulcerates over a destructive gumma in the palatal bone. These are now rare manifestations of syphilis in the mouth, but the primary syphilitic lesion, the **chancre,** is still occasionally seen, usually on the lip or tongue.

In the developing world, overwhelming bacterial cellulitis of the mouth and the destructive bacterial gingivitis known as **cancrum oris** are still occasionally seen.

Not all types of stomatitis are infective

The most common type of inflammation of the lips, tongue and buccal mucosa is that associated with **aphthous ulceration.** Tiny, painful, shallow ulcers form against a background of red mucosa (*Fig. 12.3*). The ulcer crater is covered by a creamy exudate composed of fibrin and inflammatory cells, mainly neutrophils. The ulcers are recurrent but of short duration. Large ulcers (up to 3 cm across) occasionally occur, sometimes persisting for several weeks before healing with fibrosis. However, this is a much less common variant.

Oral ulcers that are clinically and histologically identical to aphthous ulcers are a feature of **Behçet's syndrome.** There is associated ulceration of the genital mucosa, which is usually extensive and painful. In this syndrome the ulcers do not resolve quickly without treatment, and are often refractory to the treatments that normally improve ordinary aphthous ulcers. The cause of aphthous ulcers is not known.

Many common skin diseases can affect the oral mucosa

The skin diseases that most frequently involve the oral mucosa are lichen planus, erythema multiforme, discoid lupus erythematosus (DLE) and systemic lupus erythematosus (SLE), pemphigus vulgaris, and pemphigoid.

Of these, **oral lichen planus** is the most common, presenting with white lines against a background of a red buccal mucosa (*Fig. 12.4*). The disease may also affect the tongue and gingiva. Unlike lichen planus in the skin, erosion (due to separation of the epidermis) is common in the mouth. The disease may be particularly chronic, with older lesions producing patchy areas of white thickening. The histological appearances are similar to those seen in the skin (see page 488). There is a dense lichenoid inflammatory infiltrate associated with degeneration of the basal layer of the epithelium; occasional Civatte bodies represent dead basal keratinocytes. In buccal and gingival lesions the overlying epidermis is frequently very thin.

Erythema multiforme in the mouth is probably most often seen as an adverse drug reaction. However, spontaneous episodes without a drug history are seen, particularly in children and juveniles in whom no obvious causative factor can be identified, although some follow a viral illness. The lesions range from small, red mucosal areas with central blisters, to very extensive erosive blistering lesions (*Fig. 12.5*). The latter pattern is sometimes called Stevens–Johnson syndrome. Unlike the skin lesions, erythema multiforme in the mouth nearly always blisters.

Oral involvement in **SLE** and **DLE** produces ulcerated and erosive lesions that can be clinically and histologically difficult to distinguish from lichen planus.

The histological appearances of **pemphigus vulgaris** and **pemphigoid** are typical: both produce blisters and mucosal erosions.

Pigmentation of the lips and buccal mucosa is usually non-neoplastic

Most pigmented patches in the mucosa of the mouth are due to increased melanin production in dark-skinned races. Melanocytic neoplasms such as nevi and malignant melanoma are rare in the mouth.

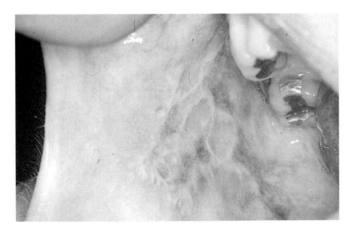

Fig. 12.4 Oral lichen planus.
The buccal mucosa shows the characteristic feature of intercepting white lines on a red background.

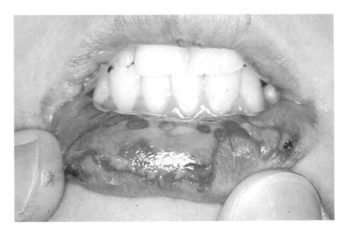

Fig. 12.5 Oral erythema multiforme.
Large, confluent, blistering lesions over the entire surface of the lower lip.

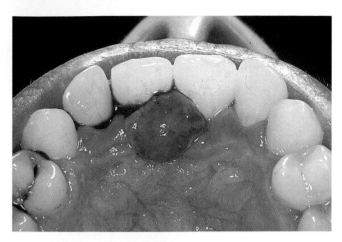

Fig. 12.6 Pyogenic granuloma.

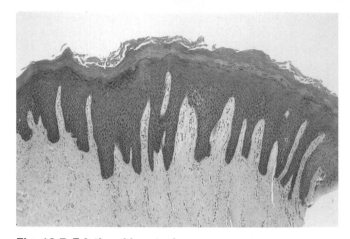

Fig. 12.7 Frictional keratosis.
The squamous epithelium is thickened and irregular, and there is an overlying thick horny layer of keratin.

Amalgam tattoo is a specific type of pigmentation that is seen only in the mouth. It is due to the deposition of metal oxides in the buccal mucosa as a result of entry of dental amalgam into the submucosa during dental procedures. The histology is characteristic, with black material being deposited on collagen fibers, in the basement membranes around vessels and nerves, and in the perimysium of any skeletal muscle.

Patches of pigmentation around the lips are a characteristic feature of the **Peutz–Jeghers syndrome** (see page 261), and pigmentation within the mouth is a now-rare manifestation of **Addison's disease** (see page 342).

Polypoid nodules of the mouth and gingiva are common

The most common type of polypoid nodule is the so-called **fibrous** or **fibroepithelial polyp**, which can form anywhere on the cheek or tongue. Those associated with the gingival margins are sometimes called **fibrous epulis**. The etiology is not known, but some may be related to chronic trauma from teeth or dentures. Macroscopically they are usually smooth-surfaced and pale pink.

Each nodule is composed of a densely compacted fibrocollagenous core covered by slightly thickened squamous epithelium. Although clinically similar to fibrous epulis, **giant-cell epulis** is often darker red in colour and occurs in the gingiva, being attached to the periodontal ligament. It is composed of large multinucleate giant cells in a fibrous stroma and is covered by squamous epithelium.

Pyogenic granulomas, which are histologically and macroscopically similar to those seen in the skin, are sometimes seen in the mouth, particularly in pregnancy (sometimes called 'pregnancy epulis') (*Fig. 12.6*).

Granular cell tumor (formerly called 'granular cell myoblastoma', but now thought to be of nerve sheath origin) is a rare tumor occasionally seen in the tongue. It usually presents as a raised, domed nodule or an even more raised polyp. Although completely benign, it will regrow if incompletely excised.

White patches in the mouth are an important physical sign

Many conditions produce white thickening of the mucosa in the mouth, including lichen planus, *Candida* infection, and chronic friction from teeth or dentures (**frictional keratosis**) (*Fig. 12.7*). In most cases the cause is not apparent, but it is mainly seen in smokers, particularly pipe smokers. It is important as a physical sign as this is one way in which pre-malignant epithelial dysplasia may present.

The most frequent tumors in the mouth are squamous cell carcinomas derived from the lining epithelium

True benign squamous tumors of the mouth are very rare; most of the lesions that have the appearance of benign squamous 'papilloma' are either viral warts or localized areas of thickened hyperkeratotic squamous epithelium secondary to chronic trauma. Invasive squamous carcinoma is the most important and common lesion.

Established invasive squamous carcinomas present as raised, nodular lesions, which develop central ulceration with a hard, raised edge. Tumors on the lip (*Fig. 12.8*) and tongue are usually recognized at an early stage and are amenable to surgery.

Squamous carcinomas in the floor of the mouth (*Fig. 12.9*) may be asymptomatic, remaining so until local invasion is extensive, and surgical removal difficult. Lesions in the cheek may also present late, mainly because patients ignore them, ascribing their development to denture trauma.

Squamous carcinomas of the mouth may arise in areas of epithelial dysplasia

Non-invasive epithelial dysplasia may precede the development of invasive squamous carcinoma. Clinically, such areas may present as thick, white patches that are raised above

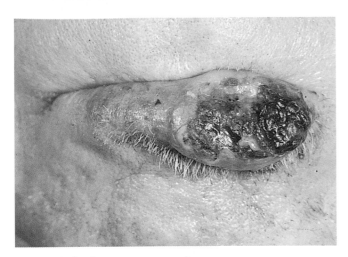

Fig. 12.8 Oral squamous carcinoma.
Squamous carcinoma of the lip, showing typical raised edges and central ulceration.

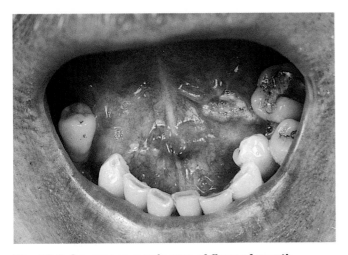

Fig. 12.9 Squamous carcinoma of floor of mouth.

KEY FACTS
Squamous cell carcinomas of the mouth

- Male preponderance.
- Affect the elderly (65+).
- Lips are the most common site (particularly lower lip).
- Actinic damage is a possible etiological factor.
- Tongue is the second most common site, usually occurring in the anterior two-thirds, on the lateral border. May present with thick white patch, eventually ulcerating.
- Floor of mouth and cheek are less common sites in UK and USA, but common in Indian subcontinent.
- Palate is the least common site.
- Most are well-differentiated and keratinizing.
- May arise in pre-existing dysplasia.
- Infiltrate locally and metastasize to regional lymph nodes in the neck.

tissues. A variant of salivary mucocele occurs beneath the tongue, in association with the ducts of the sublingual and submandibular salivary glands, forming a large, thin-walled, bluish cyst, commonly called a **ranula**.

Salivary calculi from the submandibular or parotid glands may produce a swelling in the region of the sites of emergence of their respective ducts into the mouth, i.e. sublingual and buccal regions. The swelling may be due to retained secretion or to the calculus (**sialolith**) itself.

Salivary gland tumors may occur anywhere in the mouth, but are less common than tumors in the major salivary glands

Although salivary gland tumors that occur in the mouth are less common than those in the major salivary glands, they are more likely to be malignant.

Any of the tumors that occur in the major salivary glands, such as parotid and submandibular glands (see below), can also occur in the minor salivary gland tissue of the mouth. As with the major salivary glands, **pleomorphic salivary adenoma** is the most common type of tumor, and the palate is the most common intraoral site. The one salivary tumor that almost never involves the mouth is **adenolymphoma of the parotid**. Malignant salivary tumors may also occur in the minor intraoral salivary tissue.

Salivary gland tumors are mainly benign, and most commonly affect the parotid gland

The parotid gland is the most common site for salivary gland tumors, under 25% occurring in the other large salivary glands (submandibular and sublingual) and the

the level of surrounding mucosa, or as areas of red, velvety epithelium that are level with surrounding mucosa. Such areas require biopsy to establish the presence of epithelial atypia and to exclude the development of early invasive tumor. The characteristics of dysplastic epithelium and carcinoma *in situ* are discussed and illustrated on page 89, Chapter 6.

Abnormalities of the salivary gland, including tumors, may present in the mouth

As the mouth is lined by stratified squamous epithelium, with salivary gland tissue in the submucosa, abnormalities of the salivary gland may present in the mouth.

The most frequent abnormality is a **mucocele** (or **mucous retention cyst**). These small cystic nodules on the lower lip (mucosal aspect) are the result of obstruction of the minor labial salivary gland ducts, with cystic dilatation and retention of secretions. They are frequently traumatized, with escape of mucoid secretion into the surrounding

**KEY FACTS
Salivary gland tumors**

- Most common in major salivary glands: parotid > submandibular > sublingual.
- Most commonly benign: pleomorphic salivary adenoma > Warthin's tumor.
- Salivary adenoma can occur anywhere, including the minor salivary glands in mouth.
- Warthin's tumor is almost always in the parotid.
- Adenoid cystic carcinoma is the most common malignant tumor.
- Adenoid cystic carcinoma is slow-growing but very locally invasive, spreading particularly in peri-neural spaces.

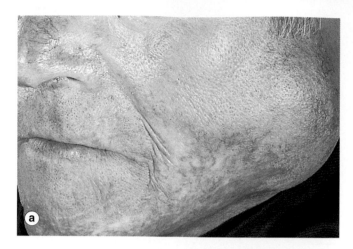

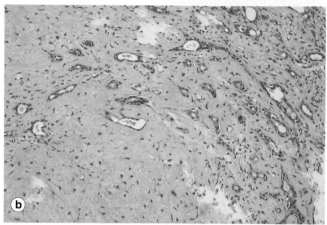

Fig. 12.10 Pleomorphic salivary adenoma.
(a) Clinical picture of an unusually large tumor in the parotid.
(b) Histology showing a mixture of adenomatous epithelial tissue and a pale myxoid stroma. The tumor is well-circumscribed and is compressing adjacent normal parotid.

minor salivary tissues of the mouth. The most common tumor is the benign **pleomorphic adenoma** (formerly called 'mixed salivary tumor'), the histological features of which are illustrated in *Fig. 12.10b*. The peak incidence is in late middle-age and beyond, the tumor presenting as a slow-growing, smooth, painless swelling. Despite its apparent encapsulation, there may be small nodules attached to the main tumor which can be left behind at surgery if the main tumor is shelled out without a surrounding zone of normal salivary gland. This can lead to apparent recurrence of this benign tumor. Adequate surgical excision in the parotid may be difficult because of the need to spare the facial nerve, which runs between the deep and superficial parts of the parotid.

The second most common tumor is the **monomorphic adenoma**. This is behaviorally identical to the pleomorphic adenoma, but has histological differences.

Warthin's tumor (adenolymphoma) is almost entirely confined to the parotid gland, usually occurring in the lower border of the parotid, near the angle of the mandible. It is most common in middle-aged men and presents as a painless, spherical, smooth-surfaced tumor, which may fluctuate in size. Larger tumors may be fluctuant because of central necrosis or due to the presence of mucin. Histologically the tumor is unusual, with an epithelial component of tall eosinophilic columnar cells forming clefts and cystic spaces within lymphoid tissue containing germinal centers (*Fig. 12.11*).

Malignant tumors of salivary tissue are rare and are particularly important in the intraoral minor salivary tissue

The most common malignant salivary tumor is the **adenoid cystic carcinoma** (*Fig. 12.12*). It can occur in the major salivary glands, such as parotid and submandibular glands, but is proportionally more common in the intraoral

salivary tissue, e.g. the palate. A slow-growing but locally invasive tumor, it frequently ulcerates in its intraoral location. Although it metastasizes late, the tumor has a poor prognosis because of its very extensive local invasion, with a particular tendency to grow in the peri-neural spaces. The tumor often extends considerably further than is apparent to the naked eye, and primary surgical excision is often unsuccessful in eradicating the tumor entirely, so further recurrence is very frequent. This, combined with poor radiosensitivity, makes management of this tumor difficult. The second operation for recurrence frequently requires radical and disfiguring orofacial surgery.

Two less common malignant tumors of salivary tissue are:

- **Mucoepidermoid carcinoma**, which arises mainly in the parotid in elderly people, occasionally developing in the palate. These lesions are of variable malignancy: some behave like pleomorphic adenoma, others are more aggressive from the outset.
- **Acinic cell carcinoma** occurs mainly in the parotid in the middle-aged and elderly, and is more common in

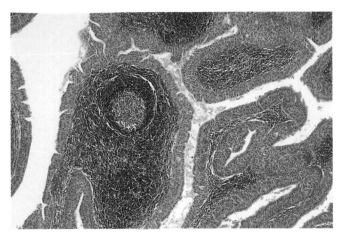

Fig. 12.11 Warthin's tumor of parotid. Histology showing a combination of glandular and lymphoid tissue.

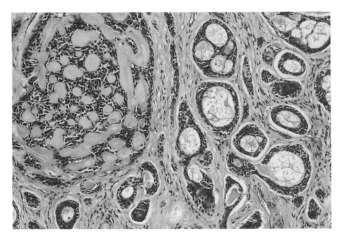

Fig. 12.12 Adenoid cystic carcinoma. This micrograph shows the typical histological appearance, the so-called cribriform pattern.

Fig. 12.13 Malignant salivary tumors
Summary table based on WHO classification

Adenoid cystic carcinoma	Most common	See text
Mucoepidermoid carcinoma	Next commonest	See text
Acinic cell carcinoma	Rare	See text
Polymorphous low-grade carcinoma	Rare	Confined to minor salivary glands in mouth, e.g. palate; good prognosis; local recurrence but metastasis rare
Myoepithelial carcinoma	Rare	Mainly in parotid in elderly
Basal cell adenocarcinoma	Rare	Low-grade locally invasive; local recurrence but metastasis rare; mainly parotid; age 50+
Carcinoma in pleomorphic adenoma	Rare	A rare complication, usually in elderly people with a long-neglected benign tumor

women than in men. It is sometimes called 'acinic cell tumor' because the majority behave in a benign fashion like pleomorphic adenoma, only rarely showing extensive local infiltration and lymph node metastasis.

Fig. 12.13 gives a summary of the malignant salivary tumors using the World Health Organization classification.

Calculus formation in the ducts of the major salivary glands leads to chronic sialadenitis

Calculi or inspissated secretions that form in the major salivary ducts lead to obstruction in the flow of salivary secretions. The back-pressure effects lead to dilatation of the ducts and atrophy of the salivary acini, associated with increased interstitial fibrosis and lymphocytic infiltrate. This is called chronic sialadenitis.

COMMON DISORDERS OF THE TEETH AND RELATED STRUCTURES

The most common disorder of teeth is dental caries

Dental caries is the result of damage to the enamel and dentine by acid formed within bacterial plaque (*Fig. 12.14*). Bacterially generated acid in the mouth is usually neutralized by the alkaline secretions of the salivary tissue. However, when the acid is made by bacteria in plaque, the physical density of the plaque prevents saliva from reaching the enamel surface of the tooth. The acid dissolves the calcium hydroxyapatite of the enamel and progressively penetrates the full thickness of the enamel, decalcifying it as it goes. This produces a visible cavity in the tooth. As the

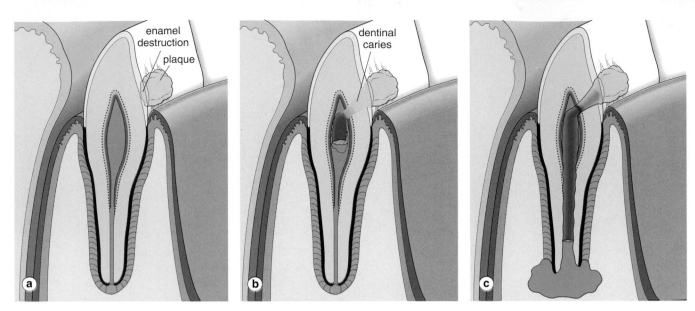

Fig. 12.14 The development of dental caries and its sequelae. (a) Acid destruction of enamel beneath plaque. (b) Dentinal caries (see *Fig. 12.15*), with acute pulpitis and pulp abscess. (c) Apical periodontal infection and abscess.

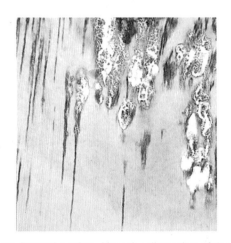

Fig. 12.15 Dental caries. Note the disruption of the dentinal structure, with large numbers of darkly stained bacteria penetrating towards the pulp cavity down the linear dentinal tubules.

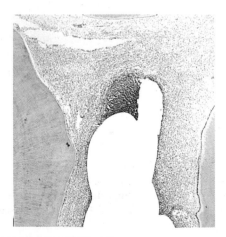

Fig. 12.16 Acute pulpitis. The pulp cavity contains an acute abscess.

cavity forms, bacteria can penetrate deeper into the tooth until the dentine is reached, and then penetrate the dentine layer through the hollow dentinal tubules (*Fig. 12.15*), which become distended with bacteria and tissue debris. This, combined with the continuing demineralizing effect of the acid, leads to liquefaction of the dentine. Eventually the dentine layer may be fully penetrated, and both bacteria and acid reach the soft central dental pulp.

Along the line of attack, the enamel and dentine are destroyed and the odontoblasts die. Although there is limited capacity for tissue reaction because the tissues are poorly cellular, in chronic lesions the odontoblasts may produce secondary dentine in an attempt at repair and restitution.

The consequences of carious attack are a pit or crater in the enamel, a penetrating destruction of the dentine and, when the dentine is fully penetrated, acute pulpitis due to bacterial and acid damage to the soft tissues of the pulp.

The most important complications of dental caries are pulpitis and peri-apical inflammation or abscess

Spread of bacteria and acid into the soft pulp space through carious penetration leads to necrosis of some of the pulp tissues, with an associated acute inflammatory reaction (mainly vessel dilatation, edema, and neutrophil infiltration). When there is extensive tissue necrosis a **pulp abscess** may form (*Fig. 12.16*). The combination of bacterial and acid necrosis with increased intrapulp pressure due to inflammatory edema leads to extensive necrosis of all the pulp tissues. Inflammatory stimulation of the nerve twigs in the pulp produces severe pain, localized or diffuse toothache being the main symptom of **acute pulpitis**.

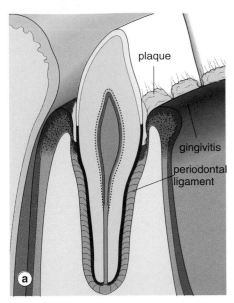 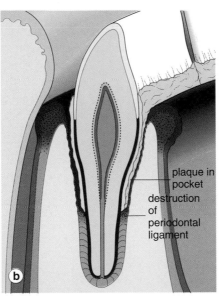 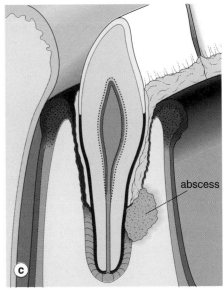

Fig. 12.17 Chronic periodontal disease and its complications. (a) Chronic gingivitis. (b) Destruction of periodontal ligament. (c) Periodontal abscess.

Where the penetration of the enamel and dentine has been through a narrow carious channel, the pulp cavity remains largely isolated from the mouth cavity (**closed pulpitis**). However, where there has been extensive destruction of the enamel and dentine, the pulp cavity may be exposed to the oral cavity (**open pulpitis**). In these cases the pulp cavity is often completely replaced by inflammatory granulation tissue, which progresses through the phases of vascular granulation tissue, fibrous granulation tissue, and fibrous scar. The scarred pulp forms a polypoid protrusion into the oral cavity, which may become re-epithelialized.

Inflammation and death of the pulp is often followed by **apical periodontal infection**, the inflammation initially being confined to the small space beneath the apex, between the tooth apex and the surrounding bone. At first the infection is acute, with a predominantly acute inflammatory reaction that is rich in neutrophils, and there is often abscess formation (peri-apical abscess). The inflammation eventually becomes chronic, with a heavy infiltrate of lymphocytes and plasma cells, and granulation tissue formation (**chronic peri-apical periodontitis**). The enlarging inflammatory mass often erodes the bone around the apex of the tooth, producing an osteolytic, rounded lesion composed of chronic inflammatory granulation tissue, which may contain small neutrophil accumulations. This is sometimes called a **peri-apical granuloma** and is the most common cause of teeth-related cystic lesions in the bone.

Expansion of acute or chronic inflammatory lesions at the apex of abnormal teeth may produce inflammation in surrounding tissues with, for example, abscesses in the mandible pointing through the skin of the neck or producing sublingual cellulitis. Similar lesions in the upper jaw can break through the floor of the maxillary sinus to produce chronic sinus inflammation.

Periodontal disease, not associated with apical abnormality, is usually a consequence of gingivitis

Some from of gingivitis (inflammation of the gums) is present in almost every mouth, and is usually the result of neglected oral and dental hygiene. **Acute gingivitis** particularly affects young men, manifesting as swelling and soreness of the gums, often with bleeding and ulceration. Large numbers of bacteria are present in the ulcerated areas, and are probably causative.

Chronic gingivitis (*Fig. 12.17a*) occurs as a result of accumulation of bacterial plaque. It usually begins in childhood, when it is asymptomatic. Regular brushing of teeth, beginning in childhood, minimizes the accumulation of bacterial plaque and reduces the likelihood of significant gingivitis in later life. Bacterial plaque becomes calcified in adults, separating the gingiva from the tooth. There is chronic inflammation in the gingival epithelium and submucosa, with large numbers of lymphocytes and plasma cells.

Chronic periodontitis results from the consequences of chronic gingival inflammation in relation to the presence of calculous plaque between the gingiva and the tooth. These are:

- **Destruction of the periodontal ligament**, leading to loosening of the tooth in its socket (*Fig. 12.17b*).
- **Progressive deepening of the pocket between tooth and gingiva**, which contains ever-increasing amounts of subgingival plaque (*Fig. 12.17b*).
- **Progressive inflammatory destruction of the alveolar bone**. leading to severe gingival recession (*Fig. 12.18*).
- **Periodontal abscess formation** (*Fig. 12.17c*) if the chronic inflammatory process becomes accelerated by

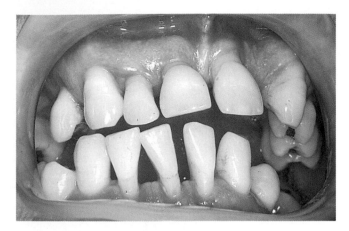

Fig. 12.18 Chronic periodontal disease.
Clinical picture showing severe gingival recession.

acute bacterial infection. This accelerates destruction of the alveolar bone, and pus may extrude into the alveolar cavity or alongside the tooth in the subgingival pocket.

Cysts related to the teeth can produce osteolytic lesions in the bones of the jaw

Dental cysts can be simply classified into those due to a developmental abnormality, and those that are secondary to inflammatory disease associated with the teeth.

Among the most important **developmental cysts** are **odontogenic keratocysts**, which usually occur in young males and are related to the mandibular molar region. They may be asymptomatic or may present with an intraoral swelling. Lined by stratified squamous epithelium, with a variable keratin layer that is sometimes parakeratotic, they may be multilocular and are occasionally multiple. Treatment is difficult, and they tend to recur after incomplete removal.

Dentigerous cysts mostly involve the third molars or the canine teeth. A typical cyst envelops the crown of an unerupted or displaced tooth and is attached to its neck. The cyst is lined by stratified squamous epithelium, usually only a few cell layers thick, supported on a thick fibrous wall. At its junction with the neck of the tooth, the cyst epithelium merges with the reduced remnants of the enamel epithelium. The cyst contains yellow fluid, which is usually clear. However, metaplasia of the squamous epithelium lining the cyst can occasionally lead to the production of keratin and mucin, which may render the cyst contents mucoid or pasty. These cysts are derived from the dental follicle of the unerupted tooth and are unilocular.

As their name implies, **lateral periodontal cysts** lie alongside the tooth. Their origin is uncertain. They are frequently asymptomatic, mainly being detected in routine dental X-rays as a round, osteolytic lesion that is discrete from, and lateral to, the root of a canine or premolar tooth. The cyst is lined by thin, non-keratinized squamous epithelium, with a surrounding fibrous wall.

The most important **inflammatory cyst** is the **radicular cyst**. It is far more common than the developmental cysts, and usually occurs in adults in association with dental caries of the permanent dentition. Most commonly involving the upper lateral incisors, it follows the development of a periapical granuloma resulting from caries. Cords of squamous epithelium grow into the chronic inflammatory mass, and central dissolution of the epithelial masses leads to cyst formation. The wall is characteristically inflamed, and cholesterol clefts are frequent, often with associated foreign body giant cells. The associated tooth dies, and the cyst may persist after extraction of the tooth. As the chronic inflammatory cyst enlarges, the surrounding bone may be eroded, producing a well-defined area of lucency on radiology.

Tumors derived from dental precursor tissues are rare

The most common tumor derived from odontogenic epithelium is the **ameloblastoma**. It is benign and does not metastasize. Tumors are mainly seen in the mandible of middle-aged adults, the vast majority developing at the angle of the mandible. They are slow-growing lesions, which locally invade the bone, tumor expansion often leading to separation of the teeth and, occasionally, to loosening. They are composed of islands of odontogenic epithelium, often with a mixed fibrous stroma. The odontogenic epithelium forms islands with peripheral, tall ameloblastic epithelial cells surrounding loose epithelium, resembling the stellate reticulum of the developing tooth. Squamous metaplasia may occur, which is a source of potential confusion with invasive squamous carcinoma. The tumor may resemble a unilocular or multilocular cyst radiologically. A summary of odontogenic tumors is given in *Fig. 12.19.*

The oropharynx is a common site of viral and bacterial infections (sore throat)

A red, inflamed, sore oropharynx is a symptom commonly encountered in family practice, and is usually due to a viral infection which also involves the nasopharynx and larynx. It is a common component of the common cold, influenza, and other viral upper respiratory tract infections, and is often severe in glandular fever (infectious mononucleosis).

Bacterial pharyngitis is much less common, and is usually due to infection by β-hemolytic streptococci; it is an important precursor of **acute post-streptococcal glomerulonephritis** and **acute rheumatic fever**.

Enlargement of the palatine tonsils as a result of inflammation is common

The mucosa-associated lymphoid tissue around the pharynx (Waldeyer's ring) comprises the palatine tonsils (tonsils), the nasopharyngeal tonsil (adenoids), and the lymphoid tissue in the submucosal region of the posterior third of the

Fig. 12.19 Summary of odontogenic tumors
Based on WHO classification

Benign

Ameloblastoma	The most common	See text
Calcifying epithelial odontongenic tumor	Fairly rare	Slow-growing, derived from odontogenic epithelium; young and middle-aged in premolar/molar region of mandible associated with unerupted tooth; locally invasive but non-metastasizing
Ameloblastic fibroma	Rare	Children and teenagers; mandible in molar/premolar region; local recurrence but non-metastasizing
Adenomatoid odontogenic tumor	Rare	Mainly maxilla in teenagers; canine/lateral incisor region; may be cystic and focally calcified
Dentinoma	Very rare	Young adults; mandible and associated with unerupted molar; composed of masses of dysplastic dentine, with strands of odontogenic epithelium
Myxoma	Rare	Young people; slow-growing lesion in mandible or maxilla, often associated with missing or unerupted teeth
Cementoma	Rare	Four main varieties: benign cementoblastoma, cementifying fibroma, gigantiform cementoma, and periapical cemental dysplasia
Squamous odontogenic tumor	Rare	Probably derived from cell rests of Malassez; resembles invasive squamous carcinoma, with which it can be confused histologically; locally infiltrative but non-metastasizing

Malignant

Malignant ameloblastoma	Extremely rare	Tumors may be histologically malignant, but metastasis is rare
Malignant change in odontogenic cysts	Extremely rare	
Intraosseous squamous cell carcinoma	Extremely rare	May be derived from residues of odontogenic epithelium in bones of jaw

tongue (lingual tonsil). As part of the immune system, the lymphoid tissue in these areas reacts to inflammation or infection in the region by undergoing lymphoid hyperplasia. The changes are most easily seen in the prominent palatine tonsils; **reactive lymphoid hyperplasia** is the most common cause of tonsillar enlargement, particularly in children and juveniles, often occurring as a response to a viral or bacterial pharyngitis.

Acute tonsillitis usually occurs as a component of a widespread acute bacterial pharyngitis, usually due to β-hemolytic streptococci. The tonsils are swollen (*Fig. 12.20*), red due to mucosal hyperemia, and partly covered by creamy acute inflammatory exudate (**acute parenchymatous tonsillitis**). Sometimes there are scattered, creamy yellow spots on the surface (**acute follicular tonsillitis**) due to beads of pus extruding from the mouths of the infected epithelial-lined

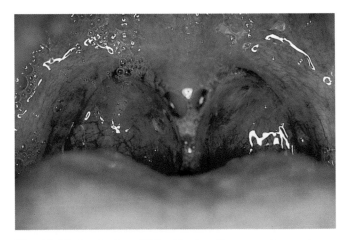

Fig. 12.20 Acute tonsillitis. The tonsils are swollen and acutely inflamed, almost meeting in the midline.

crypts. Acute streptococcal pharyngitis and tonsillitis may be complicated by the development of a peri-tonsillar abscess (**quinsy**) or, rarely, by spreading cellulitis in the neck (**Ludwig's angina**) or retropharyngeal abscess formation. Acute tonsillitis may also be a component of a severe viral pharyngitis, e.g. in glandular fever and some adenovirus infections.

In adults the tonsils usually become progressively smaller as the lymphoid component atrophies. However, in some cases the lymphoid element remains prominent, in association with enlarged crypts distended with keratin, in which numerous bacterial colonies (particularly *Actinomyces* species) are seen. This is sometimes called **chronic tonsillitis**, although the organisms are considered to be commensals.

Diphtheritic pharyngotonsillitis (due to infection by *Corynebacterium diphtheriae*) is now very rare because of immunization. Characterized by the presence of a prominent compact fibrinous acute inflammatory exudate over the inflamed structures (the diphtheritic membrane), it often causes obstructive asphyxia in children, and is responsible for the production of a bacterial exotoxin that affects the heart and nervous system.

Tumors of the tonsil are usually squamous cell carcinoma or malignant lymphoma

Benign tumors of the tonsil are very rare, and most tumors are malignant. Squamous papillomas of the tonsillar region are mainly benign viral overgrowths, and occur on the faucial pillars rather than on the tonsil.

Squamous cell carcinoma presents as a mass or an ulcer with raised edges, usually in elderly men. The tumor invades the tongue and fauces, and lymphatic spread to neck nodes occurs early. Often, late presentation means that local and lymph node spread is advanced, and complete surgical removal is impossible.

Lymphomas of the tonsil are nearly always non-Hodgkin's lymphomas. Most are high-grade lesions, which can occur in children and young adults; a smaller number are low-grade lesions, which tend to occur in elderly patients. Sometimes there is associated lymphoma in the rest of Waldeyer's ring or in the gastrointestinal tract (lymphoma of mucosa-associated lymphoid tissue; Chapter 15). Lymphoma of the tonsil has a better prognosis than squamous carcinoma because of the good response to chemotherapy.

NOSE AND NASOPHARYNX PATHOLOGY

The nose is lined by tall columnar ciliated respiratory-type epithelium, bathed in mucus produced by numerous mucus-secreting glands. The surface area is greatly increased by projections of bone (turbinates) and by the presence of communicating sinuses (maxillary, ethmoid, etc.), which are lined by identical epithelium. In the roof of the nasal cavity is a patch of specialized olfactory epithelium which is responsible for the sense of smell. The nasopharynx communicates with the middle ear via the Eustachian tube.

The skin of the nose is susceptible to a large number of dermatological disorders

The nose is heir to many skin disorders that are associated with exposure to sunlight; thus, basal cell carcinoma and solar keratoses are common (see pages 499 and 500).

Common inflammatory diseases include **rosacea** and **discoid lupus erythematosus** (see pages 509 and 534). Rosacea affecting the nose may lead to the bulbous disfigurement called **rhinophyma**, particularly in elderly men.

Pale, firm nodules in the skin of the nose are a frequent presenting symptom. The most common causes are:

- **Nodular sebaceous hyperplasia** or **sebaceous adenoma** – the nose is very rich in sebaceous glands.
- **Basal cell carcinoma** – these enlarge and eventually develop central ulceration (*Fig. 20.21*).
- **Trichoepithelioma** – a benign tumor of hair follicles.

The only certain way to distinguish a basal cell carcinoma from the other, less aggressive, lesions is to use excision biopsy.

Acquired structural deformity of the nose is almost invariably the result of trauma

Most nasal fractures will heal without therapeutic interference, but certain complications require surgical management. The complications of nasal fracture include:

- **Hematoma formation**, leading to nasal obstruction and risk of infection, with possible subsequent collapse of the cartilaginous nasal pyramid (**saddle nose**).
- **Deviation of septum** due to dislocation of the septal cartilage. This may lead to marked nasal obstruction.
- **Deviation of nose**, which is cosmetically unpleasing.

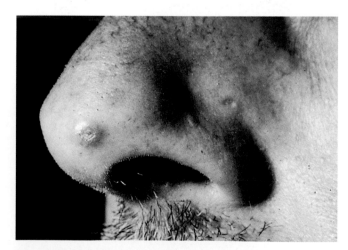

Fig. 12.21 Basal cell carcinoma of the nose.
A characteristic lesion with raised pearly edges and central ulceration.

The most common nasal symptom seen in family practice is rhinitis

Rhinitis (a runny, blocked and perhaps sore nose) is usually due either to infection or to allergy.

Infective rhinitis is usually viral in origin, e.g. common cold, influenza. Viral necrosis of surface epithelial cells is followed by exudation of fluid and mucus from the damaged surface (runny nose). Later submucosal edema produces swelling, which may lead to partial blockage of the narrow nasal airways.

In allergic rhinitis a Type I hypersensitivity reaction to inhaled materials such as grass and flower pollens produces a mixed serous–mucous exudate, and submucosal edema leads to nasal blockage. In allergic rhinitis, where the antigenic stimulus may persist for many weeks, the submucosal edema may persist and worsen. An irregular, swollen, polypoid mucosa can develop, in which one or more nasal polyps may develop (Fig. 12.22), usually bilaterally.

Typical nasal polyps are smooth-surfaced, creamy, semi-translucent, ovoid masses. They are histologically characterized by immense edema and a scattered infiltrate of chronic inflammatory cells (including plasma cells); eosinophils are often very numerous in allergic polyps.

In acute rhinitis, there is usually associated inflammation of the sinus linings

Acute maxillary sinusitis is the most important type of sinus inflammation, ethmoidal and frontal sinusitis being less significant. Swelling of the mucosa around the drainage foramen of the maxillary sinus may prevent drainage of maxillary sinus secretions into the nasal cavity, causing stasis. Stasis of maxillary secretions predisposes to secondary bacterial infection, with alteration of the retained maxillary fluid from seromucous to frankly purulent. In severe cases the infection may spread into the ethmoids and frontal sinuses, with the risk of spread of infection to the meninges.

Chronic maxillary sinusitis may follow acute sinusitis, chronic inhalational insult, or nasal obstruction

Failure of an acutely inflamed sinus to drain, even after the resolution of the acute rhinitis that initiated it, leads to chronic maxillary sinusitis, with a chronically thickened and inflamed mucosa, and persistent fluid accumulation (Fig. 12.23).

Chronic inhalation of irritant material is sometimes the result of industrial exposure, but most commonly involves cigarette smoke. Chronic rhinitis and maxillary sinusitis develop, initially as a toxic allergic reaction, but such cases are always liable to secondary bacterial infection, or exacerbation during a viral infection.

Obstruction to maxillary sinus drainage may result from a severely deviated nasal septum, or from the presence of nasal polyps.

Nosebleeds (epistaxis) and loss of smell sense (anosmia) are common complaining symptoms

The nasal submucosa is highly vascular, and bleeding from the nose (epistaxis) is common. In most cases the cause is readily apparent, e.g. trauma, especially a blow to the nose or vigorous nose-picking, or acute rhinitis (Fig. 12.24).

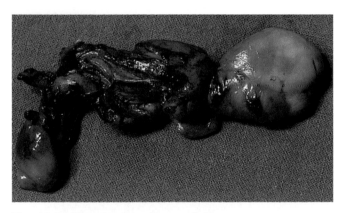

Fig. 12.22 Nasal polyp after excision.

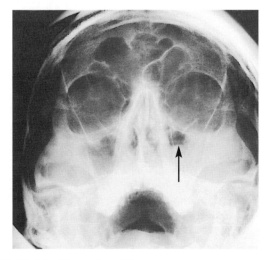

Fig. 12.23 Maxillary sinusitis.
This X-ray, taken to show the maxillary sinuses, shows a fluid level in the left sinus (arrow) due to retention of secretions.

Fig. 12.24 Causes of epistaxis	
Local disease	Little's area (particularly in acute rhinitis)
	Trauma
	Nasal malignancy
Systemic disease	Hereditary telangiectasia
	Hypertension
	Bleeding diathesis, particularly thrombocytopenia

Fig. 12.25
Causes of anosmia (loss of sense of smell)

Obstructive	Acute and chronic rhinitis (allergic and infective)
	Acute and chronic sinusitis
	Nasal polyps
	Intranasal tumors, benign and malignant
Sensorineural	Cribriform plate trauma
	Frontal lobe trauma
	Frontal lobe tumors
	Pituitary tumors

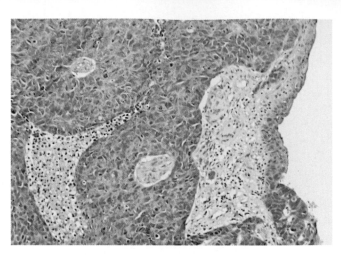

Fig. 12.26 Transitional cell carcinoma of the nose.
The tumor is composed of transitional respiratory epithelium, producing deeply invading masses.

The most common site for bleeding is a small patch on the anterior septum. This area is particularly prone, being the site of numerous submucosal anastomoses (Little's area). However, persistent nosebleeds may be an indication of significant underlying disease.

Granulomatous inflammation in the nose is an important disorder worldwide; most cases are due to leprosy, TB or fungal infections, being largely confined to the developing world. However, **sarcoidosis** may involve the nose (see page 539), and a specific form of granulomatous vasculitis, **Wegener's granulomatosis**, frequently presents with nasal lesions; Wegener's granulomatosis is considered in more detail in Chapter 10.

True benign tumors of the nose and paranasal sinuses are uncommon

The lesion most commonly mistaken for a benign tumor clinically is most often seen in the nasal vestibule, just inside the nostril, arising from the squamous epithelium of the vestibule. Although it is clinically labelled a 'squamous papilloma', histological examination shows that the vast majority of these lesions are viral warts identical to those seen on the skin.

Among the most frequently occurring benign tumors are **hemangiomas** (so-called 'bleeding polyps'). Usually located on the septum, they are responsible for repeated nosebleeds. Some are vascular chronic inflammatory lesions, resembling the pyogenic granulomas seen on the skin.

Juvenile angiofibroma is a rare tumor that occurs in male children and juveniles. It is mainly located in the nasopharynx rather than the nose. During puberty these lesions can grow quickly, mimicking a malignant tumor in their rapid growth and tendency to erode bone. They frequently ulcerate, and present with bleeding.

Transitional cell papilloma and **inverted papilloma** occur in adults. Although benign, they tend to recur or to be difficult to eradicate. Malignant change can supervene, but is rare.

The most frequent malignant tumors of the nose and sinuses are squamous and transitional cell carcinomas

The most common site for malignant tumor in the nasal cavity is in the anterior region near the nostrils; the tumor is usually squamous carcinoma. Further back in the nose there is an increasing proportion of transitional cell carcinomas (*Fig. 12.26*).

Malignant tumors of the sinuses are most common in the maxillary sinus, but some originate in the ethmoid sinus.

The major effects of tumors in the nose and nasal sinuses result from local invasion, often with destruction of the cheek, palate and, most dangerously, the orbit.

Malignant melanoma can also occur, mostly affecting the middle-aged and elderly; in the nose they are often highly pigmented.

The nasopharynx is an important site of malignant tumors

The nasopharynx is that part of the pharynx lying immediately behind the nasal cavities. It is lined by respiratory-type columnar epithelium, and there is a considerable amount of lymphoid tissue in the submucosa, which is part of the mucosa-associated lymphoid tissue (MALT). Squamous metaplasia is frequent in adults, so much of the lining epithelium eventually becomes squamous lined. Carcinoma of the nasopharynx is particularly common in China, and is usually a squamous carcinoma or an undifferentiated carcinoma. Because the nasopharynx is an inaccessible site, these tumors may remain small and undetected until after the tumor has spread to the lymph nodes in the neck (*Fig. 12.27*). The vast majority of patients with nasopharyngeal carcinoma have lymph node metastases when they first present. One of the histological characteristics of both squamous and anaplastic carcinomas is the presence of abundant lymphoid tissue in the stroma.

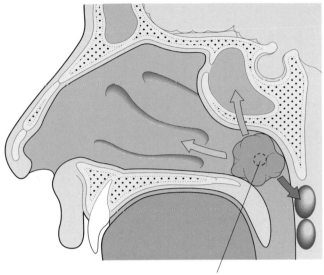

obstruction to Eustachian tube;
secretory otitis media → hearing
loss and tinnitus

diplomia due to invasion of the VI cranial nerve

nasal obstruction, epistaxis, serous nasal discharge

metastases in cervical lymph nodes

Fig. 12.27 Clinical manifestations and complications of carcinoma of the nasopharynx.

Malignant lymphoma also occurs in the nasopharynx, presumably arising from the submucosal lymphoid tissue forming part of Waldeyer's ring.

PATHOLOGY OF THE EAR

Congenital malformations of the pinna are very common

The most common congenital malformations related to the pinna are discussed in the section concerning ear disease in children (see page 241).

Acquired diseases of the pinna are frequently seen in community practice

Among the most commonly seen pinnal lesions are **keloids**; firm, dermal nodules which develop in the dermis, usually following trauma. The most common site is the ear-lobe following ear-piercing, particularly in girls of Afro-Caribbean origin. Attempts at surgical excision of these unsightly nodules are usually followed by the development of even larger keloids.

Trauma to the pinna usually the result of a violent blow, sustained during criminal assault or its socially acceptable equivalent, boxing. The most common lesion is a tense, tender hematoma, incomplete resolution of which leads to physical distortion of the pinna (**cauliflower ear**).

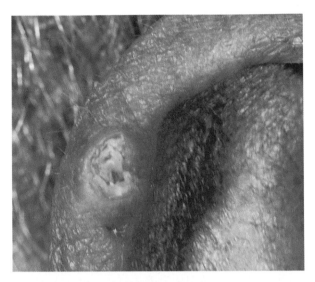

Fig. 12.28 Chondrodermatitis nodularis of the pinna.

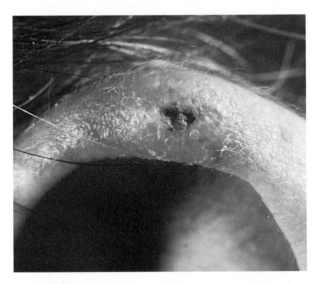

Fig. 12.29 Early squamous cell carcinoma of the pinna. In the early stage these lesions are clinically very similar to those of chondrodermatitis nodularis, and biopsy may be necessary to separate them.

Inflammatory skin disease particularly affects the back of the pinna and the groove behind the ear. **Atopic eczema** is the most common disease, particularly in children with the atopic tendency. Inflammation of the skin around the meatus is usually part of an **otitis externa** involving the full length of the meatus (see page 238).

Chondrodermatitis nodularis helicis presents as a small intractable and often tender ulcer, usually on the helix (*Fig. 12.28*). It is most common in the elderly and there may be degeneration of the pinnal cartilage beneath the ulcerated area. The cause is unknown, but it may be ischemic.

Tumors and **pre-tumorous conditions** mainly occur in the elderly. They are usually squamous cell carcinomas (*Fig. 12.29*) or basal cell carcinomas (both of which tend to be single lesions), or solar or actinic keratoses (which may be multiple). These conditions are discussed in Chapter 23.

The most common abnormalities of the external auditory meatus are wax retention and inflammation

Wax retention leading to conductive deafness (see page 240) is a frequent complaint encountered by the family practitioner. The situation is often made worse by inept attempts to remove wax, using penetrating foreign bodies such as cotton wool buds.

There are two patterns of inflammation of the external auditory meatus (**otitis externa**). Inflammation may be **localized**, due to a boil (furuncle) in the ear canal, or **diffuse**, usually due to either bacterial or fungal infection (*Fig. 12.30*). A common fungus is *Aspergillus niger*, black threads of which can be identified in the inflammatory exudate and may even be visible in the ear canal. **Allergic otitis externa** is usually a response to topical ear drops.

Viral warts, basal cell carcinomas and squamous cell carcinomas can occur in the external auditory meatus, but all are rare.

Perforation of the tympanic membrane usually results from middle ear infection, but may occasionally follow trauma

The tympanic membrane (eardrum) is a three-layered structure. There is a central sheet of fibrocollagenous support tissue containing numerous elastic fibers, covered on the external surface by stratified squamous epithelium continuous with that of the external auditory meatus, and on the inner surface by low cuboidal epithelium continuous with that lining the middle ear.

Infection (usually **acute otitis media**) is the most important cause of perforation, particularly in children. Less commonly, trauma, e.g. sustained during attempted removal of foreign bodies, may result in perforation. Most central perforations of the drum (*Fig. 12.31*) heal spontaneously.

The most important complications of a central perforation are predisposition to recurrent middle ear infection (otitis media), with impaired hearing, and failure to heal.

After perforation most eardrums heal by fibrosis

Although small central perforations heal spontaneously by fibrosis within a few days, larger perforations sometimes fail to heal and may require surgical closure using a fascial graft. A healed perforation is sometimes visible as a white scar or thinned area on the eardrum.

Acute otitis media is an important cause of earache and temporary hearing loss in children

Upper respiratory tract viral infections in children are frequently accompanied by the changes of acute inflammation in the lining of the middle ear, and in the inner lining of the tympanic membrane. Secondary bacterial infection may supervene, increasing the risk of a central perforation of the tympanic membrane. Children are particularly prone, probably because the narrow Eustachian tube can become obstructed by the hyperplastic submucosal lymphoid tissue at its lower end (**adenoids**).

The main complications of acute otitis media include persistent perforation of the eardrum, tubotympanic chronic suppurative otitis media, **otitis media with effusion** (OME or 'glue ear'), and acute mastoiditis.

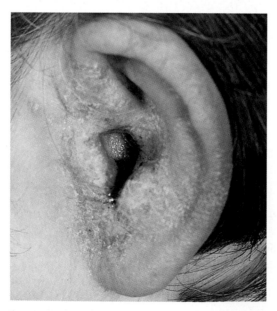

Fig. 12.30 Otitis externa.
The external auditory meatus is inflamed and covered by a scaling exudate, which spreads onto the pinna. Some of the pinnal changes are due to superimposed allergic otitis, a response to antibiotic eardrops given for the original infection.

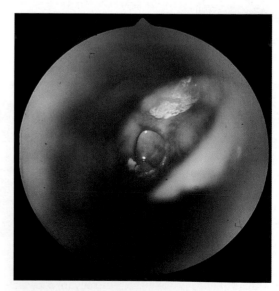

Fig. 12.31 Auroscopic view of a central perforation of the eardrum.

Acute mastoiditis is now rare

In the pre-antibiotic era, secondary bacterial infection of a viral otitis media was common, leading to acute suppurative otitis media and the risk of bacterial infection spreading to the mastoid air cells. From the mastoid air cells, suppuration could extend into the brain to cause meningitis and brain abscess. This is now rare.

Chronic suppurative otitis media usually follows permanent perforation of the eardrum

Recurrent chronic inflammation in the middle ear is an important cause of chronic earache, deafness, and persistent discharge from the external auditory meatus. It usually occurs in people with a persistent, non-healing perforation of the eardrum. Chronic suppurative otitis media (CSOM) is usually subdivided into two broad groups:

- **Tubotympanic disease**, in which the perforation is in the pars tensa of the eardrum, and the discharge is

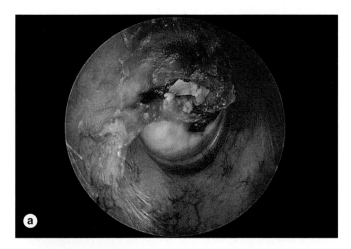

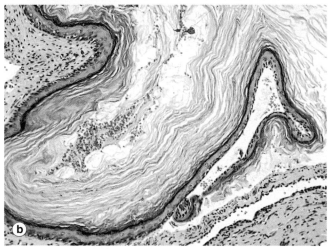

Fig. 12.32 Cholesteatoma.
In the auroscopic view of a cholesteatoma (a), the lesion is manifest as an irregular white mass. Histology (b) shows a cystic mass of keratin, which is lined by keratinizing squamous epithelium.

typically copious and mucopurulent. The mucosal lining of the middle ear becomes chronically inflamed with a heavy infiltrate of lymphocytes and plasma cells, leading to thickening and the formation of inflammatory granulation tissue, often in the form of **chronic inflammatory granulation polyps**. These inflammatory masses can protrude through the perforated tympanic membrane, and large polyps may even present at the external auditory meatus. Some chronic inflammatory polyps contain large numbers of cleft-like crystals of cholesterol esters, often surrounded by a foreign body giant cell reaction; this is called **cholesterol granuloma**. The source of the cholesterol is not known, but it may be derived from red blood cells, since cholesterol granuloma is particularly important in otitis media in which there has been hemorrhage.

- **Atticoantral disease**, in which the perforation is located in the eardrum at the attic region, and is typically associated with the development of **cholesteatoma**. Atticoantral disease is also associated with a higher risk of major complications, e.g. brain abscess and other intracranial infection.

Cholesteatoma is an important middle ear disease

Cholesteatoma is a form of epidermoid cyst. Most commonly located in the epitympanic recess (attic) and mastoid antrum, it often extends into the mastoid process. Its precise pathogenesis is disputed, but it is frequently associated with an atticoantral perforation of the eardrum. It is a cystic structure lined by squamous epithelium (*Fig. 12.32*), which constantly produces keratin. This leads to expansion of the lesion, damaging the small structures in the cavity. The area may become colonized by Gram-negative saprophytic bacteria, which probably stimulate continuing keratin formation. The enlarging keratinous mass, lined by stratified squamous epithelium, can eventually erode bone, and may destroy the labyrinth, mastoid air cells, and facial nerve. It may even erode through the skull forming the base of the middle cranial fossa. Although non-neoplastic, cholesteatomas have the same effects as a slow-growing benign tumor.

OME (glue ear) in children is commonly associated with upper respiratory tract infections

In otitis media with effusion (OME), mucoid fluid accumulates in the middle ear cavity because it is unable to drain through the child's narrow Eustachian tube. This is possibly associated with lower tube blockage due to reactive hyperplasia of the adenoid lymphoid tissue.

The fluid is sterile, and is often thick and tenacious, resembling greyish-brown liquid glue, hence the common term 'glue ear'. It is associated with conductive deafness

KEY FACTS
Causes of bleeding from the ear

- Trauma to the ear from foreign body and its attempted removal.
- Ruptured furuncle.
- Chronic inflammatory polyp.
- Traumatic perforation of the eardrum.
- Fracture of the skull forming the floor of the middle cranial fossa.

with intermittent earache. Because of the stasis of the fluid within the middle ear, there is a predisposition to acute suppurative otitis media due to secondary bacterial infection.

Tympanosclerosis is a hyaline degeneration of the eardrum submucosa. Appearing either as a crescentic white area or as chalky-looking patches, it may occur in the tympanic membrane in association with OME. It is most commonly seen after insertion of a grommet.

The most important primary disease of the small bones of the middle ear is otosclerosis

In otosclerosis the normal bone of the auditory ossicles is replaced and thickened by newly deposited woven bone (see page 511). The disease, which is usually bilateral and eventually produces deafness, may be hereditary. There is an adult female preponderance. The disease usually starts at the otic capsule between the cochlea and vestibule, and may spread to involve the footplate and limbs of the stapes. It is the involvement of the stapes and of the cochlea that leads to deafness.

The two most important diseases affecting the inner ear are Menière's disease and sensorineural deafness

Menière's disease has three components:

- **Tinnitus** (ringing or buzzing).
- **Paroxysmal vertigo**.
- **Unilateral deafness**.

Although it is usually initially unilateral, up to 50% of patients may eventually develop disease in the other ear, sometimes many years later. Its cause is unknown, but the most important abnormality is marked distension of the cochlear duct by excess fluid, such that the vestibular membrane of Reissner, which separates two fluids of different composition, bulges into the scala vestibuli (*Fig. 12.33*). This membrane may rupture, allowing the two fluids to mix. Histological study of the disease is hampered by the difficulty of obtaining untraumatized cochlea at *post mortem* examination.

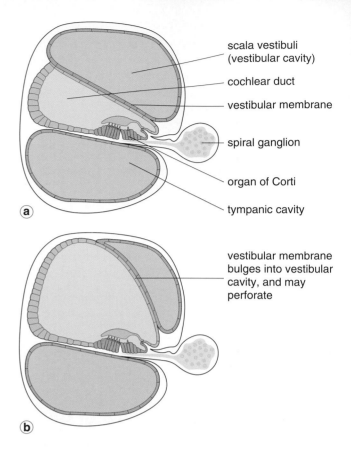

Fig. 12.33 Changes in Menière's disease. (a) Normal cochlea. (b) Affected cochlea.

Many diseases of the ear are associated with temporary or permanent hearing loss

Hearing loss can be classified as **conductive** (usually due to some abnormality in external or middle ear), **sensorineural** (usually due to some abnormality in the inner ear, auditory nerve or brain), or **mixed** (i.e. with features of both conductive and sensorineural hearing loss).

Conductive hearing loss occurs when sound waves cannot be transmitted to the inner ear

Conductive hearing loss is the most common type of temporary hearing loss encountered in family practice. In most cases it is due to occlusion of the external auditory canal by **wax**, and the hearing improves when the wax is carefully removed. Other common causes of conductive deafness are:

- **Acute otitis externa**, particularly if accompanied by marked swelling and exudate in the external auditory meatus and canal.
- **Acute and chronic otitis media and its complications**. Fluid accumulation in the middle ear in acute infection, and chronic inflammation and granulation tissue formation in chronic otitis media are important causes of conductive hearing loss. Also responsible for partial

hearing loss are erosion by cholesteatoma complicating otitis media, and accumulation of mucoid glue in otitis media with effusion.

- **Barotrauma**, e.g. after blast injuries, may lead to temporary hearing loss, which may be permanent if there is damage to the auditory ossicles. Perforation of the tympanic membrane in blast injuries is potentially recoverable.
- **Perforation of tympanic membrane by trauma or infection**.
- **Otosclerosis**.

Less common causes of conductive deafness include severe congenital malformations of the pinna and external auditory meatus, e.g. anotia.

Sensorineural deafness is due to damage to the inner ear, or to the nerve tracts transmitting messages to the brain

The most common type of permanent hearing loss is **presbyacusis**, a pattern of sensorineural hearing impairment in the elderly. There is decrease in hair cells (associated with atrophy of the epithelial tissue in the basal turn of the cochlea), atrophy of the stria vascularis, and neuronal loss in the spiral ganglia, all of which lead to a progressive sensorineural hearing loss. This type of deafness is characterized by loss of high tones combined with distortion.

The other important causes of acquired sensorineural deafness are:

- **Excessive noise**. Formerly, this was often the result of industrial exposure. However, it is now becoming an important cause in juveniles and young adults because of the use of personal stereo systems at loud volumes.
- **Ototoxic drugs**, particularly aspirin and aminoglycosides.
- **Post-infective**, e.g. non-inherited congenital deafness following maternal rubella (now rare), cytomegalovirus, and toxoplasmosis. Non-congenital post-infective deafness can follow meningitis, and this is the most common cause in children.
- **Acoustic neuroma and head injury** are important causes of acquired sensorineural deafness in adults.

There are many causes of sensorineural hearing loss, some of which are rare congenital syndromes beyond the scope of this book.

Tumors of the ear are not common, and mainly occur in the external ear

Tumors affecting the pinna have already been discussed (see page 237). Both **basal cell carcinoma** and **squamous cell carcinoma** can originate in the epithelium of the external auditory meatus, and may spread to involve the middle ear.

The most important primary tumor presenting in the middle ear is a **paraganglioma**. Derived from the glomus jugulare, it is a neuroendocrine tumor. There is a female preponderance and most patients are between 40 and 60 years old. The tumors are slow-growing and may present late, causing damage by destruction of the ossicles and perforation of the eardrum.

In children, **rhabdomyosarcoma** is an important tumor of the ear (see next section).

Schwannoma of the vestibulocochlear nerve is an important cause of unilateral hearing loss. As with paraganglioma, it is more common in women than in men, usually presenting between the ages of 30 and 50 years.

EAR DISEASE IN CHILDREN

There are many minor congenital malformations of the ear

There are many minor variations in the structure of the pinna, such as the presence of a small spur (**Darwin's tubercle**) on the helix, or prominent forward-facing ears due to a poorly formed antihelix (**bat ears**); such conditions may require surgical treatment for cosmetic reasons, but they are not associated with significant morbidity.

In the skin immediately in front of the ear a small, raised nodule or polyp may arise, situated in front of the tragus. This common malformation, which is termed an **accessory lobule**, often contains a small island of cartilage.

Pre-auricular sinus is a persistent minute pit, usually situated in the skin immediately in front of the top of the helix. They sometimes contain a small plug of keratin, causing symptoms particularly when infected, with swelling and tenderness, often associated with a persistent watery or blood-stained discharge. The pit may be the only visible surface feature of a fairly extensive branched system, and surgical eradication may be difficult.

Severe pinnal malformations (e.g. congenital absence, or the presence of only rudimentary structures) are usually associated with abnormalities of the external auditory meatus and structures within the middle ear, as a result of maldevelopment of the first and second branchial arches. The inner ear is usually normal.

Middle ear disease is common in children

Acute otitis media and otitis media with effusion (glue ear) are particularly common in children, partly as a result of the narrow Eustachian tube and the prominent adenoid lymphoid tissue at its lower end.

Infection of the external ear in children is frequently the result of the presence of an unsuspected foreign body.

Deafness in children

Temporary hearing loss is typically the result of acute otitis media or glue ear.

Permanent hearing loss, which is usually of the sensorineural type, may be congenital, due either to maternal infection or to a rare inherited disorder (see above). Acquired permanent hearing loss in children is an important complication of acute bacterial meningitis.

Rhabdomyosarcoma is the most important malignant tumor of the ear in children

Rhabdomyosarcoma is a highly malignant pleomorphic tumor composed of striated rhabdomyoblasts. It may present as a mass in the ear, but there is often a history of symptoms that have been misinterpreted as otitis media. The tumor grows rapidly and may infiltrate the para-pharyngeal tissues and the mastoid air cells, sometimes extending upwards to invade the skull and brain.

THE LARYNX AND RELATED STRUCTURES

The larynx and related structures are illustrated in *Figs 12.34* and *12.35*.

The supraglottic and glottic regions are frequently inflamed in acute pharyngitis

Viral and bacterial infections of the pharynx frequently involve the supraglottic and glottic regions, producing hoarseness and temporary voice loss. Infection usually extends into subglottic and tracheal regions, and perhaps down into bronchi, producing cough and tracheal soreness. This symptom complex, which is known as **upper**

respiratory tract infection (**URTI**), is very common but usually transient and trivial. It can have serious consequences in young children and in the elderly or debilitated.

In young children the small airway can become obstructed by mucosal and submucosal swelling (croup). Acute epiglottitis, usually due to *Haemophilus influenzae* infection, can produce fatal obstruction.

In the elderly and debilitated the cough reflex is poor, and infected material cannot be cleared from the tracheo-bronchial tree. It may pass into small peripheral bronchi and bronchioles under the influence of gravity, producing **bronchopneumonia** (see page 195, Chapter 11).

Other infective causes of laryngitis are now rare

Diphtheria is now an uncommon cause of laryngitis. Formerly the disease was frequently fatal because of the production of a thick, fibrinous membrane across the airway, leading to asphyxia.

Tuberculosis affecting the larynx usually resulted from the coughing up of tuberculous sputum from a cavitating apical abscess in adults with open pulmonary TB.

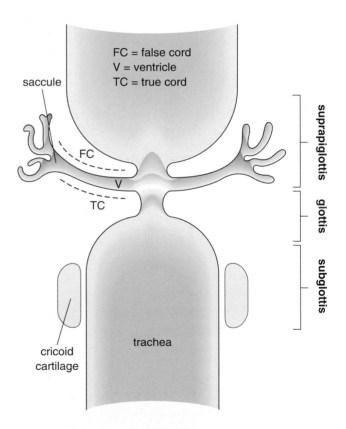

Fig. 12.35 Diagram of larynx showing supraglottic, glottic and subglottic regions.
The supraglottis includes the epiglottis, false cords, ventricles and saccules. The glottis comprises the vocal cords, anterior and posterior commissures and vocal processes of arytenoids. The subglottis is the area below the true vocal cords, as far as the level of the lower border of the cricoid cartilage.

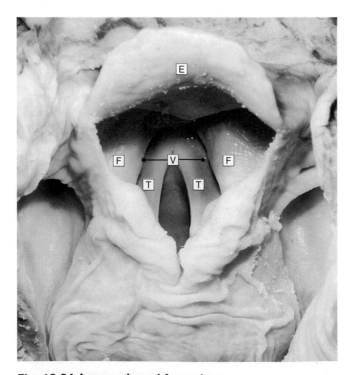

Fig. 12.34 Larynx viewed from above.
E = epiglottis; F = false cord; T = true cord; V = ventricles.

Inflammatory changes in the larynx may also result from allergic and toxic damage

Allergic pharyngolaryngeal edema can arise as a life-threatening Type I hypersensitivity reaction, which is usually associated with swelling of the face (**angioneurotic edema**). Bronchospasm may also occur as part of the same reaction, increasing the severity of the asphyxia.

Acute toxic laryngitis is rare, but is occasionally seen following the inhalation of toxic fumes during exposure in a fire (inhalation of fumes from polystyrene material being particularly important) although the direct physical effect of heat may also be responsible. Industrial exposure to toxic fumes is also an important cause.

Chronic laryngitis is most commonly seen in heavy cigarette smokers. Chronic inflammatory infiltrates are present in the larynx, and there may be thinning or keratotic thickening of the overlying epidermis. In the latter pattern, dysplastic change may occur in the basal layer. This is considered to be a predisposing factor in the eventual development of squamous carcinoma.

Benign thickenings, nodules and polyps of the larynx are a common cause of hoarseness

Chronic laryngitis may lead to permanent thickening of the laryngeal mucosa and submucosa, particularly where there is associated excess production of keratin (smoker's keratosis).

So-called **singer's nodes** are smooth, round, minute nodules located at the nodal point at the junction between the anterior third and posterior two-thirds of the vocal cords (*Fig. 12.36*). Particularly seen in singers and professional voice users, they are covered by smooth epithelium, and the submucosa shows fibrosis.

Diffuse inflammatory edema (sometimes polypoid) is the result of an unusual pattern of edema (**Reinke's edema**) with hyaline change and occasional stromal hemorrhage (*Fig. 12.37*). Histologically there is marked fibrinoid degeneration of the stroma. Excessive bleeding may lead to hematoma formation, particularly after strenuous vocal activity.

Laryngeal cysts occur most commonly in the aryepiglottic folds, rather than on the true vocal cords. These translucent structures, which are filled with thick mucus, are retention cysts resulting from blockage of the ducts of mucus glands.

Warty papillomas on the larynx are usually due to infection by the human papilloma virus (HPV II and 16)

In adults warty papilloma is usually solitary and confined to the vocal cords; its viral nature is less obvious than those in children. Clinically it may be difficult to distinguish from an early verrucous carcinoma (see page 244), and there are also histological similarities.

As the name suggests, **juvenile laryngeal papillomatosis** is largely confined to children. It consists of multiple, soft, pink papillomas on the vocal cord, also extending into other parts of the larynx, sometimes even down the trachea. These lesions have the histological features of a florid viral wart (*Fig. 12.38*). They are difficult to eradicate, often requiring repeat multiple excisions, since they are typically both persistent and recurrent.

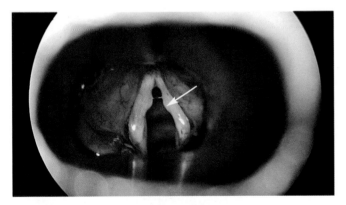

Fig. 12.36 Singer's nodules. The nodules (arrow) occur at the points of contact of the true cords.

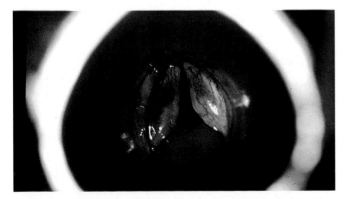

Fig. 12.37 Reinke's edema.
Diffuse swelling of the cords due to Reinke's edema.

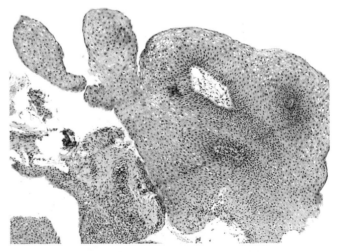

Fig. 12.38 Juvenile laryngeal papillomatosis.
Histology showing warty thickening of the epithelium due to HPV virus.

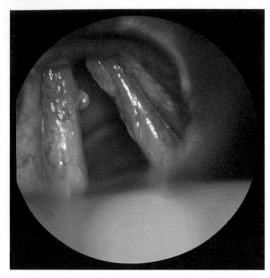

Fig. 12.39 Carcinoma *in situ* of the larynx.
The mucosa of the true cords is thickened, irregular and granular, with a small polyp. Histological examination reveals severe dysplasia of the covering epithelium. To the naked eye there is no evidence of invasion.

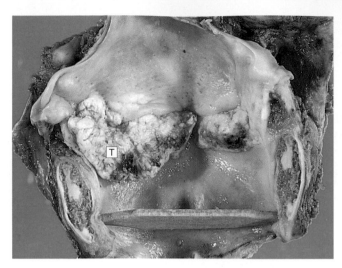

Fig. 12.40 Invasive squamous carcinoma of the larynx.
In this resected specimen of the larynx, there is extensive replacement of the left vocal cord by tumor (**T**).

Carcinoma of the larynx is an important malignancy in cigarette smokers

Carcinoma of the larynx is most common in male cigarette smokers over the age of 40 years, but is becoming increasingly common in women smokers. It is a squamous carcinoma and can occur in the **supraglottic region**, e.g. the aryepiglottic folds, false cords and ventricles; the **glottic region**, in the true vocal cords and anterior and posterior commissures; or the **subglottic region**, arising below the true vocal cords and above the first tracheal ring.

Tumors of the true vocal cords (**glottic**) are most common. They have the best prognosis if detected early (an early symptom being hoarseness), because the true vocal cords have a poor lymphatic drainage except at the commissures. The tumor remains localized to the larynx for a long time and, except in neglected tumors that have invaded local tissues widely, metastasis to lymph nodes is rare.

Supraglottic tumors can be resected with sparing of the true vocal cords. However, as these areas are better supplied with lymphatics, lymph node metastasis is more common than in glottic tumours, and may be the presenting symptom.

Subglottic tumors are the rarest type, and have a poor prognosis because of late presentation; symptoms are often manifest only when extensive growth and local spread lead to stridor and voice loss due to vocal cord involvement.

Some invasive squamous carcinomas of the larynx arise in areas of severe dysplasia and carcinoma *in situ*

Mild dysplasia of the laryngeal epithelium is a common feature of smoker's keratosis, the chronic hyperkeratotic laryngeal thickening that occurs in heavy smokers. More extensive and severe dysplasia merges with **carcinoma *in situ*** (*Fig. 12.39*), and there may be small foci suggesting microinvasion. There is some dispute as to the proportion of invasive squamous carcinomas that arise in pre-existing areas of carcinoma *in situ*, but common sense seems to suggest that, as in the colon and other sites, there is a sequence in the larynx of mild dysplasia, through moderate dysplasia, severe dysplasia and carcinoma *in situ*, culminating in invasive carcinoma (*Fig. 12.40*).

Most invasive squamous carcinomas are well-differentiated keratinizing squamous carcinomas but, occasionally, poorly differentiated forms occur, which are sometimes spindle-celled. An important variant is **verrucous carcinoma**, which usually affects one or both of the true vocal cords. Clinically it presents as an often large, warty papillary tumor, with all the clinical features of malignancy. However, histologically it appears very bland, being composed of benign-looking squamous epithelium with hyperkeratosis. Despite the innocent histology, these tumors are locally destructive and require surgical removal to prevent fatal obstruction or laryngeal destruction. Metastasis is virtually unknown, but occasionally follows attempts at radiotherapy treatment.

It is important that students know the differential diagnosis of lumps in the neck

A simple approach is based on the precise location of the lump in the neck (*Fig. 12.41*), together with its texture (solid or cystic).

The location of solid lumps can be divided into:

- **Related to thyroid gland**, e.g. multinodular goiter, solitary thyroid nodule, thyroid carcinoma, etc.
- **Related to submandibular salivary gland**, e.g. pleomorphic salivary adenoma, chronic sialadenitis.

PRIMARY TUMORS

SECONDARY TUMORS

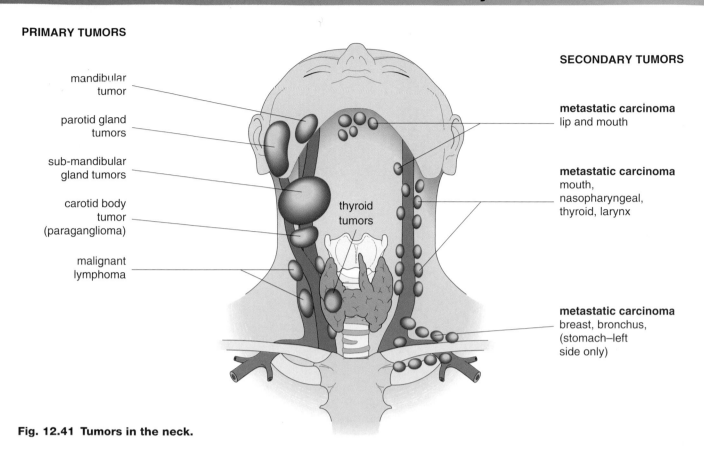

mandibular tumor

parotid gland tumors

sub-mandibular gland tumors

carotid body tumor (paraganglioma)

malignant lymphoma

thyroid tumors

metastatic carcinoma
lip and mouth

metastatic carcinoma
mouth, nasopharyngeal, thyroid, larynx

metastatic carcinoma
breast, bronchus, (stomach–left side only)

Fig. 12.41 Tumors in the neck.

- **Related to the cervical lymph node groups**. These occur mainly in the jugular chain and in the supraclavicular region.
- **Related to mandible**, e.g. mandibular cysts, abscesses and tumors of both dental and bone origin.
- **Related to carotid bifurcation**. These are almost always neuroendocrine tumors derived from the carotid body, the chemodectoma.

Tumors or lumps associated with the thyroid gland are discussed in Chapter 16, those related to the mandible on page 232, and those related to the salivary glands earlier in this chapter.

The lymph nodes in the neck frequently enlarge by benign hyperplasia in response to infection and inflammation

The lymph nodes in the neck, particularly those in the jugular region, respond to local inflammation and infection by reactive hyperplasia, which is either follicular or para-follicular in pattern (see page 306, Chapter 15). Common sources of primary infection include the tonsils, teeth, pharynx, sinuses and, occasionally, the ear. Reactive lymph node enlargement may also occur when there has been localized skin inflammation, e.g. in the scalp or behind the ear. Three important diseases may present with benign lymph node enlargement in the neck.

Infectious mononucleosis (glandular fever) is often associated with severe inflammation of the tonsils. The diagnosis can be confirmed by examination of the periph-eral blood film for atypical mononuclear cells, and by the Paul–Bunnell test, although the diagnosis can be made on histological examination of the node if it is foolishly removed surgically.

In cases of **cervical tuberculosis** the lymph nodes are often matted and inflamed. They may be slightly fluctuant, and in neglected cases they even point and discharge onto the surface ('scrofula'). Histological appearances are characteristic, with extensive caseating necrosis. It is always advisable to send part of an excised tuberculous node for culture in case the organism is an atypical or resistant mycobacterium.

Toxoplasmosis usually develops in a juvenile or a young adult. Toxoplasmic lymphadenitis is discussed and illus-trated in Chapter 15 (see pages 306 and 307). Patients with toxoplasmosis may have circulating atypical lympho-cytes, rather like patients with infectious mononucleosis. In a fully developed case the lymph node histology is very characteristic.

The lymph nodes in the neck are a common site for metastatic tumor deposition

The jugular nodes are the eventual drainage site for many of the mucosal structures in the head and neck, as well as the skin of the head and scalp. Consequently they are a common site for metastatic carcinoma deposits from sites such as the lip, tongue, mouth, nasopharynx,

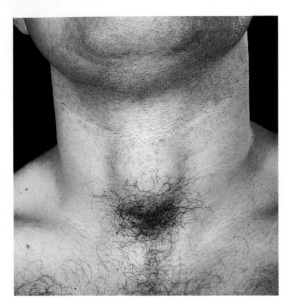

Fig. 12.42 Thyroglossal duct cyst. Note the midline location.

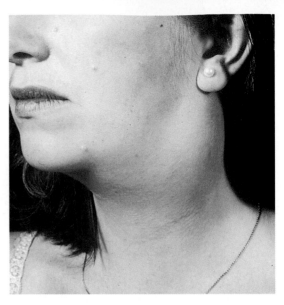

Fig. 12.43 Branchial cyst. Note the lateral location.

oropharynx, larynx, salivary glands, and thyroid. Attempts at complete surgical removal of tumors in these sites often include a block dissection of the lymph nodes of the neck on the affected side; where the primary tumor has crossed the midline, the nodes of the other side are also dissected.

The supraclavicular lymph nodes are important sites for metastatic tumor deposition from primary tumors in the bronchus, breast and (on the left side) stomach (Troisier's node).

Enlargement of one or more lymph nodes in the neck may be a presenting symptom of some types of malignant lymphoma

Malignant lymphoma, a primary malignant tumor of cells of the lymphoid system, is discussed in Chapter 15. It will not be considered in detail here. One form of Hodgkin's disease commonly presents with cervical lymphadenopathy.

Cystic or fluctuant lumps in the neck are usually either midline or lateral

The most common and important midline cystic lesion is the **thyroglossal duct cyst** (*Fig. 12.42*). This is a remnant left from the migration of the thyroid gland from the posterior part of the tongue to the neck during embryological development. It presents in young children, sometimes in the form of a cyst or, occasionally, as a persistent sinus; it may present in young adult life, when the lesions may be quite large.

Occasionally a nodule in the thyroid is fluctuant and is diagnosed as a 'thyroid cyst'. These 'cysts' are almost always benign adenomas showing central degenerative changes.

The most common and important lateral cystic lesion is the **branchial cyst** (*Fig. 12.43*). Derived from cystic remnants of the branchial arches, it produces diffuse fluctuant swelling in the lateral aspect of the neck, often beneath the angle of the mandible.

Clinical Overview

The alimentary tract extends from lips to anus, and the diseases which occur at each component of the tract vary from site to site. Diseases of the various components of the mouth as far as the oropharynx are dealt with in Chapter 12. In this chapter we deal with esophagus, stomach, small intestine, large intestine, rectum and anus.

In the esophagus the most common disorders are **reflux esophagitis** (due to exposure of the lower esophagus to gastric acid regurgitating upwards from the stomach) and **carcinoma**, both squamous and adenocarcinoma being important. In children, esophageal atresia and abnormal developmental links with the trachea are important congenital malformations.

The stomach is an important site of **peptic ulceration**, the ulceration being due to breakdown of the normal mechanisms which protect the stomach mucosa from its own acid. The recent increase in the use of endoscopy has shown that chronic gastritis is a frequent and important condition with a number of different causes, and may play an etiological role in the eventual development of adenocarcinoma of the stomach.

The small intestine is the major site of absorption of the basic food materials, and diseases of small intestinal mucosa may lead to malabsorption syndromes; an important cause is **celiac disease** (gluten enteropathy) which is an immune process leading to destruction of the small intestinal mucosa. The small intestine, particularly ileum, is the most common site for the chronic inflammatory disease called **Crohn's disease.** Acute inflammatory disorders of the small bowel are common but transient, being due to bacterial or viral infection. The stomach and colon are usually also involved (infective gastroenteritis).

Probably the most common inflammatory disease of the entire alimentary tract which requires surgical treatment is **acute appendicitis,** mainly in children and young adults, but occasionally in mature adults and the elderly where the diagnosis may be missed.

The colon may also be involved in the chronic inflammatory condition Crohn's disease, but is the main site of the chronic intermittent inflammatory disease called **ulcerative colitis**. This disease is a known predisposing factor to the development of **colorectal adenocarcinoma** which is extremely common. Other predisposing factors to colonic cancer include the development of benign neoplastic polyps in the colonic mucosa (**adenomatous polyps**). In colorectal carcinoma there is a well-recognized sequence of changes from benign polyp to invasive adenocarcinoma. Other important conditions in the colon are the mechanical abnormalities **diverticular disease** and **volvulus**. Disorders of the anus are a frequent source of medical consultations in family practice, but the disorders are mainly trivial, though with distressing symptoms (hemorrhoids, pruritus ani, anal fissure); the only life-threatening disease of the anus is squamous carcinoma.

▶

> The alimentary tract is generally susceptible to bacterial and viral infection, producing acute vomiting and diarrhea, the main source for the infection being contaminated or infected food items ('food poisoning').
>
> Vascular diseases affecting the alimentary tract are uncommon, with the exception of **arterial infarction** of the small bowel due to thrombotic or embolic occlusion of the mesenteric vessel, and **acute venous infarction** of small or large bowel due to some mechanical obstruction to normal venous drainage. The most common examples of venous infarction of the bowel are strangulation of a loop of small bowel in a hernial sac and volvulus of the large bowel.

DISEASE OF THE ESOPHAGUS AND ESOPHAGOGASTRIC JUNCTION

From its origin at the cricoid cartilage to its termination at the esophagogastric junction, the esophagus is normally lined by stratified non-keratinizing squamous epithelium.

The esophageal wall contains both striated muscle (in its upper portion) and smooth muscle (in the lower portion). A competent lower esophageal sphincter is essential to prevent the reflux of gastric contents back into the esophagus.

Reflux esophagitis is the most common abnormality of the esophagus encountered by the family practitioner

Reflux of gastric acid into the lower esophagus produces a burning pain in the centre of the lower chest or hypochondrium, commonly known as heartburn. Predisposing factors to acid reflux include those that increase intra-abdominal pressure, e.g. over-eating, pregnancy, and poor posture; and those that render the lower esophageal sphincter lax or incompetent, e.g. hiatus hernia (see page 250), smoking, and alcohol ingestion.

The normal squamous epithelium of the lower esophagus is sensitive to the effects of a gastric acid and is frequently damaged. Several complications may arise:

- **Reflux esophagitis**. The esophageal mucosa becomes acutely inflamed.
- **Peptic ulceration of lower esophagus**. Small ulcers usually develop, which become chronic, with fibrosis.
- **Lower esophageal stricture**. Chronic peptic ulceration causes progressive fibrous thickening of the lower esophagus wall. The resultant narrowing causes difficulty in swallowing.
- **Barrett's esophagus**. Persistent esophageal reflux causes metaplasia of the lower esophageal mucosa, the squamous epithelium being replaced by glandular epithelium composed of tall columnar cells (*Fig. 13.1*). This is also termed **columnar epithelial-lined esophagus** (CELO).

Barrett's esophagus predisposes to the development of adenocarcinoma

Barrett's esophagus can progress from metaplastic glandular epithelium to epithelial dysplasia (with nuclear pleomorphism and hyperchromicity), and then to frank adenocarcinoma. The columnar epithelium may show features of intestinal metaplasia, in which the epithelium resembles that of the small intestine, or may resemble that of the cardiac region of the proximal stomach.

Patients with Barrett's esophagus are kept under surveillance through repeated endoscopy and biopsy to detect early neoplastic changes. Treatment by esophageal surgery is then possible before development of invasion.

Esophagitis is rarely caused by agents other than reflux

Acute esophagitis may be caused by infective or physical agents. Bacterial infection is very rare, but fungal infection (mainly by *Candida albicans*) is an important cause of severe erosive esophagitis, particularly in immunosuppressed patients.

Viral infections of the esophagus (particularly by *Herpes simplex* and cytomegalovirus) are increasingly being seen in AIDS patients and those receiving immunosuppressive therapy.

Acute esophagitis is also produced by irradiation and by ingestion of caustic agents. Certain skin diseases, such as pemphigus, epidermolysis bullosa and Behçet's syndrome may cause esophageal ulceration, with extensive separation of the epithelium from the submucosa producing blistering, followed by erosion.

Any esophageal obstruction causes difficulty in swallowing, known as 'dysphagia'

Four main types of lesion cause obstruction:

- **Lesions in the lumen**. Swallowed foreign bodies, especially in children.
- **Lesions in the wall**. Benign neoplasm or carcinoma of the esophagus, fibrosis caused by chronic inflammation.

Disease of the esophagus and esophagogastric junction

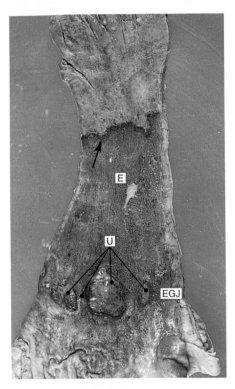

Fig. 13.1 Barrett's esophagus.
The lower esophageal mucosa (**E**) is replaced by darker columnar epithelium, with an area of ulceration (**U**) at the esophagogastric junction (**EGJ**). The arrow marks the abnormally high squamocolumnar junction.

- **Lesions outside the wall.** Esophageal diverticulum, tumors in the mediastinum (e.g. invasion by carcinoma of lung).
- **Lesions affecting function.** Achalasia (see below), Chagas' disease, motor neuron disease (see page 481).

Esophageal obstruction may be complicated by reflux of food into the airways, resulting in aspiration pneumonia (see page 197), and by malnutrition due to the inability to maintain adequate intake.

Achalasia of the esophagus is due to abnormal innervation

In achalasia, lack of coordinated muscle contraction and relaxation at the lower end of the esophagus leads to retention of the food bolus, the result of peristaltic spasms combined with sluggish relaxation at the esophagogastric sphincter. The condition is mainly seen in middle age. Over a period of time the esophagus becomes markedly dilated (megaesophagus). Its cause is unknown, but reduced numbers of ganglion cells in the muscle plexus have been noted in long-standing cases. This condition also predisposes to development of carcinoma of the esophagus.

In South America, infection by *Trypanosoma cruzi* causes a very similar condition, with destruction of myenteric plexus, termed **Chagas' disease**.

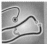
Dysphagia is commonly seen in family practice

Although esophageal stricture, achalasia and malignant tumors are the most important causes of dysphagia, they are not the most common.

In family practice, complaints of difficulty in swallowing, and the feeling of a lump in the throat, are common among young and middle-aged women. The patient describes an apparent obstruction in the cricoid region of the upper esophagus, and the swallowing problem is not directly related to food ingestion, but difficulty is particularly experienced in swallowing saliva and drinks. Called **globus pharyngeus**, the condition is associated with spasm of the cricopharyngeus muscle, identifiable on barium swallow. Although probably psychosomatic in most cases, it may be a manifestation of hiatus hernia, reflux esophagitis or peptic ulceration.

Esophageal perforation is most often caused by medical procedures

Perforation of the esophageal wall is extremely serious as it liberates secretions (including gastric juices) into the mediastinum, causing **mediastinitis**. Patients have chest pain and develop clinical shock. A chest radiograph may show air in the mediastinum.

Perforation most commonly occurs after instrumentation of the esophagus, e.g. after dilatation of stricture or endoscopy. Tearing of the lower esophagus may occur after severe vomiting with a full stomach, leading to perforation and hemorrhage from local vessels (**Mallory–Weiss tear**).

The most common malignant tumors of the esophagus are squamous carcinomas and adenocarcinomas

There is great geographical variation in the incidence of esophageal carcinoma, and it is particularly common in the Far East, especially in China and Japan. Tumors are most common in males after the fifth decade, and can be divided into two main histological types:

Squamous carcinomas are most common in the middle and lower esophagus. They mostly develop in men who are heavy alcohol drinkers or heavy smokers, and may be preceded by epithelial dysplastic change. The disease usually presents late, when the tumor has become large enough to compromise the esophageal lumen and cause dysphagia. Regional lymph node spread is early and common.

Adenocarcinomas mostly affect the lower esophagus, arising in areas of epithelial metaplasia (**Barrett's esophagus**). Some adenocarcinomas may represent a primary carcinoma of the stomach that has infiltrated into the lower esophagus. These tumors tend to metastasize via lymphatics at an earlier stage than squamous carcinomas.

The prognosis for both types of carcinoma is poor, that for squamous carcinoma being slightly better than adeno-carcinoma because it is more responsive to radiotherapy. Fewer than 10% of patients survive for 5 years.

Squamous carcinomas of the upper esophagus, located in the post-cricoid region, are very rare and are usually linked to the Plummer–Vinson syndrome, most common in middle-aged and elderly women.

Rare malignant primary tumors of the esophagus include malignant melanomas, small cell neuroendocrine carcinomas, and sarcomas.

Benign tumors of the esophagus are uncommon

Most of the rare benign esophageal tumors are leiomyomas derived from the smooth muscle of the muscularis propria. Less common are tumors derived from nerves, i.e. schwannomas and neurofibromas. They produce smooth spherical nodules projecting into the lumen, and are usually covered by intact mucosa unless they become large, at which stage ulceration of the stretched overlying mucosa can occur.

In hiatus hernia the stomach moves into the thorax

Hiatus hernia, in which the upper part of the stomach moves through the diaphragmatic esophageal hiatus into the thoracic cavity, is a common and important condition.

Patients often complain of symptoms of reflux esophagitis, and there may be peptic ulceration in the intra-thoracic part of the stomach and lower esophagus. In **sliding hiatus hernia**, the stomach herniates through the diaphragmatic hiatus through which the lower esophagus normally passes. In **paraesophageal hiatus hernia**, the stomach protrudes through a separate defect alongside the esophagus (*Fig. 13.2*).

Esophageal varices are an important cause of vomiting blood

At the lower end of the esophagus the submucosal venous plexus drains into both the systemic venous system and the portal venous system. When the pressure in the portal venous system is high, e.g. as a result of severe diffuse long-standing liver disease, the esophageal submucosal venous channels become enormously dilated to form esophageal varices, which may protrude slightly into the lumen. Rupture of the varices, or ulceration of the overlying mucosa, can produce torrential hemorrhage into the esophagus and stomach, often precipitating vomiting of blood (**hematemesis**).

The most common cause of esophageal varices is portal hypertension associated with cirrhosis of the liver (see Chapter 14).

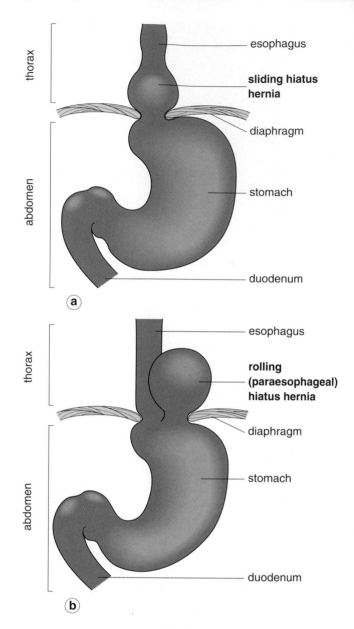

Fig. 13.2 Hiatus hernia. (a) Sliding hiatus hernia. (b) Paraesophageal hiatus hernia.

DISEASE OF THE STOMACH

The stomach has three mucosal zones: the **cardia**, which is immediately adjacent to the esophageal junction; the **body** (fundus), which contains long tubular glands secreting acid and intrinsic factor; and the **pylorus** (antrum), which contains the majority of gastrin-secreting cells. Each zone is affected by different types of pathology.

Gastritis is characterized by inflammation of the gastric mucosa

Inflammatory changes in the mucosa and submucosa of the stomach are known as **gastritis**, and may be either **acute** or

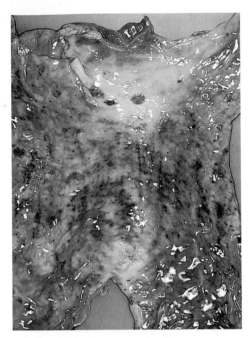

Fig. 13.3 Acute erosive gastritis.
Acute erosive gastritis is shown in the opened stomach. The mucosa appears hyperemic, and the foci of superficial ulceration are manifest as scattered, small, red areas termed **erosions**.

Diagnosis of *Helicobacter* infection

The diagnosis of *Helicobacter* infection is established using four main methods:

1 **Urea breath test.** *Helicobacter* produces the enzyme urease. If radiolabeled urea is administered and *Helicobacter* urease is present, radioactive CO_2 can be detected in the breath.
2 **Serology.** Antibodies to *H. pylori* can be detected in serum.
3 **Histology.** Organisms can be seen in biopsy material, particularly if specially stained.
4 **Culture.** *H. pylori*, a curved microaerophilic organism, can be cultured from biopsy material.

chronic. This may be assessed by endoscopic examination of the mucosa and confirmed by biopsy.

Acute gastritis is characterized by superficial acute inflammation of the gastric mucosa. It is most often caused by ingested chemicals, the most common being alcohol, aspirin, and non-steroidal anti-inflammatory drugs such as indomethacin.

Acute erosive gastritis is characterized by focal loss of the superficial gastric epithelium (*Fig. 13.3*). Patients develop dyspepsia with vomiting and, occasionally, if the erosions are numerous, hematemesis may occur. This pattern of acute gastritis is caused by shock, stress associated with severe burns or raised intracranial pressure, non-steroidal anti-inflammatory drugs, and very heavy acute alcohol ingestion.

Severe **necrotizing ulcerative gastritis** follows suicidal ingestion of strong alkalis and acids.

Chronic gastritis has been revealed by endoscopic examination to be more common than formerly thought, and carries a recognized risk of development of malignancy (see page 253).

Three main patterns of chronic gastritis are identified

1 *Helicobacter*-associated gastritis is the most common form, arising at any age. It is associated with the presence of bacterial colonies of the organism *Helicobacter pylori*. The organisms colonize the surface of the epithelium beneath the thin layer of mucus. The presence of the organisms is associated with

epithelial damage and a mixed acute and chronic inflammatory cell reaction in the lamina propria and superficial epithelium. The pyloric antrum is the most severely affected area, but damage is also seen in the fundus. Intestinal metaplasia is frequently seen, in which the normal gastric epithelium is replaced by a type similar to that seen in the small intestine.

Helicobacter is also very important in the development of duodenal inflammation and ulceration.

2 **Autoimmune chronic gastritis** is associated with an autoimmune disease (**pernicious anemia**) and is generally seen in elderly patients, in whom severe atrophy of the mucosa develops. Those affected have antibodies against gastric parietal cells (90%) and intrinsic factor (60%). The autoimmune damage to the gastric cells is associated with reduced gastric production of hydrochloric acid (hypochlorhydria) and failure of absorption of dietary vitamin B_{12}. The vitamin B_{12} deficiency leads to interference with normal erythropoiesis in the bone marrow, and the patients develop a megaloblastic macrocytic anemia (**pernicious anemia**) (see Chapter 15). This pattern of gastritis particularly affects the body of the stomach.

3 **Reactive gastritis**, also known as reflux gastritis, occurs when alkaline duodenal fluid (containing bile) refluxes into the lower part of the stomach. It is common in people who have had previous gastric surgery to the pyloric area, which presumably causes incompetence of the pyloric sphincter. However, in most cases, there is no previous history of surgery and the cause of the incompetence is not understood. This pattern of gastritis is also seen with prolonged administration of non-steroidal anti-inflammatory drugs, the common factor probably being direct toxic damage to the mucus layer.

Peptic ulceration and intestinal metaplasia are complications of chronic gastritis

Intestinal metaplasia frequently develops from chronic gastritis (particularly the autoimmune form). The normal gastric pattern of epithelium is replaced by two patterns of metaplastic epithelium: a goblet-cell pattern, similar to that seen in the small intestine; and a mucous cell pattern, similar to that seen in the pyloric antrum.

The importance of small intestinal metaplasia is its pre-disposition to undergo dysplastic change, with eventual transformation into carcinoma. An important part of the management of chronic gastritis is repeated endoscopic biopsy to detect dysplastic change before the development of malignancy.

Chronic gastritis may also be associated with the development of peptic ulceration.

Peptic ulcers may be acute or chronic

Peptic ulcers are caused by damage to the gastric lining by gastric secretions, particularly acid.

Acute peptic ulcers usually develop from areas of erosive gastritis and are predisposed by the same conditions as erosive gastritis. They may cause severe bleeding, heal without scarring, or progress to form a chronic peptic ulcer. Important causes of acute peptic ulcers are severe stress or shock (e.g. after major trauma or burns), with hypotension; acute hypoxia of the surface epithelium may be an important pathogenic mechanism.

The histology and some of the complications of chronic peptic ulcers have been discussed in Chapter 4.

The main sites of chronic peptic ulceration are the lower esophagus (due to gastric reflux), the stomach (*Fig. 13.4*), the duodenum, and gastroenterostomy sites.

The important complications of chronic peptic ulcer are:

- **Hemorrhage**.
- **Penetration**. The ulcer penetrates the full thickness of the stomach or duodenal wall, progressing into adherent underlying tissue, particularly the pancreas or liver. Penetration of the pancreas often manifests clinically as severe back pain.
- **Perforation**. This leads to peritonitis.
- **Fibrous stricture**. This is seen in peptic ulcer of the esophagus; fibrous thickening caused by healing leads to scarring of the esophagus and obstruction. In the stomach, ulcers may cause pyloric stenosis.
- **Malignant change**. This is extremely uncommon.

The most important tumor of the stomach is adenocarcinoma

Gastric adenocarcinoma is more common in men than in women, and is seen in patients after the age of 30, the incidence rising greatly after the age of 50 years.

There is marked geographic variation in the incidence of gastric cancer; compared to Western Europe and North America, it is seen more frequently in the Far East and certain parts of South America and Scandinavia. Because of

---

Peptic ulceration is due to a breakdown of normal mucosal protective mechanisms

The gastric mucosa is normally protected by a mucus barrier containing acid-resisting neutral glycoproteins and buffering bicarbonate ions. Peptic ulceration occurs when protective mechanisms are deficient, and persists because of gastric acid.

In the **esophagus** the most important cause of ulceration is reflux of acid gastric secretions onto the unprotected esophageal mucosa, hypersecretion of acid by the stomach being the most important factor in ulceration of the **duodenum**. In the **stomach** the factors that predispose to peptic ulcers include regurgitated bile in pyloric incompetence, surface epithelial damage by *H. pylori* infection, and surface epithelial damage by non-steroidal anti-inflammatory agents.

Other factors, such as chronic gastritis, smoking and genetic predisposition, are believed to play a role in the pathogenesis, although the mechanisms are poorly understood.

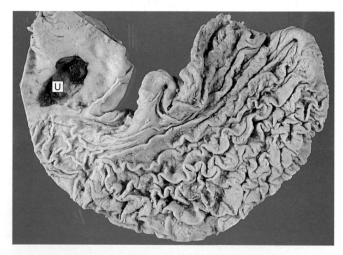

Fig. 13.4 Chronic peptic ulcer of the stomach.
A large chronic peptic ulcer (**U**) is seen in the pylorus of the stomach. Chronic ulcers may be 1–7 cm in diameter or even larger. They have sharply defined borders without any heaping up of the epithelium surrounding the ulcer crater. The floor of the ulcer is composed of fibrous scar tissue, overlaid by granulation tissue, inflammatory exudate and necrotic slough. The ulcer crater usually penetrates into the muscularis propria of the stomach, and complete healing of the ulcer leads to fibrous replacement of muscle, with regrowth of epithelium over the scar.

the great variation in geographical distribution, dietary etiological factors have been sought, but none is firmly proven. Frequent ingestion of smoked and salted preserved foods has been implicated, particularly in the generation of nitrosamines. There is an association with blood group A.

Conditions predisposing to development of gastric carcinoma are chronic atrophic gastritis and gastric adenomatous polyps (see above). At-risk groups include patients with chronic gastritis and intestinal metaplasia, postgastrectomy patients with persisting gastric inflammation, and patients in gastric cancer families (rare).

The pathogenesis of gastric carcinoma in the fundus and antrum is believed to follow a sequence from normal mucosa, through chronic gastritis, intestinal metaplasia, dysplasia and intramucosal carcinoma, to invasive carcinoma.

Carcinomas in the cardia are infrequently associated with chronic gastritis and may have another pathogenesis.

Gastric adenocarcinoma has three main growth patterns

Gastric adenocarcinoma may grow in a polypoid, ulcerating or diffuse infiltrative pattern (*Fig. 13.5*).

The **polypoid type** tends to present early because, as well as giving a feeling of gastric discomfort, the polypoid protrusion is traumatized and bleeds. Of the three types, it is the most amenable to surgical excision, and has the best prognosis.

The most common type is the **ulcerative carcinoma**. Characteristically, the ulcer has a raised edge, a necrotic shaggy base, and the radiating folds seen in benign peptic ulcers are absent.

The **diffuse infiltrative pattern** tends to present very late. The symptoms are usually those of non-specific loss of appetite, and food intolerance due to both the small capacity of the stomach and its inability to distend under a food load. Because surface ulceration is not a prominent feature, hematemesis is not common until the late stage. Metastatic spread to lymph nodes and the liver is usually present at the time of clinical presentation and, of the three types, this pattern of growth has the worst prognosis.

The term **early gastric cancer** has been used to describe tumors that are confined to the mucosa and submucosa. As these lesions may have metastases, the term 'early' can

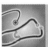

Polyps of the stomach must be biopsied

There are several benign polyps of the stomach, all of which are uncommon compared to the incidence of carcinomas of this region.

Polyps of the gastric mucosa must always be examined by biopsy to exclude the presence of a carcinoma. The main types are:

- **Hyperplastic polyps** formed by regeneration of mucosa, often at the edge of an ulcer.
- **Adenomatous polyps**, which are true benign tumors of surface epithelium, ranging up to 5 cm in size. These carry a 25–70% risk of malignant change, but are very rare.
- **Fundal polyps**, which are cystic glandular lesions seen mainly in women.
- **Hamartomatous polyps**, which occur in Peutz–Jeghers syndrome.

Other benign tumors of the stomach are derived from mesenchymal tissues, the most common being a leiomyoma. These appear as mucosal or intramural nodules and are usually asymptomatic.

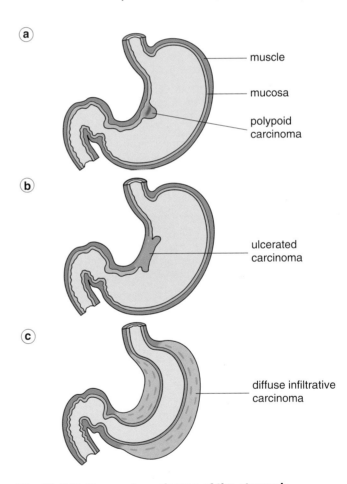

Fig. 13.5 Patterns of carcinoma of the stomach.
(a) **Polypoid**. Tumor protrudes into the stomach lumen.
(b) **Ulcerating**. A thickened localized plaque of carcinoma undergoes central ulceration to mimic benign peptic ulcer.
(c) **Diffuse infiltrative**. There is extensive spread of tumor within the mucosa and submucosa, without extensive ulceration. This diffuse infiltration produces a shrunken inexpansible rigid stomach ('linitis plastica' or 'leather-bottle stomach').

be misleading. Such tumors are generally of the polypoid type and have a better prognosis than other forms.

Histologically, adenocarcinoma of the stomach is divided into two main types. The **intestinal pattern** of tumor is composed of gland-like spaces, and the **diffuse infiltrative carcinoma** of the stomach is composed of sheets of anaplastic cells, many of which have a single vacuole of mucin, displacing the nucleus to one side (signet-ring cell).

Spread of gastric carcinoma is by four main routes

Adenocarcinoma of the stomach spreads by local, lymphatic, hematogenous and transcelomic routes.

- **Direct invasion** through the wall of the stomach leads to involvement of adjacent viscera.
- **Lymphatic spread** (the main route) is to nodes on the greater and lesser curves of the stomach, then to other nodal groups. Involvement of the left supraclavicular nodal group is well recognized (**Virchow's node, Troisier's sign**).
- **Hematogenous spread** to liver, lung and brain is common. Spread to the ovaries leads to development of **Krukenberg tumors** (see page 415).
- **Transcelomic spread** through the peritoneum results in malignant ascites.

Prognosis of gastric adenocarcinoma is poor in most cases. The 5-year survival rate in gastric carcinoma is low and depends on the stage of the tumor. Many tumors are locally advanced at diagnosis and have spread to nodes or metastasized. Prognosis after surgery is 20% 10-year survival for advanced gastric cancer, but 90% 10-year survival for lesions confined to the mucosa and submocosa, as with small polypoid tumors.

Lymphomas, neuroendocrine tumors and sarcomas are uncommon malignant tumors of the stomach

Lymphoma of the stomach accounts for about 3% of gastric tumors. This is an example of a tumor of mucosa-associated lymphoid tissue (MALT), discussed with others in Chapter 15.

Sarcomas of the stomach, which are mainly leiomyosarcomas, account for fewer than 2% of all gastric malignancies. Benign leiomyomas are more common. Derived from the smooth muscle of the stomach wall, these are smooth spherical tumors covered by stretched but intact mucosa.

Neuroendocrine tumors (carcinoid tumors) of the stomach are similar to those seen in the small bowel (see page 264).

DISEASE OF THE SMALL AND LARGE INTESTINE

Infective disorders of the intestine are common (see also Chapter 8)

Infective disorders of the bowel are common and are due to many classes of organism.

- **Viruses**: rotaviruses cause 50% of infantile diarrhea and account for some adult cases. Norwalk viruses account for 30% of adult cases of gastroenteritis.
- **Bacteria**: some bacteria cause direct damage to the bowel (e.g. *Salmonella typhi* and *Campylobacter jejuni*), while others produce enterotoxins (e.g. in salmonellosis and enteropathogenic *E. coli*). Tuberculosis may affect the gut, particularly the terminal ileum. *Yersinia* infection may cause ulceration and ileitis. *Campylobacter* infection is the commonest cause of bacterial diarrhea mainly affecting the colon.
- **Protozoa**: Giardia causes infection of the small bowel and gives rise to a malabsorption syndrome. Cryptosporidia and microsporidia may cause disease, particularly in immunosuppressed patients.
- **Fungi**: infection is virtually restricted to immunosupressed patients.
- **Helminths**: parasitization of the bowel by helminths is widespread, especially in the tropics. Many of the clinical problems are causes by immune-mediated hypersensitivity causing hypereosinophilia syndromes.

Gastrointestinal infections are common in immunosuppressed patients, particularly with AIDS. Most patients

Molecular pathology of gastric cancer

Gastric cancer is associated with a number of molecular genetic abnormalities related to oncogenes. It has been proposed that accumulated molecular abnormalities have a role in the evolution of adenocarcinoma of the stomach.

In well-differentiated gastric carcinomas, several abnormalities are commonly documented:

- Inactivation of p53 tumor suppressor gene.
- Activation of *c-met*, a receptor for hepatocyte growth factor.

In poorly differentiated carcinomas there is:

- Amplification of *Cerb-b2*, a receptor-type tyrosine kinase.
- Amplification of *K-sam*, a receptor-type tyrosine kinase.

The significance of these events in relation to prognosis or treatment is still under evaluation.

with AIDS have chronic diarrhea which can be caused by a wide range of pathogens.

Some bacterial infections cause damage by invasion

Several bacterial infections of the gut cause infection by invasion of the mucosa. Many cause diarrhea with blood and pus in the stool, termed **bacterial dysentery**. The main organisms causing this type of infection are as follows:

- *Campylobacter* invades mucosa in the jejunum, ileum and colon, causing ulceration and acute inflammation.
- *Salmonella typhi*, *S. paratyphi A, B,* and *C* are transmitted in food and water contaminated by the feces or urine of a carrier. In *S. typhi* infection organisms initially proliferate in the reticuloendothelial system. A secondary bacteremia develops and Peyer's patches become ulcerated. Patients develop fever, diarrhea, splenomegaly (75%), and a skin rash consisting of rose spots (50%).
- *Shigella* infections are mainly seen in young children. The organism invades mucosa of the colon and distal ileum causing mucosal ulceration, most marked in the sigmoid colon and rectum.
- **Enteroinvasive and enterohemorrhagic** *E. coli* cause a hemorrhagic colitis similar to *Shigella*.

Most cases of **intestinal tuberculosis** are caused by ingestion of bacteria in food (commonly milk from infected cows) or by swallowing infected sputum. The disease particularly affects the terminal ileum and cecum causing ulceration of the bowel mucosa, fibrous wall thickening and enlargement of regional lymph nodes which develop caseous graulomatous inflammation.

Whipple's disease is a rare condition caused by infection by an actinomycete called *Tropheryma whippelii*, the route of infection being unknown. It is a multisystem disorder affecting Caucasian men in the third and fourth decades with malabsorption due to small bowel involvement, lymphadenopathy, arthritis and CNS symptoms.

Some bacteria produce enterotoxins and cause disease without invasion

Bacterial enterotoxins cause disease in two circumstances. In the first, the toxin is formed in the food before it is eaten, resulting in vomiting and diarrhea about 12 hours after ingestion (e.g. staphylococcal food poisoning). In the second, the bacteria proliferate in the gut after ingestion and produce toxins which then cause intestinal disturbance; this extra growth stage means that the disease takes about 24 hours to develop after contaminated food is eaten.

Salmonella enteritidis, *S. typhimurium*, *S. hadar* and *S. virchow* produce enterotoxin-induced fluid and electrolyte disturbance. Incubation is 24–48 hours, resulting in an enterocolitis with profuse diarrhea and vomiting lasting about 48 hours.

Vibrio cholerae is acquired through water contaminated with feces. Organisms grow in the small bowel and secrete a toxin which causes uncontrolled cAMP-stimulated secretion of fluid into the gut producing severe watery diarrhea.

Pseudomembranous enterocolitis is caused by a clostridial toxin causing mucosal necrosis

In pseudomembranous colitis, *Clostridium difficile* overgrowth produces an enterotoxin that results in necrosis of the colonic mucosa. The condition is almost invariably associated with antibiotic therapy, but other diseases of the colon which allow clostridial overgrowth also predispose to its development (gastrointestinal surgery, ischemia, shock, burns). Patients develop fever, abdominal pain and diarrhea.

Important protozoans causing bowel infection are Giardia, Cryptosporidia and Entamoeba

The most important protozoa causing gut infection are:

- *Giardia lamblia*, which is a flagellate protozoan acquired from contaminated water. It infects the duodenum and upper jejunum and may cause diarrhea, abdominal pain, weight loss, or malabsorption.
- *Cryptosporidium parvum*, which is acquired from contaminated water causing a self-limiting diarrheal illness which may be severe in patients with AIDS.
- *Entamoeba histolytica*, which is acquired through water or food contaminated by cysts and causes amebic colitis.

MALABSORPTION SYNDROMES

The small intestine provides an environment for absorption of nutrients from food. There are four main elements to absorption:

- The pancreas secretes digestive enzymes into the gut lumen, which are necessary for breakdown of macromolecules.
- The liver secretes bile acids needed for solubilization and absorption of fats.
- The mucosa is specialized for absorption: transverse mucosal folds and finger-like villi provide a vast surface area.
- The mucosa is the site of a set of enzymes, located on the brush border, which hydrolyse large molecules for absorption, especially complex sugars (e.g. sucrase and lactase).

Absence of any of these elements leads to impaired digestion of food and malabsorption. This manifests as weight loss, abdominal distension, and loose, bulky stools.

If fat is not being absorbed, stools are pale, foul-smelling and characteristically float in water. Anemia is common. The main causes of malabsorption are shown in *Fig. 13.6*.

If the pancreas fails to produce or secrete the hydrolytic enzymes responsible for food breakdown, nutrients are not absorbed. The most common causes are cystic fibrosis, chronic pancreatitis, carcinoma of the pancreas, and pancreatic surgery.

The most important small intestinal cause of malabsorption in the western world is **celiac disease**; in the developing world it is probably severe **parasitic and worm infestation**.

Loss of absorptive surface of the bowel is common and is due to a number of diseases. Extensive resection of the small bowel (e.g. for infarction or Crohn's disease) reduces the absorptive area markedly. Crohn's disease, if very severe, leads to extensive submucosal edema and mucosal flattening, which reduces the surface area for absorption. Disease of the terminal ileum prevents absorption of vitamin B_{12}.

If secretion of bile into the gut is impaired, solubilization of fats cannot take place, resulting in impaired fat absorption. This is also manifest in malabsorption of fat-soluble vitamins A, D, E, and K.

Damage to enterocytes in the bowel leads to replacement by cells that lack differentiation and fail to express brush-border enzymes such as lactase or sucrase (**disaccharidase deficiency**). Disaccharides in the diet cannot be broken down, and their presence in the gut causes diarrhea, as well as bacterial overgrowth. This may become manifest after an episode of infective diarrhea.

Congenital lack of disaccharidases is also seen in infants, in the absence of mucosal damage, and is a cause of failure to thrive.

Whipple's disease is a rare but important cause of malabsorption, in which the mucosa is infiltrated by macrophages full of infective actinomycete organisms.

Celiac disease is caused by hypersensitivity to a component of gluten

Celiac disease causes atrophy of small intestinal villi due to an abnormal sensitivity to gluten, a protein in wheat flour (**gluten enteropathy**). The disease can present at any age, and in infants and children it is an important cause of failure to thrive.

Celiac disease is caused by an immune response to the protein gliadin, a component of gluten. There is an increased incidence of disease in first-degree relatives of those affected, and linkage with certain HLA groups has been shown. There is a strong association with possession of the HLA-B8 antigen, a factor also linked with the itchy, blistering skin disease, dermatitis herpetiformis (see page 496), which may occur concurrently with celiac disease. The presence of serum antigliadin antibodies is seen in the majority of cases.

Fig. 13.6
Causes of malabsorption

Common causes

Pancreatic insufficiency (e.g. chronic pancreatitis)
Celiac disease
Resection of ileum
Parasitic infestation of the gut

Frequent causes

Resection of stomach
Crohn's disease
Liver disease causing failure of bile secretion into the gut

Uncommon causes

Bacterial overgrowth in blind loops or diverticulae
Post-infective malabsorption (tropical sprue)
A-chain disease
Giardiasis
Disaccharidase deficiency (e.g. lactase)
Abetalipoproteinemia
Intestinal lymphangiectasis
Whipple's disease

Diagnosis is by biopsy of small bowel mucosa. Histologically the immune-mediated damage causes heavy lymphocytic infiltrate of lamina propria, and an increase in intraepithelial lymphocytes. There is also loss of villous architecture, ranging from blunting (partial villous atrophy) to complete flattening (total villous atrophy) (*Fig. 13.7*), and an increase in depth of crypts, which produce more epithelial cells to compensate for those lost through damage.

Complete withdrawal of gliadin from the diet (gluten-free diet) leads to gradual recovery of villous structure, which may be partial or complete.

Long-term complications of celiac disease include the development of primary T-cell lymphoma of the small intestine and, rarely, development of adenocarcinoma.

Post-infective malabsorption histologically resembles celiac disease

Malabsorption may develop in travellers who return from tropical areas, lasting for at least 2 months after an episode of infective diarrhea. There is severe folate and vitamin B_{12} deficiency, as well as weight loss. Investigation reveals crypt hyperplastic villous atrophy similar to that seen in celiac disease.

Microbiology shows colonization of the gut lumen by enterobacteria. Other causes of malabsorption in the tropics must be excluded, e.g. intestinal parasites, HIV enteropathy, and tuberculosis.

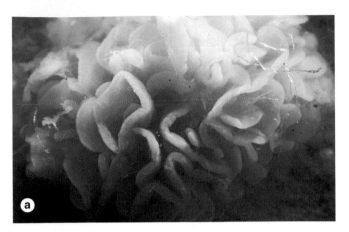

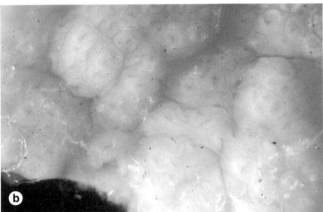

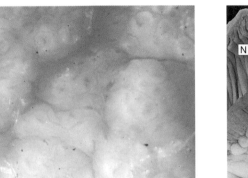

Fig. 13.7 Celiac disease.
The normal surface pattern of the jejunal mucosa viewed through the dissecting microscope is shown in (a) as a series of ridges and finger-like projections. In celiac disease the surface becomes flattened, developing a mosaic-like pattern (b).

Fig. 13.8 Crohn's disease.
The mucosa in Crohn's disease demonstrates a cobblestone pattern (a) as a result of fissured ulcers (**U**) with intervening areas of edematous mucosa (**M**). In (b) compared to normal small bowel wall (**N**), the Crohn's segment (**C**) shows wall thickening that has caused a stenosis.

CHRONIC INFLAMMATORY BOWEL DISEASE

Idiopathic chronic inflammatory bowel diseases show primary inflammation of the intestinal wall

The idiopathic inflammatory bowel diseases, of which there are two main members, have no known cause. In **Crohn's disease** there is a granulomatous inflammatory pattern of disease that affects the full thickness of the bowel wall. It is most common in the terminal ileum, but may affect any part of the gastrointestinal tract in a discontinuous pattern. With **ulcerative colitis**, a chronic inflammatory disease of the rectal mucosa, inflammation may extend to involve the whole of the colon in continuity. Importantly, both types of inflammatory bowel disease are associated with systemic manifestations outside of the intestine.

In diagnosing idiopathic inflammatory bowel disease, infective causes of inflammation have first to be excluded. Investigation is by imaging and biopsy.

Established Crohn's disease has a cobblestone-pattern mucosa

Crohn's disease is more common in women than in men, patients usually being 20–60 years old. It particularly affects the terminal ileum (synonym: **regional ileitis**), but can occur anywhere in the gut, especially in the mouth, colon, and anus.

The macroscopic appearance of the bowel in Crohn's disease varies according to the stage of the disease.

In early disease affected bowel shows marked swelling of submucosa and mucosa, mainly due to severe submucosal edema. This leads to loss of the pattern of normal transverse folds, and small superficial areas of hemorrhagic ulceration arise which, over time, develop into fissures.

In established chronic disease the bowel mucosa shows a **cobblestone pattern** due to a combination of submucosal edema and interconnecting deep fissured ulcers (*Fig. 13.8*). The bowel wall is thickened by edema and fibrosis and, commonly, there is stricture formation. Regional lymph nodes usually become enlarged. Disease is not continuous and areas of normal bowel may be present between the diseased segments (**skip lesions**). The normal bowel proximal to a segment of Crohn's disease is often dilated due to partial obstruction.

Crohn's disease shows transmural inflammation with deep fissured ulcers

Crohn's disease is histologically characterized by inflammation of all layers, submucosal edema, ulcers that extend deep into the bowel wall and form fissures, and fibrous scarring. Non-caseating granulomas may be present (*Fig. 13.9*).

Inflammation in Crohn's disease is transmural, and serosal involvement leads to inflammatory adhesion to other loops of bowel, to the parietal peritoneum of the anterior abdominal wall, or to the bladder. Deep penetration of fissured ulcers, which may extend through the full thickness of the bowel wall into the adherent viscus, causes **fistulae** (tracks between two cavities) and **sinuses** (a track from a viscus to an outside surface). This is particularly seen in the perianal region.

The direct complications of Crohn's disease are:

- Stricture formation leading to intestinal obstruction.
- Fibrous adhesions leading to intestinal obstruction.
- Perforation of the bowel by the deep fissured ulcers causing intra-abdominal abscesses.
- Perianal fistulae, fissures and abscesses.
- Increased incidence of carcinoma of the bowel after many years.
- Rarely there can be significant bleeding from areas of ulceration.

The natural history of Crohn's disease is one of remissions and relapses of inflammation, punctuated by complications caused by bowel disease. Surgery is often required to relieve intestinal obstruction and to close fistulae. Crohn's

disease is also characterized by systemic complications similar to those seen in ulcerative colitis (see page 259).

Ulcerative colitis affects the rectum and variable amounts of colon

Ulcerative colitis starts at the rectum (proctitis) and may extend for a variable distance around the colon. In the most extensive disease the whole colonic mucosa is affected. Patients typically develop diarrhea, the feces being mixed with blood, mucus and pus.

There are three clinical patterns of disease:

1 In **active acute disease** the mucosa in the rectum and affected colon shows areas of shallow ulceration, which become confluent (*Fig. 13.10*). In contrast with Crohn's disease, ulceration does not extend through

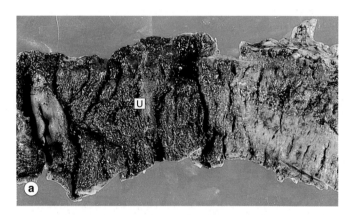

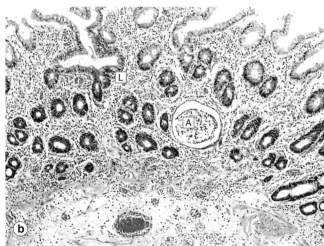

Fig. 13.10 Active ulcerative colitis.
In active disease (a) the ulcerated areas (**U**) are hemorrhagic, leading to bloody diarrhea. Intact mucosa remains as islands sitting above areas of ulceration (pseudopolyps). Histology of the intact mucosa (b) shows edema and an increase in numbers of lymphoid cells and plasma cells in lamina propria (**L**). Neutrophils are seen in lamina propria as well as in gland epithelium. Neutrophils migrate through the walls of glands to form collections, termed **crypt abscesses** (**A**), in the gland lumen. There is depletion of goblet cells and mucin from gland epithelium.

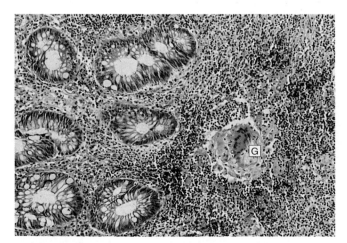

Fig. 13.9 Crohn's disease histology.
The inflammation in the wall is composed of lymphoid cells, macrophages and plasma cells. Small non-caseating granulomas (**G**), which occur in about 70% of cases, may be seen in any layer of the bowel, e.g. mucosa.

the muscularis mucosae, and inflammation is limited to the mucosa and lamina propria.

2 In **chronic quiescent or treated disease** ulceration is not prominent and the mucosa appears red, granular and thinned. Biopsy reveals chronic inflammation.

3 In **fulminant active disease** the colon shows extensive confluent mucosal ulceration. Edema and inflammation extend into the muscle layer of the colon, which progressively dilates (toxic dilatation – 'acute toxic megacolon').

Ulcerative colitis is complicated by bleeding and risk of development of fulminant disease

Ulcerative colitis has local as well as systemic effects. The direct local complications of ulcerative colitis include blood

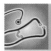

Systemic complications of ulcerative colitis

- Erythema nodosum
- Pyoderma gangrenosum
- Iritis
- Arthropathy of large joints
- Sacroiliitis
- Ankylosing spondylitis
- Chronic liver disease (4%)

Etiology of ulcerative colitis

The etiology of ulcerative colitis is unknown, but several hypotheses have been advanced, none of which is fully substantiated.

- **Psychosomatic cause.** Stress is believed to exacerbate disease in some individuals.
- **Infective cause.** Some evidence suggests that adhesive forms of enteropathogenic *E. coli* may trigger episodes of inflammation.
- **Immunological cause.** Lymphoid cells participate in inflammation.

Autoantibodies and immune complexes have been reported in some cases, but their role is uncertain. Steroids are effective in treatment of disease, suggesting that immune activation is important.

A unifying explanation is that some sort of infection triggers an inappropriate autoimmune response, which leads to destruction of colonic mucosa.

and fluid loss from extensive ulceration, both of which may be severe. Acute disease may progress rapidly to toxic dilatation and perforation and, in long-standing disease, dysplasia and neoplastic change may occur.

The systemic complications of ulcerative colitis are listed in the blue box.

The natural history of ulcerative colitis can be divided into three main patterns:

- 10% of patients develop severe disease requiring early surgery.
- 10% of patients have persistent active disease despite treatment.
- 80% of patients have chronic quiescent colitis with infrequent episodes of relapse.

In establishing a diagnosis, ulcerative colitis must be distinguished from infective colitis, Crohn's disease, ischemic colitis, and proctitis caused by sexually transmitted diseases.

Long-standing extensive ulcerative colitis predisposes to colon cancer

In chronic ulcerative colitis, regenerative changes in the rectal mucosa lead to development of dysplasia and to a risk of development of carcinoma of the colon (see page 261), which is related to extent of disease (high risk for total colitis) and duration of illness (high risk for disease of over 10 years' duration). Patients in whom disease is limited to the left side of the colon are at small risk of developing cancer.

It has been recommended that all patients over the age of 50 with total colitis should have regular screening colonoscopy every 2 years, and rectal biopsy every 6 months, to detect dysplastic changes.

TUMORS OF THE SMALL AND LARGE INTESTINE

Primary tumors of the small intestine are rare

The small intestine rarely develops primary tumors, but among those that do arise are **stromal tumors**; in particular, leiomyoma or lipoma may develop in the small bowel wall. Malignant smooth-muscle tumors (leiomyosarcomas) may also occur. An important complication of smooth-muscle or lipomatous tumors of the small intestinal wall is intussusception (see page 270).

Carcinoid (neuroendocrine) tumors, derived from the neuroendocrine cells in the small intestinal crypts, are most common in the jejunum and ileum (see page 264).

Malignant lymphomas, derived from mucosa-associated lymphoid tissue of the small bowel, are usually B-cell lymphomas. Celiac disease is a major predisposing factor in T cell lymphomas in the small bowel. Tumors may be multifocal, and spread is to local lymph nodes.

Primary adenocarcinoma of the small bowel is very rare. It usually presents as an ulcerating strictured lesion, producing small bowel obstruction. An occasional site for adenocarcinomas in the small intestine is the ampulla of Vater, the point at which the biliary and pancreatic drainage enters the duodenum.

Tumors of the large bowel are extremely common

The colon and rectum are frequently affected by both benign and malignant tumors.

- The most important and common tumors are derived from the surface epithelium of the bowel, forming **adenomata** and **carcinomas** of the colon.
- **Hyperplastic polyps** are small, flat, pale lesions, typically 5 mm in size, which occur most commonly in the rectum and sigmoid colon. They are considered to be a regenerative phenomenon and are non-neoplastic.
- **Hamartomatous polyps** occur in childhood and adolescence.
- **Neuroendocrine tumors** (carcinoid tumors) of the

large bowel occur, similar to those seen in the small bowel (see page 264).
- **Lymphomas** of the large bowel may arise, particularly in the ileocecal region, but are uncommon.
- **Stromal tumors** derived from smooth muscle, adipose tissue or Schwann cells occur, but are uncommon.

Adenomata of the large bowel appear as polyps

Adenomata derived from the glandular epithelium of the large bowel manifest as one of three different patterns of polyp (*Fig. 13.11*), categorized as **tubular**, **villous** or **tubulovillous**. Such polyps are important because they frequently develop into a carcinoma. There is much evidence to suggest that most carcinomas of the colon develop from previous adenomata, and the well-established progression from adenoma to carcinoma is the basis of the **polyp–cancer sequence** for development of carcinoma of the colon. The risk of malignant change is greatest where large lesions are present.

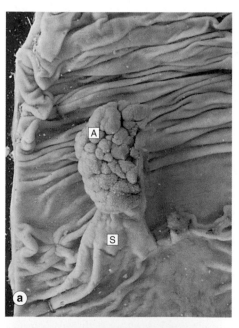

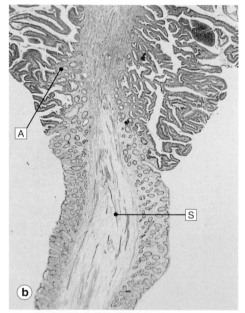

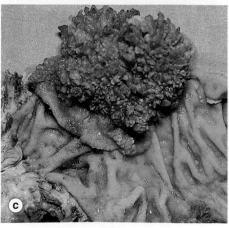

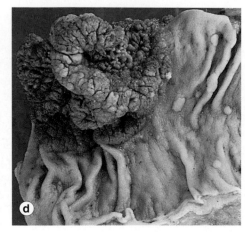

Fig. 13.11 Patterns of colonic adenoma.

(a) and (b) Tubular adenomata (**A**) are rounded lesions, 0.5–2 cm in size. They are generally red and sit on a stalk (**S**) of normal mucosa, which has been dragged up by traction of the polyp in the bowel lumen. Histologically they are composed of tubular-shaped glands. (c) Villous adenomata are frond-like lesions, about 0.6 cm thick, which occupy a broad area of mucosa, generally 1–5 cm in diameter. Rare lesions occupy very large areas of the whole circumference of the bowel. They have a velvety red appearance and, histologically, are composed of finger-like epithelial projections. (d) Tubulovillous adenomata are raised lesions, generally 1–4 cm in size. They are red and sit on a stalk of normal mucosa. Histologically they show a component identical to that of the tubular adenoma but also have a surface villous pattern that occupies between 25 and 50% of the lesion. This distinction is arbitrary as many tubular adenomata have a minor villous pattern but, by convention, are excluded from this category. Likewise, villous lesions may have a significant tubular pattern, but are excluded from a tubulovillous category if more than 50% of the lesion is villous.

Adenocarcinoma of the colon is common and may be sporadic or hereditary

Carcinoma of the colon is the second most common cause of death from neoplasia. These tumors are adenocarcinomas derived from the glandular epithelium of the large bowel mucosa.

The epidemiology of carcinoma of the colon shows great geographic variation, which has been related to environmental factors rather than genetic factors in local populations. Although there has been great interest in the role of dietary fats, fibre, processed sugar, and bile acids, none has been conclusively shown to be important in pathogenesis.

At the current level of knowledge there appear to be three types:

- Adenocarcinoma associated with familial adenomatous polyposis (FAP).
- Hereditary non-polyposis colorectal carcinoma (HNCPP).
- Sporadic colon cancer.

Carcinoma of the colon has a peak incidence in those aged between 60 and 70 years, and is rare under the age of 40. When young individuals develop the disease, inflammatory bowel disease or a genetic predisposition should be suspected.

Familial adenomatous polyposis (FAP) is an important predisposing factor to colon cancer development

Familial adenomatous polyposis is a rare autosomal dominant condition in which large numbers of adenomatous polyps develop in the colon and rectum (*Fig. 13.12*). They may begin to develop in childhood, and by the age of 30–40 years there are hundreds, of varying sizes, throughout the entire length of colon and rectum. Inevitably, one or more of these many polyps will convert into an invasive adenocarcinoma by the age of 45. Hence patients with this condition develop adenocarcinomas (often multiple) on average 20–30 years before the sporadic cases. Development of adenocarcinoma can only be prevented by a policy of frequent surveillance with removal of the entire colon at an appropriate time.

FAP and other forms of inherited polyposis syndromes are listed in *Fig. 13.13*.

FAP has been found to be associated with a mutation in a tumor suppressor gene located on the long arm of chromosome 5 (5q21); this gene is known as the APC gene (adenomatous polyposis coli gene) and mutations can be detected in screening programmes to provide early diagnosis before the polyps form.

Hereditary non-polyposis colorectal cancer (HNPCC) is much more common than FAP-associated cancer

This condition is also inherited in an autosomal dominant pattern, and is associated with an increased incidence of adenocarcinomas in the ovary, endometrium and stomach.

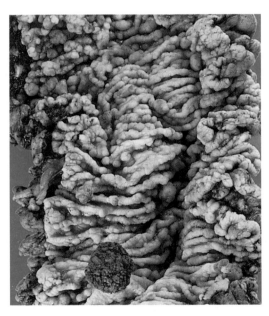

Fig. 13.12 Polyposis coli.
In polyposis coli huge numbers of adenomatous polyps develop in the large bowel. They range from a few millimeters to several centimeters in size.

Fig. 13.13 Inherited polyposis syndromes		
Name	**Clinical features**	**Carcinoma risk**
Familial adenomatous polyposis	Adenomata in colon and rectum	High risk of carcinoma
Gardner's syndrome	Adenomata in colon, rectum, as well as small bowel Osteomas of bones Soft tissue tumors	High risk of carcinoma
Peutz–Jeghers syndrome	Hamartomas in small bowel, colon, and stomach Pigmented lesions around the mouth	Small risk of carcinomas

Around 90% of carriers will develop colon cancer in their lifetime and, like FAP-associated colon cancer, the tumors develop, on average 20–30 years before the sporadic cases. It is much more common than FAP, and estimates of the frequency in the USA range from 1–5%. The colon cancers which develop in patients with this inherited tendency are often poorly differentiated and highly aggressive, with a tendency to produce large quantities of extracellular mucin ('mucoid adenocarcinoma').

Currently, four gene mutations have been identified in this condition, all involving DNA mismatch repair genes. The two most important are mutations in hMSH2 on chromosome 2p (6%) and hMLH1 on chromosome 3p (30%). Screening for these and the two other, rarer, gene mutations in people with a strong family history of colorectal cancer enables carriers to be identified and placed under regular surveillance to detect colorectal abnormalities at an early stage.

Even 'sporadic' colon cancer may have a genetic basis

Studies on sporadic colon cancers show a mixture of gene abnormalities. For example, 35–65% of non-hereditary colon cancers show allelic loss of 5q21 (APC gene), and another gene, MCC (mutated in colorectal carcinoma), which is a tumor suppressor gene, is inactivated in 15% of tumors. These gene abnormalities are noted at the 'early adenoma' stage in the adenoma–carcinoma sequence, and it is believed that a further series of gene abnormalities, e.g. activation of *K-ras* oncogene, deletion of p53 tumor suppressor gene, etc, eventually lead to the development of invasive carcinoma. Mutations in mismatch repair genes (MMR) are also often detected in sporadic colon cancer cases.

Colorectal carcinoma has several morphological patterns

There are several well-recognized morphological types of carcinoma of the colon and rectum, each associated with different clinical patterns of presentation. The main presenting features are attributable to obstruction (colicky abdominal pain and distension with later vomiting) or blood loss (acute or chronic bleeding leading to development of anemia).

- 50% of tumors occur in the rectum and sigmoid.
- 30% of tumors occur in the cecum and right colon.
- 20% of tumors occur in the descending and transverse colon.

Because the feces is fluid in the right side of the colon, a lesion may grow to a large size before causing obstruction. **Carcinomas of the right side** are mainly large, polypoid exophytic lesions, which grow into the lumen of the bowel. **Carcinomas of the left side** cause obstruction early because the feces is more solid. Left-sided lesions are of two main types: anular carcinomas, which are small but cause stenosis; and ulcerating tumors, which present mainly with bleeding.

Macroscopic and histological appearances of colorectal carcinoma are shown in *Fig. 13.14*. On the basis of cytological and architectural features, lesions can be graded from well differentiated through to poorly differentiated. As poorly differentiated lesions frequently present at an advanced stage of disease, they are associated with a poorer prognosis. Lesions that display a vigorous lymphocytic inflammatory response at the invasive edge of the tumor are thought to have a better prognosis than lesions with no host response.

Spread of carcinoma of the colon is by three main routes. There is **local spread** through the bowel wall, when invasion of the serosa of adjacent bowel or bladder may occur; **lymphatic spread** to draining nodes; and **blood spread** to the liver and other sites such as lung.

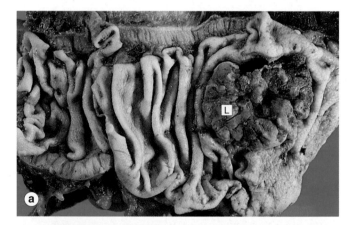

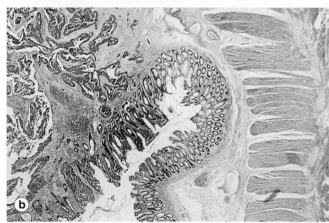

Fig. 13.14 Morphology of adenocarcinoma of the colon. Macroscopically carcinomas are raised red lesions (**L**) with a rolled edge (a) and frequent central ulceration. Lesions are composed of solid, white tissue, and invasion into the wall of the bowel may be seen. Histologically (b), the majority of lesions have a glandular pattern composed of pleomorphic neoplastic epithelial cells.

Infiltrative carcinoma of the colon is a rare pattern caused by signet-ring cell carcinoma that is virtually identical to that seen in the stomach. It is often associated with carcinoma that develops in association with inflammatory bowel disease.

Prognosis of carcinoma of the colon is related to stage

The prognosis of carcinoma of the colon is related to the stage of disease, which is assessed using a modification of a staging system originally proposed for carcinoma of the rectum by Dukes (*Fig. 13.15*). Following surgical resection, it is particularly important to determine adequacy of resection margins, particularly lateral extension to pelvic side wall or adjacent structures, which is associated with a poor outcome.

Dukes' stage	Tumor spread	5-year survival
A	Not extending through muscularis propria	> 90%
B	Extending through muscularis propria NODES UNINVOLVED	70%
C	Any involvement of bowel wall NODES INVOLVED	30%
D	Distant metastases	5–10%

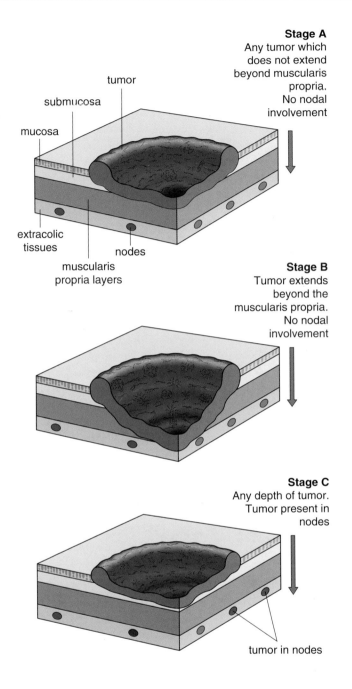

Stage A
Any tumor which does not extend beyond muscularis propria. No nodal involvement

Stage B
Tumor extends beyond the muscularis propria. No nodal involvement

Stage C
Any depth of tumor. Tumor present in nodes

tumor in nodes

Fig. 13.15 Staging of carcinoma of the colon.
Dukes' staging is shown here in its most simple and widely used form. Many modifications are in use, and some workers split stage B into B1 (extending into muscle) and B2 (extending through muscle); likewise, C1 (limited to wall with involved nodes) and C2 (through wall with involved nodes). It is important to check which modification of Dukes' staging is locally in use to avoid misunderstandings.

Molecular pathology of colonic epithelial neoplasms

As with many tumors, a sequence of molecular events in oncogenes has been identified in colonic epithelial malignancies, which seems to relate to progression of lesions from adenomata through to invasive carcinomas. Adenomata show few molecular changes, whereas advanced carcinomas have many oncogene abnormalities:

- *K-ras* on chromosome 12 is activated.

- Loss of the APC gene on chromosome 5.
- Loss of p53 from chromosome 17.
- Loss of DCC gene (deleted in colon cancer), a tumor suppressor gene, from chromosome 18.

The APC gene is lost in many sporadic carcinomas, although this is a primary gene defect in cases associated with familial adenomatosis coli (page 261).

Neuroendocrine tumors occur throughout the gut

Tumors derived from the neuroendocrine cells of the gut (carcinoid tumors) occur most commonly in the appendix and small bowel, but also arise in the stomach, colon, rectum, and esophagus. The biological behavior of the tumor appears to differ according to the site.

Lesions in the small bowel, colon and stomach are slow-growing, low-grade, and malignant (*Fig. 13.16*). Some are multicentric. Tumors appear as yellow mucosal or mural masses, and metastasis is most commonly via the portal vein to the liver.

Lesions in the rectum and appendix almost never metastasize, appearing as tumor nodules composed of firm, yellow tissue.

A small proportion of lesions in the esophagus appear as small-cell anaplastic carcinomas that are histologically identical to oat-cell carcinoma of the lung.

Depending on the nature of the neuroendocrine cells in the tumor, patients may develop a syndrome caused by hormone secretion. Some of these tumors secrete 5-hydroxytryptamine (5-HT), and its breakdown product, 5-hydroxyindolacetic acid (5-HIAA), can be detected in excess in the urine. Hepatic metastasis can produce the carcinoid syndrome, with symptoms due to excessive secretion of 5-HT (particularly facial flushing, bronchospasm and diarrhea). Tumors secreting gastrin may stimulate excess gastric acid secretion, causing peptic ulceration (Zollinger–Ellison syndrome).

VASCULAR DISEASE OF THE BOWEL

Vascular diseases of the intestine may affect small or large bowel

Interruption of the blood supply to the small bowel is most commonly seen in elderly patients with severe atherosclerosis. The arterial occlusion can be due to:

- **Emboli from intracardiac thrombosis**. Mural thrombus following a myocardial infarct, thrombotic vegetations on mitral or aortic valves, or left atrial thrombosis. The emboli lodge in the superior mesenteric artery, which supplies the entire small intestine apart from the first part of the duodenum. The extent of the bowel infarction depends upon whether the occlusion is in a proximal or distal branch (*Fig. 13.17*).

- **Thrombosis in severely atherosclerotic mesenteric artery**. This is less common than embolic occlusion but, when it occurs, it is usually located in the proximal part of the superior mesenteric artery, shortly after its origin from the aorta; the small bowel infarction is extensive and usually fatal.

- **Venous infarction due to strangulation**. Venous infarction results from occlusion of the thin-walled

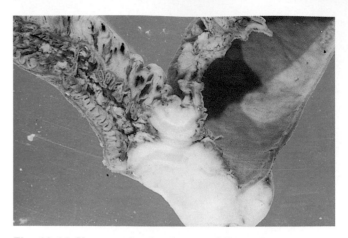

Fig. 13.16 Neuroendocrine tumor of the gut.
This is a carcinoid tumor of the ileum. It appears as a yellowish/white mural nodule and, in this instance, caused intestinal obstruction. Histologically tumors are composed of cords and nests of cells that contain neurosecretory granules best detected by immunochemical and ultrastructural techniques.

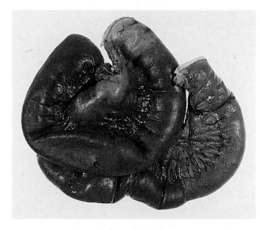

Fig. 13.17 Small bowel infarction.
This segment of small bowel was surgically resected after infarction caused by an embolus from mural thrombus in the heart. The infarcted bowel is dilated and almost black in colour.

veins draining blood from the small bowel, and is usually due to extrinsic pressure. The bowel becomes deeply congested with venous blood, which is unable to drain out. This, in turn, prevents entry of oxygenated arterial blood, so that ischemic necrosis of the bowel wall ensues. In the small intestine this pattern of venous infarction due to strangulation results from strangulation of a loop of bowel in a narrow **hernial sac** (*Fig. 13.18*), **intussusception** or, occasionally, **volvulus**. In volvulus a loop of bowel twists on itself, usually in association with fibrous peritoneal adhesions which, in turn, are usually the result of previous abdominal surgery.

- **Neonatal necrotizing enterocolitis** is discussed on page 270.

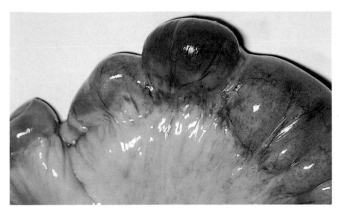

Fig. 13.18 Necrosis of bowel wall in hernia.
A segment of small bowel has been entrapped in a hernial sac. It has been strangulated, undergoing ischemic discoloration and incipient necrosis.

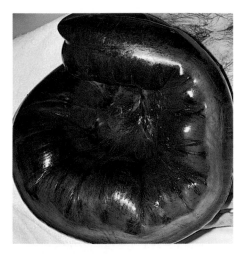

Fig. 13.19 Sigmoid volvulus.
This patient died as a result of twisting of the sigmoid colon causing venous congestion and necrosis. The affected sigmoid is greatly dilated and a dark plum colour as a result of venous infarction.

In the colon, acute ischemia is usually the result of volvulus, particularly in the sigmoid colon, where there is a large redundant sigmoid loop which twists upon itself to produce torsion of the mesentery (*Fig. 13.19*); volvulus of the cecum is usually secondary to a highly mobile cecum.

Chronic ischemic large bowel disease is most common in the elderly, but can occasionally occur in young people. Ischemic loss of the mucosa produces ulceration in the acute phase, and healing is followed by submucosal fibrosis and disruption of the fibers of the muscularis mucosae. There is frequently a chronic inflammatory infiltrate in the submucosa, in which macrophages filled with hemosiderin are a common feature. These features form the entity known as **ischemic colitis**. Fibrosis at the site of ischemia may result in stricture formation. The most common site is around the splenic flexure, at the overlap between vascular territories.

Localized ischemia in the rectal mucosa may be produced in the **mucosal prolapse syndrome** or **solitary ulcer syndrome**. Mucosal prolapse into the anal sphincter causes ischemic damage to the mucosa.

Angiodysplasia is a cause of large intestinal bleeding

Angiodysplasia is a condition in which abnormal vascular channels develop in the submucosa of the large bowel. The condition occurs in the elderly and is a cause of either occult or massive intestinal bleeding.

Clinical diagnosis is based on suspicion and is confirmed by angiography. Surgical resection of the affected bowel segment is required for treatment, and pathological diagnosis is assisted by radiographic examination of specimens after perfusion of vessels with contrast medium.

DISEASES CAUSED BY ABNORMAL GUT MOTILITY

Diverticular disease results in mucosal outpouches in the distal colon

Diverticular disease causes herniation of the mucosa of the colon through the muscularis propria, producing outpouches of the bowel lumen. There is thickening of the muscularis propria (*Fig. 13.20*).

Complications are related to stagnation of contents of the diverticula, with secondary inflammation. Acute diverticulitis is the result of acute inflammation of a diverticulum. Hemorrhage may result or the diverticulum may rupture, leading to peritonitis or the development of a paracolic abscess.

Chronic inflammation may occur, with walling off of an area of inflammation by fibrous tissue. The resulting scarring and inflammatory changes form a **diverticular mass**, which may cause large bowel obstruction and may mimic the appearances of a carcinoma of the colon on imaging.

The pathogenesis of diverticular disease has been related to abnormally high intraluminal pressure in the colon, caused by abnormal contractility of the muscularis propria. The abnormal contractility is responsible for the muscle hypertrophy. Mucosal herniation occurs at sites of penetration of the muscularis propria by blood vessels supplying the colon, along lines between the tenia coli (longitudinal muscle layers).

Intestinal pseudo-obstruction is caused by defective bowel motility

Intestinal pseudo-obstruction is manifest by abdominal pain and distension, and is caused by abnormal gut motility rather than an organic obstructive lesion.

- Primary causes, which are rare, are due to abnormalities of smooth muscle or nerve plexuses in the gut.

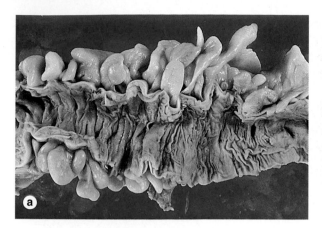

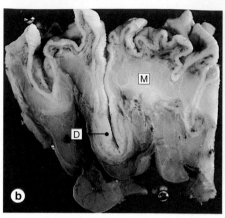

Fig. 13.20
Diverticular disease.
In diverticular disease, the outpouches of mucosa seen in the sigmoid colon appear as slit-like openings from the mucosal surface of the opened bowel (a). On sectioning the bowel (b), the diverticula (**D**) extend through the thickened muscularis propria (**M**).

KEY FACTS
Strictures in the colon

The main causes of narrowing of the colon, resulting in a stricture are:

- Carcinoma of the colon.
- Diverticular disease.
- Ischemic fibrosis caused by ischemic colitis.

- Secondary causes are common and include connective tissue diseases, particularly scleroderma, diabetic neuropathy, and amyloidosis of the gut.

Melanosis coli is associated with chronic laxative use

Patients who take laxatives for constipation sometimes develop black coloration of the mucosa of the large bowel, termed 'melanosis coli'. Histologically this is seen as accumulation of pigment-laden macrophages in the lamina propria of the colon (*Fig. 13.21*).

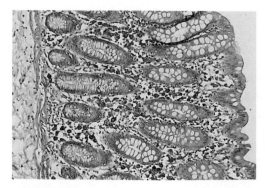

Fig. 13.21 Melanosis coli.
In melanosis coli the bowel mucosa is macroscopically black. Histologically there is accumulation of brown pigment in macrophages in the lamina propria. The pigment is *not* melanin but is a form of lipofuscin.

PATHOLOGY OF THE APPENDIX

Acute appendicitis results in severe acute inflammation of the appendix

Acute appendicitis is a common cause of abdominal pain. A predisposing factor is obstruction of the lumen of the appendix, sometimes by a fecolith, but such obstruction is not seen in all cases. The stages in the development of acute appendicitis are shown in *Fig. 13.22*.

The complications of acute appendicitis are:

- Necrosis of appendix wall (**gangrenous appendicitis**), leading to perforation, with subsequent generalized peritonitis.
- Involvement of adjacent bowel loops, causing perforation of small bowel.
- The omentum may become adherent, localizing the peritonitis to the right iliac fossa. Fibrosis and continued inflammation cause development of a mass in the right iliac fossa (**appendix mass**). This may resolve with scarring, may form an abscess that drains to the surface, or may rupture, with development of generalized peritonitis.
- Spread of infection by portal vein branches may propagate to the liver; this was formerly an important cause of portal pyemic abscesses in the liver.

Mucocele of the appendix is caused by obstruction of the lumen

A mucocele of the appendix is cystic dilatation of the appendix lumen, which contains clear mucus. There is fibrosis in the wall, and the lining is replaced by a layer of mucin-secreting goblet cells. This is caused by blockage of the proximal end of the appendix, most commonly the result of a previous episode of acute appendicitis.

Tumors of the appendix are uncommon

Adenocarcinoma of the appendix is rare. However, adeno-carcinoma of the cecum that extends into the proximal part

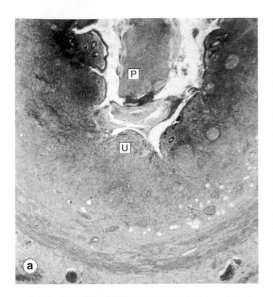

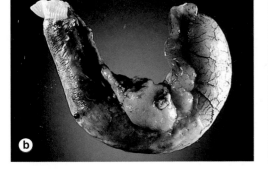

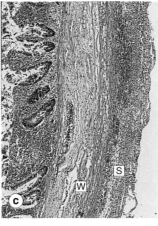

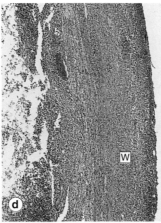

Fig. 13.22 Acute appendicitis.
In early acute appendicitis (a) there is acute inflammation of the mucosa of the appendix which undergoes ulceration (**U**). Pus (**P**) may be present in the lumen. At this stage the patient experiences an ill-defined central abdominal pain. Macroscopically (b) the appendix is usually swollen and serosal vessels are dilated. As the acute inflammation develops (c), it spreads through the full thickness of the appendix wall (**W**) to reach the serosal surface (**S**). This causes a localized acute peritonitis, which is perceived as a sharp pain, localized to the right iliac fossa. Macroscopically the appendix shows dilated serosal vessels and a rough, yellow, fibrinous exudate in the surface. If the appendicitis progresses (d), there is necrosis of the wall (**W**) of the appendix (**gangrenous appendicitis**). The muscle layer is replaced by an acute inflammatory infiltrate and necrotic muscle. The resulting weakness leads to appendix perforation, liberating bowel contents into the peritoneal cavity. This causes a generalized peritonitis and leads to a severe deterioration in clinical condition. Macroscopically the appendix is typically plum-colored or black, and a site of perforation may be seen.

An appendix mass may be caused by several disease processes

A mass localized to the region of the right iliac fossa and involving the ileum, cecum and appendix may be caused by several disease processes.

Inflammatory mass:
- Acute appendicitis
- *Yersinia* infection
- Ileocecal *Actinomyces* infection
- Ileocecal tuberculosis

Tumor mass:
- Cecal carcinoma
- Lymphoma
- Carcinoid tumor

of the appendix is not infrequent, and may be a cause of acute appendicitis in the elderly.

Carcinoid tumors may occur at the tip of the appendix and have an excellent prognosis, almost never metastasizing, mainly because of early detection.

DISEASES OF THE ANAL CANAL

The anal canal is lined by non-keratinizing squamous mucosa, and opens to the exterior at the anal orifice where the squamous epithelium becomes skin with keratinizing epidermis and skin appendages such as hair follicles and sweat glands.

Itching ('pruritus ani') and soreness are common anal symptoms in family practice

There are many causes of an itching anus, many of which are the result of skin diseases such as eczema and contact dermatitis affecting the anal region. An allergic reaction to topical applications such as anesthetic creams, deodorants, etc, is a common cause in adults, and these may also cause soreness and weeping of the skin. In children, itching and soreness around the anus should always raise suspicion of pinworm (see page 139) infestation; the tiny worms may be visible on the perianal skin, particularly at night. Perianal soreness is a common transient symptom following acute diarrhea, but only persistent soreness requires medical investigation. Rare skin diseases such as Hailey–Hailey disease, etc, may also occur in perianal skin, and often present as sore, swollen, red and weeping perianal skin. These may be the presenting symptoms of anal fissures and fistulas. Soreness and pain are the symptoms of the commonest anal problem, hemorrhoids, which are due to varicose dilatation of the submucosal venous plexuses in the anal canal with prolapse, often producing tender palpable masses protruding through the anus. Thrombosis in these is often associated with acute pain.

Infections may involve either perianal skin or the anal canal

In the perianal skin, the most common infections are fungal, mainly *Candida*, usually by local extension of Candidal infection of the vulva and perineum, particularly in diabetic women. Infection with human papilloma virus may produce perianal fleshy warts (condyloma acuminata); the highly infectious fleshy perianal warts due to *Treponema pallidum* infection in secondary syphilis are now rarely seen.

The commonest cause of infection inside the anal canal is as the result of sexually transmitted diseases, mainly in homosexual males. Gonorrhea and amebic infections are important in this group, and primary syphilitic chancres still occasionally occur.

Infection occurring in a perianal gland, the drainage neck of which is blocked, may eventually lead to a large pus-filled **ischio-rectal abscess** which requires drainage.

Anal fissure and anal fistula are common and important causes of persistent anal pain and discharge

An anal fissure is a triangular-shaped area of ulceration and inflammation at the lower end of the anal canal and mainly involving the anal mucosa, though associated inflammation may spread to the perianal skin. They are mostly located in the posterior half of the anus. Pain is particularly severe on defecation. The cause is not known in most cases and the histological features are those of chronic ulceration with inflammation.

An anal fistula is an abnormal tract running between the anal canal at the pectinate line, passing through the perianal tissues, either ending as a blind tract in the perianal connective tissue, or opening to the exterior at the perianal skin. The tract is surrounded by severe chronic inflammation, and parts of the fistula tract may contain remnants of inflamed epithelium. Again, pain is most severe on defecation.

Crohn's disease involving the colon is an important cause of both persistent anal fissure and anal fistula; anal involvement also occurs where the disease is limited to the small bowel, but it is far less common. In cases where fissure and fistula are due to Crohn's disease, the diagnosis can sometimes be made histologically by the presence of giant cell histiocytic granulomas in the chronic inflammatory tissue nearby, but foreign body giant cells are also often found when the lesions are not associated with Crohn's disease; the presence of distinct well-formed granulomas are the characteristic feature of Crohn's, not just the presence of giant cells.

The commonest tumor of the anus is squamous cell carcinoma

Squamous carcinomas at the anus may originate either in the perianal skin (in which case they are usually well differentiated and keratinizing) or from the lining of the anal canal (when they may be non-keratinizing and less well differentiated). Perianal skin carcinomas are more common in men, and tend to metastasize to inguinal lymph nodes, whereas squamous carcinomas of the anal canal are most common in women and spread to superior hemorrhoidal and lateral pelvic wall lymph nodes, as well as spreading locally into the soft tissues around the anal canal.

Carcinoma *in situ* of the perianal skin (**anal intraepithelial neoplasia – AIN**) presents as a red scaly or weeping patch in perianal skin: it often represents local extension from similar intraepithelial neoplasia affecting the perineum and vulva (VIN – see page 398). Extramammary Paget's disease (adenocarcinoma cells invading the epidermis – see page 428) may also affect perianal skin, and clinically resembles AIN.

PATHOLOGY OF THE PERITONEUM

Peritonitis may be acute or chronic

Inflammation of the peritoneal cavity (peritonitis) may be acute or chronic. Acute peritonitis is most commonly caused by extension of inflammatory processes in the abdominal cavity, particularly after perforation of the gut. Less commonly, peritonitis may be a primary infection, seen in patients with nephrotic syndrome and cirrhosis.

Histologically there is acute inflammation of the peritoneum, with fibrinous and purulent exudation. Inflammation of the serosa of the small bowel causes paralysis of gut motility, leading to dilatation, termed **ileus**. Peritonitis may be localized by adherent loops of bowel and adherence of the omentum. Organization of fibrinous adhesion by granulation tissue leads to **adhesions** by fibrous tissue. Localization of infection in the peritoneal cavity may form local abscesses, particularly in the paracolic gutters and beneath the diaphragm (subphrenic abscesses).

Chronic peritonitis may be caused by infection with tuberculosis. Granulomatous inflammation leads to organization and fibrosis, with adhesions between bowel loops (plastic peritonitis). In patients treated by ambulatory peritoneal dialysis, there may be a chronic, low-grade peritonitis caused by a mixed flora of organisms.

Peritoneal tumors are most commonly the result of metastatic spread

The peritoneal cavity is most commonly affected by metastatic tumors that have spread from one of the abdominal organs, the main primary sites being stomach, ovary, uterus and colon. Deposits of metastatic tumor are seen as small nodules seeding the peritoneum, which often cause thickening of the omentum. In disseminated mucin-secreting carcinomas the peritoneal cavity may be filled with mucinous material (pseudomyxoma peritonei). Tumors may grow as larger nodules and cause adhesions between bowel loops, resulting in bowel obstruction. Infiltration of tumor in the peritoneum may also cause accumulation of fluid in the peritoneal cavity in the form of **ascites**.

Malignant mesotheliomas may develop as primary malignant tumors of the peritoneum. As with the pleural tumors (see page 220), these are also predisposed by exposure to asbestos. Tumor causes massive thickening of the peritoneum, leading to bowel obstruction and ascites.

Accumulation of fluid in the peritoneal cavity is termed 'ascites'

The principal causes of ascites are inflammation causing peritonitis, neoplasia in the peritoneal cavity, and increased transudation of fluid from vessels due to increased pressure in the portal venous system. The main cause of this increased pressure is cirrhosis of the liver (see page 293), portal vein thrombosis, or hepatic vein thrombosis (Budd–Chiari syndrome).

GASTROINTESTINAL DISEASE IN CHILDREN

Developmental abnormalities of the bowel

The most common congenital malformations affecting the alimentary tract are:

- **Esophageal atresia with tracheo-esophageal fistula.** The most common pattern is that in which the upper end of the esophagus is intact but ends in a blind pouch (see *Fig. 5.7*). There is a central area of complete atresia and the lower esophagus is normal at the gastro-esophageal junction, but tapers proximally and communicates with the trachea.
- **Omphalocele** is the result of failure of the intestine to return to the abdominal cavity during normal rotation of the mid-gut. Development of the whole gut outside the abdominal cavity is termed 'eventration'.
- **Gastroschisis** is due to a defect in the anterior abdominal wall, resulting in protrusion of the viscera into the amniotic cavity.
- **Failure of rotation of the gut** as it returns to the abdomen causes several patterns of malformation. In non-rotation, the small bowel lies on the right of the abdomen, and the colon on the left. Other forms of malrotation lead to obstruction of bowel by twisting of the gut on itself (**volvulus**).

- **Intestinal atresia** is most common in the ileum, but also occurs higher in the bowel in the duodenum. It causes intestinal obstruction.
- **Meckel's diverticulum** is caused by an abnormality of the yolk stalk (*Fig. 13.23*). Other degrees of abnormality result in tethering of the ileum to the umbilicus by a fibrous band, development of a cyst in the fibrous band, or persistence of a sinus track between the ileum and the umbilicus.
- **Intestinal duplications** are caused by developmental abnormalities of canalization of the gut. There are two patterns: **closed cystic duplications** (most common) and **communicating tubular duplications** (unusual).
- **Imperforate anus** is more common in males than in females, and is often associated with other abnormalities. The anal canal may end blindly or, more often, opens into the urethra or vagina. A more common form is **anorectal agenesis**, in which the rectum ends blindly above the anal canal, with a fistula into the vagina or urethra. These defects are caused by defective separation of the cloaca by the urorectal septum.

Congenital pyloric stenosis is an important and common stomach disorder in infants

In pyloric stenosis, newborn infants, usually male, present with projectile vomiting, which is the result of narrowing at

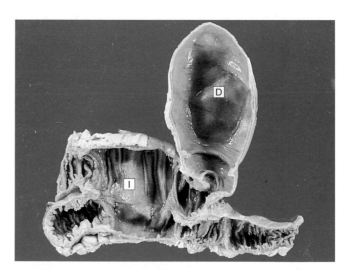

Fig. 13.23 Meckel's diverticulum.
This diverticulum (**D**) of the ileum (**I**), which occurs in 2–4% of the population, is caused by persistence of part of the yolk stalk. The diverticulum is 2–4 cm long, on the antimesenteric border of the bowel, 45 cm from the ileocecal valve. It has a muscular wall and is normally lined by small bowel epithelium, but may have gastric acid-secreting epithelium or heterotopic pancreatic tissue. If tethered to the umbilicus by a fibrous cord, the diverticulum may cause problems by acting as the apex of a volvulus. It may also be the site of inflammation similar to that seen in acute appendicitis. Alternatively, peptic ulceration may develop if acid-secreting epithelium is present.

the pylorus due to an unusually hypertrophied pyloric sphincter muscle. It occurs in about 1 in 300 live births, and is relieved by surgical transection of part of the hypertrophied pyloric sphincter muscle.

Neonatal necrotizing enterocolitis is an important type of ischemic bowel disease

Necrotizing enterocolitis affects neonatal infants and is rapidly fatal unless treated. Affected infants have bloody diarrhea and abdominal distension, often with vomiting. The bowel wall is thickened due to intense congestion, and there is extensive superficial mucosal ulceration. The pathogenesis is believed to be the result of poor perfusion of the mucosa of the bowel followed by infection.

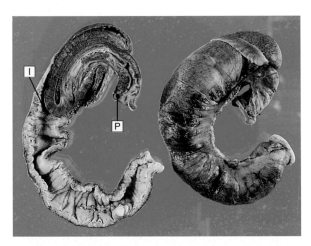

Fig. 13.24 Intussception.
This segment of bowel has invaginated in on itself. Externally the affected segment is swollen and deeply congested. On cut surface the invagination (**I**) of the bowel from the proximal end (**P**) is seen. The invaginated portion of bowel has undergone venous infarction and is deeply congested.

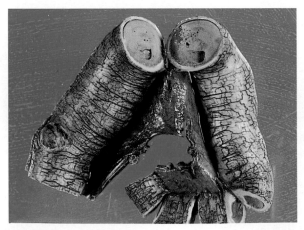

Fig. 13.25 Meconium ileus.
Microscopically the affected bowel is dilated and, on cut surface, is filled with dense gelatinous green mucoid material. Other associated complications are microcolon and intestinal atresia.

Predisposing factors are prematurity, ARDS (see page 205), Hirschsprung's disease (see page 271), and cystic fibrosis with meconium ileus.

Intussusception occurs when one segment of bowel invaginates into another

Intussusception occurs when one portion of bowel invaginates into the adjoining segment. The most common site is at the ileocecal valve, with the ileum invaginating into the cecum. This pattern is most common in children. In the rare adult cases a structural abnormality of the small intestinal wall is almost invariably responsible for precipitating the invagination, and benign tumors such as leiomyoma or lipoma are important predisposing factors.

The structural lesion is carried by peristalsis into the adjoining bowel, and the bowel segment is invaginated. This leads to venous congestion of the invaginated portion, causing bleeding from the mucosa, as well as intestinal obstruction. If the bowel remains invaginated infarction of the area takes place (*Fig. 13.24*).

Meconium ileus and rectal prolapse are manifestations of cystic fibrosis

One of the common manifestations of cystic fibrosis (see page 221) is meconium ileus, occurring in 10–20% of cases. It is caused by abnormally viscid mucin forming a mass in the bowel lumen, which cannot be expelled (*Fig. 13.25*).

Intestinal obstruction may also occur after the neonatal period, mainly due to obstruction by thick mucus at the ileocecal valve.

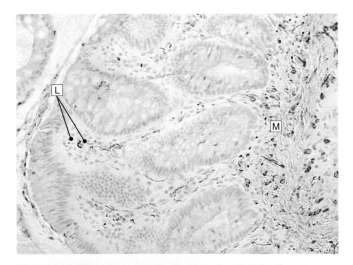

Fig. 13.26 Hirschsprung's disease (acetylcholinesterase histochemistry). In Hirschsprung's disease there is absence of normal myenteric and submucosal plexus ganglion cells. Nerve fibers in the submucosa and within the muscularis mucosa (**M**) are hypertrophied, and abnormal axons extend up into the lamina propria (**L**), visible as brown staining with histochemical stains for acetylcholinesterase.

Another common manifestation of cystic fibrosis is rectal prolapse, believed to be the result of bulky stools caused by malabsorption. Other gastrointestinal manifestations of cystic fibrosis are the result of pancreatic disease which leads to failure of the production of digestive enzymes, causing malabsorption.

Hirschsprung's disease is caused by absence of normal myenteric plexus in the bowel wall

In Hirschsprung's disease there is failure of the normal motility of the bowel due to absence of the normal myenteric plexus.

The defect always involves the rectum and may be present in continuity for a variable distance along the bowel. Some cases involve just a short segment of rectum, others the rectosigmoid segment and, in rare cases, there may be total colonic or total intestinal aganglionosis. Macroscopically the abnormally innervated bowel segment is narrowed, whereas the proximal bowel is dilated and shows hypertrophy of the muscle layers.

The disease usually presents in early childhood with failure to pass meconium or, later, with persistent constipation. Diagnosis is made by biopsy of the rectal mucosa (*Fig. 13.26*).

One form of disease is caused by mutations in the *RET* oncogene on chromosome 10. Another is linked to mutations in the endothelin-B receptor gene on chromosome 13.

Rare cases of abnormal bowel motility in childhood are caused by primary abnormalities of visceral smooth muscle (visceral myopathies) or visceral axons (visceral neuropathies).

Liver, biliary tract, and pancreas

Clinical Overview

The most frequently encountered diseases associated with the hepatobiliary system encountered in family practice are diseases of the bile duct and gallbladder, often associated with gallstones in the gallbladder or extrahepatic bile ducts. These patients present with pain beneath the right costal margin and sometimes with obstructive jaundice. Tumors of the gallbladder are rare and are usually in the elderly.

The commonest disease of the liver is associated with chronic alcoholism (**alcoholic liver disease**) which may vary in severity from mild increase in fatty change in liver cells to a chronic destructive toxic hepatitis leading eventually to the chronic liver disease, cirrhosis. Although alcohol is the most common substance to produce liver cell damage, many other toxic chemicals can produce varying degrees of liver cell damage varying from mild temporary disturbance of liver cell function (e.g. some therapeutic drugs such as methotrexate) to widespread fulminating acute fatal liver cell necrosis (e.g. an overdose of paracetamol).

Many long-term liver diseases such as alcoholic and viral hepatitis lead to the condition known as cirrhosis, in which the architecture of the various liver components is grossly distorted by destruction and fibrous scarring. This leads to progressive liver failure and portal hypertension.

The most important infections of the liver are those caused by viruses. Different hepatitis viruses cause different patterns of liver disease. Some produce acute fulminating liver cell necrosis, while others produce a more chronic progressive disease culminating in cirrhosis. Bacterial infections of the liver are uncommon. Theoretically, bacteria can gain access to the liver through the systemic arterial supply during bacteremia, through the hepatic portal venous system from a primary infected site in the gut, or by an ascending infection up the bile ducts (ascending cholangitis).

The liver is an important site of metastatic malignant tumors, important primary sites including stomach, colon, breast, bronchus and pancreas. Primary tumors of the liver parenchyma are nearly always associated with co-existing chronic cirrhosis.

The pancreas is associated with three important diseases, acute hemorrhagic pancreatitis, chronic pancreatitis, and carcinoma of the head of the pancreas.

DISEASES OF THE LIVER

Functional differences in hepatocytes exist within the hepatic lobule

All hepatocytes are not equal. Hepatocytes in different parts of the hepatic lobule have different metabolic properties, rendering each type vulnerable to different sorts of disease process.

Hepatocytes at the centre of the lobule (zone 3 of the acinus) are supplied by blood that is relatively depleted in oxygen, and these cells are most vulnerable to damage by hypoxia or poor perfusion. Hepatocytes in this central zone also have a low level of oxidative enzymes, but a high level of esterases generating metabolic intermediate substances. These are vulnerable to certain toxins, e.g. paracetamol (acetaminophen).

In contrast, hepatocytes at the periphery of the lobule (zone 1 of the acinus) are well supplied with blood and these cells resist damage by poor perfusion. Furthermore, they are not damaged by certain agents as they lack the enzymes for conversion to toxic intermediaries.

KEY FACTS
Main functions of the liver

- **Carbohydrate metabolism.** The liver is a storage site for glycogen and a main source of plasma glucose.
- **Fat metabolism.** The liver is central in the processing of dietary fats to lipoproteins, which enter the blood for peripheral metabolism.
- **Protein metabolism.** The liver is a major site of protein synthesis, particularly for plasma proteins. Important groups are albumin, coagulation factors, binding proteins for iron and copper, and certain acute-phase proteins. The liver is a major site of protein catabolism with the generation of urea. Several of the signs and symptoms of chronic liver disease are a reflection of failure of synthesis of these vital serum proteins.
- **Bile synthesis.** The liver secretes bile containing bilirubin, cholesterol, electrolytes, and bile salts. In disease, abnormal bile metabolism is the basis of jaundice.
- **Storage.** The liver stores glycogen, iron, copper, and fat-soluble vitamins, which may become pathologically excessive in disease.
- **Detoxification.** The liver detoxifies many metabolites, particularly nitrogenous compounds, hormones, and drugs.

Liver disease is manifest by four main clinical entities

The main causes of liver disease are toxins (alcohol and drug-related), infections (viruses, bacteria, parasites), disturbances of vascularity or of bile excretion, and tumors (either primary or metastatic). The resulting disease is manifest by four main clinical entities.

Acute hepatitis is seen in diseases causing necrosis of liver cells, with associated inflammation, and **chronic hepatitis** occurs when there is continued liver cell inflammation. This may be due to many causes and often results in **fibrosis**. Damage in either intrahepatic or extrahepatic bile ducts results in cholestasis.

A common end-point of long-standing liver cell destruction from any cause is the development of **cirrhosis**, in which the liver develops extensive scarring associated with nodules of regenerated liver cells. The development of this pattern of response causes distortion of liver architecture and leads to increased back-pressure in the portal blood vessels (portal hypertension) (see page 280).

Diseases of the liver usually result in abnormalities of its main functions, the most common being **jaundice**, **failure of synthesis**, and **failure of detoxification**.

Acute liver failure results in jaundice, coma, and bleeding tendency

Acute liver failure, which develops when there has been damage to the majority of hepatocytes such that liver function is critically impaired, is seen in three main clinical situations (*Fig. 14.1*):

- Following severe hepatocyte damage, e.g. as a consequence of extensive liver cell necrosis or metabolic damage.
- Following severe systemic shock as part of multiorgan failure along with ARDS and acute renal failure.
- As an acute decline in otherwise stable chronic liver disease, usually caused by chronic hepatitis (see page 287) or cirrhosis (see page 293).

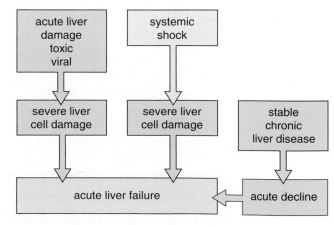

Fig. 14.1 The three main situations leading to acute liver failure.

Development of acute hepatic failure is a severe life-threatening disease, from which 80% of patients die. The features of acute liver failure are shown in *Fig. 14.2*.

JAUNDICE

Jaundice is caused by abnormalities in bilirubin metabolism and excretion

The normal metabolism of bilirubin is shown in the Key Facts box below. Abnormalities in the metabolism or excretion of bile result in development of jaundice. Biochemical jaundice can be defined as an increase in the plasma bilirubin level above the normal level of about 18–24 μmol/L (1.2 mg/dl). Clinical jaundice is evident when levels are above 50 μmol/L (2.5 mg/dl) manifesting as a yellow discoloration of the sclera and skin. Different laboratories may have different reference ranges.

Jaundice is biochemically divided into conjugated and unconjugated types

Jaundice can be caused by impaired bilirubin metabolism at several levels. It can be divided into two main biochemical types.

In **unconjugated hyperbilirubinamia** there is excessive unconjugated bilirubin in the blood. Disorders causing this pattern of disease are mainly excessive generation of bilirubin or abnormal hepatocyte metabolism, and blood levels seldom exceed 100 μmol/L.

Many disorders cause the pattern of jaundice known as **conjugated hyperbilirubinemia**, in which there is excessive conjugated bilirubin in the blood. The most common cause is obstruction of bile secretion. Disease which causes generalized damage to hepatocytes results in a predominant conjugated hyperbilirubinemia, as the main rate-limiting step in bilirubin metabolism is excretion by the canaliculi rather than conjugation. Levels often exceed 100 μmol/L.

Excessive generation of bilirubin is the most important cause of unconjugated hyperbilirubinemia

Increased bilirubin generation results from excessive destruction of red cells, the main causes of which are: hemolytic anemia (see page 320); breakdown of large hematomas; and abnormal formation of red cells (dyserythropoiesis), which is seen in megaloblastic and sideroblastic anemias (see pages 318 and 319).

The amount of bilirubin generated exceeds the capacity of the liver to conjugate and excrete it. Bilirubin circulating in the blood is unconjugated, circulates complexed to albumin, and **does not appear in the urine**. The amount of conjugated bilirubin excreted into the intestine is increased because of the increased load; some is resorbed as urobilinogen, and this is excreted in increased amounts in the urine.

Reduced uptake of bilirubin by hepatocytes can also cause unconjugated hyperbilirubinemia. This may be seen in generalized hepatocellular damage but is a less significant

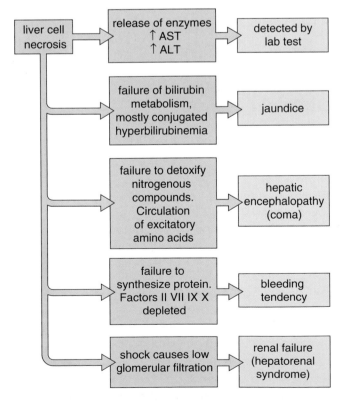

Fig. 14.2 Features of acute liver failure.

KEY FACTS
Bilirubin metabolism

- Bilirubin is derived from breakdown of hemoglobin, blood from the spleen entering the liver directly from the splenic vein into the portal vein.
- Unconjugated bilirubin is bound to albumin (cannot be excreted in urine) and circulates to the liver, where it is normally internalized and conjugated to glucuronic acid.
- Conjugated bilirubin (water-soluble) is excreted in the bile to reach the gut. In the distal gut, bacteria split the conjugate into urobilinogen, most of which exits in the feces. However, 20% is resorbed into the blood and re-excreted by the liver (enterohepatic recirculation).
- A very small amount of resorbed urobilinogen is excreted in the urine. Unconjugated bilirubin is lipid-soluble. It is therefore dangerous if present at high levels in the blood as it can enter the brain in infants and cause damage (kernicterus).

DATA SET
Obstructive jaundice

A 45-year-old woman with jaundice and right upper abdominal pain.

Plasma

Total bilirubin	163 µmol/L	(up to 70)
	9.5 mg/dl	(up to 1)
Albumin	42 g/L	(30 to 48)
Alanine transaminase (ALT)	38 U/L	(up to 50)
Alkaline phosphatase	354 U/L	(40 to 120)
γ-glutamyl transferase (GGT)	356 U/L	(up to 70)

Urine

Bilirubin positive

This pattern of elevated plasma bilirubin, alkaline phosphatase and GGT is characteristic of obstructive jaundice. Bilirubin enters the liver cells and is conjugated with glucuronic acid before regurgitating into plasma. Conjugated bilirubin is water-soluble and can therefore be excreted in urine.

In this patient, ultrasonography demonstrated a gallstone in the common bile duct.

Fig. 14.3
Causes of conjugated hyperbilirubinemia

Intrahepatic causes

Hereditary enzyme defects (Dubin–Johnson and Rotor syndromes)
Drugs causing intrahepatic cholestasis
Pregnancy-associated cholestasis
Hepatocellular damage

Extrahepatic obstruction of bile ducts

Gallstones (see page 299)
Strictures caused by inflammation or fibrosis
Carcinoma of the pancreas (see page 303)
Compression of bile ducts by extrinsic masses such as enlarged lymph nodes

contributor to jaundice than failure of excretion of conjugated bilirubin. Drugs such as rifampin interfere with bilirubin uptake.

Many of the population have impaired conjugation of bilirubin

Between 5 and 10% of the population have an inherited mild unconjugated hyperbilirubinemia that results from defective hepatic conjugation of bilirubin. One form, which is autosomal dominant, is termed **Gilbert's syndrome**. This is probably a heterogeneous condition and no precise metabolic defect has been identified. Bilirubin levels may increase in the presence of intercurrent disease, but the liver is structurally normal.

Impaired conjugation of bilirubin is also commonly seen in neonates, as activity of the enzyme, glucuronyl transferase, is low in the first 2 weeks of life (neonatal jaundice) (see page 297). Hereditary lack of glucuronyl transferase activity is seen in the congenital **Crigler–Najjar syndrome**.

Decreased transport of conjugated bilirubin causes conjugated hyperbilirubinemia and is mainly caused by biliary obstruction

Abnormal secretion or excretion of conjugated bilirubin results in accumulation of conjugated bilirubin in the blood. The key clinical features, the combination of which is also known as cholestatic or obstructive jaundice (see Data Set), are as follows:

- Jaundice.
- Bile is absent from the stools, which are pale as a result.
- Fat absorption is disturbed (development of steatorrhea) and, as a consequence, there is impaired absorption of vitamin K.
- Itching develops (pruritus) from accumulated bile salts.
- The urine contains bilirubin (dark urine), as conjugated bilirubin is soluble in water and can be excreted.

There are two main groups of causes of conjugated hyperbilirubinemia, as listed in *Fig. 14.3*.

LIVER IN DISEASE

The liver has a limited set of responses to damage

Following damage to the liver, several patterns of histological abnormality can be identified, which are the result of a limited set of pathological responses to damage. There may be fatty change, cholestasis, liver cell necrosis, fibrosis, or storage of abnormal material.

The histological diagnosis of liver disease requires evaluation of these abnormalities, and their correlation with clinical features and biochemical tests (*Fig. 14.4*).

Fatty change is most commonly caused by metabolic stresses and alcohol

Fatty change is a common response of the liver to diverse adverse stimuli (*Fig. 14.5*). (The metabolic derangements have been reviewed previously, see page 274). The main causes are:

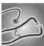

Liver disease – laboratory medicine and investigation

Biochemistry: liver function tests frequently give a good idea of the likely cause of liver disease. Certain patterns of abnormality suggest a particular type of liver disease, but none is specific.

Alkaline phosphatase: enzyme located on the cell membrane of biliary canaliculi. Very high levels indicate disease of the biliary system (intrahepatic cholestasis, extrahepatic biliary obstruction, or primary biliary cirrhosis). Moderate levels are less useful in predicting cause of liver disease.

Transaminases: enzymes located in the hepatocyte cytoplasm. High levels in blood reflect active necrosis of liver cells from any cause. ALT is more specific for the liver than AST. Low levels of increase in transaminases may be seen in cholestasis, as well as following induction of enzymes by drugs such as anticonvulsants. Elevated γ-glutamyl transpeptidase levels are a sensitive index of liver cell damage but are non-specific as to cause.

Conjugated bilirubin: secreted by liver cells. Obstruction of biliary canaliculi causes highest levels, but conjugated bilirubin also seen in association with liver cell destruction. Non-conjugated bilirubin levels increase in disorders causing excessive destruction of red cells.

Albumin: blood level reflects synthetic properties of the liver. Because of its half-life, low levels reflect long-standing liver disease, particularly cirrhosis. α-1-antitrypsin is reduced in disease caused by enzyme deficiency.

Ceruloplasmin: levels are reduced in Wilson's disease.

Transferrin: high saturation seen in hemochromatosis.

Immunology: several diseases are associated with abnormal immunological parameters. Primary biliary cirrhosis is associated with anti-mitochondrial autoantibodies and raised serum IgM levels. Autoimmune chronic hepatitis is associated with anti-smooth-muscle antibodies.

Clotting: abnormalities of clotting are commonly seen in liver disease with failure of hepatic synthesis of serum proteins. This is a feature of hepatic failure, as well as being the end-stage of chronic liver disease such as cirrhosis. The one-step prothrombin time is a sensitive index of vitamin-K-dependent clotting factors, particularly factor VII.

Imaging: imaging studies are valuable as primary investigations of patients with jaundice. Ultrasound examination may reveal dilatation of extrahepatic and intrahepatic bile ducts, or tumors as part of pre-operative assessment.

Biopsy: for the liver, percutaneous needle biopsy is usually performed. Blind biopsy of the right side of the liver is used to assess probable diffuse disease processes. CT- or ultrasound-guided needle biopsy may be used to sample discrete lesions.

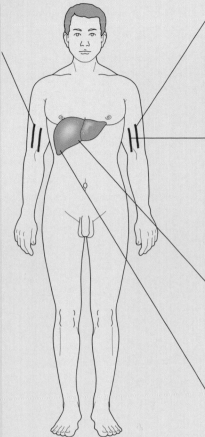

Fig. 14.4 Investigation of liver disease.
Liver disease may be investigated by imaging, blood tests and liver biopsy.

- **Metabolic stress**, e.g. hypoxia, kwashiorkor (see page 149) and diabetes mellitus (see page 540).
- **Toxins** (the most common being alcohol, see page 291) and rare drug reactions.
- **Reye's syndrome** (see page 297) causes extensive microvesicular fatty change.
- **Fatty liver of pregnancy**.

Cholestasis may be intrahepatic or extrahepatic in origin

Many of the conditions causing conjugated hyperbilirubinemia lead to the development of cholestasis. Clinically this is characterized by conjugated hyperbilirubinemia and a great increase in the serum levels of alkaline phosphatase, an enzyme normally located on the cell membranes of the biliary canaliculi. Two groups are recognized.

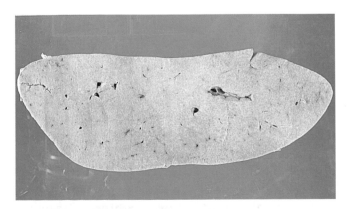

Fig. 14.5 Fatty liver.
Macroscopically the fatty liver is enlarged and, instead of appearing deep red, it is pale. Histologically, fat can be seen in hepatocytes (see page 28).

Intrahepatic cholestasis is caused by diseases affecting bile secretion in the liver, due either to abnormalities of liver cells and biliary canaliculi, or to disease of intrahepatic bile ducts (*Fig. 14.6*). Because they are generally managed by physicians, these conditions are sometimes loosely grouped as medical jaundice. Changes are apparent on liver biopsy in this type of jaundice (*Fig. 14.7*).

Extrahepatic cholestasis is caused by blockage of the main bile ducts outside the liver, discussed later in diseases of the biliary tract. As many of the conditions responsible are amenable to operative intervention, this type of problem is sometimes referred to as surgical jaundice. Extrahepatic obstruction causes distinct changes within the liver (*Fig. 14.8*).

Necrosis of liver cells can be seen in several patterns

Six main patterns of liver cell death are seen, each of which can be related to the cause of liver damage:

1 In several diseases, single liver cells die by the process of apoptosis. Dead hepatocytes form brightly eosinophilic shrunken structures known as **Councilman bodies** (see *Fig. 14.20*).

2 Death of liver cells scattered throughout the lobule, both singly and in small groups (**spotty necrosis**) of about 25 cells is seen with toxic damage and viral infections.

3 Death of liver cells confined to certain zones (**zonal necrosis**) is seen with certain diseases. For example, the centrilobular area (zone 3) is affected in paracetamol (acetaminophen) toxicity (*Fig. 14.9*) (see Data Set opposite), and the periportal area (zone 1) is involved in phosphorus toxicity.

4 **Piecemeal necrosis** describes death of liver cells in a scattered pattern immediately next to the portal tract connective tissue. This pattern is a characteristic of chronic active hepatitis.

5 Extensive patterns of necrosis that bridge between central veins, or between portal tracts and central veins, are termed **bridging necrosis**.

6 **Massive necrosis** describes necrosis of the majority of hepatocytes. This occurs with fulminant hepatic damage and is seen in some cases of viral- and toxin-induced damage.

Liver cell regeneration occurs following hepatocyte necrosis

There is normally a very low level of liver cell proliferation. After liver damage, including partial hepatectomy, regeneration of liver cells takes place in an orderly manner to

Fig. 14.6
Intrahepatic cholestasis

Intra-acinar

Viral hepatitis
Drug therapy (e.g. chlorpromazine and estrogens)
Alcoholic liver disease
Pregnancy-related cholestasis
Septicemia

Extra-acinar

Primary biliary cirrhosis
Sclerosing cholangitis
Polycystic liver disease
Tumors within the liver

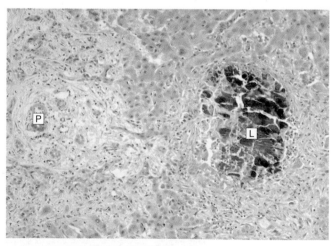

Fig. 14.8 Extrahepatic cholestasis.
In addition to plugging of biliary canaliculi by bile, a characteristic feature of this type of cholestasis is edema of the portal tracts (**P**) which are expanded. In long-standing cases there is proliferation of small bile ducts around the periphery of portal tracts. Bile may leak from canaliculi associated with hydropic degeneration of hepatocytes to cause small so-called bile infarcts or lakes (**L**).

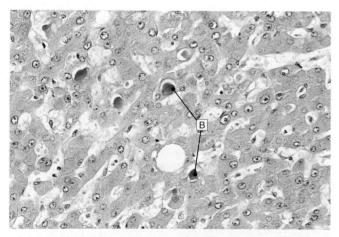

Fig. 14.7 Intrahepatic cholestasis. Bile (**B**) can be seen dilating canaliculi, predominantly in the centrilobular zones.

restore liver function. In conditions causing repeated chronic damage to the liver, regeneration may become distorted by fibrosis, resulting in cirrhosis (see page 294). In other instances, nodular hyperplasia may occur.

The cells of Ito are the source of collagen-secreting cells in liver fibrosis

The development of fibrosis is an important complication of several liver diseases, and is one of the characteristic features of cirrhosis. It is thought that growth factors, produced as part of inflammatory responses, stimulate mesenchymal cells in the liver to proliferate and differentiate

into collagen-secreting fibroblasts. The mesenchymal cells involved are the normally inconspicuous fat-storing cells of Ito, located in the space of Disse.

The liver may be involved in several storage diseases

The liver stores several substances that may become pathological in disease states. In hemochromatosis and hemosiderosis there is excessive iron storage, and excessive copper deposition is seen in Wilson's disease.

Abnormal storage of metabolic products in the liver may be seen in some of the inborn errors of metabolism. Glycogen deposition occurs in some of the glycogen storage diseases (*Fig. 14.10*) and lipids are stored in multi-system disorders of metabolism, e.g. Gaucher's disease and Niemann–Pick disease.

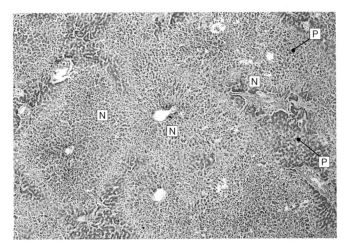

Fig. 14.9 Centrilobular (zone 3) necrosis caused by paracetamol. Following overdose of paracetamol (acetaminophen), toxic metabolites are generated in centrilobular hepatocytes, causing necrosis of this part of the lobule. Confluent necrosis (**N**) of centrilobular areas (zone 3) is seen, with surviving hepatocytes around portal areas (**P**) (zone 1).

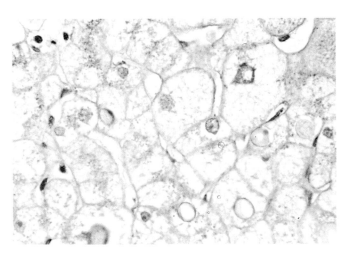

Fig. 14.10 Liver glycogenosis.
In glycogenosis Types IV, III, II and I, liver cells accumulate excess glycogen. Here, liver cells from a case of Type II glycogenosis (debrancher deficiency) show striking vacuolation of hepatocytes and liver nuclei due to the accumulation of glycogen.

DATA SET
Acute hepatic necrosis

A depressed 24-year-old man took an unknown number of paracetamol (acetaminophen) tablets. The following day he was admitted to hospital in coma following a convulsion.

Plasma

Total bilirubin	173 μmol/L	(up to 17)
	10 mg/dl	(up to 1)
Albumin	40 g/L	(30 to 48)
Alanine transaminase (ALT)	6831 U/L	(up to 50)
Alkaline phosphatase	89 U/L	(40 to 120)
γ-glutamyl transferase (GGT)	82 U/L	(up to 70)
Prothrombin time	67.6 s	(control 9.5)

Urine

Bilirubin positive

Acute hepatic necrosis is characterized by markedly raised plasma levels of alanine transaminase and aspartate transaminase, which are released from damaged hepatocytes. The prolonged prothrombin time indicates that the synthetic function of the liver is severely impaired; due to its long half-life (3 weeks) plasma albumin is an insensitive test of liver synthetic function in acute disease. Further investigations in this severely ill man should include plasma glucose and creatinine, and acid–base status. Hypoglycemia should be treated with intravenous glucose. Urgent liver transplantation may be required in patients with persistent clotting abnormalities, lactic acidosis or renal failure.

VASCULAR DISEASES OF THE LIVER

Blood is supplied to the liver via both arterial (hepatic artery) and portal venous circulations. It leaves the liver after passing through the sinusoids by the central and hepatic veins that enter the inferior vena cava. As each vascular component of the liver may be affected by disease, there are several distinct clinical and pathological syndromes.

True infarction of the liver is rare

True infarction of the liver is rare because of its dual blood supply and rich anastomosis of blood flow through the sinusoids. True infarction may be seen in five conditions:

- Surgical trauma or accidental ligation of hepatic artery.
- Therapeutic arterial embolization of the liver or therapeutic hepatic arterial ligation (performed to treat isolated neoplastic masses).
- Bacterial endocarditis.
- Eclampsia.
- Polyarteritis nodosa.

Areas of infarction appear as geographic areas of yellow necrotic tissue.

Right-sided heart failure causes passive venous congestion of the liver

Right-sided cardiac failure causes back-pressure in the systemic venous system, which is transmitted back down the hepatic vein to the central veins, causing mild increase in hepatic size. This is particularly seen in tricuspid valve incompetence, when the liver is pulsatile. The macroscopic appearance is described as nutmeg liver (see *Fig. 10.34*), properly called chronic passive venous congestion. The centrilobular sinusoids are dilated by blood, and the centrilobular hepatocytes are atrophic. If arterial hypotension complicates the right-sided cardiac failure, necrosis of the centrilobular hepatocytes may occur, with elevation of serum transaminase levels.

Portal hypertension is caused by obstruction of blood flow in the portal system

Portal hypertension is a continued elevation in portal venous pressure. This causes back-pressure in the portal vascular bed, leading to splenomegaly and ascites. New channels open up between the portal system and systemic venous system, taking the form of varicose venous channels. The main sites are the lower esophagus, where esophageal varices arise and may cause bleeding (see page 250); the umbilicus, where the channels are called 'caput medusae'; and the anus, where they are known as hemorrhoids.

The causes of portal hypertension are best considered on an anatomical basis, according to the site of obstruction to flow (*Fig. 14.11*).

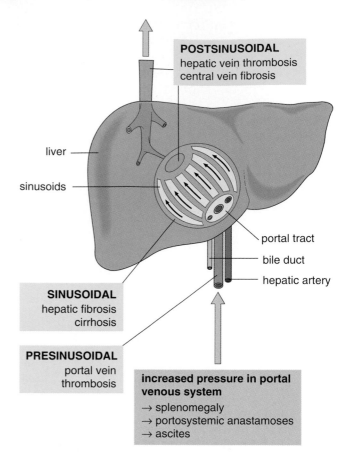

Fig. 14.11 Morphological classification of portal hypertension. The three main groups of causes for portal hypertension are:
- Presinusoidal.
- Sinusoidal.
- Postsinusoidal.

The effects that are shown in the pink box are caused by increased portal venous pressure.

- Presinusoidal – blockage of vessels before the hepatic sinusoids.
- Sinusoidal – blockage in the sinusoids.
- Postsinusoidal – blockage in the central veins, hepatic veins or vena cava.

The most common causes of portal hypertension are diseases of the liver (sinusoidal)

Hepatic disease is the most common cause of portal hypertension.

- **Cirrhosis** causes distortion and destruction of the hepatic vascular architecture.
- **Portal tract fibrosis** caused by schistosomiasis is an important cause in endemic areas.
- **Idiopathic portal hypertension** is applied to cases for which no physical cause for obstruction can be found.
- **Polycystic disease** of the liver.

Presinusoidal portal hypertension is most often caused by portal vein thrombosis

Occlusion of the portal venous system at a point before the portal tracts is usually due to portal vein thrombosis. Predisposing factors are local sepsis, polycythemia (see page 322), and pre-existing sinusoidal portal hypertension due to cirrhosis. Occlusion of intrahepatic branches causes areas of venous infarction, which are seen as congested zones with a wedge-shaped pattern. Such areas are also termed **red infarcts** or **Zahn infarcts**.

In rare circumstances, increased blood flow into the portal venous system overloads the capacity of the hepatic sinusoidal system, causing portal hypertension. This occurs in some cases of splenomegaly and with some arterio-venous malformations in the spleen and gut.

Postsinusoidal portal hypertension is caused by disease of hepatic veins and branches

Postsinusoidal portal hypertension is caused by diseases that block central veins and hepatic venous branches.

Obliteration of central veins in the liver is seen in several diseases, and causes gradual development of portal hypertension. For example, alcohol abuse may result in central venous obliteration with scarring, and some cytotoxic drugs may cause centrilobular scarring and obliteration of central veins.

Veno-occlusive disease of the liver is caused by ingestion of plants containing toxic alkaloids. These initially cause fibrosis around central veins, followed by obliteration of central veins by fibrosis. The problem is seen in Jamaica and certain areas of Africa, in those who drink herbal teas. Irradiation of the liver may also cause central venous fibrosis and development of portal hypertension.

Occlusion of the main hepatic vein produces the **Budd–Chiari syndrome**. Thrombosis is predisposed by local compression of the hepatic vein, hepatocellular carcinoma, polycythemia, pregnancy and estrogenic oral contraceptive therapy. In many cases, no predisposing factor is identified. Patients develop severe acute disease, with massive vascular congestion of the liver causing acute portal hypertension and jaundice. There is painful enlargement of the liver, with rapid development of ascites. Unless therapeutic portosystemic vascular anastomosis is performed, death results.

HEPATITIS

Inflammatory diseases of the liver are termed 'hepatitis'

Hepatitis, which may be acute or chronic, has several important causes including viral infections, autoimmune disorders, drug reactions, and alcohol.

Whatever the cause of acute hepatitis there are similar clinical features and similar histological appearances on liver biopsy.

Clinical and biochemical features of acute hepatitis

Symptoms: nausea, anorexia, low-grade pyrexia, and general malaise.

Signs: liver may become palpably enlarged and tender. Jaundice 1 week after the onset of symptoms, peaking at around 10 days.

Signs and symptoms generally recover over a period of 3–8 weeks.

Biochemical tests: bilirubin, which is mostly conjugated, is greatly elevated; levels of alanine transaminase (ALT) and aspartate transaminase (AST) are very high early in disease, reflecting liver cell necrosis, but fall with clinical recovery; serum albumin generally remains normal.

The serum alkaline phosphatase level may become mildly elevated.

Coagulation tests: may become abnormal, the one-stage prothrombin time being a sensitive indicator of severity of liver disease.

Viral infection is a common cause of hepatitis

The main so-called 'hepatitis viruses' are a group of **hepatotrophic viruses**. Although all cause a primary hepatitis, they are unrelated and belong to different viral types. The main viruses are hepatitis A and E (transmitted via a fecal–oral route), and hepatitis B, C, D and G (transmitted via a parenteral route). Several non-hepatotrophic viruses may also cause hepatitis.

Infection with a hepatitis virus may not always be followed by clinical disease, but there is a range of clinical manifestations. Following initial infection, patients may fall into the one of the patterns listed in *Fig. 14.12*.

Hepatitis A is transmitted by fecal–oral route and does not lead to chronic liver disease

Hepatitis A is an RNA enterovirus of the picorna group. Clinically, disease is transmitted by the fecal–oral route, and small epidemics may occur in nurseries or institutions. The disease has also been contracted from recreational activities in waters contaminated by sewage outfalls, and from eating sewage-contaminated shellfish. An incubation period of about 2–4 weeks is followed by fever, malaise, and anorexia (*Fig. 14.13*). Jaundice typically appears about a week later, remaining for 2 weeks or so. Patients recover fully, with recovery of abnormal liver function tests. Virus is present in the stools of affected patients about 2 weeks before and 1 week after onset of clinical jaundice. There is only a transient viremia so the risk of transmission by blood is low. The disease does not cause chronic hepatitis, and infection confers subsequent immunity by development of serum anti-HAV antibodies.

Histology of the liver shows features of acute hepatitis (see *Fig. 14.20*) but, as diagnosis is evident on clinical and virological investigation, biopsy is rarely performed.

Fig. 14.12
Clinical patterns following viral hepatitis

Pattern of disease	Viruses
Asymptomatic (frequent with hepatitis A)	A, B, C, D and E
Acute hepatitis without jaundice (anicteric hepatitis)	A, B, C, D and E
Acute hepatitis with jaundice (icteric hepatitis)	A, B, C, D and E
Massive necrosis of the liver with acute liver failure (rare)	A, B, C, D and E
One of the forms of chronic hepatitis (see page 287)	B, C and D
Chronic carrier state	B, C and D

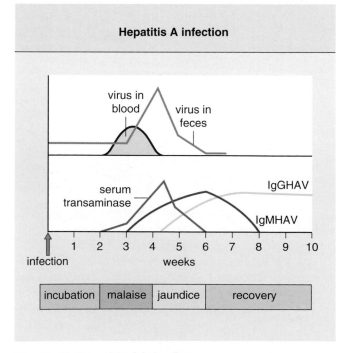

Hepatitis A infection

Fig. 14.13 Hepatitis A infection.

Hepatitis B infection is transmitted parenterally and can cause chronic liver disease

Hepatitis B virus (HBV) is a DNA virus of the hepadna group. Infective virus is transmitted in blood, semen and saliva through close physical contact, inoculation occurring through breaks in skin or mucous membranes. Hepatitis B can therefore be a sexually transmitted disease. Transmission by blood transfusion is now uncommon because of the screening of blood donations, but spread of infection among IV drug abusers via shared unsterile needles is an important mode of transmission. Vertical transmission from mother to child is also seen.

Infection causes five clinical patterns of infection (*Fig. 14.14*).

1 **Acute self-limited hepatitis** is a common outcome. Patients recover after an illness with jaundice, malaise and anorexia, and have lifelong immunity.

2 **Fulminant acute hepatitis** is very rare and causes massive necrosis of liver cells.

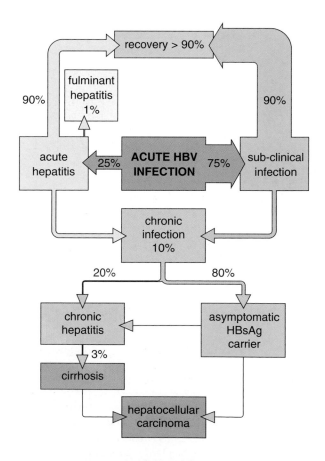

Fig. 14.14 Patterns of infection after hepatitis B infection. Flow diagram illustrating the probabilities of different clinical outcomes after hepatitis B infection. The width of the lines indicates the respective percentages. The time-scales involved are not illustrated; some stages may last for many years, others last a matter of weeks.

3 **Chronic hepatitis** affects 5–10% of cases. It may progress to cirrhosis or may recover (see *Fig. 14.14*).

4 **Asymptomatic carrier state** (may later develop chronic hepatitis).

5 **Clinically inapparent asymptomatic infection** is a sub-clinical form of infection, but it may progress to chronic hepatitis, or the patient may become a carrier.

The importance of the chronic carrier states is that patients are at risk of developing hepatocellular carcinoma. Carrier rates for hepatitis B infection show geographic variation (0.3% in western Europe and USA; 20% in southeast Asia). In adults, under 10% of patients develop a chronic carrier state, but virtually all neonates infected with HBV from the mother become chronic carriers, possibly because of an immature immune response.

Many diagnostic tests are based on identification of viral sub-units (*Fig. 14.15*).

Acute hepatitis B infection is self-limiting in most patients

In symptomatic acute infection, patients develop symptoms after an incubation period of 6–8 weeks. In the majority of patients, where the illness is self-limiting (*Fig. 14.16*), there is a rise in serum HBsAg which peaks just before the height of clinical disease, becoming undetectable after 6 months.

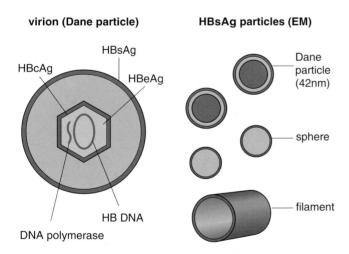

Fig. 14.15 Hepatitis B virus: sub-units of diagnostic importance. The intact hepatitis B virus is also called the Dane particle. The coat contains hepatitis B surface antigen (HBsAg), and the core contains a core antigen (HBcAg) and the e antigen (HBeAg), as well as viral DNA (HB DNA) and DNA polymerase. Detection of e antigen, viral DNA or DNA polymerase in the blood indicates circulating intact virus particles and a high degree of infectivity. By electron microscopy, spherical and filament particles can be seen, as can particles with an envelope, termed 'Dane particles'. The HBsAg particles have different antigenic determinants associated with them termed d, y, w and r. Detection of combinations of sub-units, e.g. adr, ayr, is used in viral typing in the epidemiology of infection spread.

Markers of active viral replication and infectivity also peak just before the height of clinical disease (HBcAg, HBeAg, HBV DNA, and DNA polymerase). Serum transaminase levels begin to rise just before symptomatic disease and persist until resolution of the illness. Anti-HBc is seen in blood just before onset of symptoms. With the fall in levels of HBeAg, anti-HBe appears in blood. Anti-HBs develops in blood after the acute phase of the illness is over and persists for life.

Persistent hepatitis B infection occurs when there is failure to eliminate virus from the liver

In some patients there is failure to eliminate HBV from the liver with HBsAg persisting in the blood for 6 months after initial detection. There are are two main possible consequences of this:

• Chronic carrier state associated with no active viral replication.
• Chronic liver disease associated with active viral replication.

In a proportion of cases there is no evidence of active viral replication (HBcAg, HBeAg, HBV DNA and DNA polymerase are not detected in the blood) and the patient can be classed as having a chronic carrier state. Examination of liver biopsy in such patients can reveal hepatocytes packed with HBsAG (*Fig. 14.17*). Such patients are at increased risk of developing hepatocellular carcinoma and it is believed that the HBV genome has become integrated into the host DNA.

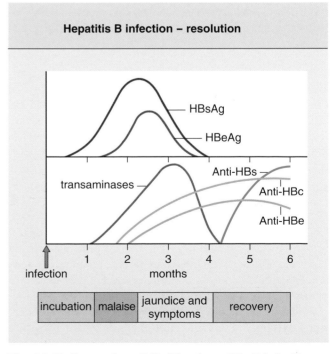

Fig. 14.16 Events in self-limiting hepatitis B infection.

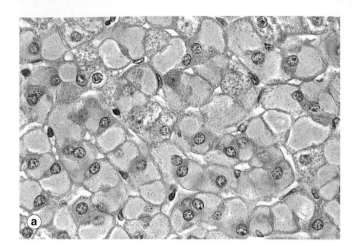

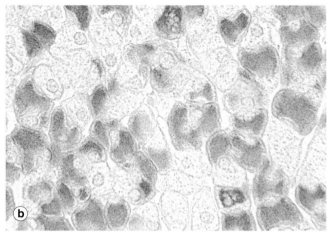

Fig. 14.17 Chronic hepatitis B infection.
In chronic hepatitis due to hepatitis B infection, liver cells accumulate HBsAg in the cytoplasm, which appears homogeneous, pale and glassy (a). These so-called 'ground glass' hepatocytes may be immunostained by antibodies to HBsAg, as shown in (b), where they are stained brown.

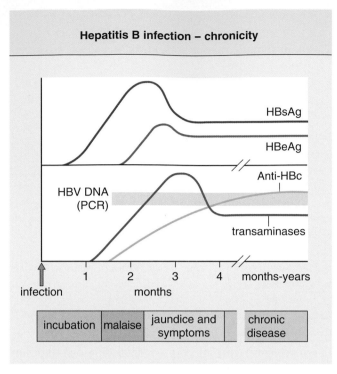

Fig. 14.18 Events in chronic hepatitis B infection.

In other patients with persistent HBV infection the presence of HBsAg is associated with the presence of HBcAg, HBeAg and HBV DNA and DNA polymerase in the blood indicative of active viral replication (*Fig. 14.18*). There is usually associated anti-HBc and sometimes anti-HBs detected in blood. The presence of HBeAg correlates with the development of chronic liver disease (chronic hepatitis and risk of development of cirrhosis).

Mutations are being increasingly recognized in the HBV genome. The importance of such mutant viruses, which can develop in the setting of chronic disease or can be acquired by infection, is that the HBeAg may not be produced and hence may be undetected in laboratory testing. HBeAg detection is therefore of less use than detection of HBV DNA in predicting infectivity in patient samples.

When anti-HBe appears in blood (termed **seroconversion**) HBeAg levels drop and there is a rise in serum transaminase levels reflecting liver cell necrosis. Patients who are HBeAg positive or in whom there is HBV DNA in

blood are candidates for treatment with interferon-α, which promotes seroconversion. The consequences of chronic active viral replication in the liver, chronic hepatitis and cirrhosis, are discussed in a later section.

Hepatitis D virus can only cause infection in the presence of HBV

Hepatitis D virus (HDV) is a hepatotrophic RNA virus. It is a defective virus, requiring the presence of HBV infection for assembly. Consequently, it can cause disease only in the presence of hepatitis B infection. Its mode of transmission is the same as that for hepatitis B infection, and it is particularly prevalent in drug abusers and dialysis patients. Chronic HDV infection seldom resolves and over 60% of affected patients will develop cirrhosis. In some patients there is rapid progression of disease over a few years.

Infection may be acquired simultaneously with HBV infection or may occur later as a superinfection. Infection is confirmed by finding serum IgM anti-D in the presence of IgM anti-HBc. HDV RNA may also be detected in blood.

Hepatitis C is clinically similar to hepatitis B infection

Hepatitis C is an RNA flavivirus. There are six sub-types with different geographic incidences. Its mode of transmission is the same as that for hepatitis B, and it is an important cause of post-transfusion hepatitis. Although it accounts for many cases of sporadic acute hepatitis, often no recognized source of infection can be identified.

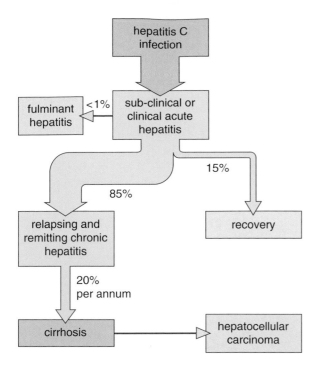

Fig. 14.19 Hepatitis C infection.
Flow diagram illustrating the probabilities of different clinical outcomes after hepatitis C infection. The width of the lines indicates the respective percentages. The time-scales involved are not illustrated.

Hepatitis C infection is responsible for the vast majority of cases of what was formerly termed **non-A non-B hepatitis**.

There is an incubation period of about 2 months, followed by acute hepatitis with fever, malaise, anorexia, and jaundice. Many patients have an asymptomatic acute infection. Some cases recover after a period of about 2 months; others have persistently abnormal liver function tests for over a year, developing a chronic hepatitis with periods of remission and relapse. Of the latter, most will develop chronic active hepatitis, and many cases progress to cirrhosis, with a risk of hepatocellular carcinoma. The course of the disease is shown graphically in *Fig. 14.19*.

Extrahepatic manifestations of disease, such as arthritis and agranulocytosis, are common. Diagnosis can be confirmed by detection of antibodies to HCV and by detection of HCV RNA in blood by PCR tests.

Hepatitis E is clinically similar to hepatitis A infection

Hepatitis E infection is caused by an RNA virus that resembles a calicivirus. Transmitted by a fecal–oral route, it is often found in contaminated water supplies and causes epidemics of acute self-limited hepatitis. It has an incubation period of about 1 month, typically causing a mild infection associated with jaundice. Infection in pregnant women may result in acute fulminant hepatitis. There is no progression to chronic hepatitis.

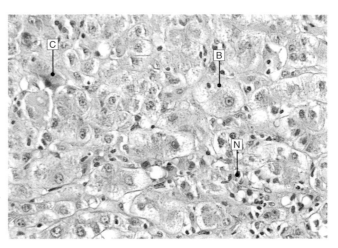

Fig. 14.20 Histology in acute hepatitis.
This is a liver biopsy from a patient with acute viral hepatitis. Many liver cells are swollen and vacuolated, a phenomenon known as 'ballooning degeneration' (**B**). Focal necrosis of hepatocytes (**N**) occurs, affecting the centrilobular areas (zone 3) most severely. Cells dying by apoptosis are seen as shrunken, eosinophilic Councilman bodies (**C**).

Hepatitis G viral infection is especially seen as post-transfusion hepatitis

Cases of hepatitis related to blood transfusion remain unexplained and the search has continued to identify new viral causes. The term HGV refers to a novel RNA virus derived from plasma of patients with chronic non A–E hepatitis. Studies have shown that HGV accounts for only a minority of cases of hepatitis without a defined viral cause: there are three to six times more cases of non-A–E hepatitis than there are HGV-related cases.

What happened to 'hepatitis F'?

In 1994, workers claimed to have transmitted an enteric agent responsible for sporadic non-A–E hepatitis to monkeys and they termed this agent HFV. However, this observation has not been confirmed, and the term HFV remains unclaimed.

The histology of acute viral hepatitis is similar for all types

Irrespective of the causative virus, the histological features of acute viral hepatitis are similar (*Fig. 14.20*):

- Hepatocytes are swollen and many undergo death by apoptosis, forming eosinophilic Councilman bodies.
- Focal infiltration of liver by lymphoid cells associated with liver cell necrosis.
- Increased number of lymphoid cells in portal tracts.
- Regeneration of liver cells produces lobular disarray.
- Mild cholestasis may be seen.

In severe cases of acute hepatitis, bridging necrosis between central veins develops. Clinical disease is usually severe but, with survival, regeneration of hepatocytes occurs. In fulminant massive necrosis the majority of liver cells undergo necrosis.

Hepatitis may be caused by other viruses

In addition to the specific hepatotrophic viruses, other viruses may cause hepatitis. For example, yellow fever is caused by a group B arbovirus, which is endemic in certain areas of Africa and central America, and transmitted by mosquito bite. The histology is similar to that of acute hepatitis. Acute hepatitis may also occur with Epstein–Barr virus and cytomegalovirus. Rubella and herpes simplex may cause severe disease in childhood. Parvovirus B19, human herpesvirus 6, togavirus, and 'mutants' of HBV and HCV are all recently described alternative causes of clinical hepatitis. A newly discovered 'TT virus' (TTV) has been implicated in hepatic disease after the use of blood products. Work suggests that many hemophiliacs have been infected with TTV and that persistent TTV infection may contribute to cryptogenic hepatic failure in hemophiliacs. More exotic viruses such as Lassa, Ebola and Marburg viruses also cause hepatitis.

NON-VIRAL INFECTIONS

The liver may be involved in several parasitic diseases

Parasitic infestation of the liver is an important problem worldwide. The main diseases involved are presented in *Fig. 14.21* and discussed in Chapter 8.

Bacterial infection of the liver is by three main routes

Bacterial infection of the liver occurs by three main routes:

- Ascending spread from colonization of the biliary tract by bacteria. This is almost always predisposed by biliary obstruction.
- Infection ascending in the portal vessels (portal pyemia) into the liver from a focus of sepsis in the abdomen, e.g. abscess caused by complicated appendicitis (see page 266).
- Systemic blood spread in septicemia. This may cause severe acute liver failure.

An important complication of bacterial infection of the liver is the development of a **liver abscess** (*Fig. 14.22*). This is a very serious condition with a high mortality if it is left untreated. Infection of the liver by *Leptospira* causes **Weil's disease**. There is fever, jaundice, purpuric skin rash, and renal failure. The liver shows focal hepatocyte necrosis

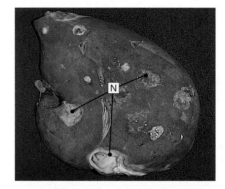

Fig. 14.22 Liver abscess. Abscesses are seen as areas of necrosis (**N**) containing purulent necrotic material. They develop after spread of bacteria to the liver by the three main routes.

Fig. 14.21
Parasitic diseases affecting the liver

Protozoa	
Amebiasis *Entamoeba histolytica*	Amebic abscess contains necrotic material resembling anchovy paste. May rupture into the abdomen or perforate the diaphragm to cause disease in the chest.
Malaria	Causes enlarged liver. Kupffer cells are hyperplastic and contain malaria pigment.
Visceral leishmaniasis	Liver is enlarged. Kupffer cells contain *Leishmania* which appear as Donovan bodies.
Helminthic infection	
Ascariasis *Ascaris lumbricoides*	Eggs from worms in the biliary tract cause cholangitis.
Schistosoma	Eggs from worms cause fibrosis in portal tracts.
Liver flukes *Clonorchis sinensis*	Flukes colonize the biliary tree and cause chronic inflammation, as well as biliary obstruction. Predispose to development of carcinoma of biliary tree.
Hydatid disease *Echinococcus granulosus*	Liver cysts develop, containing the scolices of developing worms.

and cholestasis. Syphilis may affect the liver in congenital infection, causing diffuse fibrosis of the parenchyma. In tertiary syphilis, gummatous necrosis may develop (see page 115), leading to deep scars (hepar lobatum). Tuberculous infection of the liver is seen in miliary tuberculosis (see page 56).

CHRONIC INFLAMMATORY LIVER DISEASE

Chronic destructive liver disease is caused by many different agents

Several diseases of the liver that are characterized by progressive hepatic damage over a period of many months or years have been grouped together as chronic destructive liver diseases. The most important long-term consequence of such diseases is a progressive liver cell loss, fibrosis (distorting normal lobular architecture), and regeneration of hepatocytes. When this process is diffuse and progressive, it may develop into cirrhosis (see page 293).

Chronic hepatitis is defined as inflammation of the liver persisting for more than 6 months

Chronic hepatitis it is not a single disease but a syndrome with many causes. It is clinically defined as persistent abnormal liver function tests of hepatitic type of 6 months' duration. The diagnosis of chronic hepatitis is usually made in three main situations:

- A patient is under medical follow-up (involving repeated liver function tests and serology) after an episode of acute viral hepatitis. Instead of recovering, liver function tests show continued elevation of serum transaminase levels for more than 6 months.

Fig. 14.23
Classification of chronic hepatitis

Caused by viral infections

Chronic hepatitis B
Chronic hepatitis C
Chronic hepatitis D
Chronic viral hepatitis – uncertain origin

Caused by autoimmune disease

Autoimmune hepatitis
Primary biliary cirrhosis
Primary sclerosing cholangitis

Caused by toxic/metabolic damage

Chronic drug hepatitis
Wilson's disease
α-1-antitrypsin deficiency

- A patient develops non-specific features of anorexia, malaise, and weight loss, and is discovered to have abnormal liver function tests that are suggestive of hepatitis, with raised transaminase levels. A cause for liver disease is found on investigation (viral, autoimmune or toxic/metabolic) and, as the disease persists for 6 months, a liver biopsy is performed to establish the pattern of chronic inflammation of the liver.

- Many patients are completely asymptomatic and come to medical attention only because they test HBV- or HCV-positive on routine screening, e.g. when donating blood. Investigations may then suggest a chronic hepatitis.

Chronic hepatitis is classified according to the etiology of disease

For many years, chronic hepatitis was classified on the basis of histological and clinical features into three patterns termed **chronic active hepatitis** (CAH), (also known as chronic aggressive hepatitis), **chronic persistent hepatitis** (CPH), and **chronic lobular hepatitis** (CLH). It is now realized that this scheme lacked prognostic value, artificially separated some conditions and was not of help in defining therapy. For these reasons the classification of chronic hepatitis is based on etiology (*Fig. 14.23*).

DATA SET
Chronic active hepatitis

A 35-year-old man with a history of intravenous drug abuse contracted hepatitis B. Eight months later he remained unwell.

Plasma

Total bilirubin	41 µmol/L	(up to 17)
	2.4 mg/dl	(up to 1)
Albumin	30 g/L	(30 to 48)
Alanine transaminase (ALT)	261 U/L	(up to 50)
Alkaline phosphatase	360 U/L	(40 to 120)
γ-glutamyl transferase (GGT)	233 U/L	(up to 70)
Total protein	97 g/L	(63 to 78)

Chronic hepatitis produces a variable profile of liver function tests as a result of continuing inflammation. Raised alkaline phosphatase, GGT and bilirubin indicate cholestasis; the raised ALT level is due to liver cell necrosis. Impaired liver synthetic function contributes to the hypoalbuminemia. The total protein level is nevertheless raised, due to high immunoglobulin production. Additional tests should include Hepatitis B serology, and assessment of clotting function.

Fig. 14.24
Grading and staging of chronic hepatitis

Grade of necroinflammatory lesions

Grade score	Portal	Lobular
0	None or minimal	None
1	Portal inflammation	Inflammation but no necrosis
2	Mild necrosis of periportal hepatocytes	Focal necrotic cells with acidophil bodies
3	Moderate necrosis of periportal hepatocytes	Severe focal cell damage
4	Severe necrosis of periportal hepatocytes	Damage includes necrosis of liver cells that bridges between portal tracts

Stage of fibrosis

Stage score	Severity
0	None
1	Enlarged fibrotic portal tracts
2	Fibrosis extends to periportal areas
3	Fibrosis extends into septa but no distortion of liver architecture
4	Fibrosis associated with architectural distortion corresponding to cirrhosis

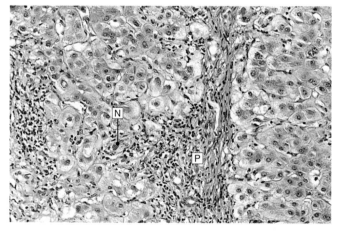

Fig. 14.25 Severe inflammation in chronic hepatitis.
Histologically there is lymphocytic inflammatory infiltration in portal tracts (**P**), which spills over into the adjacent parenchyma. Piecemeal necrosis of liver cells (**N**) is seen at the interface with the connective tissue of the portal tract. With time, this necrosis extends, star-like, from portal areas and, in late stages, progresses to bridging fibrosis between adjacent portal tracts.

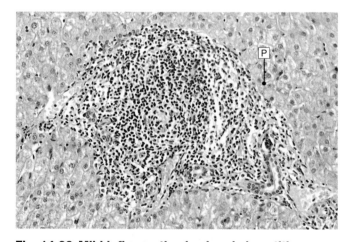

Fig. 14.26 Mild inflammation in chronic hepatitis.
In this example of chronic hepatitis, lymphoid infiltration is seen limited to the portal tract. There is no necrosis of liver cells in the lobule or adjacent to the portal tract.

Chronic hepatitis can be staged and graded according to histology of the liver

Chronic hepatitis is characterized by variable degrees of liver cell necrosis with inflammation and associated fibrosis (*Fig. 14.24*).

- Inflammation may be in the portal tracts, around the edges of portal tracts or within the hepatic lobule.

Increasing severity of inflammation is associated with necrosis of liver cells. The assessment of the severity of inflammation and liver cell necrosis in a liver biopsy is used to assess the grade of disease, active inflammation being an adverse prognostic factor (see *Figs 14.25* and *14.26*).

- Fibrosis initially develops around portal tracts, then progresses to bridge between portal tracts and later may be associated with true cirrhosis (see below). The degree of fibrosis in a liver biopsy is used to assess the stage of disease.

Chronic viral hepatitis is mainly caused by hepatitis B and C

Chronic hepatitis B infection is caused by HBV and causes a clinical hepatitis lasting longer than 6 months. Serological markers of active viral infection are present (see *Fig. 14.17*). Histologically hepatocytes may contain HBsAg visible as so-called ground glass cells (*Fig. 14.17*). Inflammatory activity varies with predominantly lymphocytic inflammation in the lobules associated with active liver cell necrosis. Liver cell necrosis can also be seen adjacent to portal tracts. In severe disease bridging fibrosis and cirrhosis can be seen.

Chronic hepatitis C infection is caused by HCV and causes a clinical hepatitis lasting longer than 6 months. Serological markers of active viral infection are present. In contrast to HBV, inflammation is characterized by the presence of lymphoid follicles and some fatty change in hepatocytes. There is also inflammatory damage to bile ducts. Chronic hepatitis due to HCV carries a much greater chance of progression to cirrhosis than that caused by HBV.

Autoimmune chronic hepatitis is associated with anti-Sm and anti-nuclear antibodies

Autoimmune chronic hepatitis, also called **lupoid hepatitis**, typically occurs in women between the ages of 20 and 40 years. It is associated with hypergammaglobulinemia, autoantibodies in the serum, and other autoimmune disorders such as thyroiditis, arthritis and Sjögren's syndrome.

The etiology is unknown and, despite the name, no autoimmune mechanism has been proven. Although anti-smooth muscle antibodies (60% of cases) and anti-nuclear autoantibodies (40–60% of cases) are found in the serum, they are not thought to cause liver cell damage. T-cell-mediated cytotoxicity directed against autoantigens on liver cells is thought to play some part in disease.

There is an insidious onset of anorexia, malaise and fatigue, and investigation reveals raised bilirubin, moderately raised transaminase levels, and slight elevation of alkaline phosphatase. ESR is commonly elevated and normochromic anemia occurs in some cases.

The disease may run a relapsing and remitting course or may progress inexorably to cirrhosis.

In establishing a diagnosis of autoimmune chronic hepatitis, other causes (e.g. viral infection, alcoholic liver disease, and primary biliary cirrhosis) need to be excluded.

Drug-related chronic hepatitis must be excluded by clinical history

Certain drugs can cause chronic hepatitis, the most common being methyldopa, nitrofurantoin and oxyphenisatin. Less common are sulphonamides, halothane, isoniazid, paracetamol, dantrolene, and etretinate. Many other drugs have been implicated, albeit rarely, so it is important to consider any drug as a potential cause of chronic hepatitis.

Fig. 14.27
Drug-induced liver damage

Liver pathology	Drugs causing damage
Fatty change	Methotrexate, tetracyclines, sodium valproate
Hepatic granulomas	Sulphonamides, allopurinol
Acute hepatitis	Isoniazid, halothane
Chronic hepatitis	Isoniazid, methyldopa
Cholestasis	Steroids, chlorpromazine
Central vein occlusion	Cytotoxic drugs
Tumors	Oral contraceptives (adenomata) Anabolic steroids (carcinomas)
Acute necrosis	Paracetamol

The mechanism is uncertain, but direct hepatotoxicity and induced autoimmune responses have been suggested.

Other forms of liver disease may result from drug ingestion (see page 291 and *Fig. 14.27*), including acute liver cell necrosis (see page 279).

Primary biliary cirrhosis is associated with anti-mitochondrial antibodies

Primary biliary cirrhosis (PBC) is characterized by chronic destruction of intrahepatic bile ducts. The incidence is 10 times higher in women than in men, and it is an important cause of chronic liver disease and cirrhosis in women over the age of 50 years.

Clinically, in the early stages of disease, patients develop pruritus and mild hyperbilirubinemia due to inflammatory destruction of intrahepatic bile ducts (see the Data Set and blue box on page 290). It is only many years later that patients develop true cirrhosis with fibrosis and regenerative nodules of liver cells. For most of the duration of the disease, patients have no histological changes of cirrhosis.

Although immune phenomena are involved, the etiology of primary biliary cirrhosis is uncertain. Liver biopsy is performed to evaluate the stage of the disease; early disease reveals obliteration of bile ducts from portal tracts, associated with small granulomas. There is infiltration of portal tracts by lymphoid cells, with destruction of adjacent hepatocytes in a manner similar to that of piecemeal necrosis. As disease progresses, there is fibrosis and proliferation of small bile ducts at the periphery of the portal tracts. In the final stages of disease cirrhosis develops. There is gradual progression over about 10 years. Treatment by drugs is ineffective and liver transplantation is often necessary.

DATA SET
Primary biliary cirrhosis

A 51-year-old woman complained of increasing generalised itching over a 12-month period.

Plasma

Total bilirubin	24 μmol/L	(up to 17)
	1 mg/dl	(up to 1)
Albumin	30 g/L	(30 to 48)
Alanine transaminase (ALT)	78 U/L	(up to 50)
Alkaline phosphatase	531 U/L	(40 to 120)
γ-glutamyl transferase (GGT)	421 U/L	(up to 70)
Total protein	91 g/L	(63 to 78)

The high alkaline phosphatase and GGT indicate cholestasis. Jaundice is not a constant finding in primary biliary cirrhosis; this patient was not visibly jaundiced. IgM levels are usually elevated, as indicated by the high total protein concentration. Further laboratory tests should include antimitochondrial antibody titers, which are characteristically high in primary biliary cirrhosis.

Primary sclerosing cholangitis is the result of inflammation and fibrosis of bile ducts and leads to cirrhosis

Primary sclerosing cholangitis (PSC) causes progressive obstructive jaundice and is characterized by chronic inflammation and fibrosis of bile ducts. It is a condition with a male predominance and a peak incidence between the ages of 25 and 40 years. It is associated with the presence of inflammatory bowel disease, 60% of patients with PSC having ulcerative colitis, and about 5% of patients with ulcerative colitis developing PSC. It is not associated with the immunological features of PBC.

PSC affects both intrahepatic and extrahepatic bile ducts. Large intrahepatic and extrahepatic ducts develop fibrous strictures with segmental dilatation. Radiological examination after injection of contrast agent up the common bile duct back into the liver (endoscopic retrograde cholangiogram) reveals a 'beaded' appearance of affected ducts (*Fig. 14.28a*).

Medium-sized ducts, and ducts in portal tracts, show inflammation and a pattern of concentric fibrosis around ducts (*Fig 14.28b*) whereas small bile ducts in portal tracts are replaced by collagenous scar (vanishing bile ducts).

Patients develop cholestatic jaundice with progression to cirrhosis over a period of about 10 years. There is an increased risk of developing cholangiocarcinoma (see page 296).

Primary biliary cirrhosis – laboratory medicine

Alkaline phosphatase: very high levels (reflecting bile duct abnormality).

Bilirubin: moderately elevated levels (despite high alkaline phosphatase levels).

AST and ALT: moderately raised.

Albumin: normal.

Prothrombin time: may be prolonged with malabsorption of vitamin K.

Immunology: anti-mitochondrial autoantibodies (titer > 1:40) in over 90% of cases. Elevated levels of serum IgM.

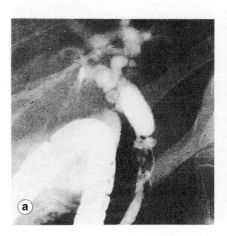

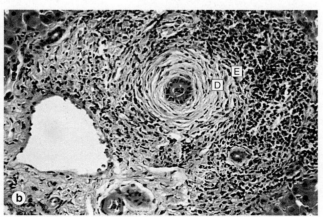

Fig. 14.28 Sclerosing cholangitis.
A beaded appearance of dilatation and stricture is seen on retrograde cholangiography (a). Histologically (b) ducts in the liver (**D**) are surrounded by a pattern of concentric fibrosis (**E**) and associated chronic inflammation, which leads to later duct obliteration.

TOXIC LIVER DISEASE

Alcohol is the most common cause of chronic liver disease

Alcohol abuse is the most common cause of liver disease in western countries, and women are more prone to alcohol-induced liver damage than men.

Alcohol is an hepatotoxin and liver damage is related to daily alcohol intake. There is no safe lower limit for alcohol ingestion, but maximum recommended daily intakes have been defined when the risk of liver damage is thought to be small (50–60 g per day in males; 30–40 g per day in females).

Toxicity of ethanol is probably due to generation of its metabolic breakdown product acetaldehyde.

Alcohol causes fatty liver, acute hepatitis and cirrhosis

Alcoholic liver damage may lead to fatty liver, in which the accumulation of fat in hepatocytes is reversible with abstinence.

In **acute alcoholic hepatitis**, ingestion of large amounts of alcohol causes a true hepatitis, with focal necrosis of liver cells. The illness resembles acute viral hepatitis, and liver function tests show raised levels of transaminases and γ-glutamyl transpeptidase (*Fig. 14.29* and Data Set box on page 294).

If a patient with alcoholic hepatitis abstains, the inflammation resolves without harm. With continued ingestion

of alcohol, fibrosis develops around central veins, and in response to continued hepatocyte necrosis. The end-result is hepatic fibrosis that may progress to cirrhosis.

Alcoholic cirrhosis affects fewer than 10% of patients suffering from chronic alcoholism. It may develop after episodes of acute alcoholic hepatitis or may be insidious in its onset, presenting only as end-stage liver disease (see *Fig. 14.33* on page 294).

Drugs are an important and common cause of liver disease

Drugs are a very common cause of liver disease, and a careful drug history is a vital part of assessment of any patient with abnormal liver function. Hepatotoxic drugs may be divided into two main groups: intrinsic hepatotoxins, which are dose-dependent, predictable, and responsible for a high incidence of toxic damage to liver; and idiosyncratic hepatotoxins, which cause liver disease in a small percentage of exposed individuals, because of either hypersensitivity or abnormal drug metabolism (see Data Set below).

All types of liver pathology may be caused by drugs, the main forms being given in *Fig. 14.27*. In view of the fact that almost any drug can cause liver disease, it is advisable to consult a specialist text when relating a drug history to potential hepatic damage.

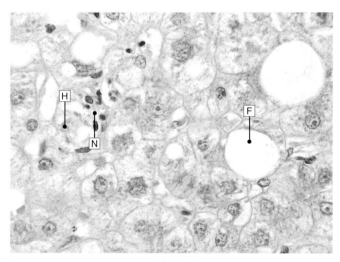

Fig. 14.29 Alcoholic hepatitis.
Liver biopsy shows fatty change (**F**) and focal necrosis of liver cells associated with neutrophil infiltration adjacent to dead cells (**N**). Mallory's hyaline (**H**) accumulates in a small proportion of hepatocytes. Composed of cytokeratin intermediate filaments, ubiquitin and αβ crystallin, it appears as brightly eosinophilic globules in liver cell cytoplasm. Although commonly seen in alcoholic hepatitis, it may also be seen in association with other forms of hepatic damage.

DATA SET
Drug hepatitis

Three weeks after commencing treatment with chlorpromazine, a 34-year-old woman with schizophrenia complained of generalized itching and yellow discoloration of her skin.

Plasma

Total bilirubin	95 μmol/L	(up to 17)
	5.5 mg/dl	*(up to 1)*
Albumin	35 g/L	(30 to 48)
Alanine transaminase (ALT)	51 U/L	(up to 50)
Alkaline phosphatase	299 U/L	(40 to 120)
γ-glutamyl transferase (GGT)	371 U/L	(up to 70)

Urine

Bilirubin positive. Idiosyncratic reactions to a number of drugs can result in intrahepatic bile statis. Routine liver function tests do not distinguish between cholestasis due to intrahepatic causes, as in this patient, and bile stasis due to obstruction of extrahepatic bile ducts. Itching is caused by high circulating levels of retained bile salts.

METABOLIC LIVER DISEASE

Hemochromatosis is caused by excessive deposition of iron in tissues

In hemochromatosis, excessive iron accumulation causes chronic damage to liver cells. Two types of disease are distinguished.

Primary hemochromatosis is inherited as an autosomal recessive trait, and leads to excessive absorption of iron from the gut. The gene is located on chromosome 6, close to the HLA locus, called HLA-H. Iron accumulates as hemosiderin in many tissues including the liver (*Fig. 14.30*), pancreas, pituitary, heart and skin. Accumulation of iron in the liver causes death of hepatocytes (possibly from the generation of free radicals) and leads to cirrhosis. Accumulation in the pancreatic islets causes diabetes mellitus, and in the cardiac muscle gives rise to a cardiomyopathy with heart failure.

Macroscopically, the liver and other affected tissues appear rusty brown due to hemosiderin in cells (hepatocytes, Kupffer cells, and biliary epithelium in the liver).

Diagnosis can be made on the finding of an extremely high saturation of transferrin in the blood, with high serum iron and ferritin levels, and is usually confirmed by liver biopsy.

Secondary hemochromatosis (also called **hemosiderosis**) is the result of excessive iron accumulation caused by other primary diseases (e.g. alcoholism) and by repeated blood transfusions for diseases with abnormalities of red cell formation, particularly thalassemia (see page 320).

Wilson's disease is an inherited disease of copper metabolism

Wilson's disease is a rare but treatable cause of chronic destructive liver disease. An inherited autosomal recessive disorder of copper metabolism, it causes excess copper to accumulate in the liver and brain. This defect is a mutation in a copper-transport ATPase gene.

Excess copper in the liver initially causes a chronic hepatitis picture clinically, and pathologically progresses to cirrhosis. Accumulation in the brain leads to psychiatric disorders, abnormal eye movements, and movement disorders resembling Parkinson's disease.

Diagnosis can be made by finding a low level of ceruloplasmin, the copper-binding protein, in the serum (as it is not released from the liver). Excess copper is demonstrable in liver biopsy material by special staining.

α-1-antitrypsin deficiency causes chronic liver disease and cirrhosis

α-1-antitrypsin deficiency (*Fig. 14.31*) is an important heritable cause of chronic liver disease, and also causes panacinar emphysema (see page 204). Affected individuals fail to produce the normal active extracellular protease inhibitor α-1-antitrypsin. Many alleles for this protease inhibitor (**Pi**) gene are known, each of which has been given a letter. The

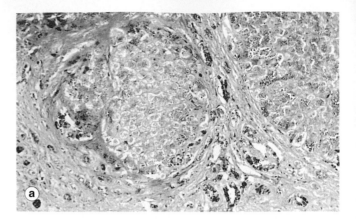

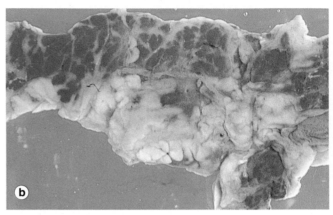

Fig. 14.30 Hemochromatosis. Perls' stain reveals iron deposition in tissues as a blue color. In (a) iron is seen in liver cells, as well as in biliary epithelium. Macroscopically, affected tissues look rusty brown, as illustrated by the pancreas in (b), taken from a patient with primary hemochromatosis.

Copper accumulation in Wilson's disease

In normal circumstances, dietary copper is taken to the liver, complexed to ceruloplasmin and secreted into the plasma. Circulating ceruloplasmin is recycled by the liver in the endosome–lysosome system, free copper being re-excreted into the bile. In Wilson's disease the liver fails to secrete the copper–ceruloplasmin complex into the plasma, thereby accumulating copper in hepatocyte cytoplasm. Free copper overspills into the blood and is deposited in the brain and cornea (Kayser–Fleischer rings).

normal phenotype is known as **PiMM**. The most significant abnormal allele is termed Z. Heterozygotes (**PiZM**) carry an increased risk of lung damage if they smoke, developing emphysema. Homozygotes (**PiZZ**) develop emphysema and liver disease.

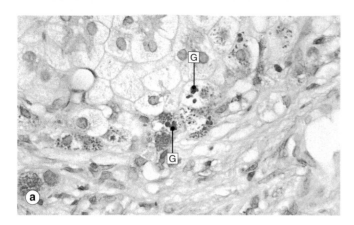

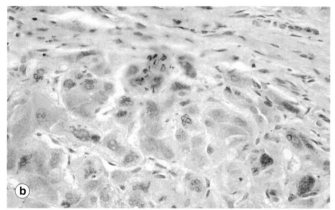

Fig. 14.31 α-1-antitrypsin deficiency.
Liver biopsy shows accumulation of α-1-antitrypsin in hepatocytes as globules (**G**) which stain with PAS (a) and can also be specifically stained by immunoperoxidase methods using antibodies to α-1-antitrypsin (b).

Disease may be manifest in neonates as a neonatal hepatitis (see page 297), although this is not an inevitable consequence of the PiZZ genotype. In adult life, disease may be discovered following investigation of abnormal liver function tests. Investigation may reveal either a chronic hepatitis or cirrhosis (see *Fig. 14.33*).

CIRRHOSIS OF THE LIVER

In cirrhosis the liver is diffusely replaced by nodules of hepatocytes separated by fibrosis

In cirrhosis the normal architecture of the liver is diffusely replaced by nodules of regenerated liver cells, separated by bands of collagenous fibrosis (*Fig. 14.33*). An irreversible form of chronic liver disease, cirrhosis is the end-stage of many processes. It has three key characteristics, namely long-standing destruction of liver cells, associated chronic inflammation that stimulates fibrosis, and regeneration of hepatocytes to cause nodules.

Fibrosis is caused by growth factors liberated from inflammatory cells, Kupffer cells, and hepatocytes. The

Fig. 14.32
Causes of cirrhosis

Common

Alcoholic liver disease
Cryptogenic (no cause found on investigation)
Chronic hepatitis caused by hepatitis B and hepatitis C viruses

Uncommon

Autoimmune chronic hepatitis and PBC
Chronic biliary obstruction (biliary cirrhosis)
Cystic fibrosis

Treatable but rare

Hemochromatosis
Wilson's disease

Rare

α-1-antitrypsin deficiency
Galactosemia
Glycogenosis Type IV
Tyrosinemia

inflammatory cells may be part of the disease process (e.g. in chronic hepatitis) or may be recruited in response to liver cell necrosis (for example in chronic alcoholism). Myofibroblast-like cells, derived from the fat-storing Ito cells are responsible for secreting collagen.

Nodules of hepatocytes form as part of the normal capacity of hepatocytes to divide and regenerate in response to damage.

Cirrhosis is best classified according to the cause of liver damage

The best way to classify cirrhosis is by its etiology. The main causes of cirrhosis (*Fig. 14.32*) are conditions known to result in chronic liver cell necrosis with fibrosis and regeneration. In early classifications two types of cirrhosis were described, based on the size of the regenerative nodules: **micronodular cirrhosis** nodules are small, ranging in size up to 3 mm; **macronodular cirrhosis** nodules are larger than 3 mm, ranging in size up to 2 cm.

This classification has little clinical relevance, although there is some inconsistent association with cause.

Cirrhosis results in liver failure and portal hypertension

The main consequences of cirrhosis are:

• Reduced hepatocyte function (decreased synthesis of proteins, failure of detoxification).

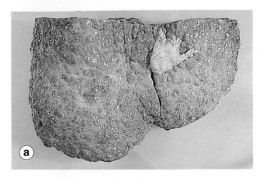
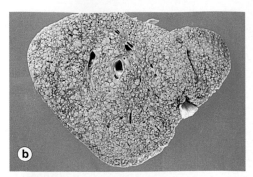
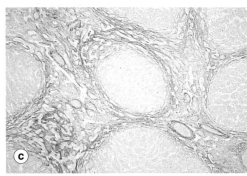
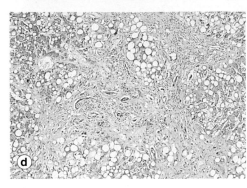

Fig. 14.33 Cirrhosis.
Macroscopically (a) the external surface of the cirrhotic liver has a bosselated appearance. On cut surface (b) the parenchyma is replaced by nodules of regenerated hepatocytes, separated by fine fibrosis. Histologically (c), nodules of hepatocytes (stained yellow in this preparation) are separated by bands of collagenous tissue (stained red). Bile ducts and portal vessels run in the fibrous septa. Some of the nodules contain a central vein, others do not. This distortion of vascular architecture leads to portal hypertension. In some cases the cause of cirrhosis can be determined from liver biopsy, e.g. alcoholic cirrhosis is frequently characterized by fatty change in hepatocytes, as shown in (d).

- Disturbance of blood flow through the liver, causing portal hypertension with all its attendant complications (see page 280).

DATA SET
Cirrhosis

A 54-year-old man with a history of alcohol abuse presented with jaundice.

Plasma

Total bilirubin	283 µmol/L	(up to 17)
	16.4 mg/dl	*(up to 1)*
Albumin	28 g/L	(30 to 48)
Alanine transaminase (ALT)	76 U/L	(up to 50)
Alkaline phosphatase	193 U/L	(40 to 120)
γ-glutamyl transferase (GGT)	549 U/L	(up to 70)

The liver function tests in patients with cirrhosis can be very variable, and are never diagnostic. In the early stages of the disease liver function tests may be normal. As the disease progresses cholestasis may occur, as in this patient, and liver cell necrosis may result in raised transaminase levels. Albumin levels are often low, due to impaired synthesis. Further tests should include plasma urea, creatinine and electrolytes, as derangements of fluid balance are common in patients with cirrhosis.

- Reduced immune competence and increased susceptibility to infection.
- Increased risk of development of hepatocellular carcinoma.
- Increased risk of development of portal vein thrombosis.

These consequences are manifest by a group of distinctive clinical features in a typical patient with cirrhosis (*Fig. 14.34*). In clinical practice, cirrhosis is encountered in one of two ways. It may develop in patients who are under follow-up for known chronic liver disease (e.g. chronic hepatitis or alcoholic liver disease), or it may first present as end-stage disease, having been entirely sub-clinical in its evolution.

Acute liver failure frequently develops in cirrhosis

Signs of chronic liver failure are seen in association with cirrhosis (see *Fig. 14.34*), and this is usually a fairly stable clinical state. Importantly, patients with chronic liver failure are at risk of an abrupt deterioration in condition that leads to acute liver failure. The main precipitating factors are alcohol binge, development of intercurrent infection, gastrointestinal bleed (e.g. from esophageal varices), portal vein thrombosis, and development of carcinoma of the liver (see page 296).

Cirrhosis may develop as a consequence of biliary obstruction

Biliary cirrhosis is the result of long-standing obstruction of bile ducts, leading to the development of obstructive

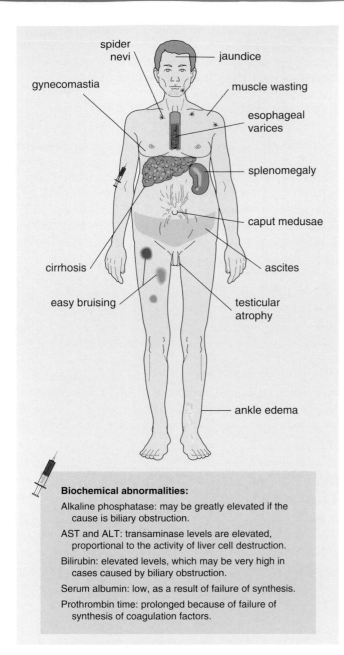

Pathogenesis of ascites in cirrhosis

Ascites is the accumulation of fluid in the peritoneal cavity (see page 268). The most common reason for ascites in association with portal hypertension is cirrhosis. Three mechanisms are involved:

1 Increased transudation of fluid caused by increased hydrostatic pressure in the portal veins.

2 Increased transudation of fluid caused by low plasma oncotic pressure (associated with hypoalbuminemia due to reduced albumin synthesis by damaged liver cells).

3 Sodium and water retention due to stimulation of abnormal renal retention by unknown mechanisms.

Biochemical abnormalities:

Alkaline phosphatase: may be greatly elevated if the cause is biliary obstruction.

AST and ALT: transaminase levels are elevated, proportional to the activity of liver cell destruction.

Bilirubin: elevated levels, which may be very high in cases caused by biliary obstruction.

Serum albumin: low, as a result of failure of synthesis.

Prothrombin time: prolonged because of failure of synthesis of coagulation factors.

Fig. 14.34 Clinical stigmata of cirrhosis.
Cirrhosis gives rise to clinical stigmata caused by failure of liver metabolism as well as those caused by portal hypertension. Testicular atrophy, spider nevi and gynecomastia are the result of impaired metabolism of endogenous estrogens. Ascites and edema are caused by low serum albumin. Varices, splenomegaly and caput medusae are caused by portal hypertension. Bruising is caused by failure to synthesize clotting factors.

jaundice, liver cell necrosis, and fibrosis with regenerative nodules. The main causes are **primary biliary cirrhosis**, unrelieved obstruction of the main extrahepatic bile ducts (also termed **secondary biliary cirrhosis**), and **sclerosing cholangitis** (see pages 278, 289 and 290).

Early in the course of biliary obstruction there is edema and expansion of intrahepatic portal tracts, with portal tract fibrosis. Bile droplets develop in biliary canaliculi, which may rupture and cause death of adjacent hepatocytes (so-called bile infarcts). Over a long period of time, liver cell death, regeneration and fibrosis result in cirrhosis.

TUMORS OF THE LIVER

Benign tumors of the liver may be derived from several cell types

Benign tumors of the liver are derived from several cell types. Many are better considered as hamartomas rather than neoplasms.

- **Hepatic adenomata** are true neoplasms, arising as well-circumscribed nodules that are up to 20 cm in size. Seen in women in the reproductive period, they are predisposed by estrogen-containing oral contraceptives. The histological appearances closely resemble those of normal liver, except that no portal structures are seen. These lesions cause problems as they may rupture and cause intra-abdominal bleeding.

- **Bile duct adenomata** are very common and are probably hamartomas. They appear as small white nodules, often beneath the liver capsule, and are composed of abnormal bile ducts in a collagenous stroma. They may be mistaken for metastatic tumor deposits at laparotomy.

- **Hemangioma of the liver** is common. It is seen beneath the capsule as a dark, almost black, lesion (typically 2–3 cm in size) which, histologically, is composed of abnormal vascular channels in a collagenous stroma.

The liver may be involved by secondary tumors

The most common malignant tumor of the liver is **metastatic tumor**. Spread to the liver is via the blood-stream, either from the portal vein in the case of tumors in the gastrointestinal tract, or by the systemic circulation for other tumors (see page 85). Clinically the liver is enlarged, feeling hard and craggy on palpation.

The lung, breast, colon, and stomach are the most common primary sites of tumors metastasizing to the liver. Many other tumors also spread to the liver, but they are numerically less frequent. There is often involvement by tumors of the lymphoreticular system, **malignant lymphomas** (see page 307), and by malignant tumors of the bone marrow, **leukemias** (see page 323).

Small deposits of tumor in the liver have little clinical effect but, when extensive, metastases cause compression of the intrahepatic bile ducts and lead to obstructive jaundice (see page 278).

Primary hepatocellular carcinoma is predisposed by cirrhosis, hepatitis B infection and mycotoxins

Primary carcinomas derived from hepatocytes are termed **hepatocellular carcinomas**, often referred to as hepatomas (*Fig. 14.35*). The predisposing factors for development are cirrhosis (independent of cause), hepatitis B and C infection with chronic carrier status, and mycotoxins contaminating food. For example, *Aspergillus flavus* produces a powerful toxin that readily causes hepatocellular carcinoma and is a frequent contaminant of stored nuts and grains in tropical countries.

The marked geographic variation seen in the incidence of this condition (very high in Africa and the Far East) is probably due to environmental levels of mycotoxins and high hepatitis B carrier rates.

Serum α-fetoprotein levels may be raised in cases of hepatocellular carcinoma and are demonstrable by immunochemistry in tumor cells. The prognosis is very poor, with a median survival of under 6 months from diagnosis.

Cholangiocarcinoma is predisposed by chronic inflammatory diseases of bile ducts

Adenocarcinomas arising from the intrahepatic bile duct epithelium are termed **cholangiocarcinomas**. They may be predisposed by chronic inflammatory diseases of the intrahepatic biliary tree, particularly sclerosing cholangitis (see page 290) and disease caused by liver flukes (see page 135). Macroscopically lesions may be single or multifocal and are associated with a very poor prognosis, most patients being dead within 6 months of diagnosis.

Angiosarcomas of the liver are caused by exposure to environmental agents

Derived from vascular endothelium, angiosarcomas are highly malignant tumors that appear as multifocal hemorrhagic nodules within the liver. Such tumors are rare unless there has been exposure to thorotrast (a radiological contrast agent used until the 1950s), vinyl chloride monomer (used in the plastic industry to make PVC), arsenic (administered in the past in certain 'tonics'), or anabolic steroids.

MULTISYSTEM DISEASE AND TRANSPLANTATION

The liver is frequently involved in multisystem disease

Liver enlargement or deranged liver function tests are commonly caused by liver involvement in systemic disease processes.

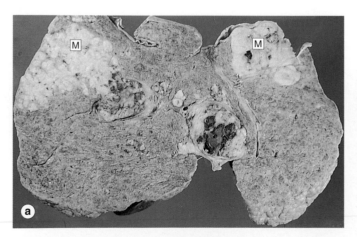
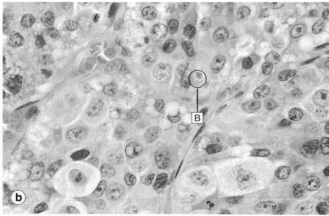

Fig. 14.35 Hepatocellular carcinoma.
Macroscopically hepatocellular carcinomas may be single or multifocal. As in (a), they usually develop in a liver already affected by cirrhosis. Tumor appears as an abnormal mass (**M**) within the liver. Histologically (b) tumor is composed of liver cells with atypical nuclear cytology and abnormal architectural arrangement. Bile secretion (**B**) by tumor cells may be seen.

- **Amyloidosis**: the liver may be involved in deposition of the abnormal protein, amyloid (see Chapter 25).
- **Sarcoidosis**: the liver is frequently involved by granulomatous inflammation as part of systemic sarcoidosis (see Chapter 25).
- **Extramedullary hemopoiesis** occurs in the liver when diseases efface the bone marrow. This is particularly seen in the myeloproliferative diseases (see page 326).
- **Cardiac failure** (see page 174).
- **Diabetes mellitus**: fatty liver and glycogen accumulation.

Liver transplants are prone to rejection as well as recurrence of original disease

Liver transplantation is being performed with increasing frequency to treat chronic liver disease, particularly that which has progressed to cirrhosis. It is also used to treat cases of fulminant hepatic failure due to extensive liver cell necrosis.

The pathological complications of transplantation are acute rejection, affecting 60% of patients in the first few weeks (treatable with steroids), and chronic rejection, affecting 15% of patients within the first year. Immune-mediated destruction of intrahepatic bile ducts and obliteration of intrahepatic vessels leads to progressive cholestatic jaundice. This is unresponsive to immunosuppression. Bile duct strictures at anastomosis sites may also complicate transplantation, and recurrent disease is seen in hepatitis B and C, and in primary biliary cirrhosis.

LIVER DISEASE IN CHILDHOOD

Biliary atresia is a cause of neonatal jaundice

In biliary atresia there is destruction of bile ducts that leads to severe jaundice in neonates. Two patterns are seen:

- **Intrahepatic atresia**, in which ducts within the liver are absent.
- **Extrahepatic atresia**, in which the main extrahepatic ducts are not patent.

These syndromes are believed to be due to intrauterine inflammatory diseases, which can also cause neonatal hepatitis, discussed next.

Liver biopsy shows striking proliferation of small bile ducts at the margins of portal tracts. Affected children develop severe jaundice. Extrahepatic atresia may be treated by surgical bypass operations. Children with severe disease develop unremitting jaundice and secondary biliary cirrhosis.

Neonatal hepatitis is a syndrome with many causes

Neonatal hepatitis is a clinical condition with many causes, presenting as neonatal jaundice.

Histologically there is hepatocyte damage, parenchymal inflammation and, in many cases, **giant-cell transformation** of hepatocytes (so-called giant cell hepatitis). The main causes are:

- Idiopathic (no cause found), accounting for 50% of cases.
- α-1-antitrypsin deficiency, responsible in about 30% of cases (see page 293).
- Viral hepatitis.
- Hepatitis due to **to**xoplasma, **r**ubella, **c**ytomegalovirus or **h**erpes simplex (TORCH group).
- Metabolic causes (galactosemia, hereditary fructose intolerance).
- Extrahepatic biliary atresia.
- Congenital hepatic fibrosis.

With the exception of cases associated with biliary atresia who require a surgical bile-drainage operation, children with neonatal hepatitis generally recover.

Jaundice in neonates can cause brain damage termed 'kernicterus'

Unconjugated hyperbilirubinemia in neonates may lead to kernicterus. Unconjugated bilirubin, which is lipid-soluble, enters the brain to cause damage to neurons, particularly in the basal ganglia. Affected children develop spasticity, choreoathetosis and mental deficiency. The most common causes are hemolysis due to rhesus incompatibility, or functional immaturity of hepatic conjugating enzyme systems.

Cystic fibrosis leads to cirrhosis in adult life in about 10% of cases

In cystic fibrosis (see page 221) affected neonates may develop obstructive jaundice due to blockage of bile ducts by abnormally viscous bile. Of those who survive to adult life, 10–15% develop chronic liver disease. This is a form of secondary biliary cirrhosis due to chronic obstruction to bile ducts by viscid bile.

Reye's syndrome is associated with microvesicular fat in liver cells

Reye's syndrome results in acute liver failure associated with cerebral edema and encephalopathy. It is seen in children and may be triggered by preceding viral infection or salicylate administration. Histologically the liver shows microvesicular fatty change. The condition is fatal in about 50% of cases.

Hepatoblastoma is a rare malignant childhood tumor

Rare malignant tumors of childhood, hepatoblastomas often replace large portions of the liver. They are composed of several cell types including fetal-pattern liver cells and mesenchymal elements. The serum α-fetoprotein is elevated.

DISEASES OF THE GALLBLADDER AND EXTRAHEPATIC BILE DUCTS

Gallstones

Stones in the gallbladder and bile duct system (**cholelithiasis**) are the most common cause of disease affecting the biliary tree. Stones form from the constituents of bile, the main components being variable proportions of cholesterol, calcium salts (phosphates, carbonates) and bilirubin (in the form of calcium bilirubinate).

Although it is recognized that most stones have several constituents, two main types of stone have been defined according to the major constituent of each: **cholesterol stones** (80% of all stones) and **pigment stones** (20% of all stones).

Cholesterol stones are predisposed by changes in cholesterol solubility in bile

Cholesterol stones (*Fig. 14.36*) occur in 20% of women and 8% of men, usually causing no problems. They form when bile becomes supersaturated with cholesterol, there being insufficient bile salts to keep the cholesterol in solution. In most cases the reasons for these changes are unclear.

The main risk factors associated with cholesterol stone formation are:

- Decreased bile acids in bile, caused by estrogen or excessive loss from gut due to malabsorption in Crohn's disease or cystic fibrosis.
- Increased cholesterol in bile caused by obesity, female sex, increasing age.

Cholesterolosis of the gallbladder occurs when the submucosa of the gallbladder is focally infiltrated by macrophages laden with cholesterol (*Fig. 14.37*). This condition is frequently associated with the development of cholesterol stones and is believed to be predisposed by the same conditions that cause decreased solubility of cholesterol in bile.

Understanding of the pathogenesis of cholesterol stone formation has led to medical treatment of stones by oral therapy with bile salts to dissolve stones.

Pigment stones are predisposed by increased hepatic secretion of bilirubin

Several clinical situations are associated with the development of pigment stones (*Fig. 14.38*), which are largely composed of calcium bilirubinate, with lesser amounts of other calcium salts and mucoproteins. It is easy to understand why patients with abnormal red-cell breakdown, generating large amounts of conjugated bilirubin, develop pigment stones. The association of pigment stones with cirrhosis and ileal resections is believed to be related to disturbance of the enterohepatic recycling of factors which regulate solubility of factors secreted in bile. Chronic biliary infections predispose to pigment gallstones by bacterial production of glucuronidases which unconjugate secreted conjugated bilirubin.

Gallstones may obstruct the biliary tract and predispose to development of carcinoma of the gallbladder

Over 70% of gallstones remain clinically silent. The main clinical complications of cholelithiasis arise from obstruction of the cystic duct or common bile duct by a stone.

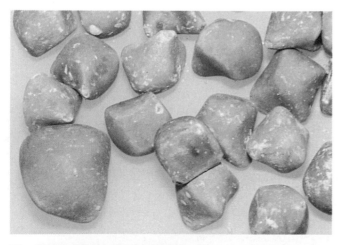

Fig. 14.36 Cholesterol stones.
Stones are round, faceted and can be 0.5–3 cm in size, but are typically large. Biochemical analysis reveals over 50% cholesterol composition, with lesser amounts of calcium salts so, strictly, most such stones are of mixed composition.

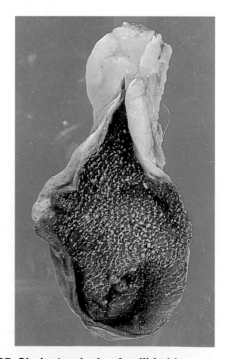

Fig. 14.37 Cholesterolosis of gallbladder.
In cholesterolosis the accumulation of lipid is seen in mucosal folds as a fine, yellow stippling.

The presence of stones in the biliary tract leads to muscle hypertrophy and thickening of the wall of the gallbladder (**obstructive cholecystopathy**). Stones impacted in the cystic duct predispose to inflammation of the gallbladder (**cholecystitis**), which may be acute or chronic (see below), and those forming in the bile ducts (**choledocholithiasis**) predispose to obstructive jaundice, cholangitis and acute pancreatitis. Stones in the gallbladder predispose to the development of carcinoma of the gallbladder (see page 300).

Gallstones may cause acute cholecystitis

Acute inflammation of the gallbladder causes pain in the right upper quadrant of the abdomen. The affected gallbladder is enlarged, red and edematous and, histologically, there is acute inflammation of the wall, with focal epithelial ulceration.

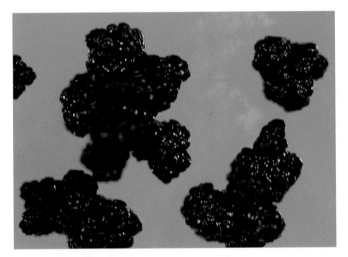

Fig. 14.38 Pigment stones.
Stones are irregular in shape. They measure up to 1 cm, being typically smaller than cholesterol stones.

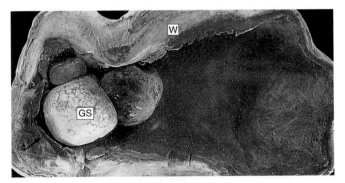

Fig. 14.39 Chronic cholecystitis.
In chronic cholecystitis there is thickening of the gallbladder wall (**W**). Histologically this is due to muscular hypertrophy, submucosal fibrosis, and chronic inflammation. Outpouches of mucosa into the wall form small cystic spaces termed 'Aschoff–Rokitansky sinuses'. In this example, stones (**GS**) are seen in the fundus, and the mucosa is inflamed.

Most cases are associated with gallstones and there is often obstruction of the cystic bile duct by a stone. Inflammation is precipitated by the chemical effects of concentrated bile in the gallbladder, but secondary infection may develop with enteric organisms such as *Escherichia coli*. Primary bacterial infection of the gallbladder, e.g. with *Salmonella*, is rare.

Acute cholecystitis can occur in critically ill patients in the absence of gallstones, when septicemic spread of infection is postulated. Complications of acute cholecystitis include perforation into the abdomen (causing **biliary peritonitis**), and secondary infection which, in severe cases, may cause **empyema** of the gallbladder, filling the lumen with pus.

Chronic cholecystitis is associated with the presence of gallstones

Chronic cholecystitis is caused by the chronic effects of gallstones. There is thickening and fibrosis of the wall, with variable chronic inflammatory infiltration of mucosa and submucosa (*Fig. 14.39*).

The pathogenesis of chronic cholecystitis is probably multifactorial. As many gallbladders that have been removed show muscle thickening and fibrosis without inflammatory changes, it may be more appropriate to call such cases **obstructive cholecystopathy**. Other cases have associated chronic inflammation and these may truly be called **chronic cholecystitis**. Development of disease has been related to contractile abnormalities of the gallbladder (stimulated by the presence of stones), to direct chemical injury to the mucosa by bile, or to the effects of repeated episodes of acute cholecystitis.

Secondary changes include extensive **calcification** of the wall of the gallbladder (porcelain gallbladder) and development of a **mucocele** of the gallbladder (*Fig. 14.40*).

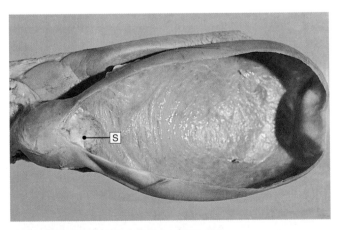

Fig. 14.40 Mucocele of the gallbladder.
Mucocele of the gallbladder is caused by obstruction of the cystic duct by stones (**S**). The bile is resorbed and the epithelium changes type to a mucin-secreting pattern, filling the gallbladder with clear mucus (emptied from this specimen). The mucosal surface is smooth and the wall is thinned.

Carcinoma of the gallbladder is associated with gallstones

Carcinoma of the gallbladder is the most common tumor of the gallbladder and is usually associated with the presence of gallstones and chronic cholecystitis. Most cases are seen in women over the age of 70 years.

Most tumors arise in the fundus and, histologically, are moderately differentiated adenocarcinomas (*Fig. 14.41*). Prognosis is poor, with a 5-year survival rate of under 5%. Infiltration of local structures, mainly the liver, makes curative surgery difficult.

Blockage of the main bile ducts causes obstructive jaundice

Obstruction of the common bile duct is most commonly due to a gallstone. Other causes include pancreatic carcinoma (see page 303), carcinoma of the ampulla of Vater (see page 260), fibrous stricture (often postoperative), and bile duct carcinoma (predisposed by chronic inflammation and liver flukes).

Microscopically the common and intrahepatic bile ducts become dilated, an important physical sign that can be readily detected by ultrasound examination. The liver becomes green, stained and enlarged.

Within the liver, features of extrahepatic cholestasis become manifest (see page 278), and secondary biliary cirrhosis may develop. An important complication is the development of secondary infection causing an ascending cholangitis that involves intrahepatic bile ducts.

DISEASE OF THE EXOCRINE PANCREAS

The normal exocrine pancreas comprises over 80% of the gland. Digestive enzymes are secreted and travel by pancreatic ducts to the duodenum.

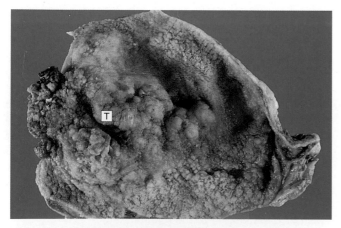

Fig. 14.41 Carcinoma of the gallbladder.
Adenocarcinoma of the gallbladder is seen as a raised, ulcerated area (**T**) in the fundus. Most tumors have invaded through the wall at the time of diagnosis. Spread is via lymphatics, as well as by direct growth into adjacent organs.

Developmental defects in the pancreas are uncommon. Heterotopic pancreatic tissue may be found in the wall of the duodenum, the stomach and in Meckel's diverticulum (see page 269).

Acute pancreatitis results in enzymic necrosis of tissues

Acute pancreatitis is an important cause of severe abdominal pain and enters the differential diagnosis of the acute abdomen (see Data Set). Severe acute inflammation and

**DATA SET
Acute pancreatitis**

A 42-year-old man with a history of alcohol abuse presented with severe abdominal pain and abdominal rigidity.

Plasma

Amylase	6470 U/L	(30 to 110)

Elevated levels of amylase in plasma are seen in a range of intra-abdominal emergencies in addition to acute pancreatitis, including perforated peptic ulcers, intestinal obstruction and biliary obstruction due to gallstones. Amylase is rapidly cleared from plasma, with a half-life of around 12 hours, and returns to normal within a few days of an attack of acute pancreatitis.

Acute pancreatitis – laboratory medicine

Full blood count: neutrophil leukocytosis.

Serum amylase: greatly elevated.

Serum albumin: falls in severe disease, due to loss in acute inflammatory exudate.

Serum calcium: falls in severe disease, due to complexing with necrotic fat and loss in exudate.

Blood sugar: hyperglycemia in severe disease, due to loss of endocrine cells.

Alkaline phosphatase: mild elevation from oedema and obstruction of lower end of bile duct.

Bilirubin: mild elevation due to oedema and obstruction of lower end of bile duct.

necrosis of the pancreas leads to liberation of the powerful digestive enzymes, resulting in extensive enzyme-mediated local tissue necrosis, particularly **fat necrosis** (*Fig. 14.42*). The main predisposing factors for pancreatitis are summarized in *Fig. 14.43*, and its pathogenesis is illustrated in *Fig. 14.44*. A complication of the development of acute pancreatitis is the conversion of the necrotic pancreas into a cyst filled with serosanguinous fluid (**pancreatic pseudocyst**).

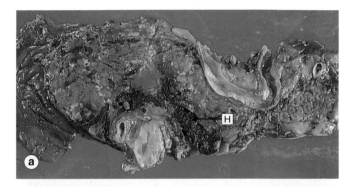

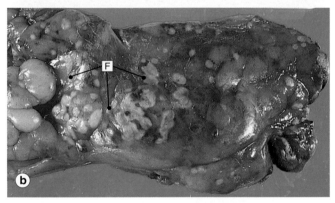

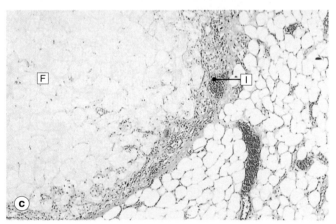

Fig. 14.42 Acute pancreatitis.

In acute pancreatitis (a) the pancreas appears edematous and is commonly hemorrhagic (**H**). Pancreatic tissue becomes necrotic and may become semi-liquid. Lipase released from the pancreatic acini causes the development of foci of fat necrosis. This is seen in (b) as white spots (**F**), typically 0.5 cm in diameter, in mesenteric and retroperitoneal fat. Histologically (c) these foci are composed of necrotic adipose tissue (**F**), with adjacent reactive inflammation (**I**).

Clinically most patients with acute pancreatitis recover. In severe disease chemical peritonitis and shock may develop. This may predispose to ARDS (see page 205).

Chronic pancreatitis is mainly caused by chronic alcohol abuse

Chronic pancreatitis results from chronic inflammation and fibrosis in the gland (*Fig. 14.45*). The four pathological features of chronic pancreatitis are continued chronic inflammation, fibrous scarring, loss of pancreatic parenchymal elements, and duct strictures and ectasia with formation of intrapancreatic calculi.

The main associations of chronic pancreatitis are shown in *Fig. 14.46*. Gallstones are not felt to play an important role in chronic pancreatitis, in contrast to their importance in acute pancreatitis.

Patients have recurrent bouts of severe abdominal pain, with eventual development of malabsorption (see page 255) and diabetes mellitus as pancreatic parenchyma is destroyed. Episodes of acute pancreatitis may complicate chronic pancreatitis.

Severe pancreatic atrophy occurs with cystic fibrosis

In cystic fibrosis (see page 221) viscid mucin occludes pancreatic ducts. Blockage results, with duct dilatation and atrophy of pancreatic acini. With time, both exocrine and endocrine parts of the pancreas are destroyed. Patients develop pancreatic insufficiency with malabsorption and diabetes mellitus.

Fig. 14.43
Predisposing factors in acute pancreatitis

Mechanical obstruction of pancreatic ducts

Gallstones
Trauma
Postoperative

Metabolic/toxic causes

Alcohol
Drugs (e.g. thiazide diuretics, azathioprine)
Hypercalcemia
Hyperlipoproteinemia

Vascular/poor perfusion

Atherosclerosis
Hypothermia

Infections

Mumps

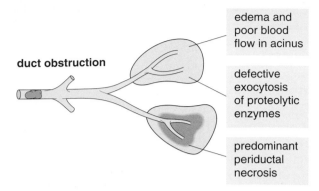

duct obstruction

edema and poor blood flow in acinus

defective exocytosis of proteolytic enzymes

predominant periductal necrosis

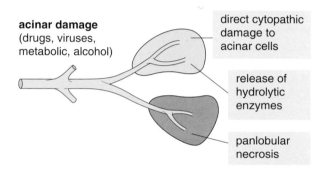

acinar damage (drugs, viruses, metabolic, alcohol)

direct cytopathic damage to acinar cells

release of hydrolytic enzymes

panlobular necrosis

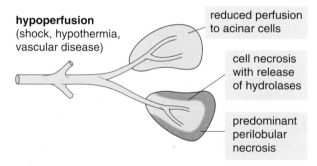

hypoperfusion (shock, hypothermia, vascular disease)

reduced perfusion to acinar cells

cell necrosis with release of hydrolases

predominant perilobular necrosis

Fig. 14.44 Pathogenesis of pancreatitis.
Three patterns of pancreatic necrosis have been defined, although in the advanced state it is hard to tell what pattern was present at the initiation as massive necrosis supervenes.

1 Periductal necrosis: necrosis takes place in acinal cells adjacent to ducts. This form is seen in conditions caused by duct obstruction, particularly associated with gallstones and alcohol.

2 Panlobular necrosis: necrosis is found affecting all portions of the pancreatic lobule. Conditions which cause direct acinar damage may initiate this pattern of damage, for example drugs, viruses, toxins and metabolic causes. Panlobular necrosis may be due to spread from initial periductal or perilobular necrosis.

3 Perilobular necrosis: necrosis takes place in the periphery of lobules. The pathogenesis is poor vascular perfusion of this zone, leading to acinar necrosis. This pattern is seen in shock and hypothermia.

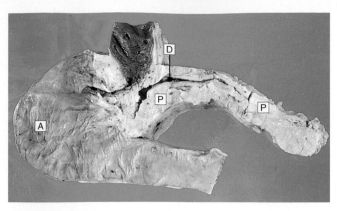

Fig. 14.45 Chronic pancreatitis.
In chronic pancreatitis the pancreas (**P**) is atrophic and replaced by rubbery, fibrous tissue, in which dilated ducts (**D**) are seen. In many cases calculi are present in the dilated ducts. In this example the duodenum is attached (**A**).

Fig. 14.46 Main associations of chronic pancreatitis	
Common	
Chronic alcoholism	Accounts for the majority of cases. Protein plugs form in ducts and become calculi. Ducts become obstructed, inflamed and scarred
Idiopathic chronic pancreatitis	Onset in old age. Often associated with peripheral vascular disease. Pathogenesis uncertain
Rare	
Cystic fibrosis	Protein plugs in ducts
Idiopathic juvenile pancreatitis	Uncertain etiology
Tropical pancreatitis	Prevalent in India and Africa. Uncertain cause

TUMORS OF THE PANCREAS

Benign tumors of the pancreas are uncommon

Benign tumors of the pancreas are rare. Cystadenomata are the most common benign tumors of the exocrine pancreas. These well-circumscribed masses are composed of multiple cystic cavities lined by serous or mucin-secreting epithelium.

Carcinoma of the pancreas is increasing in incidence

Carcinoma of the pancreas is one of the most common causes of death from cancer, with an increasing incidence in western countries. Although it is predominantly seen after the age of 60 years, there are occasional cases in younger patients.

The only environmental factor that is firmly associated with carcinoma of the pancreas is smoking. It has been speculated that dietary factors and exposure to chemical carcinogens may be contributory, but no definite risks have been determined. Diabetic women have an increased risk of development of pancreatic carcinoma.

Most carcinomas of the pancreas are adenocarcinomas. They arise with different frequencies in different parts of the pancreas (*Fig. 14.47*).

Carcinoma in the head of the pancreas tends to present early with obstructive jaundice. As a result, tumors are, on average, smaller at diagnosis than in other sites (*Fig. 14.48*).

Histologically most tumors are moderately differentiated adenocarcinomas with a prominent fibrous stroma. Less common histological variants are also described.

The main routes of spread are:

- **Local**, causing obstructive jaundice, or invasion of the duodenum.
- **Lymphatic**, spreading to adjacent lymph nodes.
- **Hematogenous**, spreading to the liver.

Pancreatic carcinoma is associated with several clinical syndromes:

- Weight loss, anorexia and chronic persistent pain in the epigastrium, radiating to the back.
- Obstructive jaundice with painless palpable dilatation of the gallbladder (Courvoisier's sign).
- Migratory thrombophlebitis, in which there is development of multiple thrombosis in superficial and deep leg veins (Trousseau's syndrome).

The prognosis for carcinoma of the pancreas is extremely poor, 90% of patients dying within 6 months of diagnosis. Palliative surgery is often performed to bypass obstruction of the bile duct (relieving jaundice) and obstruction of the duodenum. Islet-cell tumors, neoplasms derived from the pancreatic neuroendocrine cells, are discussed in the context of endocrine pathology in Chapter 16.

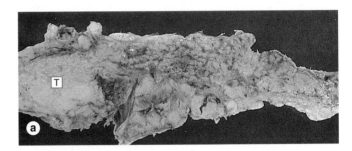

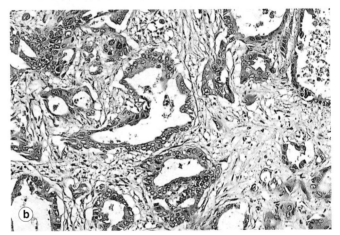

Fig. 14.48 Carcinoma of the head of the pancreas.
Tumors appear as gritty, grey, hard nodules (**T**), irregularly invading the adjacent gland and local structures (a). Histologically (b) they are usually moderately differentiated adenocarcinomas, which are composed of gland spaces in a fibrous stroma.

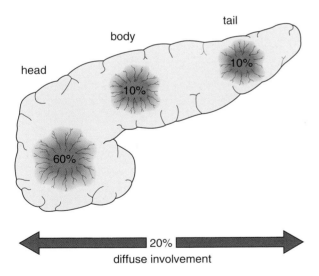

Fig. 14.47 Frequency of carcinoma of the pancreas in different parts of the gland.

Lymphoid and hemopoietic tissues

Clinical Overview

This chapter covers the pathology of the lymphoid and hemopoietic systems.

The lymphoid system incorporates the cellular systems and organs involved in mounting an immune response. Details of immunological dysfunction of this system have been presented in Chapter 7 and several multisystem diseases with an immunological pathogenesis are presented in Chapter 25. In this chapter the main structural disorders of the lymphoid system are dealt with – the commonest being the wide range of reactive proliferations seen in lymph nodes and spleen as a consequence of mounting a normal immune response to disease.

Primary tumors are the next most important disease of the lymphoid system, grouped together as the lymphomas. Taken together, reactive conditions and tumors account for the differential diagnosis of the vast majority of patients with enlarged lymph nodes.

The most important diseases of the hemopoietic system are the diseases that result in anemia and the classification and pathological consequences of these are presented. Neoplastic diseases of the hemopoietic system, resulting in leukemias, are also common conditions and understanding their classification and pathological manifestations are important for differential diagnosis. We have not gone into the fine detail of hematological disease, as we believe that students should be reading a clinical-oriented hematology text.

Lastly, the diseases which can produce splenomegaly or a mass in the thymus gland are considered. While less common clinical problems, having a working knowledge of these areas is important in differential diagnosis and planning patient investigations.

DISEASES OF THE LYMPH NODES

REACTIVE CHANGES

Reactive lymphadenopathy is the most common cause of enlarged lymph nodes

The main function of lymph nodes is to allow the interaction of antigen, antigen-presenting cells and lymphoid cells in the generation of an immune response. Different types of stimulus generate different patterns of response in lymph nodes, identification of which may be helpful in diagnosing the cause. The most common reason for patients to develop enlargement of lymph nodes is as a reaction to antigenic stimuli (reactive lymphadenopathy).

There are five main patterns of reactive response, but in most diseases a mixed pattern of responses is seen:

- **Follicular hyperplasia**: increase in B-cell germinal centres.
- **Paracortical hyperplasia**: increase in T-cell paracortical region.
- **Sinus hyperplasia**: increase in histiocytic cells in medullary sinuses.
- **Granulomatous inflammation**: formation of histiocytic granulomas in nodes.

- **Acute lymphadenitis**: acute inflammation and suppuration in lymph nodes.

Follicular hyperplasia shows increase in size and number of germinal centres

Follicular hyperplasia is a common response to most types of antigen exposure (*Fig. 15.1*). The main situations associated with this reaction are nodes draining sites of chronic inflammation (see page 51), and nodes in rheumatoid disease (see page 537). The pattern is also seen in nodes enlarged in the early stages of persistent generalized lymphadenopathy in HIV infection (see page 107).

Paracortical hyperplasia shows increase in size of T-cell areas

Expansion of the T-cell paracortical zone is associated with follicular hyperplasia as part of a reaction to chronic inflammation (*Fig. 15.2*). Relatively pure expansion of the paracortex is seen in drug hypersensitivity reactions (e.g. lymphadenopathy with phenytoin treatment) and viral infections, particularly infectious mononucleosis (caused by Epstein–Barr virus).

Histiocytic cells accumulate in medullary sinuses and may store phagocytosed material

Increase in the number of histiocytic cells in the medullary sinuses is seen in many non-specific reactions to chronic inflammation, and in nodes draining tumors. Histiocytes in sinuses may also store exogenous materials within nodes, e.g. carbon in peribronchial and hilar nodes draining the lungs.

A particular type of lymph node enlargement is seen in nodes draining inflamed skin. In these cases the medullary region is expanded by histiocytic cells that often contain melanin pigment and lipid (**dermatopathic lymphadenopathy**).

Acute lymphadenitis occurs with acute bacterial infections

Acute inflammation of lymph nodes (acute lymphadenitis) is almost exclusively seen with bacterial infections, in nodes draining the infected focus. Affected nodes enlarge rapidly and are tender. Histologically there is reactive hyperplasia of follicles, and focal infiltration of the node by neutrophils. With pyogenic organisms there may be necrosis and suppuration in the node, which may develop into an abscess.

Granulomatous inflammation in nodes may be seen in several diseases

Granulomatous inflammation in lymph nodes can present with generalized or localized lymphadenopathy; lymph node biopsy is performed to establish the cause. The main causes are:

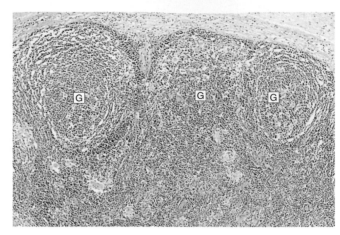

Fig. 15.1 Follicular hyperplasia.
In follicular hyperplasia there is an increase in size and number of B-cell germinal centers (**G**) in the node.

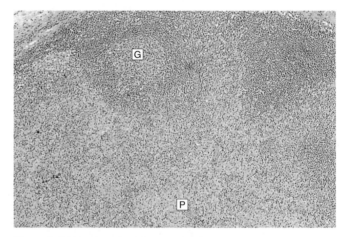

Fig. 15.2 Paracortical hyperplasia.
This lymph node shows expansion of the T-cell paracortex (**P**). Germinal centers (**G**) are pushed to the margin of the node. This example was taken from a patient with infectious mononucleosis (glandular fever).

- **Tuberculosis**: granulomas typically undergo caseous necrosis. TB must be confirmed by culture of biopsy tissue in all cases of undiagnosed lymphadenopathy.
- **Sarcoidosis** may affect regional nodes or be part of a generalized lymphadenopathy (see Chapter 25).
- **Cat scratch disease** is caused by a Gram-negative bacterium transmitted by cat scratches. It leads to a self-limited febrile illness with localized lymphadenopathy (*Fig. 15.3*).
- **Crohn's disease**: granulomas are a frequent finding in the enlarged nodes draining the bowel in Crohn's disease.
- **Toxoplasmosis**. Numerous small aggregates of histiocytic cells forming 'mini granulomas' are seen within enlarged nodes (*Fig. 15.4*).
- **Reaction to tumor**: granulomas may be found in lymph nodes draining malignant tumors.

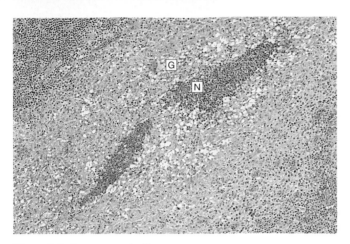

Fig. 15.3 Cat scratch disease.
In this condition, nodes show histiocytic granulomas (**G**), which contain central necrosis and neutrophilic infiltration (**N**).

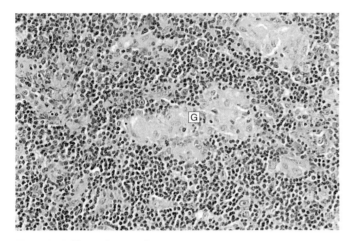

Fig. 15.4 Toxoplasmosis.
In toxoplasmosis, small granulomas (**G**) form within the lymph node and may encroach on germinal centers.

Less common causes are infections with fungi (histoplasmosis, coccidioidomycosis), *Chlamydia* (lymphogranuloma venereum) and other bacteria (*Yersinia* infection, *Brucella* infection).

Patients with HIV infection may develop lymphadenopathy at several stages of disease

At the time of seroconversion, many patients with HIV infection develop a transient lymphadenopathy. Later in the disease, lymphadenopathy is common (**persistent generalized lymphadenopathy**), with hematological and serological evidence of impaired cell-mediated immunity and reduced T-cell numbers. As clinical AIDS develops, generalized follicular hyperplasia gradually gives way to loss of follicles and depopulation of nodes of lymphoid cells.

Patients with HIV infection and AIDS are predisposed to development of lymphomas and Kaposi's sarcoma, both of which may affect nodes and cause lymphadenopathy.

NEOPLASTIC DISEASE IN LYMPH NODES

Metastatic tumor is a common cause of lymphadenopathy

The lymph nodes are a major site for metastasis of tumor by lymphatic spread. This is most commonly seen with carcinomas and melanomas, occurring less frequently with sarcomas. Clinically, development of enlarged lymph nodes may be the presenting sign of the tumor, the diagnosis being made only after histological examination of a lymph node biopsy.

Tumor cells are first seen in the subcapsular sinus; they later form solid areas, replacing the nodal structure (see page 84). With time, tumor extends outside the nodal capsule, tethering nodes to adjacent structures.

Typically, nodes involved by metastatic tumor are very hard and, in advanced cases, are fixed to other structures.

Lymphomas are neoplasms derived from lymphoid cells

The malignant lymphomas are primary neoplastic diseases of lymphoid cells, which have been divided into two main groups on the basis of clinical and pathological features.

Hodgkin's disease is characterized by neoplastic proliferation of an atypical form of lymphoid cell eponymously termed the Reed–Sternberg cell.

Non-Hodgkin's lymphomas are characterized by neoplastic proliferation of B-lymphocytes, T-lymphocytes or, very rarely, histiocytic cells. Disease typically starts in lymph nodes, spreading to involve spleen, liver and bone marrow. Other organs are commonly involved in advanced disease.

HODGKIN'S DISEASE

Hodgkin's disease is caused by proliferation of Reed–Sternberg cells

Hodgkin's disease involves proliferation of an atypical form of lymphoid cell that, until routine use of immunohistochemistry, was extremely difficult to categorize; it was hence named the Reed–Sternberg cell, after the two workers who identified its significance.

Clinically, disease presents as enlargement of a single lymph node or group of nodes, or enlarged nodes may be discovered following investigation for non-specific systemic symptoms such as weight loss, fever, or pruritus.

Macroscopically, affected nodes are enlarged (generally up to 2 cm in diameter) and are replaced by firm, rubbery, pinkish white tissue (*Fig. 15.5*). The natural history of untreated disease is one of spread to adjacent lymph node groups, with involvement of spleen, liver, and bone marrow.

Disease is initially diagnosed on lymph node biopsy. Next, the extent of disease is assessed by staging. CT scanning or MR imaging is used to detect enlarged lymph node groups and infiltration of spleen and liver. Liver biopsy

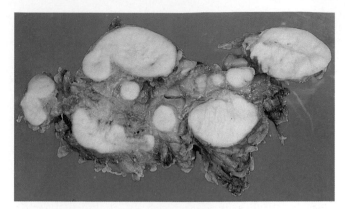

Fig. 15.5 Lymph nodes in Hodgkin's disease.
These lymph nodes are enlarged and replaced by firm, creamy white tissue. Although this example was taken from a case of Hodgkin's disease, nodes in non-Hodgkin's lymphomas may appear identical.

enables assessment of hepatic involvement, and bone marrow aspiration is used to determine marrow infiltration.

Clinical stage is described using the Ann Arbor system (*Fig. 15.6*).

Five histological sub-types of Hodgkin's disease are defined according to the histological pattern of disease

Histologically, five types of Hodgkin's disease have been defined (**WHO classification**), each with a different natural history and prognosis (*Fig. 15.7*).

Common to all types of Hodgkin's disease is the presence of Reed–Sternberg cells, the morphology of which varies in different sub-types of disease (*Fig. 15.8*). The difference between the types is in the extent and vigor of the host immune response associated with neoplastic transformation. The response is marked in lymphocyte-predominant disease, moderate in mixed cellularity, variable in nodular sclerosis, and in lymphocyte-depleted it is virtually non-existent

Nodular lymphocyte-predominant disease is mainly seen in young adult males. Histologically the nodes are replaced by reactive lymphoid cells, among which are a small population of Reed–Sternberg cells of the lymphocytic/histiocytic type. Importantly, and in contrast with the other types of Hodgkin's disease, the neoplastic cells are clearly B-cell in origin. Most patients present with Stage I or II disease.

Mixed cellularity disease mainly affects adults in later life, but any age can be affected. Lymph nodes are replaced by an infiltrate of Reed–Sternberg cells of the classic and mononuclear types, with a cellular response composed of lymphoid cells, eosinophils, plasma cells and histiocytes. Over 50% of patients present in Stage III or IV.

Nodular sclerosis is the most common type of Hodgkin's disease, mainly affecting young adults. In most cases the mediastinal nodes are involved at presentation. The key

Fig. 15.6
Ann Arbor clinical staging for Hodgkin's disease

Stage	Description
I	Disease confined to one lymph node group or Involvement of a single extranodal site (I_E)
II	Disease confined to several nodal groups on the same side of the diaphragm or With limited involvement of adjacent extranodal site (II_E)
III	Disease is present in lymph node groups on both sides of the diaphragm or With limited involvement of adjacent extranodal site (III_E) or With involvement of the spleen (III_S)
IV	Disseminated involvement of one or more extranodal tissues, such as the liver or bone marrow, with or without nodal involvement.

Notes: Disease is sub-classified according to presence or absence of systemic symptoms (e.g. fever, night sweats, weight loss)

Symptoms absent – A
Symptoms present – B

Fig. 15.7
REAL/ WHO classification of Hodgkin's disease

Nodular lymphocyte predominant Hodgkin's disease

Classic Hodgkin's disease
    Nodular sclerosis (grades I and II)
    Lymphocyte-rich
    Mixed cellularity
    Lymphocyte-depleted

feature is that the infiltrate is divided into nodules by broad bands of collagen. In nodular sclerosis grade I the infiltrate is cytologically the same as in mixed cellularity disease. In nodular sclerosis grade II the infiltrate contains pleomorphic Reed–Sternberg cells in high density.

Lymphocyte-rich Hodgkin's disease is characterized by classical Reed–Sternberg cells set in a diffuse background of lymphoid cells that do not mark as B-cells and hence are separated from nodular lymphocyte predominant disease. This entity has only recently been identified as a distinct sub-type.

Reed–Sternberg cells

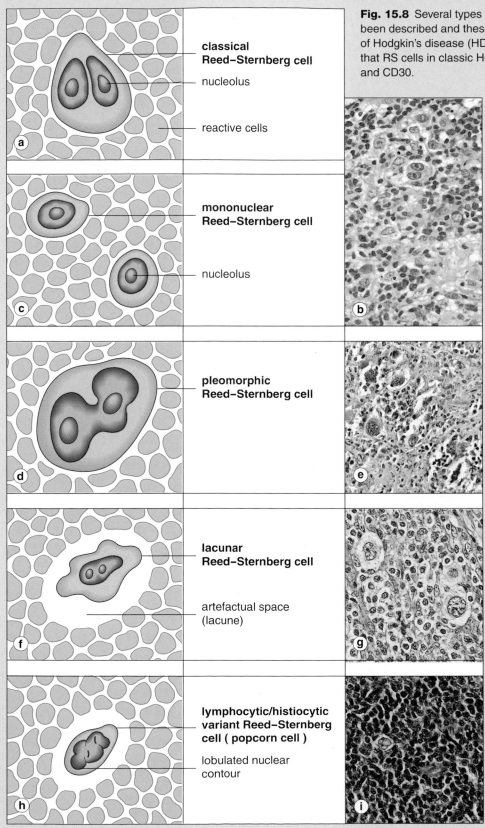

classical Reed–Sternberg cell

nucleolus

reactive cells

a

mononuclear Reed–Sternberg cell

nucleolus

c

b

pleomorphic Reed–Sternberg cell

d

e

lacunar Reed–Sternberg cell

artefactual space (lacune)

f

g

lymphocytic/histiocytic variant Reed–Sternberg cell (popcorn cell)

lobulated nuclear contour

h

i

Fig. 15.8 Several types of Reed–Sternberg (RS) cell have been described and these are found in different sub-types of Hodgkin's disease (HD). Immunohistochemistry shows that RS cells in classic Hodgkin's disease label with CD15 and CD30.

- Classical RS cells are binucleate, resembling owl eyes, and are seen in mixed cellularity and nodular sclerosis grade I HD (a and b).

- Mononuclear RS cells may be seen in any type of Hodgkin's disease but are mainly encountered in mixed cellularity disease (c and b).

- Pleomorphic RS cells have hyperchromatic large nuclei and are larger than other types of RS cell, being seen in lymphocyte-depleted and nodular-sclerosing grade II disease (d and e).

- Lacunar cells are surrounded by an artefactual space in histological sections and are characteristically seen in nodular-sclerosing grade I HD (f and g).

- The variant of RS cell seen in nodular lymphocyte predominant disease is called the lymphocytic histiocytic variant, sometimes called a 'popcorn' cell because of the bubbly outline of the nucleus (h and i). This cell type has been shown to express B-cell markers and does not express CD15 or CD30, justifying separating this type of disease from classic Hodgkin's disease.

Lymphocyte-depleted disease (*Fig. 15.8e*) is mainly seen in elderly adults. The infiltrate is composed of many pleomorphic Reed–Sternberg cells, and shows few reactive lymphoid cells. Most patients with this pattern present with Stage III or IV disease; it is associated with the poorest prognosis. Re-examination of cases previously classified as this form of disease has reclassified them as large-cell anaplastic non-Hodgkin's lymphomas often expressing a specific ALK oncogene product (see below). Thus the incidence of true lymphocyte-depleted Hodgkin's disease may be much lower than previously thought.

Prognosis in Hodgkin's disease is related to stage and sub-type

The best outcome is seen in lymphocyte-predominant disease and nodular sclerosis Type I, the worst prognosis being seen in lymphocyte-depleted disease and nodular sclerosis grade II. Mixed cellularity disease has a varied prognosis, which is largely dependent on the stage at the time of diagnosis.

Overall, the 10-year survival rate for patients with Hodgkin's disease is > 80% for the nodular lymphocyte-predominant type, 75% for nodular sclerosis Type I, 60% for the mixed cellularity type, 55% for nodular sclerosis grade II, and 5% for the lymphocyte-depleted type (40% have a 5-year survival).

Within each sub-group, factors that are associated with reduced survival and early death are advanced stage, advanced age of patient, and the presence of systemic symptoms (Type B disease – see *Fig. 15.6*).

NON-HODGKIN'S LYMPHOMAS

The non-Hodgkin's lymphomas can be grouped according to the site of origin

Non-Hodgkin's lymphomas may be classified as **nodal** (tumors originating in lymph nodes, which account for the vast majority of cases) or **extranodal** (tumors originating in specialized groups of lymphoid cells). Most extranodal lymphomas arise in specialized epithelial-associated lymphoid cells (mucosa-associated lymphoid tissue – MALT), and cases are seen in the gut and lung. Other examples develop in tissues that have been the seat of chronic lymphocytic inflammation in organs not normally noted to have a lymphoid population (e.g. testis and thyroid). Lymphomas may also develop in the brain and skin as a primary disease.

Non-Hodgkin's lymphomas originate from either B- or T-lymphocytes

Non-Hodgkin's lymphomas can be derived from either B- or T-lymphocytes. They are composed of a predominant cell type, which can be related to one of the stages of differentiation of normal T- or B-cells.

In very general terms, the growth of these tumors is related to cytology of the malignant cells: cells with small nuclei have a low rate of proliferation and are associated with a slow pace of growth; cells which have large nuclei and large nucleoli are associated with rapid proliferation and aggressive biological behavior.

On the basis of their cytology, phenotype and clinical behavior, non-Hodgkin's lymphomas can be divided into four main groups:

1 Slow-growing, indolent B-cell lymphomas (50% of cases).
2 Rapid-growing, aggressive B-cell lymphomas (30% of cases).
3 Slow-growing T-cell lymphomas (10% of cases).
4 Rapid-growing aggressive T-cell lymphomas (10% of cases).

In older classifications, histiocytic lymphomas were included. However, modern investigative techniques have shown that most of these cases were either large cell T-cell lymphomas or null-cell anaplastic large cell lymphomas with specific patterns of oncogene expression. True histiocytic lymphomas are remarkably rare.

Characterization of lymphomas gives an assessment of clinical behavior

As chemotherapy regimes differ for each pattern of lymphoma, pathological evaluation of tumor type is required for the purposes of treatment. The division of lymphomas into prognostic-related entities for clinical purposes (as opposed to academic pathological purposes) has resulted in the REAL and the latest WHO classifications (see blue box).

Immunohistochemistry is essential in diagnostic assessment of lymphoid neoplasms

Lymphocyte markers are used to discriminate between different types of lymphoid neoplasm corresponding to the CD system.

The classical reagents used to show a B-cell lineage detect CD19, CD20 and CD22. CD79a is also extensively used in this respect.

Identification of cells as being of T-cell lineage relies on detection of one or more pan-T-cell markers such as CD2, CD3, CD5, or CD7. Antibodies which detect b or d chains of the T-cell receptor can also be used.

Antibodies that detect granzyme, perforin or TIA1 can be used to characterize cells as being of NK lineage. Such cells may also express CD56, CD57 and CD16.

Antibodies which specifically detect the product of fusion oncogenes produced by translocations can be used to characterize certain types of lymphoid tumor.

Classification of lymphomas

Enthusiastic students will want to know the background to the classification of non-Hodgkin's lymphomas which has been controversial and fraught with problems of reproducibility in the hands of anyone other than the group that invented them, and sometimes having little relevance to prognosis or therapy.

In Europe and the USA in the early 1970s the Kiel/Lennert classification and the Lukes and Collins classifications divided lymphomas on the basis of morphology and immunology of cells. Tumors were divided into B- and T-cell types and related to stages in normal lymphocyte maturation. A disadvantage of this classification was that while based on a good theoretical concept it was considered by some to be difficult to relate to clinical work.

In 1982 an International Working Formulation of the National Cancer Institute (USA) divided lymphomas into three grades based on clinical behavior. This scheme used cytological features of neoplastic cells to place tumors in three groups:

• Lower grade; Intermediate grade; High grade.

Because of its clinical relevance, this scheme was widely adopted but proved problematic in that some entities behaved in a way that was not predicted by the pathological classification.

In 1994 an international group produced the Revised European American Lymphoma classification (REAL) in which problem areas were clarified and entities defined.

In 1999 the WHO proposed a new classification of lymphomas based on the REAL classification (Fig. 15.9) and this proposed classification is used in this book. Items in italics are presented later in this chapter – other entities are very rare.

Fig. 15.9
REAL/ WHO classification of lymphomas

B-cell neoplasms

Precursor B-cell lymphoblastic leukemia/lymphoma
Mature B-cell neoplasms
   B-cell chronic lymphocytic leukemia/small lymphocytic lymphoma
   B-cell prolymphocytic leukemia
   Lymphoplasmacytic lymphoma (lymphoplasmacytoid lymphoma)
   Mantle cell lymphoma
   Follicular lymphoma (follicle center lymphoma)
   Marginal zone B-cell lymphoma of mucosa-associated lymphoid tissue (MALT) type
   Nodal marginal zone lymphoma with or without monocytoid B-cells
   Splenic marginal zone B-cell lymphoma
   Hairy cell leukemia (page 325)
   Diffuse large B-cell lymphoma
   Sub-types mediastinal (thymic), intravascular, primary effusion lymphoma
   Burkitt lymphoma
   Plasmacytoma
   Plasma cell myeloma

T-cell neoplasms

Precursor T-cell lymphoblastic leukemia/lymphoma
Mature T-cell and NK-cell neoplasms
   T-cell prolymphocytic leukemia
   T-cell large granular lymphocytic leukemia
   NK-cell leukemia
   Extranodal NK/T-cell lymphoma, nasal-type (angiocentric lymphoma)
   Mycosis fungoides
   Sezary syndrome
   Angioimmunoblastic T-cell lymphoma
   Peripheral T-cell lymphoma (unspecified)
   Adult T-cell leukemia/lymphoma (HTLV1+)
   Systemic anaplastic large cell lymphoma (T- and null-cell types)
   Primary cutaneous anaplastic large cell lymphoma
   Subcutaneous panniculitis-like T-cell lymphoma
   Enteropathy-type intestinal T-cell lymphoma
   Hepatosplenic γ/δ T-cell lymphoma

Hodgkin's lymphoma (Hodgkin's disease)

Nodular lymphocyte predominance Hodgkin's lymphoma
Classic Hodgkin's lymphoma
   Hodgkin's lymphoma, nodular sclerosis (grades I and II)
   Classical Hodgkin's lymphoma, lymphocyte-rich
   Hodgkin's lymphoma, mixed cellularity
   Hodgkin's lymphoma, lymphocytic depletion (includes some 'Hodgkin-like anaplastic large cell lymphoma')

The main divisions in classification are into B-cell and T-cell types. Within each main type a division into precursor and mature lymphoid types has been made. In general, precursor lymphoid tumors are confined to childhood and adolescence.

B-CELL LYMPHOMAS

B-cell small lymphocytic lymphoma is seen in elderly patients

B-cell small lymphocytic lymphomas are low-grade tumors composed of cells that cytologically resemble small lymphocytes; there is an overlap with chronic lymphocytic leukemia, which is composed of virtually identical cells (see page 325).

The disease occurs in the elderly, typically running an indolent course over many years. It can present with enlarged nodes or anemia secondary to infiltration of bone marrow (seen in 80% cases). Immune deficiency secondary to hypogammaglobulinemia is seen in many patients, frequently leading to death by predisposing to infection. The 5-year survival is better than 60% with this type.

Histologically, lymph nodes are replaced by sheets of small lymphoid cells with little cytoplasm (*Fig. 15.10*). It is common for overspill of cells into the bloodstream to give a picture similar to chronic lymphocytic leukemia.

Lymphoplasmacytic lymphoma is seen in the elderly and runs an indolent course

Lymphoplasmacytoid lymphoma is a related form which, like B-cell lymphocytic lymphoma, is mainly seen in the elderly and runs an indolent course. Histologically it is characterized by cells with plasmacytic features, which often secrete immunoglobulin and produce a monoclonal band on serum electrophoresis. If there is production of IgM, patients may develop a hyperviscosity syndrome with poor flow of blood in small vessels and a bleeding tendency. This syndrome is termed **Waldenstrom's macroglobulinemia**.

Follicular lymphomas are B-cell lymphomas which recapitulate the function of normal follicle-center cells

Lymphomas formed from B-cells which recapitulate normal follicle center cells arrange themselves into follicles to form a follicular pattern of lymphoma.

Follicular lymphoma (*Fig. 15.11*) occurs most commonly after the sixth decade and represents one of the commonest types of disease. It is usually extensive at presentation, with involvement of bone marrow and liver. Although an indolent disease with slow progression over many years, it is difficult to cure, even with aggressive chemotherapy. Median survival is about 7–10 years. As part of the natural history of this disease, many cases transform into a high-grade diffuse lymphoma. Follicular lymphomas frequently

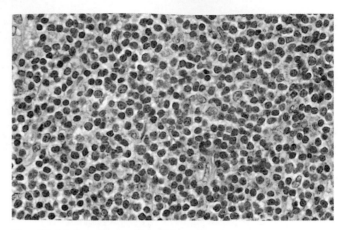

Fig. 15.10 B-cell small-cell lymphoma.
Neoplastic cells are arranged in diffuse sheets which efface the normal nodal architecture. Nuclei are small and cells have little cytoplasm.

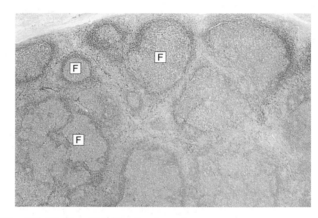

Fig. 15.11 B-cell follicular lymphoma.
In follicular lymphoma, neoplastic cells form germinal centers resembling normal follicles (**F**).

show a chromosomal translocation $t(14;18)$ that activates the Bcl-2 oncogene. The Bcl-2 protein can be detected in neoplastic follicles and this can be an aid to diagnosis.

B-cell lymphomas composed of large cells in a diffuse pattern pursue an aggressive course but respond well to therapy

Diffuse large B-cell lymphomas are common (*Fig. 15.12*). Histologically, nodes are replaced by sheets of large atypical lymphoid cells with prominent large nucleoli. Because this type of lymphoma grows so fast, enlargement of nodes is very obvious and patients notice the signs early. As a result, disease is often localized at the time of diagnosis. Presentation with extranodal disease is common, for example, with gut involvement.

This type of lymphoma affects all ages, including children, but is most common in later adult life. It may develop from progression of follicular lymphoma (secondary diffuse large B-cell lymphoma). Even when advanced, the disease

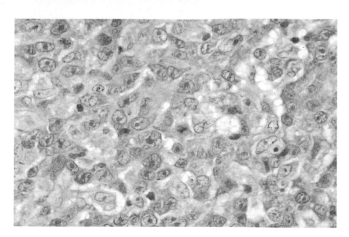

Fig. 15.12 Diffuse large B-cell lymphoma.
Neoplastic cells are large and have open nuclei with very prominent nucleoli.

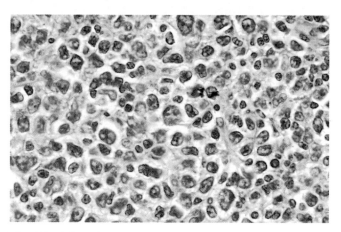

Fig. 15.14 B-cell mantle zone lymphoma.
Neoplastic cells have irregular shaped nuclei with clefts and grooves and prominent nucleoli.

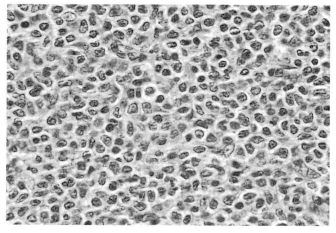

Fig. 15.13 B-cell marginal zone lymphoma.
Neoplastic cells are small- to medium-sized and have irregular nuclei and variable nucleoli. When involving a mucosal site these atypical cells infiltrate epitheli forming so-called lymphoepithelial lesions.

is curable with aggressive chemotherapy. A distinct t(14;18) translocation is seen in about 30% of cases. The Bcl-6 oncogene is rearranged or mutated in about 40% of cases.

An unusual pattern is recognized arising in the thymus of young women possibly arising from intrathymic B-cells.

Marginal zone B-cell lymphomas occur as extranodal disease arising in mucosal associated lymphoid tissue

The marginal zone lymphomas are believed to be the neoplastic counterpart of the marginal zone lymphoid cells that are normally present in lymph nodes and the spleen. These tumors characteristically arise in association with glandular epithelial tissues often in the setting of a pre-existing lymphocytic inflammatory process, being classified as lymphomas of mucosal-associated lymphoid tissue (MALT lymphomas). Histologically lymphoid cells are

medium-sized with small nucleoli (*Fig. 15.13*) and there is often a population of plasma cells in the lesion. Such lymphomas may arise in the tonsils, gut, bronchi, salivary glands, lacrimal glands or thyroid. The cells that become neoplastic continue to have the same specialized homing functions, recirculating only to the site of origin and the draining local nodes. Clinically such tumors run an indolent course. They tend not to become systematized, as it has been proposed that neoplastic cells lack adhesion molecules that would allow them to home in on other sites. Trisomy of chromosome 3 has been found in this type of tumor. Nodal and splenic forms of marginal zone B-cell lymphoma are also described.

Mantle cell B-cell lymphomas occur in adults and tend to run an aggressive course

The neoplastic cells in this form of lymphoma are believed to resemble the normal mantle zone lymphocytes found in relation to follicles in normal lymph nodes. Neoplastic cells are small- to medium-sized and have irregular shaped nuclei with deep clefts and prominent nucleoli (*Fig. 15.14*). A t(11;14) translocation is seen in this type of tumor. Disease typically presents as lymphadenopathy in adults and runs an aggressive course even with treatment.

Precursor B-cell lymphoblastic lymphomas are high-grade tumors mainly seen in childhood

Precursor B-cell lymphoblastic lymphomas are composed of cells resembling transformed lymphocytes. There is great overlap with B-cell acute lymphoblastic leukemia. There is extensive involvement of nodes and extranodal sites. This is an aggressive disease but is often curable although dictating the use of aggressive therapy (sometimes including irradiation of the neuraxis). Cells express markers of early B-cell lineage such as terminal transferase (TdT) and CD10 (CALLA).

Burkitt's lymphoma is an aggressive but curable disease mainly seen in childhood

Burkitt's lymphoma is a type of lymphoma that is endemic in Africa, but arises sporadically elsewhere, particularly affecting the jaw, ovaries, and gut (*Fig. 15.15*). In endemic Burkitt's lymphoma, Epstein–Barr virus genome is found in over 90% of cases, contrasting with under 20% of cases in sporadic disease. t(2;8), t(8;14), t(8;22) or rearrangement of the cMYC oncogene is seen in 80% of tumors.

Plasma-cell neoplasms cause lytic lesions in bone and secrete immunoglobulin

There are three tumors that can be considered as plasma cell neoplasms. These tumors retain the immunoglobulin-secreting property of mature plasma cells.

Multiple myeloma is most commonly seen after the age of 50 years. It is due to neoplastic proliferation of a single clone of bone-marrow-derived plasma cells. There are several main effects:

- Plasma cells grow within marrow, diffusely replacing normal hemopoietic tissue. Expansion may cause lytic lesions and bone pain. Bone destruction may cause hypercalcemia and pathological fractures. Lesions are most common in the vertebrae, ribs, skull and pelvis.
- Cells synthesize monoclonal immunoglobulin chains, which accumulate in the blood and may be detected by serum electrophoresis as a monoclonal band. In most cases the monoclonal immunoglobulin is IgG. When the immunoglobulin is IgM, patients may develop hyperviscosity of blood.
- Free light chains from excess monoclonal immunoglobulin may be filtered by the glomerulus to enter the urine, where they can be detected as Bence–Jones protein.
- Increased protein concentration in the blood is responsible for an elevated ESR as a result of rouleaux formation.
- Patients develop immune paresis and are susceptible to infection.
- In some cases the light chains form amyloid (see Chapter 25), which is deposited in tissues, particularly the renal glomeruli and heart.
- Renal dysfunction is common as a result of light-chain protein casts, with secondary damage to tubules and amyloid.

Diagnosis is based on examination of bone marrow aspirates, which show an excess of plasma cells (*Fig. 15.16*). It is supported by finding a monoclonal immunoglobulin band on serum protein electrophoresis, and Bence–Jones protein in urine.

Plasmacytomas are also composed of neoplastic plasma cells and may be associated with secretion of monoclonal immunoglobulin. In contrast to multiple myeloma, they are

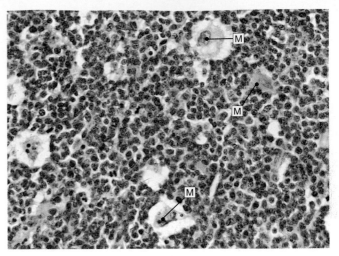

Fig. 15.15 Burkitt's lymphoma.
In Burkitt's lymphoma a characteristic feature is the presence of large macrophagic cells (**M**) scattered through the tumor, likened to a 'starry sky'.

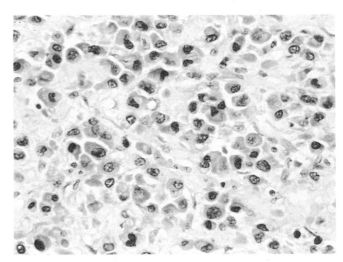

Fig. 15.16 Bone marrow in multiple myeloma.
The bone marrow shows replacement by plasma cells, many of which show cytological abnormalities with nuclear irregularities.

solitary circumscribed lesions. In bone they may form osteolytic lesions. They may also develop in soft tissue. Many cases develop multiple myeloma after a period of years.

Benign monoclonal gammopathy is a term applied to patients who have a monoclonal immunoglobulin band on serum electrophoresis, but have no pathologically demonstrable plasma-cell abnormality. The natural history is for many patients to develop myeloma after a period of years.

T-CELL LYMPHOMAS

T-cell lymphomas commonly affect the skin or other extranodal tissues

Mycosis fungoides and **Sezary syndrome** are two types of indolent, slowly progressing T-cell lymphoma which affect

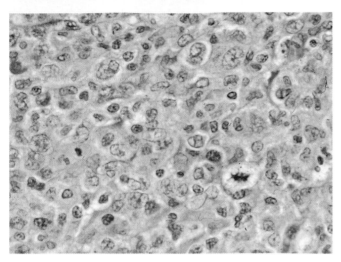

Fig. 15.17 Peripheral T-cell lymphoma.
In this peripheral T-cell lymphoma neoplastic cells are large with moderate amounts of cytoplasm. Although cells superficially resemble histiocytes (which in times past caused such tumors to be incorrectly classed as histiocytic lymphomas), immunohistochemical techniques reveal them to be T-cells.

the skin and draining lymph nodes. The T-cells have been termed cerebriform because the nuclear membrane is very convoluted, resembling the gyri of the brain. In mycosis fungoides and Sezary syndrome, neoplastic T-cells migrate into the epidermis, causing an erythematous rash (see page 508). In Sezary syndrome these atypical cells also circulate in the blood. Lymph nodes can become affected. With progression of disease, the skin develops thick plaques of lymphoma and there is visceral involvement. A rare form of T-cell lymphoma is characterized by dominant involvement of subcutaneous tissues leading to the term **subcutaneous panniculitis-like T-cell lymphoma**.

Angio-immunoblastic T-cell lymphoma presents in the elderly, with systemic features of malaise, fever and skin rashes. There is generalized lymphadenopathy. Investigations reveal polyclonal hypergammaglobulinemia and hemolytic anemia. Histologically, nodes show proliferation of small T-cells, which attract a considerable population of reactive cells (plasma cells, eosinophils, histiocytes) through secretion of lymphokines. The disease pursues an aggressive course and may transform into a high-grade T-cell lymphoma.

One form of T-cell lymphoma, termed **angiocentric lymphoma**, grows by invading the walls of blood vessels. This type of disease is common in Asia and often presents as disease affecting the nose or skin, Histologically atypical T-cells can be seen invading and occluding vessels, leading to the common finding of necrosis of both normal and neoplastic tissues. Immunochemistry may show that these cells have a T-cell/NK-cell phenotype.

Enteropathy-type intestinal T-cell lymphomas are especially seen as a complication of coeliac disease (page 256). The small bowel shows thickening of the mucosa by neoplastic T-cells. There is frequent ulceration of the bowel and this may be complicated by perforation. This type of disease runs an aggressive course.

Peripheral T-cell lymphomas have diverse clinical and pathological patterns

With the wider use of immunohistochemistry peripheral T-cell lymphomas have been increasingly recognized, but even so such tumors only account for a small proportion of lymphomas. There is a degree of pathological heterogeneity in many of these conditions and although a 'splitting' classification of peripheral T-cell lymphomas has been proposed it has low reproducibility. For practical purposes the peripheral T-cell neoplasms are grouped together under the term **peripheral T-cell lymphoma, unspecified**. In addition to the presence of atypical neoplastic T-cells (*Fig. 15.17*), such tumors often recruit a substantial population of reactive cells, presumably related to the ability of neoplastic T-cells to secrete appropriate cytokines.

In addition to the group of 'unspecified' peripheral T-cell lymphomas there are a group of distinctive types:

- In children and adolescents, **precursor T-cell lymphoblastic lymphoma** is an aggressive but curable form of disease. Characteristically there is dominant involvement of the mediastinal nodes or thymus gland and disease usually presents with leukemic features. Extensive colonization of nodal and extranodal sites dictates the use of aggressive therapy including irradiation of the neuraxis.

- **T-cell prolymphocytic lymphoma** is usually of T-helper cells (CD4) and, in contrast to the B-cell variant of small lymphocytic lymphoma, is a more aggressive disease. Neoplastic proliferation of large granular lymphocytes may also occur, more often with a leukemic picture, and in such cases cells may have features of either T-cells or NK cells.

- Although uncommon in the western world, in the Caribbean and Asia T-cell lymphoma is more common due to causation by human T-cell leukemia virus Type 1 (HTLV-1). In resulting **adult T-cell lymphoma/leukemia** (*Fig. 15.17*) there is frequent extensive disease with skin involvement, hypercalcemia and leukemia.

- **Large-cell anaplastic lymphoma** is composed of large cells with a superficial resemblance to epithelial cells. They express CD30 (formerly called Ki 1) and epithelial membrane antigen. Cells have either a T-cell or null cell phenotype. A t(2;5) translocation has been seen in many cases leading to expression of the ALK oncogene. Detection of this oncogene product is possible using immunohistochemistry and this has led to increased recognition of such lymphoid tumors, including small-cell types, which appear to have similar biological properties. The term 'ALKoma' has been used to group such tumors.

Investigation of lymphomas

The management of lymphoma has developed into a specialized area of clinical practice. It is essential that the oncologist, surgeon, radiologist and pathologist discuss cases at all stages in the diagnostic process.

Histological evaluation of biopsy tissue is central to diagnosis and subsequent management. It is essential to use immunohistochemical markers for different lymphoid cell types, especially for B-cells and T-cells as previously described (page 310). In some circumstances, establishing that a lesion is malignant depends on showing that a cell proliferation is monoclonal by demonstrating clonal immunoglobulin gene rearrangement (B-lymphocytes) and clonal T-cell receptor gene rearrangement (T-lymphocytes). Cytogenetic investigation may demonstrate the presence of a specific chromosomal marker, e.g. the translocations seen in follicular lymphomas (see page 312) and Burkitt's lymphomas (see page 314).

In cases of suspected lymphoma, tissue removed for biopsy is now received fresh in the laboratory and carefully divided to allow a detailed morphological and molecular analysis.

Etiological factors in lymphomas

Although several factors have been implicated in development of lymphomas, e.g. they may be caused by Epstein–Barr (EBV) virus or HTLV-1, in most cases a cause is not known.

Lymphomas may develop in the setting of long-standing chronic immune-mediated disease. This may be autoimmune disease (thyroiditis, see page 336, Sjogren's disease, or a reaction to exogenous antigen, e.g. celiac disease). It is thought that continued immune activation predisposes to neoplastic change.

The incidence of lymphomas increases in patients with immune deficiency, be it congenital or acquired, when they are associated with EBV infection.

SURVIVAL AND PROGNOSIS IN LYMPHOMA

Survival for all types of treated non-Hodgkin's lymphoma evens out after 10 years because low-grade disease is hard to cure

The survival for patients with non-Hodgkin's lymphoma varies according to the grade of disease and its extent. Paradoxically, patients with rapidly growing aggressive tumors may be cured, whereas many patients with slow-growing lesions suffer late relapses. Patients who have clinically aggressive disease are often encountered at an early stage and may be cured by aggressive chemotherapy. Patients with slow-growing, indolent tumors often have extensive dissemination at diagnosis and, although disease may be controlled by therapy, cure is seldom achieved.

Although there is around a 70% 5-year survival for the indolent types of non-Hodgkin's lymphoma, with a 40% 5-year survival for initially aggressive disease, survival at 10 years is still about 40% for both types, reflecting continued deaths in patients with indolent forms of disease. Patients who tend to die early with non-Hodgkin's lymphoma include the elderly, those who have extensive dissemination with hematological abnormalities, and those with systemic symptoms or weight loss and fever.

DISEASES OF THE THYMUS

The normal thymus

The thymus is composed of lymphoid cells and specialized epithelial cells. It is the site for development and maturation of T-lymphocytes, as well as clonal deletion of self-reactive T-lymphocytes. Normally the thymus regresses after puberty. Failure of development of the thymus results in deficient T-cell-mediated immunity (see page 106).

The thymus is a site of development of several different types of tumor

Several different types of tumor occur in the thymus, usually presenting as an anterior mediastinal mass. These may be detected on chest radiograph as an incidental finding, or may produce disease by compression of adjacent structures. Occasionally attention is drawn to the thymus because of an autoimmune disease such a myasthenia gravis (see Chapter 21). The main tumors of the thymus are as follows:

- Lymphomas, particularly T-lymphoblastic lymphoma, nodular sclerosing Hodgkin's disease, and some B-cell lymphomas.
- Germ-cell tumors (teratoma and seminoma) account for about 20% of mediastinal tumors. They display a similar histological spectrum to that seen in the testis (see pages 385–389).
- Neuroendocrine tumors are composed of neuroendocrine cells and resemble those seen elsewhere. Clinically they may be associated with Cushing's syndrome.
- Thymomas are derived from thymic epithelial cells (spindle-cell or round-cell types) with an infiltrate of reactive lymphoid cells. They may be associated with

myasthenia gravis, red cell aplasia, and non-organ-specific autoimmune diseases (see page 111). Although 80% of thymomas are benign, 20% of these lesions behave as low-grade malignant tumors, infiltrating local structures with metastatic spread in about 10% of cases.

Thymic hyperplasia can be associated with autoimmune disease

Thymic hyperplasia is uncommon. Histologically, lymphoid follicles composed of B-cells develop in the thymic medulla, and there may be associated increase in the size of the thymus. This may also be associated with the development of autoimmune disease, particularly myasthenia gravis (see page 472).

DISEASES OF THE SPLEEN

The normal spleen weighs 100–200 g. Its two main functions are trapping and presenting antigens circulating in the blood and culling effete red cells from the circulation.

Hypersplenism is associated with enlargement of the spleen

A common physical sign, enlargement of the spleen may have many causes, the main types of which are summarized in *Fig. 15.18*. Irrespective of the cause, enlargement may result in development of hypersplenism. This syndrome is associated with two main problems: sequestration of red cells, white cells and platelets, and premature destruction of red cells. Hypersplenism therefore leads to reduction in the levels of red cells, white cells and platelets in the blood (pancytopenia) and, as a compensatory response, hyperplasia of the bone marrow. Splenectomy leads to clinical and hematological improvement. Another important complication of an enlarged spleen is that it is vulnerable to traumatic rupture, e.g. in glandular fever or malaria.

Hyposplenism increases the risk of serious bacterial infection by capsulated organisms

Lack of splenic function is clinically encountered in three main circumstances: surgical removal (for disease or trauma),

Fig. 15.18
Causes of splenomegaly

Infective causes	
Bacterial	For example, typhoid, tuberculosis, brucellosis, infective endocarditis
Viral	Infectious mononucleosis
Protozoal	Malaria, leishmaniasis, trypanosomiasis, toxoplasmosis
Vascular causes	
Portal hypertension	Main cause is cirrhosis (see page 293)
Neoplastic causes	
Lymphomas	Hodgkin's disease and non-Hodgkin's lymphoma
Leukemias	Particularly chronic leukemias, less common in acute types
Extramedullary hemopoiesis	Seen in myeloproliferative diseases and diseases with diffuse marrow replacement by tumor
Metastases	Splenic metastases from solid tumors are rare
Hematological causes	
Hemolytic anemias	Hereditary spherocytosis, β thalassemia, autoimmune hemolysis
Autoimmune thrombocytopenia	Destruction of platelets in spleen results in accumulation of foamy histiocytes in sinuses
Immunological causes	
Felty's syndrome	Follicular hyperplasia in the spleen associated with hypersplenism with rheumatoid disease
Sarcoidosis	Spleen infiltrated by granulomas (see Chapter 25)
Amyloidosis	Spleen infiltrated with amyloid (see Chapter 25)
Metabolic causes	
Storage disorders	Due to heritable enzyme deficiencies, e.g. Gaucher's disease and Niemann–Pick disease, which result in storage of material in splenic macrophagic cells

sickle-cell disease (microvascular occlusion causes ischemic atrophy, known as 'autosplenectomy'), and celiac disease (splenic atrophy).

As a consequence patients become susceptible to recurrent bacterial infections, particularly by capsulated bacteria (*Streptococcus pneumoniae*, *Haemophilus influenzae*, *Neisseria meningitidis*, *Escherichia coli*), and develop severe septicemia, intravascular coagulation, and multiorgan failure.

There are also abnormalities of red cells, which develop inclusion bodies (Howell–Jolly bodies) and abnormal shape (schistocytes and target cells). Usually, abnormal red cells are removed from the spleen as they squeeze through the splenic sinusoids.

DISEASES OF THE BLOOD

RED CELL DISORDERS

Reduction in the mass of circulating red cells is termed anemia

Anemia can be defined as a reduction in the mass of circulating red cells; it is detected by analysis of peripheral blood (low hemoglobin, low red cell count, low hematocrit).

To compensate for the lack of oxygen-carrying capacity, several changes take place in anemia. Biochemical changes

---

Fig. 15.19
Pathological classification of anemia

Reduced production of red cells

Deficiency of hematinics
Iron deficiency
B_{12} and folate deficiency

Dyserythropoiesis (production of defective cells)
Anemia of chronic disorders
Myelodysplasia
Sideroblastic anemia

Marrow infiltration

Aplasia (failure of production of cells)
Aplastic anemia
Red-cell aplasia

Increased destruction or loss of red cells

Bleeding

Hemolytic anemia
Red-cell abnormalities (membrane, enzymes, hemoglobinopathies)
Abnormalities outside red cells (immune, microangiopathic, parasitic)

Hypersplenism

---

in red cells reduce the affinity of hemoglobin for oxygen, and there is increased cardiac output, together with attempted increased red cell production.

The causes of anemia can be classified according to etiology (*Fig. 15.19*). In clinical practice the most common cause is iron deficiency, followed by the anemia of chronic disorders and deficiency of vitamins B_{12} and folate. All of the other causes are much less common.

ANEMIA DUE TO DEFICIENCY OF HEMATINICS

Iron deficiency is the most common cause of anemia

The main causes of iron-deficiency anemia are impaired intake, excessive blood loss (most common cause in adults), or increased demand (e.g. pregnancy and lactation).

The peripheral blood shows a hypochromic microcytic pattern (*Fig. 15.20*). There is a low total serum iron and increased total iron-binding capacity; a decreased serum ferritin level reflects reduced total body iron stores.

In addition to signs and symptoms of anemia, some patients with iron-deficiency anemia may develop angular cheilitis, atrophic glossitis, esophageal webs, koilonychia and brittle nails.

Chronic blood loss is the most common cause of iron-deficiency anemia

If blood loss has been slow, anemia can be severe. The most important causes are diseases of the gastrointestinal tract, particularly peptic ulceration, carcinoma of the stomach and carcinoma of the colon (especially cecum), menorrhagia, and loss of blood from lesions in the urinary tract.

Patients with unexplained iron-deficiency anemia require careful screening for an occult cause of blood loss.

Deficiency of vitamin B_{12} and folate causes macrocytic megaloblastic anemia

Megaloblastic anemia is the result of impaired DNA synthesis in marrow precursor cells. This type of anemia is due

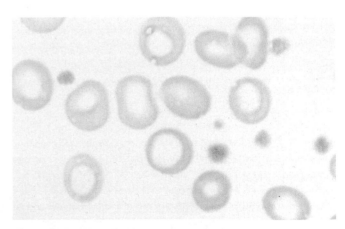

Fig. 15.20 Hypochromic, microcytic red cells.

to deficiency of vitamin B_{12} and folic acid. Vitamin B_{12} is normally absorbed from the diet by binding to intrinsic factor (IF), a glycoprotein secreted by gastric parietal cells. The B_{12}-IF complex binds to cells in the terminal ileum, where B_{12} is absorbed. The most common cause of B_{12} deficiency is lack of production of IF, resulting in pernicious anemia. In the stomach this is associated with autoimmune atrophic gastritis or can occur after surgical gastrectomy. Disease or surgical removal of the absorption site in the terminal ileum may also cause B_{12} deficiency.

Folic acid deficiency is most commonly due to inadequate dietary intake (folic acid is normally found in vegetables, meat and eggs). Deficiency is commonly encountered in alcoholics and in patients with malabsorption.

In the marrow, lack of B_{12} or folate causes development of abnormally large red-cell precursors (megaloblasts), which develop into abnormally large red cells (macrocytes). Because much erythropoiesis results in formation of defective cells that are prematurely destroyed, the marrow compartment is expanded and normally fatty marrow in the long bones becomes active. Patients have anemia, neutropenia and thrombocytopenia. In vitamin B_{12} deficiency, but not folate deficiency, neurological disease may occur, with the development of subacute combined degeneration of the spinal cord. Patients may also develop impaired cardiac function.

ANEMIA DUE TO FAILURE OF PRODUCTION

Aplastic anemia is due to failure of hemopoietic stem cells

In aplastic anemia there has been failure of marrow stem cells. Patients develop a pancytopenia and have a severe life-threatening disease. The marrow is depopulated of cells and is replaced by fat. Many cases are idiopathic, but others follow a known insult to the marrow (*Fig. 15.21*).

Pure red-cell aplasia is caused by specific suppression of red-cell production

In contrast to aplastic anemia, in which all formed elements of blood are affected, pure red-cell aplasia is characterized by suppression of red-cell progenitor cells. Patients develop anemia, but other formed elements of marrow are unaffected.

There are three groups: **acute self-limited** red-cell aplasia, which occurs after parvovirus infection or exposure to certain toxins; **chronic acquired** red-cell aplasia, which is autoimmune and may be associated with thymomas (see page 316); and **chronic constitutional** red-cell aplasia, which is due to a hereditary defect in progenitor cells.

ANEMIA DUE TO DYSERYTHROPOIESIS

Anemia of chronic disorders is the second most common cause of anemia

Patients with underlying diseases such as non-organ-specific autoimmune diseases (e.g. rheumatoid disease and SLE), chronic infective diseases (e.g. tuberculosis, malaria, schistosomiasis), or neoplasia (lymphoma and some carcinomas) may develop a normochromic or hypochromic anemia.

There are three main abnormalities found in such anemias – iron stored in macrophages is not released for use in bone marrow, circulating red cells have a reduced life span, and the marrow shows lack of response to erythropoietin.

Serum iron and serum iron binding capacity are low, but serum ferritin is normal or raised (compare iron-deficiency anemia, see page 318).

Myelodysplastic syndromes cause refractory anemia and predispose to leukemia

Myelodysplastic syndromes are diseases of late adult life, in which there is production of abnormal clones of marrow stem cells. The products of abnormal clones are defective and prematurely destroyed; thus, depending on severity, anemia and pancytopenia may develop. The presence of genetically abnormal clones in the marrow predisposes to the development of leukemia in about 40% of cases. The main problem is an indolent anemia that requires treatment with transfusions over several years but does not respond to administering hematinics (refractory anemia).

Histologically the marrow shows normal or increased cellularity with megaloblastic cells. Abnormal red-cell precursors containing iron (ringed sideroblasts) may be seen, and abnormal myeloblasts may be found. Based on the numbers of myeloblasts and abnormal red-cell precursors, five sub-types of myelodysplasia have been defined in a French-American-British (FAB) classification (*Fig. 15.22*).

Fig. 15.21
Factors associated with development of aplastic anemia

Radiation
Antineoplastic chemotherapeutic agents
Drugs: chloramphenicol, gold, NSAIDs
Toxins: benzene
Viruses: papovavirus, HIV-1
Fanconi's anemia: autosomal recessive

Fig. 15.22
FAB classification of myelodysplastic syndromes

Refractory anemia
Refractory anemia with ring sideroblasts
Refractory anemia with excessive blasts
Refractory anemia with excessive blasts in transformation
Chronic myelomonocytic leukemia

Sideroblastic anemias are characterized by defective heme synthesis in red-cell precursors

The sideroblastic anemias are characterized by abnormal red-cell progenitor cells that accumulate excess iron in their cytoplasm, forming cells termed ring sideroblasts. These cells have defective heme synthesis and result in anemia. There are two main groups of disease:

- **Secondary sideroblastic anemias**, which are drug-related (isoniazid), toxic-related (lead, alcoholism) or neoplasia-related (hematological malignancies).
- **Primary sideroblastic anemia** (myelodysplastic syndrome).

Marrow infiltration may result in leukoerythroblastic anemia

Extensive infiltration of the bone marrow may cause obliteration of normal hemopoietic elements. Extramedullary hemopoiesis then commonly develops. Patients develop leukoerythroblastic anaemia, which is characterized by circulating erythroblasts and primitive white cells.

The main conditions causing extensive infiltration of bone marrow are disseminated carcinoma, disseminated lymphoma and myelofibrosis (see page 326). A leuko-erythroblastic picture may also develop after massive hemorrhage, severe hemolysis and severe infections.

ANEMIA DUE TO DESTRUCTION OF RED CELLS

Hemolytic anemia is characterized by reduced red-cell survival in the blood

In hemolytic anemia, chronic increased red-cell destruction causes development of anemia with increased reticulocytes in blood, splenomegaly, erythroid hyperplasia resulting in expansion of bone marrow, and unconjugated hyperbilirubinemia. There are two main groups of factors causing hemolysis. Intrinsic defects in red cells result in abnormal erythrocyte fragility.

- **Membrane defects**, e.g. hereditary spherocytosis.
- **Enzyme defects**, e.g. glucose-6-phosphate dehydrogenase.
- **Defects outside red cells** causing red-cell lysis, autoimmune and mechanical trauma to cells.

Red-cell destruction takes place in the spleen and by reticuloendothelial cells in the liver.

HEMOLYSIS DUE TO DEFECTS IN RED CELLS

The most common red-cell membrane defect causing hemolysis is hereditary spherocytosis

Hemolytic anemia may be caused by membrane defects in red cells. The most common disease is hereditary spherocytosis. Red cells have an abnormal cell-membrane-associated cytoskeleton, which is caused by abnormalities of the red-cell membrane-bracing proteins ankyrin, spectrin or band 4.2 protein. In some cases a defect in one of the spectrin genes has been documented.

Patients with this disease have jaundice, splenomegaly and hemolytic anemia. Red cells are spherical on blood film (*Fig. 15.23*) and are abnormally fragile, undergoing lysis in the spleen. There is expansion of the hemopoietic marrow and splenomegaly. Splenectomy is performed to prevent hemolysis.

Enzyme defects in red cells may predispose to hemolysis

Hemolytic anemia may be also be caused by enzyme defects that render red cells susceptible to damage by oxidant stress. Glucose-6-phosphate dehydrogenase deficiency is an X-linked condition, in which hemolytic crises are precipitated by infections or administration of certain drugs (quinine, phenacetin, aspirin). Pyruvate kinase deficiency causes a chronic hemolytic anemia.

Thalassemia is the result of quantitative abnormalities of synthesis of globin chains of hemoglobin

Thalassemia syndromes are caused by defective synthesis of the α- or β-globin chains of hemoglobin. Disease is inherited and is common in the Mediterranean, Middle and Far East, and Southeast Asia, where carrier rates of 10–15% are found. The main pathological features are the consequence of increased requirements for red-cell production (caused by red-cell destruction):

- Increased intramedullary hemopoiesis causes deformed bones (increased size and bossing of the skull).
- Increased extramedullary hemopoiesis causes hepatosplenomegaly.

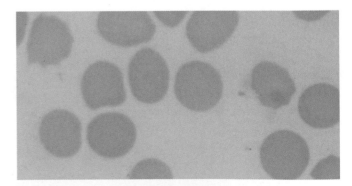

Fig. 15.23 Hereditary spherocytosis.
Spherocytes are abnormal red cells which have a convex instead of a bi-concave shape. In a normal blood film, the center of red cells is slightly paler than the periphery. In spherocytes, the center of the cell is darker than the periphery. Such cells are abnormally fragile and prone to hemolysis.

- Consequences of excess iron deposition in tissues, derived from transfusions with hemolysis (affects heart, liver and pancreas).

In severe forms of disease there is a hypochromic microcytic anemia associated with hemolysis of red cells. The most severe form of disease is that which results from abnormality of the β-globin chain.

Normal adult hemoglobin (HbA) is composed of two α-globin chains and two β-globin chains ($\alpha_2\beta_2$). In thalassemia, one or more of the genes responsible for synthesis of α- or β-globin chains is abnormal. Depending on which chain is affected, an α thalassaemia or β thalassemia results.

In β thalassemia over 90 different mutations have been described, leading to either reduced or absent synthesis of β-globin chain, one of which is present on each copy of chromosome 11. Heterozygotes develop a mild disease termed 'thalassemia minor' (thalassemia trait), whereas homozygotes develop 'thalassemia major', which is associated with a severe hemolytic anemia. In some instances, no β-globin is produced (β^0) while in other β-globin chains are markedly reduced (β^+).

In α thalassemia, disease is mainly caused by deletion (rather than mutation) of parts of the globin genes. Each individual has four α-globin genes (a pair of α-globin genes is present on each of the copies of chromosome 16), thus there are four possible degrees of a thalassemia, dependent upon how many genes are abnormal. Hemolysis is less severe in α thalassemia than in β thalassemia. Features of thalassemia syndromes are summarized in *Fig. 15.24*.

Sickle-cell disease causes increased destruction of red cells associated with an abnormal hemoglobin

In sickle-cell disease a point mutation in the gene coding for the β-globin chain results in an abnormal form of hemoglobin, termed HbS ($\alpha_2\beta S_2$). This form of hemoglobin polymerizes at low oxygen saturations, causing abnormal rigidity and deformity of red cells, which assume a sickle shape. As a result, red cells are abnormally fragile (undergoing hemolysis), and sludge in small vessels (causing vascular occlusion).

In sickle-cell trait, individuals are heterozygous for the β-globin gene abnormality and 30% of the hemoglobin is HbS, resulting in no significant clinical abnormality.

In patients with sickle-cell disease (homozygous for the abnormal β-globin gene), over 80% of hemoglobin is HbS, the rest being HbF and HbA_2. There are three patterns of acute deterioration, termed sickle-cell crises:

1 **Sequestration crises**. In the early years of sickle-cell anemia, sudden pooling of red cells in the spleen may develop, causing a rapid fall in hemoglobin concentration, which can lead to death.

2 **Infarctive crises**. Obstruction of small blood vessels occurs, leading to infarcts. Commonly affected tissues are bone (especially femoral head), spleen (leading to splenic atrophy), and skin (leading to ankle ulcers).

3 **Aplastic crises**. Splenic atrophy caused by infarction predisposes to infection leading to depression of red-cell

Fig. 15.24
Summary of thalassemia

Clinical disease	Globin chains present	Features
β thalassemia		
Thalassemia major	Homozygous β^0/β^0 Homozygous β^+/β^+	Hypochromic microcytic anemia. Severe haemolysis, hepatosplenomegaly, marrow hyperplasia causing skeletal deformities. Iron overload develops with repeated transfusions
Thalassemia minor	Heterozygous β^+/β Heterozygous β^0/β	Moderate reduction in HbA, increase in HbA2 ($\alpha_2\delta_2$). Mild anemia with hypochromic cells
α thalassemia		
Silent carrier	$-\alpha/\alpha\alpha$	Asymptomatic with no structural blood abnormality
α thalassemia trait	$--/\alpha\alpha$ $\alpha-/\alpha-$	Asymptomatic but mild hemolytic anemia with some microcytic cells
Hemoglobin H disease	$--/\alpha-$	Moderate hemolytic anemia with hypochromia and microcytosis, HbH forms from tetramers of β chain
Lethal (hydrops fetalis)	$--/--$	Lethal *in utero*

production. This precipitates a rapid fall in hemoglobin concentration in the face of continued hemolysis.

In addition to development of crises, abnormalities occur in many organs (*Fig. 15.25*). Other mutations of the β-globin gene form hemoglobins C, D and E, which also result in hemolysis.

HEMOLYSIS CAUSED BY DEFECTS OUTSIDE RED CELLS

Hemolysis may be caused by immune-mediated destruction of red cells in autoimmune hemolytic anemias

Antibodies binding to antigens on red cells may cause premature destruction of red cells. The three main types of disease in which this happens are warm-antibody hemolytic anemia (80% of cases), cold-antibody hemolytic anemia (20% of cases) and isoantibody hemolytic anemia (rare) (*Fig. 15.26*).

Hemolysis may be caused by mechanical destruction of red cells

Mechanical damage to red cells may lead to reduced life span and hemolysis. There are three main groups of mechanical hemolysis:

- **Macroangiopathic**. Prosthetic cardiac valves.
- **Microangiopathic**. Fragmentation by fibrin strands in small vessels, as seen in disseminated intravascular coagulation. In this condition there is activation of the coagulation system in small vessels, causing microthrombi. This results in depletion of coagulation factors and platelets (increased risk of bleeding) and in mechanical fragmentation of red cells (hemolysis).
- **Splenic**. Hypersplenism caused by enlargement of the spleen is associated with hemolysis. Red cells are sequestered in the spleen and are prematurely destroyed.

Increase in the red cell mass is termed 'polycythemia'

Polycythemia, also termed erythrocytosis, is characterized by an absolute increase in the mass of circulating red cells, detectable by a rise in the hematocrit.

Secondary polycythemia occurs in conditions that give rise to arterial hypoxia, the two main causes being chronic lung disease and cyanotic congenital heart disease. In these circumstances, hypoxia stimulates expansion of red cell mass. A similar phenomenon is seen in people who live at high altitudes, such as in the Andes. Uncommonly, abnormal secretion of erythropoietin causes polycythemia, e.g. in renal disease or cerebral hemangioblastoma.

Primary polycythemia occurs in a condition termed **polycythemia rubra vera**, which is one of the myeloproliferative disorders (see page 326).

At a hematocrit above 50%, hyperviscosity of blood predisposes to vascular thrombosis, e.g. causing cerebral infarction.

Fig. 15.25
Systemic complications of sickle-cell disease

Lungs	Pulmonary infarction, development of acute chest syndrome (characterized by decreased pulmonary function, which may be fatal).
Brain	Cerebral infarction.
Kidneys	Papillary necrosis caused by vascular occlusion in vasae rectae.
Bone	Salmonella osteomyelitis is predisposed by small infarcts in bone caused by vascular occlusion.
Immune	Hyposplenism increases susceptibility to bacterial infection.
Hepatobiliary	Pigment gallstones due to hemolysis. Secondary hemosiderosis due to iron overload in transfused patients.
Eye	Blindness caused by small vessel occlusion and ischemic retinopathy.

Fig. 15.26
Causes of immune hemolytic anemias

Warm-acting antibodies:
IgG class, destruction of red cells in spleen

Idiopathic (50%)
CLL
Lymphocytic lymphoma
SLE
Viral infections
Drug-induced hemolysis (α-methyl-dopa, quinidine)

Cold-reacting antibodies:
IgM class, destruction of red cells by Kupffer's cells in liver

Idiopathic
Lymphoma-related
Mycoplasma pneumonia
Infectious mononucleosis

Isoimmune

Hemolytic disease of the newborn (Rhesus incompatibility)
Transfusion reactions

DISORDERS OF CIRCULATING WHITE BLOOD CELLS AND MARROW

The two main reasons for an increase in numbers of white blood cells (leukocytosis) are **reactive changes** in the number of circulating white cells (associated with different types of disease, see Key Facts), and **neoplastic diseases** of white cells.

White cell function may be impaired because of too few cells or because of abnormal function

White cell function may be qualitatively impaired or there may be reduced numbers of circulating cells.

Reduced neutrophil function predisposes to bacterial infections, particularly those causing ulceration in the mouth and oropharynx. The main causes of reduced numbers of neutrophils (**neutropenia**) are:

- Generalized abnormalities of marrow function (associated with disorders of red cells and platelets).
- Marrow hypoplasia, which is commonly acquired due to therapeutic irradiation or chemotherapy, B_{12} or folate deficiency, and some overwhelming infections. Reduced marrow cellularity is seen on bone marrow biopsy.
- Abnormal destruction of neutrophils (drug-induced, autoimmune, hypersplenism). This is associated with increase in neutrophil precursors on bone marrow biopsy.

Among the main causes of defective neutrophil function are systemic disturbances, particularly diabetes mellitus, corticosteroid therapy, renal failure and alcoholism. Rare

KEY FACTS
Changes in circulating white cells in blood

- **Neutrophil leukocytosis** most commonly occurs as a response to bacterial infection or to tissue necrosis (infarction).
- **Eosinophilia** is seen as a response to parasitic infections, in hypersensitivity responses, associated with neoplasia (chronic granulocytic leukemia and Hodgkin's disease) and in hypereosinophilia syndromes, with vasculitis and pulmonary infiltration.
- **Lymphocytosis** is seen in viral infections, particularly glandular fever (infectious mononucleosis), and less commonly in infections such as typhoid and brucellosis.
- **Monocytosis** is uncommon but may be seen in infective endocarditis and with some protozoal infections (malaria, trypanosomiasis).

congenital causes may lead to defects in phagocytosis and bacterial killing.

Numbers of lymphoid cells (**lymphopenia**) are reduced with age, but this is also seen in association with SLE (see Chapter 25), steroid therapy, and immune-deficiency states (see Chapter 7).

NEOPLASTIC DISEASES OF WHITE CELLS

Neoplastic diseases of white blood cells are divided into four main groups:

- **Malignant lymphomas** are diseases of tissue-based and nodal lymphocytes (see page 307).
- **Leukemias** and myeloproliferative disorders are malignant neoplasms derived from cells of the bone marrow. Neoplastic cells may circulate in the blood, secondarily colonizing other tissues.
- **Plasma cell tumors** are neoplasms derived from terminally differentiated B-cells derived from bone marrow (see page 314).
- **Histiocytoses** are neoplasms derived from histiocytic cells, particularly Langerhans' cells.

Certain of these diseases overlap with each other, for example some lymphomas also have a leukemic pattern.

Leukemias are the most common neoplastic disease of white cells

The most common neoplastic disease of white cells is leukemia, the incidence of which is 9 per 100 000. The disease may be acute or chronic. The general characteristics of leukemias include: neoplastic proliferation of marrow cells, forming one or more cell lines; circulation of neoplastic cells in peripheral blood in most but not all cases; and suppression of other marrow elements, leading to symptoms due to lack of normal red cells, white cells and platelets.

Acute leukemias are characterized by proliferation of immature cells known as blast cells. Typically there is rapid progression of disease which, without treatment, is fatal in a short period of time.

Chronic leukemias are characterized by proliferation of more mature cells. Typically there is slow progression of disease, but this type may also transform into a more aggressive pattern.

Common to all leukemias is expansion of the bone marrow and infiltration by neoplastic white cells (*Fig. 15.27*).

Acute leukemias are divided into lymphoblastic or non-lymphoblastic groups

Acute leukemias are divided into those derived from lymphoid cells, **acute lymphoblastic leukemia** (ALL), and those derived from myeloid, monocytic, erythroid, and megakaryocytic cells, which are grouped as the **acute non-lymphoblastic leukemias** (ANLL).

In acute leukemia, replacement of the bone marrow by blast cells causes anemia due to loss of red cells, susceptibility to infection due to loss of normal white cells, and susceptibility to bleeding due to loss of platelets.

Patients develop fever, malaise, bleeding (petechial hemorrhages), and mouth ulcers due to infections. The peripheral blood shows an increased white cell count (including blast cells) in about 50% of cases; importantly, in many cases the white cell count may be normal or reduced.

The diagnosis of acute leukemia is based on examination of bone marrow aspirate and histology (*Fig. 15.28*). Acute leukemias frequently show infiltration of many organs, especially the brain and gonads. Splenomegaly and lymphadenopathy are not usually prominent, except in some cases of acute lymphoblastic leukemia.

Acute lymphoblastic leukemia (ALL) most commonly affects children, only rarely occurring in young adults. The prognosis is related to the type of leukemia as defined by the FAB classification (*Fig. 15.29*).

Acute non-lymphoblastic leukemia (ANLL) is most commonly seen in adults and encompasses several different types of disease as categorized by the FAB classification (*Fig. 15.30*). M1–M3 are myeloblastic in type. They are separated according to the degree of differentiation, which

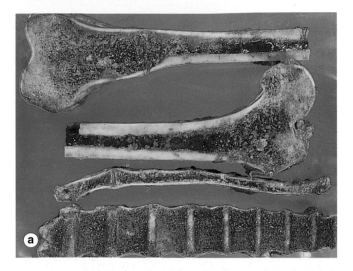

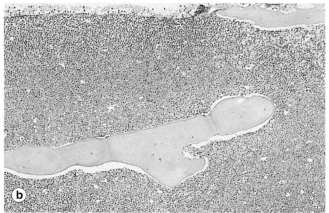

Fig. 15.27 Leukemic infiltration of marrow.
In leukemia, neoplastic cells replace normal red (hemopoietic) and yellow (inactive) bone marrow. Vertebrae, ribs and long bones show diffuse replacement of marrow space by pale, cellular, neoplastic cells (a). Histologically (b), the normal marrow is replaced by abnormal, monotonous, leukemic cells.

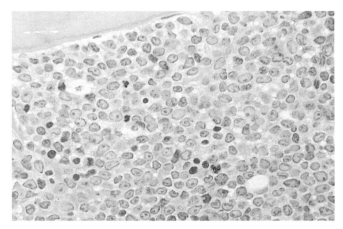

Fig. 15.28 Acute leukemia histology.
Marrow in acute leukemia is extensively replaced by neoplastic cells, which efface normal marrow. There is hypercellularity, large numbers of blast cells characterized by large nuclei and mitoses, and reduced amounts of normal hemopoietic elements. This example is from a case of acute lymphoblastic leukemia.

Fig. 15.29 ALL classification
ALL is classified by morphology into groups L1–L3. Using immunochemistry, the nature of the cells can be further defined, and this is related to prognosis. Patients with L3 morphology, a high white count, and mature B-cell type have worst prognosis.

FAB type	Cytology	Phenotype	Incidence (%)	Prognosis
L1	Small lymphoid cells	Null cell ALL (early B-cell)	12	intermediate
L2	Large lymphoid cells	Common ALL (pre-B-cell)	75	good
		T-cell ALL	12	intermediate
L3	Large lymphoid cells with vacuolated cytoplasm	Mature B-cell ALL	1	poor

is assessed by cytochemical detection of myelocyte markers. M5 is composed of monoblasts, and M4 is an overlap between myeloblastic and monoblastic types. Although M6 is termed 'erythroblastic leukemia' both myeloblastic and erythroblastic cells are seen.

Chronic leukemias are divided into lymphocytic, myeloid and hairy-cell types

Chronic leukemias are mainly seen in adults over the age of 40 years, but can develop in childhood.

Accounting for about 30% of all cases of leukemia, **chronic lymphocytic leukemia** (CLL) is mainly seen in patients over the age of 50 years. It is characterized by neoplastic proliferation of small mature lymphocytes (*Fig. 15.31*). The vast majority of cases of CLL are of the B-cell type, with only about 5% of cases of T-cell type. The bone marrow is infiltrated by abnormal clusters of lymphocytes, initially sparing normal hemopoietic elements, but later effacing the marrow. The peripheral blood contains large numbers of circulating abnormal lymphoid cells. Lymphadenopathy is common and is often a presenting feature of disease; affected nodes show the same histological picture as that of small-cell diffuse lymphocytic lymphoma (see page 312). Splenomegaly is also commonly seen. Autoimmune hemolytic anemia and thrombocytopenia are present in about 10% of cases, and a paraproteinemia is found in about 5% of cases. Prognosis in disease is related to clinical staging (*Fig. 15.32*).

Hairy-cell leukemia is a form of B-cell leukemia in which cells have many fine surface projections. Typically, there is diffuse marrow involvement and the spleen is very large with hypersplenism and pancytopenia, but lymphadenopathy is uncommon. Increase in circulating white cells is not marked. As several of the clinical problems are derived from hypersplenism, splenectomy may alleviate many of the symptoms. Many cases also respond to interferon treatment.

Chronic myeloid (granulocytic) leukemia (CGL) is also considered as one of the myeloproliferative disorders (see page 326). It is most common in adults between 30 and 40 years, accounting for about 20% of all cases of leukemia. Affected patients develop hepatosplenomegaly, with massive enlargement of the spleen due to infiltration by leukemic cells. The peripheral blood shows a leukocytosis with an excess of neutrophils, myelocytes and metamyelocytes. There is usually a moderate anemia, but thrombocytopenia

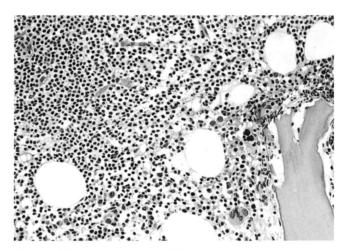

Fig. 15.31 Bone marrow in CLL.
The bone marrow is replaced by small mature lymphoid cells. In early stages of disease this replacement is focal, allowing normal platelet and red-cell production.

Fig. 15.30 ANLL classification		
FAB type	**Cytology**	**Incidence**
M0	Undifferentiated myeloblastic	Uncommon
M1	Acute myeloblastic leukemia (without differentiation)	50% of all cases
M2	Acute myeloblastic leukemia (with differentiation)	
M3	Acute promyelocytic leukemia	Uncommon
M4	Acute myelomonoblastic leukemia	30% of all cases
M5	Acute monocytic leukemia	Uncommon
M6	Acute erythroblastic leukemia	Uncommon
M7	Acute megakaryocytic leukemia	Uncommon

Fig. 15.32 Clinical staging of CLL	
Poor prognosis, with survival of about 2 years, is associated with low hemoglobin < 11 g/dl or platelet count < 100 × 10⁹/L at presentation	
Stage 0	Lymphocytosis of blood and marrow.
Stage 1	Lymphocytosis and enlarged nodes.
Stage II	Lymphocytosis and enlarged liver or spleen.
Stage III	Hemoglobin < 11 g/dl, with features of Stage 0, I or II.
Stage IV	Platelet count < 100 × 10⁹/L, with features of Stage 0, I, II or III.

Cytogenetic changes in chronic myeloid leukemia

Patients with chronic myeloid leukemia commonly have an abnormal chromosome in leukemic cells, termed the **Philadelphia chromosome** (Ph1). This is a reciprocal transformation between the long arms of chromosome 9 and 22 t(9;22)(q34;q11). It results in the formation of the *bcr-abl* fusion gene, which produces a protein with tyrosine kinase activity. Around 90% of cases of CGL are Ph-positive-associated, with a median survival of around 4 years. The remaining 10% are Ph-negative-associated, with a median survival of around 1 year.

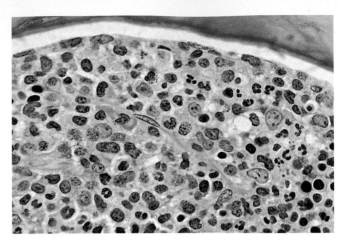

Fig. 15.33 Bone marrow in CGL. The bone marrow is replaced by myeloid cells in varying stages of differentiation.

is not marked. Basophils may be increased in number. The bone marrow shows increased cellularity, with marrow replaced by neutrophil precursors (*Fig. 15.33*). The natural history of the disease is for transformation into an acute leukemia: 75% transform into acute myeloblastic leukemia, and 25% into acute lymphoblastic leukemia. The onset of transformation is usually associated with the development of increasing numbers of blast cells in the marrow, together with increasing anemia and thrombocytopenia, but in some patients is abrupt. Most patients die within 6 months of blast transformation.

MYELOPROLIFERATIVE DISEASES

Myeloproliferative diseases are caused by abnormal marrow stem-cell proliferation

Myeloproliferative disorders are characterized by proliferation of marrow stem cells, which differentiate into erthyroid, granulocytic, megakaryocytic or fibroblastic cells. There is frequent overlap between diseases, with transformation of one into another, and termination of disease as ANLL.

Included in this group of diseases is **polycythemia rubra vera**, which mainly occurs after the age of 40 years, causing polycythemia with all its complications, particularly vascular thrombosis. The marrow contains increased numbers of erythroid precursors, as well as increased numbers of megakaryocytes and fibroblasts. Splenomegaly is common, and 15% of patients develop myelofibrosis, 10% developing ANLL. With treatment, overall survival is about 10 years.

In **primary thrombocythemia** there is thrombocytosis associated with bleeding tendency or thrombosis. Splenic infarction and secondary hyposplenism are common.

Myelofibrosis is characterized by proliferation of fibroblasts in the marrow, which is a response to growth factors secreted by abnormally proliferating myeloid cells. As the marrow is replaced by fibroblasts and collagen, extramedullary hemopoiesis develops in the spleen and liver,

causing hepatosplenomegaly. Clinically, patients develop anemia and the signs and symptoms of a massively enlarged spleen. The peripheral blood shows anemia with abnormally shaped red cells and a leukoerythroblastic picture. Patients typically survive for about 3 years, with approximately 10% developing ANLL.

Chronic granulocytic leukemia is also a form of myeloproliferative disease with splenomegaly, anemia, and neutrophilia.

HISTIOCYTOSES

The Langerhans'-cell histiocytoses are proliferations of histiocytic cells

The Langerhans'-cell histiocytoses are a group of diseases characterized by proliferation of histiocytic cells with markers and structural features of Langerhans' cells. These disorders were formerly called histiocytosis-X. Normal Langerhans' cells are found in the skin and lymph nodes, where they act as dendritic antigen-presenting cells. The spectrum of severity in this condition has three main clinical patterns (overlaps are also seen).

Eosinophilic granuloma (unifocal Langerhans histiocytosis) is a localized collection of Langerhans' cells associated with many reactive eosinophils. Lesions may develop in bone (pathological fractures, bone pain, radiographic finding) or soft tissues (swelling). Local removal of lesions is curative.

Hand–Schuller–Christian disease (multifocal Langerhans histiocytosis) is characterized by multiple deposits of Langerhans' cells associated with reactive cells (principally eosinophils) in bone, lung, skin and pituitary gland. Deposits cause local tissue destruction and, in the lung, restrictive lung disease.

The classic clinical triad is diabetes insipidus, exophthalmos, and bone defects on skull radiograph.

Letterer–Siwe disease (acute disseminated Langerhans' cell histiocytosis) is mainly seen in young children. It is manifest by skin rash, lymphadenopathy and hepato-splenomegaly. Infiltration of bone marrow causes thrombocytopenia, anemia and predisposition to infections. It is rapidly fatal unless treated.

DISEASES OF COAGULATION AND PLATELETS

Reduced platelets in blood lead to increased susceptibility to bleeding

Reduced platelet numbers or defects in function result in a bleeding tendency. Patients develop petechial hemorrhages and bruising in skin, bleeding into mucosal surfaces and, sometimes, severe bleeding into tissues after trauma. The main causes are abnormal platelet production due to marrow disease, or increased destruction of platelets.

Defective production is seen in megaloblastic anemias, marrow infiltration, and after marrow suppression by chemotherapy.

Idiopathic thrombocytopenia (ITP) is due to auto-immune destruction of platelets, which are coated with anti-platelet antibodies. Disease may be acute or chronic, the acute form being seen mainly in children after viral infection that generally recovers spontaneously. The chronic form is seen mainly in adult females and is associated with autoimmune disease or drugs. Platelet destruction occurs in the spleen, and splenectomy prolongs platelet survival.

Consumption of platelets and coagulation factors is seen in **disseminated intravascular coagulation, thrombotic thrombocytopenic purpura**, and **hemolytic uremic syndrome**. The common mechanism is formation of microvascular thrombi that consume platelets.

Platelet dysfunction is seen in several systemic disturbances, e.g. uremia, chronic liver disease, myeloma, and with administration of anti-platelet drugs. Congenital disorders of platelet function are uncommon.

Increase in platelet numbers may be due to neoplasia (thrombocythemia) or a reactive process (thrombocytosis). **Primary thrombocythemia** is one of the myeloproliferative diseases, patients developing both thrombotic as well as bleeding tendency. **Reactive thrombocytosis** is seen after splenectomy, in association with systemic neoplasia, and with systemic inflammatory responses.

Coagulation disorders lead to increased risk of serious bleeding

Abnormalities of coagulation lead to increased risk of serious bleeding (see page 152 *et seq.*). The main causes are iatrogenic administration of anticoagulants, hereditary defects in coagulation factors (e.g. hemophilia, von Willebrand's disease), and liver disease causing impaired production of clotting factors.

The main pathological consequences of poor blood coagulation are bleeding after surgical procedures such as biopsy, bleeding into joints after minor trauma, and intracranial hemorrhage; the predisposition to subdural hemorrhages is particularly increased.

Disseminated intravascular coagulation results in tissue ischemia, hemorrhage, and red-cell hemolysis

Disseminated intravascular coagulation results from activation of the coagulation system in small vessels throughout the body. This has several main effects:

- Platelets are consumed, resulting in a low platelet count.
- Fibrin thrombi are deposited in small vessels in brain, kidney, lungs and other organs, causing ischemic changes.
- Coagulation factors are consumed and there is activation of the fibrinolytic system; fibrin-degradation products acting as inhibitors of coagulation are generated.
- Red cells are fragmented by passage through vessels occluded by thrombi, and there is destruction of red cells (microangiopathic hemolysis).

Patients develop ischemia and dysfunction of major organs, bleeding into tissues, and hemolytic anemia. The main precipitating causes of this syndrome are septicemia, systemic shock, and obstetric disorders (toxemia, placental abruption, amniotic fluid embolism).

BONE MARROW TRANSPLANTATION

The graft-versus-host reaction is a problem in bone marrow transplantation

In bone marrow transplantation, commonly used to treat hematological malignancies, the patient's own immune system is destroyed following cytotoxic or radiotherapeutic destruction of bone marrow cells. When healthy bone marrow cells are transplanted into the recipient, there is a danger of a **graft-versus-host reaction** (GVH), which may be acute or chronic.

In the GVH reaction, transplanted immunologically competent bone marrow cells (including T-lymphocytes) may mount an immune response against various components of the recipient's tissues, which bear antigens that the transplanted immune cells recognize as foreign.

Acute GVH occurs within 3 months of graft in up to 70% of recipients. It produces features of diarrhea, dermatitis, malabsorption, and jaundice. The proliferating transplanted immune-competent cells destroy epithelial cells in the gut, liver and skin. This is a potentially life-threatening condition, the risk of which is minimized by careful HLA matching. Although recent efforts to remove T-cells from donor marrow have reduced the risk of GVH reactions, they have increased the risk of graft failure.

Chronic GVH occurs 3–15 months after transplantation in about 40% of recipients. It produces a syndrome similar to progressive systemic sclerosis (see Chapter 25).

16 Endocrine system

The most important and frequently occurring disease associated with the endocrine system is one of the patterns of **diabetes mellitus**, that associated with an abnormality of the endocrine islets of Langerhans in the pancreas. However, this disease has such widespread systemic effects that it is dealt with in the chapter on 'Important Systemic Disorders' – Chapter 25.

The importance of the endocrine system in disease is largely confined to disorders in which there is either over-production or under-production of the relevant hormones, producing severe systemic metabolic disturbances. The most common endocrine organ to produce pathology is the thyroid gland, which can either over-produce (**hyperthyroidism**) or under-produce (**hypothyroidism**) the thyroid hormones which regulate the body's metabolic rate. The thyroid is also important in that it is the only endocrine gland which is close to the surface and in a site where any increase in size is easily visible, and the patient is aware that the gland is abnormally large. **Multinodular colloid goiter** is a frequent abnormality in the thyroid in the middle-aged and elderly, who seek medical advice and treatment because of the cosmetic effects of the swelling.

In the thyroid there are a number of conditions which can lead to both excessive and reduced hormone output, but in the other endocrine organs such as the adrenal glands, parathyroid and pituitary, the commonest cause of excess hormone output is the presence of a benign hormone-secreting tumor, i.e. **adrenal cortical adenoma**, **parathyroid adenoma** and **pituitary adenoma**. Excess hormone can also be produced by **hyperplasia** of the endocrine glands, but this is less common and is usually a reactive compensatory response to a low level of the hormone or some other substance in the blood. Under-secretion of hormone is usually due either to surgical extirpation of the gland (e.g. **hypoparathyroidism**) or to autoimmune destruction of the endocrine tissue, (e.g. **Hashimoto's disease**, **Addison's disease**). The pituitary gland controls the secretions of many of the other endocrine glands, and central failure of pituitary hormone secretion can lead to reduced hormone production in other organs.

In general, neither infections nor vascular disease are common in endocrine glands, and malignant tumors are extremely rare with the exception of the thyroid gland, where they are relatively common but produce no hormonal effects. There are three common types of thyroid carcinoma, **papillary**, **follicular**, and **anaplastic** types, all of which present as palpable or visible lumps in the neck. When the lump has been identified as originating in the thyroid, it is important to distinguish whether it is due to one of these malignant tumors or one of the benign lumps of the thyroid, mainly part of a multinodular colloid goiter or a solitary benign **thyroid adenoma**. Preoperative diagnosis can often be made by examining the cytology of a sample of the cells from the lump obtained by fine-needle aspiration.

The endocrine system produces hormones, which act as chemical messengers, passing in the bloodstream to their target tissues

The endocrine system can be divided into:

- Endocrine organs, which are entirely dedicated to the production of hormones, e.g. pituitary, adrenal, thyroid, parathyroid.
- Endocrine components in mixed organs, which are discrete endocrine cell clusters within organs that also have another function, e.g. pancreas, ovary, testis.
- Diffuse endocrine system, which comprises scattered cells within another organ or tissue, e.g. endocrine cells in gut and bronchial mucosa. Because the hormones produced act locally on adjacent cells, not normally entering the systemic circulation, these cells are not truly endocrine, and are sometimes called 'paracrine'.

The most important diseases of the endocrine glands are associated with over- or under-production of hormones

The control of hormone secretion by the various components of the endocrine system is normally finely tuned by a combination of neural and chemical feedback mechanisms. Loss of this control, due to either primary or secondary disease affecting the endocrine organ, produces metabolic and structural abnormalities. Many examples are given later in this chapter. Tumors occurring within endocrine glands may be hormonally active (functioning) or inactive (non-functioning).

PITUITARY

The pituitary gland has two components, the adenohypophysis and the neurohypophysis

The **adenohypophysis** synthesizes and secretes a number of hormones, most of which act on other endocrine glands, e.g. adrenocorticotrophic hormone (ACTH) stimulates adrenal cortex to produce cortisone, and thyroid stimulating hormone (TSH) stimulates thyroid to produce thyroxine.

The **neurohypophysis** is in direct continuity with the hypothalamus, storing and secreting antidiuretic hormone (ADH) and oxytocin synthesized in the neurons of the hypothalamus (*Fig. 16.1*).

Many of the functions of the pituitary gland are controlled by neural and chemical stimuli from the hypothalamus, diseases of which cause secondary abnormalities in pituitary function.

The most common and important diseases of the pituitary gland are tumors of the adenohypophysis (pituitary adenomata)

Pituitary adenomata, although benign in that they do not metastasize, can be life-threatening by virtue of their position and ability to secrete excess hormone.

Non-functioning adenomata progressively enlarge until they break out of the sella turcica in an upwards direction, often compressing the optic chiasma. This produces a characteristic visual disturbance known as **bitemporal hemianopia** (*Fig. 16.2*). The tumor may destroy the normal functioning adenohypophysis, producing symptoms and signs of hypopituitarism (see page 331).

Functioning adenomata (*Fig. 16.3*) may, in theory, produce any of the adenohypophyseal hormones, but the majority produce either prolactin or growth hormone (*Fig. 16.4*); a few produce ACTH.

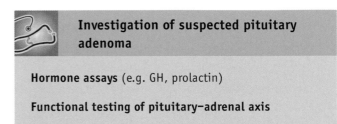

Investigation of suspected pituitary adenoma

Hormone assays (e.g. GH, prolactin)

Functional testing of pituitary–adrenal axis

Imaging, usually MRI scan and CT scan

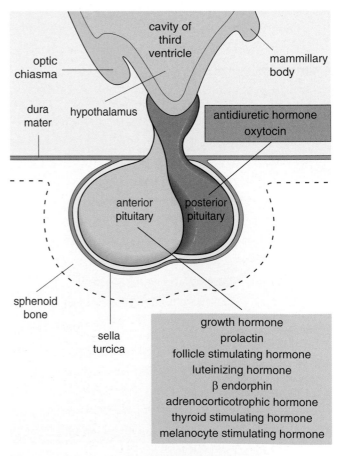

Fig. 16.1 Pituitary and hypothalamus and their hormones. The hormones secreted by the anterior pituitary (adenohypophysis), hypothalamus and posterior pituitary (neurohypophysis) are shown.

In general, functioning pituitary tumors present earlier than the non-functioning variety, and may be very small, despite producing significant metabolic abnormality (microadenomata).

Reduced output of all anterior pituitary hormones is termed 'panhypopituitarism'

Defective production of anterior pituitary hormones (panhypopituitarism), which may result from either pituitary or hypothalamic disease, is rare. The most important **pituitary causes** are:

- Surgical removal of a pituitary tumor.
- Obliteration of normal pituitary by a primary pituitary tumor or metastatic tumor, e.g. metastatic breast carcinoma.
- Ischemic necrosis of adenohypophysis, due to hypotensive shock. This may occur as a result of *intrapartum* or *post partum* hemorrhage (**Sheehan's syndrome**).

Fig. 16.3
Functioning pituitary adenomata

	Clinical features
Prolactin-producing	Menstrual disturbances and infertility in women
	Endocrinologically asymptomatic in men
Growth-hormone-producing	Before puberty: giantism
	After puberty: acromegaly
ACTH-producing	Adrenal cortical hyperplasia (Cushing's disease) (see page 341)

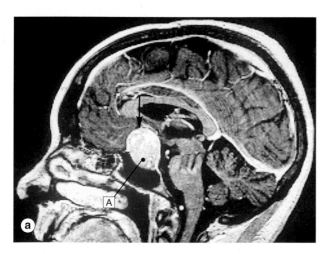

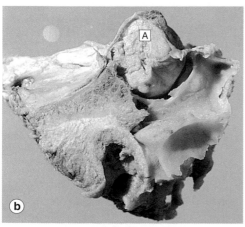

Fig. 16.2 Large pituitary adenoma (A) expanding upwards to compress optic chiasma (arrow).
This large tumor presented with visual disturbance and was not hormone-producing. Macroscopically (b), adenomas are soft fleshy tumors (**A**). This is in a *post mortem* specimen of pituitary fossa.

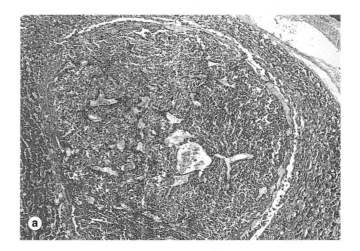

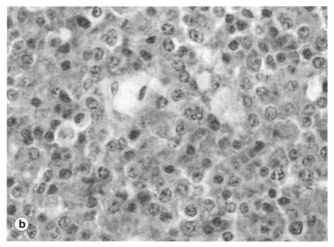

**Fig. 16.4 Pituitary adenoma. (a) H & E.
(b) Immunochemistry.** Pituitary adenomas have solid and trabecular patterns (a). Immunochemistry can be used to ascertain hormone production; here, growth hormone is stained brown.

Very rare causes include inflammation (autoimmune adenohypophysitis, sarcoidosis) and traumatic disruption following skull fracture.

Hypothalamic causes of panhypopituitarism include destruction of the hypothalamus by:

- primary brain tumor, e.g. glioma or craniopharyngioma
- infarction
- inflammation, e.g. sarcoid (see Chapter 25).

Diseases of the neurohypophysis are very rare

Most failures of ADH and oxytocin production are the result of damage to the hypothalamus, usually due to tumor invasion or infarction.

Failure of ADH production leads to **diabetes insipidus**, in which lack of ADH prevents resorption of water from the glomerular filtrate in the renal collecting ducts. Large quantities of very dilute urine are excreted (polyuria), and risk of body water depletion must be counteracted by greatly increasing water intake (polydypsia). The main causes of diabetes insipidus are: surgical extirpation of pituitary or its stalk – usually in the course of tumor removal, and inflammatory or neoplastic lesions in hypothalamus, the most common inflammatory cause being sarcoidosis. In about 30% of cases of diabetes insipidus, no structural cause is found.

Inappropriate ADH secretion, independent of disease in pituitary or hypothalamus, may occur in association with some tumors, particularly oat-cell carcinoma of the lung, and some neuroendocrine tumors. It is also a frequent transient phenomenon after head injury, neurosurgery for tumor, and some lung diseases, producing a low serum sodium and water imbalance, with the risk of water intoxication.

THYROID GLAND

The thyroid gland secretes two different types of hormone from two cell types

The thyroid gland is a pure endocrine gland composed of two cell types, which secrete two types of hormone.

The **thyroid follicle cells**, which make up the bulk of the gland, are arranged in a follicular pattern. They produce the hormone **thyroxine** (T_4) and its more potent deiodinated product **tri-iodothyronine** (T_3). Most T_3 is produced by removal of an iodine atom from T_4 in the peripheral tissues. Both hormones affect many metabolic processes, almost always by increasing their activity, thus increasing the basal metabolic rate.

The **parafollicular or 'C' cells** are a minority population of cells, occurring mainly in small clusters in the interstices between follicles. They produce the hormone **calcitonin**, which is involved in **calcium homeostasis**, possibly inhibiting osteoclastic bone resorption (compare parathormone, page 338).

The thyroid follicle cells synthesize and secrete T_4 and T_3 under the control of thyroid stimulating hormone (TSH) from the pituitary

T_4 is synthesized by the thyroid follicle cells, which preferentially take up iodine and link it to tyrosine. The iodotyrosines are then stored in the follicle acini and linked with protein to form **thyroglobulin** (**thyroid colloid**). This is removed as required from the colloid store, as a result of pinocytosis by the same follicle cells, which then split off the linked protein by lysosomal breakdown and convert the hormone into active components T_3 and T_4. These are then secreted into the adjacent thyroid capillaries to pass into the circulation.

The term 'goiter' is used to describe any swelling of the thyroid gland

Traditionally the word 'goiter' has been used to describe any enlargement of the thyroid. Thyroid enlargement can have many causes and may sometimes be associated with metabolic disorder due to decreased or increased thyroid hormone output. The term 'toxic goiter' is sometimes used to describe enlarged thyroids associated with increased thyroid hormone output (thyrotoxicosis), and the term 'non-toxic goiter' is applied to an enlarged thyroid when thyroid hormone levels are normal. As both terms are imprecise and imply no specific pathology, they are best avoided.

Increase in size of the thyroid may be diffuse or nodular

Enlargement of the thyroid gland produces a palpable and often visible swelling in the front of the neck. The increase in size may be diffuse or nodular, and nodular enlargement may involve all or part of the gland. The distribution and palpation characteristics of the swelling often give valuable clues to the underlying pathology:

- **Irregular multinodular enlargement of the entire thyroid** is the most common cause of thyroid enlargement, and is particularly seen in the elderly. This pattern is also called **multinodular goiter.**
- **Focal nodular enlargement within the thyroid** may be due to a thyroid tumor. This pattern of enlargement must be investigated (usually by excision and histological examination), as the tumor may be either benign or malignant.
- **Symmetrical slightly nodular (bosselated) firm enlargement of the whole thyroid** is characteristic of Hashimoto's disease (see page 336).
- **Symmetrical diffuse enlargement of the thyroid** is usually associated with evidence of hyperthyroidism, e.g. in Graves' disease (see below), and is sometimes called **parenchymatous goiter**. This pattern of enlargement is also seen as a physiological response in women at puberty and in pregnancy.

With the exception of tumors and Hashimoto's disease, most forms of thyroid enlargement are due to **hyperplasia** of the thyroid follicles and their cells. The increase in cell numbers may also be associated with an increase in cell function, with excessive production and secretion of T_4 and T_3 leading to the clinical features of **hyperthyroidism**.

Multinodular goiter is the most common cause of thyroid enlargement in the elderly

At *post mortem* examination many elderly people are found to have nodular distortion of thyroid architecture. However, only in cases in which the enlargement is great do patients seek treatment, usually for **cosmetic reasons** (the thyroid enlargement producing an unsightly swelling in the neck) and because **compression symptoms** may develop due to pressure on the trachea. Compression symptoms are particularly likely when the main enlargement is in the thyroid isthmus, with the large nodule passing behind the manubrium (**retrosternal goiter**).

Multinodular goiter produces irregular hyperplastic enlargement of the thyroid due to the development of well-circumscribed nodules of varying size. As many of the larger nodules are filled with brown gelatinous colloid, the larger goiters are often called **multinodular colloid goiters** (*Fig. 16.5*). A few nodules may show evidence of hemorrhage and fibrous scarring. Sometimes, there are smaller, creamy coloured, fleshy nodules, which contain little colloid and are mainly composed of thyroid follicle cells.

Most patients with multinodular goiter have normal thyroid function but, occasionally, one of the nodules becomes functionally, as well as structurally, hyperplastic and secretes excess T_3 and T_4. The cause of multinodular colloid goiter is uncertain, but it may represent the uneven responsiveness of various parts of the thyroid to fluctuating TSH levels over a period of many years.

Diffuse smooth enlargement of the thyroid is usually due to follicle-cell hyperplasia

The structural hyperplasia responsible for enlargement of the organ as a whole may be associated with normal (**euthyroid**), increased (**hyperthyroid**) or reduced (**hypothyroid**) secretion of thyroid hormones, according to the stimulus producing the hyperplasia.

The symmetrical diffuse pattern of enlargement may be caused by **dietary thyroid deficiency (endemic goiter)**, which is the result of low iodine levels in the local water and soil. Iodine deficiency leads to low levels of T_3 and T_4 in the blood, initiating increased TSH secretion from the pituitary gland. This stimulates compensatory hyperplasia of the thyroid follicular cells throughout the organ, producing the characteristic pattern of enlargement. Formerly seen in small communities in the inland mountainous areas of parts of Europe (giving rise to names like 'Derbyshire neck'), this is now rare in the western world. Despite the attempted compensatory hyperplasia, patients are hypothyroid.

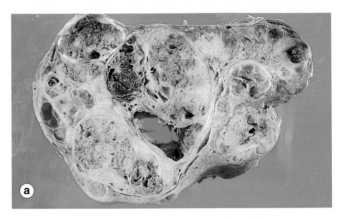

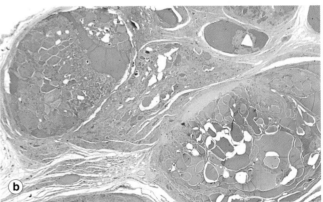

Fig. 16.5 Multinodular colloid goiter. (a) Gross. (b) Low-power histology. The nodules in multinodular goiter are composed of hyperplastic thyroid acini. Many contain gelatinous colloid, others are solid and cream coloured. Cystic degeneration and fibrosis are common.

Congenital enzyme deficiency may also be responsible for parenchymatous goiter. It arises in certain very rare disorders in which there is failure of normal T_3 and T_4 synthesis. Patients are thus hypothyroid despite the attempted compensatory hyperplasia.

The most common cause, however, is **autoimmune thyroiditis**. There are two patterns, one of which (**Graves' disease**) is particularly associated with hyperthyroidism. The other pattern (**Hashimoto's disease**) is associated with eventual reduced secretion of hormone, often after passing through transient hyperthyroid and euthyroid states. These two important diseases are discussed in more detail later.

Thyroiditis is usually due to either viral or autoimmune inflammation

Inflammation of the thyroid gland, which is termed **thyroiditis**, may be viral or autoimmune.

Viral thyroiditis is rare, the most common clinical pattern being **de Quervain's thyroiditis**. Seen in young and middle-aged women as a slight diffuse tender swelling of the thyroid, it usually occurs in association with a transient febrile illness, often during various viral epidemics.

Many of the patients are young mothers whose children are concurrently suffering with or recovering from mumps, measles or other viral illnesses. Inflammatory destruction of follicles is often associated with a giant-cell granulomatous reaction to leaked colloid, hence the synonym 'giant cell thyroiditis' or 'granulomatous thyroiditis'.

Autoimmune thyroiditis encompasses Graves' disease and Hashimoto's disease, both of which are discussed in more detail below. Progressive lymphocytic infiltration of the thyroid is noted in patients as they age, and may be a normal aging change. However, some patients have focal lymphocytic infiltration in excess of what would be expected for their years, and this condition has sometimes been called **focal lymphocytic thyroiditis**.

Excessive secretion of thyroid hormones (TH) produces hyperthyroidism

Hyperthyroidism is caused by excessive secretion of TH. Most of the clinical features (collectively known as **thyrotoxicosis**) (*Fig. 16.6*) are manifestations of a permanently raised metabolic rate, and the pathological changes that occur include loss of subcutaneous fat, reduction of skeletal muscle bulk and, sometimes, cardiomyopathy. In addition, there may be a visible or palpable enlargement of the thyroid gland (goiter).

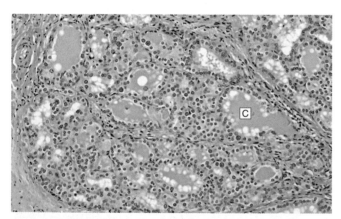

Fig. 16.6 Thyrotoxic hyperplasia.
The epithelial cells are increased in number and size, and the edges of the colloid (**C**) are scalloped, indicating active removal of stored colloid for processing into thyroxine.

Fig. 16.7
Clinical features of hyperthyroidism

Feeling hot
Increased sweating
Weight loss, with proximal muscle weakness
Rapid heart rate, palpitations
Atrial fibrillation (occasionally)
Diarrhea
Anxiety and restless hyperactivity

Thyrotoxicosis may result from an autonomous nodule of hyperactive thyroid tissue that is out of TSH control. This autonomous 'hot' nodule may be a solitary thyroid adenoma, or may be a component of a multinodular enlargement of the thyroid (multinodular goiter).

Diffuse thyroid hyperactivity due to **Long-Acting Thyroid Stimulator (LATS)** secretion in autoimmune thyroiditis (Graves' disease) may also be responsible, and is discussed below.

Graves' disease is the most important cause of hyperthyroidism

Graves' disease is a form of autoimmune thyroiditis that presents with symptoms of hyperthyroidism (*Fig. 16.7*), diffuse enlargement of the thyroid gland, and exophthalmos (protuberant, staring eyes due to expansion of retro-orbital soft tissue, mainly expansion of adipose tissue) (*Fig. 16.8*).

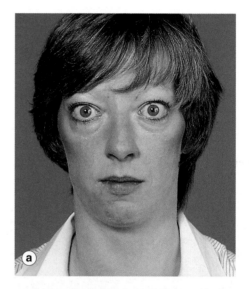

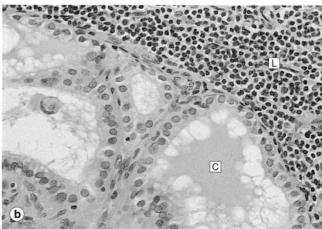

Fig. 16.8 Graves' disease. (a) Clinical photo.
(b) Histology. In this disease the thyroid is focally infiltrated by lymphoid cells (**L**). Antibody-stimulated hyperplastic thyroid acini are enlarged, with large nuclei and a scalloped appearance to the colloid (**C**).

The disease is due to the presence of an IgG antibody called **LATS** which acts directly on thyroid follicle cells, stimulating them to divide (to produce increased cell numbers – hyperplasia) and to synthesize and secrete TH continuously, out of the control of TSH from the pituitary. TH is therefore synthesized and secreted irrespective of the requirement, and the normal feedback mechanism is bypassed. The thyroid shows diffuse, fleshy enlargement, and the follicles are lined by large, active follicle cells, the follicle lumina containing virtually no stored colloid (*Fig. 16.8*). Another histological feature of the disease is the presence of increased numbers of lymphoid aggregates, including some lymphoid follicles. There is a high incidence of the HLA antigen HLA-DR3 in patients with Graves' disease.

Reduced output of thyroid hormone produces the symptoms and physical signs of hypothyroidism

In infants, hypothyroidism produces the clinical syndrome called **cretinism**, which produces a puffy face and enlarged tongue, coarse features, a protuberant abdomen, and delayed physical and mental developmental milestones. The main causes of cretinism are:

- **Untreated maternal hypothyroidism**. This is now rare, due to better prevention, recognition and treatment of maternal hypothyroidism. It is still a problem in some areas of the world where endemic goiter due to dietary iodine deficiency is seen.

- **Inherited enzyme defect**. This produces sporadic cretinism and is due to failure of normal T_3 and T_4 synthesis.

In adults, hypothyroidism manifests as the syndrome called myxedema, which is due to reduced metabolic rate. There is progressive slowing of physical and mental activity, increasing lethargy and sensitivity to cold, puffy face, coarse dry skin, thinning of hair (particularly of the eyebrows), hoarseness and deepening of voice, and various internal abnormalities, particularly heart failure and a predisposition to hyperlipidemia and hypothermic coma. The main causes of myxedema are:

- **Surgical ablation of the thyroid gland**, which is usually as a result of total thyroidectomy for malignant disease, or aggressive subtotal thyroidectomy for hyperthyroid Graves' disease.
- **Hashimoto's disease** (see below).
- **Some drug therapy**, e.g. lithium.

However, many patients with myxedema present for the first time in old age, and only a few have a history of previous thyroid surgery or disease. At *post mortem* examination, these patients have a uniformly shrunken fibrous gland with very little residual follicular tissue and often only a scanty lymphocytic infiltrate, representing an end-stage thyroid.

There are no clues in either the history or the histology as to the etiology of the thyroid shrinkage, but some patients have demonstrable anti-thyroid antibodies. These cases are sometimes called **primary atrophic thyroiditis**. It is speculated that some patients with so-called focal lymphocytic thyroiditis may progress to this state, as may patients with sub-clinical Hashimoto's disease or previous de Quervain's thyroiditis.

DATA SET
Hyperthyroidism

A 34-year-old shop assistant complained of night sweats and palpitations. She had lost 10 kg in weight over the previous 6 months.

Free thyroxine	42 pmol/L	(12–26)
Free tri-iodothyronine	12 pmol/L	(3.3–7.5)
Thyroid stimulating hormone	< 0.1 mU/L	(0.4–6.3)

This patient has Graves' disease, characterized by high free thyroxine levels which suppress pituitary secretion of thyroid stimulating hormone. The condition is caused by autoantibodies which bind to TSH receptors in the thyroid gland. It is seldom necessary to measure the titer of these antibodies in order to make the diagnosis. Autoantibodies to thyroid microsomes and thyroglobulin are simpler to measure, and are frequently present at high titers in Graves' disease, although they are not specific for this condition.

DATA SET
Hypothyroidism

A 44-year-old woman was seen by her GP complaining of lack of energy.

Free thyroxine	4 pmol/L	(12–26)
Thyroid stimulating hormone	56 mU/L	(0.4–6.3)

This patient has primary hypothyroidism, with low levels of thyroid hormone secretion in spite of the massively raised output of TSH from the pituitary gland. A raised plasma TSH is a sensitive early marker of thyroid insufficiency, and measurement of TSH is valuable in monitoring the adequacy of thyroid hormone replacement therapy.

Hashimoto's disease is a destructive autoimmune thyroiditis that leads to hypothyroidism

Hashimoto's disease is most common in middle age, affecting women more than men. It is an example of organ-specific autoimmune disease (see page 112). The most common autoantibodies are an anti-microsomal antibody and an antibody against thyroglobulin. Hashimoto's disease is particularly seen in patients with the HLA antigen, HLA-DR5.

The initial clinical manifestations include diffuse enlargement of the thyroid, occasionally with a preliminary phase of hyperthyroidism, but by the time most patients seek medical attention they have passed through hyperthyroid and euthyroid phases and are becoming progressively hypothyroid.

On clinical examination, the thyroid is usually symmetrically enlarged and firm, with a bosselated surface. As a result of the disappearance of brown (iodine-rich) colloid, and its replacement by lymphocytes, the cut surface (*Fig. 16.9*) is white rather than the normal brown colour.

It may be that some Hashimoto thyroids proceed to primary atrophic thyroiditis. Laboratory demonstration of the anti-thyroid antibodies forms the basis of the diagnosis of Hashimoto's disease, rendering biopsy unnecessary.

Patients with Hashimoto's disease (and Graves' disease) show a high incidence of other autoimmune diseases (e.g. vitiligo, SLE, etc.).

Solitary nodules in the thyroid usually require excision to confirm their nature

Because most malignant epithelial tumors of the thyroid initially present as a solitary thyroid nodule, complete surgical excision with a safe margin of normal thyroid tissue is usually necessary. However, an accurate preoperative diagnosis can often be made after cytological examination of cells obtained by **fine-needle aspiration** of the nodule.

Solitary palpable thyroid nodules may be due to a:

- **Disproportionately prominent nodule** in a multinodular goiter.
- **Solitary thyroid adenoma** (*Fig. 16.10*), which may either be full of colloid or have a more

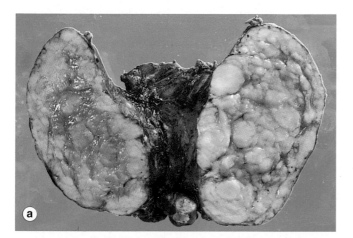

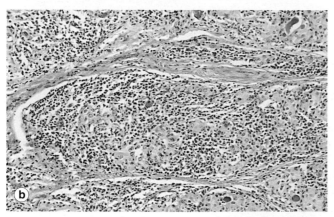

Fig. 16.9 Hashimoto's disease.
The thyroid is diffusely enlarged and slightly bosselated (a), with a fleshy, white cut surface due to the lymphocytic infiltrate and the replacement of brown colloid. Histology (b) shows follicular and diffuse lymphocytic infiltration, with replacement of thyroid follicles.

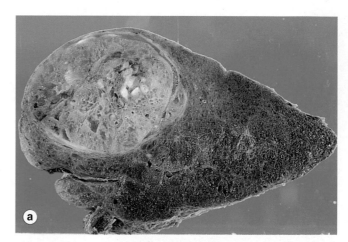

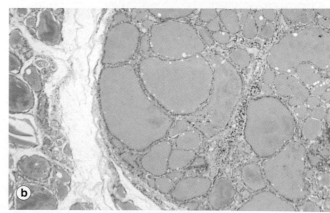

Fig. 16.10 Solitary thyroid adenoma.
A single, well-circumscribed, ovoid nodule, partly brown but with flecks of white calcification, occupies one pole of the thyroid (a). Histology from the edge of the nodule (b) shows at least part of the adenoma to be composed of large colloid-filled acini (colloid adenoma). Other variants may be more cellular.

cellular follicular pattern. The latter may appear fleshy on cut surface.

- **Malignant thyroid tumor** (mainly carcinomas derived from the follicle epithelium). Only histological examination can distinguish these tumors from solitary thyroid adenomata with the more cellular follicular pattern.

There are three main types of malignant tumor derived from thyroid follicle cells

The three main types of malignant tumor derived from thyroid follicle cells (*Fig. 16.11*) have very different natural histories, behavior and prognosis. The most common type is **papillary carcinoma**, a well-differentiated tumor that arises most frequently in young adults. It is often multifocal

within the thyroid, and tends to metastasize via lymphatics to nodes in the neck. It is slow-growing and has an excellent prognosis; even metastatic tumors grow slowly and can be cured by surgical resection.

Follicular carcinoma most commonly affects middle-aged people. Metastasizing via the bloodstream, it is one of the tumors that characteristically spreads to bone. Patients may occasionally present with a spontaneous fracture due to metastatic disease, before the primary tumor is detected. It has a good prognosis.

Entirely confined to the elderly, **anaplastic carcinoma** grows very rapidly, extensively invading tissues near the thyroid, such as the trachea and soft tissues of the neck. It may present with a rapidly enlarging thyroid mass causing tracheal compression or jugular vein invasion. The prognosis

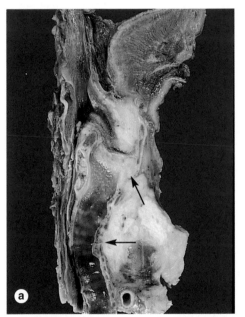

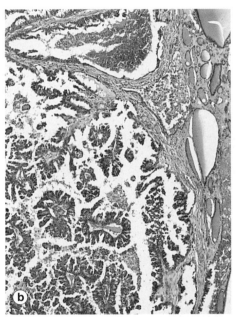

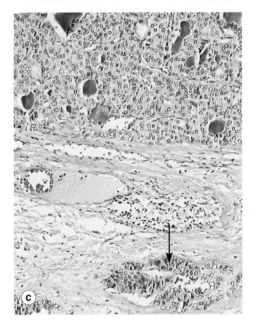

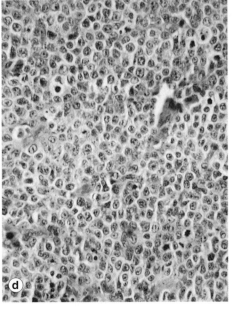

Fig. 16.11 Thyroid carcinoma.

(a) This gross specimen shows a thyroid carcinoma which is showing extensive local spread. The upper arrow shows its upwards extension to involve the larynx, and the lower arrow shows its backward growth to infiltrate, compress and distort the trachea. This pattern of growth is characteristic of anaplastic carcinoma in the elderly. This patient had symptoms for only 8 weeks before death.

(b) This photomicrograph shows typical papillary carcinoma of the thyroid with the tumor cells on a vascular core producing the characteristic papillary pattern. Sometimes the stromal core contains small calcific spherules ('psammoma bodies').

(c) This photomicrograph shows typical follicular thyroid carcinoma in the upper half. Although the tumor attempts to reproduce the follicular pattern of the normal thyroid, it is much more cellular with less colloid (pink) being formed. The arrow shows where the tumor has invaded into a nearby blood vessel, an important indication that the tumor is malignant rather than a benign adenoma.

(d) Histology of anaplastic carcinoma. The tumor is composed of undifferentiated small round cells arranged in sheets, with no evidence of follicular or papillary differentiation. Histologically it may be difficult to distinguish this type of tumor from a lymphoma without the aid of immunocytochemistry.

is very poor. The cells of the tumor, which are usually small, undifferentiated and round, must be distinguished histologically from **malignant lymphoma**; the latter can also affect the thyroid in the elderly, but is more responsive to treatment.

The only significant abnormality of the parafollicular or 'C' cells of the thyroid is the tumor known as 'medullary carcinoma'

Medullary carcinoma has the features of a neuro-endocrine tumor, being composed of small cells containing neuroendocrine granules. An unusual feature is the occasional presence of amyloid in the supporting stroma. Occurring in the middle-aged and elderly, these tumors are occasionally seen in children and young adults, as a component of the multiple endocrine neoplasia (MEN) Type II syndrome (see below).

The tumors are slow-growing, metastasize to local lymph nodes (*Fig. 16.12*) and have a good prognosis. Those arising in patients with the MEN syndrome are sometimes more aggressive and are associated with a poorer prognosis. However, the poor prognosis is usually due to the adverse

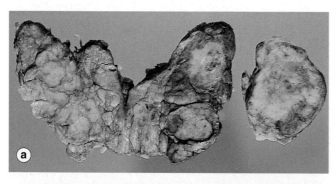

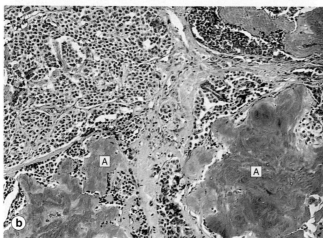

Fig. 16.12 Medullary carcinoma of the thyroid.
The tumor in (a) presented as a solitary nodule in the thyroid, but there was metastatic tumor in a neck lymph gland at the time of presentation. Histology (b) shows a neuroendocrine pattern of growth, with tumor cells and large masses of amyloid in the stroma (**A**).

affects of the other endocrine tumors rather than that in the thyroid. The tumors secrete calcitonin, and the diagnosis can be supported by the demonstration of raised plasma calcitonin levels. The increased calcitonin produces no systemic manifestations.

PARATHYROIDS

The parathyroid glands are small endocrine glands whose sole function is the secretion of parathormone

There are usually four, and sometimes up to eight, parathyroid glands, which are usually located close to the thyroid gland. Two glands are close to the upper poles of the right and left lateral thyroid lobes, and the others are situated near to the lower poles, but their position is variable; there may be parathyroid glands within the thyroid gland tissue and in the thymic fat remnant below the thyroid and in the mediastinum. This variable location is clinically important because the most important parathyroid diseases are treated surgically, and the glands may be difficult to find, particularly since normal parathyroids are so small (approximately $5 \times 3 \times 2$ mm).

Parathormone (PTH), the parathyroid hormone, is important in calcium balance, acting at two sites:

- **The bone surface**, where it mainly stimulates the resorption of mineralized bone by osteoclasts, with the release of calcium into the bloodstream.

- **The renal tubules**, where it stimulates the preferential resorption of calcium ions from the urine, minimizing phosphate ion resorption. It also catalyses the production of 1.25 dihydroxyvitamin D from a less active precursor (see page 514).

Overall, increased PTH secretion increases serum calcium levels, and reduced secretion lowers serum calcium levels. Variations in serum calcium level are usually kept within the normal physiological range by limited variation in PTH secretion; inappropriate increase or decrease in PTH secretion leads to pathological increase (**hypercalcemia**) or decrease (**hypocalcemia**) in serum calcium levels. The bone changes produced by excess PTH activity are discussed in Chapter 24.

Increased PTH secretion is usually due to the presence of a benign parathyroid adenoma

Parathyroid adenoma is usually a solitary tumor that affects only one of the parathyroids, the other parathyroids often showing atrophy. The tumors are usually small and are very rarely palpable in the neck, the main presenting symptoms being due to excessive secretion of parathyroid hormone (**primary hyperparathyroidism**), which produces the symptoms and signs of **hypercalcemia**. The histological appearances of parathyroid adenoma are shown in *Fig. 16.13*.

Malignant parathyroid tumors, with invasion and metastatic spread, are very rare, although some parathyroid adenomata may show considerable pleomorphism and nuclear and cytoplasmic atypia.

Primary parathyroid adenoma is only one of the possible causes of hypercalcemia (see *Fig. 16.14*). Rarely, primary hyperparathyroidism is the result of diffuse hyperplasia of the parathyroids rather than a solitary tumor.

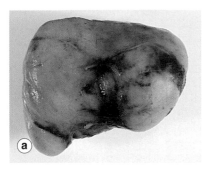 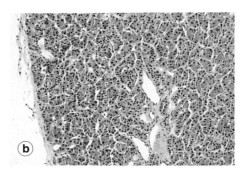 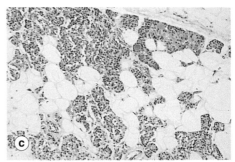

Fig. 16.13 Parathyroid adenoma. (a) A 1 cm parathyroid adenoma removed at operation from a patient with hypercalcemia. (b) The edge of a parathyroid adenoma showing a solid mass of parathyroid cells. (c) The normal parathyroid shows that the hormone-producing cells normally comprise only a small part of the gland, the rest being adipose tissue.

Hypercalcemia

Fig. 16.14a
Causes of hypercalcemia

Widespread metastatic tumor in bone	Destruction of cancellous bone by tumor releases calcium
Parathyroid adenoma	Increased PTH secretion releases calcium from bone by osteoclastic resorption
Multiple myeloma	Plasma-cell tumors in medullary bone release calcium by eroding bone
Ectopic PTH secretion	Some tumors, e.g. oat-cell carcinoma of bronchus, secrete PTH
Vitamin D intoxication Sarcoidosis Milk–alkali syndrome	Rare

Fig. 16.14b
Pathological effects of hypercalcemia

Deposition of calcium in kidney tubules (nephrocalcinosis)
Renal calculi
Excessive calcification of blood vessels
Corneal calcification

DATA SET
Primary hyperparathyroidism

A 42-year-old man with recurrent renal calculi.

Plasma

Calcium	2.92 mmol/L	(2.2–2.6)
	11.6 mg/dl	(8.5–10.3)
Phosphate	0.51 mmol/L	(0.7–1.4)
Albumin	43 g/L	(35–50)
	4.3 g/dl	(3.5–5.0)
Alkaline phosphatase	270 U/L	(80–280)
Parathyroid hormone	75 ng/L	(10–55)

Hyperparathyroidism and malignant disease are the two commonest causes of hypercalcemia, and can be distinguished by measurement of parathyroid hormone (PTH) in plasma. Levels are suppressed in hypercalcemia due to malignant disease, and high or high normal in patients like this man with hyperparathyroidism. Plasma phosphate may be low in either condition, but phosphate levels are raised in patients with renal impairment of any cause. Alkaline phosphatase levels are raised in a minority of patients with primary hyperparathyroidism.

Diffuse hyperplasia of all parathyroid glands is usually a compensatory response to persistently low serum calcium levels

The most common cause of compensatory parathyroid hyperplasia is in renal failure, in which excessive urinary loss of calcium leads to a persistent serum hypocalcemia (*Fig. 16.15*).

The parathyroid hyperplasia produces increased PTH secretion, which mobilizes calcium from bone by stimulating increased osteoclastic activity. However, the calcium so released only brings the serum calcium level closer to normal, never producing hypercalcemia. This compensatory device is called **secondary hyperparathyroidism**

DATA SET
Secondary hyperparathyroidism

An 83-year-old man who lived alone seldom cooked for himself, eating mainly bread and biscuits.

Plasma

Calcium	1.97 mmol/L	(2.2–2.6)
Phosphate	0.50 mmol/L	(0.7–1.4)
Albumin	36 g/L	(35–50)
Alkaline phosphatase	410 U/L	(80–280)
PTH	85 ng/L	(10–55)

Hypocalcemia, due in this patient to dietary vitamin D deficiency, causes secondary hyperparathyroidism. The resulting increase in osteoblastic activity is reflected in the raised alkaline phosphatase levels. Suppression of renal phosphate resorption causes hypophosphatemia.

and is associated with a normal or low serum calcium. Very rarely, an autonomous parathyroid adenoma may arise in one of the hyperplastic parathyroids (**tertiary hyperparathyroidism**).

Hypoparathyroidism is most commonly the result of surgical removal of the parathyroid glands

The parathyroid glands may be removed inadvertently or deliberately during surgery on the thyroid gland. If not surgically excised, they may be severely damaged by operative trauma or by interference with their blood supply.

Much less commonly, the parathyroid glands may be damaged by an autoimmune disease process (autoimmune parathyroid disease) associated with the presence of an autoantibody; this usually occurs in patients who have another autoimmune endocrine disease, e.g. Hashimoto's disease (see page 336) or Addison's disease (see page 342).

Reduced PTH secretion leads to a reduction in the serum calcium, with a corresponding increase in serum phosphate levels. Hypoparathyroidism is only one of the causes of hypocalcemia (see *Fig. 16.16*).

ADRENAL

The adrenal gland has two distinct endocrine components: the cortex and the medulla

The adrenal cortex (*Fig. 16.17*) synthesizes, stores and secretes three main groups of hormone, all of which are steroid hormones synthesized from cholesterol:

- **Glucocorticoid hormones**, e.g. hydrocortisone from zona fasciculata and zona reticularis.

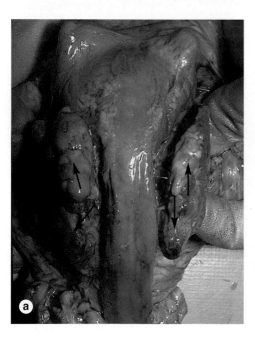

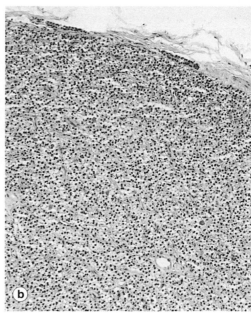

Fig. 16.15 Parathyroid hyperplasia.
(a) A photograph of the posterior aspect of the thyroid gland taken at *post mortem* examination, showing enlargement of all parathyroids (arrows). (b) The hyperplastic parathyroid is histologically almost identical to the parathyroid adenoma in *Fig. 16.13(a)*; compare the cellularity with that of the normal parathyroid shown in *Fig. 16.13(c)*.

- **Mineralocorticoid hormone** (aldosterone), from the zona glomerulosa.
- **Sex steroids**, from zona reticularis.

The adrenal medulla is derived embryologically from neural crest ectoderm and is part of the sympathetic nervous system. It synthesizes and secretes the vasoactive amines, **adrenaline** and **noradrenaline** (**epinephrine** and **norepinephrine**).

Excessive production of adrenal cortical hormones usually results from hyperplasia or tumor

Production of adrenal cortical hydrocortisone and sex steroids is controlled by ACTH secreted by the pituitary gland; aldosterone secretion is controlled by renin production by the juxtaglomerular apparatus in the kidney (see page 351). Excessive ACTH production, for example by an ACTH-secreting adenoma of the pituitary, stimulates an increase in the number, size and secretory activity of the adrenal cortical cells, leading to adrenal cortical hyperplasia (*Fig. 16.18*), which may be diffuse or nodular.

The uncontrolled excessive production of adrenal cortical hormones may produce Cushing's or Conn's syndromes (see Key Facts).

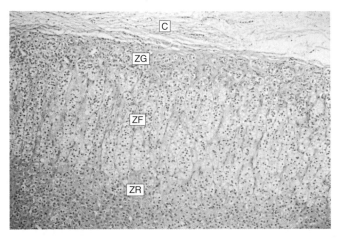

Fig. 16.17 Normal adrenal cortex.
Micrograph showing the three distinct zones of the adrenal cortex: the zona glomerulosa (**ZG**), the zona fasciculata (**ZF**) and the zona reticularis (**ZR**). They are enclosed by a capsule (**C**).

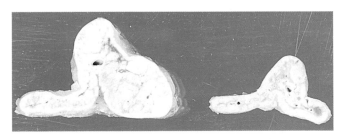

Fig. 16.18 Adrenal cortical hyperplasia. The adrenal on the right is normal, that on the left shows hyperplasia.

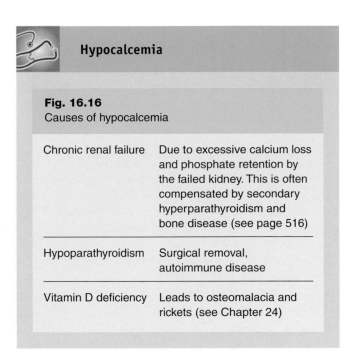

Hypocalcemia

Fig. 16.16
Causes of hypocalcemia

Chronic renal failure	Due to excessive calcium loss and phosphate retention by the failed kidney. This is often compensated by secondary hyperparathyroidism and bone disease (see page 516)
Hypoparathyroidism	Surgical removal, autoimmune disease
Vitamin D deficiency	Leads to osteomalacia and rickets (see Chapter 24)

KEY FACTS
Cushing's syndrome

- Due to excess glucocorticoids, with the most common cause being therapeutic administration of corticosteroids. May also result from pituitary adenoma (causes excess ACTH secretion), adrenal adenoma, ectopic ACTH secretion (e.g. from bronchial carcinoma), and adrenal cortical carcinoma.
- Affects most systems, including: typical facies (moon face), with acne and hirsutism; severe osteoporosis, with vertebral collapse common, myopathy (muscle weakness and wasting); skin fragility and poor wound healing; trunk obesity with stria; peptic ulceration, hypertension and diabetes; hypokalemia; and psychiatric disturbances.
- Diagnosis is based on clinical features and demonstration of raised plasma cortisol level.
- Elucidation of cause is through dexamethasone suppression test, MRI and CT scan visualization of pituitary and adrenal glands, and through analysis of blood ACTH level (high – pituitary adenoma or ectopic ACTH source; low – primary adrenal tumor).

KEY FACTS
Conn's syndrome

- Due to excessive secretion of the mineralocorticoid, aldosterone, which is autonomous (primary aldosteronism). Excessive secretion of aldosterone due to excess plasma renin levels (secondary aldosteronism) is more common, e.g. in hepatic cirrhosis, nephrotic syndrome.
- Primary aldosteronism almost invariably caused by adrenal cortical adenoma.
- Effects include retention of sodium and water (in combination this leads to systemic hypertension), and excessive urinary potassium loss (leads to risk of cardiac arrhythmias).
- Diagnosis is based on establishing the presence of hyperaldosteronism by blood electrolyte estimations (high Na+, low K+, metabolic alkalosis), and is confirmed by detection of raised plasma aldosterone levels and by visualization of adrenal cortical adenoma by CT scan or MRI. Plasma renin level is low in Conn's syndrome and high in secondary aldosteronism.

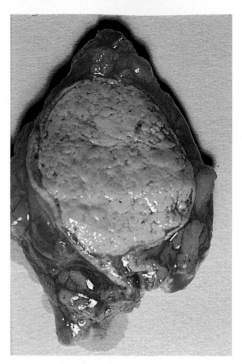

Fig. 16.19 Adrenal cortical adenoma.
The adrenal contains a solitary, well-circumscribed, yellow adenoma derived from the cortex.

Adrenal cortical adenoma is a well-circumscribed, yellow tumor (*Fig. 16.19*) in the adrenal cortex, which is usually 2–5 cm in diameter. The colour of the tumor, as with the adrenal cortex as a whole, is due to the stored lipid (mainly cholesterol), from which the cortical hormones are synthesized. These tumors are frequent incidental findings at *post mortem* examination, and appear to have produced no significant metabolic disorder; only a very small percentage produce Cushing's syndrome. Nevertheless, these apparently 'non-functioning' adenomata are most often encountered in elderly obese people who are often hypertensive. There is some debate that they may really represent nodules in diffuse nodular cortical hyperplasia.

Very occasionally, a true adrenal cortical adenoma is associated with the clinical manifestations of Conn's syndrome, and can be shown to be excreting mineralocorticoids.

Adrenal cortical carcinoma is rare, and virtually every case is associated with excessive production of hormones, usually glucocorticoids and sex steroids. As a result the patients usually have features of Cushing's syndrome mixed with androgenic effects, which are particularly noticeable in women. The tumors are usually large and yellowish white, and local invasion and metastatic spread are common.

Ectopic ACTH secretion may be associated with non-adrenal tumors, particularly oat-cell carcinoma of the bronchus and some carcinoid tumors. In cases of the highly malignant bronchial tumor the symptoms are mainly metabolic, with hypokalemia, alkalosis and impaired glucose tolerance. The patient rarely survives long enough to develop the physical features of Cushing's syndrome, although these and hypertension may develop if the inappropriate secretion is due to a less rapidly fatal tumor.

Chronic adrenal cortical insufficiency produces Addison's disease

Addison's disease is caused by chronic adrenal cortical insufficiency due to lack of glucocorticoids and mineralocorticoids. The main features of the disease are: low serum sodium and high serum potassium with chronic dehydration; hypotension, often markedly postural; lethargy and weakness; vomiting and loss of appetite; and brownish pigmentation of skin and buccal mucosa.

The most common cause is destruction of the cortex of both adrenals by autoimmune adrenalitis, often associated with autoimmune thyroid disease (see pages 334 and 336), autoimmune gastritis and other endocrine organ autoimmune disease. Other causes are bilateral adrenal tuberculosis, fungal infections and adrenal destruction by tumor, but all are rare.

Acute adrenal cortical failure is usually due to hemorrhagic infarction, but may be iatrogenic

Bilateral hemorrhagic necrosis of the adrenals is usually associated with disseminated intravascular coagulation. It is a feature of severe septicemia, particularly meningococcal

DATA SET
Chronic adrenal cortical failure

A 45-year-old woman with a history of progressive lassitude and weight loss over a period of months was seen by her general practitioner.

Plasma

Sodium	129 mmol/L	(135–145 mmol/L)
Potassium	6.2 mmol/L	(3.5–5.3 mmol/L)
Urea	9 mmol/L	(1.0–6.5 mmol/L)
Creatinine	125 µmol/L	(60–120 mmol/L)
Plasma cortisol	4–22 µg/dl	(110–607 nmol/L) am
	3–17 µg/dl	(83–469 nmol/L) pm

Mineralocorticoid deficiency due to adrenal cortical failure causes loss of sodium from the distal renal tubules, resulting in hyponatremia. Associated loss of water leads to dehydration and reduced renal blood flow, reflected in the mild uremia. Potassium and hydrogen ions are retained in the distal tubules, and hyperkalemia and metabolic acidosis are common findings. Glucocorticoid deficiency may result in hypoglycemia.

A short Synacthen test was performed:

Basal	Plasma cortisol	54 nmol/L

Synacthen 250 µg given intramuscularly

30 minutes post-Synacthen	Plasma cortisol	71 nmol/L

Synacthen is a synthetic analog of ACTH. A normal response to Synacthen shows a rise in plasma cortisol of at least 200 nmol/L above baseline. The absence of an adequate response in this patient confirms the diagnosis of adrenal insufficiency.

---

septicemia, in which it is known as the 'Waterhouse–Friderichsen syndrome' (*Fig. 16.20*). There is hypovolemic and hypotensive shock, with hypoglycemia, and high risk of sudden death.

Iatrogenic acute adrenal cortical failure may occur when prolonged high-dose therapeutic corticosteroid therapy is abruptly stopped. Prolonged corticosteroid therapy leads to suppression of normal endogenous steroid production by the adrenal cortex, which becomes markedly atrophied. Sudden cessation of exogenous steroid therapy produces acute adrenal cortical failure (**adrenal crisis**), with hypovolemic and hypotensive shock, hypoglycemia, and risk of sudden death.

Tumors of the adrenal medulla may produce excess adrenaline/noradrenaline or their breakdown products

The two principal types of tumor of the adrenal medulla are **pheochromocytomas** (occurring in adults) and **neuroblastomas** (occurring in children). Neuroblastomas are dealt with in a later section on page 347.

Pheochromocytoma is a tumor of the adrenaline- and noradrenaline- (epinephrine- and norepinephrine-) secreting cells of the adrenal medulla. It produces high levels of both hormones and their breakdown products, vanillylmandelic acid (VMA) and homovanillic acid (HVA), both of which are excreted in the urine and can be estimated as a diagnostic test.

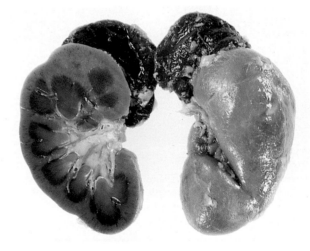

Fig. 16.20 Waterhouse–Friderichsen syndrome.
Taken from a child with meningococcal septicemia, both adrenals show acute hemorrhagic necrosis leading to acute adrenal failure.

The tumor is usually spherical (*Fig. 16.21*) and less than 5 cm in diameter. It has a pale, creamy cut surface that changes to dark brown almost instantly when exposed to air, due to oxygenation of tumor pigments. Despite the fact that the tumor is usually small and non-metastatic, it is a hazardous condition with high perioperative mortality.

The excessive amine production produces hypertension that is often initially paroxysmal and associated with severe

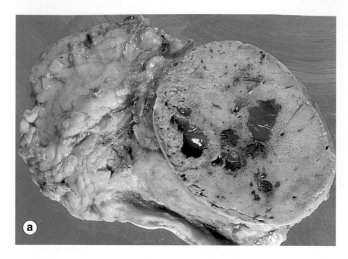

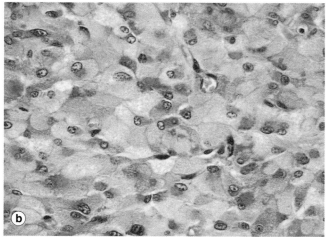

Fig. 16.21 Pheochromocytoma.
(a) The adrenal contains a well-circumscribed, spherical, brown tumor with small foci of hemorrhage. (b) Histology shows a typical neuroendocrine tumor with cells resembling those of the normal adrenal medulla.

**DATA SET
Pheochromocytoma**

A 38-year-old woman complained of panic attacks. Her blood pressure was high (170/105), and was not controlled by conventional doses of α-blocking antihypertensive medication.

24-hour urinary catecholamine excretion:

Adrenaline (epinephrine)	170 nmol/day	(up to 200)
Noradrenaline (norepinephrine)	2967 nmol/day	(up to 530)
VMA	47 µmol/day	(up to 35)

Excessive catecholamine secretion from a pheochromcytoma results in increased urinary excretion of noradrenaline and/or adrenaline, and the catecholamine metabolite VMA (vanillylmandelic acid, or 3-methoxy-4-hydroxymandelic acid). Measurement of catecholamines in plasma is useful if the sample can be obtained during an attack.

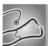

Diagnosis of pheochromocytoma

History: headaches, unexplained cardiac failure.

Examination: irregular systemic hypertension.

Laboratory investigations: raised urinary VMA (24-hour collection).

Visualization: adrenal mass on MRI or CT scan.

headaches, but the hypertension eventually becomes constant. There may be intractable, and often unexplained, cardiac failure. Pheochromocytoma is one of the causes of surgically treatable systemic hypertension.

Bilateral tumors are more commonly seen in patients with the relevant MEN syndrome (see page 346).

Pheochromocytoma may rarely occur in extra-adrenal sympathetic tissue, mainly in the retroperitoneal area alongside the abdominal aorta (organ of Zuckerkandl).

PANCREATIC ENDOCRINE TISSUE

Most of the endocrine tissue in the pancreas is located in discrete islands

Islands of endocrine cells, the **islets of Langerhans**, are scattered throughout the head, body and tail of the pancreas, embedded in the enzyme-secreting exocrine component. The islets are nests of endocrine cells with pink granular cytoplasm containing neuroendocrine granules; each nest has an intimate capillary network, into which the secretions of the islets are discharged. There is a minor endocrine component, with scattered endocrine cells in the ducts leading from the exocrine acini, particularly the smaller ducts.

The endocrine cells secrete the following hormones:

- **Insulin,** which permits transfer of blood glucose into cells and stimulates the synthesis of glycogen in liver and skeletal muscle. Insulin lowers the blood sugar level, and in the absence of insulin, the blood glucose level rises and cells become depleted of glucose.

- **Glucagon**, which opposes the functions of insulin.
- **Somatostatin**, which has many functions and is found widely throughout the body. In the pancreas it inhibits the release of insulin and glucagon from the islets; in other organs, e.g. the stomach and hypothalamus, it has other functions.
- **Pancreatic polypeptide**, which is a minor secretion, the function of which is not known.
- **Amylin (IAPP)**, which has an unknown function.

Well over 60% of the cells in the islets are associated with insulin production; about 20% are associated with glucagon secretion. The nomenclature of the islet cells has been complex. However, as the use of immunocytochemical techniques allows the identification of the product of an individual cell, it is now best to label the cell types by their secreted product, e.g. 'insulin-secreting'.

The most common and important disease associated with the endocrine pancreas is a form of diabetes mellitus

Diabetes mellitus due to autoimmune damage to the insulin-secreting cells of the islets is a common and significant disease associated with the endocrine pancreas.

Diabetes mellitus is a clinical syndrome resulting from disorders in carbohydrate, lipid and protein metabolism due to an intracellular lack of glucose. This lack can be due to either severe primary insulin deficiency in the blood, leading to failure of transport of glucose into the cells; or to failure of glucose to enter the cells as a result of resistance of the cell membranes to the effects of what may be normal levels of circulating insulin.

The former pattern is termed **Type I (insulin-dependent) diabetes mellitus (IDDM)**, and the latter is called **Type II (non-insulin-dependent) diabetes mellitus (NIDDM)**. Type I diabetes is the pattern associated with autoimmune damage to the insulin-secreting cells of the islets of Langerhans, which leads to a deficiency of insulin secretion, producing high blood glucose levels.

Although some of the features of both types of diabetes mellitus are the result of gross biochemical disturbance, many of the clinical features producing severe morbidity and mortality are structural complications that affect many tissues and organs throughout the body. A detailed description of diabetes mellitus is therefore given in the chapter concerned with systemic disease processes (Chapter 25).

The only other important condition resulting from abnormality in the endocrine component of the pancreas is islet-cell tumour

Tumours of the islet cells of the pancreas are examples of neuroendocrine tumors. Most are benign, producing their symptoms through excess secretion of a specific hormone, usually insulin. The tumors are usually solitary, but in the MEN syndromes most are multiple (*Fig. 16.22a*).

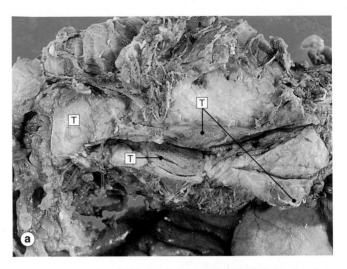
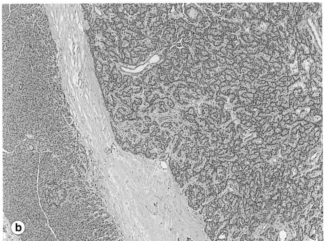
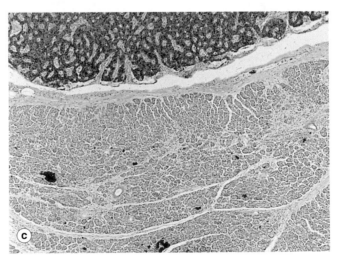

Fig. 16.22 Islet-cell tumor of the pancreas.
This surgically resected specimen of the pancreas (a) was taken from a patient with MEN I syndrome, and shows a number of separate islet-cell tumours (T). Histologically (b), tumours are composed of cords and nests of neuroendocrine cells in contact with adjacent pancreatic tissue. Immunohistochemistry (c) showed that the neuroendocrine cells were producing insulin (brown color). In this case, the patient presented with recurrent hypoglycemic attacks.

Insulinoma produces hypersecretion of insulin, leading to hypoglycemic attacks that are often severe enough to produce coma; pre-coma symptoms include confusion and behavioral disturbance (sometimes aggressiveness).

Glucagonoma is very rare. The excess secretion of glucagon is often asymptomatic, although patients may be anemic and develop an unexplained secondary diabetes. A bizarre characteristic skin rash called necrolytic migratory erythema sometimes occurs.

Very rarely, islet-cell tumors may secrete unusual hormones such as vasoactive intestinal peptide (VIP) and gastrin (producing the Zollinger–Ellison syndrome of recurrent and multiple peptic ulcers in stomach and proximal small intestine), or may even produce ACTH.

OVARY AND TESTIS

The ovary is an important endocrine organ, producing estrogens and progesterones

The ovary cyclically produces estrogen and progesterone under the influence of cyclical production of follicle-stimulating hormone (FSH) and luteinizing hormone (LH) by the pituitary which, in turn, is stimulated by hypothalamic gonadotrophin-releasing hormones.

- **Estrogens**, produced by the ripening **ovarian follicle**, stimulate the proliferation of the endometrium and are responsible for the development and maintenance of secondary sexual characteristics, e.g. in the breast. Estrogens are also produced in small amounts by other components of the ovary, e.g. the stroma and the hilar cells.
- **Progesterones**, produced by the **luteinizing follicle**, stimulate secretory changes in the endometrium. Persistence of the corpus luteum after conception leads to persistence of progesterone secretion, which is essential for the development of the decidua and for the maintenance of pregnancy. It also has an influence on breast structure and function.

Imbalance of oestrogens and progesterones can have significant pathological effects on the uterus and breasts, leading to menstrual abnormalities, infertility, spontaneous abortion, irregular breast enlargement, and breast lumps. Imbalance has been implicated in the development of breast cancer and endometrial cancer. Many of these conditions are discussed in Chapters 19 and 20.

The ovary can sometimes produce abnormal amounts of androgens, leading to masculinization

Although the ripening follicles mainly produce estrogens, they (and the hilus cells) can also produce androgens. These are normally produced in such minute amounts that there is no significant clinical impact, but some rare diseases of follicles or hilus cells (Stein–Leventhal syndrome and

Sertoli–Leydig cell tumors, see Chapter 19) can be associated with excessive androgen secretion. This leads to masculinization, with cessation of menstruation, infertility, loss of female secondary sexual characteristics, and acquisition of male characteristics such as hirsutism. Excess estrogens are also secreted, but they are usually overwhelmed by the androgen effects.

The endocrine component of the testis secretes testosterone

The interstitial or **Leydig cells** form the endocrine component of the testis. These cells secrete testosterone, the hormone responsible for the initiation of spermatogenesis in childhood and for its maintenance in adult life. It is also responsible for the maintenance of structure and function of the male genital ducts (e.g. vas deferens) and the accessory secretory glands (e.g. the prostate), and for the development and maintenance of the male secondary sexual characteristics.

Testosterone depletion is rare, although the amount secreted decreases in old age

Pathological testosterone depletion produces loss of masculine characteristics and reduction of spermatogenesis. It is rare as a spontaneous disease, but will inevitably follow bilateral orchidectomy, which is sometimes undertaken medically to control advanced cancer of the prostate (see Chapter 18). The undescended testis continues to produce testosterone, even though it may be incapable of spermatogenesis (see page 383). The Leydig cells are also capable of secreting estrogens, but normally do so in such small amounts that they are overwhelmed by the testosterone effect. However, rare tumors of the Leydig cells (interstitial cell tumor, see page 390) frequently secrete abnormal quantities of estrogens, and may present with features of feminization such as loss of libido, loss of body hair, and gynecomastia.

The pineal gland and thymus both secrete hormones

Although the pineal gland and thymus both secrete hormones, diseases of these organs that produce hormone effects are very rare. The thymus gland is discussed in Chapter 15.

In the multiple endocrine neoplasia (MEN) syndromes patients develop tumors in a number of endocrine organs

In those affected by the MEN syndromes, there is usually a strong family history of multiple endocrine tumors with autosomal dominant inheritance. Patients are younger than those who develop single sporadic tumors.

In **MEN I syndrome** patients usually show a combination of parathyroid hyperplasia, pancreatic islet-cell tumors (often multiple), and pituitary adenomata. These are the most common features, but there may also be parathyroid adenomata, hyperplasia of the parafollicular calcitonin-secreting cells in the thyroid, and adrenal cortical hyperplasia.

Patients with the **MEN IIa syndrome** have a combination of pheochromocytoma (sometimes bilateral) and medullary carcinoma of the thyroid (which may be multifocal). Occasionally there is hyperparathyroidism due to parathyroid hyperplasia. A small sub-group, **MEN IIb** (sometimes called **MEN III**), also shows large numbers of neuromas and ganglioneuromas in the dermis and submucosal regions throughout the body.

The medullary carcinoma of the thyroid in *Fig. 16.12* and the islet-cell tumor in *Fig. 16.22* were from patients with MEN II and MEN I syndromes, respectively.

The most common disease of the diffuse neuroendocrine system is tumor formation

Through advances in immunocytochemical methods, many scattered cells in epithelial surfaces and solid organs have been identified as being neuroendocrine in nature. In addition many of their peptide and protein hormones have been identified. Under normal circumstances these cells are **paracrine**, i.e. produce hormones that act locally and do not enter the blood circulation. However, some tumors pass excessive amounts of the hormone into the circulation and can produce systemic effects, e.g. carcinoid tumor of the small intestine and the **carcinoid syndrome** (see page 264, Chapter 13).

ENDOCRINE DISEASE IN CHILDREN

Deficiency of growth hormone in children leads to pituitary dwarfism

Children with pituitary dwarfism are perfectly formed, but very small, and fail to grow at the usual rate. Bone age is delayed, the voice is high-pitched, and the genitalia are small (most noticeable in boys). Those affected are prone to recurrent attacks of hypoglycemia. The pituitary abnormality may be a familial deficiency of growth hormone, or there may be a tumor replacing the pituitary (e.g. a large pituitary adenoma or a craniopharyngioma); in the case of tumors, there is deficiency of other anterior pituitary hormones.

Hypothyroidism in children leads to cretinism

Cretinism is discussed earlier in this chapter (see page 335). It may be endemic, and is due either to maternal hypothyroidism associated with iodine lack, or to a congenital enzyme deficiency.

Transient hyperthyroidism is common in girls at the time of puberty

Transient hyperthyroidism is usually associated with a mild, diffuse enlargement of the thyroid gland. It occurs so frequently that it may almost be regarded as a transient physiological response. Symptoms of hyperthyroidism are usually minimal and disappear in a short time, but the thyroid enlargement occasionally persists, and the hyperthyroid state may become permanent.

Adrenal cortical disorders in children are rare

Adrenal cortical tumors are very uncommon in children, most children with Cushing's syndrome having a pituitary tumor or a tumor resulting from exogenous steroid therapy. An important condition that occurs in children is **congenital adrenal hyperplasia**, an autosomal recessive disorder associated with lack of 21-hydroxylase in the adrenal cortex. 21-hydroxylase is involved in the production of both aldosterone and cortisone from precursors; in its absence the precursors are instead converted into testosterone. The patients thus have cortisone and aldosterone deficiency, but testosterone excess; this manifests itself as precocious sexual development in boys, and as virilization in girls (with masculinization of the female external genitalia, e.g. clitoral hyperplasia). Because the plasma cortisone levels are low, the anterior pituitary is stimulated by the feedback mechanism to secrete excess ACTH, which leads to marked adrenal cortical hyperplasia. The clinical features are called the **adrenogenital syndrome**. Patients may also develop electrolyte abnormalities, including excessive salt loss, due to aldosterone deficiency.

Neuroblastoma of the adrenal medulla is an important malignant tumor in children

Adrenal neuroblastoma is an example of an 'embryonal tumor' and is derived from primitive neuroblasts. Tumors arise from the adrenal medulla and from the sympathetic ganglia of the autonomic nervous system. It is one of the group of peripheral primitive neuroectodermal tumours (PNETs). Most tumors occur in children under the age of 3 years, the majority occurring in children under the age of 1 year.

Macroscopically, neuroblastomas range from small nodules to enormous masses (*Fig. 16.23a*), although in most cases the tumor is already large at first diagnosis, the most common presenting symptom being a palpable abdominal mass. Metastatic spread is via the bloodstream and the tumor has a predilection for spread to bone. Some cases present with symptoms due to bone metastasis.

Histologically the tumors are composed of mitotically active small primitive neuroblastic cells which exhibit variable degrees of neuronal maturation (*Fig. 16.23b*); occasionally, characteristic 'rosettes' can be seen comprising a ring of neuroblasts with fine neurofilaments in the lumen. Some tumors even contain mature ganglion cells in addition to the primitive neuroblastic areas, in which case they are called **ganglioneuroblastomas**.

Prognosis in neuroblastoma is highly dependent on the age of onset of disease, with survival rates at 2 years as follows: neonates (70%), cases aged under 1 year (30%), cases aged between 1 and 2 years (20%), and cases aged over 2 years (5%).

Tumor stage also has an important bearing on prognosis. Staging is based on whether tumor is confined to the adrenal, on whether it crosses the midline, on evidence of lymph node involvement and on evidence of bloodstream spread. An important stage of neuroblastoma is defined as **stage 4S**, in which there is a localized primary tumor with metastasis to skin and liver, with minimal marrow involvement; this is confined to children under the age of 1 year.

Paradoxically, **stage 4S** is associated with a very good prognosis and **spontaneous regression of tumor** with little or no treatment.

The natural history of untreated neuroblastoma is for local and metastatic spread resulting in death. With treatment, many tumors show partial or complete response to therapy.

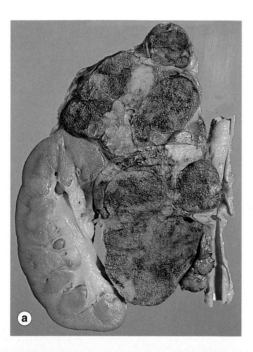

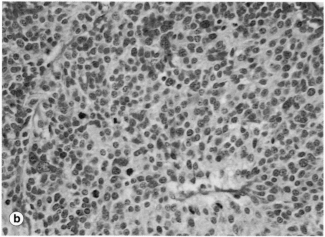

Fig. 16.23 Neuroblastoma.
(a) An advanced neuroblastoma which has arisen from the adrenal at the upper pole of the kidney and has spread to produce a large mass on one side of the aorta, with para-aortic lymph nodes. The brown, hemorrhagic cut surface appearance is characteristic. (b) Histology showing predominantly small, undifferentiated cells (neuroblasts), with a small amount of intervening stroma in the form of nerve fibers.

Neuroblastoma – laboratory medicine

- Neuroblastomas secrete catecholamines and so elevated levels of metabolites may be found in the urine. Markers measured are vanillylmandelic acid (VMA), homovanillic acid (HVA) and dopamine (see Data Set below).
- Diagnosis of neuroblastoma must always be based on tissue diagnosis: either biopsy of primary tumor, or based on cells seen in bone marrow aspiration or trephine biopsy.
- Genetic analysis of neuroblastoma has shown frequent presence of deletion of the short arm of chromosome 1, or amplification of the N-*myc* oncogene, or loss of alleles from chromosome 14, or a combination. Tumors with N-*myc* amplification have a worse prognosis (10% 3-year survival) than those with one copy of this gene (50–90% 3-year survival).

DATA SET
Neuroblastoma

A 3-year-old boy had been unwell for several weeks. On examination, a large mass was palpable on the right side of the abdomen and flank.

Urinary catecholamines:

Adrenaline (epinephrine)	18 nmol/mmol of creatinine (up to 30)
Noradrenaline (norepinephrine)	360 nmol/mmol of creatinine (up to 120)
Dopamine	96 165 nmol/mmol of creatinine (up to 900)

Neuroblastomas commonly secrete dopamine, which is excreted in urine. Alternatively, the dopamine metabolite HVA (homovanillic acid) can be measured in urine.

17

Diseases of the urinary system

Clinical Overview

In essence the kidney can be considered to be a length of small blood vessel lying in close proximity to an epithelial-lined cylinder, the proximity allowing interchange of content between vessel and cylinder. The system allows waste material to pass from the blood into the cylinder and also allows homeostatic control of the composition of the fluid in the epithelial-lined cylinder, by selective reabsorption of certain components back into the blood vessel. The contents of the epithelial-lined channel then pass into a system of conducting vessels (the lower urinary tract) where they are temporarily stored in a reservoir (the bladder) before being excreted in the form of urine.

It is obvious, therefore, that most diseases of the kidney will be associated with abnormalities of either the blood vessel system or the epithelial-lined tubule system, often both since they are so interdependent. The kidney is particularly vulnerable to any type of vascular disease, including the consequences of severe large vessel atheroma, but particularly the vessel abnormalities associated with **diabetes mellitus** and **benign** and **accelerated hypertension**.

The kidney is also sensitive to various types of immune reactions in which immune complexes are deposited in one form or another in the walls of the small blood vessels forming the glomerulus. This group of disorders are called '**the glomerulonephritides**' and are an important cause of failure of all or some of the kidney functions. When any component of the vascular system is occluded, the epithelial-lined tubular system undergoes atrophy, since it is dependent on oxygen for its function; thus vascular disease leads to temporary or permanent destruction of the tubular system.

The tubular system in the kidney is very metabolically active because of the high energy demands involved in pumping ions and water across the barriers into the adjacent blood vessel. They are therefore extremely vulnerable to hypoxia, and anything which produces inadequate blood perfusion through the kidney's vascular system will lead to necrosis of the tubular epithelial cells. This is the commonest cause of **acute renal failure**, but the changes are reversible if perfusion can be re-established.

The conducting system which carries the tubular fluid away is in communication with the outside at the urethra. This lower urinary tract is predisposed to bacterial infection which may spread backwards into the kidney's tubular system to produce infection of the kidney itself (**acute pyelonephritis**). Urine is essentially a concentrated aqueous solution of solutes, some of which are sometimes precipitated out to form **calculi** which can obstruct the urinary drainage system leading to numerous complications.

▶

> Only two types of tumor commonly occur in the kidney, one of which occurs in adults (**renal adenocarcinoma**), the other affecting only children (**nephroblastoma**). The lower urinary tract is lined by a specialized transitional epithelium called urothelium which is a frequent site of the malignant tumor, **transitional cell carcinoma**, which can occur anywhere along the urothelial-lined lower urinary tract. It may be multifocal, and is one of the forms of cancer which may follow industrial exposure to certain chemical carcinogens.
>
> Congenital malformations of the kidney and lower urinary tract are common, although many (such as horseshoe kidney and duplex ureter) are asymptomatic and do not disturb renal function. However, some lead to renal failure at birth (e.g. **renal agenesis**) or later in life (**polycystic disease**).

The urinary system can be divided into the upper and lower urinary tracts.

The **upper urinary tract** comprises the kidney, which is responsible for the ultrafiltration of blood (to remove the waste products of the body's metabolic processes in the form of urine), and for the maintenance of water and electrolyte homeostasis. Impaired kidney function is evident as a variety of metabolic disturbances and, according to the severity, is termed either **partial renal failure** or **total renal failure**.

The **lower urinary tract** comprises the pelvicalyceal systems, ureters, bladder and urethra, which are responsible for the collection, transportation, storage and ultimate voiding of urine.

The kidney develops from part of the mesodermal mass, the metanephric blastema, high on the posterior abdominal wall on either side of the midline. The pelvicalyceal system and ureters are derived from the ureteric bud, which is an outgrowth of the primitive mesonephric duct. The bladder and urethra develop from the urogenital sinus.

KIDNEY

The kidney has numerous metabolic functions

The **glomerulus** is responsible for filtration of urine, retaining proteins and other large molecules in the blood. The property of selective filtration lies in the structure and ionic charge of the glomerular basement membrane (GBM). Structural abnormalities in the membrane and neutralization of anionic sites cause it to lose this property.

The **tubular and ductular systems** have several main functions, each of which is dependent upon normal cellular function of tubular epithelial cells. These systems are responsible for resorption of glucose and amino acids filtered by the glomerulus, selective resorption of water under the control of ADH, and selective resorption or secretion of sodium, potassium, calcium, phosphate and hydrogen ions to maintain homeostasis.

Erythropoietin is secreted by the kidney and is essential for the normal production of red blood cells by the marrow.

Renin is secreted by the juxtaglomerular apparatus and is responsible for activating angiotensin, which stimulates the secretion of aldosterone by the adrenal cortex. Aldosterone then acts on tubules to re-absorb sodium ions and water from the glomerular filtrate, thereby maintaining plasma volume and blood pressure.

The main functioning unit of the kidney is the nephron

The structure of the nephron is given in simplified diagrammatic form in *Fig. 17.1* The main components are:

- **The pre-glomerular blood vessels**, which are responsible for supplying blood to the glomerulus.
- **The glomerulus**, which is a highly specialized capillary system. The basement membrane of the lining endothelium is fused to that of surrounding epithelium to create a highly selective filtration barrier. The glomerular capillary tuft is situated within **Bowman's capsule**, which collects the ultrafiltrate and passes it into the next component of the nephron:
- **The tubular system**, which is divided into several parts. The **proximal tubules** are mainly involved in the selective resorption of various components of the glomerular filtrate, the **loop of Henle** is involved in creating an ionic concentration gradient in the renal medulla, and the **distal tubule** is mainly involved in acid–base balance and sodium- and potassium-ion resorption.
- **The collecting tubules and ducts**, which are responsible for the resorption of water from the dilute urine under the control of anti-diuretic hormone (ADH).
- **The post-glomerular vasculature** has two main functions: it provides oxygenated blood for the tubular epithelium, and also participates in homeostasis; ions, water, and other small molecules pass between the tubular and ductular parts of the nephron and the

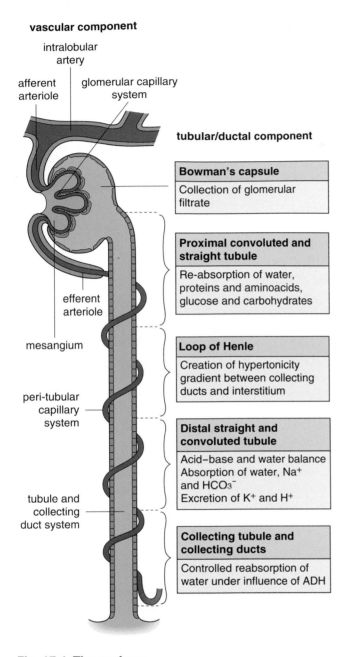

Fig. 17.1 The nephron.
The main functional unit of the kidney is the nephron.

vascular component

intralobular artery

afferent arteriole

glomerular capillary system

efferent arteriole

mesangium

peri-tubular capillary system

tubule and collecting duct system

tubular/ductal component

Bowman's capsule
Collection of glomerular filtrate

Proximal convoluted and straight tubule
Re-absorption of water, proteins and aminoacids, glucose and carbohydrates

Loop of Henle
Creation of hypertonicity gradient between collecting ducts and interstitium

Distal straight and convoluted tubule
Acid–base and water balance
Absorption of water, Na^+ and HCO_3^-
Excretion of K^+ and H^+

Collecting tubule and collecting ducts
Controlled reabsorption of water under influence of ADH

post-glomerular vasculature. The post-glomerular (peri-tubular) capillaries are therefore in very close association with the tubular and ductular system.

Glomerular diseases are caused by disturbances of structure, whereas tubular diseases are mainly caused by metabolic disturbances

Functionally, the activity of the glomerulus is mostly determined by the integrity of its structure. In contrast, the activity of the renal tubule is mostly determined by the metabolic activity of the lining epithelial cells.

Glomerular function tends to be disrupted by diseases that alter glomerular structural arrangements (seen with structural damage to basement membrane, endothelium, epithelium or mesangium), and tubular function tends to be disrupted by metabolic insult to the tubular cells (e.g. hypoxia or toxins).

As both glomerular and tubular function are highly dependent on adequate perfusion by blood, if this is disrupted both functions are impaired. Once function is disturbed in one part of the nephron, secondary abnormalities often develop in other parts because of the close structural and functional relationships in the nephron.

The kidneys have a considerable degree of functional reserve, but when disease processes damage sufficient numbers of nephrons to exceed the compensatory ability of those remaining, renal failure ensues.

Partial renal failure syndromes affect only some elements of renal function

There are two main types of partial renal failure: the nephritic syndrome and the nephrotic syndrome.

The **nephritic syndrome** is the result of disturbance of glomerular structure that involves reactive cellular proliferation. This causes reduced glomerular blood flow (leading to reduced urine output – **oliguria**), leakage of red cells from damaged glomeruli (**hematuria**), and consequent retention of waste products (**uremia**). The low renal blood flow activates the renin–angiotensin system, with fluid retention and mild hypertension. Small amounts of proteins are also lost in the urine, but this is usually trivial. The hematuria is not gross and is usually manifest as a smoky brown discoloration of urine.

The **nephrotic syndrome** is the result of abnormality in the glomerular basement membrane or mesangium, such that the glomerulus loses the capacity for selective retention of proteins in the blood. This leads to loss of very large amounts of protein, mostly albumin, in the urine (**proteinuria**), with consequent loss of protein from the blood (**hypoalbuminemia**) leading to **edema**. There is **susceptibility to infections** because of low levels of immunoglobulins and complement, **susceptibility to thrombosis** because of increased levels of fibrinogen in the blood, and **hyperlipidemia** due to reduced levels of serum apolipoproteins.

Other indications of renal abnormality are **intermittent hematuria** and **persistent proteinuria** which can be thought of as early partial renal failure. The latter may precede the development of a nephrotic syndrome.

Acute renal failure is characterized by widespread abrupt cessation of nephron function

Acute renal failure is a form of total renal failure in which the majority of nephrons suddenly and simultaneously stop working. Clinically this causes a dramatic fall in urine production (**oliguria**), which is often total (**anuria**). With little opportunity for metabolic compensation, problems of disturbed fluid and electrolyte balance and failure of elimination develop rapidly. There is an increase in serum potassium level and metabolic acidosis, and nitrogen retention with uremia (see Data Set).

Several diseases can produce acute renal failure, all operating by causing sudden generalized cessation of all functions of all nephrons. There are many causes which can be divided into:

- **Central perfusion failure** – conditions such as hypovolemic shock, sudden and profound hypotension (due, for example, to massive hemorrhage or central pump failure in myocardial infarction) lead to inadequate perfusion of the kidneys. The most sensitive component of the nephron to poor perfusion and consequent anoxia are the epithelial cells of the proximal and distal convoluted tubules, which may undergo extensive necrosis (**acute tubular necrosis**). Combined with insufficient glomerular perfusion for ultrafiltration to take place, this leads to failure of the entire nephron. This is the most common cause of reversible acute renal failure.

- **Tubular and interstitial disease** – due to hypoxic, toxic or infective damage, for example, acute pyelonephritis (see page 370).

- **Glomerular diseases** – immune-mediated damage to glomeruli sometimes causes acute renal failure when all glomeruli are damaged severely at the same time.

Occlusion of glomerular capillaries prevents ultrafiltration, and also prevents blood flowing through the efferent arterioles to the peri-tubular capillary system to provide vital oxygen for the highly oxygen-dependent tubular epithelial cells.

Acute renal failure is often reversible if the damaging stimulus is removed, allowing restoration of normal structure in the kidney through regeneration of damaged elements, particularly tubular epithelial cells. Where there has been very severe generalized necrosis of the kidney, recovery may not be possible.

Chronic renal failure occurs with slow progressive destruction of individual nephrons over a long period of time

Chronic renal failure is a form of total renal failure caused by progressive destruction of individual nephrons over a long period of time. As more and more nephrons are destroyed, renal function becomes progressively more impaired. However, in contrast to acute renal failure there is opportunity for metabolic compensation.

Among the main consequences of chronic renal failure are progressive retention of nitrogenous metabolites (**uremia**) and progressive failure of tubular function. The latter produces early inability to concentrate urine (**polyuria**) and abnormalities in biochemical homeostasis (including salt and water retention, compensated metabolic acidosis, and other electrolyte imbalances, particularly hyperkalemia). Sodium and fluid retention may cause hypertension.

DATA SET
Acute renal failure

A 24-year-old man sustained severe intra-abdominal injuries in a motor cycle accident. At laparotomy he was found to have a ruptured spleen and liver and extensive intraperitoneal hemorrhage. Over the next 24 hours he passed only 200 ml of urine.

Plasma

Sodium	135 mmol/L	(135 to 145)
Potassium	6.1 mmol/L	(3.5 to 5.3)
Bicarbonate	15 mmol/L	(23 to 33)
Urea	32 mmol/L	(1.0 to 6.5)
Creatinine	427 µmol/L	(60 to 120)
Osmolality	309 mmol/Kg	(285 to 295)

Urine

Na	58 mmol/L
Osmolality	310 mmol/Kg

Acute renal failure is associated with raised levels of urea and creatinine in plasma, due to decreased filtration at the glomeruli. Retention of potassium and hydrogen ions results in hyperkalemia and metabolic acidosis, reflected in the low plasma bicarbonate.

Tubular damage impairs sodium resorption, resulting in urinary sodium loss, usually at concentrations in excess of 20 mmol/L. The plasma osmolality is high due mainly to the high urea concentration. The ability of the damaged renal tubules to dilute or concentrate urine is impaired, and consequently the urinary osmolality approximates that of plasma.

Failure of renal activation of vitamin D causes secondary hyperparathyroidism and bone disease, (**renal osteodystrophy** – see page 514), and destruction of renal parenchyma leads to reduced erythropoietin levels which, together with the direct suppressive effect of uremia on

marrow, results in anemia. Uremia also causes defective platelet function and a bleeding tendency.

Several diseases can produce chronic renal failure, all of which cause slow, progressive, irreversible generalized destruction of nephrons (both glomeruli and tubules). The main causes of chronic renal failure are vascular disease (long-standing hypertension), disease of glomeruli (glomerulonephritis and diabetic glomerular disease) and disease of tubules and interstitium (infective, toxic and obstructive damage to tubules and renal papillae).

In contrast to many cases of acute renal failure, chronic renal failure is not reversible because there has been destruction of nephrons. A kidney in which all nephrons have been irreversibly damaged is macroscopically small and shrivelled and is known as an **end-stage kidney** (see page 368, *Fig. 17.17*). The main clinical and biochemical features of the four main renal impairment syndromes are summarized in *Fig. 17.2* and the Data Sets.

**DATA SET
Chronic renal failure**

A 46-year-old man with insulin dependent diabetes mellitus since the age of 16.

Plasma

Sodium	133 mmol/L	(135 to 145)
Potassium	5.5 mmol/L	(3.5 to 5.3)
Bicarbonate	16 mmol/L	(23 to 33)
Urea	44 mmol/L	(1.0 to 6.5)
Creatinine	637 μmol/L	(60 to 120)

24-hour urine

Protein	1.1 g/day	(up to 0.1)

Proteinuria is an early indicator of renal damage in patients with diabetes. Chronic renal failure develops over months to years, with progressive rises in plasma urea and creatinine as glomerular filtration falls. Regular monitoring of the rising plasma creatinine level enables the physician to anticipate the need for dialysis or renal transplantation. Electrolyte imbalance causing hyperkalemia and hyponatremia is a relatively late development. Metabolic acidosis due to impaired renal hydrogen ion excretion causes hypobicarbonatemia.

**KEY FACTS
Renal failure**

¥ There are two syndromes of total renal failure: **acute renal failure** and **chronic renal failure**.
¥ There are two main syndromes of partial renal failure: **nephritic syndrome** (oliguria, hematuria and uremia) and **nephrotic syndrome** (proteinuria, hypoproteinemia, edema).
¥ Chronic renal failure is irreversible, as it is caused by permanent destruction of nephrons.
¥ Acute renal failure sometimes recovers when the

Fig. 17.2
Renal failure syndromes

Pattern	Total/partial	Mechanism	Effects
Nephrotic syndrome	Partial	Glomerular permeability increase	Severe protein loss in urine, leading to hypoalbuminemia and edema
Nephritic syndrome	Partial	Glomerular perfusion failure (usually transient)	Rising blood pressure and urea, hematuria, mild edema
Acute renal failure	Total	Acute glomerular perfusion failure and tubular epithelial failure (often reversible)	Oliguria/anuria, nitrogen retention (uremia), acidosis, potassium retention
Chronic renal failure	Total	Chronic irreversible nephron failure, both glomerular and tubular failure	Nitrogen retention (uremia), hydrogen ion retention (acidosis), potassium retention, reduced erythropoietin, impaired vitamin D metabolism

VASCULAR DISEASE AND THE KIDNEY

As has been emphasized, renal function is dependent upon a normal vascular supply. Vascular disease therefore has a great impact on renal function. The main problems stem from ischemic changes induced by **hypertension**, and from occlusion of renal vessels by emboli, causing **infarction**.

Several vascular diseases have a major impact on the capillaries of the glomerular tuft, particularly vasculitis and conditions associated with intravascular thrombosis.

Reduction in blood flow to the kidneys, for example in prolonged hypotension, commonly results in necrosis of renal tubular epithelium, termed **acute tubular necrosis**. This is discussed in the later section on tubulointerstitial diseases (see page 371).

Diseases affecting pre-glomerular vessels may produce either chronic or acute renal failure

Normal renal function is dependent on adequacy of renal blood supply, with sufficient flow to maintain glomerular filtration, as well as oxygenation of the tubular and ductal parts of the nephron. Diseases of pre-glomerular vessels, or central pump failure, have a major impact on the function of the kidney.

In general, **slowly progressive disease of the vessels** leads to slowly progressive destruction of nephrons, ischemic glomerular filtration failure and ischemic tubular atrophy, culminating in chronic renal failure and a small, shrunken end-stage kidney.

The initial effect of **rapidly progressive disease of vessels** or **severe central pump failure** is sudden reduction of glomerular filtration, and the development of hypoxic necrosis of tubular epithelium. This leads to acute renal failure with oliguria or anuria, and the affected kidney is usually swollen.

Renal artery stenosis causes renal ischemia and may result in secondary hypertension

Generalized atherosclerosis particularly affects the aorta and the origin of the renal artery, but in severe cases may extend into the main renal arteries and the major branches. In most cases the atherosclerotic occlusion of the renal artery is most severe at its origin from the aorta. This **renal artery stenosis** can lead to chronic ischemia of the affected kidney, with reduction in function of all nephrons on that side, producing an end-stage shrunken kidney. The unaffected kidney undergoes compensatory hypertrophy, so renal function is largely unaffected in most cases (*Fig. 17.3*). Renal artery stenosis is also caused by **arterial fibromuscular dysplasia**.

Renal artery stenosis may lead to **renovascular hypertension**, thought to result from abnormal activity in the renin–angiotensin system in the chronically ischemic kidney. It is important in that it is one of the recognized causes of hypertension that is amenable to surgical correction.

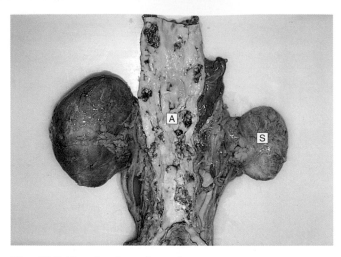

Fig. 17.3 Renal artery stenosis.
Severe atheroma of the aorta (**A**) has caused occlusion of the lumen of one of the renal arteries. This has caused ischemia to the kidney, which is shrunken (**S**). The ischemic kidney can then precipitate hypertension by oversecretion of renin. Loss of function of this irreversibly damaged kidney is compensated for by the other kidney, which undergoes hypertrophy (leading to enlargement) and takes on double the workload.

Benign hypertension produces thickening of the wall of renal vessels, with persistently reduced flow

In long-standing benign hypertension, changes in muscular renal arteries and renal arterioles lead to reduced flow of blood to glomeruli (*Fig. 17.4*). Renal artery branches within the kidney show thickening of the wall due to a combination of fibroelastic intimal proliferation, elastic lamina reduplication, and muscular hypertrophy of the media (see page 167). Afferent arterioles undergo hyalinization, their muscular walls being replaced by an amorphous material, which is rigid and inelastic (see page 167). These thickenings of the vessel wall lead to reduction in the size of the lumen and reduced blood flow.

Chronic and progressive reduction in blood flow to the nephron leads to chronic ischemia, with slow conversion of individual glomeruli into a mass of hyaline tissue devoid of capillary lumina. As the blood supply to the tubule is derived from flow through the glomerulus into the efferent arteriole and peri-tubular capillaries, ischemic destruction of the associated tubule occurs. This process picks off individual nephrons over a period of many years, with no initial clinical symptoms. Biochemically a gradual increase in blood levels of urea and a reduction in creatinine clearance occur.

Eventually, sufficient numbers of nephrons become non-functioning for the patient to develop manifestations of chronic renal failure. This sequence of changes, called **benign hypertensive nephrosclerosis**, is an important complication of long-standing benign hypertension, chronic renal failure being one of the important sequelae of benign hypertension.

In accelerated 'malignant' hypertension the renal vessel walls are acutely damaged

In accelerated hypertension the rise in blood pressure is very rapid, causing a pattern of renal damage different from that seen in benign hypertension. Larger muscular vessels respond with a loose fibroelastic proliferation of the intima, but the afferent arterioles exposed to the sudden high pressures frequently undergo necrosis, often with fibrin in their damaged walls (**fibrinoid necrosis**, see page 171). Similarly, the glomerular capillary network may also undergo **segmental tuft necrosis**. When sufficient nephrons are rendered non-functional because of damage to glomerular tufts and afferent arterioles, the patient may develop acute renal failure.

The renal changes seen in benign and accelerated hypertensive nephrosclerosis are summarized in *Fig. 17.4.*

Large renal infarcts are usually due to thromboemboli in the systemic circulation

The most common cause of renal infarction is the passage of emboli down renal arterial branches. Typical embolic infarcts in the kidney are usually wedge-shaped subcapsular areas of necrosis, with the broad base at the capsular surface. Infarcts initially appear red and slightly raised above the capsular surface, but after 4–5 days they develop a yellowish white centre with a rim of hyperemia. Old infarcts appear as narrow, wedge-shaped, depressed scars. The most common causes are emboli from a mural thrombus formed over a recent myocardial infarct, thrombotic vegetations on mitral and aortic valves, thrombus on a mitral or aortic valve prosthesis, or thrombus from the left atrium of patients with atrial fibrillation.

Complete occlusion of a renal artery due to thrombosis leads to infarction of the whole kidney. However, except as a complication of arterial surgery during renal transplantation, this is a rare occurrence.

Diseases such as microscopic polyarteritis, accelerated hypertension and Henoch–Schönlein purpura (and other disorders in which there is destruction of small vessel walls) produce **micro-infarcts**, which are usually multiple ('flea-bitten kidney'). When the disease is limited to very small vessels, the necrosis is confined to segments of the glomerular capillary tuft (**tuft necrosis**).

Renal cortical necrosis is an unusual pattern of renal infarction associated with clinical conditions resulting in severe hypotension. The most common clinical situations in which it occurs are hypovolemic shock, severe sepsis, and eclampsia seen in pregnancy (see page 417). Macroscopically necrosis is confined to the outer part of the renal cortex which, in the acute stages, is pale and focally hemorrhagic. The condition results in acute renal failure and, with the extent and pattern of damage, there is no functional recovery. The mechanism of necrosis is uncertain, but diffuse spasm in renal blood vessels is thought to play a major part in precipitating ischemic damage.

renal muscular artery   **glomerulus**

normal

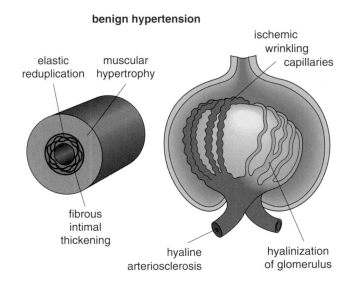

benign hypertension

malignant hypertension

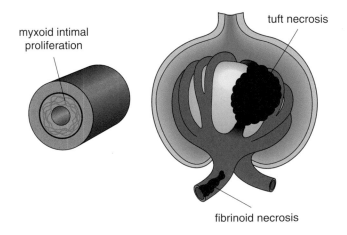

Fig. 17.4 Hypertensive renal disease.
In hypertensive damage to the kidneys the main effects are on small muscular arteries, afferent arterioles, and glomerular tufts.

Intravascular coagulation may precipitate renal failure

When disseminated intravascular coagulation (see page 327) occurs, fibrin thrombi form and there is intravascular hemolysis of red cells. This most commonly occurs in cases of septicemia, but it is also seen in systemic inflammatory response syndrome (see page 40). In the kidney this causes occlusion of renal glomerular capillaries by fibrin/platelet thrombi. Factors from degranulated platelets stimulate mesangial proliferation and there may be associated tuft necrosis, causing acute renal failure.

When renal failure is associated with evidence of intravascular coagulation and microangiopathic hemolysis, the clinical syndrome is termed **hemolytic–uremic syndrome**.

GLOMERULAR DISEASES

The glomerulus is the target of many disease processes, leading to temporary or permanent impairment of function

As a highly specialized component of the blood circulatory system, responsible for ultrafiltration, the glomerulus can be damaged by: **generalized vascular disease**, particularly hypertension (see page 355) vasculitis, and diabetes mellitus (see page 540); **immunological disorders**, particularly where immune complexes are deposited in glomerular capillary walls; and **depositions of foreign material**, e.g. amyloid (see Chapter 25).

The term **glomerulonephritis** is traditionally used to describe the group of diseases in which the primary pathology is some sort of structural abnormality in the glomerulus. Despite the suffix-*itis*, most are not characterized by inflammatory changes. Damage to the glomerulus may be severe, leading to permanent scarring, in which case the associated tubule atrophies. Alternatively some conditions produce temporary abnormality and, following resolution, there is restoration of nephron function.

Glomerular disease is classified according to the histological pattern of damage seen on renal biopsy, hence a knowledge of this aspect of histopathology is needed to understand disease. This arrangement is supplemented by further classification according to etiology of disease. In many cases the cause of glomerular disease is uncertain and some types of glomerular disease are considered idiopathic.

Most glomerular diseases are due to abnormalities at the glomerular filtration barrier

Ultrafiltration of the blood occurs in the glomerulus, producing an ultrafiltrate which passes into Bowman's capsule and thence into the tubular system where selective absorption and secretion of various components occurs, followed by concentration to produce urine. Ultrafiltration occurs across the **glomerular filtration barrier** which is composed of:

- The fenestrated thin **endothelial cell layer** which forms the internal lining to the glomerular capillary (red in *Fig. 17.5*).
- An unusually thick **glomerular capillary basement membrane** (blue in *Fig. 17.5*).
- The **epithelial cells** or 'podocytes' which form an outer coating to the glomerular capillary. These cells (green in *Fig. 17.5*) are in contact with the outer surface of the basement membrane via a series of foot processes. At the vascular hilum of the glomerulus, these epithelial cells are continuous with the flattened epithelial cells lining Bowman's capsule.
- A high **polyanionic charge** on the epithelial surface of the basement membrane and on the inner surfaces of the podocytes (indicated by minus signs in *Fig. 17.5*).

Another important component of glomerulus structure is the **mesangium**, which is the supporting 'mesentery' to the capillary (*Fig. 17.6*). It comprises mesangial cells (phagocytic support and secretory cells) and their amorphous secretory product, the mesangial matrix. The role

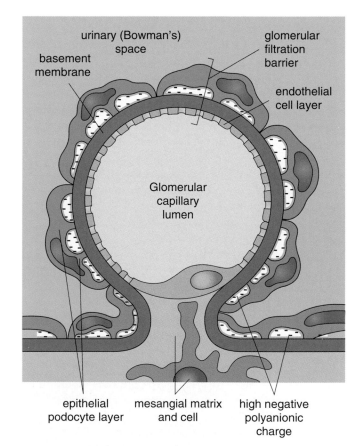

Fig 17.5 The glomerular filtration barrier.
The glomerular filtration barrier comprises the fenestrated endothelial cell layer (red), the glomerular capillary basement membrane (blue), the endothelial podocyte layer (green) and the high polyanionic charge on the outer surface of the basement membrane and the inner layers of the podocytes (indicated by minus signs).

of the mesangium in ultrafiltration is not known, but abnormalities of the mesangium are an important component of acute and chronic glomerular disease.

The glomerulus has a limited set of histological responses to damage

Five main patterns of response to damage are seen in the glomerulus, combinations of which describe all types of glomerular disease.

Proliferation of endothelial cells leads to occlusion of capillary lumina, often with neutrophils present. This proliferation reduces the flow through glomeruli and correlates with oliguria and uremia.

Proliferation of mesangial cells which is usually associated with increased production of matrix, is a common feature of many glomerular diseases. In some cases this may regress once the acute episode is over; in others the production of excess mesangial matrix over many years eventually leads to sclerosis (hyalinization) of all or part of the glomerular tuft, with loss of capillary lumina.

Basement membrane thickening may be due to the deposition of an abnormal substance (immune complexes or amyloid), synthesis of new basement membrane material, insinuation of mesangial cytoplasm and matrix, or a combination of these causes.

Capillary wall necrosis, usually fibrinoid necrosis (see *Fig. 17.14*), occurs in diseases in which there is severe acute capillary wall damage, e.g. necrotizing vasculitis and accelerated (malignant) hypertension.

Crescent formation is an important reaction to severe glomerular capillary damage, stimulated by leakage of blood and fibrin into the urinary space. Crescents are formed by proliferation of the epithelial cells that line Bowman's capsule, which crush the glomerulus, and lead to permanent loss of the whole nephron (see *Fig. 17.15*). The presence of widespread crescents is a poor prognostic sign, relating to severe and usually rapidly progressive disease.

Glomerular disease may not affect all glomeruli in a uniform manner

Most glomerular disease affect different glomeruli to varying degrees, with only a small number of diseases affecting all glomeruli in a uniform manner. This explains how some glomerular diseases cause sudden acute renal failure (disease affects all glomeruli in a uniform manner), whereas others cause a selective partial renal failure syndrome (disease affects small areas in a small proportion of glomeruli). A nomenclature has been agreed for the various patterns of disease (*Fig. 17.7*).

Thus a glomerular disease may be described as 'diffuse global', 'diffuse segmental', 'focal global' or 'focal segmental'. The vast majority are either 'diffuse global' or 'focal segmental'.

Clinical features of glomerulonephritis broadly relate to histological findings

Although learning the clinical patterns of disease that relate to each of the several types of glomerulonephritis seems daunting, there are four general rules-of-thumb which, albeit not absolute, explain the vast majority of cases.

1 Structural change in the GBM (generally associated with thickening) or deposition of excessive mesangial matrix leads to abnormal loss of protein in the urine or to **nephrotic syndrome**.
2 Glomerular damage associated with proliferation of endothelial or mesangial cells is associated with development of microscopic hematuria or **nephritic syndrome**.
3 If there is both damage to basement membrane and cell proliferation, a **mixed nephritic/nephrotic syndrome** is likely.
4 If damage to glomeruli is rapid, features of acute renal failure develop.

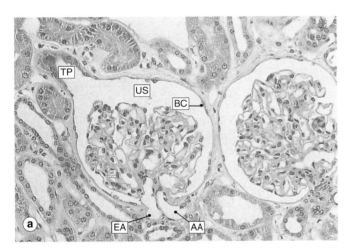

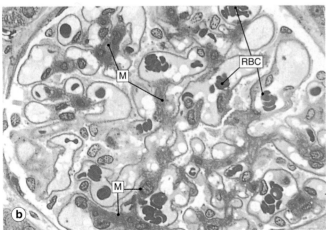

Fig. 17.6 The normal glomerulus. (a) Paraffin H&E (3 μm). (b) Resin – Toluidine blue (1 μm).
The glomerulus has four main components; endothelial cells, basement membrane, epithelial cells, and mesangium. Key: TP = tubular pole; EA and AA = efferent and afferent arterioles; BC = Bowman's capsule; US = urinary space; M = mesanguim; RBC = red blood cells in glomerular capillary lumen.

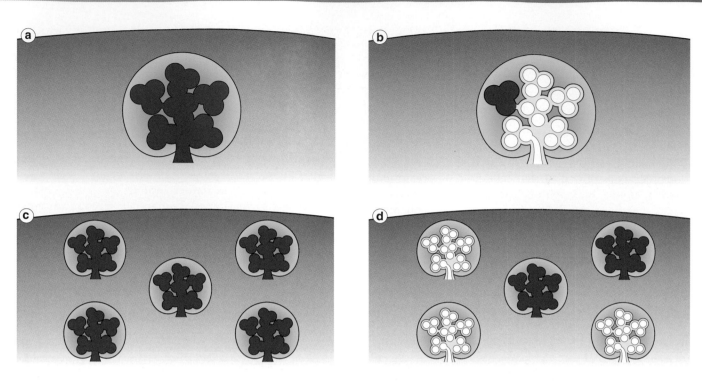

Fig. 17.7 Patterns of glomerular disease.
(a) **Global**: affecting the whole of the glomerulus uniformly. (b) **Segmental**: affecting one glomerular segment, leaving other segments unaffected. (c) **Diffuse**: affecting all glomeruli in both kidneys. (d) **Focal**: affecting a proportion of glomeruli, with others unaffected.

 Immune mechanisms in glomerular disease

Many glomerular diseases are caused by immune-mediated damage, with three main mechanisms involved.

1 **Circulating immune complexes**. In the most common pattern of immunological disease, immune complexes circulating in the blood are trapped or deposited at the basement membrane or the mesangium, or both. The pattern of glomerular disease depends on the nature, quantity and distribution of the immune complexes, and the pattern of the reaction to their presence (cell proliferation, necrosis and membrane thickening). In some cases the reason for the circulating immune complexes is known (e.g. response to a recent infection or tumor), in others it is undetermined.

2 **Trapped circulating antigen**. It is speculated that in some diseases a circulating antigen becomes trapped in the glomerulus, subsequent circulating antibodies then binding to the trapped antigen. This is believed to occur in certain cases of the autoimmune disease systemic lupus erythematosus (SLE) (see page 535), when free DNA in the blood is trapped in the glomerular basement membrane (GBM), subsequently binding to anti-DNA antibodies. It is also thought to occur in cases of hepatitis B viral infection, in which viral DNA is deposited in the glomerular basement membrane, predisposing to immune complex formation.

3 **Anti-GBM antibodies**. In an uncommon form of immune-mediated damage, there are autoantibodies directed to a component of the GBM (anti-GBM disease). This is the basis of **Goodpasture s syndrome**, in which antibodies cause direct damage to the basement membrane (see page 364). The nature of the antigen involved has been determined. Type IV collagen, a major constituent of basement membrane, is composed not of a single protein but of a family of at least five chains (termed $\alpha 1$–$\alpha 5$), each of which contains a non-collagenous domain. The Goodpasture antigen is the non-collagenous domain of the $\alpha 3$ Type IV collagen chain, which is the target for anti-GBM autoantibodies in patients with Goodpasture s syndrome.

▶

In some of these immune-mediated glomerular disease there is secondary activation of complement, leading to attraction of neutrophils and activation of the coagulation system.

In other types the reason for the cellular reaction to immune complex is uncertain. In assessing renal disease it is important to identify the site, type, and pattern of immune complexes and complement within the glomerulus by immunohistochemistry and electron microscopy.

The different patterns point to different diagnoses,

The renal biopsy

The diagnosis and management of renal disease has been greatly enhanced by routine use of percutaneous needle biopsy of the kidney.

Needle biopsy is carried out under local anesthetic, under radiological control. A core of renal tissue, 2 cm long and 0.2 cm wide, is removed.

Histological examination of glomeruli and tubules is performed to identify structural abnormalities and to characterize patterns of glomerular, tubular and interstitial damage.

Immunohistochemical examination is required to identify immunoglobulins and complement components in immune glomerular disease, and **electron microscopic examination** is required for fine detail of glomerular structure, including the site of immune complexes within the glomerulus.

Another common conceptual hurdle is understanding how someone with a partial renal failure syndrome, such as a nephrotic syndrome, eventually develops total chronic renal failure. In most glomerular diseases, the damage causing the nephritic or nephrotic syndrome also eventually causes glomeruli to become completely scarred (hyalinized), leading to loss of individual nephrons.

Glomerular hyalinization is the result of excessive production of mesangial matrix by the mesangial cells, over a long period of time. The expanding mesangial matrix mass slowly but progressively crushes the sophisticated glomerular architecture out of existence, until no blood flows through the glomerular capillaries, and no oxygenated blood passes into the efferent arterioles and peri-tubular capillary systems. The tubules are deprived of oxygenated blood, tubular epithelial cells die irrevocably and become atrophic. Thus the destruction of the glomerulus leads to destruction of the entire nephron unit.

As more and more nephrons are destroyed, the partial renal failure syndrome (nephritic or nephrotic) develops into the total renal failure syndrome of chronic renal failure.

This is associated with progressive shrinkage of the kidney to form a small, scarred organ, termed '**end-stage kidney**'.

IMPORTANT TYPES OF GLOMERULONEPHRITIS

Acute diffuse proliferative glomerulonephritis usually presents as the nephritic syndrome

Acute proliferative glomerulonephritis is a diffuse global disease of glomeruli. It is caused by deposition of immune complexes in glomeruli, which is stimulated by a preceding infection. Although infection is most commonly streptococcal, a range of bacterial, viral and protozoal infections can also stimulate this pattern of disease.

Histologically, there is increased cellularity of the glomerulus, with four main features (*Fig. 17.8*):

- **Proliferation of endothelial cells** produces occlusion of capillary lumina, leading to reduced glomerular filtration, with rising blood pressure and blood levels of nitrogenous components (urea and creatinine).
- **Presence of immune complexes** in lumps on the epithelial side of GBM.
- **Presence of neutrophil polymorphs** in capillaries.
- **Mild mesangial cell proliferation.**

In children the illness is usually clinically mild and transient. As there has been cell proliferation, patients develop features of the nephritic syndrome, with oliguria, hematuria, hypertension and peri-orbital edema. Supportive treatment is required until the nephritic syndrome resolves, usually over 3–6 weeks, as the immune complexes are cleared from the GBM. With resolution of disease, the proliferating endothelial cells are shed, mesangial cell increase regresses, capillary lumina become patent again, and renal function returns to normal.

A small percentage of cases do not resolve completely, but persist, with evidence of **rapid progression to renal failure**. These cases develop epithelial crescents, which compress the glomeruli, and rapidly progressive renal failure ensues (**rapidly progressive glomerulonephritis**). This is more common in adults than in children. The pathology is presented on page 367.

Alternatively, in rare cases there is **slow inexorable deterioration in renal function** over a period of many years. Although the patient appears to recover from the acute nephritic syndrome, urine testing reveals persistent proteinuria. This is associated with persistent enlargement of the mesangium, which fails to regress when the endothelial proliferation regresses. Over the years the mesangial cells produce excess matrix, eventually producing large hyaline masses that compress the glomerular capillaries and ultimately replace the entire tuft. Throughout this period the patient is asymptomatic until the increasing urinary protein loss leads to the nephrotic syndrome. When all glomeruli have become hyalinized by this diffuse global process, chronic renal failure develops.

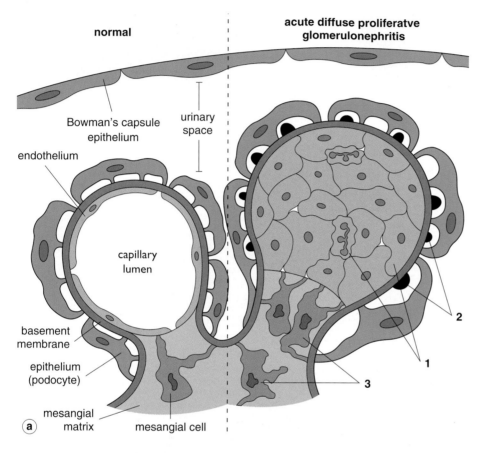

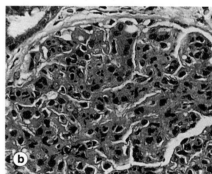

Fig. 17.8 Diffuse acute proliferative glomerulonephritis.

(a) In diffuse acute proliferative glomerulonephritis there is endothelial proliferation with neutrophils (1), sub-epithelial lumpy immune complex deposits (2), and mesangial cell increase (3). (b) The glomerulus is hypercellular due to proliferation of endothelial and mesangial cells. Glomerular capillary lumina cannot be identified because they are obliterated by the proliferating endothelial cells. The immune complex deposits can only be seen by electron microscopy.

Pathogenesis of acute diffuse proliferative glomerulonephritis

The most common cause of acute diffuse glomerulonephritis is pharyngeal infection with β-hemolytic *Streptococci* of Lancefield group A. Not all strains cause this disease and there are certain so-called nephritogenic strains (Griffith s types 12, 4, 1, 25 and 49). Children are most commonly affected, with onset 1—2 weeks after the primary infection. Immune complexes develop and circulate in the blood to be filtered out in the glomerulus. Immunofluorescence shows granular deposition of IgG and C3 in the GBM and mesangium. Ultrastructurally these deposits are sited beneath the epithelium.

The activation of complement is the reason for attraction of neutrophils into the glomerulus.

These degranulate and damage endothelial cells, stimulating their proliferation. Mesangial cell proliferation is mediated by factors derived from complement and platelets, and is accompanied by increased expression of PDGF and PDGF-receptor proteins, resulting in an autocrine mechanism of cell proliferation.

If damage to the glomerular capillaries is severe, fibrin and blood leak into Bowman s space and stimulate epithelial cell proliferation, resulting in a crescent which permanently effaces the glomerulus. If 80% of glomeruli have crescents, this is associated with rapid progression to renal failure with a poor prognosis (see page 367).

KEY FACTS
Diffuse proliferative glomerulonephritis

¥ Caused by immune complexes in glomerulus, often after streptococcal infection.

¥ Causes nephritic syndrome, with proliferation of endothelium and mesangium and recruitment of neutrophils.

¥ Most cases recover, but a minority may rapidly progress to renal failure or slowly develop chronic renal failure after apparent recovery.

Membranous nephropathy presents with proteinuria and the nephrotic syndrome

Characterized by the presence of immune complex deposits in the basement membrane of all segments of all glomeruli, membranous nephropathy is diffuse and global. The etiology of immune complexes in membranous disease is uncertain (see pink box on page 362). Unlike diffuse proliferative glomerulonephritis, there is no inflammation or associated endothelial or epithelial proliferation, although the mesangium may be increased. The disease passes through three pathological stages (*Fig. 17.9*):

1 Immune complex deposited on epithelial side of basement membrane.

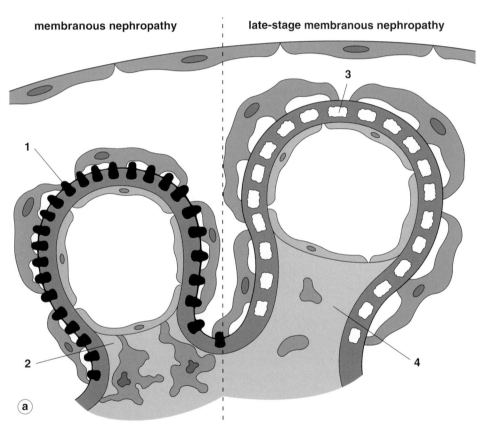

membranous nephropathy | late-stage membranous nephropathy

(a)

Fig. 17.9 Membranous nephropathy.
(a) In membranous nephropathy there are electron-dense deposits on the epithelial side of the basement membrane (1), and slight mesangial increase (2). In late-stage disease there is removal of deposits, leaving a thick 'lacy' membrane (3), and increasing mesangial matrix deposition (4). (b) Electron micrograph of a basement membrane thickened by deposition of antigen–antibody complexes on the epithelial side of the basement membrane, from a patient with membranous nephropathy who presented with the nephrotic syndrome. (c) Methenamine silver staining shows mesangial matrix and basement membrane material. In membranous nephropathy, new basement membrane material is deposited around immune complexes, and can be seen as spaced black spikes and dots on the outer surface of the membrane (arrows).

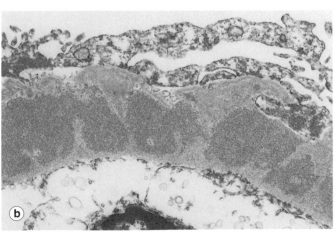

(b)

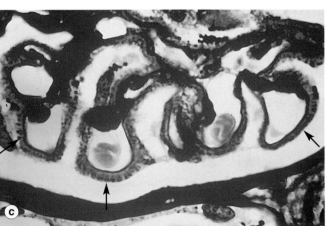

(c)

Pathogenesis of membranous nephropathy

In membranous nephropathy, sub-epithelial immune complexes develop in the glomeruli (mainly IgG with a small amount of complement). In most cases, circulating immune complexes cannot be demonstrated in the blood, and the concept that pre-formed circulating complexes are filtered out in the glomerulus seems doubtful in this pattern of disease. It is more likely that the immune complexes form *in situ*, with a circulating antigen becoming trapped in the glomerulus, followed by deposition of antibody. This *in situ* formation may explain why, in contrast to diffuse

proliferative glomerulonephritis, there is little complement and no inflammatory or proliferative responses. The precise reason why the presence of immune complexes causes basement membrane thickening is, at present, unknown. The basement membrane becomes abnormally leaky as its composition changes, and there is reduction in the normal polyanionic sites, which normally repel proteins and keep them from filtering into urine.

In cases with a drug-related, neoplastic or infective cause, treatment of the underlying condition removes the source of

---

2 New basement membrane deposited around immune complex deposits.

3 Immune complex deposits disappear, leaving thickened 'lacy' basement membrane.

The abnormality of the basement membrane renders it unusually permeable; it no longer selectively retains proteins, leading to heavy proteinuria and the **nephrotic syndrome**. With time, the abnormal glomeruli develop increase in mesangial matrix produced by the mesangial cells. This, together with membrane thickening, causes gradual hyalinization of the glomeruli and death of individual nephrons. This process takes place over many years and, from a nephrotic syndrome, the patient may develop chronic renal failure with uremia. The natural history of the disease is variable. In crude figures, about 25% of patients develop remission, 25% develop stable, persisting proteinuria, and 50% develop chronic renal failure over a period of about 10 years.

Membranous nephropathy is one of the most important causes of the nephrotic syndrome in adults, and patients can be divided into two groups:

- 80–90% of cases have no apparent reason for development of immune complexes, and are classed as primary or idiopathic membranous nephropathy.
- 10–20% of cases have a reason for development of immune complex disease, as they have abnormal circulating antigens:
  — **Infective**: hepatitis B, malaria, syphilis.
  — **Drug-related**: gold therapy, penicillamine, captopril, heroin.
  — **Tumor-associated**: lung cancer and lymphomas.
  — **SLE**: 10% of renal involvement in lupus is of the membranous pattern.

In some cases, where there is a recognizable cause, successful treatment of the cause (e.g. withdrawal of drug or the complete excision of the lung tumor) leads to spontaneous remission of the membranous nephropathy.

KEY FACTS
Membranous nephropathy

- ¥ Mainly seen in adults as a common cause of nephrotic syndrome.
- ¥ Caused by immune complexes forming in glomerulus.
- ¥ Basement membrane is thickened and abnormally permeable.
- ¥ Leads to chronic renal failure over many years in 50% of cases.
- ¥ 80—90% are idiopathic, 10—20% are secondary to circulating abnormal antigens.

Diffuse membranoproliferative ('mesangiocapillary') glomerulonephritis often presents as a nephrotic or a mixed nephritic/nephrotic syndrome

Membranoproliferative glomerulonephritis (MPGN), also called **mesangiocapillary glomerulonephritis**, is a pattern of glomerular reaction to complement abnormalities. Some are secondary to systemic disorders, such as SLE, infective endocarditis, malaria and infected ventricular CSF shunts, but the major group is idiopathic, divided by clinical and pathological features into two types (Type I and Type II), each with a particular pathogenesis.

As the name implies, the common factors in this process are **mesangial proliferation** and **basement membrane thickening** as the main structural abnormalities.

The basement membrane abnormality is responsible for the clinical symptoms of proteinuria or a full nephrotic syndrome. Because there is cellular proliferation, patients may also develop hematuria or a nephritic syndrome. A mixed nephrotic/nephritic syndrome is seen in some cases.

Type I MPGN accounts for 90% of cases and is mostly seen in adolescents and young adults. There is accentuated lobularity of glomerular segments (*Fig. 17.10a*), which is caused by proliferation of mesangial cells. Capillaries are greatly thickened due to sub-endothelial deposits of immune complex containing IgG or IgM and C3. Thickening is also due to in growth of mesangial cell cytoplasm between the endothelium and basement membrane, with formation of a double-contour or tram-track basement membrane (*Fig. 17.10b*). A very rare variant of Type I MPGN (sometimes called **Type III**) has deposits in other parts of the basement membrane.

Typically there is progressive deterioration in renal function over a period of about 10 years, resulting in chronic renal failure.

Type II MPGN accounts for 10% of cases and is also seen in children and young adults. There is marked thickening of GBM, but mesangial proliferation is usually not so prominent as in Type I. The characteristic feature is large, continuous, ribbon-like, dense deposits within the basement membrane, giving rise to the alternative name of **dense deposit disease** (*Fig. 17.10c*). By immunohistochemistry these deposits contain no immune complexes and are composed of complement factor C3. The pathogenesis of this disease has been related to activation of the alternative complement pathway (see pink box). Some cases are associated with partial lipodystrophy.

This type has a poor prognosis, with development of chronic renal failure. The disease commonly recurs in transplanted kidneys.

Fig. 17.10 Membranoproliferative glomerulonephritis.
In this pattern of disease (a) there is apparent exaggeration of the lobularity of the glomerulus by mesangial increase. (b) and (c) show mesangial cell proliferation (1), basement membrane thickening due to mesangial cytoplasm intrusion into membrane (2) and complement deposition (3), which in Type I is sub-endothelial (b) and in Type II takes the form of linear dense deposits (c).

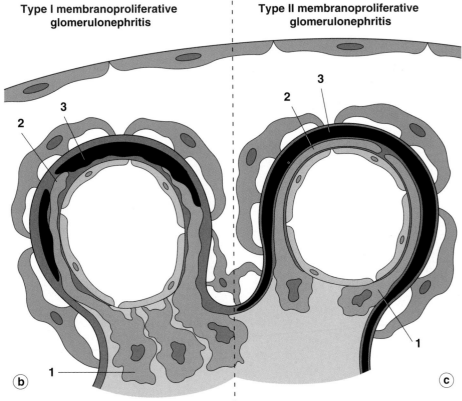
Type I membranoproliferative glomerulonephritis — Type II membranoproliferative glomerulonephritis

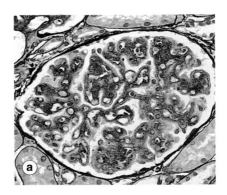

Pathogenesis of MPGN

Membranoproliferative glomerulonephritis is basically the result of abnormalities of complement deposition and handling in the glomerulus.

In **Type I MPGN**, complement deposition in the GBM is supplemented by an immune complex disease component, circulating complexes being present in up to 50% of cases. The main complement found in glomerular deposits is C3, and immunoglobins include IgG, IgM and occasionally IgA. The presence of C1q and C4 in deposits supports the contention that activation of the classic complement pathway plays a part in the pathogenesis. Complement activation causes consumption of serum complement, and serum levels of C3 are reduced in 60% of cases.

▶ In **Type II MPGN** there are no immune complexes and the dense deposits of C3 in the basement membrane are caused by abnormal activation of the complement system. This is mediated by a circulating autoantibody to C3 convertase, which prevents its normal breakdown. Normally, C3 convertase activates C3, but has a very short half-life. The autoantibody, termed **C3 nephritic factor**, stabilizes C3 convertase, allowing continued activation of C3. The absence of C1q and C4, the early components of the classic pathway, is explained by direct action of C3 convertase. The complement activation may cause consumption of serum complement and serum levels of C3 are markedly reduced in

KEY FACTS
Membranoproliferative glomerulonephritis

¥ Mainly seen in adolescents and young adults.

¥ May cause hematuria, nephrotic syndrome or mixed nephritic/nephrotic syndrome.

¥ Mesangial proliferation and basement membrane thickening. Serum complement is low.

¥ Idiopathic Type I (90% cases): complement deposition, usually with added immune complex deposition.

¥ May be idiopathic or secondary to systemic disease, e.g. SLE.

¥ Idiopathic Type II (10% cases): primary complement activation in glomeruli, without immune complexes. Also known as dense deposit disease .

¥ Results in progression to renal failure over many years

Focal segmental proliferative glomerulonephritis can be either primary or secondary

In almost every case, focal glomerulonephritis is also 'segmental', only occasional lobules of the glomerular tuft being involved in disease. In this type of reaction, there is cellular proliferation affecting only one segment of the glomerular tuft and occurring in only a proportion of all glomeruli. As there is cellular proliferation, patients tend to present with hematuria or the nephrotic syndrome with proteinuria. In some cases the focal glomerulonephritis can be a stimulus for crescent formation (see page 367).

This reaction is caused by several different diseases, divisible into two groups: **primary types** (IgA mesangial disease and Goodpasture's syndrome), and those associated with other systemic diseases, which are classed as **secondary** focal segmental glomerulonephritis. In the evaluation of these cases, electron microscopy and immunohistochemistry are essential to establish the deposition of immune complexes characteristic of different types.

Of the primary types, **IgA mesangial (Berger's) disease** is the most common cause of glomerulonephritis in adults. It usually presents with recurrent hematuria or persistent proteinuria. In a small proportion of cases there is a nephritic syndrome.

There is segmental and focal proliferation of glomerular tuft, and electron microscopy shows deposits of IgA in the mesangium and at the junction between the mesangium and the basement membrane (paramesangial). Tuft proliferation is followed by mesangial matrix deposition and eventual sclerosis of the damaged segment (*Fig. 17.11*). Around 25% of patients progress to eventual chronic renal failure over a period of many years, when sufficient segments of sufficient glomeruli have been damaged to lead to glomerular sclerosis and nephron death.

The pathogenesis of the disease is uncertain. The IgA that is deposited in the mesangium almost certainly comes from bone marrow rather than from mucosal sites. Consequently, previous suggestions that chronic mucosal allergies predispose to the condition are unlikely to be correct.

Goodpasture's syndrome is a very rare cause of primary proliferative glomerulonephritis, and is characterized by the presence of autoantibody to Type IV collagen in GBM (anti-GBM, see page 358), seen as linear deposition of IgG and C3 by immunohistochemistry. In advanced disease, glomeruli are diffusely affected. As the autoantibody also reacts with alveolar basement membrane, there is also pulmonary alveolar hemorrhage.

Secondary focal proliferative glomerulonephritis, often with tuft necrosis, can occur in **connective tissue disorders** such as SLE, and focal segmental glomerulonephritis is seen with frequent tuft necrosis in cases of **vasculitis affecting the kidneys**, e.g. microscopic polyarteritis and Wegener's arteritis. Other secondary types occur with infective endocarditis and Henoch–Schönlein nephritis.

Infective endocarditis is associated with focal segmental glomerulonephritis in about 20% of cases. There is segmental proliferation associated with immune complex deposition, and tuft necrosis is often seen.

Henoch–Schönlein nephritis is usually seen in childhood in association with other manifestations of Henoch–Schönlein disease such as skin purpura, arthralgia and abdominal pain; nephritis manifests as hematuria. IgA is seen in affected glomeruli.

In some types of focal segmental proliferative glomerulonephritis, tuft necrosis stimulates crescent formation, particularly in Goodpasture's syndrome and the secondary types of disease.

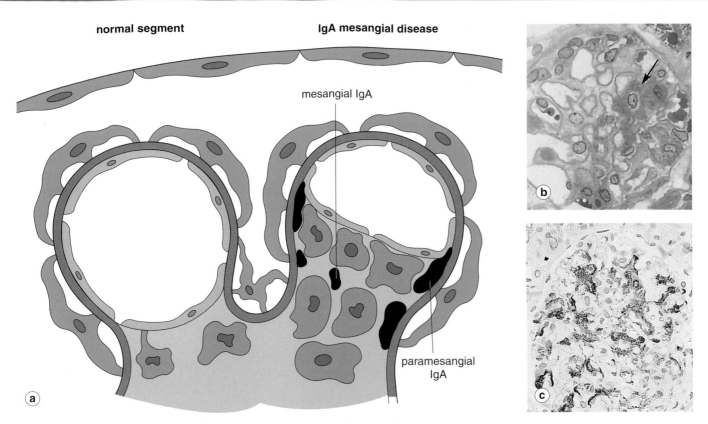

normal segment   IgA mesangial disease

mesangial IgA

paramesangial IgA

Fig. 17.11 Focal segmental proliferative glomerulonephritis (IgA disease).
In focal segmental proliferative disease, proliferative change in glomerular tufts is followed by sclerosis. Histologically (b), this micrograph shows a glomerulus in a thin resin section stained by Toluidine blue. The right half of the glomerulus (arrow) is abnormal due to deposition of immune complex (IgA), with associated mesangial increase and compression of the glomerular capillaries. On the left the glomerular segments are normal with widely patent capillaries. The most common type is due to deposition of IgA in the mesangium, shown as brown staining in this immunoperoxidase preparation (c).

KEY FACTS
Focal segmental proliferative glomerulonephritis

¥ Several different diseases result in one pattern of response, in which segments of a few glomeruli are affected by cell proliferation. Immunohistochemistry and electron microscopy are needed to distinguish them.

¥ Results in hematuria or persistent proteinuria or nephritic syndrome.

¥ IgA mesangial disease is the most common primary type and causes progressive development of renal failure over many years.

¥ As well as primary types, there are types secondary to systemic disease.

¥ Goodpasture s disease is caused by anti-glomerular antibodies.

¥ Secondary causes include infective endocarditis, vasculitis and connective tissue diseases.

Minimal change disease is a common cause of nephrotic syndrome in childhood

Minimal change disease is mainly seen in children under the age of 6 years, in whom it causes proteinuria and nephrotic syndrome. In adults the condition is less common, but still accounts for 10–15% of cases of nephrotic syndrome.

The characteristic feature, and the reason for the name, is that by light microscopy there is nothing abnormal to see in the glomeruli. By electron microscopy there is fusion of the foot processes of podocytes (*Fig. 17.12*). Immune complexes and deposits are not seen. Tubules may show accumulation of lipid in lining cells, giving rise to the old-fashioned alternative name of **lipoid nephrosis**, which is sometimes still used.

Treatment with steroids usually brings about remission of disease within 2 weeks, although relapse is frequent when steroids are stopped.

An immune pathogenesis is suggested by the response of the disease to steroid therapy, and it has been proposed that minimal change disease is caused by non-complement-fixing antibodies to antigens on the glomerular epithelial cell membrane. Detailed study of the basement membrane has shown that it becomes depleted of polyanionic charges,

normal | minimal change nephropathy

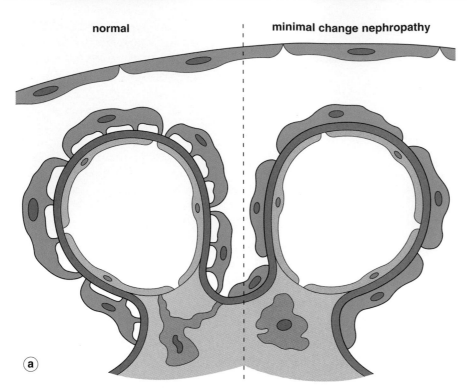

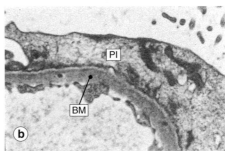

Fig. 17.12 Minimal change glomerulonephritis.
Shown diagrammatically (a), normal foot processes are regularly spaced, but in this pattern of disease they become fused. In (b), which is a biopsy from the kidney of a child with the nephrotic syndrome, the complex secondary foot process arrangement is lost and the primary foot processes (**PI**) lie directly on the basement membrane (**BM**).

leading to failure of retention of proteins. In adults, disease has been associated with the presence of tumors such as lymphomas and renal cell carcinomas.

Focal glomerulosclerosis accounts for many cases of nephrotic syndrome and has a poor prognosis

Focal glomerulosclerosis is a common cause of nephrotic syndrome or persistent proteinuria. Numerically it accounts for 10% of cases of nephrotic syndrome in childhood and for 20% of cases in adults. There is focal hyalinization in glomeruli, which is caused by increase in mesangial matrix; granular IgM and C3 are seen with immunohistochemistry.

In children and young adults, focal glomerulosclerosis is seen as an idiopathic disease, accounting for most cases of nephrotic syndrome that fail to respond to steroid therapy.

In later adult life, it is seen secondary to other disorders. Increasingly this pattern of glomerular damage is being seen in association with HIV infection as part of HIV nephropathy.

Focal glomerulosclerosis has a poor prognosis. There is progression of disease over many years, with hyalinization of glomeruli and loss of functioning nephrons leading to chronic renal failure.

Immunological damage to glomeruli occurs in systemic connective tissue diseases, the most important of which is SLE

Glomerular disease is seen in several of the connective tissue disorders (see Chapter 25), but most frequently occurs in SLE.

The glomerulus is affected in several ways in SLE, mimicking the various patterns of primary glomerulonephritis, including:

- **Diffuse membranous nephropathy**. This pattern is similar to normal membranous nephropathy, but characterized by the presence of IgG, IgM, IgA, C3 and C1q, known as a 'full-house' of deposits (after the excellent hand in the card game poker, comprising three cards of one kind, e.g. three 10s, and two of another, e.g. two 8s), in the sub-epithelial region, sometimes forming so-called 'wire-loop' lesions (*Fig. 17.13*). In addition, there may be less conspicuous intramembranous, sub-endothelial, and mesangial immune complex deposits. This pattern is associated with nephrotic syndrome and slow progression to chronic renal failure.

- **Diffuse mesangial** or **membranoproliferative glomerulonephritis** often with large immune complex deposits in a sub-endothelial position (mainly C3 and some IgG). Intramembranous and mesangial deposits may also be seen. This pattern is associated with rapid progression to renal failure.

- **Focal segmental proliferative glomerulonephritis** with segmental mesangial proliferation and often fibrinoid tuft necrosis; this pattern is associated with hematuria, proteinuria and slow progression.

Systemic scleroderma (progressive systemic sclerosis) may be associated with fibrinoid necrosis of afferent arterioles and some segments of the glomerular tufts. Small arteries and large arterioles show a characteristic 'onion-skin thickening' of the intima, similar to that seen in malignant or accelerated hypertension.

Polyarteritis nodosa affecting large arteries produces multiple small infarcts in the kidney; **microscopic polyarteritis nodosa** affects arterioles and the glomerular tuft, producing infarction of entire glomeruli or segments, visible as fibrinoid necrosis (see *Fig. 17.14*).

Wegener's granulomatosis (see page 169) involves the kidneys in 90% of cases, giving rise to rapidly progressive renal failure, with a nephritic syndrome.

Rheumatoid arthritis mainly involves the kidney when there is associated amyloidosis (see page 543), or occasionally as a result of tubular damage associated with treatment (e.g. gold therapy, penicillamine). Occasionally, patients develop rheumatoid vasculitis, which can lead to glomerular segmental tuft necrosis (see *Fig. 17.14*).

Epithelial crescent formation is a reaction to severe glomerular capillary tuft abnormalities and characterizes rapidly progressive disease

An epithelial crescent is caused by overgrowth of epithelial cells lining Bowman's capsule (*Fig. 17.15a*). The stimulus for epithelial proliferation is believed to be serum proteins and fibrin in Bowman's space. As epithelial cells proliferate and crescents enlarge, they compress the glomerular tuft, which shrivels and becomes non-functional (*Fig. 17.15b*). In the evaluation of cases of proliferative glomerulonephritis, the presence of large numbers of glomeruli with crescents indicates a poor prognosis, with usually rapid progression to renal failure.

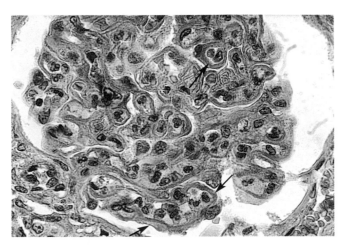

Fig. 17.13 Lupus nephropathy.
This pattern of lupus glomerular involvement is similar to that in membranous nephropathy, forming wire-loop lesions (arrows).

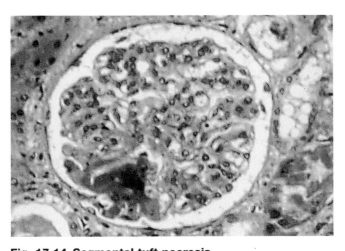

Fig. 17.14 Segmental tuft necrosis.
This glomerulus shows one segment where the normal structure has been completely destroyed by red-staining fibrinoid tuft necrosis. This is an important glomerular feature in a range of diseases in which there is acute damage to small blood vessels.

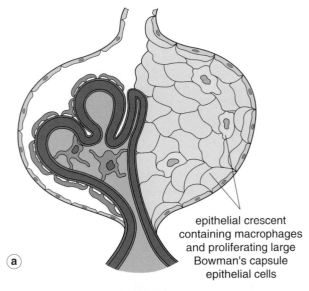

epithelial crescent containing macrophages and proliferating large Bowman's capsule epithelial cells

(a)

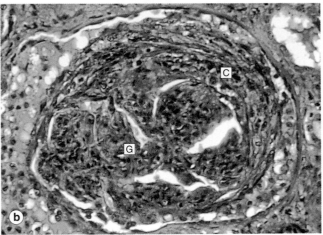

(b)

Fig. 17.15 Crescentic glomerulonephritis.
(a) The rapidly proliferating epithelial crescent crushes the glomerular tuft, which may show a range of changes including focal proliferative glomerulonephritis, segmental tuft necrosis, mesangiocapillary glomerulonephritis, or acute proliferative glomerulonephritis. (b) This photomicrograph shows a glomerulus (**G**) being compressed by a proliferating crescent (**C**); the crescent is squashing the damaged glomerular tuft out of existence.

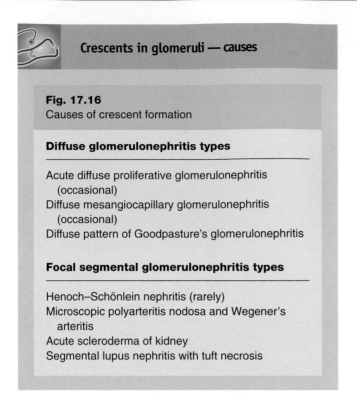

Crescents in glomeruli — causes

Fig. 17.16
Causes of crescent formation

Diffuse glomerulonephritis types

Acute diffuse proliferative glomerulonephritis
(occasional)
Diffuse mesangiocapillary glomerulonephritis
(occasional)
Diffuse pattern of Goodpasture's glomerulonephritis

Focal segmental glomerulonephritis types

Henoch–Schönlein nephritis (rarely)
Microscopic polyarteritis nodosa and Wegener's
arteritis
Acute scleroderma of kidney
Segmental lupus nephritis with tuft necrosis

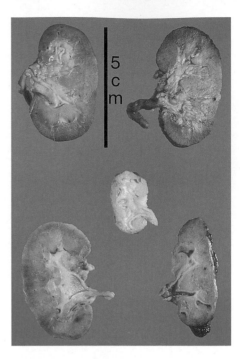

Fig. 17.17 End-stage kidneys.
Five different kidneys showing end-stage changes, all greatly
reduced in size with great reduction in the cortex. A normal
kidney is approximately 10–12 cm long. The cause of this
end-stage kidney state is different in each of the five; in three
the shrinkage is symmetrical and regular, therefore probably
due to diffuse glomerular disease. The centre and bottom right
kidneys are irregularly shrunken, and are probably due to
either vascular disease or chronic inflammatory destruction.

The formation of an enlarging epithelial crescent is a
non-specific reaction to severe glomerular capillary tuft
damage, characterized by tuft necrosis and proliferation
of cells in the glomerulus. The main diseases causing
crescent formation are shown in *Fig. 17.16*. Crescents are
not, therefore, a feature of membranous nephropathy, in
which there is absence of such cellular reactions. When
crescent formation is established, the particular type of
underlying glomerular abnormality can be determined only
in those glomeruli in which crescent formation has not yet
occurred.

An end-stage kidney which is small and shrunken may be caused by many diseases

When there has been nephron loss due to either
glomerular or vascular disease and development of chronic
renal failure, the kidney becomes small and shrunken (see
Fig. 17.17).

Macroscopically, affected kidneys are small and there is
granularity of the external surface, reflecting fine scarring
due to nephron hyalinization. The pelvicalyceal system
is normal, an important distinction from cases of end-
stage kidney due to chronic pyelonephritis (see page 370).
Histologically, there is hyalinization of glomeruli, tubular
atrophy, and interstitial fibrosis.

The term 'chronic glomerulonephritis' is sometimes
inappropriately used when a patient has chronic renal failure
with small contracted kidneys in which all the glomeruli
are hyalinized. Because renal glomeruli are destroyed, it is
often not possible to ascertain the cause.

It is likely that many patients who present for the
first time with established end-stage renal failure and
hyalinization of the majority of glomeruli have had IgA
mesangial disease.

DIABETES AND AMYLOID

The kidney is frequently affected in diabetes mellitus

As patients with diabetes mellitus frequently suffer renal
disease, monitoring of renal function is an important
part of follow-up.

Diabetes is now one of the most common causes of
end-stage renal failure. The associated renal disease can
be divided into three forms: complications of diabetic vascular disease, diabetic glomerular damage, and increased
susceptibility to infection and papillary necrosis.

Diabetes causes increased severity of atherosclerosis
in large, medium and small arteries, predisposing to renal
ischemia. In addition, diabetes causes hyaline arteriolosclerosis in afferent arterioles, resulting in ischemic
glomerular damage.

Diabetic glomerular damage involves diffuse thickening of the glomerular capillary basement membrane

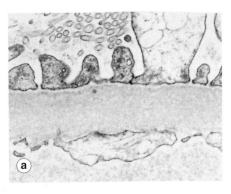
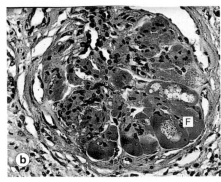
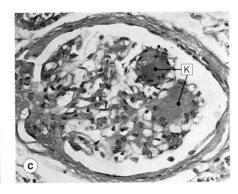

Fig. 17.18 Diabetic renal disease. (a) Basement-membrane thickening. (b) Exudative lesions. (c) Nodular glomerulosclerosis. Diabetes causes basement-membrane thickening, seen on electron microscopy (a). Exudative lesions (b) are seen as fibrin-like material (**F**) over the tips of glomerular capillary loops. In nodular glomerulosclerosis (c), rounded hyaline areas develop in glomeruli, termed 'Kimmelstiel–Wilson nodules' (**K**).

(*Fig. 17.18a*), leading to an increase in permeability, protein-uria and, occasionally, the nephrotic syndrome. Exudative lesions due to a combination of thick permeable basement membrane and abnormal mesangium may be visible as masses of red-staining coagulated fibrin protein (fibrin caps) on the surface of the glomerulus (*Fig. 17.18b*). Changes in mesangium lead to excess mesangial matrix formation. This initially occurs in an even pattern throughout the glomerulus (**diffuse diabetic glomerulosclerosis**), but later takes the form of laminated spheres, which are known as 'Kimmelstiel–Wilson nodules' (**nodular diabetic glomerulosclerosis**) (*Fig. 17.18c*).

Diabetic glomerulosclerosis causes progressive hyaliniza-tion of glomeruli, with obliteration of capillary loops and death of individual nephrons. Over a period of years this leads to chronic renal failure.

Among the other features of kidney involvement in diabetes is **predisposition to bacterial infection**. Acute pyelonephritis is an important and common complication of diabetes mellitus, being the result of relative immune suppression seen in diabetics, together with reduced neu-trophil function.

Another feature is **papillary necrosis**, in which the tips of the papillae undergo necrosis and may be shed in the urine, causing acute renal failure (*Fig. 17.19*). This is fre-quently seen in association with severe acute pyelonephritis and is thought to be caused by inflammatory thrombosis in vasa recta supplying the renal papillae. Renal papillary necrosis may also occur in association with:

- Severe acute pyelonephritis, when it is thought to be caused by inflammatory thrombosis in vasa recta supplying the renal papillae.
- Obstructive uropathy, with or without associated infection.
- Analgesic nephropathy (see page 372); phenacetin was formerly the major cause, but is no longer prescribed or available.

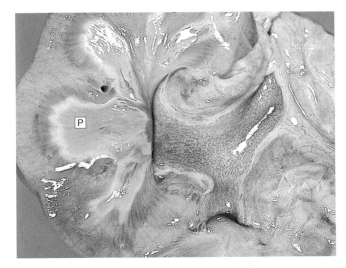

Fig. 17.19 Renal papillary necrosis.
Renal papillae (**P**) are pale with a line of demarcation from the adjacent viable kidney. The tips of papillae are later shed.

KEY FACTS
Diabetic renal disease

- ¥ Basement-membrane thickening.
- ¥ General renal ischemia caused by atheroma affecting aorta and renal arteries.
- ¥ Diabetic hyaline arteriolosclerosis causes glomerular ischemia.
- ¥ Diabetic glomerulosclerosis (diffuse and nodular types) causes proteinuria and leads to progressive glomerular hyalinization and eventual chronic renal failure.
- ¥ Increased risk of pyelonephritis.
- ¥ Increased risk of papillary necrosis.

The most important infiltrative disease of the glomerulus is amyloidosis

The kidney is a target organ in amyloidosis, a condition in which extracellular fibrillar protein is deposited in a variety of tissues. For a more detailed discussion, see Chapter 25. The amyloid is deposited as fibrils in the GBM and in the mesangium. As amyloid is deposited in the basement membrane, the membrane thickens and its permeability is increased, so that the first manifestation is **proteinuria**. With heavy deposition of amyloid, the protein loss increases until the patient develops features of the **nephrotic syndrome**.

Amyloid is an important cause of the nephrotic syndrome in adults. Heavy amyloid deposition in the mesangium, in combination with increased mesangial matrix formation, can eventually lead to expansion of the mesangium, ultimately leading to compression of the glomerular capillary system, and transition into **chronic renal failure**. Amyloid is also deposited in the walls of intrarenal vessels, particularly afferent arterioles.

DISEASE OF RENAL TUBULES AND INTERSTITIUM

Disease of renal tubules and interstitium accounts for a large number of cases of renal failure. The main causes of disease are infections, ischemia, and toxic and metabolic disorders. The main types of disease are **pyelonephritis** (acute and chronic), **acute tubular necrosis**, and **interstitial nephritis** (acute and chronic).

The most important and common type of tubulointerstitial inflammation is acute pyelonephritis due to bacterial infection

Acute pyelonephritis is caused by bacterial infection with organisms entering the kidney by two routes:

- **Ascending infection from the lower urinary tract** (most common). Predisposing factors that lead to ascending urinary tract infection are pregnancy, diabetes mellitus, stasis of urine, e.g. due to lower urinary tract destruction by a calculus, enlarged prostate, or malignant invasive tumor in the pelvis, structural defects of the urinary tract, and reflux of urine from bladder into ureters (vesicoureteric reflux).

- **Bloodstream spread in bacteremic or septicemic states** (unusual). Although less common, this seems to be the most likely cause in elderly patients who develop pyrexia of unknown origin, often with rigors, and acute renal failure.

Clinically patients develop fever, rigors and pain in the back, often associated with signs of a lower urinary tract infection. Diagnosis is made by examination of urine, especially culture to demonstrate the organism responsible. Most cases of infection are caused by *E. coli*, other enteric organisms being seen less frequently.

KEY FACTS
Nephrotic syndrome in adults

The main causes of nephrotic syndrome in adults are:

- ¥ Diabetes, SLE, amyloidosis, and other systemic disorders (40%).
- ¥ Membranous glomerulonephritis (20%).
- ¥ All forms of proliferative glomerulonephritis (15%).
- ¥ Minimal change glomerulonephritis (10%).
- ¥ Focal glomerulosclerosis (10%).
- ¥ Membranoproliferative glomerulonephritis (5%).

KEY FACTS
Nephrotic syndrome in childhood

The main causes of nephrotic syndrome in children are:

- ¥ Minimal change glomerulonephritis (60%).
- ¥ Focal glomerulosclerosis (10%).
- ¥ All forms of proliferative glomerulonephritis (10%).
- ¥ Membranoproliferative glomerulonephritis (10%).
- ¥ Membranous glomerulonephritis (5%).
- ¥ Secondary to systemic disorder (5%).

Macroscopically the kidneys show variable numbers of small, yellowish white cortical abcesses, which are usually spherical, under 2 mm in diameter, and are sometimes surrounded by a zone of hyperemia; the cortical abscesses are often most prominent on the sub-capsular surface, after the capsule has been stripped away (*Fig. 17.20a*). In the medulla the abscesses tend to be in the form of yellowish white linear streaks that converge on the papilla. The pelvicalyceal mucosa may be hyperemic or covered with a fibrinopurulent exudate. Histologically the kidney shows focal infiltration with neutrophils (*Fig. 17.20b*).

If untreated, infection may spread to cause Gram-negative septicemia with shock. In severe infections, particularly in diabetics, there may be renal papillary necrosis caused by inflammatory thrombosis of vasa recta supplying the papillae. **Perinephric abscess** may develop if infection spreads to perinephric fat, and pyonephrosis (distension of the pelvicalyceal system with pus) may be present if there is obstruction at the pelviureteric junction or lower.

Chronic pyelonephritis is characterized by chronic interstitial inflammation associated with large scars of the kidney

Chronic pyelonephritis is a common cause of end-stage chronic renal failure, accounting for about 15% of all cases.

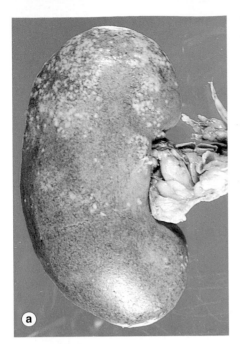
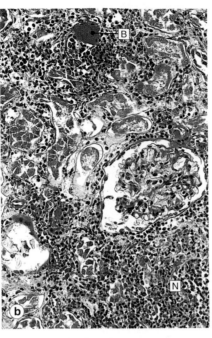

Fig. 17.20 Acute pyelonephritis. Macroscopically, small microabscesses are visible as white spots beneath the renal capsule (a). Histologically (b), the kidney is infiltrated with neutrophils (**N**) with occasional bacterial colonies (**B**) visible.

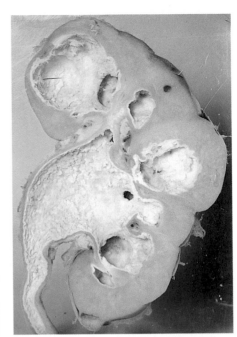

Fig. 17.21 Tuberculous pyelonephritis. Caseous material fills the renal pelvis and calyces.

The disease is characterized by interstitial chronic inflammation and scarring, which destroys nephrons. The areas of scarring are associated with distortion of the pelvicalyceal system of the kidney. Renal-induced hypertension may develop and hypertensive-induced vascular damage (page 355) can increase renal damage.

There are two forms of chronic pyelonephritis: reflux-associated and obstructive.

In the most common form, **reflux-associated chronic pyelonephritis**, reflux of urine from the bladder up the ureters predisposes to recurrent bouts of inflammation, leading to scarring. This occurs in childhood, and disease becomes manifest in early adult life, with progressive impairment of renal function.

In **obstructive chronic pyelonephritis**, recurrent episodes of infection occur in a kidney in which there is obstruction to the pelvicalyceal drainage. The obstruction, which can be at any level in the lower urinary tract, may be due either to anatomical abnormality or to renal tract stone.

Kidneys have irregular areas of scarring, seen as depressed areas, 0.5–2 cm in size. The scars are sited over a club-shaped distorted renal calyx and are associated with fibrous scarring of the renal papilla. The most common site for these areas of scarring is the renal calyces at the poles of the kidney.

Histologically the kidney has irregular areas of interstitial fibrosis with chronic inflammatory cell infiltration. Tubules are atrophic or may be dilated and contain proteinaceous material. Glomeruli show periglomerular fibrosis and many demonstrate complete hyalinization.

Tuberculous pyelonephritis may lead to destruction of the whole kidney

Tuberculous pyelonephritis is characterized by white caseous material filling the pelvicalyceal system, which may be unilaterally or bilaterally affected (*Fig. 17.21*). Infection is initially renal but, over a period of months or years, enlarges and ruptures into the pelvicalyceal system, releasing tubercle bacilli into the lower urinary tract. This can lead to the development of tuberculous ureteritis, cystitis and, in the male, prostatitis and epididymoorchitis.

With time, extension of caseous granulomatous inflammation leads to destruction of cortex and medulla, so that at the end-stage of the disease the kidneys are reduced to cystic masses of partially calcified caseous material; if both kidneys are affected, chronic renal failure results.

This pattern of renal involvement in TB is distinct from renal involvement in rapidly progressive **miliary TB**, in which the kidney is just one of many organs that receive large numbers of tubercle bacilli, spread from a fulminating lung infection. In miliary TB there are very large numbers of small tuberculous granulomas scattered throughout both kidneys. The patient usually dies before the individual granulomas can enlarge and show much caseation.

Acute tubular necrosis is a common and important cause of reversible acute renal failure

In acute tubular necrosis (ATN), metabolic or toxic disturbances cause necrosis of renal tubular epithelial cells. Although the tubular epithelial cells die and are shed, regeneration is possible if the damaging stimulus is corrected, since residual viable tubular epithelial cells can proliferate to re-populate the tubules. It is this regenerative capacity of the tubular epithelial cells that permits adequate tubular functioning after renal transplantation following a prolonged period of hypoxia of the graft.

There are two main groups of causative factors: ischemic and toxic. **Ischemic tubular necrosis** is caused by failure of renal perfusion. This is usually the result of hypotension and hypovolemia in shock, or may occur after extensive acute blood loss. Clinical situations that carry a high risk of developing ischemic ATN are major surgery, severe burns, hemorrhage, and causes of severe hypotension and shock.

Toxic causes of ATN are uncommon and are summarized in *Fig. 17.22*. There are three phases to ATN:

1 **Oliguric phase**. A damaging stimulus causes necrosis of renal tubular epithelium. There is blockage of renal tubules by necrotic cells, and a secondary reduction in glomerular blood flow (caused by arteriolar constriction) reduces glomerular filtration. Macroscopically, kidneys are diffusely swollen and edematous (*Fig. 17.23*). Patients develop acute renal failure and oliguria. Supportive measures are required to prevent hyperkalemia and fluid overload.

2 **Polyuric phase**. Over 1–3 weeks, regeneration of renal tubular epithelium takes place, with removal of dead material by phagocytic cells, as well as in the form of casts in urine. As tubules open up and glomerular blood flow increases, patients develop polyuria. This is because the regenerated tubular cells are undifferentiated and have not developed the specializations necessary for resorption of electrolytes and water. Replacement of fluid and electrolytes is needed to compensate for excessive loss from urine.

3 **Recovery phase**. Tubular cells re-establish differentiation and there is restoration of homeostatic renal function.

Interstitial nephritis is an inflammatory disease of renal interstitium and tubules

Interstitial nephritis is characterized by inflammation in the interstitium, associated with tubular atrophy or damage. There are many causes, the main one of which is exposure to drugs, particularly certain analgesics and antibiotics. Less commonly, physical agents such as irradiation cause a similar pattern of tubulo-interstitial damage.

Drug-induced acute interstitial nephritis presents 2–3 weeks after exposure to a causative agent, with fever, hematuria, proteinuria and elevated blood urea. In some cases acute renal failure develops. There is edema of the interstitium, associated with lymphocytic and eosinophil inflammatory infiltration. Tubules may show epithelial degeneration or necrosis. It is thought that an immune reaction to drugs is the underlying mechanism. Recovery usually takes place on withdrawal of the causative agent.

Drug-induced chronic interstitial nephritis is characterized by development of chronic renal failure after exposure to a causative agent. There is interstitial fibrosis, chronic inflammation, and atrophy of tubules. Many cases of diagnosed chronic interstitial nephritis have no determinable cause and are regarded as idiopathic.

Analgesic nephropathy is a form of tubulo-interstitial disease caused by administration of analgesic agents, particularly phenacetin and NSAIDs. It is also associated with renal papillary necrosis. After long-term exposure to the causative agent, patients develop renal tubular failure with polyuria, metabolic acidosis and, ultimately, chronic renal failure. Analgesic nephropathy is associated with an increased risk of development of carcinoma of the urothelium (see page 378).

Radiation nephritis is seen after kidneys are included in the field of radiation used to treat malignancy. There

Fig. 17.22	
Toxic causes of acute tubular necrosis	
Endogenous products	Hemoglobinuria and myoglobinuria
Heavy metals	Lead, mercury
Organic solvents	Chloroform, carbon tetrachloride
Drugs	Antibiotics, NSAIDs, cyclosporin
Other toxins	Paraquat, phenol, ethylene glycol, poisonous fungi

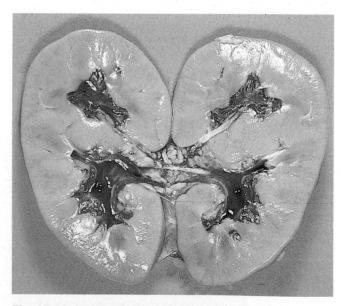

Fig. 17.23 Acute tubular necrosis. In acute tubular necrosis, kidneys are swollen and pale, particularly the cortical regions.

is hyalinization of glomeruli and small vessels, with later ischemic tubular atrophy and interstitial fibrosis.

Metabolic abnormalities may cause secondary tubular damage

Urate nephropathy is seen in a small proportion of patients with hyperuricemia. Precipitation of urate crystals occurs in the renal collecting ducts, causing tubular damage, inflammation and later scarring.

Nephrocalcinosis is caused by persistent hypercalcemia. Calcification occurs in the renal parenchyma, particularly tubular basement membrane, with tubular damage and later fibrosis. During development of this condition there is failure of tubular function, with development of polyuria.

Myeloma (see page 314) causes casts of secreted Bence–Jones protein to precipitate out in renal tubules, causing physical obstruction of tubules. Amyloid may develop in glomeruli (see Chapter 25) and, if the myeloma is associated with hypercalcemia from bone destruction, there may be superimposed nephrocalcinosis. Urography with certain contrast agents may precipitate acute tubular blockage and acute renal failure.

RENAL TRANSPLANTATION

Renal transplantation is increasingly being performed as a treatment for end-stage renal failure. After transplantation, several complications may occur, including thrombosis of the surgical vascular anastomosis leading to ischemia in the graft, transplant rejection, or recurrence of disease in transplanted kidney, e.g. membranoproliferative glomerulonephritis.

Four patterns of renal transplant rejection are recognized

The four patterns of rejection seen after renal transplantation are hyperacute rejection, acute rejection, accelerated acute rejection, and chronic rejection.

Hyperacute rejection occurs within a very short time of the organ being perfused by the host's blood. It takes the form of widespread intravascular thrombosis in small vessels, with focal necrosis and neutrophil infiltration. It is the result of pre-formed host antibodies reacting instantly with antigens in the graft, and in the past was almost entirely due to host antibody against donor blood group substances; it was therefore nearly always the result of blood-group incompatibility. More recently, it is due to pre-formed anti-HLA antibodies in recipient blood, formed by prior exposure to blood transfusions, or from previous grafts. Although a problem in early renal transplants, since testing recipients for the presence of antibodies to donor lymphocytes became routine practice, hyperacute rejection is now almost never seen.

Acute rejection occurs within a week or so of the graft being inserted, but may also appear after cessation of immunosuppressive therapy. It is termed 'acute' because it typically progresses rapidly, being mediated by both humoral and cell-mediated mechanisms.

- The cellular component of acute rejection is mediated by T-cells reacting against donor HLA antigens, particularly class II. The graft becomes infiltrated by lymphocytes, most of which are T-cells, and the lymphocytes destroy various components of the graft, including tubules.

Rare functional disturbances of tubules

Several functional disorders of renal tubular transport are described, which lead to metabolic disturbances. Some of these are acquired secondary to tubular damage, whereas others are inherited metabolic diseases.

Failure to resorb water is seen in chronic renal failure, nephrocalcinosis, and hypokalemia. It is also seen in nephrogenic diabetes insipidus (a rare disease). **Fanconi s syndrome** is a generalized disorder of renal tubular transport, in which there is glycosuria, aminoaciduria and renal tubular acidosis. Although it may be primary, it is more often seen secondary to tubulo-interstitial diseases such as toxic tubular damage.

Aminoaciduria syndromes result in excretion of abnormal amounts of amino acids in the urine.

This may be due to elevated blood levels, but may be caused by primary defects in tubular transport as, for example, in cystinuria.

Renal tubular acidosis Type I results in defective function of distal tubules and failure to acidify urine.
This may be acquired, being seen in tubulo-interstitial diseases, or (rarely) may be inherited as a disorder of metabolism.

Renal tubular acidosis Type II results in defective function of the proximal tubule due to defective bicarbonate resorption. It is usually seen as part of Fanconi s syndrome.

Vitamin D resistant rickets is an X-linked dominant disease caused by defective tubular resorption of phosphate.

- The humoral component of acute rejection is characterized by vasculitis with endothelial necrosis, neutrophil infiltration of vessel walls, and damage to the intima and elastic lamina of the larger arteries in the graft.

Parenchymal damage caused by the cellular acute rejection usually responds rapidly to immunosuppressive therapy, whereas damage caused by vascular pathology associated with the humoral component may be permanent. A typical case of acute rejection has a mixture of both components.

Accelerated acute rejection can occur in a patient who has had a previous unsuccessful graft and is therefore already sensitized to donor antigens.

Chronic rejection occurs slowly and progressively over some months. The result of slow breakdown of the host's tolerance to the graft, it may be due to inadequate immune suppression. Histologically, there is intimal fibrosis in arteries in the graft, leading to secondary ischemic damage to the parenchyma. The interstitium is infiltrated by plasma cells and eosinophils.

TUMORS OF THE KIDNEY

Benign tumors of the kidney are commonly seen as an incidental finding and are of little clinical significance. The main tumors of the kidney in adults are renal adenocarcinomas; metastatic tumors are seen, but they are uncommon. Transitional cell carcinomas of the renal pelvis are considered in the section on disease of the lower urinary tract. The only other common renal tumor is nephroblastoma (Wilms' tumor), which is seen almost exclusively in early childhood.

Benign tumors of the kidney are frequent incidental findings

Benign tumours of the kidney are common incidental findings at *post mortem* examination and may also be encountered as incidental findings on imaging.

Renal adenomas are benign epithelial tumors derived from renal tubular epithelium. Their histological appearances overlap with those of renal cell carcinomas, making them very difficult to distinguish. In order to separate adenomas from carcinomas, an arbitrary cut-off of 3 cm in size has been adopted. Some small lesions suspected of being adenomas may be carcinomas, going on to metastasize.

Renal oncocytomas are benign epithelial tumors composed of large cells with eosinophilic cytoplasm filled with mitochondria. They are best considered as a variant of adenoma.

Angiomyolipomas are tumors composed of smooth muscle, fat, and large blood vessels. They are seen in association with tuberose sclerosis (see page 359).

Renal fibromas are very common small benign tumors of spindle cells. Typically 3–10 mm in size, they are of no functional significance and are found in the medulla. They may be hamartomas rather than true neoplasms.

KEY FACTS
Renal transplantation complications

¥ Thrombosis of vascular graft.

¥ Recurrence of original renal disease.

¥ Hyperacute rejection (now rare) happens immediately after transplant. Caused by blood-group incompatibility or pre-formed anti-HLA antibodies.

¥ Acute rejection happens 2—3 weeks after transplant, or after stopping immunosuppression. Caused by humoral and cell-mediated mechanisms.

¥ Chronic rejection occurs over a period of months, causing permanent loss of nephrons.

Renal adenocarcinoma is the most common malignant tumor of the kidney

Renal adenocarcinoma, derived from the renal tubular epithelium, accounts for 90% of primary malignant renal tumors in adults.

Usually seen after the age of 50 years, they present with hematuria and loin pain, although occasionally the presenting symptom is a mass in the loin or a pathological fracture due to metastases in bone. Renal carcinomas are often also associated with paraneoplastic syndromes of hypercalcemia, hypertension, polycythemia, or Cushing's syndrome caused by ectopic or inappropriate hormone secretion. Renal adenocarcinomas account for around 3% of all carcinomas in adults.

Macroscopically these tumors are usually rounded masses, with a yellowish cut face marked with areas of hemorrhage and necrosis (*Fig. 17.24*). There are several histological patterns of renal adenocarcinoma, the most common being the 'clear-cell pattern', in which the tumor cells have clear cytoplasm due to the high content of glycogen and lipid (*Fig. 17.25*). Tubular and papillary carcinomas are characterized by epithelial cells with a granular cytoplasm.

The tumor spreads by local expansion (breaking through the renal capsule into perinephric fat) and by blood-borne metastasis (involving lungs, bone, brain and other sites as a result of tumor invasion of the renal vein). A characteristic behavioral feature is that large tumors may grow as a solid core along the main renal vein, even entering the inferior vena cava.

Prognosis depends on the stage at presentation: if tumor is confined within the renal capsule, there is a 70% 10-year survival; however, prognosis is very poor if metastases are present at diagnosis.

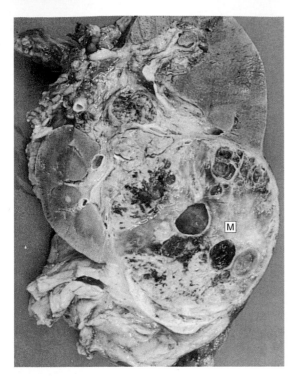

Fig. 17.24 Adenocarcinoma of the kidney.
A renal carcinoma appears as a yellow mass (**M**), with areas of necrosis and hemorrhage.

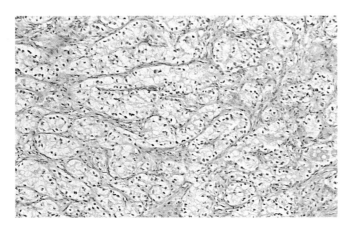

Fig. 17.25 Renal adenocarcinoma. Clear-cell carcinoma of the kidney is composed of uniform vacuolated cells.

Etiology and molecular pathology of renal carcinoma

The incidence of renal carcinoma is increased in von Hippel–Lindau syndrome (familial hemangioblastomas in central nervous system, see page 360), which is inherited as a gene on chromosome 3.

There is a rare familial form of renal cell carcinoma, the gene for which is also located on chromosome 3, separate from the gene for von Hippel–Lindau syndrome.

The majority of renal carcinomas occur as sporadic events. Recent work has revealed common cytogenetic abnormalities, which relate to specific histological sub-types of tumor.

- The most common non-papillary clear-cell renal cell carcinomas are characterized by the loss of chromosome 3p sequences and loss of chromosome 14q sequences.

- Papillary renal cell tumors can be divided into two groups: trisomy of chromosome 17 is seen in papillary renal cell adenomas, whereas tumors with additional trisomies, e.g. trisomy 16, 20 or 12, are papillary renal cell carcinomas.

- Some tumors, known as 'chromophobe renal cell carcinomas', show several allelic losses not seen in the other types, together with re-arrangement of mitochondrial DNA.

Although these different cytogenetic findings do not appear to correlate with the stage, grade or biological behavior of tumors, they are opening the way for a molecular, rather than a histological, classification of this type of carcinoma, with a view to understanding etiology.

KEY FACTS
Renal carcinoma

- Male : female incidence is approximately 3 : 1.
- Incidence is greatest in those over 50 years, and increases with age.
- Common presenting symptoms include hematuria, loin pain, loin mass.
- Occasional presenting symptoms include bone metastasis, brain metastasis, polycythemia.

- Local spread through renal capsule into perinephric fat.
- Lymphatic spread to para-aortic and other nodes.
- Bloodstream spread to lungs, bone, brain, liver.
- Prognosis depends on stage at presentation, e.g. tumor confined within renal capsule has 70% 10-year survival, but very poor prognosis if metastases present at diagnosis.

Nephroblastoma is one of the common malignant tumors of childhood

Nephroblastoma (Wilms' tumor) is an embryonal tumor derived from the primitive metanephros. Although it does occasionally occur in adults, it is predominantly a tumor of young children, with a peak incidence between the ages of 1 and 4 years.

Tumor presents as an abdominal mass or, less frequently, with hematuria. Macroscopically, tumors are rounded masses that replace large amounts of the kidney, appearing as solid, fleshy, white lesions with frequent areas of necrosis (*Fig. 17.26*). Histologically, there are various combinations of four elements, these being primitive small-cell blastomatous tissue resembling the developing metanephric blastema, immature-looking glomerular structures, epithelial tubules, and stroma composed of spindle cells and striated muscle.

Prognosis is related to spread of tumor at diagnosis. The presence of histological features of anaplasia in tumors is associated with poor prognosis. Although these tumors grow rapidly and there is often evidence of spread at the time of diagnosis, treatment by a combination of radiotherapy and intensive chemotherapy achieves a high cure rate.

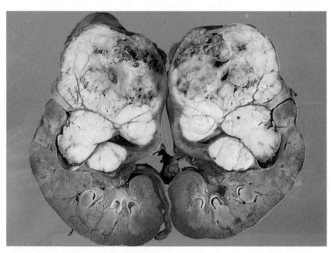

Fig. 17.26 Nephroblastoma.
The kidney is extensively replaced by fleshy, white tumor.

Molecular pathology of Wilms tumor

Wilms tumor appears to represent more than one genetic entity. At least three different genes seem to be important in the origin of Wilms tumor, the best characterized being WT1, a tumor-suppressor gene on chromosome 11. Mutations in this gene may be associated with congenital loss of iris (aniridia), and it is likely that development of Wilms tumor follows a two-hit model for tumor suppressor genes (see Chapter 6) in that there are cases in which both copies of the gene are defective or lost.

DISEASES OF THE LOWER URINARY TRACT

The lower urinary tract extends from the calyces in the kidney to the distal end of the urethra, and is structurally adapted to transmit urine from the kidney to the exterior, the bladder being modified to act as a reservoir. The lower urinary tract is lined by urothelium (**transitional-cell epithelium**), which is capable of resisting the osmotic stresses of contact with urine.

There are five main groups of disorders in the lower urinary tract: **infection**, which is often secondary to stasis of urine, following obstruction to flow; **obstruction** by intrinsic occlusion or extrinsic pressure; **stone formation**, which is often secondary to stasis of urine combined with infection; **tumor formation**, i.e. neoplasia of transitional-cell epithelium; and **developmental abnormalities**.

INFECTION

Infections in the lower urinary tract are predisposed by obstruction and stasis

Lower urinary tract infection is usually due to Gram-negative coliform bacilli, e.g. *E. coli* and *Proteus*, which are normally commensals in the large bowel; because they have a short urethra, women are particularly prone to developing ascending infections. In men, lower urinary tract infection is usually associated with structural abnormalities of the lower urinary tract and stasis due to obstruction.

Diabetes mellitus also predisposes to infection. In most cases the lower urinary tract infection remains localized to the urethra and bladder, but organisms may ascend the ureter and enter the pelvicalyceal system, particularly when there is an obstructive lesion. An **acute bacterial urethritis** and **cystitis** may lead to an ascending **ureteritis** and **pyelitis** (inflammation of the renal pelvis and calyces). In this way, organisms may gain access to the renal parenchyma to produce **acute pyelonephritis** with the formation of abscesses in the renal medulla and cortex (see page 370).

The main complications of lower urinary tract infection are acute and chronic pyelonephritis (see page 370), pyonephrosis (distension of the pelvicalyceal system with pus, usually the result of infection superimposed on obstruction, often at the pelviureteric junction), and papillary necrosis in severe infections, particularly in diabetics. The main causes of papillary necrosis are shown in *Fig. 17.27*.

OBSTRUCTION

Obstruction of the drainage of urine from the kidney causes hydronephrosis

Obstruction, one of the most important consequences of disease of the lower urinary tract, may occur at any place in the tract:

- **Renal pelvis** – calculi, tumors.
- **Pelviureteric junction** – stricture, calculi, extrinsic compression.
- **Ureter** – calculi, extrinsic compression (pregnancy, tumor, fibrosis).
- **Bladder** – tumor, calculi.
- **Urethra** – prostatic hyperplasia or carcinoma, urethral valves, urethral stricture.

If obstruction occurs in the urethra, the bladder develops dilatation and secondary hypertrophy of muscle in its wall. This predisposes to development of outpouching of the bladder mucosa (diverticula).

If obstruction occurs in a ureter, there is dilatation of the ureter (**megaureter**), with progressive dilatation of the renal pelvicalyceal system, termed **hydronephrosis** (*Fig. 17.28a*). Fluid entering the collecting ducts cannot empty into the renal pelvis and there is intrarenal resorption of fluid.

At this stage, if the obstruction is relieved, renal function returns to normal. However, if obstruction persists, there is atrophy of renal tubules, glomerular hyalinization, and fibrosis. As an end-stage, the renal parenchyma becomes severely atrophic and renal function is permanently impaired (*Fig. 17.28b*). Usually, the end-stage of hydronephrosis develops only with unilateral obstruction of a ureter, as renal function is maintained by the non-obstructed kidney. With bilateral obstruction, most usual with lesions in the bladder base or retroperitoneal tissues, renal failure develops before severe atrophy of both kidneys does. The causes of hydronephrosis are shown in *Fig. 17.29*. Urinary tract obstruction also predisposes to infection and stone formation.

Hydronephrosis

Fig. 17.29 Causes of hydronephrosis
Hydronephrosis can be caused by obstruction to the drainage of the kidney at many levels

Idiopathic obstruction at the pelviureteric junction

Extrinsic compression of ureter (tumor or retroperitoneal fibrosis)

Tumor in renal pelvis or ureter (transitional cell carcinoma)

Calculus in ureter

Congenital ureteric abnormality (ureterocele)

Disease at base of bladder (carcinoma)

Compression of prostatic urethra (hyperplasia or carcinoma)

Urethral obstruction (urethral stricture or valves)

Fig. 17.27
Causes of papillary necrosis

Lower urinary tract obstruction without infection

Urinary tract infection with or without obstruction

Diabetic nephropathy with or without infection

Analgesic abuse, usually associated with phenacetin (an uncommon cause since the pathogenesis was recognized)

Sickle-cell disease

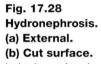

**Fig. 17.28
Hydronephrosis.
(a) External.
(b) Cut surface.**
In hydronephrosis (a) there is dilatation of the renal pelvis (**P**). In advanced disease (b) there is severe loss of renal parenchyma around a grossly dilated renal pelvicalyceal system.

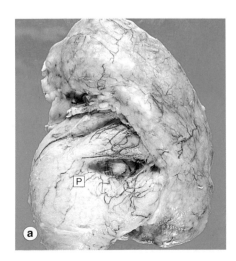

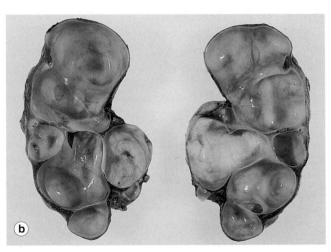

URINARY CALCULI

Most renal calculi are composed of calcium oxalate and phosphate

Urinary calculi may form anywhere in the lower urinary tract (**urolithiasis**), the most common sites being the pelvicalyceal system and bladder. The two main predisposing factors for stone formation are increased concentration of solute in urine (low fluid throughput or primary increase in metabolite), and reduced solubility of solute in urine (due to persistently abnormal urinary pH). Conditions that cause these factors to operate are low fluid intake, urine stasis, persistent urinary tract infection, and primary metabolic disturbances.

The most common urinary stones, accounting for 80% of cases, are composed of calcium oxalate or phosphate. Half of these cases are associated with idiopathic hypercalciuria, with only about 10% being caused by hypercalcemia. Other cases may be caused by hyperoxaluria, which has several associations, e.g. inflammatory bowel disease. The second most common type of calculi, accounting for 15% of cases, are those composed of magnesium, ammonium, and calcium phosphates (**struvite**). They are associated with infection in the lower urinary tract as a result of urea-splitting organisms, which make urine permanently alkaline.

Uric acid stones account for about 5% of cases and are predisposed by conditions causing hyperuricemia, e.g. gout. However, 50% of patients with uric acid stones do not have hyperuricemia, and it is suggested that production of persistently acid urine is the predisposing factor.

Cystine stones are rare, accounting for under 1% of cases. They are seen in heritable tubular transport defects causing cystinuria.

Stones at different sites in the urinary tract have different appearances

Stones formed at different sites in the urinary tract have different morphological appearances. For example, calculi in the pelvicalyceal system are often multiple and may be small, taking the form of gravel. However, large, branching **staghorn calculi** occasionally form by the constant accretion of calcium salts, conforming to the contours of the pelvicalyceal system (*Fig. 17.30*).

The presence of calculi in the pelvicalyceal system predisposes to persistent pelvicalyceal infection, pyonephrosis and perinephric abscess, and development of squamous metaplasia in the urothelium. Squamous cell carcinoma may occasionally occur in the metaplastic areas.

Most stones in the ureter have developed in the renal pelvis, secondarily passing down the urinary tract. Often this is associated with intense loin pain, termed **ureteric colic**, which may be associated with ureteric obstruction and hydronephrosis. In the bladder the stones are usually spherical and laminated, and may reach a large size. The main predisposition for stone formation in the bladder is stasis and chronic infection. The presence of bladder calculi

KEY FACTS
Urinary calculi

- ¥ Due to increased concentration of solute in urine or reduced solubility of product in urine.
- ¥ Infection, stasis, and metabolic abnormalities are the main underlying causes.
- ¥ Most commonly composed of calcium oxalate and phosphate, 10% of such stones being caused by hypercalciuria or hyperoxaluria.
- ¥ The second most common are triple-phosphate stones caused by chronic infections.
- ¥ Uncommon types are urate and cystine stones.

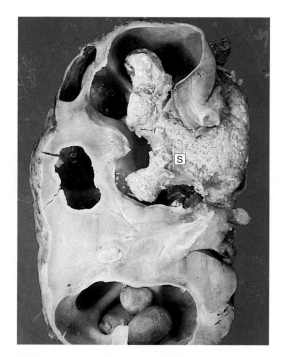

Fig. 17.30 Renal staghorn calculus.
The renal pelvis is filled with a large calculus that is shaped to its contours, resembling the horn of a stag (**S**). The calyceal system at the lower pole contains separate rounded calculi.

causes squamous metaplasia in the urinary bladder and may be associated with development of squamous carcinoma.

TUMORS OF THE LOWER URINARY TRACT

Tumors of the lower urinary tract are derived from the transitional cells of the urothelium

Most tumors of the lower urinary tract arise from transitional-cell epithelium and are mainly caused by environmental agents excreted in high concentration in the

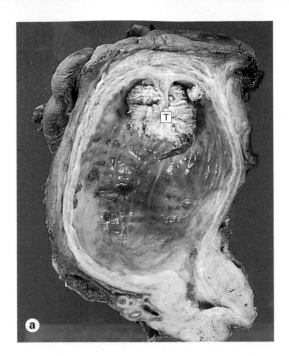

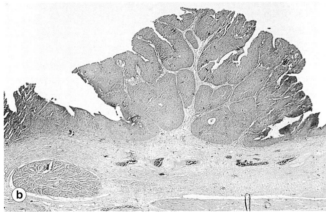

Fig. 17.31 Transitional-cell carcinoma.
A papillary transitional-cell carcinoma is seen arising from the dome of the bladder (a) as a fronded cauliflower-like lesion (**T**). Histologically (b), lesions are composed of papillae covered with transitional epithelium.

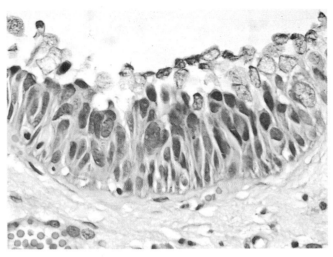

Fig. 17.32 Carcinoma *in situ* of transitional-cell epithelium. *In situ* transitional-cell carcinoma is a flat lesion, characterized by marked cytological atypia of cells in the absence of invasion.

urine (see pink box on page 380). A field change takes place in the whole of the urothelium, such that all areas, from renal pelvis to urethra, are at risk of development of neoplasia. For this reason, multiple tumors are common. Transitional-cell tumors are most common in men, but are also fairly common in women.

The majority of tumors derived from the transitional-cell epithelium occur in the bladder and have a papillary growth pattern (**papillary transitional-cell carcinomas**) (*Fig. 17.31*). The epithelium covering the papillae can vary from histologically bland (low grade) to cytologically abnormal (moderate grade). All papillary transitional-cell tumors are regarded as carcinomas, regardless of how bland the epithelium appears on histological examination. Transitional-cell carcinomas exhibiting severe cytological abnormalities (high grade) tend not to have a papillary pattern, growing as solid, ulcerating lesions instead. It is well documented that patients can start with a low-grade tumor which, over time, develops progressive cytological atypia and turns into a high-grade tumor.

Transitional-cell carcinomas are histologically graded from I to IV on the basis of cellular and nuclear pleomorphism and mitoses. The grade of tumor relates to biological behavior.

About 80% of tumors encountered are non-invasive low-grade papillary tumors. After resection, about 70% of such lesions recur locally and, of these, a quarter will be a higher grade lesion and a tenth will have become invasive.

About 20% of tumors encountered are invasive moderate- or high-grade lesions, with a mixed solid and papillary growth pattern (already invasive at first diagnosis). A distinction must be made between non-invasive papillary transitional-cell carcinomas and the entity called **carcinoma *in situ*** of transitional-cell epithelium. Macroscopically, the latter is a flat, red lesion, often with marked cytological atypia, in the absence of invasion (*Fig. 17.32*). This type of flat, non-invasive lesion has a sinister reputation for development into high-grade, solid, invasive carcinoma.

When invasive, transitional-cell carcinomas spread by local, vascular and lymphatic routes. Staging of carcinoma of the bladder divides tumors into *in situ*, papillary non-invasive, superficially invasive, deeply invasive and metastatic categories.

Transitional-cell carcinomas in the renal pelvis (*Fig. 17.33*), ureter and urethra are histologicaly similar in nature to those seen in the bladder. Importantly, following on from the concept of a field change seen in transitional-cell neoplasia, a patient who has had a tumor in one site is at risk of developing a second tumor in another site in the urothelium.

Carcinogenesis in transitional-cell carcinoma

Transitional-cell carcinomas of the lower urinary tract can develop from exposure to environmental agents excreted in high concentration in the urine. This is sometimes the result of occupational exposure to a carcinogen, and some cases of transitional-cell carcinoma are regarded as industrial diseases that are liable for compensation. The main carcinogens responsible are associated with cigarette smoking, aniline dyes, and the rubber industry (car-tire plants).

Half of the population inherit two deleted genes for glutathione S transferase M1 (GSTM1), the enzyme that normally acts to detoxify many carcinogens. Studies have shown that the deleted 0/0 genotype for GSTM1 increases the risk of development of transitional-cell carcinoma in patients exposed to the carcinogenic effects of cigarette smoke; it has been estimated that this common genetic predisposition underlies about 25% of cases of transitional-cell carcinoma.

Molecular genetic studies have shown several abnormalities in transitional-cell carcinoma. Monosomy and loss of heterozygosity for chromosome 9 suggest that a specific tumor suppressor gene is missing in a high proportion of tumors, and the hunt is on to characterize the gene responsible. Mutation of the p53 gene is seen in many tumors and is associated with tumor progression and invasion. Abnormal expression of several other oncogenes has been documented and these are also associated with tumor progression.

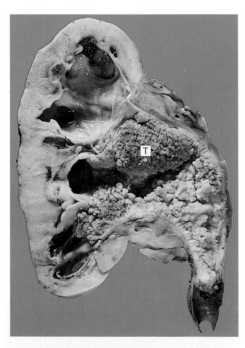

Fig. 17.33 Transitional-cell carcinoma of renal pelvis. Papillary transitional cell carcinoma (**T**) fills the renal pelvis with dilatation of the renal calyces caused by urinary obstruction.

Squamous cell carcinoma and adenocarcinoma of the bladder are uncommon lesions with special etiology

Non-transitional-cell carcinomas of the bladder, which account for about 15% of all tumors, can be broken down into squamous cell carcinomas, pure adenocarcinomas, mixed tumors (transitional-cell and adenocarcinomas), undifferentiated carcinomas, and spindle-cell carcinomas.

Squamous cell carcinomas of the lower urinary tract are most often seen in the bladder and renal pelvis. They are derived from metaplastic epithelium, most commonly associated with chronic irritation from a calculus. In endemic areas an important cause of squamous metaplasia and subsequent carcinoma is **schistosomiasis.**

Adenocarcinomas of the bladder are uncommon, but are usually seen in the dome region, where they are believed to derive from persistent glandular tissue in urachal remnants. In some cases these tumors spread along a remnant track to the umbilicus. The rare congenital condition of exstrophy of the bladder, which is due to failure of closure, predisposes to later development of adenocarcinoma.

CONGENITAL DISEASES OF THE KIDNEY AND LOWER URINARY TRACT

DEVELOPMENTAL DISEASES OF THE URINARY TRACT

Congenital diseases of the kidneys are often seen associated with other abnormalities of development

Congenital renal disease is a common clinical problem, often found in association with other congenital abnormalities. The main developmental abnormalities of the kidney can be classified as: agenesis, failure of differentiation (renal dysplasia), abnormal anatomic development, abnormalities of renal tubular transport, and developmental abnormalities of structural elements.

Bilateral renal agenesis occurs as part of Potter's syndrome. Affected infants have abnormal facies and, frequently, abnormalities of lower urinary tract, lungs and nervous system. Characteristically, because the kidneys are not present to contribute to amniotic fluid, there is oligo-hydramnios in pregnancy.

During development, there may be failure of differentiation of metanephric tissues, leading to **renal dysplasia**. This may affect a whole kidney or just one segment, and may be unilateral or bilateral. The affected areas are replaced by solid and cystic masses in which cartilage is usually prominent (see *Fig. 5.4* and page 63).

Renal development may be anatomically abnormal, leading to **horseshoe kidney** (*Fig. 17.34*) in which the two kidneys are fused across the midline, and pelvic kidney in which the kidney is sited low in the pelvis.

Several congenital metabolic defects affect the kidney. These are usually defects in transport of amino acids across tubular epithelium, such that they are excreted in the urine.

Alport's syndrome causes renal failure and is due to a defect in Type IV collagen

Alport's disease, an inherited condition, is characterized by progressive nephritis leading to renal failure in the second decade. It is associated with sensorineural hearing loss and eye diseases (corneal dystrophies and lens abnormalities). In the majority of families, inheritance is X-linked dominant transmission. The main defect is within the GBM, which shows splitting.

There is now substantial evidence that X-linked Alport's syndrome is due to defective Type IV collagen, involving mutations in a gene for the alpha 5 chain of Type IV collagen on the X chromosome (COL4A5). This form of Type IV collagen is an important constituent of the basal lamina in glomeruli, the lens, and the organ of Corti.

CYSTIC DISEASE OF THE KIDNEY

Several cystic diseases of the kidney produce chronic renal failure

There are several cystic diseases of the kidney, some of which produce renal failure by causing disturbance of renal structure. Importantly, some conditions are heritable.

Adult polycystic disease is inherited in an autosomal dominant pattern, generally becoming clinically manifest in adult life. Increasingly, disease is detected in childhood, with family screening and ultrasound examination. Cysts develop and progressively enlarge over a number of years, but remain asymptomatic until the number and size of the cysts is so great that the patient becomes aware of abdominal masses (*Fig. 17.35*).

At about the same time, the replacement and compression of functioning renal parenchyma by the cysts leads to slowly progressive impairment of renal function, and patients develop chronic renal failure and hypertension.

Patients with adult-type polycystic renal disease may also develop cysts in the liver, lung and pancreas. There is an association with berry aneurysms of the cerebral arteries (page 436) which, with development of hypertension, predisposes to intracranial hemorrhage.

There are two genes associated with this condition: 90% of cases are associated with PKD1, which is located on chromosome 16, and 5–10% with PKD2, located on chromosome 2. As yet, the gene sequences and functions are unknown.

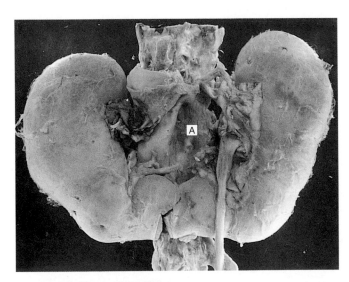

Fig. 17.34 Horseshoe kidney.
The kidneys are fused across the midline in front of the aorta (**A**). The ureters are kinked over the joining segment, and this may be an unusual cause of hydronephrosis.

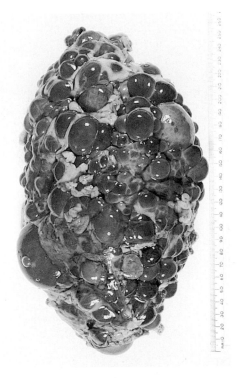

Fig. 17.35 Adult polycystic disease.
The kidney is converted into a mass of large cysts. Hemorrhage into cysts is common, leading to bloodstained contents.

Nephronophthisis complex describes two diseases: familial juvenile nephronophthisis (NPH) and medullary cystic disease (MCD). Both are inherited causes of cysts at the corticomedullary junction of the kidney, and are associated with interstitial fibrosis leading to early-onset chronic renal failure. The conditions account for 10–25% of cases of end-stage renal failure in the first three decades. Although virtually identical clinically and pathologically, NPH presents around the age of 11 years as an autosomal recessive disease, and MCD around the age of 20 years as an autosomal dominant trait.

Medullary sponge kidney is a condition in which multiple cysts develop in renal papillae. Renal function is not impaired and the main clinical problem is development of renal stones, which predispose to renal colic and infection.

Infantile polycystic disease is uncommon and is encountered at birth. Children develop severe renal failure, with compression of the lungs due to massive enlargement of the kidneys.

Simple renal cysts are the most common form of renal cystic disease and must be distinguished from the congenital types discussed above. They are widely held to be acquired abnormalities, incidence increasing with age. They contain clear, watery fluid and have a smooth lining. Simple cysts may be single or multiple and vary in size, generally being no larger than 5–6 cm. They have no effect on renal function, but may rarely become infected or develop hemorrhage.

Acquired cystic disease is seen in kidneys left *in situ* while patients are treated by dialysis or transplantation for chronic renal failure.

Developmental abnormalities of lower urinary tract

Developmental abnormalities in the lower urinary tract often accompany complex congenital malformation syndromes. They may also occur as isolated abnormalities, the most clinically significant being:

- **Ureteric defects** forming bifid or double ureters. These may be associated with vesicoureteric reflux, and predispose to recurrent infections.

- **Ureterocele** is a cyst of the lower ureter, sited at its passage through the bladder wall. The cyst bulges into the bladder and causes obstruction of the ureter, leading to hydroureter and hydronephrosis. The majority of cases (90%) are unilateral.

- **Persistent urachus** leads to a vesicoumbilical fistula, urachal cysts, and urachal sinuses.

- **Exstrophy of the bladder** (ectopia vesicae) is uncommon and is caused by failure of closure of the bladder, associated with a defect in the pelvis and abdominal wall. The bladder lining is exposed and infants develop recurrent infections, leading to metaplasia of the transitional-cell epithelium to a glandular type. This condition predisposes to the development of adenocarcinoma of the bladder.

- **Posterior urethral valves** are folds of lining mucosa in the urethra that cause obstruction leading to hydronephrosis. They are more common in males than in females, and predispose to ascending pyelonephritis in children.

18 Male genital system

Clinical Overview

The most important diseases of the male genital system are the highly malignant tumors which occur in the prostate gland and in the testis. Carcinoma of the prostate gland affects middle-aged and elderly men, often presents late such that the tumor is already well advanced when medical advice is sought, and can be difficult to treat. One main problem is that the tumor spreads to bone, particularly the vertebrae. Tumors of the testis occur in young and middle-aged men, usually presenting as a painless intrascrotal swelling. The most common tumors are derived from germ cells and are highly malignant, although recent advances in tumor monitoring and the use of chemotherapy have greatly improved the prognosis.

However, these tumors comprise only a comparatively small part of family practice; conditions such as congenital maldescent of the testis and torsion of the testis (in children), sexually transmitted infections such as gonorrhea and penile warts (in young and middle-aged men), and benign prostatic hyperplasia leading to obstruction to urinary drainage with all its attendant complications (in elderly males) are very much more frequent. Most disorders of the penis are skin diseases which just happen to occur on the penis; common examples are contact dermatitis, lichen planus and squamous carcinoma.

Intrascrotal swellings are a frequent presenting symptom, but many are due to herniation of small bowel into the scrotum, rather than a primary abnormality of intrascrotal components. Other important causes of intrascrotal swelling include hydrocele (accumulation of fluid in the scrotum) and varicocele (varicose enlargement of the pampiniform plexus of veins). It is important to distinguish these benign causes of intrascrotal swelling from malignant tumors in the testis.

TESTIS, EPIDIDYMIS AND PARATESTICULAR TISSUES

The testis is the source of male gametes, the spermatozoa, but also acts as an endocrine organ, producing male sex hormones. In development the testis may fail to descend into the scrotum, therefore failing to function. The testis may be involved in infective and inflammatory disorders, which usually also affect the adjacent epididymis. Disease that leads to destruction of the testis may produce infertility or endocrine disturbance, or both. The most important diseases of the testis are the testicular tumors, many of which occur in men in the first four decades of life.

Maldescent of the testis gives rise to cryptorchidism and increased risk of development of testicular tumors

In the embryo the testis develops high on the posterior abdominal wall from the genital ridge, and the germ cells migrate to the genital ridge from the endoderm of the yolk sac. At about 7 months' gestation, the testes migrate down the posterior abdominal wall and through the inguinal ring into the scrotum, guided by a cord (the gubernaculum). Occasionally, this migration fails to occur and the testis becomes arrested somewhere along its normal route, most commonly at or near the inguinal ring or in the inguinal canal.

The temperature in these locations is sufficiently high to prevent normal germ-cell development and the testis remains small, with seminiferous tubules lined only by Sertoli cells; in these circumstances the testis is termed **cryptorchid**. In a maldescended testis, germ cells never develop properly and the testis remains incapable of producing effective spermatozoa. Some function may be achieved if, at an early stage, the testis is surgically pulled down into the scrotal sac, an operation called an 'orchidopexy'. Cryptorchidism is unilateral in 75% of cases (bilateral in 25%). Detection and correction of testicular maldescent is important, as an undescended testis has a greatly increased chance of developing a malignant tumor (see page 385).

Infections of the testis commonly also involve the epididymis

Infection of the testis (orchitis) is often associated with an infection that enters through the epididymis (epididymitis), resulting in **epididymo-orchitis**. The most important infections of the testis and epididymis are acute bacterial epididymo-orchitis, viral orchitis, and tuberculous epididymo-orchitis.

Acute infection is usually due to gonococci and *Chlamydia* (sexually transmitted) or *Escherichia coli* and other Gram-negative bacilli. Infection spreads from the urethra and lower urinary tract. Clinically the testis and epididymis are greatly enlarged and very tender. Histologically there is extensive infiltration of the seminiferous tubules and interstitium by neutrophils, later followed by lymphocytes and plasma cells; interstitial edema is considerable, and there is often patchy hemorrhage. Successful treatment with antibiotics is followed by healing and scarring, but there may be permanent damage to seminiferous tubules and epididymis, with consequent impairment of fertility.

Viral orchitis is usually the result of infection by the mumps virus after puberty. The disease is usually unilateral, and is associated with tender enlargement of the testis. The inflammatory infiltrate is mainly composed of lymphocytes and plasma cells. In a small proportion of cases, bilateral disease after puberty can result in reduced fertility.

Tuberculous epididymitis may be the result of bloodstream spread of mycobacteria to the testis during a phase of active pulmonary TB. It may also be caused by spread of infection from the kidney and lower urinary tract. The bacteria are sequestered in the epididymis, and produce slowly progressive caseous destruction over a period of many years, often continuing long after the initial pulmonary tuberculous lesion has healed (*Fig. 18.1*).

The testis is rarely involved in tertiary syphilis, being the site of gumma formation. **Granulomatous orchitis**, a condition of unknown etiology, is an inflammatory disease in which there is a histiocytic and giant-cell inflammatory reaction associated with seminiferous tubule destruction.

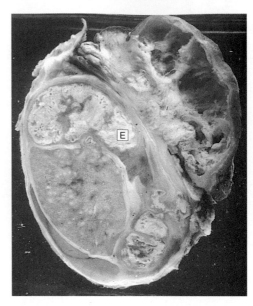

Fig. 18.1 Tuberculous epididymitis. The epididymis (**E**) is converted into a mass of caseous necrosis, and there is often associated tuberculous prostatitis and cystitis.

Torsion of the testis causes venous infarction

Torsion of the testis, which is mainly seen in children and adolescents, occurs when the testis twists on its pedicle, obstructing the venous return. Blood continues to enter the testis and, with venous return mechanically obstructed, venous infarction occurs (see page 160). A torted testis is swollen and painful and, clinically, may simulate orchitis in the early stages. With advanced torsion, the testis is swollen and almost black in color because of the vascular congestion. As such cases are non-viable, surgical removal is required to treat advanced disease. Early detection and surgical relief of torsion is required to save testicular viability. Similar clinical features may be caused by torsion of hydatids of Morgagni.

The ductal system from the testis is mainly affected by cysts, inflammatory disorders and, rarely, tumor

There are few important disorders that affect the tubular system between the epididymis and the prostatic urethra. Among the most common are epididymal cysts (**spermatoceles**), which are cystic dilatations of the head of the epididymis (*Fig. 18.2*). The cyst is usually thin-walled and translucent, containing watery or slightly milky fluid, in which spermatozoa can be identified. **Varicoceles** are composed of a dilated pampiniform plexus of veins, which expands within the scrotal sac.

Benign tumors of support tissues (e.g. lipoma, fibroma) may occur, particularly in tissues of the spermatic cord. Lipomas are the most common, followed by fibromas.

Sperm granuloma is a tender, indurated nodule, usually found alongside the vas deferens. Histologically it shows a

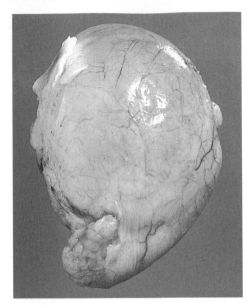

Fig. 18.2 Spermatocele. Spermatoceles (epidermal cysts) are thin-walled, attached to the epididymis, and contain opalescent fluid.

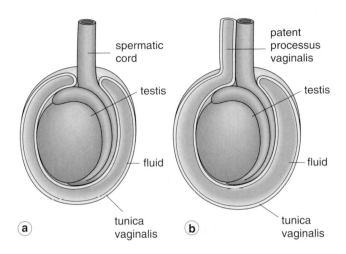

Fig. 18.3 Hydrocele.
(a) In a **hydrocele** the tunica vaginalis surrounding the testis is distended by fluid. (b) In **congenital hydrocele** there is associated patency of the processus vaginalis, with continuity with the peritoneal cavity.

chronic inflammatory reaction to remnants of spermatozoa, and is thought to represent a reaction to spermatozoa that have leaked out of the ductular system. It may also be found in the region of the head of the epididymis, but a location close to the vas deferens is most common. These lesions are often seen as nodules at the site of operative vasectomy.

Adenomatoid tumor is a benign neoplastic growth, which develops in or close to the epididymis. The tumor is a small, well-circumscribed, firm, white nodule, most commonly arising in middle-aged men. These lesions are thought to be of mesothelial origin.

Paratesticular sarcomas are uncommon tumors that develop from support tissues of the epididymis, especially in childhood. The most common are rhabdomyosarcoma and leiomyosarcoma.

Inflammation of the ductular system may occur secondary to urinary tract infection or specifically in association with gonorrhea.

The most common disease of the tunica vaginalis is hydrocele

The tunica vaginalis and tunica albuginea are invested with mesothelial cells and may be the site of fluid accumulation, inflammation or, uncommonly, tumor formation.

Hydrocele which is the most common cause of swelling within the scrotum, is the result of fluid accumulating in the cavity bounded by the tunica vaginalis. Congenital patency of the processus vaginalis may be a cause in childhood, other causes being inflammatory and neoplastic disorders of the testis or epididymis (*Fig. 18.3*). Blood accumulating in the tunica is termed **hematocele**.

Benign proliferations of the mesothelial cells lining the tunica may occur. These may be reactive or may form adenomatoid tumors. Rarely, malignant mesothelioma (see page 220) may develop within the tunica sac.

Testicular tumors are common in early adult life

Tumors of the testis are important, as they account for a high proportion of tumors seen in early adult life; they are particularly significant in those aged between 20 and 45 years. The two main groups of testicular tumors are: germ-cell tumors (97% of all cases), which are derived from the multipotential germ cells of the testis, and sex-cord stromal tumors (3% of all cases), which are derived from the specialized and non-specialized support cells of the testis.

Testicular germ-cell tumors are predisposed by maldescent and a chromosomal abnormality

In recent years the incidence of testicular germ-cell tumors has been increasing in western countries. Although they occur at a rate of 2 per 100 000 of the population, the rising incidence has given cause for concern that an environmental agent is responsible.

An important predisposing factor is testicular maldescent leading to cryptorchid testis. There has been recent speculation that exposure to estrogenic agents in the environment *in utero* may impair testicular descent and maturation, predisposing to later development of neoplasia.

An abnormality of chromosome 12 (an isochromosome of the short arm called i (12p)) is found in 90% of testicular

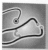

Classification and nomenclature of germ-cell tumors

The most important testicular tumors are those derived from the germ cells lining the seminiferous tubules; they comprise 90–95% of all malignant testicular neoplasms. Germ cells form four main types of neoplastic tissue:

1 Totipotent germ cells differentiating to spermatocytic tissue form tumors called 'seminomas'.
2 Primitive totipotent germ cells with no differentiation.
3 Primitive totipotent germ cells differentiating to somatic embryonal tissues such as epithelium, cartilage, and smooth muscle.
4 Primitive totipotent germ cells differentiating to extraembryonic tissues such as trophoblast and yolk sac.

Depending on the type of histological differentiation seen in germ-cell tumors, they are given different names.

In the **WHO classification** (*Fig. 18.4*) a rigorous definition of teratoma is adopted, in that a teratoma is considered to be composed of somatic differentiated elements (endoderm, mesoderm, ectoderm).

Tumors composed of undifferentiated cells are termed 'embryonal carcinomas' and are regarded as more primitive than a teratoma.

Tumors with differentiation to extraembryonic tissues (trophoblast and yolk sac) are not considered conceptually to be teratomas.

The UK classification of testicular tumors is no longer used and has been entirely replaced by the WHO classification and nomenclature (*Fig. 18.4*). For reference, the equivalent names of germ-cell tumors in the current WHO and defunct UK classifications is given in *Fig. 18.5*.

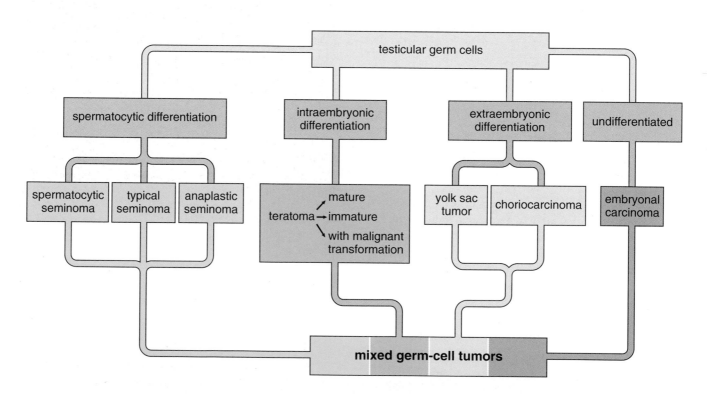

Fig. 18.4 WHO classification of germ-cell tumors of the testis.

germ-cell tumors, and other abnormalities of 12p are found in the other 10%. An abnormality at this locus is present in all testicular germ-cell tumors, irrespective of histological type, and is also seen in the ovarian germ-cell equivalent tumors.

In some patients a precursor of invasive germ-cell neoplasia is the presence of *in situ* germ-cell neoplasia. Detectable in biopsy material, the seminiferous tubules are packed with atypical germ cells, without evidence of breach in the basement membrane.

Fig. 18.5

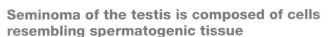

Comparison of the UK and WHO classifications of non-seminomatous germ-cell tumors

British	WHO
Teratoma differentiated (TD)	Mature teratoma
Malignant teratoma intermediate (MTI)	Immature teratoma, or mixed teratoma and embryonal carcinoma
Malignant teratoma undifferentiated (MTU)	Embryonal carcinoma
Malignant teratoma trophoblastic (MTT)	Choriocarcinoma
Yolk-sac tumor	Yolk-sac tumor
Mixed germ-cell tumor	Mixed germ-cell tumor

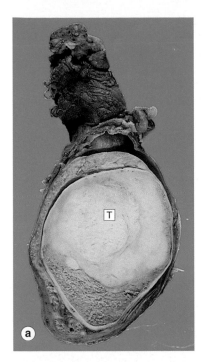

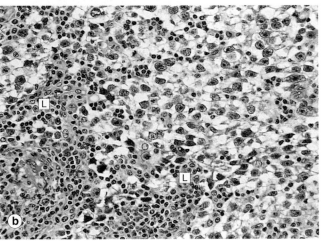

Fig. 18.6 Seminoma. Macroscopically (a) the testis is replaced by firm, white tumor (**T**). Histologically (b). neoplastic cells are polygonal, with clear cytoplasm and large nuclei. Septa containing lymphoid cells (**L**) are a prominent feature.

Seminoma of the testis is composed of cells resembling spermatogenic tissue

Seminoma of the testis is the most common malignant testicular tumor, accounting for about 50% of all malignant germ-cell tumors. It is most common in those aged between 40 and 50 years, characteristically presenting with a painless, progressive enlargement of one testis; bilateral involvement is rare.

Macroscopically the normal, pale-brown testicular tissue is replaced by a homogeneous creamy-white tumor mass (*Fig. 18.6a*). In contrast to other types of germ-cell tumor, there is no evidence of cyst formation or hemorrhage; necrosis occurs only in the largest, neglected tumors.

The most common histological type of seminoma is termed **classic** (or typical) **seminoma**. Histologically these tumors are composed of sheets of regular, tightly packed cells that have small, dark-staining central nuclei and clear cytoplasm.

A characteristic feature is the presence of fibrous septa, in which numerous lymphocytes are found (*Fig. 18.6b*). Seminoma shows immunoreactivity for placental alkaline phosphatase (PLAP).

Other histological variants of seminoma include **anaplastic seminoma**, in which the cells show marked pleomorphism and increased mitotic activity and **spermatocytic seminoma**, which is composed of larger than normal tumor cells with central, round, dark-staining nuclei and abundant eosinophilic cytoplasm; some small cells, which resemble spermatocytes, are also present. This variant tends to occur in patients over the age of 50 years and has a better prognosis than classic seminoma and anaplastic seminoma.

Seminomas with trophoblastic (human chorionic gonadotrophin-containing) giant cells are encountered in 10% of cases, but the biological relevance of the trophoblastic tissue is uncertain. Such tumors may be associated with increased blood levels of human chorionic gonadotrophin (HCG) secreted by trophoblast.

Seminoma may be found in association with other germ-cell elements, forming mixed germ-cell tumors.

Testicular teratomas composed entirely of mature somatic elements behave in a benign fashion

Testicular germ cell tumors composed of fully differentiated somatic tissues are the least common of the teratoma variants. Usually seen in young children, these are true teratomas (mature teratoma), with representatives of all three embryonic layers present; all tissues are well differentiated and fully matured, so that a wide range (e.g. skin, hair, cartilage, and bone) can be identified (*Fig. 18.7*). These mature teratomas almost always behave in a very benign way, but a thorough histological examination of each tumor should be made in order to exclude the presence of undifferentiated tissues.

Immature testicular teratomas consist of representatives of all three embryonic layers, but haphazardly arranged and incompletely differentiated

Although the teratomatous components are incompletely differentiated, they are still identifiably glandular epithelium, cartilage, neural tissue, etc, though with little or no attempt at organized arrangement in the main, although small foci of better differentiated, semi-organoid tumor may be found, resembling mature teratoma. Also, there may be foci in which one of the teratomatous elements is cytologically and histologically malignant, for example a focus of squamous cell carcinoma or adenocarcinoma.

Germ-cell tumors containing undifferentiated elements (embryonal carcinoma) are common as pure tumors, or mixed with other elements

Some testicular germ-cell tumors contain sheets of immature cells in solid, tubular or papillary patterns. When in a pure form these tumours are termed 'embryonal carcinoma' (WHO). These tumors tend to occur in those between the ages of 20 and 30 years.

Macroscopically these tumors tend to have a variegated appearance, with fleshy and cystic or necrotic areas (*Fig. 18.8a*). Histologically, cells are pleomorphic and there are typically many mitoses (*Fig. 18.8b*).

In other germ-cell tumors, undifferentiated elements are seen in association with differentiated somatic elements. These are considered mixed germ-cell tumors in the WHO

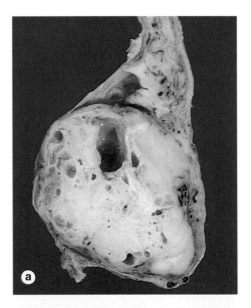

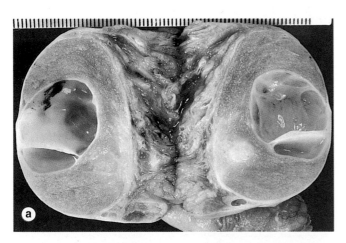

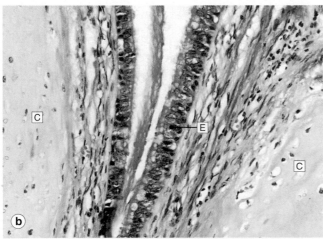

Fig. 18.7 Teratoma composed of mature elements.
Macroscopically, differentiated teratomas are usually cystic (a). Histologically (b), a variety of differentiated elements such as epithelium (**E**) and cartilage (**C**) are seen.

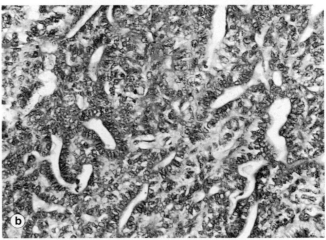

Fig. 18.8 Testicular germ-cell tumor with no differentiation. Germ-cell tumors that consist of undifferentiated elements are composed of solid and cystic soft tumor in which areas of necrosis and hemorrhage are common (a). Histologically (b), sheets of pleomorphic undifferentiated cells are seen. This is termed 'embryonal carcinoma' (WHO).

classification. Macroscopically these lesions have both solid and cystic areas, as well as areas of necrosis centered on the undifferentiated elements. Germ-cell tumors composed predominantly of undifferentiated cells often also contain yolk-sac tumor or trophoblastic tissue.

Yolk-sac tumor is a form of highly malignant germ-cell tumor and secretes alpha fetoprotein

One of the extraembryonic elements that may develop in a germ-cell tumor is differentiation to resemble embryonic yolk sac (also called 'endodermal sinus tumor'). This may be present in a pure form, particularly in children in the first 3 years of life, but is more often encountered as a component of a mixed germ-cell tumor, most commonly mixed with undifferentiated cells.

Yolk-sac elements have characteristic histological appearances, forming solid, papillary and microcystic patterns. This type of germ-cell tumor can also be identified by immunohistochemical detection of **alpha fetoprotein** (AFP) (*Fig. 18.9*), which is also secreted into the blood and can be detected as a tumor marker.

These tumors are highly malignant and spread rapidly. When trophoblastic or yolk-sac elements are seen in association with other elements, they confer a worse prognosis.

Testicular choriocarcinoma is highly malignant and secretes HCG

Testicular germ-cell tumors that are composed of trophoblast (choriocarcinoma in the WHO classification) contain recognizable syncytiotrophoblast and cytotrophoblast, as would be seen in placental tissue. Tumors may be entirely composed of trophoblastic tissue, or trophoblast may be seen as part of a mixed germ-cell tumor. This element can be identified by immunohistochemical detection of HCG, which may also be detected in the blood as a tumor marker.

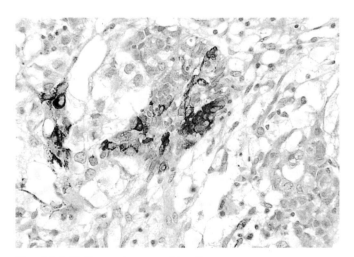

Fig. 18.9 Yolk-sac tumor of testis.
In this immunohistochemical preparation, yolk-sac tumor is shown to express AFP (brown stain).

Although seminomas may contain trophoblastic giant cells, this does not make them mixed tumors, and the biological significance of their presence is uncertain.

Seminomas tend to spread to nodes, whereas non-seminomatous germ cell tumors (NSGCT) tend to spread via the bloodstream

Seminomatous tumors tend to spread to lymph nodes in the iliac and para-aortic groups, bloodstream spread being a late feature. In contrast, non-seminomatous germ-cell tumors (NSGCT) tend to spread via the bloodstream at an early stage, and in some tumors (particularly trophoblastic germ-cell tumors) there may be widespread metastases before the patient becomes aware of any particular testicular enlargement. Metastatic disease may be widespread, but the lung is a particularly common site. Nodal spread also occurs.

Prognosis in germ-cell tumors is related to histological type, as well as to tumor stage. The prognosis in NSGCT has improved greatly since the use of cytotoxic chemotherapy. In general, germ-cell tumors containing trophoblastic, yolk-sac and undifferentiated elements have the worst prognosis.

Use of tumor cell markers in testicular tumors

The serum levels of AFP and β-unit of HCG should be measured before and after removal of any suspected testicular tumor, as these proteins are produced by many testicular germ-cell tumors.

- Trophoblastic germ-cell tumors have elevated levels of HCG.
- Yolk-sac tumors have elevated levels of AFP.
- 90% of patients with MTU/embryonal carcinoma have elevated AFP/HCG or both.
- 50% of patients with teratoma (immature/MTI) have elevated AFP/HCG or both.
- 10% of patients with seminoma have elevated HCG.

If tumor is confined to the testis (stage I), levels of marker will drop after orchidectomy. If levels do not fall, there is an indication of metastatic disease. In follow-up after treatment, increasing levels of a marker protein are an indication of tumor recurrence, often before tumor can be detected by imaging.

Lactic dehydrogenase (LDH) is a useful marker of tumor bulk, although the enzyme is ubiquitous and not specific for testicular germ-cell tumors. Serial LDH measurements allow the monitoring of the effects of therapy on tumor bulk.

Sex-cord and stromal tumors of the testis are less common than germ-cell tumors

Tumors may be derived from the non-germ-cell components of the testis (the interstitial Leydig cells and the Sertoli cells), but these are much less common than germ-cell tumors and account for about 5% of all cases. The testis may also be a site for development of primary lymphoma.

Leydig-cell tumors (also termed **interstitial cell tumors**) may occur at any age from childhood to late adult life. In childhood, tumors may cause precocious development of secondary sexual characteristics; in adults they often cause loss of libido and gynecomastia, reflecting secretion of either testosterone or estrogen, or both. Macroscopically, tumors appear circumscribed and are yellow (*Fig. 18.10*). They are composed of cells that resemble normal Leydig cells. Although the majority of tumors are benign, tumors over 5 cm in diameter, and those with mitoses, may behave in a malignant fashion.

Sertoli-cell tumors (also called **androblastoma**) may arise at all ages, including infancy, but have a peak incidence in the fourth decade. Typically, tumors are well circumscribed and are composed of cells resembling the normal Sertoli cells of the tubules. Most lesions are benign, but tumors with many mitoses may behave in a malignant fashion.

Primary lymphoma of the testis is mainly seen after the age of 50 years. Tumors are generally high-grade non-Hodgkin's lymphomas.

Spread of other tumors to the testis may be seen, particularly acute leukemias.

Testicular disease may result in male infertility

Male infertility is the result of failure of the production of mature motile spermatozoa. Initial tests involve analysis of a sample of semen for the presence of spermatozoa.

In some cases no spermatozoa are seen in the ejaculate. A number of conditions are recognized as being responsible, the most common being: destruction of testicular tissue

or scarring in ducts as a result of inflammatory disease, e.g. following infection; congenital absence of vas deferens or seminal vesicles; or the presence of cryptorchid testes. The chromosomal disorder, **Klinefelter's syndrome** (XXY), is associated with severe atrophy of testicular tubules and absent germ cells. Serum levels of FSH are elevated in cases of failure of the testis, in which case no function can be expected.

Other disorders are associated with abnormally small numbers of spermatozoa. Endocrine causes, particularly disease of the hypothalamic/pituitary axis and estrogen excess (endogenous or exogenous), must always be suspected. Germ cells are very sensitive to abnormal environment and are easily damaged; they are particularly sensitive to the effects of systemic chemotherapy and irradiation. For normal germ-cell development and maturation to take place, the testicular temperature should be lower than core temperature. Exposure to high temperature, either through maldescent or due to an environmental cause, may result in infertility.

In some cases the cause of reduced spermatozoa production is uncertain after investigation, and testicular biopsy may be performed for diagnosis. Sometimes the seminiferous tubules show a complete absence of germ cells, being lined only by Sertoli cells. Alternatively, early stages of spermatogenesis may be normal, but the late stages leading to the formation of mature spermatozoa are defective (so-called **maturation arrest**).

PROSTATE GLAND

The main diseases of the prostate are inflammatory disorders, hyperplasia and carcinoma

There are three important conditions of the prostate: **prostatitis** (which may be acute or chronic), **benign prostatic hyperplasia**, and **prostatic adenocarcinoma**. In younger men, disease of the prostate is mainly due to infections, some of which are sexually transmitted diseases. In older men, enlargement of the prostate is an almost universal phenomenon, most commonly due to prostatic hyperplasia, and leads to obstruction of the urinary outflow through the prostatic part of the urethra. Occasionally, clinically apparent prostatic urethral obstruction may be caused by development of carcinoma.

Prostatitis is mainly caused by infections that gain access from the urethra

Acute inflammation of the prostate usually follows acute infection in the bladder or urethra, and is particularly common following surgical instrumentation of the urethra. The usual causative organisms in older males are those that infect the bladder and urethra, particularly *E. coli* and *Proteus*. Sexually transmitted diseases may also cause prostatitis, particularly gonococcus and *Chlamydia* (a cause of

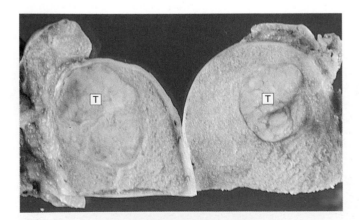

Fig. 18.10 Leydig-cell tumor of the testis.
A Leydig-cell tumor is seen as a well-circumscribed tumor (**T**), with a yellow cut surface.

non-gonococcal urethritis). Acute infections are characterized by the presence of a heavy neutrophilic infiltrate, often with abscess formation.

True infective chronic prostatitis is also associated with lower urinary tract infection, and results from inadequately treated acute prostatitis. A further cause of chronic prostatitis is TB, cases usually being associated with renal or epididymal TB. Chronic prostatitis usually shows an admixture of neutrophils with lymphocytes and plasma cells; in tuberculous cases there is a giant-cell histiocytic reaction, with focal caseation.

An uncommon pattern of chronic inflammation in the prostate is termed **malacoplakia**. This is due to infection by Gram-negative bacteria and there is an exuberant inflammatory response dominated by numerous macrophages and plasma cells. Organisms are phagocytosed by histiocytes, forming intracellular residual bodies which become calcified (Michaelis–Gutmann bodies). The exuberant inflammatory response may clinically simulate a tumor.

Benign prostatic hyperplasia affects most males over the age of 70 years

Benign prostatic hyperplasia is the most common disorder of the prostate. It affects almost all men over the age of 70 years, but is found with increasing frequency and severity from about the age of 45 years onwards. Clinically it presents with difficulty with micturition, due to compression of the prostatic urethra by the enlarging prostate gland. In most cases it is the two lateral lobes that are markedly enlarged. However, in some cases the posterior lobe shows the greatest enlargement, which may obstruct the urinary outflow tract at the internal urinary meatus at the bladder neck. Prolonged prostatic obstruction is the most common cause of chronic obstructive uropathy, and may lead to marked hypertrophy of the bladder wall, with trabeculation of bladder muscle, and acute or chronic retention of urine in the bladder. In such cases the failure to empty the bladder may lead to reflux of urine into the pelvicalyceal system, producing mega-ureter and hydronephrosis and predisposition to infection.

The pathogenesis of benign prostatic hyperplasia is not known, but it is believed to be due to androgen–estrogen imbalance (see pink box below). The area that is hormone sensitive, and that undergoes this pattern of hyperplasia, is the peri-urethral group of prostatic glands, not the true prostatic glands at the periphery. Continuing enlargement of the peri-urethral glands compresses the peripheral true prostatic glands, leading to their collapse, leaving only their fibrous supporting stroma behind.

Macroscopically the hyperplastic component of the prostate shows a nodular pattern of hyperplastic glandular acini separated by fibrous stroma (*Fig. 18.11*). Some of the nodules are cystically dilated and contain a milky fluid. Other nodules contain numerous calcified concretions (corpora amylacea). Histologically the acini are hyperplastic and tightly packed, lined by tall columnar epithelial cells with small basal nuclei, and the epithelium is sometimes thrown up into irregular papillary folds. Another component of the prostatic enlargement is muscular hypertrophy, particularly in the region of the bladder neck.

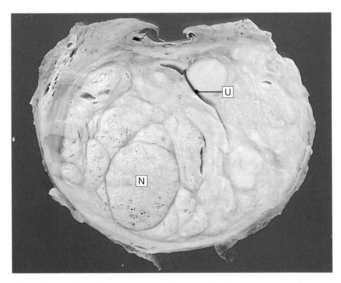

Fig. 18.11 Benign prostatic hyperplasia.
In prostatic hyperplasia the prostate is replaced by nodules of glandular tissue (**N**), which compress the prostatic urethra (**U**).

 Pathogenetic factors in prostatic hyperplasia

A metabolite of testosterone called **dehydrotestosterone** (DHT) is thought to be the main stimulator of growth of prostatic glands and stroma. This active testosterone derivative is produced focally in the prostate, probably in the stromal cells, by the action of an enzyme, 5α reductase, on circulating testosterone. DHT acts on both stromal and epithelial cells in the prostate to increase mitotic activity, probably by binding to nuclear receptors and stimulating the transcription of growth factors. Clinical studies with a 5α reductase inhibitor has shown a reduction in prostatic size in a percentage of cases. However, there are obviously many other factors involved including the possible role of estradiol levels, which increase with old age.

Carcinoma of the prostate is the second most common type of cancer in males

Carcinoma of the prostate is an important and common cause of malignancy in men, occurring with increasing frequency over the age of 55 years.

Carcinoma of the prostate is an adenocarcinoma with varying degrees of differentiation, which arises in the true prostatic glands at the periphery of the prostate. Local spread is therefore most likely to occur through the prostatic capsule, before the tumor infiltrates medially towards the urethra. For this reason, attempts to obtain biopsy samples of prostate to establish a diagnosis of malignancy by using the transurethral route may give false negative results; a needle biopsy of the outer prostate using a trans-rectal approach is more likely to be successful.

The etiology of this type of tumor is uncertain and, although tumors are often under endocrine control by testosterone, there is no evidence that endocrine imbalance is a primary causative factor. In the absence of any firm causative factors, no primary preventive strategies offer themselves for carcinoma of the prostate; efforts are therefore being directed to develop strategies for screening to detect early-stage disease.

Because of its peripheral origin, prostatic cancer is often well-established before the patient develops symptoms of difficulty with micturition due to urethral obstruction, and some tumors may remain silent, even in the presence of widespread metastases. Prostatic cancers can be divided into three groups on the basis of their behavior:

- **Invasive prostatic carcinomas.** Clinically important since they invade locally and metastasize.
- **Latent prostatic carcinoma.** These are small foci of well-differentiated carcinoma, frequently an incidental finding in the prostatic glands of elderly men. They appear to remain confined to the prostate for a long period.
- **Occult carcinomas** are clinically not apparent in the primary site, but present as metastatic disease.

Macroscopically, carcinomas of the prostate appear as diffuse areas of firm, white tissue, which merge into the fibromuscular prostatic stromal tissues. Distortion and extension outside the capsule of the prostate is common, producing a firm, craggy mass that can be palpated on rectal examination. Histologically, most lesions have a differentiated glandular pattern (good prognosis), a smaller proportion being composed of poorly differentiated sheets of cells having no acinar pattern (poor prognosis) (*Fig. 18.12*).

Carcinoma of the prostate metastasizes to bone and nodes and invades the bladder base

Prostatic carcinomas spread by three main routes:

- **Direct spread** to base of bladder and adjacent tissues. This causes obstruction of the urethra (difficulty in

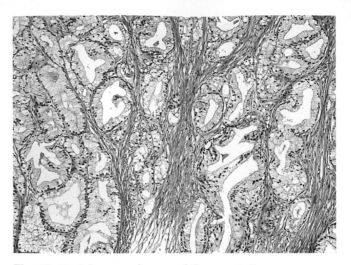

Fig. 18.12 Adenocarcinoma of the prostate.
This moderately differentiated adenocarcinoma of the prostate is composed of epithelial cells with clear cytoplasm, forming gland-like spaces.

micturition) and may block the ureters, causing hydronephrosis (see page 377).
- **Lymphatic spread** to pelvic and para-aortic nodes.
- **Vascular spread** to bone. Bone metastases by prostatic carcinoma may be sclerotic with bone production (dense on radiograph), rather than lytic with bone destruction.

Occasionally, the first manifestation of disease is from metastatic spread, for example compressing the spinal cord after vertebral metastasis. The pathological diagnosis of metastatic prostatic carcinoma is assisted by immuno-histochemical detection of prostate-specific antigen and prostate-specific acid phosphatase in biopsy material. These may also be used as serum markers for disease, levels being particularly raised when there is metastatic disease.

As many prostatic carcinomas are dependent on testosterone for growth, orchidectomy, or treatment with estrogenic drugs or agonists of luteinizing hormone-releasing hormone, may induce tumor regression.

PENIS AND SCROTUM

The penis and scrotum are sites for developmental, infective, dermatological, and neoplastic diseases

Malformations of the penis and penile urethra may occur, which are particularly associated with maldescent of the testes. Etiology is uncertain, but exposure to estrogens *in utero* has been suggested as a potential cause. For example, in **hypospadias** there is abnormal opening of the urethra onto the ventral surface of the penis, and in **epispadias** there is abnormal opening of the urethra onto the dorsal surface of the penis.

The penile urethra, which is lined by transitional-cell epitheliums, is part of the lower urinary tract, as well as being the conducting system for ejaculate from the genital system. The main abnormalities of the urethra are infections causing urethritis.

Gonococcal urethritis is caused by *Neisseria gonorrhoeae*, acquired as a sexually transmitted disease. It causes a purulent urethral discharge. If untreated, scarring may lead to development of a urethral stricture.

Non-gonococcal urethritis is mainly caused by *Chlamydia trachomatis* and *Ureaplasma urealyticum*. It causes a purulent urethral discharge and, in rare cases, disease may lead to development of Reiter's syndrome (arthritis, urethritis and conjunctivitis).

Phimosis is a condition in which the foreskin is abnormally tight and does not retract easily over the glans penis. A complication is inability to release the foreskin after it has been retracted, causing painful swelling of the glans (**paraphimosis**). Inflammation of the glans, which is termed **balanitis**, may be caused by a variety of bacterial organisms, being predisposed by poor hygiene or phimosis.

The penis is prone to develop a number of skin diseases, e.g. lichen planus, psoriasis, viral warts, and molluscum contagiosum. Some of these skin diseases are discussed in Chapter 23.

In **balanitis xerotica obliterans** (BXO) the foreskin becomes abnormally thickened and scarred, resulting in phimosis. This is a primary inflammatory skin condition, identical in pathology to the vulval and skin disease **lichen sclerosus** (see page 396).

The penile mucosa is the site of original infection in **sexually transmitted diseases** such as syphilis (the chancre, see page 115). and *Herpes genitalis*. In the latter, typical herpetic blisters form on the glans penis. A particular type of viral infection seen on the penis and around the perineum is **condyloma acuminatum**, caused by one of the human papilloma viruses; the warts have a cauliflower-like appearance. Although uncommon in western countries, ulcerated lesions on the penis may be caused by *Haemophilus ducreyi* (chancroid), *Calymmatobacterium granulomatis* (granuloma inguinale) and *Chlamydia trachomatis* (lymphogranuloma venereum).

The most important neoplastic lesion of the penis is **squamous cell carcinoma**. This develops either as a well-differentiated keratinizing invasive form, usually seen in elderly men, or as the non-invasive carcinoma *in situ* form (Queyrat's erythroplasia), presenting as a red patch or indurated plaque, similar to intraepidermal carcinoma of the skin. There is a spectrum of changes from dysplasia to carcinoma *in situ*, grouped together as **penile intraepithelial neoplasia** (PIN); many cases are associated with human papillomavirus infection. Invasive squamous cell carcinoma occurs most commonly in uncircumcized men, presenting as a warty cauliflower-like growth that bleeds easily. It tends to grow slowly, but is often neglected because of patient embarrassment; the most common site of spread is to the inguinal lymph nodes via lymphatics.

The skin of the scrotum is a common location for a number of skin disorders including epidermal cysts, nodular calcinosis cutis, and some inflammatory skin diseases such as psoriasis. It is the site of an unusual type of superficial venous infarction known as 'Fournier's gangrene'.

The most important tumor of the scrotum is invasive squamous carcinoma. This is now rare, but was of importance historically because of its known association with the occupation of chimney sweep.

Gynecological and obstetric pathology

Clinical Overview

The normal functioning and diseases of the female genital tract form a large component of clinical practice. Students in training will experience the factors involved in antenatal care, normal delivery (spontaneous and assisted), postnatal care, and probably the techniques of assisted artificial conception. Understanding these requires a knowledge of anatomy, physiology and biochemistry, but little in the way of pathology. However, not all conceptions, pregnancies and deliveries run a smooth normal course, and a section in this chapter (**Obstetric pathology** – see page 415) outlines the main clinical problems and their underlying pathology.

Abnormalities of the female genital tract which are not directly related to conception, pregnancy or childbirth are called **gynecological pathology,** and form the bulk of this chapter. A large part of a gynecologist's clinical practice is associated with bleeding from the genital tract and pain, usually due to disorders of menstruation which can have many causes (e.g. benign abnormalities of endometrium or myometrium), but sometimes due to the important tumors **carcinoma of the endometrium** (in post-menopausal women) and **carcinoma of the uterine cervix** (mainly in pre-menopausal women).

Early detection of carcinoma of the uterine cervix before it becomes an invasive tumor is based upon the regular microscopic examination of smears taken from the surface epithelium of the cervix (**cervical cytology**). There are, however, many other simple benign causes of non-menstrual bleeding from the female genital tract, particularly benign **polyps** of the endometrium and uterine cervix.

The main pathological conditions affecting the ovaries are benign and malignant cysts and solid tumors. Hormonal dysfunction of the ovaries is usually manifest as disorders of menstruation or problems with conception and pregnancy.

The vulva is composed of skin, and is heir to many of the diseases of skin at other sites, including allergic and contact dermatitis, psoriasis, epidermal cysts, benign nevi, viral warts, and the malignant tumor **squamous cell carcinoma**. Three skin conditions which are particularly common in the vulva are **lichen sclerosus**, **lichen planus** and **lichen simplex chronicus**. Most inflammatory skin diseases of the vulva present clinically with itching, soreness and irritation.

The vagina is relatively free of pathology, with the exception of infections including sexually transmitted diseases.

GYNECOLOGICAL PATHOLOGY

DISEASES OF THE VULVA

The vulva is frequently affected by skin diseases, often not recognized or diagnosed by gynecologists

The labia majora and minora are skin, and subject to a wide range of skin diseases, particularly inflammatory skin disease, causing pruritus and soreness. One of the most frequent, and often misdiagnosed, is **acute contact dermatitis** (**allergic dermatitis**, *Fig. 19.1*) following the use of topical applications such as deodorants, creams and ointments used for the treatment of vulval irritation and soreness (particularly antiseptic or disinfectant solutions and creams).

There is an enormous range of materials which can cause contact dermatitis in the vulva, including soap, detergents in shower gels and bubble baths, detergents used in washing underwear, and constituents of various cosmetics including perfumes, etc. Even rubber and chemicals in contraceptives and nail varnish may produce an allergic type of dermatitis as may, ironically, local anesthetic creams and topical steroids given as treatment.

Other types of inflammatory skin disease can also affect the vulva, e.g. psoriasis, (see page 489), seborrheic dermatitis (see page 488), drug rashes of various types (see page 497) and blistering diseases (see page 493). Careful history taking, combined with examination of the rest of the skin will often enable a diagnosis to be made. Unfortunately, gynecologists rarely examine the rest of the patient, and often miss the diagnosis.

Lichen simplex chronicus is a pattern of chronic dermatitis which produces thickening of the vulval skin

Constant repeated frictional trauma, almost always due to the repeated scratching of a chronically itching vulva, causes thickening of the epidermis by proliferation of squamous keratinocytes (acanthosis), thickening of the overlying keratin layer (hyperkeratosis), and fibrosis of the underlying dermis – for clinical and histological details see page 487 and *Fig. 23.2*. This condition is erroneously called 'hypertrophic vulval dystrophy' by gynecologists and gynecological pathologists, a term which should be abandoned. Proper management is based on the investigation and treatment of the underlying cause of the original itching, often a contact or allergic dermatitis, or one of the specific inflammatory skin diseases which particularly affect the vulva, lichen sclerosus or lichen planus.

Lichen sclerosus is an important skin disease and commonly affects the vulva

Lichen sclerosus results in epidermal atrophy and densely collagenous upper dermal fibrosis. The condition has a particular predilection for the skin in the genital area, occurring frequently in the vulva, and less commonly in the penis (balanitis xerotica obliterans, see page 393). It presents as white papules or confluent patches, which are covered by atrophic epidermis in which telangiectatic blood vessels are prominent (*Fig. 19.2*). The histology is identical to that seen in affected skin elsewhere, with compact hyalinization of the upper dermis with an underlying lymphocytic infiltrate.

Long-standing inadequately treated lichen sclerosus may lead to severe scarring and narrowing of the introitus,

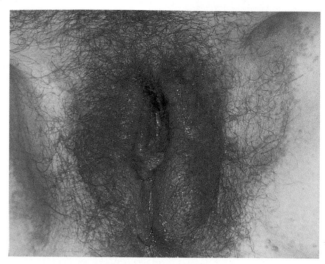

Fig. 19.1 Acute contact dermatitis.
The labia majora and minora are red, swollen and sore-looking, and the redness also involves the groin. This is due to a local contact dermatitis to a disinfectant solution.

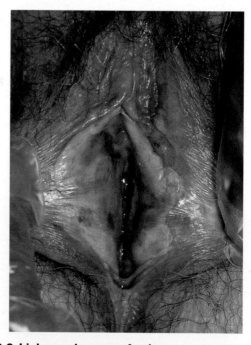

Fig. 19.2 Lichen sclerosus of vulva.
This vulva shows extensive, thick, white patches due to collagenous thickening, overlaid by an atrophic epithelium.

and is a predisposing factor to the eventual development of squamous carcinoma. Chronic scratching of lichen sclerosus lesions may produce co-existent lichen simplex chronicus, a combination inaccurately called 'mixed vulva dystrophy', another term to be dispatched to oblivion.

Lichen planus is a common inflammatory condition of the skin which frequently affects the vulva; the diagnosis is often missed

In the vulva, the lesions may resemble those seen in the skin at other sites, raised purplish plaques and patches, particularly on the labia majora. However, on the labia minora it is frequently clinically different, producing very sore superficial red weeping erosions (see *Fig. 19.3*). This pattern can also be seen in the other common orificial site of lichen planus, the mouth. The disease may be confined to the vulva, but careful history taking and examination of the skin elsewhere will usually reveal current skin lesions or evidence of past skin or oral involvement with lichen planus.

Like lichen sclerosus, lichen planus is curable with strong topical steroids if diagnosed clinically and histopathologically; hence vulval biopsy to establish or confirm an accurate diagnosis is an important part of the management of such cases. Also like lichen sclerosus, some cases of vulval lichen planus are clinically and histologically modified by lichen simplex chronicus due to repeated scratching. Long-standing under-treated lichen planus may also predispose to the development of squamous carcinoma.

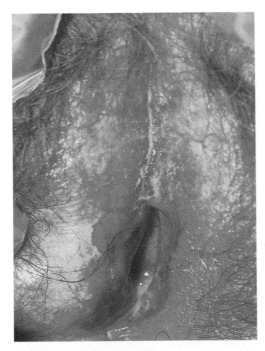

Fig. 19.3 Erosive lichen planus.
The labia show reddening and there is an area of red denudation of mucosa, producing an erosion. This is typical of the erosive pattern of lichen planus.

Most infections of the vulva are caused by viruses or fungi

The vulval skin is frequently involved with infective disease, usually due to viruses and fungi. Viral infections of the vulval skin are due either to herpes virus or to the human papillomavirus (HPV). Fungal infections are usually caused by superficial dermatophytes or *Candida*.

Herpes vulvitis produces initially painless blisters, which subsequently break down to form a painful, sore, eroded area. The herpes virus is acquired through sexual contact, and the disease is therefore mainly seen in young women.

HPV (human papillomavirus) is also sexually transmitted and may be associated with thickening of vulval skin and mucosa in the labia minora (**flat condyloma**), or may present as multiple protuberant warts (**condylomata acuminata**), which are either sessile or pedunculated. HPV strains 6 and 11 are responsible for most vulval lesions. There is a strong link between HPV infections of the vulva and intraepithelial neoplastic change in the vulva (see page 398) and cervix (see page 401).

Fungal infections of the vulva are mainly due to *Candida albicans*. There is usually associated fungal vaginitis, presenting with a copious vaginal discharge and vulval reddening and soreness. The infection and its manifestations are often severe in diabetics. Infection of vulval skin with dermatophytic fungi also produces similar superficial inflammation and soreness.

Sexually transmitted disease affecting the vulva can be caused by a number of different types of organisms

In addition to sexually transmitted herpes virus and HPV, a number of other organisms can produce vulval lesions as a result of sexually transmitted infection, although many of them are confined to tropical countries. Among the most important are *Calymmatobacterium granulomatis*, which causes **granuloma inguinale** and produces ulcerating nodules on the vulva, and *Chlamydia trachomatis*, which causes **lymphogranuloma venereum** with ulcerating vulval papules and enlarged inguinal lymph nodes.

Haemophilus ducreyi causes **chancroid**, with multiple tender papules and ulcerating nodules on the vulva, associated with tender enlargement of the inguinal lymph nodes.

Treponema pallidum is the causative organism of **syphilis**. The lesions are small, indurated vulval or vaginal papules (chancre) in the first stage (representing the site of entry of the organism), and multiple moist, warty, vulvovaginal and perineal lesions (condylomata lata) in the second stage.

Benign cysts on the vulva are common and may be derived from skin or Bartholin's glands

The hair-bearing skin component of the vulva may be the site of formation of benign keratin-filled epidermal cysts similar to those seen elsewhere in the skin. Bartholin's glands are mucus-secreting glands in the posterior part of the labia majora. They discharge their secretions into the vestibule through short ducts that are normally lined by transitional-cell epithelium, although squamous-cell metaplasia is common. Cystic dilatation of the ducts and glands may result from duct obstruction, the cysts being lined by mucus-secreting columnar epithelium, transitional or squamous epithelium, or a mixture.

The most important malignant tumor of the vulva is squamous-cell carcinoma

Squamous carcinoma of the vulva, which usually occurs in elderly women, may show extensive local invasion

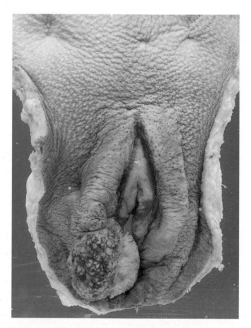

Fig. 19.4 Verrucous carcinoma of the vulva. This radical vulvectomy specimen shows a verrucous carcinoma that has invaded the right labium majus.

and metastases in inguinal lymph nodes. One variant in very old women, **verrucous carcinoma**, produces a large, warty, cauliflower-like growth that grows slowly, invading local tissues, but almost never metastasizes (*Fig. 19.4*). Well-differentiated squamous carcinomas of the vulva have a good prognosis provided that they are confined to the vulva and inguinal nodes; the prognosis is worse if there is local invasion to other pelvic organs (e.g. bladder, rectum), metastatic tumor in iliac lymph nodes, or evidence of blood-borne metastasis.

Although most invasive squamous carcinomas of the vulva appear to arise *de novo*, some arise in epithelium in which there is severe dysplasia amounting to carcinoma *in situ* (*Fig. 19.5*). This phenomenon, **vulval intraepithelial neoplasia** (**VIN**), is generally seen in patients younger than those with invasive tumors, and there may be co-existent evidence of HPV warty change in the affected and adjacent epithelium. Furthermore, HPV16 can be demonstrated in many cases of VIN. Although invasive carcinoma and VIN do occasionally co-exist in elderly women, it is thought that progression of VIN to invasive carcinoma is not common.

Other neoplastic lesions of the vulva are mainly melanocytic lesions or skin appendage tumors

Apart from squamous-cell carcinomas, other tumors arising in the vulva are derived from melanocytes or skin appendages. Benign intradermal and compound nevi are common on the vulval skin, and the labia majora are an important site for the development of malignant melanoma. The features of both benign nevi and malignant melanoma are identical to those occurring in the skin (see Chapter 23). Although any of the skin-appendage tumors described in Chapter 23 can occur in the skin of the vulva, only **papillary hidradenoma** (derived from the eccrine ducts) is frequently seen.

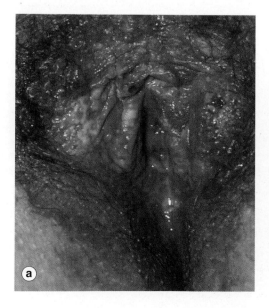
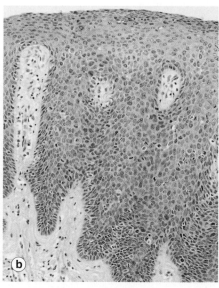

Fig. 19.5 Vulval intraepithelial neoplasia (VIN).
In (a) there is very extensive red thickening of the vulva, extending onto the perineum and peri-anal region. This is due to extensive VIN. In the micrograph (b) the full thickness of the vulval epithelium shows dysplastic squamous cells, with many mitoses (VIN III).

Rarely, Paget's disease of the vulva may occur, representing intraepidermal spread of a carcinoma derived from an adenocarcinoma of skin appendages. It is histologically similar to the disease of the nipple.

DISEASES OF THE VAGINA

The most important diseases of the vagina are infections (vaginitis)

The vagina can become infected by the same agents that cause vulvitis, e.g. herpes simplex virus, HPV, *Candida albicans*, *Gardnerella vaginalis*. The vagina has an abundant natural bacterial flora, the principal organism in which is *Lactobacillus acidophilus*. This produces lactic acid by the breakdown of glycogen in the surface vaginal epithelium, thereby creating an acid environment in which most other organisms cannot proliferate. However, this barrier only works effectively against bacteria. Infective vaginitis is usually sexually transmitted, presenting with vulvovaginal soreness and discharge.

Trichomonas vaginalis is a common cause of vaginitis in young women and is usually sexually transmitted. The vaginal mucosa becomes red and inflamed, with a frothy white discharge on its surface.

Gardnerella vaginalis is a very common cause of nonspecific vaginitis, commonly associated with a thin, milky white vaginal discharge.

Herpes simplex produces erosive vaginal lesions, and the organism may be transmitted to the fetus during passage through the birth canal. Usually, there are associated vulval herpetic lesions.

Candida albicans is a normal commensal in the vagina, but its proliferation is usually suppressed by the normal vaginal flora. Clinical infection can occur when the vaginal flora is destroyed, e.g. by antibiotics. White plaques of fungal hyphae develop on an inflamed vaginal mucosa, and there is vaginal discharge associated with severe vulval irritation. Infection may be severe in patients with diabetes mellitus.

Less common causes of vaginal infection include the gonococcus (usually secondary to gonococcal cervicitis), *Mycoplasma*, and HPV (usually associated with extensive vulval and perineal condylomata which extend up the vagina at a late stage), and some forms of staphylococci. Staphylococci are usually introduced into the vagina with a tampon, and proliferation of bacteria in a neglected or retained tampon may lead to production of bacterial exotoxins, giving rise to the **toxic shock syndrome**.

Primary tumors of the vagina are very rare

Primary tumors of the vagina in adults are exceptionally rare, but the vagina is frequently the site of metastases, particularly from malignant tumors of the cervix, endometrium and ovary. Vaginal bleeding after hysterectomy for uterine or ovarian malignancy should always be investigated and biopsied because of the frequency of metastatic tumor in the residual vaginal vault.

The main primary vaginal tumors are **squamous-cell carcinomas** and, even more rare, adenocarcinomas. Clear-cell carcinoma of the vagina is seen in women exposed *in utero* to the synthetic estrogen diethylstilboestrol, preceded by replacement of normal vaginal epithelium by glandular epithelium, termed vaginal adenosis.

In childhood the vagina may be the site of development of **rhabdomyosarcoma**, which macroscopically appears as a polypoid, gelatinous mass protruding into the vagina.

DISEASES OF THE CERVIX

The cervix is an important site of pathology, particularly in women of reproductive age. The ectocervix is covered by squamous epithelium, and the endocervical canal by mucus-secreting columnar epithelium, which shows glandular downgrowths. At various stages in a woman's reproductive life, the junction between the squamous and columnar epithelium migrates onto the convexity of the ectocervix, then back into the endocervical canal. This **squamocolumnar junction** is the seat of most of the epithelial diseases that occur in the cervix.

The original squamocolumnar junction is usually located in the region of the external os, but its precise location at birth is influenced by exposure to maternal hormones *in utero*.

Around puberty, hormonal influences cause extension of the columnar epithelium onto the ectocervix, forming an **ectropion** or **cervical erosion** (*Fig. 19.6*). This process is augmented by a first pregnancy, particularly when it occurs shortly after menarche.

Before puberty, the pH of the vagina and cervix is alkaline, but afterwards bacterial breakdown of glycogen in the vaginal and cervical squamous epithelium renders it an acidic environment, the pH being about 3.

Exposure of the sensitive columnar epithelium of the ectropion to the post-pubertal acidic environment of the vagina induces squamous metaplasia and a transformation zone between the endocervical columnar epithelium and the ectocervical squamous epithelium. This zone is composed of new squamous epithelium in an area previously occupied by columnar epithelium.

Thus the squamocolumnar junction is of variable size, but its site always approximates to the external os. In older women it may retreat into the endocervical canal.

The most important diseases of the cervix are listed in *Fig. 19.7*.

Chronic cervicitis is produced by the same organisms responsible for infective vaginitis

The term 'chronic cervicitis' is sometimes applied inaccurately by clinicians when the area of ectocervix around the external os is red and irregular; in most cases this is not inflammation, but represents the extension of columnar epithelium onto the external os, sometimes called **ectropion** or, inaccurately, a 'cervical erosion'.

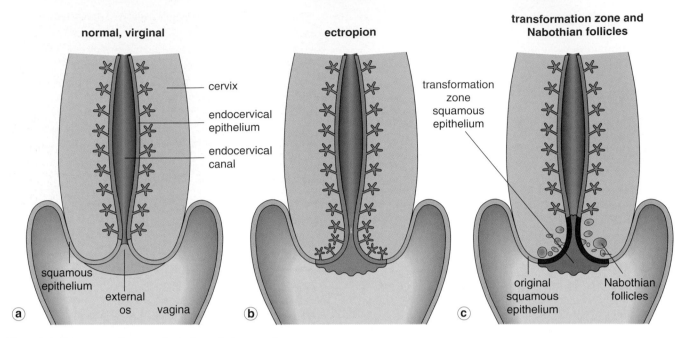

Fig. 19.6 Squamocolumnar junction of the cervix.
The mobility of the squamocolumnar junction, the development of ectropion, and the formation of the transformation zone are illustrated. (a) The squamocolumnar junction is originally situated in the region of the external os. (b) At puberty the endocervical epithelium extends distally into the acid environment of the vagina, forming an ectropion. (c) A transformation zone forms as squamous epithelium regrows over the ectropion. The openings of the crypts may be obliterated in the process, which leads to the formation of mucus-filled Nabothian follicles.

Fig. 19.7
The most important diseases of the cervix

Chronic cervicitis
Cervical polyp
Microglandular endocervical hyperplasia
Leiomyoma
Wart-virus change due to HPV
Intraepithelial neoplasia
Invasive carcinoma of the cervix
Adenocarcinoma of the endocervix

Acute cervicitis with erosion may be seen in herpes simplex infection, and there is usually herpetic disease of the vulva and vagina. Genuine chronic endocervicitis, with a heavy lymphocytic and plasma cell infiltrate, may be found in association with infections of the vagina by *Trichomonas*, *Candida*, *Gardnerella* and the gonococcus.

Microglandular endocervical hyperplasia is mainly seen in pregnancy and in women taking oral contraceptives with a progestogen component

Microglandular endocervical hyperplasia is a common cervical change, which is induced by hormonal changes. It is a pattern of endocervical proliferation in which the cervical crypts multiply and become architecturally disordered,

sometimes associated with decidual change in the stroma. This change is seen particularly during pregnancy, and is the result of progestogen stimulation of the endocervix; however, the changes may persist after the removal of the causative stimulus. It is also seen in women taking oral contraceptives containing progestogen.

The lesion may be asymptomatic, but there is often a complaint of an excessive mucous vaginal discharge, and in severe cases the cervix looks to be the seat of numerous small endocervical polyps.

Cervical polyps are a common cause of intermenstrual bleeding

Cervical polyps are common abnormalities which, through erosion and ulceration, may cause intermenstrual bleeding. They are seen in about 5% of women. Macroscopically they appear smooth, rounded or pear-shaped, and are typically 1–2 cm in diameter. The polyps derive from the endocervix, protruding from the cervix through the external os. They are composed of endocervical stroma and glands, the latter often being distended with mucus. The surface of the polyp may show ulceration and inflammation and, if long-standing, there may be surface squamous metaplasia.

Benign tumors of the cervix are uncommon, the most frequent being leiomyomas

True benign neoplasms of the cervix are uncommon, most nodules associated with the cervix being endocervical polyps. Leiomyomas may occur in the cervix, but are less common at this site than in the uterus (see page 409, *Fig. 19.19*). Derived from the smooth muscle of the cervix wall, they expand the cervix asymmetrically, producing distortion and compression of the endocervical canal.

HPV infection is common in the ectocervical epithelium and is an important etiological agent in cervical cancer

HPV infection of the cervix is sexually acquired. Over 70 sub-types of HPV have been defined, each of which has been allocated a number.

Occasionally, HPV infection may produce papillary lesions of cervical squamous epithelium (**condyloma acuminatum**), which are similar to those seen on the vulva (see page 397). They are usually located on the ectocervical squamous epithelium or on the squamous epithelium of the transformation zone, and may be multiple.

More often, HPV infection causes **flat condylomas**. These cannot normally be seen with the naked eye, but may be recognizable on colposcopic examination after painting the cervix with dilute acetic acid, which turns them white.

Histologically the epithelium in flat condylomas is abnormal, with binucleate cells (particularly in the upper layers of the epithelium), and so-called 'koilocytic change' in the most abnormal epithelial cells (*Fig. 19.8*). These viral changes can be recognized on cervical-smear cytology. Both patterns of wart-virus involvement of the cervical squamous epithelium are most frequent in the transformation zone epithelium, and may co-exist with changes of intraepithelial neoplasia.

Different types of HPV are differently associated with invasive carcinoma of the cervix:

- HPV 16 and 18 are frequently associated.
- HPV 6 and 11 are rarely associated.
- HPV 31, 33, and 35 are uncommonly associated.

Despite the frequent association of HPV 16 and 18 with development of carcinoma, it must be emphasized that of all women harbouring these infections, only a small minority go on to develop carcinoma.

Cervical intraepithelial neoplasia is an important precursor of invasive malignancy

The metaplastic epithelium of the transformation zone is susceptible to change during reproductive life. Mild degrees of nuclear enlargement can be seen in response to chronic inflammation, in reparative epithelium, and in association with HPV infection. However, more severe atypia is now regarded as a pre-neoplastic proliferation and is called **cervical intraepithelial neoplasia** (CIN) (*Fig. 19.9*). This change takes place in the metaplastic epithelium of the transformation zone of the cervix and is usually associated with infection by HPV.

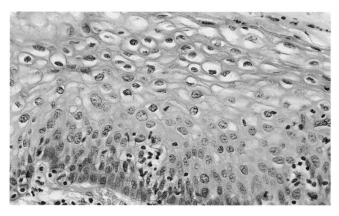

Fig. 19.8 Wart-virus change in the cervix.
The cervical epithelium shows the characteristic features of wart-virus change in a 'flat condyloma' from the transformation zone; the epithelium is atypical, with koilocytes in the upper layers of the epithelium.

Three grades of severity are recognized, dependent upon what proportion of the thickness of the cervical epithelium is replaced by atypical cells.

CIN I corresponds to mild dysplasia. Atypical cells are confined to the lower third of the epithelium, the upper two-thirds showing normal differentiation and maturation with flattening of cells.

CIN II corresponds to moderate dysplasia. Atypical cells occupy the lower half of the epithelium, but evidence of differentiation and maturation with flattening of cells is seen in the upper half. Nuclear abnormalities may extend through the full thickness of the epithelium, but are most marked in the lower half, where there may be increased mitoses with some abnormal forms.

CIN III corresponds to severe dysplasia and carcinoma *in situ*. Atypical cells extend throughout the full thickness of the epithelium, with minimal differentiation and maturation on the surface. Mitotic figures and abnormal mitoses are present through all layers, and there may be extension of the change along endocervical crypt necks, and foci of true microinvasion.

Histological appearances of typical CIN patterns are shown in *Figs 19.9b* and *c*.

These abnormal epithelial changes occur in the transformation zone, but may extend over the ectocervical surface and up the endocervical canal. In about 10% of cases, atypia termed **cervical glandular intraepithelial neoplasia** (CGIN) is also seen in endocervical epithelium.

The presence of abnormal epithelial cells can be detected by cytological examination of a smear of surface epithelial cells removed from cervix; this is the basis of screening for disease (see blue box on page 402).

CIN I is associated with a small risk of progression to carcinoma, CIN II and CIN III being associated with higher risk of development of carcinoma. The natural history of CIN is important, as it determines how often screening is required to detect progression of disease.

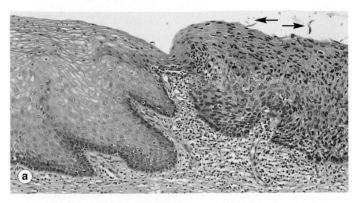

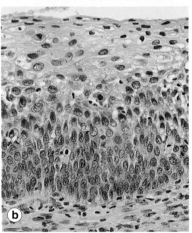
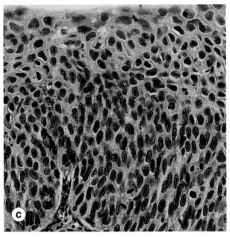
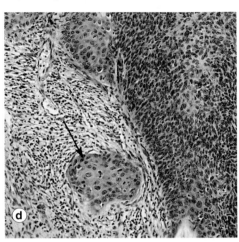

Fig. 19.9 Cervical intraepithelial neoplasia.
(a) shows the junction between normal ectocervical epithelium and severe full-thickness CIN. Note the ease with which the abnormal epithelial cells from the atypical epithelium can desquamate (arrows); this forms the basis of diagnostic exfoliative cytology. (b) shows mild/moderate atypia of cervical epithelium (CIN I–CIN II). The atypical cells are confined to the deeper parts of the epithelium but cells at the surface show maturation with flattening. (c) shows moderate/severe atypia of cervical epithelium (CIN II–CIN III). Atypical cells with pleomorphism and mitotic activity extend through the full thickness of the epithelium. (d) shows foci of early microinvasion (arrow) arising in an area of CIN III.

Diagnostic cervical cytology

The development of abnormalities in the cervical epithelium is an important factor in the prevention of subsequent invasive carcinoma of the cervix. Detection of abnormal cells is based on the presence of abnormal cytology. Using a specially shaped spatula, cells are scraped from the ectocervix and lower cervical canal and smeared onto a slide. They are fixed in a preservative solution and sent to a pathology laboratory for cytological examination after the addition of Papanicolaou stain (the origin of the term 'Pap smear'). In CIN, the exfoliated cells have an increased nuclear:cytoplasmic ratio and a clumped, irregular chromatin pattern, being termed **dyskaryotic** (*Fig. 19.10*).

If atypical epithelial cells are detected in a cervical smear, patients are recalled. The site of abnormal epithelium is identified by colposcopy, and the diagnosis confirmed by biopsy of the abnormal area. If the lesion is non-invasive and completely visible, not extending high up into the endocervical canal, ablation of the atypical area can be performed using laser or cryotherapy.

If the topmost edge of the lesion cannot be seen in the endocervical canal, the lesion has to be removed as part of an excision biopsy.

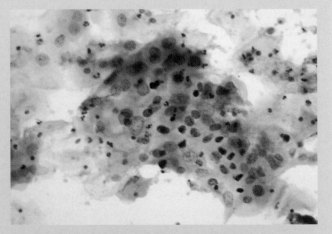

Fig. 19.10 Cervical cytology smear in CIN.
This cytology preparation shows a clump of cervical epithelial cells demonstrating moderate and severe dyskaryosis.

- 50% of patients with CIN I have spontaneous regression of disease.
- 30% of patients with CIN I have persistent low-grade atypia.
- 20% of patients with CIN I progress through CIN II to CIN III over a period of about 10 years.
- 20% of patients with CIN III progress to develop invasive carcinoma of the cervix within 10 years.

It has been suggested that smears repeated every three years are adequate for the purposes of population screening. Despite this frequency, it is still possible for some individuals to progress from CIN I to invasive carcinoma in a short space of time.

Invasive carcinoma of the cervix is most commonly squamous-cell carcinoma

Invasive carcinoma of the cervix may occur at any time during the reproductive and post-menopausal years, but the average age of development is about 50 years. It accounts for 3–5% of cases of carcinoma in females.

Macroscopically, early lesions appear as areas of granular irregularity of the cervical epithelium, progressive invasion of the stroma causing abnormal hardness of the cervix. Late lesions appear as fungating, ulcerated areas, which destroy the cervix (*Fig. 19.11*).

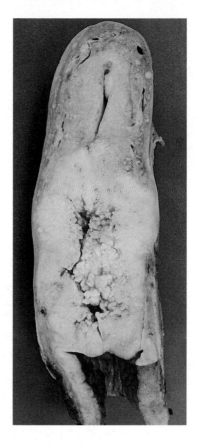

Fig. 19.11 Invasive squamous carcinoma of the cervix.
In this hemi-section through the uterus, cervix and upper vagina, a fungating lesion has completely destroyed the cervix and is invading the lower part of the body of the uterus.

Risk factors in cervical squamous-cell carcinoma

Sexual intercourse: very low incidence in virgins; more frequent in married women than in single women.

Age at first intercourse: higher incidence in women who have intercourse before the age of 17, and in those who marry early (presumably also a reflection of earlier intercourse).

Sexually transmitted diseases: higher incidence in women with a history of sexually transmitted disease, and also in prostitutes (see HPV below).

Socioeconomic status: incidence higher in the lower social groups, but this may be related to life-style and sexual habits rather than any other factor.

Smoking: epidemiological studies suggest a link between heavy smoking and cervical carcinoma, particularly CIN. Although it is difficult to rule out other factors such as different social and sexual life-styles in smoking and non-smoking women, depression of local immune surveillance by Langerhans' cells has been suggested as important.

Male factors: to explain the importance of sexual intercourse, carcinogenic agents have been sought in smegma, spermatozoa and other components of the semen, but no definite evidence of a chemical carcinogen has been found.

HPV: the co-existence of HPV with CIN and invasive carcinoma, seen frequently in cone biopsy and colposcopy specimens, suggests a link. Furthermore, the identification of DNA from HPV types 16, 18 and 33 in more than 60% of cervical carcinomas strongly suggests a link and possible causative factor. This is currently an area of intense research. Proteins produced by HPV inactivate products of tumor suppressor genes, thereby facilitating tumor development.

HIV infection: carcinoma of the cervix is predisposed by immunosuppression and has increased in incidence as a consequence of AIDS.

Other infective agents: attempts to prove a role for infective agents such as *Chlamydia* and *Herpes simplex* have been inconclusive, the link usually being no stronger than the fact that both diseases are the result of sexual intercourse.

The vast majority of carcinomas of the cervix are **squamous-cell carcinomas**, arising from the transformation zone or ectocervix. Lesions fall into three histological patterns: keratinizing squamous-cell carcinoma, non-keratinizing large-cell squamous carcinoma, and non-keratinizing small-cell squamous carcinoma.

Although squamous-cell carcinoma of the cervix is predisposed by a variety of factors, the common denominator is sexual activity, suggesting that exposure to environmental agents (particularly infection) is most important.

Adenocarcinoma of the cervix is less common than squamous carcinoma, but may be increasing in incidence

Adenocarcinoma of the cervix is almost always derived from the mucus-secreting columnar epithelium lining the endocervical canal, and may be preceded by adenocarcinoma *in situ*. Both invasive and *in situ* carcinoma can be detected by cervical smear cytology. Invasive adenocarcinomas comprise 5–10% of all primary malignant tumors of the cervix; there is evidence of an apparent increase in incidence, but this may be largely explained by a reduction in the incidence of invasive squamous carcinomas. Compared with invasive squamous carcinoma, adenocarcinoma tends to metastasize to lymph nodes earlier and to be less radiosensitive; it is generally regarded as having a worse prognosis.

Prognosis of squamous cell carcinoma of the cervix is related to stage at diagnosis

The common presenting symptom is vaginal bleeding in the early stages, but advanced neglected tumors may cause urinary obstruction due to bladder involvement.

The histological type of the tumor is less important for prognosis than is the staging at diagnosis. Microinvasive carcinomas show minute foci of very superficial invasion, only detected histologically, and have a very good prognosis after local excision. Invasive carcinomas are staged according to the degree of local invasion, and survival is related to stage (*Fig. 19.12*). Invasion of paracervical and external iliac nodes occurs early.

DISEASES OF THE ENDOMETRIUM

The endometrium lines the uterus, responding to cyclical hormonal stimulation during the menstrual cycle. The morphology of the endometrium can be used as a reliable index of the phase of the menstrual cycle. The main diseases of the endometrium include morphological changes in response to endocrine effects, inflammatory diseases causing endometritis, polyps, hyperplasia (divided into several types and important in predisposing to neoplasia), tumors (epithelial tumors, mostly carcinomas and rarer tumors of endometrial stroma), endometriosis (a condition in which endometrium grows outside the uterus), and adenomyosis (a condition in which endometrium grows down into the muscle of the uterine wall).

Fig. 19.12
Stage and 5-year survival for carcinoma of the cervix

Stage	5-year survival	Degree of local invasion
I	90%	Confined to cervix
II	75%	Invasion of upper part of vagina or adjacent parametrial tissues
III	30%	Spread to pelvic side wall, lower vagina or ureters
IV	10%	Invasion of rectum, bladder wall or outside pelvis

Morphological changes reflecting endocrine defects are commonly seen in the endometrium

Histological examination of the endometrium is frequently undertaken as part of the investigation of disordered menstruation or infertility. The histological pattern of endometrium is correlated with the stated last date of menstrual period and with any relevant drug therapy.

Among the most common abnormalities encountered in clinical practice is **senile atrophy**, seen after the menopause. Glands are simple, lined by inactive cuboidal cells and may form large cystic spaces. There is no evidence of mitotic activity, reflecting lack of estrogenic stimulation.

Anovulatory cycles are common at the start and end of reproductive life. They are associated with irregular menstruation. The effects of excessive estrogen stimulation are manifest in the endometrium as proliferation of glands.

Luteal-phase defect or irregular ripening is associated with infertility. This may be caused by failure of production of progesterone by the corpus luteum, or by defective receptors for progesterone within endometrium. Examination of the endometrium in the second half of the menstrual cycle shows inadequate or absent development of secretory changes in the endometrium.

Persistence of the corpus luteum at the end of the normal menstrual cycle causes failure of normal endometrial shedding, leading to abnormal uterine bleeding. Examination of the endometrium reveals a mixed pattern of menstrual-phase, secretory-phase and proliferative-phase patterns.

Oral contraceptive pills cause changes in the structure of the endometrium, which is greatly reduced in bulk. Glands become small and inactive, with poor development of the stroma.

Intrauterine contraceptive devices (IUCDs) are sometimes associated with chronic endometritis and *Actinomyces* infection.

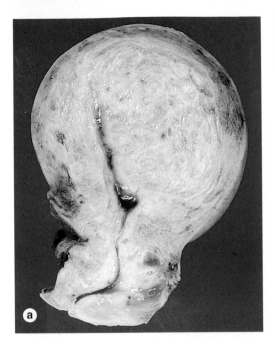

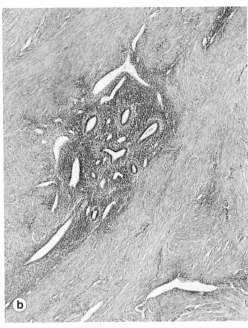

Fig. 19.13 Adenomyosis of the uterus.
(a) In this uterus, removed because of heavy, irregular and painful periods, the myometrium is expanded as a result of severe adenomyosis, particularly posteriorly. The islands of endometrium can be seen as yellowish brown areas surrounded by hypertrophied smooth muscle (nodular adenomyosis). (b) Histology of an area of endometrial glands and stroma within hypertrophied myometrium, taken from the specimen in (a).

Metaplasia of the endometrium is usually seen in post-menopausal women, arising less commonly in normal cycling endometrium. The main types are squamous metaplasia and metaplasia to epithelial patterns resembling tubal or endocervical epithelium.

Acute endometritis is usually encountered as a complication of pregnancy

Acute endometritis is characterized by infiltration of endometrial glands by neutrophils. Caused by bacterial infection, it is usually seen as a complication of parturition or miscarriage. The organisms most commonly responsible are streptococci, staphylococci and clostridia, which are often associated with anaerobic organisms when there is retained dead tissue within the uterine cavity *post partum*.

In severe cases of acute inflammation, a **pyometra** may develop when the uterine cavity is filled with pus. This is the consequence of obstruction of the cervical os, complicated by infection of the uterine cavity. The main reasons for obstruction of the cervix are tumors, and scarring as a result of previous surgical intervention.

Chronic endometritis is usually associated with recent gestation, pelvic inflammatory disease, or IUCDs

Chronic endometritis may be associated with menstrual irregularities, but is also found in women who are being investigated for infertility. Histologically the endometrium shows lymphoid infiltration, with formation of plasma cells. The majority of cases are associated with a definite clinical risk factor for developing inflammation. The condition occurs after recent pregnancy, miscarriage or instrumentation in 50% of cases, in association with pelvic inflammatory disease (e.g. salpingitis) in 25% of cases, and

in association with previous use of IUCDs in about 20% of cases. In the remaining 5% of cases without a defined risk factor, chronic endometritis may be caused by gonococcal or chlamydial infection, or TB.

In tuberculous endometritis, because granulomas form only in secretory endometrium, they may not be seen in samples taken from early in the cycle. The condition is commonly part of more widespread infection involving fallopian tubes.

In adenomyosis, endometrium burrows deep within the wall of the uterus

Adenomyosis is a condition in which endometrium grows down to develop deep within the myometrium. The condition may cause enlargement of the uterus and is sometimes associated with menstrual abnormalities and dysmenorrhea.

Macroscopically, small, irregular, pink areas, some with small cysts, are seen in the affected myometrium (*Fig. 19.13a*). Histologically, islands of endometrium are seen deep within muscle (*Fig. 19.13b*). If traced, these deep islands are found to be in continuity with surface endometrium. This process may affect the myometrium diffusely or may occur focally, producing apparently circumscribed nodules of hypertrophied muscle and deep endometrium (**nodular adenomyosis**).

Ectopic growth of endometrium outside the uterus is termed 'endometriosis'

Endometriosis is a condition in which ectopic endometrium develops outside the uterine cavity. It affects 1 in 15 (7%) women of reproductive age, with associated infertility in about 30% of cases. The pathogenesis is discussed in the pink box on page 406.

Pathogenesis of endometriosis

The reason for the development of endometriosis remains uncertain, but there are three main theories:

1 **Retrograde menstruation.** In normal women it is well documented that fragments of endometrium migrate into the peritoneal cavity along the fallopian tube at the time of menstruation. It has been proposed that this material implants in some cases, causing endometriosis, and that although in normal women the immune system destroys such implanted endometrium, in women susceptible to endometriosis the immune surveillance is absent.

2 **Metaplasia of peritoneal epithelium** may cause it to differentiate to form endometrium. Metaplasia may also cause development of tubal-pattern epithelium, causing the related condition of endosalpingosis. The stimulus for such metaplasia remains uncertain.

3 **Metastatic spread of endometrium.** This theory suggests that endometrium found in nodes, pleura, lung and umbilicus has been spread by lymphatics or blood vessels.

None of these hypotheses alone explains endometriosis in all of its manifestations, and it is likely that all three mechanisms are operative to differing degrees.

It is well established that endometriosis is dependent on estrogen for continued growth and proliferation, with disease becoming inactive after oophorectomy or onset of the menopause. This is the rationale for treatment that induces a hypo-estrogenic state by suppression of the hypothalamic–pituitary–ovarian axis with analog of gonadotrophin-releasing hormone (GnRH).

The common sites for ectopic endometrial growth are ovaries, fallopian tubes, round ligaments, and pelvic peritoneum. Less common sites are intestinal wall, bladder, umbilicus, and laparotomy scars. Rarely, involvement of lymph nodes, lung and pleura is seen.

The ectopic endometrium still responds to cyclical hormonal stimulation, with phases of proliferation and breakdown with bleeding. The bleeding and breakdown stimulate the formation of fibrous adhesions and accumulation of hemosiderin pigment.

Macroscopically, foci of endometriosis appear as cystic and solid masses, which are characteristically dark brown from iron pigment accumulated as a result of repeated bleeding. Histologically, endometrial glands and stroma are seen, together with fibrosis and macrophages containing iron pigment.

Endometrial tissue growing in abnormal sites stimulates fibrosis and may cause fibrous adhesions between adjacent organs. When peritoneum is involved, adhesions may cause bowel obstruction. The condition usually presents with cyclical pelvic pain, dysmenorrhea, and infertility. When it affects the fallopian tubes and ovaries, the whole of the fallopian tube and ovary may be converted to a cystic mass containing brown, semi-liquid material (chocolate cyst).

Treatment by endocrine manipulation of endometrial growth is usually effective.

Endometrial polyps are localized overgrowths of endometrial glands and stroma

Endometrial polyps are very common and are usually seen in the peri-menopausal age range. They are thought to be caused by over-proliferation of glands in response to

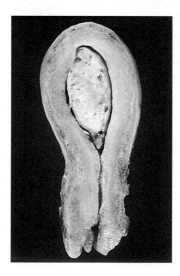

Fig. 19.14 Benign endometrial polyp. The microcystic appearance is due to cystically dilated endometrial glands within the polyp.

estrogenic stimuli. Macroscopically they vary in size but are usually 1–3 cm in diameter and are usually sited in the uterine fundus. They appear as firm smooth nodules within the endometrial cavity (*Fig. 19.14*), occasionally prolapsing through the cervical os.

Histologically they are made up of cystically dilated endometrial glands in a vascular stroma. They are clinically associated with menstrual abnormalities and dysmenorrhea, but may develop ulceration or undergo torsion.

Endometrial hyperplasia is caused by estrogenic stimulation and may be pre-neoplastic

Endometrial hyperplasia is seen in response to estrogenic stimulation. An endogenous response may be seen with

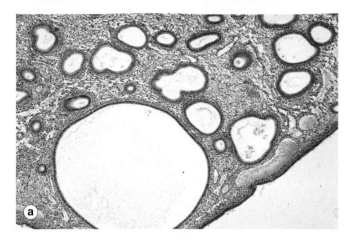

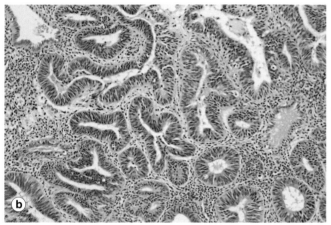

Fig. 19.15 Endometrial hyperplasia.
(a) This endometrium shows simple hyperplasia, with cystic dilatation of glands showing no other architectural or cytological atypia. (b) This endometrium shows complex atypical hyperplasia, with irregular branching glands and dark-staining epithelium due to cytological atypia.

successive anovulatory cycles or estrogen-secreting tumors, and an exogenous response with estrogen-containing drugs.

The importance of endometrial hyperplasia is that it is associated with an increased risk of development of adeno-carcinoma of the endometrium. There are several histo-logical types, **simple hyperplasia** being the most common pattern, diffusely affecting the whole endometrium. Proliferation of glands can be seen, with evident mitoses and stratification of cells. Glands grow in a regular tubular pattern, but are often dilated (*Fig. 19.15a*); however, there is no cytological atypia of the nuclei. This type is associated with a very slightly increased risk of malignancy after a long period of time, typically over 10 years.

Complex hyperplasia is almost always seen focally within the endometrium. There is obvious proliferation of epithelium, evident by mitotic figures, but the glands grow in an irregular pattern, with branched irregular contours and little intervening stroma. The cells forming the glands do not show cytological atypia. This type is associated with a slightly increased risk of development of malignancy.

Complex atypical hyperplasia is commonly seen only focally within the endometrium. Like complex hyperplasia, there is proliferation of epithelium, evident by mitotic figures, and the glands grow in an irregular pattern, with branched irregular contours (*Fig. 19.15b*). However, the cells forming the glands show cytological atypia, with pleo-morphism and hyperchromatism. About 30% of cases with this pattern of hyperplasia will develop a carcinoma of the endometrium, usually within 5 years of diagnosis.

Endometrial carcinoma is the most common cancer of the female genital tract

Carcinomas of the endometrium are nearly all adeno-carcinomas, with several histological sub-types. This type of carcinoma is the most frequent invasive malignancy in the female genital tract, accounting for about 7% of all tumors in women. Endometrial carcinoma can be divided into two main groups:

- Tumors that occur at a time close to menopause, associated with endometrial hyperplasia and abnormal estrogenic stimulation of the endometrium. This is the largest group and is associated with a generally good prognosis.
- Tumors that occur in older, post-menopausal women, not associated with estrogenic stimulation or endometrial hyperplasia. Tumors in this group are more often associated with a poor prognosis.

Macroscopically, small tumors appear as diffuse, solid areas or polypoid lesions in the endometrium, whereas larger tumors fill and distend the endometrial cavity with soft, white, friable tissue (*Fig. 19.16a*). Necrosis of tumor is common and leads to a frequent presenting feature of post-menopausal bleeding.

Most tumors associated with estrogenic excess are **endometrioid adenocarcinomas** (60% of all cases). These can be graded (I–III) according to the amount of glandular and solid pattern with tumor (*Fig. 19.16b*). A high grade is associated with worse prognosis. In some cases, areas of squamous metaplasia or true squamous carcinoma (**adenosquamous carcinoma**) are also present.

Two other main types of tumor are seen, mostly in the non-estrogen-related post-menopausal group. **Uterine papillary serous carcinoma** is a highly aggressive tumor. Even in the absence of significant myometrial or vascular invasion, recurrence, widespread metastasis and death may occur. **Uterine clear-cell carcinoma** also behaves in a highly malignant fashion.

Spread of carcinoma of the uterus is mainly by local inva-sion. In cases of **direct invasion** a factor that has a close correlation with prognosis is invasion into the myometrium. Tumors with a small depth of invasion have a better prognosis than those showing involvement of most of the thickness of the myometrium. Progressive local invasion leads to parametrial involvement and later spread to bladder and rectum.

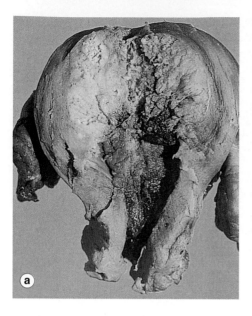

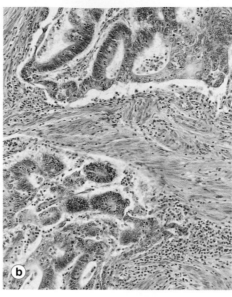

Fig. 19.16 Endometrial adenocarcinoma.
(a) The endometrial cavity is distended by soft, friable endometrial adenocarcinoma, showing necrosis and hemorrhage. There is considerable depth of invasion, the tumor being close to penetrating the serosal surface at the fundus of the uterus. (b) Histology of the tumor in (a) shows a moderately differentiated endometrioid type of adenocarcinoma (the most common type) extensively invading the smooth muscle of the myometrium.

Fig. 19.17
Surgical stage of endometrial carcinoma, and outcome after treatment with surgery and radiotherapy

Stage	Proportion of cases		5-year survival
I	80%	Corpus of uterus only	75%
II	5%	Corpus and cervix	52%
III	5%	Invasion confined to pelvis	30%
IV	10%	Invasion outside pelvis or involves bladder or rectal mucosa	10%

Spread along lumen of fallopian tubes leads to frequent involvement of ovaries, and with **venous and lymphatic invasion** there may be involvement of the vagina and para-aortic nodes. Widespread hematogenous metastasis is uncommon, except with papillary serous carcinomas and clear-cell carcinomas. The prognosis of carcinoma of the uterus is related to stage, as outlined in *Fig. 19.17*.

Tumors of endometrial stroma may be pure or seen as part of mixed tumors

Under 2% of all uterine tumors involve neoplastic proliferation of the stromal element of the endometrium. These tumors are thought to be derived from primitive Müllerian cells that can variably differentiate into endometrial stroma, epithelium, or support tissues. Tumors present as expansile masses within the uterine cavity, causing post-menopausal bleeding; with the more malignant tumors, there is evidence of dissemination.

Pathogenesis of endometrial carcinoma

In the peri-menopausal age group, the majority of endometrial adenocarcinomas are associated with hyperestrogenism and endometrial hyperplasia. Hyperestrogenism may be exogenous or endogenous in origin.

Clinical associations carrying a higher risk of development of adenocarcinomas are obesity (due to endogenous production of estrogen in adipose tissue), diabetes mellitus, nulliparity, and hypertension.

An increased incidence of endometrial carcinoma is also seen in some families, in which it is associated with an increased risk of breast cancer, and the occurrence of dominant-acting oncogenes seems likely in this group. Mutation of K-*ras* oncogene is a common event in the development of about 10% of sporadic endometrial cancers. Abnormality in p53 is also a common event.

Endometrial stromal sarcoma is composed of malignant stromal spindle cells and can be graded from low to high.

Adenosarcoma contains malignant stroma and a histologically benign epithelial component. Tumors commonly recur after hysterectomy.

Carcinosarcoma (malignant mixed Müllerian tumor) has both malignant stromal and epithelial components. Often the stromal component contains tissues not normally seen in the uterus, e.g. cartilage, fat and skeletal muscle. This typically occurs in elderly women and has an extremely poor prognosis (*Fig. 19.18*).

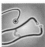

Diagnosis of endometrial disease

The diagnosis of endometrial disease is aided by several imaging and histological techniques.

- **Transvaginal ultrasonography** can indicate lesions within the uterus, and establish the thickness of endometrium.
- **Hysteroscopy** may identify endometrial polyps or submucosal myomas.
- **Endometrial biopsy** is frequently performed, for example, to distinguish anovulatory from ovulatory bleeding and to exclude a hyperplastic condition or a carcinoma.

Endometrial biopsy by pipette aspiration removes a small sample. This procedure may be performed as a clinic or office procedure without anesthetic.

Cervical dilatation and curettage (D and C) of endometrium is a means of obtaining a large sample of endometrium, but requires a general anesthetic. Material may be sent for culture (establishing cause of endometritis) or histology.

In the evaluation and staging of tumors, **MR imaging** is increasingly being used to establish the extent of tumor spread preoperatively.

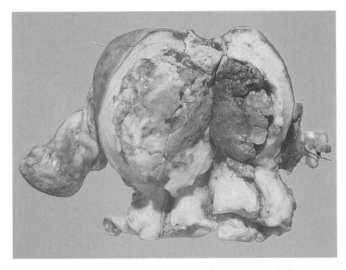

Fig. 19.18 Malignant mixed Müllerian tumor of the endometrium. The endometrial cavity is greatly distended by a soft, fleshy, partly necrotic and hemorrhagic tumor. This old lady presented with post-menopausal bleeding, abdominal distension and pain, and had pulmonary and peritoneal metastases at the time of diagnosis.

DISEASES OF THE MYOMETRIUM

The myometrium is composed of smooth muscle. Apart from changes in pregnancy, the myometrium is affected in adenomyosis (see page 405) and by tumors (either leiomyomas or, rarely, leiomyosarcomas and adenomatoid tumors).

Leiomyomas (fibroids) are the most common tumors of the uterus

Leiomyomas, also called fibroids, are the most common benign tumors of the female genital tract. They affect over half of all women over the age of 30, usually becoming symptomatic in the decade before the menopause.

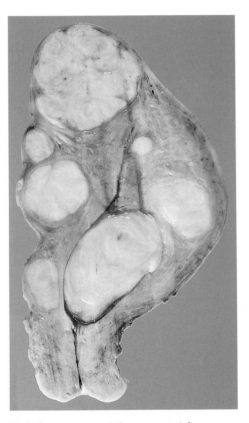

Fig. 19.19 Leiomyomas of the myometrium.
This patient presented with heavy, irregular, painful periods. The uterus is distorted by multiple well-circumscribed benign leiomyomas in intramural, subserosal and submucosal sites.

Macroscopically, leiomyomas appear as rounded, rubbery, pale nodules, which have a whorled appearance on cut surface. They may arise in several locations within the uterus (e.g. intramural, submucosal and subserosal) and are very commonly multiple (*Fig. 19.19*).

Leiomyomas vary in size, ranging from under 1 cm in diameter to giant lesions that are 20–30 cm in size. The typical diameter for lesions responsible for clinical problems is 2–4 cm.

Histologically, tumors are composed of smooth-muscle cells and intervening collagenous stroma. Importantly, there is no cellular atypia and very few mitoses are seen. Several uncommon histological variants of leiomyoma are also described, characterized by unusual cellular or stromal patterns, e.g. myxoid change.

Degenerative changes and complications occur in these tumors. For example, tumors may outgrow their blood supply, becoming replaced by hyaline material, as well as undergoing calcification. In pregnancy, and less commonly at other times, tumors may develop ischemic degeneration in which lesions become soft and uniformly dark red (so-called 'red degeneration'). Pedunculated tumors may undergo torsion, developing venous infarction.

Clinically these tumors are associated with abnormal menstrual bleeding, dysmenorrhea, or infertility. Occasionally they cause problems because of their effects as a large abdominal mass, e.g. compressing the bladder. During pregnancy, leiomyomas may cause complications such as spontaneous abortion, premature labor, and obstruction of labor.

Uterine leiomyomas depend on the trophic action of estrogen for maintenance of size, and tumors usually shrink after the menopause. Treatment with GnRH-agonists, which induce hypoestrogenism, is being used to cause shrinkage of the uterus and fibroids to allow easier surgical removal by myomectomy. For most women who no longer wish to conceive, the treatment is to have a hysterectomy.

Leiomyosarcomas of the uterus are a tumor of the post-menopausal age group

Overall, leiomyosarcomas of the uterus are uncommon, accounting for about 2% of all tumors in the female genital tract. They arise most frequently in the post-menopausal age group.

Macroscopically tumors are typically large, fleshy masses within the myometrium, which may be necrotic. They are usually around 10–15 cm in diameter. Histologically tumors are composed of smooth-muscle cells but, in comparison with a benign tumor, there is greater cellularity, with mitoses and nuclear hyperchromatism. The single most useful assessment in deciding whether a smooth-muscle tumor is benign or malignant is to perform a mitotic count. Lesions with high mitotic counts are regarded as being biologically malignant. In between those lesions with very high or very low counts are borderline lesions termed 'smooth-muscle tumors of uncertain malignant potential'.

As with most sarcomas, leiomyosarcomas of the uterus tend to metastasize preferentially by vascular spread, particularly causing pulmonary metastases.

DISEASES OF THE FALLOPIAN TUBES

The fallopian tubes run from the endometrial cavity, through the wall of the uterus, forming the fimbriated end applied to the ovaries, which is responsible for guiding released ova into the uterus.

The main diseases of the fallopian tubes are inflammatory diseases (e.g. salpingitis), uncommon tumors of the epithelium and smooth-muscle wall, and ectopic pregnancy (see page 417). Post-inflammatory scarring and obliteration of the fallopian tube is an important and common cause of infertility.

Salpingitis is an important cause of late tubal obstruction and infertility

Salpingitis is nearly always caused by infection that has gained access by ascending from the uterine cavity. Most cases result in acute salpingitis with acute inflammation, but others result in a chronic inflammatory reaction. The main associations for salpingitis are following pregnancy and endometritis, IUCD use, sexually transmitted disease (*Mycoplasma*, *Chlamydia* and gonococcus), TB and *Actinomyces*.

In cases of acute salpingitis, the tubes are macroscopically swollen and congested, with a red, granular appearance to the serosal surface, due to vascular dilatation. Histologically the lumen may contain pus and there is infiltration of the tubal epithelium by neutrophils. With resolution, chronic inflammation may supervene, associated with distortion of mucosal plicae, fibrosis and occlusion of the tubal lumen. A **pyosalpinx** occurs when there is massive distension of the tubal lumen by pus.

Chlamydial colonization of the tubal mucosa is increasingly being recognized as a cause of impaired tubal function in infertile women and a common cause of ectopic pregnancy. This is usually in the absence of symptoms and laparoscopic signs of active infection. The histological correlates of such infection are uncertain.

Tuberculous salpingitis is acquired by hematogenous spread from a site outside the genital tract. The tubes develop multiple granulomas in the mucosa and wall, causing adhesions to adjacent tissues (especially ovary). In advanced cases the tube may be converted to a cavity filled with caseous necrotic material.

Infection by *Actinomyces* is predisposed by colonization of the female genital tract in association with IUCD use. The pus in the tubal lumen contains colonies of *Actinomyces*, visible macroscopically as 'sulfur granules'.

In many cases of infection of the fallopian tube, adhesions form between the tube and the ovary, and infection involves the tube, ovary and adjacent parametrial tissues. This situation gives rise to a matted clump of tissue and fibrosis, referred to as a **tubo-ovarian mass**, in which individual components are hard to discern.

Hydrosalpinx is dilatation of the fallopian tube, with flattening of the mucosa, the lumen being distended by

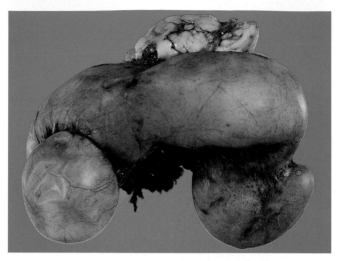

Fig. 19.20 Fallopian tube showing hydrosalpinx.
The fallopian tube is distended, very thin-walled, and contains clear fluid. It is convoluted and distorted by fibrous scarring, the result of healing of previous inflammation (salpingitis).

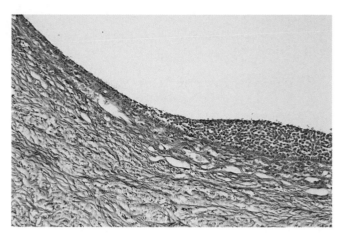

Fig. 19.21 Follicular ovarian cyst.
This micrograph shows part of the wall of a small follicular cyst, in which follicle granulosa cells can be seen lining the wall.

clear, watery fluid. This is believed to be a sequel to previous inflammatory damage to the tube, acquired with healing of previous inflammation (*Fig. 19.20*).

Tumors of the fallopian tube are very uncommon

Neoplastic lesions of the fallopian tube are rare, but among those that do occur are benign adenomatoid tumors, encountered in the mesosalpinx, and primary adenocarcinomas, seen in post-menopausal women. As the latter are usually seen at an advanced stage, they generally have a poor prognosis.

In addition, tumors of the endometrium may spread up the tubal lumen, and metastatic disease in the pelvic peritoneum may involve the tubal serosa. Small cysts at the fimbrial end of the fallopian tube are common and, generally, clinically silent.

DISEASES OF THE OVARIES

The ovaries are paired organs attached to the back of the broad ligament. The important components of the ovary are surface 'germinal' epithelium, stroma responsible for production of many steroid hormones, and follicles containing the germ cells.

The main diseases of the ovary are non-neoplastic cysts, stromal hyperplasia, and tumors (there is a wide variety of benign and malignant lesions derived from epithelium, stroma, or germ cells).

Non-neoplastic cysts of the ovaries are common

Non-neoplastic cystic lesions in ovaries are extremely common, the majority arising from development of Graafian

follicles, others being derived from surface epithelium. Among the main types are **mesothelial-lined inclusion cysts**, which are small lesions ranging from microscopic up to 3–4 cm in diameter. They are lined by cells that are the same as those of the ovarian surface epithelium, and are filled with clear fluid.

Follicular cysts are derived from ovarian follicles and are lined by granulosa cells, with an outer coat of thecal cells (*Fig. 19.21*). Cysts are, by definition, over 2 cm in diameter. In some cysts the thecal coat becomes luteinized. Although most cysts are clinically insignificant, some may be a cause of hyperestrogenism.

Corpus luteum cysts are caused by failure of involution of the corpus luteum. Cysts are typically 2–3 cm in diameter, with a thick, yellow lining of luteinized granulosa cells. There is continued production of progesterone, resulting in menstrual irregularity.

Theca-lutein cysts are usually seen as multiple bilateral cysts, up to 1 cm in diameter, filled with clear fluid. They are caused by high levels of gonadotrophin, which precipitates follicle development (e.g. in hydatidiform mole and drug treatment).

Endometriosis may be the cause of cystic ovarian lesions filled with dark brown, iron-containing fluid (see page 405).

Stromal hyperplasia is a cause of virilization in post-menopausal women

Hyperplasia of the ovarian stroma associated with luteinization is commonly seen in the ovaries of post-menopausal women. Ovaries are usually enlarged and have a firm texture, being replaced by proliferated stromal cells. Clinically, affected women often show virilization, as the stromal cells produce androgens.

Hyperplasia of the stroma is also seen in association with a variety of neoplastic and non-neoplastic growths within the ovary, and may be associated with endocrine effects.

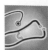

Polycystic ovary syndrome (Stein–Leventhal syndrome) is a common cause of infertility

The polycystic ovary syndrome is an important and common cause of infertility. Patients are obese, hirsute, and have acne and menstrual abnormalities (amenorrhea or irregular periods). The ovaries show thickening of the capsule, and multiple follicular cysts with stromal hyperplasia (*Fig. 19.22*).

The pathogenesis of this syndrome is still uncertain. Patients have a persistent anovulatory state, high levels of LH and estrogen, low levels of FSH with high levels of circulating androgen produced by the ovary. There is insulin resistance and hyperinsulinism. The high estrogen levels may cause endometrial hyperplasia and increase the risk of development of endometrial carcinoma.

It is not uncommon to see luteinizing hormone-driven ovarian hyperandrogenism, acne, anovulation, oligomenorrhea, and large, multifollicular ovaries in early to mid puberty, arising as a self-limited maturational stage in development. However, it is not possible to tell if this is a precursor of polycystic ovary syndrome in a proportion of cases.

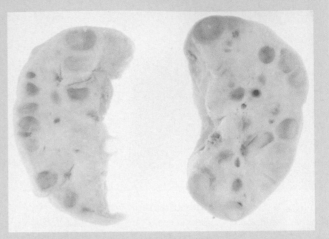

Fig. 19.22 Polycystic ovary syndrome (Stein–Leventhal syndrome). These ovaries from a patient with Stein–Leventhal syndrome show enlargement by multiple follicular cysts, which are particularly arranged around the periphery, together with thickening of the ovarian stroma.

NEOPLASTIC DISEASE OF THE OVARIES

Primary tumors of the ovary may be derived from any of the normal cellular constituents of the ovary. They are divided into those derived from surface epithelium (70%), those from sex-cord and stromal cells (10%), and those from germ cells (20%).

In addition to primary tumors, the ovary is frequently involved in metastatic disease from other sites. Malignant tumors of ovary spread locally and particularly seed to peritoneum, when ascites is an important complication.

Epithelial tumors of the ovary can differentiate into several types

The epithelial tumors of the ovary are derived from the surface epithelium which is, in turn, derived from embryonic coelomic epithelium. Tumors with this origin differentiate into a variety of tissues.

- **Endocervical differentiation:** mucinous ovarian tumors.
- **Tubal differentiation:** serous ovarian tumors.
- **Endometrial differentiation:** endometrioid and clear-cell ovarian tumors.
- **Transitional differentiation:** Brenner tumors.

In histological assessment of epithelial tumors of the ovary, it can be difficult deciding which lesions are benign and which are malignant. In between those tumors that are obviously benign or malignant are some cases in which there are histological features of atypical cells and abnormal tissue architecture, but no evidence of invasion. Such lesions are termed '**tumors of borderline malignant potential**'. Most borderline tumors behave in a benign fashion, the remainder behaving as low-grade malignant tumors.

Serous tumors of the ovary contain watery fluid and are often bilateral

Benign serous tumors of the ovary (70%) are termed **serous cystadenomas** (*Fig. 19.23a*). These thin-walled, unilocular cysts contain watery fluid and are bilateral in about 10% of cases. Histologically they are lined by a cuboidal, regular epithelium in which small papillary projections may be seen. A related tumor, termed an **adenofibroma**, is a benign, sometimes solid and sometimes cystic (cystadenofibroma) tumor, composed of benign serous epithelium and spindle-cell stroma.

Malignant serous tumors of the ovary are termed 'serous cystadenocarcinomas' (*Figs 19.23b* and *c*). These are the most common form of ovarian carcinoma and are bilateral in about half of all cases. Macroscopically, tumors may be cystic, mixed solid and cystic, or largely solid in appearance. Histologically they are composed of cystic cavities lined by columnar and cuboidal cells, with papillary proliferations of cells and solid areas. Cells are pleomorphic and mitoses are seen. Importantly, invasion of the ovarian stroma does occur, confirming the malignant character. These lesions are associated with an overall 20% 5-year survival.

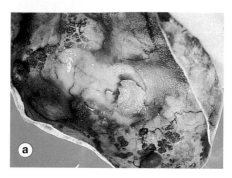
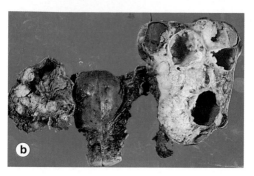
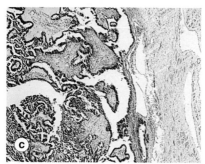

Fig. 19.23 Serous tumors of the ovary.
Benign serous cystadenomas are thin-walled, unilocular cysts bearing small papillary projections (a). The malignant counterpart of (a) is the serous cystadenocarcinoma (b), showing a mixed solid and cystic pattern. Note that the tumors are bilateral, a frequent feature. Histology of the tumor in (b) shows the papillary pattern of adenocarcinoma (c), with papillary fronds covered by pleomorphic atypical epithelium.

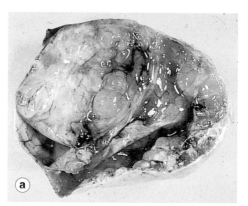
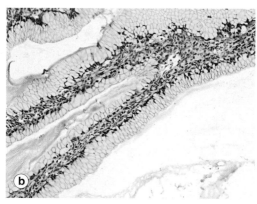
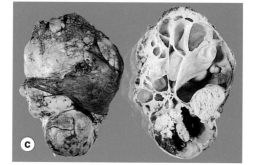
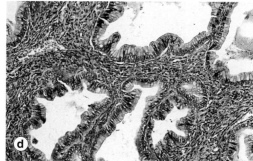

Fig. 19.24 Mucinous tumors of the ovary.
In (a) a fresh, unfixed, benign mucinous tumor of the ovary has a characteristic multilocular cystic appearance and a shiny mucoid content. Histology of a cyst wall shows well-differentiated, tall, columnar epithelium (b), with basal nuclei, and luminal cytoplasm distended with mucin, which is also present in the cyst cavity space. Like the benign tumor in (a), the malignant mucinous cystadenocarcinoma in (c) is multilocular, but the solid areas in the walls of some cysts are malignant. Histology from one of the solid areas in (c) shows that the epithelium is much more pleomorphic and less well differentiated (d) than that seen in the benign tumor (b).

Borderline serous tumors of the ovary are bilateral in about 30% of cases. Macroscopically, tumors may be cystic, or mixed solid and cystic. Histologically they are composed of cystic cavities lined by columnar and cuboidal cells, with papillary proliferations of cells and solid areas. Cells are pleomorphic and mitoses are seen. However, invasion of the ovarian stroma does not occur, despite the presence of cellular atypia. These lesions are associated with an overall 75% 10-year survival.

Mucinous tumors of the ovary are usually multilocular and contain gelatinous material

Benign mucinous tumors of the ovary are multilocular cystic lesions that contain glutinous viscid mucoid material

(*Figs 19.24a* and *b*). They are bilateral in only 5% of cases. Histologically the cysts are lined by a single layer of columnar, mucin-secreting cells with regular nuclei and no atypical features or mitoses.

Malignant mucinous tumors of the ovary, termed **mucinous cystadenocarcinomas** (*Figs 19.24c* and *d*) are bilateral in 25% of cases. These tumors may occur in young women, and the median age at diagnosis is 35 years. Macroscopically they are multilocular cystic lesions that contain viscid or gelatinous mucoid material. They may grow to a very large size. Solid areas may be seen in the walls of some cysts. Histologically the tumors are composed of columnar, mucin-secreting cells, which show heaping of nuclei, solid areas, pleomorphism and mitoses. Importantly, invasion of ovarian stroma is seen, confirming the malignant nature of the lesion. Overall survival is 34% at 10 years.

Borderline mucinous tumors of the ovary are bilateral in 10% of cases. Apart from the fact that there is no evidence of invasion of ovarian stroma, they resemble mucinous cystadenocarcinomas macroscopically and histologically. Overall survival is 90% at 10 years.

Endometrioid tumors of the ovary are usually malignant and often bilateral

Benign and borderline endometrioid tumors are uncommon, the vast majority of cases being malignant (**endometrioid carcinomas**). These account for 20% of ovarian carcinomas and are bilateral in about 40% of cases. Clear-cell carcinomas of the ovary are a variant of endometrioid carcinomas, characterized by cells that have clear cytoplasm and contain abundant glycogen. Overall, endometrioid carcinomas have a 40% 5-year survival.

Mixed Müllerian tumors are composed of both epithelial and stromal elements, including cartilage and skeletal muscle. These lesions are also considered a variant of endometrioid carcinoma and have an extremely poor prognosis.

Brenner tumors of the ovary contain transitional-type epithelium, as well as a spindle-cell stroma

Brenner tumors are composed of nests of epithelium resembling transitional cell epithelium of the urinary tract, associated with a spindle-cell stroma. Macroscopically,

lesions are solid and have a firm, yellowish white cut surface. Histologically, nests of transitional cell epithelium are separated by a spindle-cell stroma. The epithelial component may vary from histologically benign to highly atypical, allowing pathological classification into benign, borderline, and malignant Brenner tumors.

There are several forms of sex-cord stromal tumors of the ovary

About 10% of ovarian tumors are derived from the stromal cells and sex-cord cells of the ovary. As several of this group secrete estrogen, patients may develop endometrial hyperplasia and a predisposition to endometrial neoplasia.

Fibromas are benign tumors, usually seen in postmenopausal women. They are tough, whorled, white lesions composed of spindle cells and collagen. This type of tumor may be accompanied by ascites and pleural effusion in under 1% of cases (**Meigs' syndrome**).

Thecomas are solid tumors composed of the spindle cells of the ovarian stroma. These stromal cells are commonly functional, producing estrogen. Macroscopically, tumors are yellow due to the cellular content of lipid (*Fig. 19.25*). The vast majority of lesions are benign.

Some lesions show features of fibroma with focal areas developing features of thecoma (**fibrothecoma**). This reflects a common origin of both fibroma and thecoma from the spindle cells of the ovarian stroma.

Granulosa-cell tumors are composed of the granulosa cells derived from follicles. Around 75% secrete estrogen and present with signs of hyperestrogenism. Macroscopically, tumors are soft and yellow, and can vary in size from a few centimeters to large masses. If confined to the ovary, they are associated with an excellent prognosis. If tumors are large

Molecular pathology of ovarian carcinoma

Like many carcinomas, ovarian carcinomas are associated with several oncogene abnormalities, which increase in number with high-grade tumors. For example, p53 and *Ki-ras* mutations are not seen in benign epithelial tumors, but are seen in high-grade carcinomas. Over-expression of *c-erb-B2* oncogene is associated with greater biological aggressiveness and an unfavourable course of disease.

Some cases of carcinoma of the ovary are associated with a penetrant dominant genetic predisposition. Clinical suspicion should be aroused by the presence of several affected members in a family, patients with both ovarian and breast cancer, and families in which there are multiple cancers in both males and females. Many families with this pattern of disease have an abnormality in a gene termed '*BRCA1*' (on chromosome 17), which is also an important cause of familial breast cancer.

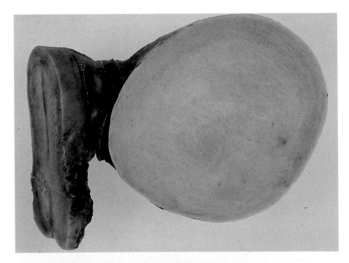

Fig. 19.25 Fibrothecoma of the ovary.
A large, well-circumscribed, spherical tumor with a whorled cut-surface appearance replaces one ovary. The slightly yellow tinge is a reflection of accumulated lipid within the plump spindle cells of the thecoma component. On the left is the cut surface of the attached uterus.

or extend outside the ovary, they are more likely to behave in an aggressive manner, with local recurrence or metastasis.

Sertoli–Leydig cell tumors (androblastomas) are very uncommon and most are small benign lesions confined to the ovary. They may cause masculinizing effects from secreted hormones.

Germ-cell tumors of the ovary may be benign or malignant, histologically resembling those seen in the testis

Germ-cell tumors account for 20% of ovarian neoplasms, occurring from childhood onwards. The classification of these lesions closely follows that for germ-cell tumors of the testis (see page 386).

Benign cystic teratomas (dermoid cyst of ovary) are the most common ovarian germ-cell tumors, accounting for about 10% of all neoplasms of the ovary. Macroscopically the affected ovary is replaced by a cyst lined by skin with skin appendage structures, particularly hair (*Fig. 19.26*). Teeth, bone, respiratory tract tissue, mature neural tissue and smooth muscle are other common elements. Lesions can vary in size from 2–3 cm up to masses that are 10–20 cm in diameter. These lesions are benign, but are bilateral in 10% of cases. A small number of cases develop secondary malignant change in one of the elements of the teratoma, commonly squamous-cell carcinoma of the epidermal component.

Solid teratomas are very uncommon and are seen mainly in adolescents. These large, solid lesions are composed of a variety of tissue components such as squamous epithelium, cartilage, smooth muscle, respiratory mucosa, and neural tissue. In most cases, small areas of primitive embryonal tissue are also seen, or other types of germ-cell tumor are encountered (classifying the lesions as 'malignant immature teratoma' or 'mixed malignant germ-cell tumour with a propensity for metastasis', respectively). In cases in which only mature tissues are seen, there is a good prognosis after removal.

Struma ovarii is composed of mature thyroid tissue. Considered by many to be a teratoma with only one line of maturation, it may cause hyperthyroidism.

Dysgerminomas of the ovary are similar to seminomas of the testis. Affected ovaries are enlarged and replaced by soft, white tumor with histological appearances like those seen in seminoma

Yolk-sac tumor is a rare, highly malignant form of germ-cell tumor, usually seen in women under the age of 30 years. Lesions are typically large and necrotic, secreting α fetoprotein detectable in the blood as a tumor marker.

Choriocarcinoma is a rare form of germ-cell tumor composed of trophoblastic cells. It is highly malignant, with a propensity for vascular spread. Tumors secrete HCG, which can be used as a tumor marker.

Metastatic tumors of the ovary are usually from the breast and gastrointestinal tract

Tumors often metastasize to the ovary, the most common sites of origin being breast, stomach, and colon. A so-called **Krukenberg tumor** is an ovary enlarged by metastatic signet-ring-cell adenocarcinoma (commonly from the stomach), which stimulates stromal hyperplasia. Such tumors are usually bilateral. Ovaries are commonly involved with Burkitt's lymphoma and in acute leukemias.

OBSTETRIC PATHOLOGY

It is not our purpose to provide a detailed text on obstetric pathology here, but rather to offer an outline of the important pathology related to common or significant conditions likely to be encountered in community obstetric practice, and some pathology relating to conditions met in hospital obstetric practice.

Pregnancy is associated with a number of important abnormalities, among which is **hyperemesis gravidarum**. Although nausea and occasional vomiting are common in early pregnancy, true hyperemesis gravidarum, with uncontrollable persistent vomiting leading to hemoconcentration and electrolyte abnormalities, is rare. Its cause is not known, but the rapid rise in estrogens and progesterone in early pregnancy is thought to be important.

Anemia of two types may occur, namely iron deficiency and folate deficiency. In both cases the most common cause is increased requirement due to the additional burden of the growing fetus, particularly in multiple pregnancies. Occasionally, reduced intake may be a factor. This is usually as a result of inadequate diet due to poverty or to poor food intake, or the consequence of the repeated vomiting associated with hyperemesis.

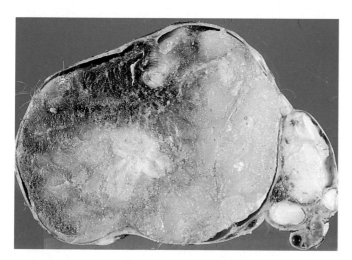

Fig. 19.26 Benign cystic teratoma of the ovary (dermoid cyst). The ovarian cyst cavity contains a partly gelatinous and partly 'buttery' material in which some hairs can be seen. The cyst is lined largely by skin epithelium with skin appendages, including hair follicles.

Pregnant women are prone to develop **urinary tract infection** because of stasis in the bladder and urinary tract, possibly associated with dilatation and kinking due to relaxation of smooth muscle under the influence of increased progesterone levels. This may be augmented by an obstructive element due to the enlarging uterus compressing the bladder and ureters in late pregnancy. About 2% of women develop clinically manifest acute urinary tract infection, a further 5% having asymptomatic bacterial colonization of urine.

Skin rashes in pregnancy are usually the result of drugs taken for anemia or urinary tract infection. Specific pregnancy-related skin rashes include a blistering skin eruption of unknown cause and **herpes gestationis**. The latter occurs in the second and third trimesters, presenting as urticated spots that then blister, usually on the abdomen and trunk.

Hypertension in pregnancy is usually due to mild preeclamptic syndrome. However, pregnancy may unmask a latent tendency to develop benign essential hypertension. Rarer causes include underlying glomerular disease and a previously asymptomatic pheochromocytoma of the adrenal medulla. The dangers of hypertension in pregnancy are cardiac failure and predisposition to cerebral hemorrhage.

Preeclamptic toxemia syndrome comprises raised blood pressure, proteinuria and peripheral edema

Preeclamptic toxemia is common in the United Kingdom, occurring in about 10% of all pregnant women. Seen particularly in association with multiple pregnancies, primigravidae and women over the age of 35 years, it is a syndrome characterized by increased blood pressure, proteinuria and peripheral edema.

Most cases are mild, with the blood pressure under 100 mmHg diastolic and no proteinuria; in severe cases the diastolic pressure is consistently above 100 mmHg, and there is proteinuria and severe peripheral edema.

The preeclamptic syndrome has hazards for both mother and fetus, but maternal problems are rare, being largely confined to severe preeclampsia, which may progress into full-blown eclampsia (see below). A feature of preeclampsia is reduced placental blood flow; this may lead to fetal hypoxia in late pregnancy, particularly during labor, with increased risk of perinatal mortality. The fetus may also suffer intrauterine growth retardation and have low birth weight. The mechanisms thought to be involved in the genesis of hypertension, proteinuria and edema in the preeclamptic syndrome are outlined in *Fig. 19.27*.

Pathogenesis of preeclampsia

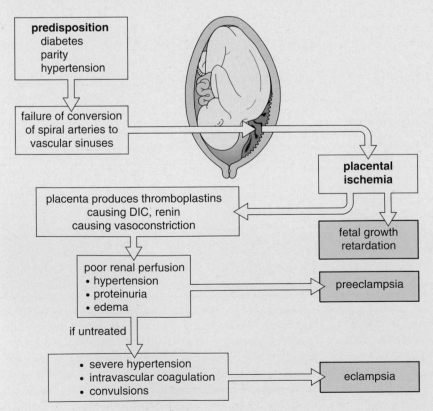

Fig. 19.27 Preeclampsia is predisposed by maternal factors of parity, diabetes and hypertension. First pregnancy carries most risk. A main factor in development is failure of conversion of narrow spiral arteries to low-resistance vascular sinuses in the placenta. Placental ischemia results in poor fetal growth and liberation of substances which cause vasoconstriction and promote hypertension. In the kidney, endothelial cells become swollen, with deposition of fibrin in glomeruli, leading to proteinuria. If untreated severe hypertension and intravascular coagulation occur with development of cerebral ischemia and fits.

Eclampsia is now a rare complication of pregnancy

Rarely, a small proportion of patients with severe pre-eclampsia develop eclampsia. Patients develop severe systemic disturbance, experiencing frontal headaches, rapid and sustained rise in blood pressure, shock, anuria and fits. They develop disseminated intravascular coagulation, with widespread occlusion of blood vessels, fibrinoid necrosis of vessel walls, and, in fatal cases, widespread microinfarcts in brain, liver, kidney and other organs. Fatal eclampsia is now rare due to treatment of the preeclamptic syndrome.

Spontaneous abortion is very common, often occurring before a woman is aware of her pregnancy

Many fertilized ova fail to implant successfully, and it has been estimated that more than 40% of conceptions fail to convert into recognizable pregnancies; of those which do, 15% terminate as clinically recognized spontaneous abortion. There are many causes of spontaneous abortion throughout the gestation period, the causes differing at different stages:

- **First trimester causes.** The majority are associated with abnormal fetuses, most being linked to abnormal chromosome karyotypes, particularly X0 (Turner's syndrome). Structural developmental abnormalities, such as neural tube defects, are also important. Maternal systemic lupus erythematosus (SLE) and the presence of circulating antiphospholipid antibodies are a recognized cause of repeated spontaneous abortion in the first trimester, and the disease may be clinically undiagnosed. Transplacental infection, e.g. *Brucella*, *Listeria*, rubella, *Toxoplasma*, cytomegalovirus and herpes, may lead to spontaneous abortion early in pregnancy.

- **Second trimester causes** include chorioamnionitis, rupture of membranes, placental hemorrhages and structural abnormalities of the uterus (e.g. congenital uterine malformations), large submucosal leiomyomas, and incompetence of the cervix. Abortions due to abnormal placentation may occur in this period, but are more common in the third trimester.

- **Third trimester causes** are mainly the result of maternal abnormality such as uncontrolled hypertension or eclampsia. The various types of placental abnormality, e.g. placental hemorrhage, abruption and infarction, are important causes in this trimester.

In ectopic pregnancy the fertilized ovum implants in an abnormal site

Ectopic gestation occurs when a fertilized ovum implants outside the uterine cavity. The most common site is implantation in a fallopian tube. A common cause is infection by chlamydial organisms. Tubal ectopic pregnancy is also likely when there is some structural abnormality of the fallopian tube, usually scarring resulting from previous episodes of salpingitis, although an increasingly common predisposing factor is previous tubal surgery for contraceptive purposes.

The fertilized embryo implants in the tubal mucosa and submucosa, and proliferation of trophoblast erodes submucosal blood vessels, precipitating severe bleeding into the tubal lumen (*Fig. 19.28*). Many tubal ectopic pregnancies present as an acute abdominal emergency, with severe lower abdominal pain that is usually localized to the side of the ectopic pregnancy; however, some tubal ectopics rupture, leading to bleeding into the peritoneal cavity, in which case the pain is less well localized. Rupture usually occurs in the early stages of pregnancy, and the patient may not be aware that she is pregnant; occasionally, ectopic pregnancies do not cause early hemorrhage and may be sustained for some weeks, during which the endometrium develops decidual changes.

Other sites of abnormal implantation are very rare but include peritoneal cavity, ovary and cervix.

Abnormal development of gestational trophoblast may lead to hydatidiform mole

Several disorders of abnormal trophoblast development are recognized, ranging from abnormal proliferative conditions through to highly malignant tumors. These are grouped under the term **trophoblastic diseases**. Many of these disorders follow a preceding abnormal gestation and are associated with cytogenetic abnormalities.

Hydatidiform mole is a benign abnormal mass of cystic vesicles derived from the chorionic villi (*Figs 19.29a* and *b*). Hydatidiform moles may be partial or complete:

- In **partial mole** the vesicular degeneration of the chorionic villi affects only part of the placenta.

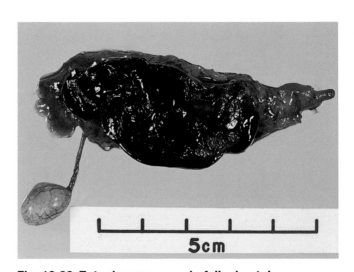

Fig. 19.28 Ectopic pregnancy in fallopian tube.
The distal fallopian tube is distended by blood clot in which there are chorionic villi eroding the tubal wall; fetal parts are rarely seen.

Fetal parts and some normal placental villi are present, along with the abnormal trophoblastic tissue. This has a low risk of subsequent development of malignancy.

- In **complete mole** no normal placenta is identified and the mole forms a bulky mass, which can fill the uterine cavity. No fetal parts or normal placental villi are present. This has a low risk of subsequent development of malignancy.

In both cases a characteristic feature of the mole is atypical hyperplasia of the syncytiotrophoblast and cytotrophoblast cells on the surface of the distended villi. The incidence of both types of mole is about 1 in 2000 in the UK and USA. However, they occur far more frequently in some parts of Asia, South America and Africa, the incidence in Taiwan, for example, being 1 in 400 pregnancies.

A small proportion (probably about 10%) of both partial and complete moles show invasion of the myometrium by the molar component, but this is not evidence of development of malignant neoplasm.

Evacuation of both complete and partial moles from the uterus may not be complete; some residual trophoblastic tissue is frequently left behind, particularly where there is deep invasion of the myometrium. Detection of such cases is by ultrasound imaging, as well as by demonstrating continued elevated levels of HCG secreted by trophoblast. These cases should be regarded as having **persistent trophoblastic disease**, and require chemotherapy to eradicate the residual trophoblastic tissue.

In some cases of persistent trophoblastic disease, there is a risk of subsequent development of malignant tumor of trophoblast, choriocarcinoma.

Choriocarcinoma is a malignant tumor of trophoblastic tissue

Around 50% of choriocarcinomas develop from a hydatidiform mole, only 20% arising after a normal pregnancy. The time-lag between pregnancy and the development of choriocarcinoma is very variable; it is usually a matter of a few months, but may occasionally take many years. It is rare in the UK and USA (approximately 1 in 50 000 pregnancies) but, like mole, is more common in Asia, South America and Africa.

The tumor forms hemorrhagic masses in the endometrial cavity, with a peripheral rim of viable tumor surrounding extensively necrotic and hemorrhagic debris. Histologically

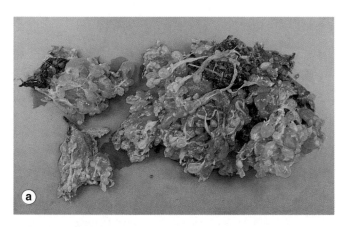

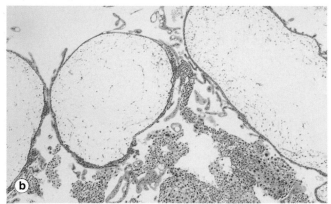

Fig. 19.29 Hydatidiform mole. The uterine contents in a hydatidiform mole are entirely composed of abnormal cystic vesicles (a). No normal placenta or fetal parts are identified. This is a complete mole. (b) Histology shows the cystic vesicles to be enormously enlarged. There are edematous chorionic villi, with hyperplasia of the surface trophoblast cells.

Cytogenetics of hydatidiform mole

In some cases it is difficult to be certain of the nature of hydropic villi with abnormal trophoblastic proliferation. Cytogenetic analysis of molar tissue has offered an insight into the possible origin of these diseases, as well as a means of assisting diagnosis.

The majority (80%) of complete hydatidiform moles are 46XX, both X chromosomes being derived from paternal spermatozoa. The implication is that a single haploid spermatozoon has penetrated an 'empty' ovum (i.e. monospermic or homozygous) or, alternatively, two single haploid sperms, both bearing the X chromosome, have penetrated (i.e. dispermic or heterozygous). It is claimed that the dispermic moles are more likely to lead to persistent trophoblastic disease than the monospermic moles.

A small percentage of complete moles have a chromosome constitution 46XY, both the X and Y chromosomes being derived from paternal spermatozoa; this is probably the result of penetration of an empty ovum by two haploid spermatozoa, one bearing an X chromosome, the other a Y chromosome.

Most partial moles have a chromosome constitution 69XXY, i.e. they are triploid.

(*Fig. 19.30*) it is composed of masses of cytotrophoblastic cells, often covered by a rim of pleomorphic syncytio-trophoblast; there is no evidence of structured villus formation. Trophoblastic tissue has a propensity for invading vessel walls, and blood-borne metastases occur early to many sites, particularly lung and brain. Formerly rapidly fatal, this tumor responds to cytotoxic chemotherapy, and the prognosis with correct treatment is now excellent (particularly if post-treatment monitoring of HCG levels is carried out).

Placental abruption is due to abnormal premature separation of a normally located placenta

Premature separation of the placenta is termed **placental abruption** and is an important cause of *ante partum*

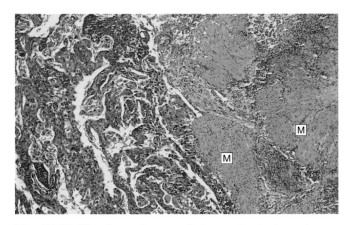

Fig. 19.30 Choriocarcinoma of uterus. In choriocarcinoma the uterine cavity contains masses of pleomorphic trophoblast, which invades myometrium (**M**). To the naked eye, this appears as a hemorrhagic and necrotic mass resembling a blood clot.

hemorrhage (see below), which may lead to stillbirth and even maternal death. The mechanisms of premature separation are not known, but it is particularly likely to occur in women who have a history of abruption, a history of many previous pregnancies, hypertension, or polyhydramnios and premature rupture of membranes.

In most cases, placental separation is manifest as abdominal pain with vaginal bleeding. However, the hemorrhage may occasionally be concealed, the blood being contained within the placental bed. In such cases the patient develops lower abdominal pain, rapidly followed by hypotension and clinical manifestations of shock.

There are two main causes of *ante partum* hemorrhage

Ante partum hemorrhage is bleeding from or into the female genital tract after the twenty-eighth week of pregnancy and before delivery. The main causes are **placental abruption** and **placenta previa**. The above account for two-thirds of all cases and have a roughly equal incidence. In the remaining one-third the cause is not apparent, but some trivial cause in the lower genital tract, e.g. a cervical polyp, may occasionally be responsible.

Placenta previa is implantation of the placenta low in the uterus so that it encroaches on the lower segment

The lower segment of the uterus does not contract during labor, but becomes passively stretched as the uterus enlarges. In placenta previa the fact that the placenta overlies the lower segment may lead to *ante partum* hemorrhage or an obstructed labor, depending on the precise location of the placenta. Four grades of placenta previa are recognized (*Fig. 19.31*):

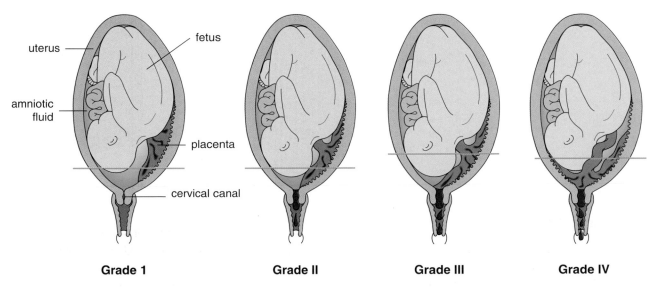

Fig. 19.31 Grades of placenta previa.
Normally the placenta does not extend into the lower uterine segment (below the blue line in diagram). In placenta previa, different grades of severity are associated with increasing encroachment of placenta on the lower segment and cervical os.

- **Grade I.** The edge of the placenta encroaches on the lower segment, but does not reach the internal os.
- **Grade II.** The placenta occupies the lower segment, with its edge reaching the internal os but not covering it.
- **Grades III/IV.** The placenta is implanted in the lower segment and either partly (Grade III) or completely (Grade IV) covers the internal os.

All grades are likely to present with *ante partum* hemorrhage, as the lower segment stretches before delivery.

Grades III and IV are particularly likely to lead to an obstructed labor, the placenta preventing the passage of the presenting fetal part into the os, thus necessitating cesarean section.

In addition to leading to *ante partum* hemorrhage, placenta previa is particularly likely to lead to *post partum* hemorrhage because the stretched lower segment of the uterus contracts less than the rest of the uterus after delivery, allowing continued seepage of blood from the placental bed.

Breast disease

Clinical Overview

The female breast depends on a variety of hormones for its normal activity, and exhibits considerable structural and functional variation throughout life, particularly during puberty, pregnancy, lactation, the normal menstrual cycle, and at the menopause. This hormone-regulated growth also gives rise to the most common form of breast disease, that due to abnormal proliferation, termed **fibrocystic change**. As its name implies a cystic component is frequent in this disease, which is the commonest cause of a fluctuant cystic breast lump.

Inflammatory diseases of the breast are rare: acute infection occurs only in the lactating breast. The most common chronic inflammatory lesion is that which follows trauma, with a foreign body giant cell and fibrous reaction developing to lipid released from traumatized adipocytes (**fat necrosis**).

An important and common breast lump in young women is the well-circumscribed rubbery-textured **fibroadenoma** which contains both epithelial and fibrous elements; this may be a hamartoma or nodular hyperplasia rather than a true tumor.

The most important disease of the breast is **carcinoma** and, as most breast diseases present as a palpable lump, it is most important to distinguish promptly cases of breast cancer from the many forms of benign breast disease. Although the true nature of a breast lump can only be ascertained by histological examination of many areas of the excised lump, a good idea of its nature before surgery can be obtained by a combination of its clinical features (size, outline, texture, relation to adjacent tissues, etc), mammographic examination of the affected breast, and cytological examination of the epithelial cell component of the lung obtained by fine-needle aspiration.

INFLAMMATORY DISORDERS OF THE BREAST

Mastitis and breast abscess are seen as a complication of lactation

Infections of the breast are associated with lactation, the organisms (commonly *Staphylococcus aureus* and *Streptococcus*) gaining access through cracks and fissures in the nipple and areola. The initial infection causes an acute mastitis, with painful tender enlargement of the breast, which generally resolves after treatment with appropriate antibiotics.

Without antibiotic therapy, bacterial mastitis is often followed by the development of a breast abscess, which may require surgical drainage.

Chronic inflammation of the breast is rare, but may develop after incomplete resolution of an acute mastitis. Tuberculous mastitis may occur, but is uncommon in western countries.

Fat necrosis follows trauma and can clinically mimic neoplastic disease

Following episodes of trauma, localized areas of inflammation of the breast may occur as a result of fat necrosis.

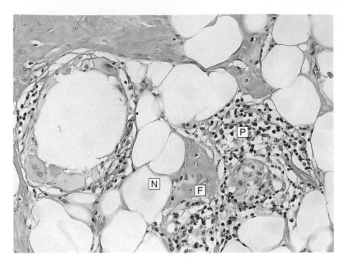

Fig. 20.1 Fat necrosis.
In the response to fat necrosis (**N**) there is an initial acute inflammatory reaction, followed by a chronic inflammatory response in which numerous plasma cells are seen (**P**). Macrophages phagocytose lipid released from adipocytes, forming multinucleate giant cells, as well as foam cells (**F**), also termed 'lipophages'.

The trauma causes necrosis of adipose tissue, precipitating an inflammatory and reparative response to the dead fat cells (*Fig. 20.1*).

Organization with fibrous repair takes place, producing a hard, irregular breast lump. The main clinical significance of this condition is that patients may not be able to recall a history of trauma, and these lesions often clinically resemble a breast carcinoma, e.g. the presence of skin tethering.

Duct ectasia is caused by inflammatory destruction of support tissues around ducts

Mammary duct ectasia is a disease of uncertain pathogenesis. There is abnormal progressive dilatation of large breast ducts, which accumulate retained secretory products and shed epithelium. The disease is mainly seen in parous women in the peri-menopausal age range.

Although the precise cause is uncertain, it is thought that an important abnormality is inflammatory destruction of the normal elastic-containing support tissues around ducts, which then allows dilatation. The inflammatory component has led to the alternative term of 'periductal mastitis' for this condition.

Clinically, patients develop a firm breast lump, which may resemble a carcinoma, or there may be a nipple discharge. Macroscopically, affected areas of breast show distended ducts, up to 1 cm in diameter, filled with inspissated creamy material.

Histology shows dilated ducts containing proteinaceous material and phagocytic macrophages distended with lipid. There is fibrosis around ducts, associated with non-specific chronic inflammation.

BENIGN PROLIFERATIVE DISEASES OF THE BREAST

Fibrocystic change is the most common disorder of the female breast

The most frequent disorder of the female breast is fibrocystic change. This produces clinical symptoms in 10% of all women, being present asymptomatically in about 40%. It is common in the breasts of mature women, with an increasing incidence towards the menopause, after which few cases are seen. This condition has also been known by a variety of other terms including 'fibroadenosis', 'cystic mammary dysplasia', 'cystic hyperplasia', 'cystic mastopathy' and 'chronic mastitis', but these terms are now no longer preferred.

Fibrocystic change is characterized by hyperplastic overgrowth of components of the mammary unit, i.e. lobules, ductules and stroma. There is **epithelial overgrowth** of lobules and ducts, often termed **adenosis** or **epitheliosis**, and **fibrous overgrowth** of specialized hormone-responsive lobule-supporting stroma.

Unequal growth of epithelial and stromal elements occurs, giving rise to a range of solid and cystic nodules within the breast, broadly termed **fibroadenomatoid hyperplasia** or **fibroadenosis**. This presents as palpable thickening and nodularity of breast tissue, but may also result in the development of single breast lumps. The most important clinical aspects of fibrocystic disease are that it must be distinguished from malignancy and that, in a small proportion of cases, it increases the chances of later development of carcinoma of the breast. It must be emphasized that in the majority of cases, patients with fibrocystic disease in the absence of epithelial hyperplasia are not at increased risk from later development of carcinoma of the breast.

The cause of fibrocystic disease is uncertain. Most believe that it is due to disturbances of cyclical ovarian estrogen and progesterone levels, accompanied by altered responsiveness of breast tissues in women approaching the menopause.

Fibrocystic disease has several histological patterns

Macroscopically, areas of fibrocystic disease appear as firm, rubbery replacement of breast tissue, in which cysts may be visible. There are many histological variations within fibrocystic disease.

In many cases the epithelium lining hyperplastic ducts undergoes metaplasia to a form similar to that of normal apocrine glands (**apocrine metaplasia**) (*Fig. 20.2*).

Cysts are a prominent component, increasing in incidence with the approach of the menopause. They range in size from those detectable only by histology to palpable lesions 1–2 cm in diameter. Cysts are lined by flattened epithelium derived from the lobular–ductal unit and are

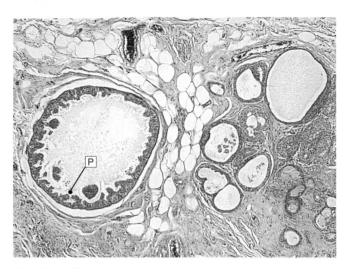

Fig. 20.2 Fibrocystic disease.
In fibrocystic disease there is proliferation of ducts, lobular tissue and stromal support tissues to form a mass of cystic spaces and fibrous tissue. The epithelium of some ducts is replaced by bright, pink-staining epithelium (**P**) resembling normal apocrine glands.

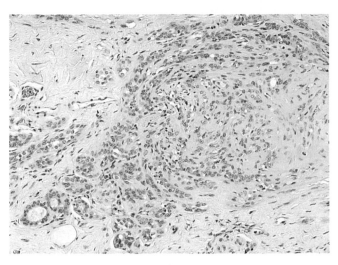

Fig. 20.3 Sclerosing adenosis.
In sclerosing adenosis there is proliferation of stromal and myofibroblastic cells, as well as of small breast ducts. The stromal component compresses the ducts into narrow ribbons and slits, mimicking the appearances of an invasive carcinoma.

filled with watery fluid. As some carcinomas of the breast may be associated with cysts, it is not safe to assume that a lesion is benign because it has a fluid-filled cyst. Cytological examination of fluid aspirated from breast cysts may be useful in diagnosis.

In some cases, there is marked proliferation of specialized hormone-responsive stromal tissue and myoepithelial cells, separating and compressing acinar and ductal structures into narrow ribbons of cells. This change, known as **sclerosing adenosis**, may be difficult to distinguish, both radiologically and histologically, from some patterns of invasive carcinoma (*Fig. 20.3*). Despite the potential for confusion, this pattern of disease is not associated with development of carcinoma.

Epithelial hyperplasia within proliferated ducts and lobules may be seen in a minority of cases of fibrocystic disease; this is important since this type of change is associated with an increased risk of later development of carcinoma. In most cases, the cytology and architecture of the proliferated epithelium give no cause for concern, and lesions are classified as **hyperplasia of usual type**.

In other cases, abnormalities in cell cytology and architecture have some, but not all, of the features of carcinoma *in situ*, in which instances the term **atypical hyperplasia** is used. For patients who have simple epithelial hyperplasia (about 25% of all cases of fibrocystic disease), the risk of subsequent development of carcinoma is increased two-fold. For those who have atypical epithelial hyperplasia (about 5% of cases), the risk of subsequently developing a carcinoma increases five-fold.

Fibrocystic disease may be manifest as replacement of breast tissue by dense fibrous tissue, termed **mammary fibrosis**, particularly in women after the menopause.

KEY FACTS
Fibrocystic disease

- Caused by abnormal response of breast to ovarian hormones.
- Is a form of hyperplasia involving epithelial as well as stromal elements.
- Overgrowth of ducts and acini, fibrosis and cysts are main features.
- Increased risk of subsequent development of carcinoma is related to the presence of epithelial hyperplasia, particularly atypical hyperplasia.
- Sclerosing adenosis can be clinically and radiologically confused with carcinoma.

Sclerosing lesions of the breast are commonly seen in radiographic screening

Several lesions of the breast are characterized by a predominant fibrous component that forms a localized area of irregular, stellate, collagenous sclerosis in which epithelial elements are also present. These lesions have become significant in modern clinical practice, as they can be confused with a carcinoma on mammographic screening. The main types are:

- **Sclerosing adenosis.** This may present as a solitary, palpable lesion in young women, in addition to being seen in areas of fibrocystic change in older women.

- **Radial scars and complex sclerosing lesions** are composed of collagenous and elastic tissue enclosing distorted ductules. Careful histological examination of these lesions is required, as some forms of carcinoma (tubular carcinoma) can adopt this pattern of growth.

Fibroadenoma presents as a mobile lump in the breast of young women

One of the lesions most commonly responsible for causing a lump in the breast is the **fibroadenoma**, a benign, localized proliferation of breast ducts and stroma. There is debate as to whether this lesion is a true neoplasm or actually represents a nodular form of hyperplasia. Fibroadenomas are seen most frequently in women aged 25–35 years as solitary discrete lesions, but histologically identical areas may also be a component of fibrocystic disease. The fibroadenoma is therefore best regarded as a form of hormone-dependent nodular hyperplasia, rather than a true benign tumor.

Macroscopically, fibroadenomas are typically 1–4 cm in diameter, appearing as firm, rubbery, well-circumscribed, white lesions that are mobile in the breast. They have a glistening cut surface and a tough texture.

There are two histological components (*Fig. 20.4*): the **epithelial component**, which forms gland-like structures lined by duct-type epithelium, and the **stromal component**, which is a loose, cellular fibrous tissue around the epithelial areas.

A specialized type of fibroadenoma, termed a **juvenile fibroadenoma**, occurs in adolescents, forming huge masses that are frequently the same size or larger than the original breast. Histologically they resemble normal fibroadenomas.

NEOPLASTIC BREAST DISEASES

BENIGN BREAST TUMORS

Benign tumors of the breast are less common than malignant tumours

There are several benign tumors of the breast, in addition to nodular lesions due to proliferative diseases. Many workers still consider fibroadenoma to be a benign tumor rather than a form of nodular proliferation. The breast may also be the site of development of benign tumors of support tissues, e.g. lipomas and leiomyomas. The main benign tumors of the breast are breast hamartomas, adenomas, duct papillomas, and phyllodes tumors.

Hamartomas of the breast are seen on mammographic screening

Mammographic screening is currently revealing a greater number of benign lesions of the breast than ever before. These are coming to the attention of pathologists as they are now being excised or biopsied. Hamartomas macroscopically resemble fibroadenomas. They are composed of a mass of fibrous stroma, which encloses lobular and ductal structures.

Duct papillomas are a common cause of a blood-stained nipple discharge

Papillomas of mammary duct epithelium may arise as solitary or multiple lesions. **Solitary papillomas** are usually located in the larger lactiferous ducts near the nipple. They are most common in middle-aged women and are a common cause of a bloody nipple discharge (*Fig. 20.5*). Lesions are usually 1–2 cm in size and consist of a delicate

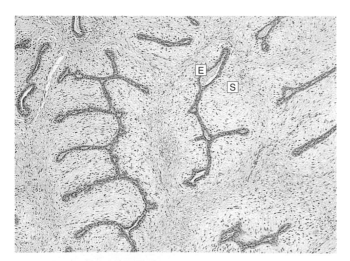

Fig. 20.4 Fibroadenoma.
The fibroadenoma is composed of both epithelial (**E**) and stromal (**S**) components. Although lesions form localized, circumscribed lumps, they are believed to be hyperplastic rather than neoplastic.

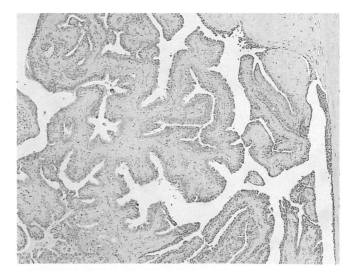

Fig. 20.5 Papilloma of the breast.
A breast papilloma is shown within a dilated duct. It is composed of fronds of tissue, with a vascular stroma covered by a two-layered ductal epithelium.

supporting stroma covered by a double layer of cuboidal or low columnar epithelial cells, resembling the lining of a duct; with larger lesions, the duct is often dilated. Malignant change is rare.

Multiple papillomas are far less common than solitary lesions and are usually located in smaller ducts deeper in the breast in young women. This type is associated with increased risk of later development of breast carcinoma.

True adenomas of the breast are uncommon primary tumors

Compared to nodular proliferative lesions such as fibroadenomas and sclerosing lesions, true adenomas of the breast are uncommon.

Tubular adenomas occur in young women and are composed of regular tubular-shaped glands and a minimal stroma. There is no associated risk of developing carcinoma.

Adenoma of the nipple commonly presents as ulceration and reddening of the nipple, clinically confused with Paget's disease of the nipple (see page 428). These lesions are composed of duct-like structures associated with a collagenous stroma.

Phyllodes tumors are composed of both epithelial and stromal elements

A phyllodes tumor is composed of epithelial-lined, cleft-like spaces surrounded by a cellular spindle-cell stroma (*Fig. 20.6*). These lesions were previously called 'cystosarcoma phyllodes' or 'giant fibroadenomas', names that are no longer recommended.

Clinically, tumors present as a breast lump and can be seen at any age following puberty, although most are encountered after the age of 40 years. Macroscopically they are rubbery, white lesions in which a whorled pattern of slit-like spaces and solid areas can be seen.

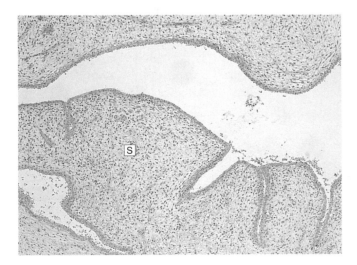

Fig. 20.6 Phyllodes tumor.
Phyllodes tumors are composed of a spindle-celled stroma (**S**), containing clefts lined by epithelium.

The histological appearance of these lesions is variable and it is possible to classify phyllodes tumors as benign, of borderline malignant potential, or definitely malignant.

In 90% of cases both epithelial and stromal elements are bland and give no cause for concern. However, in the remaining 10% of cases there are atypical features to the stromal element, with pleomorphism and mitoses, leading to a borderline or malignant classification.

Biologically the majority of phyllodes tumors are benign, but about 10% recur locally. Tumors with atypical histological features are particularly prone to recur, and the very small minority with marked atypical histological features (classified as malignant) may spread, with development of metastases.

MALIGNANT TUMOURS OF THE BREAST

Carcinoma of the breast affects up to 1 in 10 women

Malignant tumors of the female breast are extremely common, accounting for 20% of all malignancies in women. In the UK, 1 in 12 women will develop carcinoma of the breast at some time in their life (1 in 10 women in the USA). Breast cancer may occur at any age outside childhood, but has a low incidence in the first three decades, rising steeply thereafter.

Most tumors are **invasive adenocarcinomas**, which arise from the terminal ducts and lobular units, forming **invasive lobular carcinomas** or **invasive ductal carcinomas**. Carcinoma of the breast may also be encountered at a stage prior to invasion, carcinoma *in situ* of mammary ducts or lobules (**intraduct** and **intralobular carcinoma**), and this is a risk factor for later development of invasive breast carcinoma.

In addition to the two main groups of ductal and lobular carcinoma, there are less common, special types of breast carcinoma, which are often associated with a better prognosis, e.g. tubular carcinoma and mucinous carcinoma.

Breast carcinoma presents in four main ways:

1 A palpable lump in the breast, increasingly being detected by patients themselves as a result of health education.
2 Abnormality detected on mammography as a result of developing breast-screening programmes.
3 Incidental histological finding in breast tissue removed for another reason.
4 First manifest as metastatic disease (see page 428).

Intraduct carcinoma of the breast is a form of carcinoma *in situ*

Non-invasive intraduct carcinoma may present as a breast lump or be detected as a mammographic abnormality. It accounts for about 5% of cases presenting clinically as a palpable breast lump, but for up to 20% of cases identified by radiological screening. It is most common in women between the ages of 40 and 60 years.

Histologically, tumor cells fill and distend small- and medium-sized ducts (*Fig. 20.7*). There are four main histological types: **solid**, in which ducts are packed with solid masses of cells; **comedo**, in which there has been necrosis of the cells in the center of the ducts; **cribriform**, in which cells form gland-like structures within the ducts; and **micropapillary**, in which cells form papillary projections into ducts.

It has been estimated that if left, about 30% of cases would progress to invasive carcinoma. If treated by mastectomy, intraduct carcinoma has an excellent prognosis.

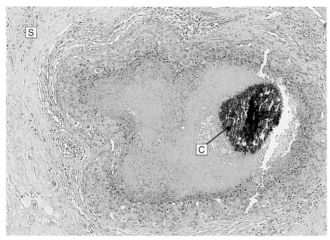

Fig. 20.7 Ductal carcinoma *in situ* of the breast.
A breast duct is lined by large tumor cells with large atypical nuclei. The basement membrane of the duct is intact and there is no invasion of stroma (**S**). The central area of tumor has become necrotic, with calcification (**C**) which may be seen on mammograms (see *Fig. 20.14*).

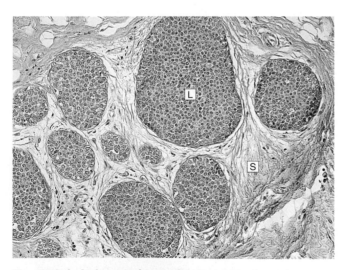

Fig. 20.8 Lobular carcinoma *in situ* of the breast.
In non-invasive lobular carcinoma the normal lobular architecture is maintained, but lobules (**L**) are increased in size, being packed with atypical cells that fill and expand them. The basement membrane remains intact and there is no evidence of invasion of the stroma (**S**).

Lobular carcinoma *in situ* increases risk of invasive breast cancer in both breasts

Lobular carcinoma *in situ* accounts for about 6% of all cases of breast cancer. It does not usually present as a palpable mass, often being encountered as a histological finding in breast tissue removed for another reason, e.g. fibrocystic disease. Histologically, abnormal cells fill the mammary lobules (*Fig. 20.8*).

The importance of this disease is that it carries a high risk of subsequent development of invasive carcinoma. It has been estimated that about 20% of patients with lobular carcinoma *in situ* will develop invasive carcinoma after 20 years. The risk of neoplasia is present for both breasts, not just the breast carrying the *in situ* disease, and either lobular or ductal invasive carcinoma may develop.

Invasive carcinoma of the breast is divided into six main histological types, only two of which are common

There are six main types of invasive breast carcinoma, which are named according to their histological pattern and occur with varying frequency (*Fig. 20.9*). In contrast to *in situ* neoplasia, there is invasion into local tissues, with the possibility of metastatic spread.

The macroscopic appearance of invasive carcinoma is mainly determined by the non-neoplastic stromal component

An invasive carcinoma of the breast can vary in size from less than 1 cm in diameter to masses occupying the whole of a breast; however, the majority of lesions are 1–3 cm in

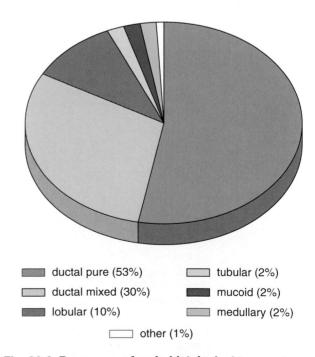

- ductal pure (53%)
- ductal mixed (30%)
- lobular (10%)
- tubular (2%)
- mucoid (2%)
- medullary (2%)
- other (1%)

Fig. 20.9 Frequency of main histological types of invasive carcinoma of the breast.

diameter at the time of diagnosis. Macroscopically the appearance of a carcinoma of the breast is mainly determined by the quality and quantity of its induced stromal component.

Most carcinomas of the breast excite a fibrous stromal reaction (desmoplastic response) and appear as irregular areas of gritty, firm yellowish white tissue with the consistency of an unripe apple (*Fig. 20.10*).

Tumors which have little in the way of a desmoplastic response are composed of neoplastic cells with scant fibrous stroma, appearing soft and fleshy.

Some carcinomas secrete large amounts of mucin into the stroma, and appear white with a gelatinous consistency (mucoid or colloid carcinoma).

The most common types of invasive carcinoma of the breast are ductal and lobular

Invasive ductal carcinoma is the most common type of breast cancer. It may occur as a pure form or may be mixed with another pattern of carcinoma, most commonly lobular carcinoma. Tumor cells invade breast tissue and there is usually a desmoplastic response, creating a dense fibrous stroma (*Fig. 20.11*). A minority of tumors are low-grade lesions, the majority being either intermediate or high-grade poorly differentiated types. When ductal carcinoma is mixed with specialized tumors that have a good prognosis (e.g. tubular or colloid carcinoma). the prognosis is slightly better than for the pure ductal tumor.

Invasive lobular carcinoma is the second most common type of breast cancer. Importantly, tumor is often multifocal within the breast, and this type is associated with a high frequency of bilateral breast involvement relative to other sub-types. Tumor cells invade breast tissue, with a desmoplastic response. Characteristically, tumor cells are compressed into narrow cords, described as 'Indian file' pattern of invasion (*Fig. 20.12*).

Although uncommon, some specialized carcinomas of the breast are associated with a better prognosis

Although they account for under 10% of all invasive breast cancers, certain specialized histological types of invasive carcinoma are associated with a better prognosis than the ductal and lobular types.

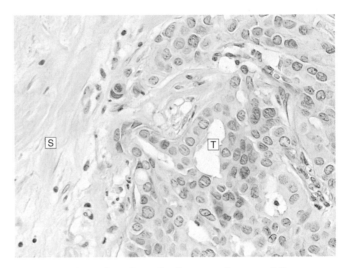

Fig. 20.11 Invasive ductal adenocarcinoma of the breast. In this example of a moderately differentiated invasive ductal adenocarcinoma of the breast, tumor islands have invaded adjacent stroma (**S**). The tumor still forms tubule-like structures (**T**).

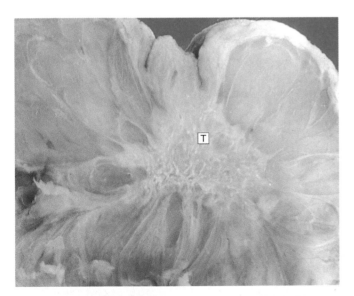

Fig. 20.10 Invasive breast cancer with abundant stroma. On cut surface an area of invasive carcinoma of the breast is seen as an irregular yellowish white area (**T**). Because of the stromal response, these are sometimes termed 'scirrhous carcinomas'. The stromal fibrous response has caused dimpling of the overlying skin.

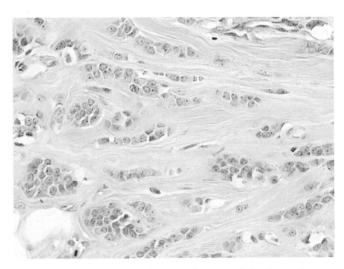

Fig. 20.12 Invasive lobular carcinoma of the breast. Lobular carcinoma is characterized by invasion in narrow cords of cells, termed 'Indian file' invasion. Cells are smaller than those seen in typical ductal carcinomas.

Tubular carcinomas are composed of well-differentiated cells that form regular tubular structures resembling small ducts. Although they represent 2% of all invasive carcinomas, they account for about 20% of cases detected by mammography. There is usually a desmoplastic response, with fibrous stroma forming a stellate pattern. Because cells are so well differentiated, this pattern is associated with a very good survival.

Mucoid carcinoma (also termed 'colloid carcinoma') is most commonly seen in post-menopausal women. Cells in the lesion secrete mucin into the stroma, giving tumors a soft, slimy texture. This pattern of tumor is associated with a very good survival compared to ductal carcinomas of a similar size.

Medullary carcinomas of the breast are most commonly seen in post-menopausal women. They form apparently well-circumscribed masses and, lacking much of a desmoplastic response, are soft and fleshy. The neoplastic cells are generally large and highly pleomorphic, with numerous mitoses. A characteristic feature is a dense infiltrate of reactive lymphoid cells at the tumor periphery, representing a host response to tumor. These lesions are associated with only a slightly better survival than similarly sized ductal carcinomas.

Paget's disease of the nipple is a pattern of spread of breast cancer to the epidermis

Paget's disease of the nipple is a pattern of spread of a ductal carcinoma of the breast. Patients develop reddening and thickening of the skin of the nipple and areola, sometimes followed by ulceration resembling eczema. Histologically the epidermis of the nipple and areola is infiltrated by large pale pleomorphic neoplastic epithelial cells, termed 'Paget's cells' (*Fig. 20.13*). Eczematous or inflammatory conditions of the nipple must always be regarded with suspicion, and biopsy should be performed to exclude Paget's disease.

Carcinoma of the breast spreads in a characteristic fashion

Carcinoma of the breast spreads in a characteristic fashion, which explains several of the common clinical manifestations of disease. Metastatic disease and recurrence of tumor may be a late event, occurring many years after local treatment of disease.

Local spread is into adjacent breast, into overlying skin (skin tethering), and deeply into pectoral muscles (deep fixation of tumor).

Lymphatic spread is into local lymphatics in the breast. When lymphatic drainage of the skin is involved, this gives rise to a *peau d'orange* appearance. Spread to axillary lymph nodes and nodes in the internal mammary chain is caused by embolization of tumor to nodes.

Vascular spread leads to dissemination of tumor to distant sites. The preferred sites for metastasis are **bone** (pathological fractures, hypercalcemia, leukoerythroblastic anemia, spinal-cord compression), **lung** (breathlessness), **pleura** (effusion and breathlessness), and **ovary** (Krukenberg tumor, see page 415). Other sites are commonly involved but with less consistency.

Prognostic factors can be used to predict survival in breast cancer

Breast cancer is not one disease and there is great variation in survival following treatment. The factors related to prognosis in breast cancer are clinically important as they allow informed counselling of patients.

Stage of tumor is widely regarded as the most powerful prognostic factor. Several staging systems are in use including the TNM classification (see page 88). Although staging systems vary in precise criteria, there are common features:

- Large primary tumor size (> 2 cm) or fixation to local tissues is associated with poor prognosis.

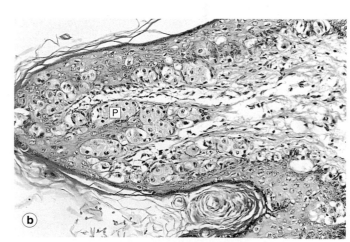

(a)   (b)

Fig. 20.13 Paget's disease of the nipple.
Macroscopically (a) Paget's disease appears as a red, scaling rash around the nipple. Histologically (b) the lower part of the epidermis is replaced by large, pale cells with pleomorphic nuclei (**P**). These are breast carcinoma cells that have spread along the mammary and nipple ducts to invade the epidermis. In the underlying breast there is either intraduct or invasive ductal carcinoma.

- Spread to nodes is associated with significant reduction in 5-year survival from around 80% to 60%.
- Vascular spread is associated with a poor prognosis and a 5-year survival of about 10%.

The link between early stage and good clinical outcome is one of the main reasons for promoting breast-screening programmes.

Grade of tumor assessed by looking at degree of gland formation, pleomorphism and numbers of mitoses, provides additional prognostic data. Carcinomas can be assigned to three groups, which are related to survival at 10 years:

- Grade I (85%).
- Grade II (60%).
- Grade III (45%).

In some recent series, grade of tumor (when carefully assessed according to objective criteria) is considered to allow more accurate prediction of survival than stage.

Histological type of tumor is another prognostic factor, some specialized types of carcinoma of the breast (tubular, mucoid) being associated with better prognosis than the common ductal and lobular types, as they have a low propensity for metastasis.

Molecular biological prognostic factors in breast cancer

In addition to the factors of stage, grade, histological type and hormone receptor status, recent work has concentrated on the relation of prognosis to more fundamental aspects of tumors.

- **Cell proliferation.** It is possible to determine cell-proliferation rates in tumors. Tumors with high proliferation rates have a worse prognosis than those with low rates. This is still significant, independent of conventionally determined grade of tumor, which looks at mitotic figures.

- **Expression of oncogenes.** Within each grade and stage of breast cancer there is still some variation in survival rates. Expression of oncogenes is being investigated to see if it explains such variation. In keeping with many other tumors, breast cancer is associated with several oncogene abnormalities, particularly abnormalities of p53 (see page 94). However, studies show that such factors do not contribute to determining survival. The expression of the *neu* oncogene (also called '*HER*-2' or '*c-erb*-B2') has shown a small contribution to survival in several studies.

Prognosis can also be related to **hormone receptor status.** Patients with breast tumors that express receptors for estrogen and progesterones have a longer disease-free survival than those that do not. This is a reflection of tumor differentiation and likely response to anti-hormone therapy.

The cause of breast cancer is uncertain, but there are several defined risk factors

Epidemiological studies have shown that breast cancer is related to several risk factors, although the cause is uncertain.

Geographical. The incidence of disease is five times greater in developed western countries than in less developed areas.

Familial breast cancer. There is an increased genetic risk of developing breast cancer in about 5% of all cases (see pink box below).

Familial breast cancer

Approximately 5% of cases of carcinoma of the breast are associated with a penetrant dominant genetic predisposition. Clinical suspicion is warranted in the presence of several affected members in a family, patients with early onset of disease, patients with bilateral breast cancers, patients with both ovarian and breast cancer, and families in which there are breast, ovarian, endometrial and colon cancers, or sarcomas in both males and females.

There have been several advances in the genetics of breast cancer, revealing underlying genetic abnormalities.

- Of all families with a strong familial history of breast cancer, many have an abnormality in the BRCA1 gene on chromosome 17. This is also associated with development of carcinoma of the ovary and prostate.

- About 5% of families with breast cancer have a mutation of the p53 tumor-suppressor gene on chromosome 17. Family members develop a wide range of other tumors in addition to breast cancer.

- Another familial breast cancer syndrome is associated with a gene on chromosome 13 termed BRCA2.

Other breast cancer genes are being actively sought. Through detection of these abnormal genes, it is now possible to use molecular genetic techniques to identify individuals at risk of developing breast cancer, although the best way to manage such patients clinically is still uncertain.

Proliferative breast disease. Epithelial hyperplasia is associated with an approximately two-fold increased risk of development of carcinoma. Atypical hyperplasia is associated with a five-fold increased risk in women with no family history of breast cancer, but the risk increases 11-fold in women with a family history of breast cancer.

Early onset of menarche (10 years rather than 15 years) carries a three-fold increased risk.

Late birth of first child (35 years rather than 20 years) carries a three-fold increased risk.

Late menopause (55 years rather than 45 years) carries a three-fold increased risk.

Nulliparous state. Breast cancer is more frequent than in multiparous women.

Exogenous hormones. Marginal increase in patients on hormone-replacement therapy after menopause. No conclusive association with use of oral contraceptives.

Dietary factors. Increased risk of development of breast cancer has been linked to obesity in the pre-menopausal period and also to a high alcohol intake.

Diagnosis of breast cancer

The diagnosis of breast cancer is made using a combined clinical, imaging and pathological approach (so-called 'triple approach').

Clinical. No woman should be allowed to have a lump in the breast without a firm diagnosis. Public health education has resulted in more women practicing regular self-examination, and all lumps discovered should be investigated.

Imaging. Some types of breast cancer do not usually produce palpable lumps (notably lobular carcinoma *in situ*), and others produce a lump only when relatively advanced. Mammographic screening of the breast may detect subtle lesions by microcalcification or altered patterns of soft-tissue shadowing (see *Fig. 20.14*). MR imaging with enhancement is being used in some centers to screen patients at high risk of developing carcinoma; lesions can thus be detected at the earliest stage.

Fine-needle aspiration with cytology. To obtain diagnostic information about a breast lesion, it can be sampled by aspirating cells using a fine needle. Smear preparations are assessed cytologically (*Fig. 20.15*), giving high confidence in accurate diagnosis in experienced centers.

Needle biopsy. In some cases, biopsy using a cutting needle is performed, providing a histological diagnosis.

Lump excision biopsy. After diagnosis with aspiration cytology or biopsy, some lesions can be treated by excision biopsy. For lesions that are not palpable, a guide wire must be inserted into the lesion under radiological control to lead the surgeon to the abnormal area.

Fig. 20.14 Breast mammogram.
A mammogram is a soft tissue X-ray of the breast. Here, the speckles of white calcification are strongly suggestive of a carcinoma.

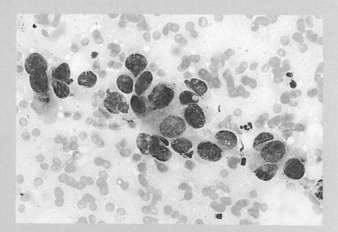

Fig. 20.15 Fine-needle aspiration cytology.
Aspiration of breast tumors by needle can produce cytological preparations that are reliable in diagnosis of the nature of the lesion. In this case, large nuclei with an abnormal chromatin pattern indicate a carcinoma.

Carcinoma of the breast in men is uncommon

Adenocarcinoma of the breast in men accounts for only 1% of all cases of breast cancer. Lesions fall into the same spectrum as those seen in the female breast, with the exception of lobular carcinoma *in situ* (as the male breast contains no lobular tissue). Paget's disease (see page 428) may also be seen in the male, and any rash of the nipple should be viewed with the same suspicion as in the female.

The prognosis of carcinoma of the male breast is similar to that for females. Invasion of the chest wall is seen more often in males, possibly because of the small size of the breast, and so lesions are more often locally advanced at diagnosis. Squamous carcinoma of the nipple may also be seen in men, but it is a very uncommon tumor.

In the breast, malignant tumors other than carcinomas are uncommon

Malignant tumors other than carcinomas are uncommon in the breast. Mention has already been made that **phyllodes tumors** may be malignant (see page 425) and can result in local invasion and metastatic disease.

Primary sarcomas in the breast are uncommon, usually only being recognized as such following biopsy (often in the belief that a lesion is probably a carcinoma). The main types are angiosarcoma, malignant fibrous histiocytomas, and fibrosarcomas.

Lymphomas may occur in the breast as primary disease or as part of a systemic lymphoma.

Gynecomastia of male breast is most commonly idiopathic, but may be a sign of underlying endocrine disturbance

The male breast is normally rudimentary and inactive, consisting of fibroadipose tissue containing atrophic mammary ducts. Enlargement of the male breast, which is termed **gynecomastia**, may be unilateral (70% of cases) or bilateral. In most cases it is idiopathic. Other causes include:

- Klinefelter's syndrome (see page 69).
- Estrogen excess (cirrhosis, puberty, adrenal tumor, exogenous estrogens).

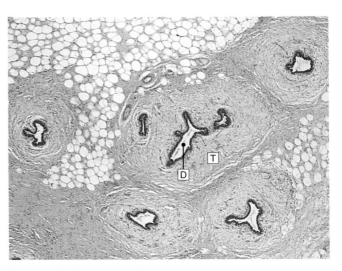

Fig. 20.16 Gynecomastia.
In gynecomastia the simple mammary ducts (**D**) become enlarged, often with thickening of the epithelial layer, and there is an increase in periductal fibrous tissue (**T**), which may be markedly collagenous.

- Gonadotrophin excess (testicular tumor).
- Prolactin excess (hypothalamic or pituitary disease).
- Drug-related (spironolactone, chlorpromazine, digitalis).

There is enlargement of the breast as a firm, raised, rubbery mass beneath the nipple (*Fig. 20.16*).

Accessory nipple and breast tissue are the most common developmental abnormalities of the breast

Accessory breast tissue (polymastia) may develop anywhere along the embryological milk line. The most common site is in the axilla. Such areas are composed of specialized breast tissue, which respond to normal trophic hormonal influences, increasing in size with pregnancy and lactation.

Accessory nipples (polythelia) may develop anywhere along the embryonic milk line. They are seen on the chest wall, abdominal wall, inguinal region, or vulva.

Nervous system and muscle

Clinical Overview

Diseases affecting the normal functioning of the brain are a very common complaint in family practice, but most are probably the result of biochemical abnormalities, e.g. depression, hypomania, bipolar disorder and schizophrenia, are not associated with visible structural pathology, and are therefore not dealt with in this chapter.

Trauma to the brain, particularly following road traffic accidents and falls, are an important part of specialist hospital practice, and may involve the surgical removal of blood clots and the management of brain swelling. These traumatic lesions affect all ages from infancy to extreme old age. **Cerebrovascular disease**, leading to stroke, is very common and important in the elderly population, but **subarachnoid hemorrhage** may affect younger adults with minor arterial disease.

With the increasing age of the general population, more people are surviving to extreme old age and developing dementing disorders due to neuronal degeneration and loss, such as **Alzheimer's disease**. This area of neuropathology is attracting considerable research attention, since the problem is likely to increase markedly in the next decade.

Infections involving the central nervous system are most commonly bacterial and confined to the meninges (**bacterial meningitis**), or viral and affecting the brain parenchyma (**viral encephalitis**); fungal infections and parasitic infestations are uncommon. All brain infections are more common and severe in the immunosuppressed.

Tumors of the brain are common. The most common primary tumors of the brain are those derived from the glial support tissues, but the brain is also a favored site for **metastatic tumor** deposits from other primary sites.

The nervous system is also prone to unique disorders which are specific to certain structural components, for example, the destruction of myelin in the group of primary demyelinating diseases such as **multiple sclerosis**.

Our knowledge of skeletal muscle disorders has been greatly improved by the more frequent use of skeletal muscle biopsies and the application of special laboratory techniques. Not only have these enabled an accurate tissue diagnosis to be made in most cases, it has revealed that a very limited set of clinical symptoms and physical signs can be caused by a wide range of pathological causes. Many of these disorders are heritable diseases.

INTRODUCTION

The nervous system is affected by general pathological processes, such as inflammation and infarction, but it is also the site of specific diseases of the specialized tissues of the nervous system, such as neurodegenerative diseases and demyelinating disorders.

The main cell types of pathological significance in the nervous system are: **neurons**; **astrocytes**, which act as specialized support cells; **oligodendrocytes**, which form myelin; and **microglia**, which are resident cells of the monocyte/macrophage type.

The compact anatomy of the nervous system means that even small lesions may produce severe functional disturbances. Importantly, any neurons that are lost cannot be replaced, as they lack the capacity for cell division.

RESPONSES OF THE NERVOUS SYSTEM TO INJURY

The nervous system has several pathological responses to injury that are not seen in other tissues.

Neuronal chromatolysis is a reparative response of neurons following damage to the axon (*Fig. 21.1*). The neuronal cell body swells due to accumulation of neuro-filaments and there is peripheral migration of the Nissl substance, associated with nuclear swelling. Chromatolysis is part of the regenerative response whereby neurons can regrow a severed axon (see page 465).

Phagocytosis. Following cell death, removal of damaged tissues is achieved by phagocytic resident microglial cells, which are supplemented by recruitment of monocytes from the blood. These phagocytic cells become vacuolated by accumulated lipid from dead cells, forming foam cells.

Gliosis. Astrocytes become activated, proliferating to fulfil metabolic roles in protecting neurons. Following

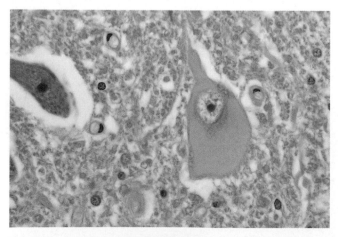

Fig. 21.1 Neuronal chromatolysis.
This neuron shows central chromatolysis. The neuron is swollen with no visible Nissl substance. The nucleus is large, centrally placed with an open chromatin pattern.

death of cells, and removal by phagocytes, damaged areas are replaced by proliferation of astrocytes, which form a **glial scar**. In large areas of damage, astrocytic gliosis may not entirely replace a defect, and an area remains that is partly cystic and partly gliotic.

Cerebral edema is accumulation of tissue fluid in between the cells of the nervous system. Seen after damage from many different causes, it is the result of breakdown of the blood–brain barrier due to ischemia, trauma, inflammation, and metabolic disorders. This breakdown also occurs around tumors.

Severe cerebral swelling is associated with a rise in the pressure within the skull (**raised intracranial pressure**).

Expanding intracranial lesions cause raised intracranial pressure

The cranial cavity is divided into three spaces by the falx and tentorium cerebelli. If a lesion expands within the brain substance, there is only a limited amount of room within the skull to accommodate it. Initially, reduction in the size of the ventricles and subarachnoid space occurs, but once this volume is used, further increase in the size of a lesion is associated with increase in intracranial pressure.

Swellings within the brain are particularly dangerous when they lead to rapid local expansion of one part, causing it to shift from one brain compartment to another, a process termed **cerebral herniation**. There are four types of cerebral herniation (*Fig. 21.2a*):

Transtentorial herniation is caused by lesions expanding in one cerebral hemisphere. There is herniation of the medial part of the temporal lobe down over the tentorium cerebelli to compress the upper brain stem (*Fig. 21.2b*). The third cranial nerve becomes first stretched, then compressed on the side of the lesion, giving rise to a fixed dilated pupil. Branches of the posterior cerebral artery are also compressed as the brain herniates, causing secondary infarction of the occipital lobe. As the midbrain is distorted by compression, small vessels are torn and secondary hemorrhage occurs into the brain stem leading to death.

Cerebellar tonsillar herniation is caused by expanding lesions in the posterior fossa. There is herniation of the lower part of the cerebellum (cerebellar tonsils), which pushes down into the foramen magnum and compresses the medulla; this process is also known as coning. As the medulla is compressed, it causes cessation of respiration and death. This may be precipitated by performing a lumbar puncture in a person with a mass in the brain. Withdrawal of CSF allows a pressure gradient to develop and there is rapid coning with death. Lumbar puncture should never be performed until the possibility of a mass lesion in the cranial cavity has been excluded.

Cingulate gyrus (subfalcial) herniation is caused by a lesion in one of the cerebral hemispheres, resulting in movement of the cingulate gyrus beneath the falx cerebri. This is often associated with compression of the adjacent anterior cerebral artery, leading to secondary cerebral infarction.

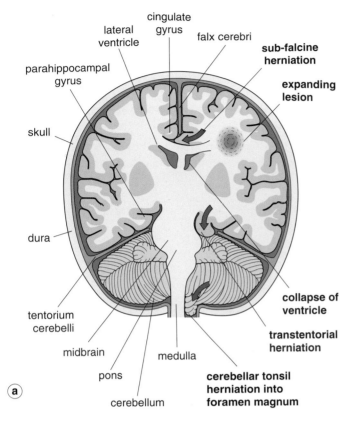

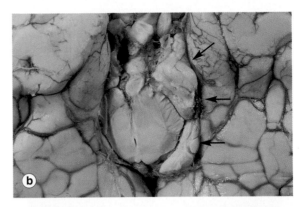

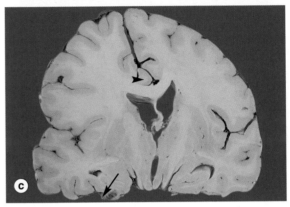

Fig. 21.2 Cerebral herniation. (a) If there is expansion of a lesion on one side of the brain, for example a tumor or a hematoma, a pressure gradient develops. The cingulate gyrus may move beneath the falx cerebri and the parahippocampal gyrus may herniate through the tentorial hiatus. If pressure increases in the posterior fossa, herniation of the cerebellar tonsils into the foraman magnum may occur. (b) Herniation of the parahippocampal gyrus through the tentorial hiatus. The free edge of the tentorium cerebelli has indented the cerebrum (arrows) along the margin of the herniated brain tissue. (c) Herniation contusions (arrow) may be visible where the uncus or parahippocampal gyrus has been pressed against the edge of the tentorium, in this case by a subdural hematoma (not visible in figure). Histologic examination of the contusions reveals focal necrosis and small hemorrhages. The subdural hematoma has also displaced midline structures and caused subfalcine herniation of the cingulate gyrus (arrowhead).

Clinical features of raised intracranial pressure

Patients with raised intracranial pressure may develop symptoms and signs due to an expanding cerebral lesion. In slowly expanding lesions, compensation takes place and signs develop slowly. In rapidly expanding lesions, signs and symptoms can develop within minutes.

There may be **vomiting** due to movement of the medulla and stimulation of vomiting centers, **headache** due to stimulation of pain-sensitive nerve endings associated with stretched vessels, and **papilledema** due to impaired flow of axonal cytoplasm in the optic nerves, caused by increased pressure of the CSF in the optic nerve sheath.

If a lesion expands rapidly, there is danger of cerebral herniation. It is usual to observe patients carefully on a regular basis to detect the earliest signs of an enlarging brain lesion. This is usually done after head trauma to detect any developing cerebral pathology.

- The pupils are observed. A sluggish pupillary reaction to light is seen when there is stretching of the third cranial nerve in early transtentorial herniation. A fixed dilated pupil indicates crushing of the nerve and is seen in more advanced herniation.
- Conscious level is assessed. As the brain stem is compressed, there is progressive reduction in conscious level.

In the late advanced stages of raised intracranial pressure, **bradycardia**, **hypertension** and **neurogenic pulmonary edema** develop. These are usually seen only in patients who are close to death from a cerebral mass lesion.

Diencephalic herniation is caused by generalized swelling of both cerebral hemispheres. There is compression of the ventricles, with descent of the thalamus and midbrain through the tentorial hiatus. This causes tearing of vessels in the midbrain, with secondary hemorrhage.

CEREBROVASCULAR DISEASE

Cerebrovascular diseases are the third most common cause of death in western countries. The most frequent manifestation of disease is a sudden episode of neurological deficit termed a stroke, which is the result of cerebral hemorrhage or cerebral infarction in the majority of cases.

Arteriovenous malformations predispose to intracranial hemorrhage

Arteriovenous malformations (AVMs) are developmental abnormalities of blood vessels (both arteries and veins) in which leashes of unusually fragile vessels are formed. They occur most commonly in relation to the cerebral hemispheres, but other sites (including the cord) are affected. Macroscopically, lesions may involve the meninges, extend deep into the brain, or be mixed in pattern. They vary in size, but are typically 3–4 cm in diameter. Lesions have several feeding arterial vessels and several draining channels, making surgical removal very difficult.

Clinically, AVMs are a cause of epilepsy and of other focal neurological signs. The major problem is that the fragile vessels bleed, causing life-threatening intracranial hemorrhage. Hemangiomas also occur in the brain as cavernous or capillary lesions.

Cerebral blood vessels are prone to atheroma, arteriolosclerosis and amyloid deposition

The cerebral arteries are prone to the general pathological processes that affect systemic arteries.

Atheroma principally affects the main named cerebral arteries. It is generally more severe in the basilar artery than in the anterior and middle cerebral vessels. The main complications of atheroma are thrombosis and aneurysm formation. Atheroma is particularly important in the extracranial cerebral arteries, the carotid and vertebral vessels in the neck. It is now appreciated that the majority of cerebral ischemic events are caused by disease in the extracranial vessels, especially in the region of the carotid bifurcation.

Arteriolosclerosis affects the small vessels that penetrate the brain and is caused by long-standing hypertension or diabetes. Vessels show replacement of the muscular media by hyaline material, which weakens the walls and predisposes to intracerebral hemorrhage. Reduction in the size of the lumen of small vessels also predisposes to very small cerebral infarcts (**lacunar infarcts**).

Amyloid (see Chapter 25), especially that derived from Aβ peptide (as seen in Alzheimer's disease), is frequently deposited in the cerebral vessels of the elderly, causing amyloid angiopathy. This predisposes to intracerebral hemorrhage in a peripheral distribution in the cerebral hemispheres; it is the cause of cerebral hemorrhage in about 10% of cases in patients over the age of 70 years.

Berry aneurysms are the most common type of aneurysm of cerebral arteries

Berry aneurysms are small saccular aneurysms that occur in about 2% of the population. Macroscopically they appear as rounded swellings arising from the cerebral arteries (*Fig. 21.3*). Although they can be 0.2–3 cm in diameter, most are under 1 cm. Occurring particularly at the branch points of vessels around the circle of Willis, they are frequently multiple.

- 45% arise in the region of the anterior communicating cerebral artery.
- 30% arise from the middle cerebral artery as it divides deep in the Sylvian fissure.
- 20% arise in the region of the internal carotid arteries, usually at the origin of the posterior communicating artery.
- 5% arise elsewhere in the cerebral circulation.
- Aneurysms are prone to rupture, with consequent subarachnoid hemorrhage (see page 440).

Berry aneurysms arise because of developmental defects in the internal elastic lamina of vessels. The stress of the systolic waves causes herniation of the intima, with formation of saccular aneurysms. This is accentuated by hypertension, and aneurysms are commonly seen in association with coarctation of the aorta and adult polycystic renal disease.

Less common are **atherosclerotic** and **infective (mycotic) aneurysms**. Atherosclerotic aneurysms are most common in the basilar artery, where they tend to be fusiform (*Fig. 21.4*). Infective (mycotic) aneurysms arise

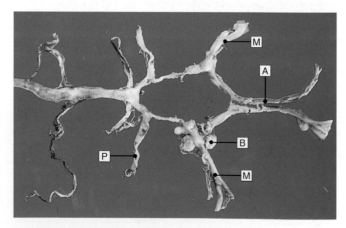

Fig. 21.3 Berry aneurysm.
This is the circle of Willis, with anterior (**A**), middle (**M**) and posterior (**P**) cerebral arteries linked by communicating vessels. Berry aneurysms (**B**) are seen arising where the internal carotid bifurcates into middle and anterior cerebral vessels.

in cases of infective endocarditis, when a small segment of arterial wall is acutely inflamed and dilates due to local bacterial infection from a small septic embolus.

Stroke is common in the general population

Stroke occurs in 2 per 1000 of the general population. A clinical diagnosis with several pathological causes, it is mainly seen in the elderly population.

The **clinical diagnosis of stroke** is defined as a sudden onset of non-traumatic focal neurological deficit that causes death or lasts for over 24 hours.

The terms **minor stroke** and **reversible ischemic neurological deficit** (RIND) are used when recovery of clinical features occurs after a period of time, usually defined as 7 days.

Transient ischemic attacks (TIA) are defined as episodes of non-traumatic focal loss of cerebral or visual function lasting no more than 24 hours.

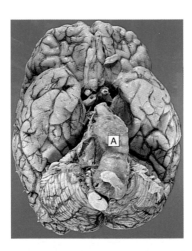

Fig. 21.4 Fusiform atherosclerotic aneurysm.
The basilar artery is replaced by a large fusiform aneurysm (**A**) caused by atherosclerosis.

The causes of stroke can be divided into two main groups: **ischemic** (85%), caused by cerebral infarction; and **hemorrhagic** (15%), caused by intracerebral and subarachnoid hemorrhage.

Hemorrhages and ischemic lesions caused by trauma are discussed later in this chapter (see page 441 *et seq.*).

BRAIN ISCHEMIA AND INFARCTION

There are four types of ischemic stroke: large vessel, small vessel, venous and global

The four main types of ischemic stroke are classified according to the pathogenesis of reduced blood flow to the brain.

Large vessel disease causes regional infarction, the main mechanisms being embolism and thrombosis in named cerebral arteries. Infarcts correspond to territories of supply of named cerebral arteries and their main branches.

Small vessel disease causes microinfarcts known as lacunar infarcts. These are caused by arteriolosclerosis predisposed by hypertension and diabetes. The main sites for this type of infarction are the pons and the basal ganglia/internal capsule region.

Venous infarction causes hemorrhagic necrosis. Due to thrombosis in a main cerebral venous sinus, it is associated with abnormal predisposition to thrombosis, e.g. polycythemia or dehydration.

Global ischemia causes widespread neuronal necrosis and can lead to laminar cortical necrosis. It is seen when there is reduction in cerebral blood flow as, for example, with cardiorespiratory arrest. When blood flow is reduced but not completely absent (as in severe hypotension), infarction at arterial boundary zones occurs, sometimes termed 'watershed infarction'.

Mechanisms of hypoxic and ischemic damage

Hypoxic and ischemic damage to the brain results in failure of supply of energy sources. Neurons have small metabolic reserves and are extremely sensitive to energy deprivation. This situation is seen in: **failure of blood oxygenation**, which occurs in severe respiratory disease, asphyxiation and carbon monoxide poisoning; **failure of blood flow**, which may be either focal (as occurs in occlusion of a cerebral artery) or generalized (as occurs with a cardiac arrest); and **severe hypoglycemia**, which causes energy deprivation to the brain despite an adequate supply of blood and oxygen.

Failure of supply of energy substrates to the brain causes death of neurons, with sparing of vessels and support cells, which are more robust. The neurons that

are most vulnerable are the large cells in the hippocampus and those in the cerebellar cortex (Purkinje cells).

Total irreversible cessation of blood flow leads to cerebral infarction in the territory supplied by the artery involved. This affects all cell types including glial cells and vessels.

An important event in ischemic damage is **activation of glutamate receptors**, which causes uncontrolled entry of calcium into neurons, leading to cell death. This concept, termed excitotoxicity, is believed to be a common factor in many types of neuronal death, including that seen in severe epilepsy. Use of drugs that block certain types of glutamate receptor can prevent neuronal death following ischemia.

Regional cerebral infarction is caused by occlusion of named cerebral arteries

Regional cerebral infarcts are caused by occlusion of main named arteries supplying the brain. The most common causes originate outside the cranial cavity, e.g. emboli from the heart, aorta or carotid vessels, and thrombosis in the carotid or vertebral arteries (*Fig. 21.5*), predisposed by atheroma. Less common causes of infarction are seen in younger stroke patients (see blue box).

Cerebral infarcts correspond to the territory of supply of the occluded arteries. It is difficult to see an infarct in the first 24 hours, as changes are limited to focal swelling and blurring of the normal demarcation between gray and white matter, termed a **pale or anemic infarct**. If there is lysis of an occlusive thrombus, the infarcted area may be reperfused with blood, resulting in a hemorrhagic infarct (*Fig. 21.6*).

By about 1 week the infarcted area becomes macroscopically soft and is infiltrated by macrophages, which remove dead tissue. Proliferation of astrocytes occurs around the margins of the infarct, and these partly replace the dead tissue, usually being well established by about 2 weeks. Larger regional areas of infarction invariably heal as fluid-filled cystic spaces bounded by gliosis (*Fig. 21.7*).

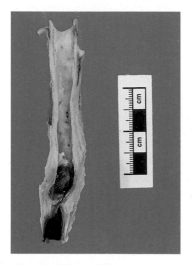

Fig. 21.5 Carotid artery thrombosis. This is the carotid artery dissected from the neck of a patient who died of cerebral infarction. There is complete occlusion by thrombus complicating an established atheromatous plaque at the level of the bifurcation.

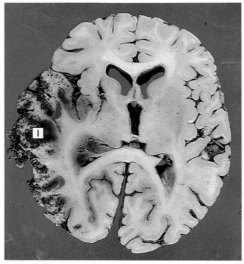

Fig. 21.6 Recent hemorrhagic cerebral infarct. This is a transverse axial slice through a brain, in the same plane as seen in routine CT scans. A large infarct, corresponding to the territory of the middle cerebral artery is seen as an area of swollen hemorrhagic brain (**I**). The hemorrhage was caused by reperfusion after lysis of an occluding thrombus.

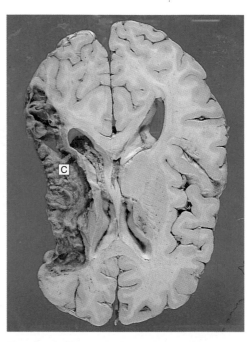

Fig. 21.7 Old healed cerebral infarct. This is a transverse axial brain slice. With time, a regional cerebral infarct is replaced by a cystic gliotic cavity (**C**).

Stroke in younger patients

The causes of strokes in younger patients are different from those seen in the elderly.

- 40% are the result of non-traumatic intracerebral hemorrhage, the main causes being hypertension, berry aneurysms, AVMs, and bleeding into tumors. Cocaine and heroin abuse also predisposes to hemorrhage.

- 20% of cases have subarachnoid hemorrhage, the majority being due to ruptured berry aneurysms or vascular malformations.

- 40% of cases have cerebral infarction. In 30% of these cases no cause is ascertained. In the other 70% there are diverse and sometimes unusual causes including **vascular occlusion** (cardiogenic emboli, premature atherosclerosis, vasculitis, arterial dissection), **vascular spasm** (migraine-associated, recreational drugs), **increased thrombolic tendency** (oral contraceptives and pregnancy, alcohol and smoking, antiphospholipid antibodies), and **heritable conditions** (congenital lack of inhibitors of coagulation).

Although a number of clinical syndromes related to occlusion of individual arteries are described, the most important practical distinction is between those affecting the **carotid territory** (frontal, temporal, parietal lobes or basal ganglia/internal capsule) and those affecting the **vertebrobasilar territory** (occipital lobe, cerebellum or brain stem).

Large cerebral infarcts may cause death by associated cerebral swelling, leading to herniation, and brain stem compression. Infarcts in critical sites, particularly brain stem infarcts, may interfere with vital functions and lead to death. Immobility and difficulty in swallowing lead to development of pneumonia in many patients.

Lacunar infarction is caused by arteriolosclerosis of small vessels

Lacunar infarcts are small, often slit-shaped, areas of infarction that are less than 1 cm in maximum diameter. They are an important form of cerebral infarct, particularly in patients with hypertension and diabetes, being caused by **hyaline arteriolosclerosis**.

Macroscopically, lesions are usually multiple and are seen in the sites normally supplied by fine perforating branches, such as the basal ganglia, internal capsule, thalamus and pons (*Fig. 21.8*).

Clinically, lacunar infarcts can be asymptomatic or may cause very restricted neurological deficits such as monoparesis. Multiple lacunar infarcts in the basal ganglia cause a syndrome of rigidity and abnormal gait, which superficially resembles Parkinson's disease, termed vascular pseudo-Parkinsonism. Lacunar infarction is also associated with ischemic white-matter degeneration, an important cause of dementia. Because hypertension and diabetes are risk factors for ischemic heart disease and atheroma, lacunar infarcts are often seen in association with regional infarcts caused by large vessel disease.

Cortical laminar necrosis is caused by generalized failure of perfusion

Diffuse necrosis of cerebral cortical neurons is the pattern of infarction seen in generalized failure of blood flow or oxygenation as seen, for example, following cardiac arrest, with severe hypoglycemia, and after carbon monoxide poisoning.

Changes develop 24 hours after resuscitation from the damaging episode. There is widespread damage to the cerebral cortex, with death of the majority of cortical neurons. With time, there is phagocytosis of dead neurons with astrocytic gliosis.

Macroscopically the cerebral cortex is shrunken and there is extensive loss of axons from the brain, causing white matter loss (*Fig. 21.9*).

Patients who survive global laminar necrosis generally have severe brain damage, existing in a vegetative state devoid of higher cortical functions. Lesser degrees of hypoxia or cerebral perfusion failure result in similar damage, limited to the particularly vulnerable areas of the hippocampus and cerebellar cortex.

Venous infarction is caused by venous sinus thrombosis

Venous infarction is the least common pattern of cerebral infarction. It occurs when there is occlusion of the venous sinuses and cerebral cortical veins by local thrombosis (*Fig. 21.10*).

Predisposing factors include dehydration in children, spread of infection from adjacent foci in the head (nasal sinus and middle ear) and disorders that cause hypercoagulability of blood, particularly polycythemia, oral contraceptive therapy and pregnancy.

Macroscopically the affected brain shows severe hemorrhagic infarction caused by vascular congestion.

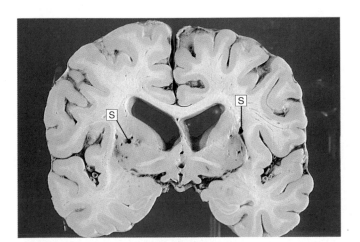

Fig. 21.8 Lacunar infarcts of brain.
Lacunar infarcts are seen as small slit-shaped cavities (**S**), a few millimeters in size, in the basal ganglia on both sides. They are caused by disease of small perforating vessels.

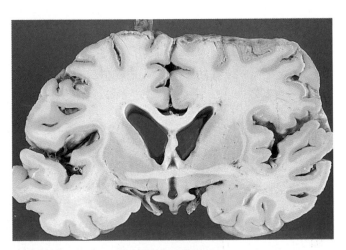

Fig. 21.9 Cortical laminar necrosis.
The cortex is replaced by a band of yellow gliotic tissue, most evident in the superior part of the brain compared to the temporal lobes.

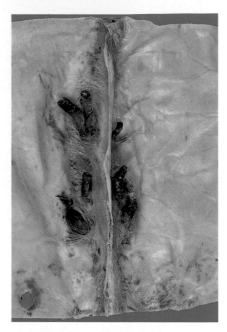

Fig. 21.10 Sagittal sinus thrombosis. This shows the inside of the dura from the skull. The sagittal sinus is thrombosed with propogation of thrombus down cortical veins that have been stripped off with the dura.

SPONTANEOUS INTRACRANIAL HEMORRHAGE

Spontaneous intracranial hemorrhage accounts for about 15% of all strokes and is caused by intracerebral hematoma and subarachnoid hemorrhage. Petechial hemorrhage is a less common pattern. Hemorrhage caused by trauma is considered in a later section (see page 442).

Cerebral hematomas are most commonly caused by hypertensive vascular damage

The most common cause of cerebral hemorrhage is hypertensive vascular damage. Prolonged hypertension results in arteriosclerosis and in the development of small microaneurysms (Charcot–Bouchard aneurysms), which predispose to vessel rupture, resulting in a hematoma. The common sites for hypertensive intracerebral hematoma are those supplied by fine perforating vessels (basal ganglia, internal capsule, thalamus, cerebellum and pons).

In patients over the age of 70 years, 10% of cerebral hemorrhages are caused by the presence of cerebral artery amyloid, which is composed of Aβ peptide (see page 543). This causes hematomas, seen in the periphery of cerebral hemispheres (lobar hemorrhages). This type is associated with a better clinical outcome than the deep bleeds associated with hypertension.

Less common causes of a cerebral hematoma are bleeding into a tumor, rupture of vascular malformations, cerebral vasculitis, bleeding associated with disordered coagulation, and bleeding occurring in association with leukemias.

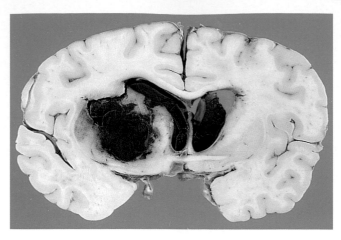

Fig. 21.11 Intracerebral hematoma.
A large hematoma effaces the basal ganglia, with compression of adjacent brain. Blood has ruptured into the ventricles.

Macroscopically, hematomas appear as a large blood clot, causing compression and damage to adjacent brain (*Fig. 21.11*). Large hematomas in the basal ganglia or thalamus often rupture into the ventricular system. If the patient survives a bleed, the hematoma is removed by phagocytic cells; astrocytic gliosis takes place, leaving a cavity stained yellow-brown with hemosiderin. Large bleeds that cause raised intracranial pressure, and those that rupture into the ventricular system, are usually fatal.

Subarachnoid hemorrhage is most often caused by a ruptured berry aneurysm

Bleeding into the subarachnoid space (between the arachnoid and the pia) is termed **subarachnoid hemorrhage**. A cause of stroke from adolescence to old age, it accounts for about 5% of all cases. In most cases, the cause of subarachnoid bleeding is rupture of a berry aneurysm; less common causes are rupture of an intracerebral hematoma into the subarachnoid space or rupture of a vascular malformation.

Macroscopically a layer of blood is present over the brain surface in the subarachnoid space (*Fig. 21.12*). Blood is therefore present in the cerebrospinal fluid (CSF) and can be detected on lumbar puncture. There are two effects of subarachnoid hemorrhage:

- Blood around vessels causes vascular spasm and leads to widespread cerebral ischemia and brain swelling.
- There may be blockage of CSF resorption, causing acute hydrocephalus.

About 30% of patients die immediately; others who present with headache and signs of meningeal irritation may have surgical intervention and clipping of the aneurysm. In the absence of operative intervention, 30% of patients have a rebleed within 1 year, most within 1 month of their first bleed. A long-term complication is development of hydrocephalus caused by blockage and fibrosis in the CSF pathways.

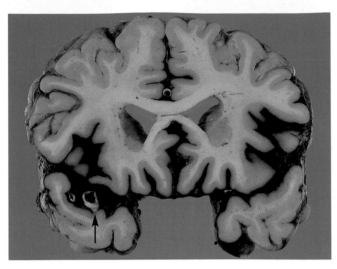

Fig. 21.12 Subarachnoid hemorrhage.
Owing to rupture of a berry aneurysm just visible in the sylvian fissure (arrow), blood is present in the subarachnoid space over the cerebral hemispheres.

Diffuse petechial hemorrhage in the brain is caused by damage to small vessels

The least common form of cerebral hemorrhage is multiple petechial hemorrhages scattered throughout the brain. These are 1–2 mm in size and are concentrated in the white matter. They are caused by disease that disrupts the walls of small cerebral blood vessels, allowing extravasation of red cells. Patients with this pattern of disease tend to present with confusion and decreased conscious level, rather than with focal neurological signs. The main causes are acute hypertensive encephalopathy, fat embolism, vasculitis of small cerebral vessels (e.g. polyarteritis), cerebral malaria and acute hemorrhagic leukoencephalitis (allergic vasculitis of cerebral vessels).

TRAUMA TO THE CENTRAL NERVOUS SYSTEM

Head injury is one of the most common causes of disability and death in young men, mainly sustained during road traffic accidents and falls. Injury is divided into two types:

- **Non-missile trauma** (closed head injury) is the result of acceleration/deceleration forces to the head, and the resultant rotational and shearing forces on the brain, which cause movement of the brain within the skull. This happens when the head is violently thrown forward or when a head travelling at speed is suddenly brought to a halt (motor cyclist's head in contact with road). This is the most common pattern of head trauma encountered clinically.

- **Missile trauma** (open head injury) is caused by penetration of the skull or brain by an external object such as a bullet.

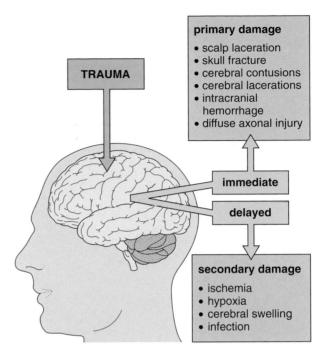

Fig. 21.13 Closed head injury. Primary and secondary damage related to non-missile head injury.

Brain pathology from head injury may be divided into two groups: primary or secondary

Brain pathology from head injury may be primary (i.e. the immediate consequence of impact damage) or secondary (i.e. occurring as a delayed consequence of brain swelling, bleeding and hypoxia) (*Fig. 21.13*).

There are two main patterns of primary brain damage in closed head injury.

1 **Cerebral contusions** occur when the brain moves within the cranial cavity, causing parts of the brain to be crushed by violent contact with the skull or dural membranes. For the most part, these occur adjacent to the site of impact (*coup* lesions) and diagonally opposite (*contrecoup* lesions). The most common sites for this pattern of damage are the underside of the frontal lobes, the tips and inferior aspects of the temporal lobes, the occipital poles, and the cerebellum (*Fig. 21.14*). Early contusions appear as petechial hemorrhage into cortical gray matter and underlying white matter. Over a period of several hours there is oozing of blood, and contusions become hemorrhagic, with severe swelling of the brain (*Fig. 21.15*). Severe contusions may be associated with extensive intracerebral, subarachnoid and subdural hemorrhage. Contusions heal by gliosis, which is often associated with brown hemosiderin deposition (caused by the associated hemorrhage).

2 **Diffuse axonal injury** is the result of shearing of axons due to acceleration/deceleration/torsional forces, leading to severe damage to white matter tracts.

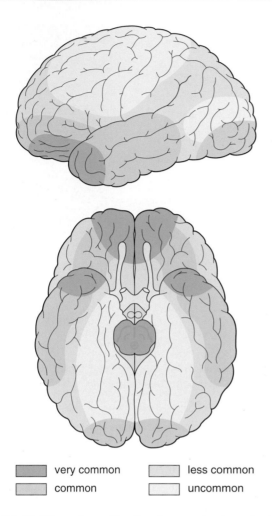

very common

common

less common

uncommon

Fig. 21.14 Sites of predilection for cerebral contusions.

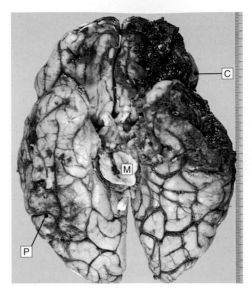

Fig. 21.15 Cerebral contusions. Primary impact damage has caused severe hemorrhagic contusion of the left frontal lobe (**C**) – *coup* lesion, with smaller contusions on the right parietal lobe (**P**) – *contrecoup* lesion. Swelling of the left side of the brain has caused cerebral herniation with compression of the midbrain (**M**).

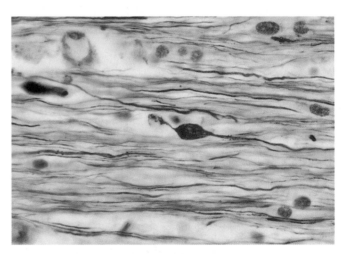

Fig. 21.16 Diffuse axonal injury.
If silver stains are used on white matter normal axons are seen as long thin black-stained structures. Axonal swellings can be seen as oval-shaped structures and have been caused by axonal damage in head injury.

Patients with this pattern of damage who survive are generally severely disabled. Most of the changes are seen histologically only, consisting of axonal tearing visible as swellings of the torn ends of nerve fibers (axonal retraction balls) (*Fig. 21.16*). Petechial hemorrhages may also occur in the corpus collosum and brain stem, and their detection at these sites is a useful indicator of this type of severe head injury.

Secondary brain damage occurs after the immediate impact. Head injury is often associated with widespread trauma, which leads to problems maintaining blood oxygenation and blood pressure. As a consequence, head injury is often complicated by the development of secondary hypoxic brain damage and cerebral edema.

Tearing of blood vessels with trauma leads to four main types of cerebral hemorrhage: **intracerebral hematoma**, caused by tearing of vessels within the brain parenchyma; **subarachnoid hemorrhage**, caused by tearing of vessels adjacent to the subarachnoid space; **subdural hemorrhage**, caused by tearing of veins (discussed below); and **extradural hemorrhage**, caused by tearing of vessels in the skull (discussed below).

Extradural hemorrhage is caused by tearing of vessels running outside the dura

Extradural hemorrhage causes a hematoma in the potential extradural space between the skull and the dura (*Fig. 21.17*) and is almost always the result of skull fracture, which tears an artery or a main venous sinus running outside the dura. A vessel commonly involved is the **middle meningeal artery** (associated with fracture of the temporal bone).

The extradural hematoma appears as a gelatinous layer of blood clot outside the dura. This accumulation causes

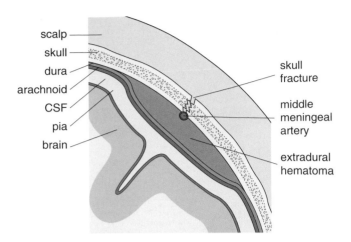

Fig. 21.17 Extradural hemorrhage.

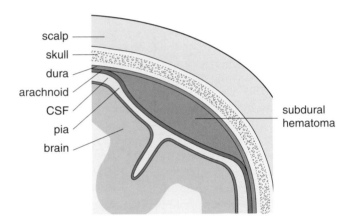

Fig. 21.18 Subdural hemorrhage.

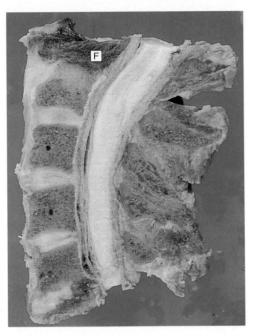

Fig. 21.19 Spinal cord trauma. Fracture of a vertebra (**F**) is associated with narrowing of the spinal canal and compression of the cord, which appears slightly yellowed and swollen at the site of injury.

compression of the brain and development of transtentorial herniation. In many cases, high-pressure arterial blood accumulates rapidly, leading to an acute decline in conscious level with raised intracranial pressure. In other cases, blood accumulates over a period of hours and it is not uncommon to have a history of head trauma followed by gradual development of drowsiness, leading to coma and death.

Some subdural hematomas are caused by minor head trauma and have a chronic pattern of evolution

Subdural hemorrhage results in a hematoma developing in the subdural space between the dura and the arachnoid (*Fig. 21.18*). It is caused by traumatic tearing of venous vessels that traverse the subdural space. There are two patterns.

Acute subdural hematomas are usually seen after a severe head injury and are associated with other types of brain injury. They cause rapid accumulation of blood, leading to acute neurological deterioration as a result of raised intracranial pressure.

Chronic subdural hematomas usually occur as a result of minimal trauma and are mainly seen in the very young (including childhood non-accidental injury) and the elderly. Blood typically accumulates slowly over a period of days or weeks, becoming localized by a membrane of fibrovascular granulation tissue. In addition to the osmotic effects of degenerating blood clot drawing in fluid from the CSF, increase in the size of the hematoma occurs with further bleeding. Clinical symptoms and signs may only become obvious weeks after an apparently trivial injury, as a result of raised intracranial pressure.

Macroscopically a subdural hematoma is seen as a layer of gelatinous blood clot (acute type) or as an organized layer of dark liquefied clot surrounded by membranes (chronic type), which flattens and compresses the underlying brain, staining the outside of the arachnoid with hemosiderin.

Trauma to the spinal cord is a common cause of disability in young men

Most spinal cord injuries occur in young males as a result of road traffic accidents, falls and sport.

Injury is mainly caused by fracture and dislocation of the vertebral column, causing compression of the spinal cord by distortion of the spinal canal (*Fig. 21.19*). Minor contusions of the cord result in transient recoverable neurological abnormality. Severe contusions cause damage to ascending and descending tracts, as well as necrosis of neurons at the segments damaged.

The consequence of cord damage depends on the spinal level of the injury; cervical lesions cause tetraplegia, whereas

Fig. 21.20
Causes of spinal cord compression

Prolapse of intervertebral disc

Osteophytes caused by spondylosis

Bone disease (rheumatoid or Paget's)

Extradural tumor or abscess, or meningeal fibrosis

Intradural tumor (schwannoma, arteriovenous malformation, meningioma)

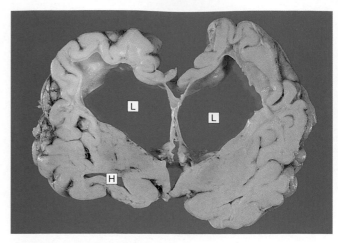

Fig. 21.21 Hydrocephalus.
The lateral ventricles (**L**) including the temporal horns (**H**) are dilated. In this case the cause was obstruction of CSF flow through the cerebral aqueduct.

lower thoracic lesions cause paraplegia. Denervated muscles undergo atrophy, with secondary contractures and deformities in limbs. Denervation of the bladder leads to problems with micturition, urinary stasis and recurrent infections.

Penetrating injuries of the spinal cord are uncommon, but may be seen after stabbings or shootings. Complete transection of the cord may occur, hemisection giving rise to a Brown–Séquard syndrome.

In addition to trauma, the spinal cord and nerve roots are vulnerable to damage by non-traumatic compression, the main causes of which are summarized in *Fig. 21.20*.

HYDROCEPHALUS

Excess CSF in the intracranial cavity is termed 'hydrocephalus' and most cases are caused by obstruction of the flow of CSF

The term hydrocephalus is used to describe conditions in which there is increase in the CSF volume within the brain, with expansion of the cerebral ventricles. The most common type, which is termed **non-communicating hydrocephalus** or **obstructive hydrocephalus**, is caused by blockage of the CSF pathway from the ventricles to the subarachnoid space. A less common type is communicating hydrocephalus, in which there is impairment of resorption of CSF at the arachnoid villi along the dural venous sinuses, usually precipitated by previous infection or bleeding into the subarachnoid space.

Among the main causes of obstructive hydrocephalus is **congenital hydrocephalus**, seen in about 1 in 1000 births. Some cases have stenosis of the aqueduct of Sylvius, some have associated Arnold–Chiari malformation (see page 457), and some are inherited as an X-linked trait.

Tumors may obstruct the ventricular system, particularly those located in the brain stem, cerebellum, or pineal region which block the cerebral aqueduct or fourth ventricle.

Scarring and **blockage of the CSF exit foramina** at the base of the brain are common complications of meningitis or subarachnoid hemorrhage.

Hemorrhage in the brain or subarachnoid space may obstruct CSF drainage pathways.

Macroscopically, there is dilatation of the ventricular cavities of the brain proximal to the site of obstruction (*Fig. 21.21*). The effects of hydrocephalus depend on the speed of development of disease and age of the patient.

In **acute hydrocephalus**, swelling of the brain may be rapid and may cause death due to cerebral herniation.

In **chronic hydrocephalus**, signs and symptoms develop slowly and there are clinical features of raised intracranial pressure. When hydrocephalus develops in children, before fusion of the skull bones, there is progressive enlargement of the head circumference. In adults, where the skull is rigidly fused, prolonged disease causes thinning of the skull vault. In the absence of treatment, long-standing disease causes axonal damage and gliosis in the white matter. In children this leads to mental subnormality and in adults can lead to the development of a dementia syndrome, with early gait disturbance and incontinence as prominent features.

Treatment of hydrocephalus involves placement of a permanent shunt to drain CSF into the peritoneal cavity. This leads to other pathological complications because shunts become periodically blocked, leading to acute attacks of hydrocephalus. Shunts also become infected with low-virulence organisms, producing signs and symptoms of infection, as well as immune-mediated glomerular disease.

SYRINGOMYELIA

A syrinx is a fluid-filled cavity in the cord or brain stem

A syrinx is a fluid-filled, slit-like cavity that develops in the spinal cord (**syringomyelia**) or brain stem (**syringobulbia**), causing compression of the white matter tracts and resulting in neurological disability. Most syringeal cavities are secondary to trauma or ischemia, or are associated with tumors of the spinal cord. Less commonly, a syrinx may be a primary developmental phenomenon. Syringeal cavities are most frequent in the cervical spinal cord and may extend over many segments.

Clinical manifestations of syringomyelia are due to compression of the spinal cord tracts and include wasting of the intrinsic muscles of the hand, spastic weakness in the legs, and loss of pain and temperature sensation, with preservation of touch.

INFECTION OF THE CENTRAL NERVOUS SYSTEM

Infection of the central nervous system (CNS) is an extremely common clinical problem, which can be caused by most classes of infecting organism. There are four main patterns of associated inflammation, corresponding to the primary seat of the infective process:

1 **Meningitis** (inflammation of the meninges) is divided into leptomeningitis (inflammation centered on the subarachnoid space) and pachymeningitis (inflammation centered on the dura).
2 **Cerebritis** and **cerebral abscess** (focal inflammation of the brain).
3 **Encephalitis** (diffuse inflammation of the brain) or **myelitis** (diffuse inflammation of the cord).
4 **Meningoencephalitis** (combination of diffuse inflammation of the brain and inflammation of leptomeninges).

Leptomeningitis

Leptomeningitis is a form of inflammation centered on the subarachnoid space. Infecting organisms circulate and spread by the CSF route. Initial infection is nearly always the result of blood-borne spread of the infecting organism, but infection may also be caused by direct spread from infection in the middle ear, mastoid, nasal sinuses, and dural venous sinuses. Penetrating wounds, including fracture of skull, can also predispose to leptomeningitis.

Leptomeningitis can be divided into three main groups: **acute purulent meningitis**, which is mainly caused by bacterial infection; **lymphocytic meningitis**, which is mainly caused by viral infection; and **chronic** and **granulomatous meningitides**, which are caused by TB and unusual organisms (see Chapter 8).

Acute purulent meningitis is almost always caused by bacterial infection

Acute purulent meningitis is a severe infection that is nearly always caused by bacterial infection. Patients are severely unwell and have signs of infection, neck stiffness and photophobia. CSF examination shows turbid fluid with many neutrophil polymorphs and a low sugar; bacteria may be seen on special staining.

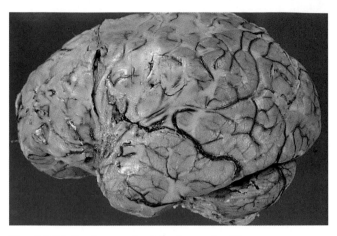

Fig. 21.22 Acute purulent leptomeningitis.
The subarachnoid space contains a creamy purulent exudate caused by bacterial meningitis. This is an acute inflammatory exudate that is rich in neutrophils.

Macroscopically, the subarachnoid space contains a cream-coloured acute inflammatory exudate that is rich in neutrophils (*Fig. 21.22*). The severe inflammation causes secondary thrombosis of superficial vessels and cerebral ischemic damage. If treated early, there may be resolution of disease. However, complications caused by organization of the inflammatory exudate may lead to obstruction of the CSF drainage pathways and to development of hydrocephalus.

The main causes of acute purulent meningitis vary according to age. In neonates *Escherichia coli*, *streptococci* and *Listeria monocytogenes* are responsible, and in children *Haemophilus influenzae* and *Neisseria meningitidis* are the principal causes. *Neisseria meningitidis* and *Streptococcus pneumoniae* type 3 are involved in adults, and in the elderly the main causative organisms are *Streptococcus pneumoniae* type 3 and *Listeria monocytogenes*.

Lymphocytic meningitis is usually caused by viruses and is a benign self-limited disease

Lymphocytic meningitis is a self-limited disease caused by several viral infections. In most cases patients have clinical malaise and meningism, and require investigation to exclude the presence of a bacterial meningitis. Typically the CSF is clear, has a normal glucose level, but has a mild elevation of protein and contains an increase in lymphoid cells.

The cause of infection is ascertained by virological or serological examination of CSF and blood. The most common causes are infection by the mumps, Coxsackie, ECHO, Epstein–Barr, lymphocytic choriomeningitis and polio viruses. No organism is detected in many cases.

Chronic and granulomatous meningitides are severe inflammatory diseases that lead to meningeal fibrosis and cranial nerve lesions

Chronic and granulomatous meningitides are forms of severe productive chronic inflammation and fibrosis. The

CSF is typically opalescent, with a raised protein level, reduced glucose level, and an increased lymphocyte count with the presence of plasma cells. The important causative organisms are *Mycobacterium tuberculosis*, *Treponema pallidum* (syphilis), *Cryptococcus neoformans*, and *Borrelia burgdorferi* (Lyme disease).

Macroscopically, there is thickening and opacity of the leptomeninges, with marked thickening and fibrosis in advanced disease. Histologically, there is lymphocytic and plasma-cell infiltration of the meninges with fibrosis. The cause of chronic meningitis may be apparent on examination. In tuberculous meningitis, caseating granulomas are seen, and mycobacteria may be visible on Ziehl–Neelsen (ZN) staining. In cryptococcal infection, fungi are usually clearly visible.

Meningeal fibrosis and inflammation have two main effects: they lead to obstruction of the drainage pathways for CSF, causing hydrocephalus (see page 444), and vascular lesions cause infarction and cranial nerve and spinal root palsies.

Pachymeningitis is mainly caused by direct spread of infection from a focus in the skull

Pachymeningitis is a pattern of inflammation caused by infection centered on the dura. In the vast majority of cases, it is the result of direct spread from a focus of infection in the adjacent skull, e.g. penetrating wounds with fracture of skull, osteomyelitis of vertebra or skull, or infection in the middle ear, mastoid, nasal sinuses, and dural venous sinuses.

The main causative organisms are *streptococci* and *Staphylococcus aureus*, Gram-negative organisms also being involved, as well as anaerobic organisms.

One of the main complications of pachymeningitis is epidural abscess. This may cause septicemia, spread to cause leptomeningitis, or act as a mass compressing nervous tissue. Another complication is subdural empyema with spread of infection in the subdural space, often causing thrombosis of cerebral venous channels.

Cerebritis and cerebral abscess are examples of severe focal infection of the brain caused by a wide range of organisms

Focal inflammation of the parenchyma of the brain, termed **cerebritis**, frequently leads to formation of a cerebral abscess. These patterns of inflammation develop in four main ways:

1 Secondary to meningitis and caused by the same types of organism.
2 Local extension from sepsis in the middle ear or mastoid cavities.
3 Hematogenous, particularly associated with bacterial endocarditis, cyanotic congenital heart disease, and pulmonary bronchiectasis.
4 Trauma following open injuries to the CNS.

Areas of brain affected by cerebritis appear as ill-defined areas of swelling, which are congested and soft on cut surface, being composed of necrotic brain infiltrated by neutrophils. An abscess is a rounded cavity, typically 1–2 cm in diameter, filled with pus and walled off both by gliosis and by fibroblasts derived from tissue adjacent to blood vessels (*Fig. 21.23*). Certain brain areas are preferred sites for abscess formation, according to etiology. For example, infection of the middle ear causes abscesses in temporal lobe or cerebellum, nasal sinus infection causes abscesses in frontal lobes, chronic lung sepsis tends to cause abscesses in frontal lobes, and septic emboli tend to cause abscesses in parietal lobes.

Microbiology usually reveals mixed bacterial organisms in cerebral abscesses, including a high frequency of anaerobic bacteria. TB may form a localized caseous abscess termed a '**tuberculoma**'. Cerebral abscesses may also be caused by fungal infection, e.g. *Candida*, *Aspergillus* and amebas, and some cases of cerebritis and abscess are due to *Toxoplasma*, predisposed by immunosuppression.

With the exception of viral meningitis, all forms of meningitis can lead to development of cerebritis or cerebral abscess. If they are not excised or drained surgically, abscesses may rupture to cause meningitis or ventriculitis.

Encephalitis and myelitis are diffuse inflammatory processes leading to neuronal death and brain swelling

Diffuse inflammation of the brain (**encephalitis**) and cord (**myelitis**) is caused by viral, rickettsial and certain bacterial organisms (mainly *Listeria*, *Treponema*, and *Borrelia*). The main viral organisms responsible for this pattern of infection are herpes simplex, polio and rabies. Clinically, diffuse inflammation causes neurological dysfunction manifest by myelopathy (motor and sensory signs) or encephalopathy (confusion and reduced level of consciousness).

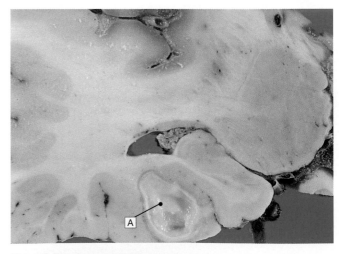

Fig. 21.23 Cerebral abscess.
An abscess (**A**) containing yellow pus is seen in the temporal lobe. This was caused by spread of infection from the middle ear.

Macroscopically, there is hyperemia of the meninges, petechial hemorrhages in the brain, and brain swelling due to edema. In some types, e.g. encephalitis due to herpes simplex, there is extensive brain necrosis. The results of encephalitis or myelitis are death of neurons, cuffing of cerebral blood vessels by lymphoid cells, and astrocytic gliosis. Depending on the cause, viral cellular inclusion bodies may be seen. For example, cytoplasmic Negri bodies are seen in rabies, and nuclear viral inclusion bodies are seen in herpes encephalitis.

VIRAL DISEASES OF THE NERVOUS SYSTEM

Viral diseases of the nervous system are seen in four main patterns:

- **Viral meningitis**, characterized by the development of lymphocytic meningitis (see page 445).
- **Cytolytic**, in which there is cell destruction producing encephalitis or myelitis. This is the most clinically severe pattern of involvement, most commonly seen with herpes simplex (*Fig. 21.24*).
- **Latent**, in which virus is integrated into the host cells, with the potential for reactivation as a cytolytic infection. This is extremely common with herpes zoster, causing shingles.
- **Persistent**, in which there is slow, smouldering degeneration of neuronal tissues caused by viral infection in the absence of elimination by immune responses, e.g. measles virus infection causing subacute sclerosing panencephalitis.

The main viral infections of the CNS are summarized in *Fig. 21.25*. Diffuse parenchymal infections lead to headache, drowsiness, and, in severe cases, coma. In addition to direct infection, systemic viral infections can predispose to immune-mediated demyelinization or vasculitis in the nervous system.

AIDS commonly affects the nervous system

One of the most common causes of viral infection of the nervous system is HIV. Not only does HIV directly affect the brain and spinal cord, AIDS also predisposes to several complications due to immunosuppression.

The **AIDS dementia complex** (**HIV cognitive/motor complex**) is a clinical syndrome that has elements of intellectual impairment, and behavioral and motor changes. Several pathologically defined changes underlie this clinical syndrome.

Lymphocytic meningitis is seen in patients around the time of seroconversion and is defined as occurring in the absence of any demonstrable opportunistic pathogens.

HIV encephalitis is a multifocal process characterized by inflammatory foci including multinucleate giant cells, mainly seen in white matter, basal ganglia and brain stem.

HIV leukoencephalopathy is characterized by myelin loss, gliosis, phagocytic macrophages and scattered multinucleate giant cells in white matter. There is little or no inflammatory infiltration.

Diffuse poliodystrophy is the term applied to neuronal loss, microglial activation and gliosis in CNS gray matter.

Vacuolar myelopathy is the term used to describe vacuolation in myelin sheaths, with myelin loss in the spinal cord.

Cerebral vasculitis is seen most prominently in childhood HIV disease of the brain.

Clinically, patients with mild cases of cognitive impairment and motor slowing have myelin pallor and gliosis corresponding to HIV leukoencephalopathy, whereas those with severe cognitive impairment and motor slowing tend to have HIV encephalitis. Patients with clinical signs of spinal cord disease have vacuolar myelopathy. The cerebral atrophy often seen on imaging correlates with neuronal loss and diffuse poliodystrophy.

The immunosuppression induced by AIDS predisposes to several opportunistic infections of the CNS, particularly

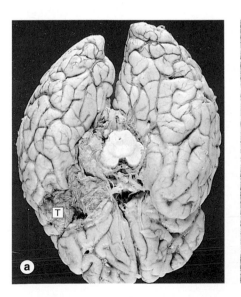
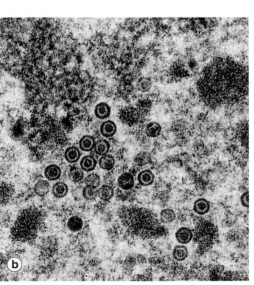

Fig. 21.24 Herpes encephalitis. In herpes simplex encephalitis (a) necrosis of the temporal lobes (**T**) is a typical development. Brain biopsy is useful in diagnosis when the virus can be seen by electron microscopy (b) as rounded particles with a dense core. Virus can also be identified by immunostaining or culture. In early cases, PCR can be used to identify viral DNA in CSF samples.

Fig. 21.25
Main viral infections of the CNS

Virus	Notes
Herpes zoster	Causes shingles in peripheral nerve dermatomes from latent infection of CNS dorsal root ganglion cells. Causes a vasculitis of the CNS.
Herpes simplex (HSV)	HSV-I causes necrotizing encephalitis affecting temporal lobes (*Fig. 21.24*). HSV-II causes meningitis and neonatal necrotizing encephalitis.
HIV-1	The causative virus of AIDS causes HIV encephalitis and myelopathy of spinal cord (see page 447).
Poliovirus	This is a picorna enterovirus. Most infections are sub-clinical. May cause lymphocytic meningitis or paralytic poliomyelitis with motor neuron death.
Cytomegalovirus	Causes encephalitis in immunosuppressed patients, e.g. AIDS. Also causes congenital infection of the CNS *in utero*, resulting in microcephaly and cerebral calcification.
Rubella	Causes infection of the brain *in utero* and leads to microcephaly.
HTLV-1	Causes tropical spastic paraparesis, a form of demyelination of the spinal cord.
Rabies virus	Rhabdovirus, transmitted by animal bite, travels in peripheral nerves to CNS, causing severe meningoencephalitis with a high fatality rate. Negri bodies are viral inclusions seen in nerve cells.
Measles	Causes subacute sclerosing panencephalitis in childhood, characterized by neuronal death and gliosis.
JC virus	A papovavirus causing progressive multifocal leukoencephalopathy (multiple foci of demyelination in immunosuppressed patients).
Arbovirus infections	Vertebrate hosts and mosquito vectors, causing epidemic encephalitis with a high mortality (Eastern and Western equine encephalitis, Venezuelan encephalitis, Japanese B and Murray Valley encephalitis).

atypical mycobacteria, cryptococcal meningitis, cytomegalo-virus (CMV) (microglial nodular encephalitis describes the pattern of cortical inflammation seen due to CMV), herpes zoster encephalitis, toxoplasmosis, progressive multifocal leukoencephalopathy due to papovavirus, and *Candida* and *Aspergillus* infection.

AIDS patients are at risk of developing primary cerebral lymphomas (see page 464).

Spongiform encephalopathies are caused by an unconventional protein-only agent and can be genetic as well as transmissible

Creutzfeldt–Jakob disease (CJD) is an uncommon nervous system disorder. It is characterized by accumulation of a modified normal cell-membrane protein, termed **prion protein** (PrP). The precise way in which the protein is modified is unknown.

The disease is associated with a rapidly progressive dementia in humans, with histological vacuolation in the brain, known as **spongiform encephalopathy** (*Fig. 21.26*). It is similar to kuru in humans, scrapie in sheep and bovine spongiform encephalopathy (BSE) in cattle, which are also

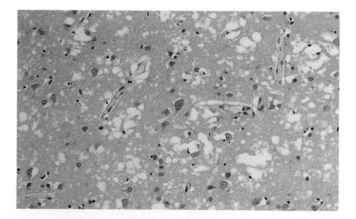

Fig. 21.26 Spongiform encephalopathy.
This shows cerebral cortex with large areas of coarse as well as fine vacuolation, characteristic of spongiform encephalopathy.

characterized by accumulation of PrP. As these diseases were once thought to be caused by a virus with a long incubation, they were formerly termed slow-virus diseases. It is now recognized that this is a protein-only infective disorder, a biologically unique phenomenon.

New variant CJD has been caused by transmission of the agent causing BSE in cattle to man, by ingestion of contaminated meat in the diet. This disease is characterized by early psychiatric symptoms followed by sensory symptoms, cerebellar ataxia and only late dementia. The brain shows prominent accumulation of PrP amyloid plaques (*Fig. 21.27a*). Importantly in this condition PrP also accumulates in the lymphoid tissues in affected patients allowing diagnosis by tonsil biopsy in life (*Fig. 21.27b*).

Although most human disease is sporadic, cases have resulted from transplantation of tissue from an affected person, as well as from administration of growth hormone derived from cadavers. Identical and transmissible disease can result from hereditary mutations in the gene coding for the prion protein in man (hereditary CJD and Gerstmann–Straussler syndrome, causing familial cases of ataxia and dementia).

FUNGAL INFECTIONS OF THE CNS

Fungal infection of the nervous system is usually seen in patients who are immunosuppressed

Infection of the nervous system by fungi is frequently seen in patients who are immunosuppressed (most commonly following organ transplantation or anti-cancer chemotherapy, or with HIV infection and AIDS).

Candidiasis causes multiple small cerebral abscesses in the CNS, usually secondary to septicemia caused by primary *Candida* infection elsewhere. *Aspergillus* is another organism that affects the brain from hematogenous spread, usually from primary lung involvement, leading to formation of fungal abscesses.

Phycomycoses (mucormycosis, zygomycosis) infect the brain by local spread from primary infection of the paranasal sinuses. Fungi typically invade along vessels, causing vascular thrombosis and cerebral infarction.

Cryptococcosis is due to a yeast-like organism that most commonly causes a fungal meningitis in immunosuppressed patients but may also affect patients with normal immune function (see page 125 and *Fig. 8.16*).

PARASITIC INFECTION OF THE NERVOUS SYSTEM

Parasitic infection of the nervous system by protozoa and metazoa is increasing in western countries

Infection of the nervous system by protozoa was formerly uncommon in western countries, but is being seen increasingly because of international travel and increased risk of infection in patients with immunosuppression.

Toxoplasma can cause a congenital infection resulting in hydrocephalus and cerebral calcifications. It is also now frequently seen in patients with AIDS, causing cerebritis and brain abscesses (see page 446 and *Fig. 21.23*).

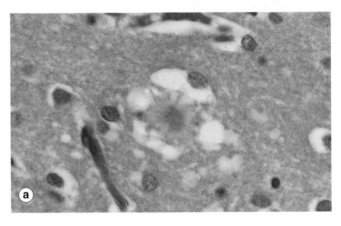

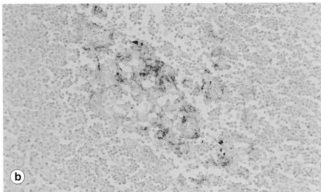

Fig. 21.27 New variant CJD.
(a) An amyloid plaque composed of PrP in the brain from a patient with new variant CJD. (b) Tonsillar tissue stained with an antibody that detects PrP. This has accumulated in the follicle center in the lymphoid tissue. Similar PrP accumulates in other lymphoid sites such as spleen, nodes and appendix. This does not happen in sporadic CJD.

Worldwide, **malaria** is the most common protozoan disease to involve the brain (particularly infection with *Plasmodium falciparum*), causing vascular thromboses with petechial hemorrhages (cerebral malaria) (see page 133). **Trypanosomiasis** may be associated with an encephalomyelitis in acute disease.

Entamoeba histolytica can cause an amebic abscess by spread from the gut, whereas a meningitis is caused by free-living amebas such as *Naegleria*, usually acquired by swimming in contaminated pools in warm climates.

The two main metazoan parasites to infect the brain are *Echinococcus granulosus* (causing hydatid disease) and the larval form of the pork tapeworm, *Taenia solium* (causing cysticercosis) (see page 137).

TUBERCULOSIS OF THE BRAIN

Infection of the nervous system with TB may cause meningitis or abscess

Infection of the CNS by *Mycobacterium tuberculosis* is by blood spread from a site of primary infection, most commonly the lung. There are two main types of infection.

Meningitis is characterized by numerous granulomas in the leptomeninges, with features of a chronic meningitis (see page 445). Infection is most marked around the base of the brain and, even when infection is treated, there is often development of meningeal fibrosis to cause hydrocephalus.

Tuberculous abscess (tuberculoma) forms with infection of the brain parenchyma. A tuberculoma is typically a firm, lobulated mass of granulomatous inflammation with central caseous necrosis, up to several centimeters in diameter, and walled off by fibrous tissue. Lesions occur within the cerebral hemispheres, but are most common in the cerebellum. Treatment with antibiotics is usually ineffective and surgical excision is required.

DEMYELINATING DISEASES

The demyelinating disorders are diseases in which the main abnormality is damage to CNS myelin. Myelin loss is seen in many disease processes after axonal loss, but this type of secondary myelin loss is not considered as part of the group of demyelinating diseases. The most important condition causing demyelination is **multiple sclerosis**.

Multiple sclerosis is an immune-mediated disease of uncertain cause

Multiple sclerosis (MS) is a disease in which there are relapsing episodes of immunologically-mediated demyelination within the CNS. Loss of myelin leads to failure of axonal function and neurological dysfunction.

The lesions of MS are confined to the brain and spinal cord. Areas of demyelination are termed plaques, best seen at the angles of the lateral ventricles, in the cerebellar peduncles, and in the brain stem, although they can occur at any site in the CNS.

Areas of active recent demyelination appear as salmon-pink granular patches of softening in white matter. Histologically, there is myelin loss associated with lymphocytic cuffing of small vessels. Macrophages enter the lesion and phagocytose damaged myelin, accumulating lipid and forming foam cells. Astrocytes around plaque margins become enlarged.

Areas of old myelin loss appear as sharply demarcated patches of firm, gelatinous, greyish-pink discoloration (*Fig. 21.28*). These inactive plaques, sometimes called burnt-out plaques, show loss of myelin, very few inflammatory cells, and are occupied by astrocytes.

Although the axons that span a plaque are mostly preserved, there is clear-cut evidence of loss of a small proportion of axons from plaque areas.

Most patients who develop MS are aged between 20 and 40 years. The early common clinical symptoms are limb weakness, blurring of vision, incoordination, and abnormal sensation. There is great variation in outcome. Some patients have a benign form of disease, experiencing minor

Etiology and pathogenesis of multiple sclerosis

MS has a peak incidence between the ages of 20 and 40 years, with a slight female predominance. Many theories have been advanced to explain the disease, but the etiology of the condition is uncertain.

Although viral infection has been postulated, none has been consistently detected or directly implicated in disease. Immunological mechanisms are central to disease pathogenesis, and an active immunological response is present in areas of demyelination. The cause of the immune response remains uncertain. An association with certain HLA antigens (HLA-DR2) has also been demonstrated. It is likely that the disease is the result of a genetic susceptibility, predisposing to mounting an inappropriate immune response to viral infections.

In the region of active plaques, microglial cells show enhanced expression of Class II major histocompatibility antigens, suggestive of immune activation. Lesions are infiltrated by T-cells, B-cells and macrophages, again emphasizing immune activation. Trials with cytokine agents which modulate the immune response are under evaluation.

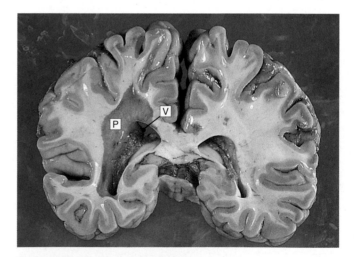

Fig. 21.28 Multiple sclerosis.
A large plaque (**P**) is seen adjacent to the lateral ventricle (**V**). Histologically, areas of myelin loss are revealed on myelin stains.

disability and few episodes of demyelination. Others have frequent repeated episodes of myelin loss, progressing such that in the late stages of disease they are rendered blind, paraplegic and incontinent, with cognitive dysfunction caused by loss of hemispheric white matter.

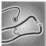

Diagnosis of multiple sclerosis

The diagnosis of MS is based on clinical evaluation and on exclusion of other causes of focal neurological disease. Several diagnostic procedures are particularly helpful.

Electrophysiology shows increased time for conduction in CNS tracts, measured by showing increased latency for visual and auditory evoked responses.

Magnetic resonance imaging can show even small areas of demyelination within the brain and spinal cord, particularly if gadolinium enhancement is used.

CSF examination usually shows a mild increase in lymphoid cells, and a mild increase in protein with a normal glucose level. Activation of the immune system in the CNS can be identified by demonstrating oligoclonal bands of immunoglobulin in the CSF by electrophoresis.

Myelin loss is seen in several diseases as a secondary process

Demyelination is a prominent component of several diseases.

Leukodystrophies are inborn errors of metabolism in which there is abnormal formation or metabolism of myelin, sometimes termed **dysmyelination**. The main types are metachromatic leukodystrophy due to aryl sulfatase A deficiency, and adrenoleukodystrophy caused by metabolic defects in peroxisomal metabolism of long-chain fatty acids.

Binswanger's disease is caused by ischemic damage to myelin as a result of widespread cerebral arteriolosclerosis. There is loss of hemispheric myelin, leading to cognitive decline.

Progressive multifocal leukoencephalopathy is caused by infection with papovavirus, seen in patients who are immunosuppressed (see page 127).

NEURODEGENERATIVE DISEASES

The neurodegenerative diseases are common disorders in which there is degeneration of specific groups of neurons or brain areas, causing characteristic clinical syndromes. The incidence of these diseases rises with age, particularly after the age of 65 years and, increasingly, many are recognized as familial. The main clinical syndromes caused by neurodegenerative disease are dementia syndromes with cognitive decline, movement disorders (particularly defects of cerebellar and extrapyramidal systems), motor weakness, and autonomic failure.

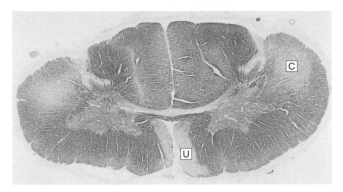

Fig. 21.29 Motor neuron disease. The crossed (**C**) and uncrossed (**U**) corticospinal tracts in the cervical spinal cord show pallor due to loss of axons (Luxol fast blue/cresyl violet).

Motor neuron disease (amyotrophic lateral sclerosis) causes paralysis due to death of motor neurons in the motor cortex, brain stem and spinal cord

Motor neuron disease is a progressive neurodegenerative disease. It is mainly seen in old age, a small number of patients presenting in middle age. Disease typically begins as mild weakness in one limb. There is then progression to severe paralysis, with loss of swallowing and respiration leading to death in 2–3 years. The cause of the disease is unknown.

Different sub-types relate to the loss of different groups of motor neurons:

- **Amyotrophic lateral sclerosis** is the most common pattern, showing loss of both cortical motor neurons and lower motor neurons in the spinal cord and brain stem.
- **Progressive bulbar palsy** is common and shows loss of brain stem motor neurons.
- **Progressive muscular atrophy** is uncommon and shows loss restricted to spinal lower motor neurons.
- **Primary lateral sclerosis** is rare and shows loss of neurons restricted to the motor cortex.

There is loss of motor neurons from cortex, brain stem and spinal cord, and gliosis with secondary degeneration of motor tracts (*Fig. 21.29*). Inclusion bodies containing the protein ubiquitin are found in surviving neurons.

Parkinson's disease results from loss of neurons from the substantia nigra

Parkinson's disease is a movement disorder that mainly affects patients over the age of 45 years. It is clinically characterized by disturbance of movement with rigidity, slowness of voluntary movement (bradykinesis), and rest tremor. Severity of disease is related to loss of the neuromelanin-containing nerve cells from the substantia nigra in the midbrain; these cells normally produce dopamine, their loss reducing the amount of dopamine in the basal ganglia.

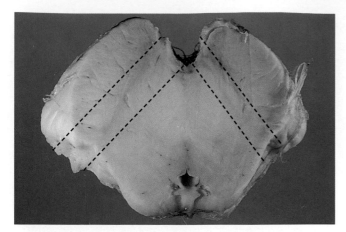

Fig. 21.30 Parkinson's disease. In this section through the midbrain, pigmented neurons have been lost from the substantia nigra (between lines), which is abnormally pale.

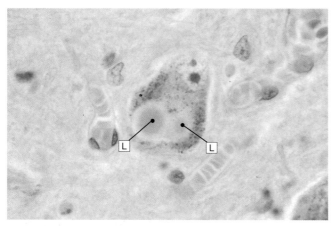

Fig. 21.31 Lewy body in Parkinson's disease.
Lewy bodies (**L**) are spherical inclusions seen in the melanin-containing neurons in Parkinson's disease. Typically they have a hyaline core and a pale halo. They are based on aggregated neurofilaments and α synuclein.

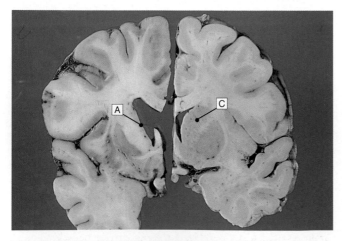

Fig. 21.32 Huntington's disease. This shows slices from two brains. On the right is a normal brain with normal caudate (**C**); on the left the brain from a patient with Huntington's disease shows severe atrophy of the caudate (**A**).

Macroscopically, there is loss of pigment from the substantia nigra, which is the result of death of the melanin-containing dopaminergic cells (*Fig. 21.30*). The surviving cells in the substantia nigra contain spherical inclusions termed **Lewy bodies** (*Fig. 21.31*).

The cause of Parkinson's disease is unknown but rare cases are familial. The disease may be symptomatically treated by administration of drugs that correct the neurotransmitter imbalance, e.g. L-dopa. The natural history of the disease is for patients to develop failure of response to treatment, with death eventually occurring from wasting and poor nutritional intake.

Huntington's disease is an autosomal dominant disease causing chorea and dementia

Huntington's disease is a neurodegenerative disease causing choreiform movements and dementia, with onset in middle life. The disease is an autosomal dominant disorder with a prevalence of approximately 1 in 20 000; the gene has been characterized at its location in the short arm of chromosome 4 (see pink box below).

Macroscopically the brain shows atrophy of the caudate and putamen due to cell loss and gliosis (*Fig. 21.32*), and careful measurements have shown subtle loss of neurons from the cerebral cortex.

Molecular genetics of Huntington's disease

The gene for Huntington's disease is located on chromosome 4. The cause of the disease is an abnormally long, tandemly repeated trinucleotide (CAG). In normal individuals this gene has between 9 and 34 repeats, whereas in Huntington's disease patients have around 70 repeats. The protein produced by the gene, which has been named **huntingtin**, is expressed in many tissues but has no homology with other proteins; its function is at present unknown. Protein accumulates inside neuronal nuclei forming inclusions as well as accumulating inside some nerve cell processes.

The age of onset of disease is related to the length of the repeat sequence; patients with large repeat sequences have early onset. With passage of the gene through generations, the repeat sequence increases in length, resulting in progressively earlier ages at presentation, a phenomenon termed **anticipation**.

Now that the gene has been identified, confident genetic testing for the disease is possible, with all the attendant ethical and social implications.

The natural history of this disease is for affected individuals to develop progressive cognitive decline, with increase in severity of the movement disorder. Patients die as a result of their severe mental and physical incapacity.

Alzheimer's disease is the most common cause of dementia

Alzheimer's disease is the most common neurodegenerative disease and the most common cause of dementia. Clinically, patients develop progressive failure of memory, degeneration of temporal and parietal association cortex (causing dyspraxia and dysphasia) and, frequently, disturbances in emotion. With progression of disease over many years, patients become immobile and emaciated, death commonly being due to the development of a pneumonia.

The cause of the disease is unknown, but there are well-defined genetic predispositions (see pink box below).

The brain in Alzheimer's disease is smaller than normal and brain weight is reduced, evident as shrinkage of gyri and widening of sulci of the cerebral hemispheres (*Fig. 21.33*). Atrophy is most evident in the temporal lobe, particularly the parahippocampal gyrus, but also in frontal and parietal regions. The occipital lobe and the motor cortex are generally spared.

Histologically, there are several main abnormalities seen in Alzheimer's disease. **Amyloid**, composed of Aβ-peptide, is deposited in the cerebral cortex as spherical deposits

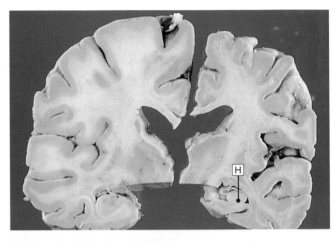

Fig. 21.33 Alzheimer's disease.
This shows slices from two brains. On the left is a normal brain from a 70-year-old; on the right is the same region from a 70-year-old with Alzheimer's disease. The diseased brain is atrophic with loss of cortex and white matter, most marked in the hippocampal region (**H**).

Molecular pathogenesis of Alzheimer's disease

It is possible to divide cases of Alzheimer's disease into four main clinical groups, each of which is beginning to be associated with molecular genetic abnormalities that have been linked to genes on chromosomes 21, 19, 1 and 14:

- Sporadic late onset (most common).
- Familial late onset (uncommon).
- Familial early onset (rare).
- Associated with Down's syndrome.

Molecular analysis of the amyloid of Alzheimer's disease shows that it is derived from a normal cell-membrane protein of unknown function, coded on chromosome 21 and termed **Alzheimer precursor protein** or **APP**. Defects in this protein explain some cases of early-onset familial disease, as well as the association of Alzheimer's disease with Down's syndrome (trisomy 21). The protein found in the amyloid is a fragment of APP, referred to as Aβ protein or A4 protein. Mutation in the APP gene accounts for under 5% of the rare early-onset cases of familial Alzheimer's disease, hence a minute overall number of cases of Alzheimer's disease.

The presence of apolipoprotein apoE4, a normal form of apolipoprotein, is believed to account for linkage of

Alzheimer's disease to chromosome 19. ApoE4 predisposes to the development of familial late-onset Alzheimer's disease, as well as sporadic late-onset cases. In the 3% of the population who are homozygous for this apolipoprotein variant, the risk of developing Alzheimer's disease is believed to be 90%, whereas the 25% of the population who are heterozygous are at high risk of developing disease. This is likely to account for susceptibility for development of disease in the majority of cases, although the mechanism for this increased susceptibility is at present uncertain.

The gene responsible for linkage to chromosome 14 is termed presenilin-1 and mutations in it account for the majority of cases of early-onset familial Alzheimer's disease. A homologous protein termed presenilin-2 is coded for by a gene on chromosome 1, mutations in this gene also causing some cases of familial early-onset Alzheimer's disease. The presenilin proteins are involved in the metabolism of APP. Mutations result in increased production of Aβ protein in a form that readily forms amyloid. Detailed molecular investigation of metabolism of the proteins in tangles (see page 454), mainly consisting the microtubule-binding protein Tau, has as not yet revealed why they form.

termed **senile plaques** (*Fig. 21.34a*). Intraneuronal inclusions comprising bundles of abnormal filaments termed **neurofibrillary tangles** develop in cortical neurons (*Fig. 21.34b*). Tangles are frequently flame-shaped and occupy much of the space within the neuronal cytoplasm, being largely composed of a microtubule-binding protein called Tau protein. Cortical nerve-cell processes become twisted and dilated (**neuropil threads**) due to accumulation of the same filaments that form the tangles. Neurofibrillary tangles and plaques can be seen in the brains of cognitively normal elderly individuals, one interpretation being that they are in an early stage of disease at the time of death. The pathological diagnosis of Alzheimer's disease is based on the presence of lesions in high density in a patient with clinical dementia.

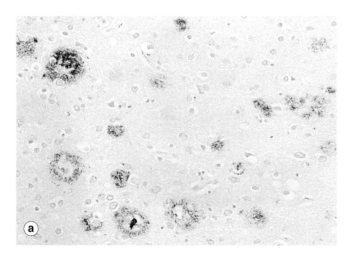

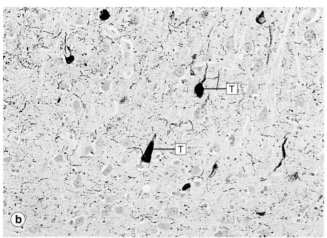

Fig. 21.34 Alzheimer's disease. (a) Plaques (immunochemistry – Aβ protein). (b) Tangles and neuropil threads (immunochemistry – Tau protein).
Immunohistochemical staining can identify the accumulations of abnormal proteins in the brain in Alzheimer's disease. Amyloid plaques composed of Aβ peptide are seen scattered in the cortex (a). In (b) tangles (T) composed of Tau protein can be seen as flame-shaped structures in neurons. The fine brown linear staining is nerve-cell processes filled with Tau protein, termed neuropil threads.

The neurochemical analysis of brains from patients with Alzheimer's disease has shown widespread neurotransmitter defects, particularly loss of acetylcholine from the cortex. Treatment protocols that supplement cholinergic transmission have shown promising results in trials.

Dementia may be associated with Parkinsonism or frontal lobe degeneration

Dementia with Lewy bodies is the second most common cause of dementia and has clinical features that overlap with those of Alzheimer's disease and Parkinson's disease. Patients have a cortical dementia resembling Alzheimer's disease, but also have mild features of rigidity and bradykinesia (slowness). Lewy bodies, the neuronal inclusions characteristic of Parkinson's disease, are seen in both the substantia nigra and the cerebral cortex.

Frontal dementias account for about 10% of all cases of dementia and are characterized by the development of impaired frontal lobe function, with memory impairment in combination with a syndrome of disinhibition and mutism. Macroscopically, there is atrophy of the frontal and temporal lobes of the brain, and histological examination reveals neuronal loss, with some sub-types having neuronal inclusions. The importance of frontal patterns of dementia is that many cases are late-onset autosomal dominant conditions, with genes that are at present mostly unknown. Mutation in the Tau protein gene is responsible in some families.

Neuronal system atrophies are neurodegenerative diseases affecting several neuronal groups

A number of uncommon neurodegenerative diseases show loss of neurons from several nuclei in the brain, brain stem, cerebellum and spinal cord, and are given names according to the pattern of involvement. There are large numbers of such syndromes, each having different genetic and pathological causes. Clinically, patients have symptoms and signs that relate to the neuronal groups involved, including rigidity, chorea, cognitive decline and weakness.

Among the main types of multisystem atrophy are **spinocerebellar degenerations**, a group of familial diseases with several inheritance patterns, which are characterized by loss of cerebellar cortical neurons and degeneration of spinal cord tracts. The best known of these is **Friedreich's ataxia**, a spastic cerebellar ataxia with degeneration of posterior columns and corticospinal and spinocerebellar tracts which is an example of a triplet-repeat expansion genetic disorder caused by GAA triplet repeat expansions of between 200 and 900 copies in the first intron of the frataxin gene.

Cerebellar cortical atrophies are diseases in which the main abnormality is loss of Purkinje cells from the cerebellar cortex, with lesser involvement of other neuronal groups. Patients present with cerebellar ataxia, usually in the third decade. Many cases are familial with defined gene mutations (*Fig. 21.35*).

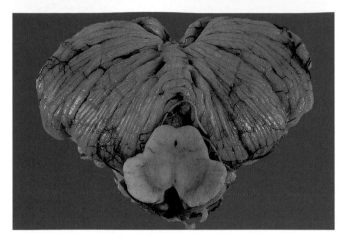

Fig. 21.35 Cerebellar atrophy.
There is marked atrophy in the vermis of the cerebellum.

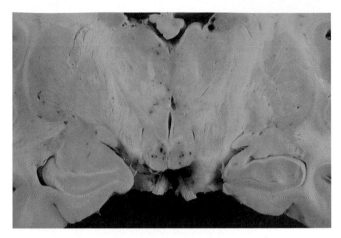

Fig. 21.36 Wernicke's encephalopathy.
In this coronal section of brain the mamillary bodies show petechial hemorrhages characteristic of acute Wernicke's encephalopathy caused by thiamine deficiency.

In multiple system atrophy, patients have prominent cerebellar ataxia, extrapyramidal rigidity and bulbar paresis, caused by loss of neurons from the cerebellar cortex, substantia nigra and pons respectively. Characteristic inclusions are seen in glial cells.

Idiopathic orthostatic hypotension (Shy–Drager syndrome) is a disorder dominated by the presence of orthostatic hypotension. This may occur in isolation, or, more usually, as part of multiple-system atrophy involving the substantia nigra, motor neurons and cerebellum. The basis of hypotension is loss of neurons from the intermediolateral column in the thoracic spinal cord.

METABOLIC AND TOXIC DISEASE

Metabolic and toxic disorders of the nervous system are common causes of neurological disease

Several major diseases of the CNS have a metabolic or toxic causation, a reflection of the vulnerability of the nervous system to injury. The main causes are vitamin deficiency states, liver failure, carbon monoxide poisoning, and alcohol abuse.

Several **vitamin deficiency states** are associated with damage to the nervous system. Vitamin B_1 (thiamine) deficiency causes **Wernicke's encephalopathy**. Vitamin B_{12} deficiency is commonly associated with **pernicious anemia** (see page 318). In the nervous system this causes degeneration of the lateral and posterior columns of the spinal cord, termed subacute combined degeneration of the cord, leading to paresthesias, ataxia, and sensory abnormalities.

Hepatic encephalopathy is a clinical state that arises in patients with severe liver failure. Patients develop impaired consciousness, which may progress to coma. Disease is thought to be due to the presence of excitatory transmitter substances in the blood, which have not been detoxified by the liver, e.g. GABA.

Carbon monoxide poisoning is commonly encountered, either as an accident (usually involving faulty heating equipment) or as a result of attempted suicide. In patients who survive the acute poisoning and are resuscitated, delayed damage to the brain may occur, signs usually becoming apparent 24–36 hours after exposure to carbon monoxide. There is necrosis of the globus pallidus, demyelination of the hemispheric white matter and, frequently, diffuse cortical laminar necrosis (see page 439).

The brain and peripheral nerves are frequently damaged in chronic alcoholism

Acute alcohol intoxication causes neuronal depression and may lead to death through cessation of respiration.

Chronic alcoholism is associated with several diseases of both the central and the peripheral nervous system. It has been difficult to determine whether this is due to direct toxicity or whether it is caused by the nutritional and vitamin deficiencies commonly seen in patients dependent on alcohol.

The brains of alcoholic patients show generalized **cerebral cortical atrophy**, which sometimes causes cognitive decline. Cerebellar ataxia in patients with alcoholism is usually caused by **cerebellar degeneration** associated with severe atrophy of the cerebellar cortex.

Wernicke's encephalopathy is caused by thiamine deficiency, commonly seen in patients dependent on alcohol. It presents clinically as a triad of confusion, ataxia, and abnormal eye movements with ophthalmoplegia. Pathologically, there are petechial hemorrhages from small vessels in the mammillary bodies (see *Fig. 21.36*), which are associated with necrosis and loss of neurons, leading to eventual shrinkage and gliosis. Acute Wernicke's encephalopathy may prove fatal unless B-complex vitamins (including thiamine) are administered. Damage to the limbic system from repeated episodes of Wernicke's encephalopathy causes a permanent impairment of recent memory, termed **Korsakoff's psychosis**.

Exposure of the fetus to alcohol, when the mother is dependent, leads to growth retardation and cerebral malformations (fetal alcohol syndrome).

DEVELOPMENTAL ABNORMALITIES

Developmental abnormalities of the CNS are common, affecting 1% of newborns. They can be divided into two main groups: primary developmental abnormalities, which are the direct result of a genetic abnormality, and secondary developmental abnormalities, which are due to disruption of development by an intrauterine disease process such as infection or ischemia, or toxic factors.

The majority of malformations of the nervous system have no ascertainable cause

Establishing the cause of a developmental abnormality of the nervous system is important from the perspective of reproductive counseling for parents. Unfortunately, 60% of developmental abnormalities of the nervous system have no identifiable causative factor. Of the remainder, 20% are mixed environmental and genetic, 5% are due to single gene defects, 5% are due to chromosomal abnormalities, and 10% are due to exogenous factors such as infection,

toxins, or poor nutrition. *Fig. 21.37* lists the main causative factors and associated malformations.

Neural-tube defects are the most common form of developmental abnormality of the CNS

Defects in the closure of the neural tube are the most common cause of congenital malformation of the nervous system. Such defects may affect either the cranial or the spinal closure of the neural tube, and may be an open defect or one closed by meninges and skin.

The most severe and common form of cranial neural-tube defect is **anencephaly**. The cranial vault is generally not formed, although the face and eyes are usually well developed. The brain is replaced by a disc of abnormally developed neural tissue. A less severe cranial neural-tube defect is development of an **encephalocele**, in which a defect in the bone of the skull is associated with cystic outpouching of meninges, which may contain brain.

Neural-tube defects of the spinal cord are most common in the lumbar region. The severity of the defect is variable (*Fig. 21.38*). The main defects include:

- **Spina bifida occulta.** Abnormal development of the bony arch of the spinal column. Meninges and cord normal. There may be an associated sinus track to the skin surface, or subcutaneous lipoma.
- **Meningocele.** Abnormal development of the bony arch of the spinal cord, with cystic outpouching of

Fig. 21.37
Causes of developmental abnormalities of brain

Chromosomal abnormalities

Down's syndrome (trisomy 21)	Abnormal gyral formation and defective arborization of neuronal processes
Trisomy 13–15 (Patau's syndrome)	Forebrain abnormalities with midline facial clefts
Trisomy 17–18 (Edwards' syndrome)	Gyral maldevelopment

Single gene abnormalities

Autosomal recessive gene	Meckel syndrome (encephalocele)
	Roberts' syndrome (encephalocele)

Multifactorial

Genetic and environmental	Anencephaly, meningocele, encephalocele

Infections

Rubella	Microcephaly, focal necrosis of brain areas
Cytomegalovirus	Necrosis and developmental failure
Toxoplasmosis	Necrosis and developmental failure

Teratogens

Thalidomide	Anencephaly and meningomyelocele
Aminopterin	Anencephaly and encephalocele

meninges covered by skin. Spinal cord may be normally or abnormally formed.

- **Meningomyelocele.** Abnormal development of the bony arch of the spinal cord, with cystic outpouching of meninges including nerve roots and incorporating abnormally developed spinal cord.
- **Myelocele.** Abnormal development of the bony arch of the spinal cord, with exposure of abnormally developed spinal cord.

The neurological deficit associated with spinal neural-tube defects is related to the degree of severity of abnormality of the spinal cord and nerve roots. Other developmental abnormalities may be present, particularly hydrocephalus caused by Arnold–Chiari malformation (see page 444).

Patients with spinal neural-tube defects commonly have paraplegia with urinary and fecal incontinence. Without surgical correction, they develop spinal and limb deformities. A major complication is recurrent urinary tract infection leading to chronic pyelonephritis and renal failure.

Diagnosis can be made *in utero* by ultrasound scanning or by detecting raised levels of α fetoprotein (AFP) in serum or amniotic fluid.

The Arnold–Chiari malformation Type II is the second most common developmental abnormality of the CNS

In Arnold–Chiari Type II malformations there is herniation of the brain stem and the lower part of the cerebellum into the foramen magnum, blocking drainage of CSF and causing hydrocephalus. This abnormality is nearly always associated with development of a lumbar meningomyelocele. Less common abnormalities of the CNS are summarized in *Fig. 21.39*.

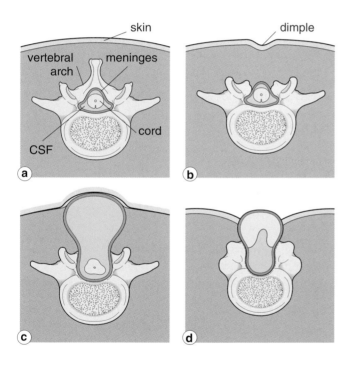

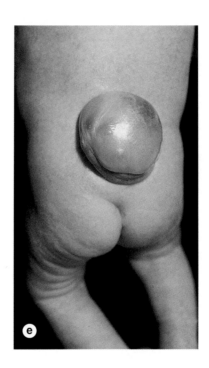

Fig. 21.38 Spinal neural tube defects.
(a) Normal.
(b) Spina bifida occulta.
(c) Meningocele.
(d) Meningomyelocele.
(e) Meningocele in a newborn child.

Fig. 21.39
Developmental abnormalities of the CNS

Agyria and pachygyria	Brain is smooth or has few gyri due to failure of migration of neuroblasts into developing brain
Heterotopia	Ectopic foci of gray matter due to premature arrest of migrating neuroblasts in developing brain
Holoprosencephaly	Single large ventricle with non-division of forebrain
Porencephaly and schizencephaly	Cystic cavities in the brain with gliosis following infarction caused by intrauterine vascular occlusion
Ulegyria	Gliotic shrunken gyri caused by hypoxic necrosis
Microcephaly	Small brain with many causative factors

Hypoxia is a major cause of perinatal brain damage

The neonatal brain is vulnerable to a wide variety of injurious agents, the most important being hypoxia associated with the trauma of birth. The two main abnormalities found are hemorrhage and necrosis.

Perinatal hypoxia is a major cause of neurological damage in the newborn, with an incidence of about 3 per 1000 live term births. Although many die, around one-third develop cerebral palsy, epilepsy or mental retardation.

Hypoxic ischemic encephalopathy is the term applied to brain damage caused by neonatal asphyxia. The main lesions encountered are: hemorrhages into the brain and ventricles from the germinal matrix adjacent to the lateral ventricles, necrosis of brain leading to cystic gliosis (ulegyria, porencephaly, hydranencephaly), and necrosis of white matter in cerebral hemispheres (peri-ventricular leukomalacia).

Birth trauma may cause tearing of dural veins, leading to subdural hematoma.

INBORN ERRORS OF METABOLISM

The nervous system is involved in several inborn errors of metabolism, either primarily or as a consequence of systematized disease. The main disorders in this group are those of myelin formation, termed **leukodystrophies**, and **storage disorders** (see Chapter 25) due to lack of normal enzyme activity causing accumulation of a metabolic product in nerve cells.

Leukodystrophies are genetically determined defects in myelin metabolism

Leukodystrophies generally present in childhood as cognitive or motor decline, but can also be seen, although less commonly, in adult life. They are caused by genetically determined metabolic abnormalities in the formation or metabolism of myelin. Macroscopically, brains are small and there is loss of myelin with gliosis (*Fig. 21.40*). The main types of leukodystrophy are:

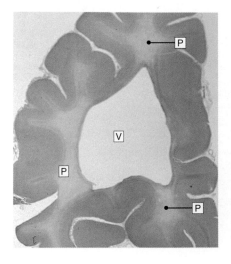

Fig. 21.40 Leukodystrophy. In this section from the frontal lobe of a child with leukodystrophy there is massive loss of myelin from the white matter, leaving it palely stained (**P**). The lateral ventricle (**V**) is dilated as a compensation for loss of cerebral tissue.

- **Adrenoleukodystrophy.** X-linked recessive disease caused by deficiency of peroxisomal enzymes involved in oxidation of long-chain fatty acids.
- **Metachromatic leukodystrophy.** Autosomal recessive disease caused by lack of activity of aryl sulfatase A.
- **Krabbe's disease (globoid-cell leukodystrophy).** Autosomal recessive disease caused by galactocerebroside β-galactosidase deficiency.

The diagnosis of these metabolic defects in myelin formation is made by assay of enzymes detectable in blood leukocytes or cultured fibroblasts.

Neurometabolic storage disorders are genetic diseases causing accumulation of abnormal material in the brain

Several of the inborn errors of metabolism (see Chapter 25) are characterized by storage of abnormal material in the nervous system. This type of disease most commonly arises in childhood, when it presents as cognitive or motor decline. Among the main types are as follows:

- **Gangliosidoses** are autosomal recessive disorders causing neuronal storage of gangliosides, e.g. Tay–Sachs disease.
- **Mucopolysaccharidoses** cause abnormal storage of mucopolysaccharides in brain and other tissues, the main types being Hurler's syndrome (gargoylism) and Hunter's syndrome.
- **Gaucher's disease** is caused by deficiency of β-glucocerebrosidase resulting in accumulation of glucocerebroside in brain and macrophages in other organs.
- **Ceroid lipofuscinoses** are disorders in which there is neuronal storage of lipofuscin-like lipids. The commonest types are due to abnormalities in the gene encoding palmitoyl-protein thioesterase which are normally involved in the catabolism of lipid-modified proteins. The main type is Batten's disease.
- **Niemann–Pick disease** is caused by deficient sphingomyelinase activity, only some varieties having neurological involvement.

Diagnosis of neurometabolic storage diseases is made by showing the abnormal enzyme activity in lymphocytes or cultured fibroblasts. Some forms of ceroid lipofuscinoses not yet associated with a gene defect can be morphologically diagnosed by demonstration of abnormal lipid material in the rectal ganglion cells on rectal biopsy.

Wilson's disease is an autosomal recessive disorder of copper metabolism that causes neuropsychiatric disease or movement disorders

Wilson's disease is an autosomal recessive disorder in which there is excessive copper accumulation in the brain, liver and kidneys. Neurological disease usually presents in adolescence with psychiatric disease (onset of psychosis), movement disorder (spasticity, rigidity, dysarthria, painful muscle spasms) or odd eye movements.

Advanced cases of neurological disease are now uncommon because of effective treatment. In severe cases, there is shrinkage of the basal ganglia, with loss of nerve cells and gliosis. The gene, which is located on chromosome 13, codes for a copper transport ATPase.

PHACOMATOSES

The phacomatoses are familial disorders in which there are developmental abnormalities associated with hamartomatous or neoplastic growths. The main types of disease are: neurofibromatosis 1 (NF1), neurofibromatosis 2 (NF2), tuberous sclerosis, and von Hippel–Lindau syndrome.

NF1 is an autosomal dominant disease that causes multiple benign tumours of peripheral nerves

NF1, formerly called 'von Recklinghausen's syndrome', is an autosomal dominant disorder affecting 1 in 4000 individuals. The main clinical features are development of benign tumors of peripheral nerves, termed **neurofibromas** (see page 467), and the presence of pigmented skin lesions called **cafe au lait spots**. Less prominent are hamartomas of the iris, optic-nerve gliomas, and bone abnormalities. Patients characteristically develop multiple polypoid skin nodules, which can vary from 1 mm up to 5 cm in diameter. There is a risk of development of malignant nerve tumors (**neurofibrosarcomas**). The gene defect in NF1 is located on chromosome 17 (see pink box).

NF2 is an autosomal dominant disease that causes tumors on the acoustic nerves

NF2 is an autosomal dominant disorder affecting 1 in 100 000 individuals. The clinical features are development of bilateral benign tumors (also termed **schwannomas**) of the eighth cranial nerve, which are also known as **acoustic neuromas**, hence the alternative name of bilateral acoustic neurofibromatosis (BANF). There is also a tendency to develop other brain tumors, meningiomas and gliomas. Patients present with tinnitus, deafness, or signs of a mass lesion compressing the lower cranial nerves and brain stem. The gene defect for NF2 is located on chromosome 22 (see pink box).

Tuberous sclerosis is an autosomal dominant disease causing epilepsy and mental retardation associated with hamartomas of the brain

Tuberous sclerosis is an autosomal dominant condition affecting 1 in 100 000 individuals. Affected patients develop epilepsy, mental retardation, skin lesions called angiofibromas and retinal hamartomas. A minority of patients develop cardiac tumors termed **benign rhabdomyomas**, as well as renal tumors (**angiomyolipomas**). *Formes frustes* of tuberous sclerosis are common in which a full clinical phenotype does not develop.

The brain shows characteristic lesions termed tubers (after which the syndrome is named), which appear as firm,

Genetics of neurofibromatosis syndromes

Neurofibromatosis was once regarded as one disease, but is now considered to be two diseases, termed NF1 and NF2.

NF1, or von Recklinghausen's disease, is caused by mutation in a gene on chromosome 17. The gene codes for neurofibromin, which is a guanidine-triphosphatase-activating protein (GAP protein). These proteins normally convert the proto-oncogene p21-*ras* from an active GTP-bound form to an inactive GDP-bound form. The *ras* proteins usually act to modulate cell proliferation, and their overactivity has been implicated in tumor formation. In NF1 it is likely that mutant forms of protein cannot inactivate *ras* and that activated *ras* therefore accumulates to promote cell growth.

NF2 is caused by mutation in a gene on chromosome 22, which codes for a protein that has been termed **schwannomin** or **merlin** by different workers.

The schwannomin protein acts as a tumor suppressor, but its mechanism of action is uncertain. It has similarities with cytoskeletal proteins linking to the spectrin–actin complex (which normally braces the cell membrane), suggesting that lack of the protein causes abnormal cell-to-cell contact and interferes with normal contact-dependent inhibition of cell growth. Screening of patients with NF2 has shown several different mutations in the gene, each predicted to result in synthesis of a truncated form of schwannomin. Interestingly, mutations in this gene have been seen in meningiomas from patients not affected by NF2, raising the possibility of its involvement in sporadic cases of meningioma.

The identification of these genes means that patients and families may be screened for mutations and given appropriate counseling.

white nodules, 1–3 cm in size, at the crest of gyri. The tubers are hamartomatous overgrowths of neurons and astrocytes. There is more than one genetic cause for this phenotype. A gene for tuberous sclerosis is located on chromosome 16, and codes for a protein termed tuberin, which has homology with a GTPase-activating protein, GAP-3. Another gene has been located for a protein termed 'hamartin' which is not homologous for any other proteins. It is believed that hamartin and tuberin associate together to form a function complex rather than being involved in separate pathways.

von Hippel–Lindau disease causes multiple benign hemangioblastomas and predisposes to renal carcinoma

von Hippel–Lindau disease is a familial disorder in which affected individuals are genetically predisposed to develop multiple benign tumors of the brain and spinal cord, termed hemangioblastomas. Angiomas of the retina may also be present, and there is predisposition to development of carcinoma of the kidney and pheochromocytoma of the adrenal.

The von Hippel–Lindau disease tumor-suppressor gene has been identified by positional cloning and is located on chromosome 3, the inferred gene product showing no homology to other human proteins. Mutations and deletions in the gene have been detected in patients with von Hippel–Lindau disease, as well as in some sporadic renal-cell carcinomas. Patients with this diagnosis require intense follow-up for multiple and recurrent tumors.

Hemangioblastomas are well-circumscribed tumors that most commonly develop in the cerebellum, but also develop in brain stem and spinal cord. These lesions may secrete erythropoietin and cause polycythemia.

TUMORS OF THE NERVOUS SYSTEM

Primary neoplasms of the CNS are important as they commonly affect young patients; in incidence they are second only to the leukemias, accounting for about 10% of cancer deaths in those aged between 15 and 35 years. Overall, they account for only about 2% of all deaths from cancer and, in general, are uncommon. Tumors are derived from the various tissues that make up the CNS:

- **Metastases.** Overall, the most common cause of a neoplasm affecting the brain.
- **Meningeal.** Tumors derived from epithelial cells of the meninges, termed 'meningiomas'.
- **Neuroepithelial.** Tumors loosely termed 'gliomas', which are derived from astrocytes, oligodendrocytes, ependyma, neurons or primitive embryonal cells.
- **Non-neuroepithelial.** Tumors including cerebral lymphomas, germ-cell tumors, cysts and tumors extending from local growth in the skull and pituitary.

METASTASES TO CNS

Metastatic tumors are commonly seen in the brain and vertebral column

Metastases to the CNS are very common; outside specialist clinical neuroscience units they are encountered more often than primary brain tumors.

As well as focal neurological signs, metastases to brain cause signs of raised intracranial pressure. The main primary sites of metastatic tumor to brain are lung, breast and skin (melanoma). Macroscopically, metastases are often multiple and commonly begin as lesions at the junction of the cortex and white matter. Cerebral edema is often extensive around metastases, accounting for the main problem of raised intracranial pressure.

Metastatic tumor commonly affects the spinal cord as extradural deposits, causing compression. The most common are metastases from carcinomas of the prostate, kidney, breast and lung, together with lymphoma and myeloma.

TUMOURS OF MENINGEAL ORIGIN

Meningiomas are benign tumors derived from epithelial cells of the meninges

Meningiomas are tumors derived from meningothelial cells, the epithelial cells of the meninges. They are common intracranial tumors, and have a female preponderance.

Meningiomas are typically rounded lesions that arise from the dura and grow slowly to compress underlying brain (*Fig. 21.41*). Most are fleshy and rubbery in consistency, but a minority are tough and fibrous. Tumors can vary in diameter from 1 or 2 cm up to 7 cm. Although most lesions are solitary, they may be multiple. Infiltration of the skull by tumor may occur, causing local bony thickening. Meningiomas typically present with either focal neurological signs or with features of raised intracranial pressure.

Tumors arise anywhere in the meninges, the most frequent sites being next to the falx, over the cerebral convexities, or

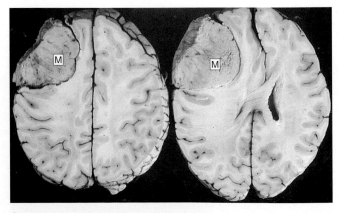

Fig. 21.41 Meningioma.
These two sections from different levels in the same brain show a meningioma (**M**) compressing the frontal lobe and distorting underlying brain.

over the sphenoid wings. Less commonly, meningiomas arise from the spinal dura and compress the spinal cord.

Histologically, tumors are composed of meningothelial cells, which may have a wide variety of histological patterns. A characteristic feature is the presence of small foci of calcification (**psammoma bodies**). The natural history of these tumors depends on the histological pattern.

- The vast majority are classed as benign meningiomas. These are slow-growing expansile lesions with a low risk of recurrence after surgical removal.

- A small proportion are classed as atypical meningiomas, have many mitoses, cell pleomorphism and necrosis, and an increased risk of local recurrence after surgery.

- A rare group are classed as malignant meningiomas. These are rapidly growing tumors that behave as locally invasive malignant tumors resembling sarcomas.

TUMORS OF NEUROEPITHELIAL ORIGIN

Tumors of neuroepithelial origin are common primary brain tumors, broadly grouped under the term **gliomas**. The main types are derived from astrocytes, oligodendrocytes, ependyma, choroid plexus, neurons, and embryonal cells. Tumors range from benign, slow-growing lesions to malignant, rapidly growing tumors known as **anaplastic gliomas**. Gliomas have a tendency for diffuse infiltration of adjacent brain, which makes surgical removal difficult and leads to frequent local recurrence.

Astrocytomas are diffuse lesions that range from benign to highly malignant

Astrocytomas may arise in the cerebral hemispheres, brain stem, spinal cord or cerebellum, and are derived from astrocytic cells. They vary from tumors with no histological features of atypia and a slow pace of growth (**astrocytoma**) to lesions with high cellularity, mitoses, pleomorphism and a rapid pace of growth (**anaplastic astrocytoma**).

Macroscopically, astrocytomas appear as ill-defined, pale areas of softening in the tissue of the nervous system, which blend into adjacent normal brain (*Fig. 21.42*).

These tumors may arise in children or adults, most presenting with focal neurological signs or raised intracranial pressure. Because of the diffuse nature of most astrocytomas, complete surgical removal is rarely possible and treatment by surgical debulking and radiotherapy is usual. Tumors do not metastasize, but can spread locally by diffuse infiltration of adjacent brain. Low-grade tumors are associated with many years' survival, anaplastic astrocytomas having a survival of 4–5 years. Low-grade tumors usually evolve into high-grade tumors with time.

Pilocytic astrocytomas are a special type of astrocytoma, usually seen in the cerebellum in childhood. They have an excellent prognosis following surgical removal. Typically they are seen as a cystic lesion with a solid nodule of tumor in the cyst wall.

Glioblastomas are highly malignant tumors derived from glial cells

The most common form of glioma, glioblastomas are highly malignant astrocytic glial tumors with a rapid pace of growth. The incidence is greatest around the age of 65 years, but lesions also occur less commonly in childhood and adolescence.

Macroscopically, tumors are necrotic hemorrhagic masses, arising principally in the cerebral hemispheres (*Fig. 21.43*), less frequently in the brain stem, and only rarely in the

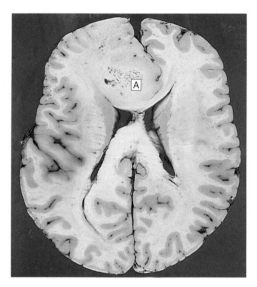

Fig. 21.42 Low-grade astrocytoma.
A low-grade astrocytoma (**A**) has arisen in the frontal lobe, distorting surrounding brain. It is extremely difficult to tell where tumor starts and ends because of the diffuse infiltrative nature of such lesions, precluding surgical removal in most cases.

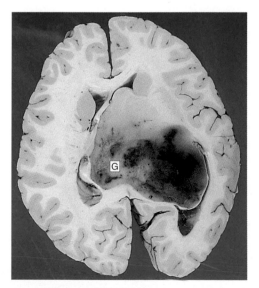

Fig. 21.43 Glioblastoma.
A large glioblastoma (**G**) arises from one cerebral hemisphere and has grown to fill the ventricular system. Such malignant tumors are associated with necrosis and hemorrhage.

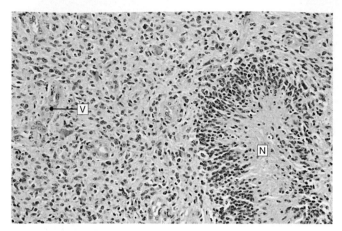

Fig. 21.44 Glioblastoma. Glioblastomas are composed of pleomorphic cells. A characteristic feature is necrosis (**N**), with cell nuclei pallisaded around the necrotic material. Growth factors secreted by tumor cause proliferation of endothelium in vessels (**V**).

cerebellum or spinal cord. Tumors are composed of a mixture of astroglial cell types with many mitoses and nuclear pleomorphism. Necrosis is always present, as this is the feature that delineates this type of lesion from the anaplastic astrocytoma (*Fig. 21.44*).

Tumors may present as glioblastomas or may have evolved into glioblastoma from a previously diagnosed lower-grade astroglial tumor. They usually cause death by rapid local growth, but may also spread within the neuro-axis. They have a median survival of around 10 months from diagnosis.

Oligodendrogliomas usually occur in the cerebral hemispheres of adults

Oligodendrogliomas and anaplastic oligodendrogliomas are glial tumors composed of cells resembling oligodendro-cytes. They arise in the cerebral hemispheres and have only rarely been described in the brain stem, cerebellum or cord. Macroscopically, tumors are very similar to astrocytomas, arising as ill-defined greyish white lesions that merge with adjacent brain. Histologically, tumors are composed of cells with rounded nuclei and pale vacuolated or pink-staining cytoplasm resembling oligodendrocytes (*Fig. 21.46*). These lesions may be divided into low-grade and anaplastic oligo-dendrogliomas on the basis of cellularity, mitoses, pleo-morphism, and vascular proliferation. It is not uncommon to find mixed glial lesions with both astrocytic and oligo-dendroglial features (**oligoastrocytomas**). There are dis-tinct cytogenetic changes in this type of glioma which distinguish them from astrocytic tumors.

Low-grade tumors in the temporal lobe have a favorable prognosis, whereas high-grade tumors recur locally and can also invade the meninges and spread in the CSF path-ways. Anaplastic oligodendrogliomas have been found to respond to chemotherapy.

Cell biology of gliomas

Progression of tumors with time from low-grade astrocytomas to anaplastic astrocytoma through to glioblastoma is well established. This progression has been related to the development of serial molecular genetic defects, each contributing to further derangement of growth control (*Fig. 21.45*).

In the histological diagnosis of brain tumors, it is often difficult to give an accurate assessment of the grade of an astroglial tumor. It is hoped that characterization of gliomas by their molecular genetic abnormalities may lead to better assessment of likely behavior.

Fig. 21.45
Oncogene defects seen in astroglial tumors

Low-grade astrocytoma	p53 mutation. Loss of alleles from chromosome 17.
Anaplastic astrocytoma	p53 mutation. Loss of alleles from chromosomes 17 and 19.
Glioblastoma	p53 mutation. Loss of alleles from chromosomes 17, 19 and 10 EGF-R amplification.

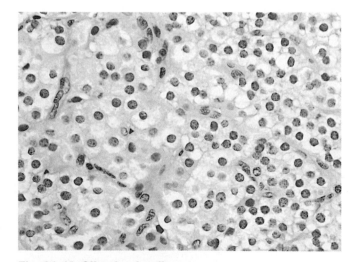

Fig. 21.46 Oligodendroglioma.
Oligodendrogliomas are composed of cells with rounded nuclei and vacuolated cytoplasm. Despite the name and the morphological resemblance to oligodendroglia, cell biological studies show no markers for oligodendrocytes in such tumors. The name is retained for historical reasons.

Ependymomas, most commonly seen in childhood, often occur in the spinal cord and ventricles

Ependymomas and anaplastic ependymomas are tumors derived from ependymal cells. They are most common in the first two decades of life, accounting for around 10% of all intracranial tumors in childhood. The most common sites are the spinal cord and the region of the fourth ventricle.

Histologically, ependymomas form tubules resembling the central canal of the spinal cord (*Fig. 21.47*). Although most ependymomas demonstrate no cellular atypia, anaplastic ependymomas show cells with mitoses, pleomorphism, and vascular endothelial proliferation, and are associated with a worse prognosis.

Myxopapillary ependymomas are a variant of ependymoma seen in the filum terminale of the spinal cord. They behave as locally infiltrative lesions.

Choroid plexus tumors are mainly benign papillomas

The most common tumor of the choroid plexus is the choroid plexus papilloma, derived from epithelial cells. Arising most frequently in childhood, these papillary, frond-like tumors most often develop in the lateral ventricle. Choroid plexus papillomas are benign and closely resemble normal choroid plexus, whereas the less common choroid plexus carcinomas are invasive malignant epithelial tumors with both solid and papillary areas.

Tumors containing neuronal elements are mainly benign

Several tumors of the nervous system contain neuronal cells; lesions may be solely composed of neuronal elements or may be mixed tumors with both neuronal and glial elements.

Gangliocytoma and **ganglioglioma** are neoplasms mainly seen in childhood. These well-circumscribed lesions are usually seen in the temporal lobe, where they can present as temporal-lobe epilepsy. Histologically, tumors contain differentiated neuronal ganglion cells and have a good prognosis after removal.

Central neurocytoma is a tumor that occurs in the lateral ventricles of young adults. It is composed of small neuronal cells and has an excellent prognosis after removal.

Embryonal tumors of the CNS are rapidly growing malignant lesions

The embryonal tumors of the CNS are common in childhood, forming a large proportion of primary tumors. They are composed of primitive small cells, which resemble the multipotential cells of the developing fetal brain, and are also called **primitive neuroectodermal tumors**

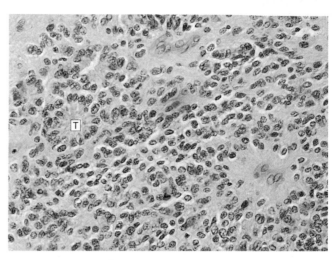

Fig. 21.47 Ependymoma. These tumors form tubular structures (**T**) resembling the central canal of the spinal cord.

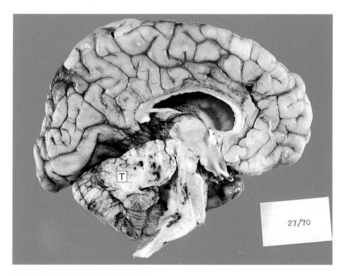

Fig. 21.48 Medulloblastoma.
Medulloblastomas arise in the cerebellum and appear as masses of soft, white tissue (**T**), often in the vermis (as here).

(**PNETs**). As a group, they are rapidly growing lesions composed of small cells with many mitoses. As well as being prone to local spread, they have a tendency to spread via CSF pathways.

The main tumor in this group is the **medulloblastoma**, which arises in the cerebellum and is composed of primitive small cells with multiple lines of differentiation (*Fig. 21.48*). As a result of modern treatment with surgery, radiotherapy and chemotherapy, the 10-year survival rate is over 50%.

Histologically, tumors are composed of sheets of small anaplastic cells with rod-shaped and rounded nuclei (*Fig. 21.49*). Evidence of neuronal and glial differentiation may be seen. Less common PNETs are cerebral neuroblastomas (composed of primitive neurons) and ependymoblastomas (composed of primitive ependyma).

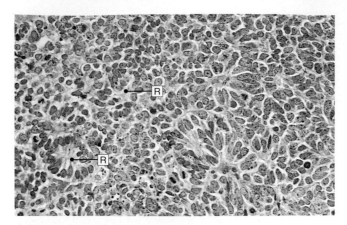

Fig. 21.49 PNET.
Primitive neuroectodermal tumors are composed of small cells with a high mitotic rate. In some, neuroblastic rosettes (**R**) form, indicating primitive neuronal maturation.

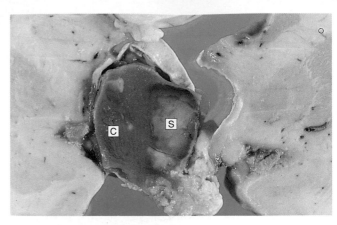

Fig. 21.50 Craniopharyngioma.
A craniopharyngioma has both solid (**S**) and cystic (**C**) areas. The cyst is filled with thick fluid containing lipid derived from breakdown of the lining epithelium.

NON-NEUROEPITHELIAL TUMORS OF THE CNS

Lymphomas of the nervous system are increasing in incidence as a complication of immunosuppression

Primary lymphomas of the nervous system are usually high-grade non-Hodgkin's lymphomas of B-cell type. These tumors may arise sporadically, but are increasing in incidence and are associated with immunosuppression, particularly in patients with AIDS.

Lesions are ill-defined and multifocal, usually being seen deep in the hemispheric white matter. Histology shows brain infiltrated by atypical lymphoid cells. These tumors have a very poor prognosis, with most patients dead 5 years after diagnosis.

Solitary plasmacytomas may also arise in the brain. These lesions are composed of sheets of plasma cells and may be associated with monoclonal light chains in CSF or serum.

The nervous system is a site for the origin of germ-cell tumors, mainly from the pineal gland

Germ-cell tumors identical to those seen in the ovary and testis may arise in the brain, most occurring in the pineal gland. The full range of germ-cell tumors is seen, i.e. germinoma, embryonal carcinoma, yolk-sac tumor, choriocarcinoma, teratoma and mixed germ-cell tumors. Most are malignant and are prone to spread via the CSF pathways, requiring treatment by radiotherapy and chemotherapy. Treatment may be monitored by detection of tumor markers in the CSF.

Developmental cysts of the nervous system may present as space-occupying lesions

Many different types of cysts and tumor-like lesions involve the CNS. For example, **dermoid** and **epidermoid cysts** are lined by squamous epithelium and filled with keratin. They are slowly expanding cysts, common in the temporal lobe region.

Colloid cysts of the third ventricle are solitary cysts lined by columnar epithelium. Filled with mucoid material, they arise in the third ventricle, commonly producing hydrocephalus by blocking the foramen of Monro.

Arachnoid cysts arise from the leptomeninges and are filled with CSF. They cause compression of underlying brain.

Craniopharyngiomas are infiltrative epithelial tumors arising from the region of the pituitary fossa

Composed of squamous-cell-like epithelium, craniopharyngiomas are derived from remnants of Rathke's pouch, the embryological source of the anterior pituitary gland. Accounting for 3% of intracranial tumors, they are most common in childhood. Tumors compress the pituitary gland and damage the overlying hypothalamus and optic chiasm, presenting with either hypopituitarism or visual problems. Macroscopically, lesions have cystic and solid areas, frequently growing into adjacent brain and around major blood vessels (*Fig. 21.50*), often with calcification.

Although craniopharyngiomas are benign, local recurrence is often a problem because of inability to completely excise infiltrative tumors.

DISEASES OF PERIPHERAL NERVES

Peripheral nerves are composed of several fascicles, each surrounded by the peri-neurium, which is composed of epithelial-like peri-neural cells. Within the peri-neurium, individual axons are supported by Schwann cells, which may form myelin.

Clinical features of peripheral nerve diseases

Diseases of peripheral nerves are termed **neuropathies** and are clinically manifest by sensory or motor abnormalities, which may be predominantly motor, predominantly sensory, or mixed, depending on which diameter of nerve fibers is affected by a disease process.

Clinically, several terms are used to describe peripheral nerve disease. The term 'neuritis' is often used, but it does not usually imply an inflammatory pathology.

- **Polyneuropathy** is generalized symmetrical involvement of peripheral nerves.
- **Focal peripheral neuropathy** is disease affecting peripheral nerves in a haphazard manner, the term 'mononeuropathy' being applied when one nerve is affected, and 'multiple mononeuropathy' being used to describe asymmetrical disease of several nerves.
- **Radiculopathy** is disease affecting a nerve root.

Disease of peripheral nerves is clinically investigated by electrophysiology. When diagnosis is uncertain, nerve biopsy may be performed; the most common site is from the sural nerve in the foot, as it leaves no significant neurological deficit.

There are three main pathological types of damage to peripheral nerves: primary axonal degeneration, primary demyelination, and destruction of both axon and myelin.

Provided that the cell body of the nerve remains intact, damage to the peripheral axon or myelin may be repaired by regeneration.

Peripheral nerve damage can be divided into axonal damage or demyelination

In **axonal degeneration** nerve-cell bodies are unable to maintain long axonal processes. The result is degeneration of axons, starting at the periphery and progressing up towards the neuronal cell body. This process is often termed a **dying back neuropathy** and is commonly due to toxic and metabolic damage to nerve-cell bodies. Loss of axons can be inferred by reduced amplitude of nerve impulses when measured electrically from affected nerves.

In **segmental demyelination** the disease process spares axons but damages Schwann cells and myelin. Loss of myelin can be inferred by slowing of conduction velocity when measured electrically. Loss of myelin is mainly seen in immune-mediated disease, as well as with several toxins.

Regeneration in the peripheral nervous system

The sequence of events that follows sectioning of axons in a nerve is termed **Wallerian degeneration** and, under favorable circumstances, this is followed by axonal regeneration.

1   When an axon is severed or damaged, the axon and myelin distal to the injury degenerate. The degenerate myelin and axon are removed by macrophages and Schwann cells. The target tissue, e.g. muscle, is denervated and atrophies.

2   Schwann cells in the distal nerve proliferate and enlarge within the still-intact basement membrane tube enclosing them.

3   The nerve-cell body becomes swollen, the nucleus enlarges and there is an increase in the quantity of cytoplasmic intermediate filaments, termed **central chromatolysis** (a structural change reflecting regeneration). The stump of the proximal axon swells and several small axon sprouts grow out down the column of proliferated Schwann cells, which acts as a guide for the regenerating axon. The axons grows 2–3 mm per day, eventually re-innervating the denervated tissue.

4   The axon is remyelinated, but new myelin segments between nodes of Ranvier are shorter than in the original nerve.

Axons' capacity for regeneration allows surgical repair of peripheral nerves by nerve anastomosis after severance. Grafting of a portion of nerve is required when there has been scarring, as axons can only grow down the intact basement membrane tubes of Schwann cells, not through a collagenous scar.

Provided that the cell body is intact, and that there is no scarring in the nerve, axons and myelin may regenerate, allowing recovery from damage to peripheral nerves (see pink box).

The main infections of nerves are herpes zoster and leprosy

In herpes zoster infection, virus lies dormant in the neuronal cell bodies of dorsal root ganglia, but becomes reactivated and tracks down nerves to cause infection of the skin in the sensory dermatome (**shingles**).

Mycobacterium leprae mainly affects peripheral nerves in the tuberculoid form. Destruction of both axons and myelin occurs by granulomatous inflammation, particularly in cutaneous nerves, predisposing to skin ulceration and loss of digits because of loss of sensation.

Laceration, compression and entrapment are common mechanical causes of nerve dysfunction

One of the most common causes of peripheral nerve dysfunction is mechanical trauma. Laceration of nerves is seen after penetrating trauma and is associated with some bone fractures. The nerve distal to the laceration undergoes Wallerian degeneration. If surgical anastomosis is performed, axons may regrow to re-innervate the denervated tissues.

Entrapment and compression of nerves is commonly seen in several sites:

- Nerve roots are compressed in intervertebral foramina by prolapsed intervertebral discs or osteophytes due to osteoarthritis of the spine.
- The median nerve is compressed by swellings in the carpal tunnel at the wrist.
- The ulnar nerve can become compressed in the flexor carpal tunnel at the medial epicondyle of the humerus.
- The common peroneal nerve can be compressed at the neck of the fibula.

Compressed nerves develop segmental demyelination and abnormal conduction but, with prolonged damage, there is additional axonal degeneration.

Acute immune-mediated demyelination is the most common cause of an acute peripheral neuropathy

Guillain–Barré syndrome, also known as **acute post-infectious polyradiculoneuropathy** is the most common form of acute neuropathy. It is an immune-mediated demyelination of peripheral nerves, usually seen 2–4 weeks after a viral illness, but also triggered after a variety of infective processes. Histologically, nerves show infiltration by lymphoid cells, with phagocytosis of myelin by macrophages.

Widespread demyelination in peripheral nerves causes motor weakness, often leading to respiratory failure, with less prominent sensory changes. Remyelination usually occurs over a period of 3–4 months and is associated with recovery in most cases.

Chronic demyelinating polyradiculoneuropathy is a chronic form of immune-mediated demyelination in which repeated episodes of demyelination and remyelination cause proliferation of Schwann cells, often leading to physical swelling of peripheral nerves (hypertrophic neuropathy).

Peripheral neuropathy may occur as a paraneoplastic syndrome, several cases being due to formation of autoantibodies to the tumor, which cross-react with myelin.

Neuropathies may be caused by toxins, causing either demyelination or axonal degeneration

Many toxins cause damage to peripheral nerves, either by damaging myelin or by causing damage to neurons, leading to axonal degeneration:

- **Chronic alcohol abuse** is a common cause of peripheral neuropathy, which may be due to the direct toxic effects of alcohol as well as the effects of vitamin deficiency.
- **Drugs**, e.g. isoniazid, sulfonamides, vinca alkaloids, dapsone and chloroquine, are important causes of neuropathy.
- **Occupational exposure to chemicals** such as lead, arsenic, mercury and acrylamide.

Most toxins produce a dying back axonal neuropathy that results in symmetrical sensory/motor neuropathy with a 'glove and stocking' distribution, reflecting loss of the ends of the longer axons.

Diabetes is the most common metabolic disorder causing neuropathy

Several metabolic disorders are associated with the development of a peripheral neuropathy, the most common being diabetes.

Diabetes mellitus is associated with four main patterns of neuropathy: symmetrical predominantly sensory peripheral polyneuropathy, autonomic neuropathy, proximal painful motor neuropathy, and cranial mononeuropathy (mainly third, fourth and sixth nerves).

The sensory and autonomic neuropathy is mainly due to a combination of axonal degeneration and segmental demyelination, whereas the motor neuropathy and cranial mononeuropathy are caused by vascular disease in blood vessels supplying nerves.

Vitamin deficiency is an important cause of peripheral neuropathy, particularly B_1 (thiamine) and B_{12}.

Amyloid (see Chapter 25) may infiltrate peripheral nerves and cause a neuropathy. In addition to secondary amyloid associated with systemic inflammatory diseases or myeloma, several types of familial amyloid cause a specific neuropathy due to a defect in the gene coding for transthyretin (prealbumin).

Vascular disease is a common cause of peripheral nerve damage

Vascular disease is an important cause of peripheral nerve disease, resulting in focal necrosis of major nerve trunks and loss of myelinated axons.

The most common causes of vascular damage to nerves are **atherosclerosis** and **arteriosclerosis**, particularly affecting arteries supplying nerves in the lower limbs of patients who have critical ischemia. This is most common in patients with diabetes.

Vasculitis may cause nerve infarction, presenting as a multiple mononeuropathy in, for example, polyarteritis nodosa, SLE, Wegener's granulomatosis and rheumatoid disease.

Hereditary diseases are uncommon but important causes of peripheral neuropathy

Several peripheral neuropathies have a hereditary basis, many of which are of known cause. The mechanism for development of neuropathy varies in each case. Porphyria, Fabry's disease, leukodystrophies, abetalipoproteinemia and familial amyloidosis syndromes are all hereditary diseases that can be associated with peripheral neuropathies.

Charcot–Marie–Tooth (CMT) syndrome is one of the most common inherited neurological diseases. It comprises a group of genetically determined polyneuropathies, which are divided into several types on the basis of clinical pattern of disease. CMT Type 1A is an autosomal dominant demyelinating disease caused by a mutation in the gene coding for peripheral myelin protein-22, a vital component of normal myelin.

Hereditary neuropathy with a tendency to pressure palsies is an autosomal dominant disease in which there are recurrent focal neuropathies caused by minor pressure on nerves. This is believed to be caused by monosomy for the gene for peripheral myelin protein-22. Several other familial neuropathies are linked to mutations in genes coding for myelin proteins.

The main tumors of peripheral nerve are benign nerve-sheath tumors, neurofibromas and schwannomas

The main tumors of peripheral nerve arise from the nerve sheath and are termed schwannomas and neurofibromas. Uncommonly, malignant peripheral nerve-sheath tumors can develop (neurofibrosarcomas and malignant schwannomas).

Schwannomas which are usually solitary tumors, can occur on any peripheral nerve. They are rounded lesions, typically 1–2 cm in diameter when removed, composed of spindle-shaped cells with features of Schwann cells. Schwannomas affecting the eighth cranial nerve are termed acoustic neuromas and may be part of the neurofibromatosis 2 syndrome (see page 459).

Neurofibromas which may be solitary or multiple, are nodular or plexiform in type. Nodular neurofibromas are discrete tumors that form a defined mass, whereas plexiform neurofibromas diffusely affect nerves over a wide area, making surgical removal very difficult. Nodular neurofibromas are fusiform or rounded tumors composed of spindle cells that resemble peri-neural cells. Plexiform neurofibromas often appear as boggy areas of ill-defined swelling and are composed of nerves expanded by a proliferation of peri-neural cells and extracellular matrix material. Multiple neurofibromas are seen as part of the neurofibromatosis 1 syndrome (see page 459).

Malignant nerve-sheath tumors may arise *de novo* or may occur as malignant change in an existing benign tumor, usually in cases of neurofibromatosis. They behave as soft-tissue sarcomas (discussed in Chapter 24).

Post-traumatic neuroma is a regenerative phenomenon of attempted axonal sprouting

When a nerve is severed, by either trauma or surgery, the cut end develops a collagenous scar associated with attempted regeneration of axons. In most cases this is asymptomatic, but in some instances the attempt at regeneration forms a nodule that is painful to pressure. Histologically the nodule consists of collagen, proliferated Schwann cells and sprouting axon terminals. This common clinical problem, termed an amputation neuroma, sometimes arises in the stumps of leg amputations as a cause of pain when using a limb prosthesis.

The same collagenous scarring prevents successful regrowth of axons down a nerve after trauma; such lesions have to be surgically removed and the cut ends of nerve anastomosed, often with a nerve graft, to allow re-innervation.

MUSCLE DISEASES

Diseases of muscle fall into three main groups

In clinical practice, most non-neoplastic diseases of muscle present because of weakness, wasting, or pain in muscle. There are three main groups.

Muscular dystrophies are inherited diseases of muscle, which generally result in progressive degeneration. They are classified according to inheritance pattern, clinical pattern of muscle groups involved and, as the genes responsible become characterized, increasingly by molecular genetic techniques.

Myopathies are a group of conditions of diverse etiology, grouped together because of a predominant impact of disease on the muscle. There are four main sub-groups:

- Inflammatory myopathies, in which there is a primary inflammation of muscle, often amenable to therapy (very common).
- Secondary myopathies, in which a systemic disease process causes pathology in muscle, often amenable to therapy (common).
- Metabolic myopathies, in which a primary metabolic problem has a major impact on muscle function (uncommon).
- Congenital myopathies, which are distinguished from the dystrophies in that they are generally non-progressive (rare).

Neurogenic disease, particularly disease of peripheral nerves or motor neurons, causes secondary atrophy of skeletal muscle.

Muscle biopsy

Biopsy of muscle is an important investigation in certain neuromuscular diseases in which there are clinical features of weakness, muscle wasting, or muscle pain (myalgia). The two main techniques of biopsy are **open excision biopsy**, which provides a large sample but is relatively invasive, and **percutaneous needle biopsy**, which provides a small sample but can be repeated if needed.

The main biopsy sites are the vastus lateralis, deltoid or gastrocnemius muscles. As it requires specialized techniques, histological examination of a muscle biopsy is not performed in most clinical laboratories. The sample needs rapid transport to the laboratory while fresh. Preservation by snap-freezing in liquid nitrogen then allows histological sections to be cut for enzyme histochemical staining, enabling delineation of

fiber types. Electron microscopy is used to look for mitochondrial abnormalities as well as the structural changes that can take place in some of the congenital muscle diseases, so small samples need immediate glutaraldehyde fixation.

Muscle enzymes

In the investigation of muscle disease it is possible to estimate the level of activity of muscle fiber necrosis by looking at the **serum creatine kinase** level. This enzyme is present in skeletal muscle and is liberated in the blood in muscle disease. As there are several isoenzymes of creatine kinase, estimation of the muscle-specific enzyme gives some specificity. The level of this serum enzyme is also elevated following necrosis of cardiac muscle after myocardial infarction.

KEY FACTS
Skeletal muscle

- Skeletal muscle is composed of individual striated muscle fibers, which can be divided into two main sub-types. Type 1 fibers contain abundant mitochondria and are specialized for aerobic metabolism. Type 2 fibers contain abundant glycogen and are specialized for anaerobic metabolism. Fiber types are identified by enzyme histochemistry.
- A normal muscle is composed of a mixture of the two types of fiber, which are arranged randomly.
- Innervation of muscle is at specialized motor end-plates that have acetylcholine receptors on the muscle surface.

Skeletal muscle has only a limited repertoire of pathological responses

Atrophy of muscle fibers occurs mainly with disuse, ischemia, denervation, steroid therapy, and malnutrition. It may affect one sub-type of fiber preferentially, usually Type 2.

Hypertrophy of muscle fibers occurs to compensate for loss or atrophy of other muscle fibers due to a disease process.

Change in fiber type distribution is detected by histochemical staining. It is usually seen in association with

change in muscle innervation, when muscle fibers come to be arranged in groups rather than a random checker-board pattern.

Necrosis of muscle is usually seen in single fibers and is a feature of many of the primary muscle diseases. Less commonly, large areas undergo necrosis, usually due to vascular pathology in main vessels.

Phagocytosis of dead muscle fibers by macrophages occurs following necrosis.

Regeneration of skeletal muscle fibers can take place from the population of muscle stem cells (satellite cells).

Fibrosis, often accompanied by infiltration with adipose tissue, occurs following organization of large areas of necrosis, as well as being the end-result of individual cell necrosis, and is characteristic of many types of muscular dystrophy.

Primary inflammation occurs in the inflammatory myopathies.

Given that skeletal muscle has a limited set of responses, the histological diagnosis of muscle disease is based on evaluation of the combination of different types of pathological responses.

Muscle disease can be divided into two main groups according to the pathology. In **dystrophic and myopathic disease**, there is hypertrophy and atrophy of fibers, with single fibers undergoing degeneration, necrosis, and phagocytosis. There is variable fibrosis.

In **neurogenic disease**, atrophy of fibers is seen in groups, with fibers elsewhere showing compensatory hypertrophy. Fiber-type grouping is often seen on histochemical staining.

Congenital myopathies are a cause of childhood hypotonia

The congenital myopathies usually present in childhood as hypotonia (floppy baby syndrome) or muscle weakness. The majority of congenital myopathies are named after the structural abnormalities seen on muscle biopsy, e.g. central core disease, nemaline body myopathy, myotubular myopathy, congenital fiber-type disproportion. They are generally non-progressive, which distinguishes them from muscular dystrophies. Inheritance is variable, with both sporadic and heritable types. Although many types are compatible with a long life expectancy, others may cause disability because of secondary skeletal deformities or respiratory muscle involvement.

Muscular dystrophies are progressive, genetically determined, degenerative diseases of muscle

The muscular dystrophies are a group of genetically determined degenerative diseases of muscle. Pathologically, they are characterized by the destruction of single muscle cells over a prolonged period of time, with fiber regeneration and the development of fibrosis. The muscular dystrophies are classified according to the pattern of muscle groups involved, the pattern of inheritance (*Fig. 21.51*) and, increasingly, defined molecular genetic abnormalities. It has recently become apparent that diagnosis of muscular dystrophy simply on the basis of the pattern of muscle

involvement is unreliable, as several different muscle diseases can present with identical clinical features.

Duchenne dystrophy is the most common form of muscular dystrophy in childhood

Duchenne dystrophy is an X-linked recessive disorder, hence it is almost exclusively seen in males. It is caused by mutation in the gene coding for **dystrophin**, a protein that normally helps anchor the internal cytoskeleton of muscle fibers through the cell membrane and to the extracellular matrix. Lack of this protein renders fibers liable to tearing with repeated contraction. The onset of clinical features is in early childhood, affected children showing muscle weakness with a high serum creatine kinase level (caused by necrosis) and clinical calf hypertrophy (due to fatty replacement of muscle). The disease has a very poor prognosis, most affected individuals dying in their late teens. Heart muscle is also affected, leading to cardiomyopathy.

Molecular pathology of Duchenne dystrophy

The molecular basis of the disorder is a mutation in a very long gene on the short arm of the X chromosome, coding for the protein **dystrophin**. This protein mediates anchorage of the actin cytoskeleton of skeletal muscle fibers to the basement membrane via a membrane glycoprotein complex. The dystrophin molecule is a long, rod-shaped protein, one end binding to the membrane glycoprotein, the other to actin, with a middle rod region.

Several mutations in the dystrophin gene give rise to different degrees of severity of muscle disease:

- Mutations causing frame shifts in the gene lead to complete failure of production of dystrophin and to severe Duchenne dystrophy.
- Mutations causing abnormalities in the binding sites for the membrane or actin mean that anchorage is inefficient, causing moderate to severe forms of Duchenne dystrophy.
- Mutations in the middle rod region still allow anchorage of muscle to basement membrane, and a mild form of dystrophy develops called **Becker's dystrophy**.

The complete lack of dystrophin in severe Duchenne dystrophy means that poorly anchored fibers tear themselves apart under the repeated stress of contraction. Free calcium then enters muscle cells, causing cell death and fiber necrosis.

Fig. 21.51
Muscular dystrophies

Type of dystrophy	Inheritance	Muscle involved in initial stages
Duchenne type	X-linked recessive	Pelvic girdle
Becker type	X-linked recessive	Pelvic girdle
Limb girdle	Autosomal recessive	Pelvic girdle
Fascioscapulohumeral	Dominant	Face, shoulder girdle, arm
Scapulohumeral	Autosomal recessive	Shoulder girdle and arm
Oculopharyngeal	Dominant	External ocular and pharynx
Myotonic dystrophy	Dominant	Face, respiratory, limbs

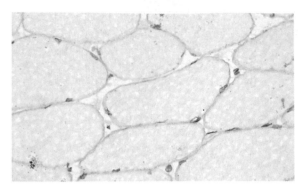

Fig. 21.52 Dystrophin abnormalities. This shows staining of muscle for dystrophin (brown). In Duchenne dystrophy this staining would be absent as no protein is produced. In Becker's dystrophy, staining is reduced or patchy.

Histologically, there is muscle fiber necrosis, phago-cytosis of dead fibers, and replacement of muscle by fibrous and fatty tissue. Immunostaining for dystrophin reveals that it is absent from fibers (*Fig. 21.52*). Diagnosis can be assisted by performing molecular genetic analysis of the dystrophin gene.

Myotonic dystrophy is an autosomal dominant disorder

Myotonic dystrophy is the most common inherited muscle disease of adults, affecting 1 in 8000 of the population. It is characterized by muscle weakness, myotonia (inability to relax muscles), and several non-muscle features including cataracts and frontal baldness in males, cardiomyopathy, and low intelligence. Patients also show neurofibrillary tangles similar to those seen in Alzheimer's disease (see page 454) in the brain with aging. It is inherited as an autosomal dominant disorder and usually becomes appar-ent in adolescence with facial weakness and distal weakness in the limbs. Death is commonly due to involvement of the respiratory muscles.

The gene for myotonic dystrophy is located on chromo-some 19, coding for a protein kinase (see pink box). Histologically, affected muscles show abnormalities of fiber size, with fiber necrosis, abundant internal nuclei, and replacement by fibro-fatty tissue.

Patients with a limb girdle syndrome may have one of several diseases

Patients who have weakness in pelvic girdle and proximal leg muscles or in shoulder girdle and proximal arm muscles are said to have a **limb girdle syndrome**. On investigation, most patients with this clinical pattern of weakness have metabolic or neurogenic muscle disease or a late-onset Becker's dystrophy. Other cases have a true limb girdle muscular dystrophy, which is associated with several differ-ent patterns of inheritance, and in many cases defined gene mutations.

Molecular pathology of myotonic dystrophy

Myotonic dystrophy is an autosomal dominant neuromuscular disease. The gene for the disorder is on chromosome 19; the mutation has been identified as an unstable trinucleotide CTG repeat in a sequence related to a gene coding for a cAMP-dependent protein kinase, widely expressed in many tissues. The mechanism through which this mutation causes myotonia is unknown.

The CTG repeat varies in length between affected siblings, generally increasing through generations in parallel with increasing severity of the disease. This is the basis of **anticipation**, whereby clinical disease is more severe in later generations of an affected family as a result of progressive increase in size of the gene expansion. Congenital myotonic dystrophy, a severe disease of the newborn, is exclusively maternally inherited.

Fascioscapulohumeral weakness may be caused by several diseases

True fascioscapulohumeral muscular dystrophy presents with weakness in the face and shoulder, and is associated with a slow clinical progression. Onset is generally in the third decade. All cases presenting with this pattern of weakness require investigation, as a variety of metabolic, inflammatory, neurogenic and myopathic disorders may be responsible.

Inflammatory myopathies are diseases with an underlying abnormal immune response

The inflammatory myopathies are characterized by primary inflammation of muscle, with resulting fiber necrosis. The inflammatory infiltrate is mainly composed of T-cells and monocytes as part of an abnormal autoimmune response. There are three main types of inflammatory myopathy.

Polymyositis presents clinically with weakness of proxi-mal limb muscles and facial muscles, ptosis, and dysphagia. Although the precise stimulus causing disease is unknown, there are well-recognized clinical associations, the most common being the presence of connective tissue diseases such as SLE, rheumatoid disease or scleroderma (see Chapter 25). Polymyositis may also be a non-metastatic manifestation of malignancy, in which case it may be part of the clinical syndrome of dermatomyositis in which muscle disease is accompanied by a characteristic skin rash.

Muscle biopsy shows lymphocytic infiltration of muscle with fiber necrosis. Disease may respond to immuno-suppressive treatment with steroids or azathioprine.

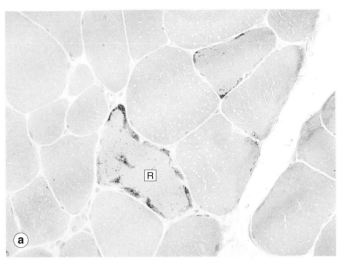
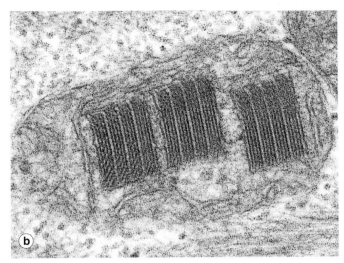

Fig. 21.53 Mitochondrial myopathy. (a) Trichrome stain. (b) Electron microscopy.
In affected muscle (a), aggregates of mitochondria can be seen by light microscopy, staining red with special stains, hence the term 'ragged red fibers' (**R**). Ultrastructure (b) often shows crystalline inclusions in mitochondria, termed 'parking-lot inclusions', because of their orderly pattern.

Inclusion body myositis is clinically similar to polymyositis, but occurs mainly in elderly patients. Muscle biopsy shows inflammation of muscle, fiber necrosis and the presence of vacuoles and filamentous inclusions in fibers (seen by electron microscopy). Diagnosis of this disorder is important because it is slowly progressive and has a poor response to immunosuppressive treatment.

Sarcoidosis may affect muscle, but it is relatively uncommon compared to other types of inflammatory myopathy.

Secondary and metabolic myopathies are common in clinical practice

Diseases of muscle secondary to either systemic disease or metabolic abnormality are seen frequently in clinical practice. There are many types and only the clinically most common are presented.

Type 2 fiber atrophy myopathy is the most common pathological finding in biopsies from patients with muscle weakness. The Type 2 fibers undergo selective atrophy, which can be detected on histochemical staining. This pattern of muscle abnormality is non-specific and may be secondary to several problems, the main ones being disuse, malignancy, steroid administration, Cushing's disease, thyroid disease and connective tissue diseases.

Endocrine myopathy describes the association of muscle weakness and wasting with endocrine disease. The main cause is corticosteroid excess (therapeutic or in Cushing's disease), which results in atrophy of Type 2 fibers. Similar changes can occur with thyroid disease.

Carcinomatous myopathy describes the association of muscle weakness and wasting with systemic neoplasia. The tumor may cause non-metastatic manifestations in muscle through Type 2 fiber atrophy myopathy, the development of polymyositis or dermatomyositis, or denervation due to a paraneoplastic neuropathy.

Mitochondrial myopathy is due to heritable genetic abnormalities affecting mitochondrial function. Diseases are due to either mitochondrial (maternal inheritance) or nuclear genetic abnormalities (Mendelian inheritance). Disease syndromes are characterized by muscle weakness, particularly extraocular muscles, with or without other neurological and metabolic disturbances. Muscle biopsy reveals abnormal pleomorphic mitochondria, often with crystalline inclusions on electron microscopy (*Fig. 21.53*). Molecular genetic analysis may show specific abnormalities in the mitochondrial genome, but the nuclear genetic causes are as yet uncharacterized. This is now recognized to be an important and common cause of disease, which can have onset at all ages.

Glycogenoses may affect muscle. The two main types of glycogenosis affecting muscle are acid maltase deficiency (Type 2) and McArdle's disease (myophosphorylase deficiency, Type 5). Both are diagnosable on muscle biopsy.

NEUROGENIC DISORDERS OF MUSCLE

Neurogenic disorders may present as muscle disease

Clinically, weakness of muscle may be caused by denervation due to disease either of peripheral nerves or of anterior horn cells. Denervation is easily recognized on muscle biopsy as it causes atrophy of large groups of fibers. If re-innervation occurs, the normal random distribution of Type 1 and Type 2 fibers is replaced by large groups of a single fiber type, termed **fiber-type grouping**.

Spinal muscular atrophy is a heritable degeneration of spinal motor neurons

The childhood spinal muscular atrophies (SMA) constitute the second most common autosomal recessive disorder after cystic fibrosis. Disease is manifest by muscle weakness and wasting due to degeneration of the anterior horn cells in the spinal cord, resulting in denervation of muscle. Inheritance is autosomal recessive due to a defective gene located on chromosome 5. Based on age of onset and severity of disease, three main clinical patterns of disease are recognized, thought to be due to different mutations in the gene.

Type I and II **Werdnig–Hoffman disease** presents as a floppy baby at birth. In the severe acute form, affected children usually die in the first year of life; an intermediate form is associated with longer survival. Muscle biopsy shows large groups of abnormally small muscle fibers that have never been innervated (*Fig. 21.54*)

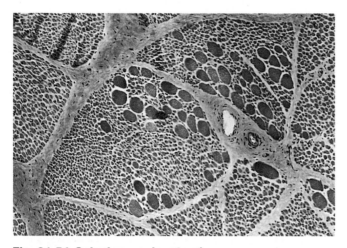

Fig. 21.54 Spinal muscular atrophy.
In biopsy, large areas of muscle are composed of minute non-innervated fibers, contrasting with larger pink fibers that have been innervated.

Type III **Kugelberg–Welander syndrome** is a less severe form of infantile SMA, with onset in the first 2 months of life. Affected babies have proximal limb girdle weakness with slow deterioration over time. Muscle biopsy shows large groups of atrophic fibers in keeping with the denervation.

Juvenile- and adult-onset spinal muscular atrophies are uncommon, presenting in later life, with limb girdle weakness. There is a dominant pattern of inheritance, not linked to chromosome 5. These must be distinguished from other causes of a limb girdle syndrome by investigation. Muscle biopsy shows features of neurogenic atrophy, with fiber-type grouping indicative of re-innervation.

DISORDERS OF MUSCLE FUNCTION

Myasthenia gravis is an autoimmune disease caused by antibodies to the acetylcholine receptor

Myasthenia gravis is a disease characterized by muscle weakness, ptosis and dysphagia. A main differential diagnosis is with an inflammatory myopathy, which can have identical clinical features. It is an autoimmune disease caused by generation of autoantibodies to the acetylcholine receptor located in the post-synaptic membrane of muscle motor end-plates. These antibodies prevent synaptic transmission by blocking the receptor sites.

Diagnosis can be made by giving a therapeutic trial of a short-acting anti-cholinesterase drug, which increases acetylcholine concentrations in the synaptic cleft and allows transmission.

An important association with this condition is pathology of the thymus gland. About 25% of cases have a thymoma (see page 316), others having thymic gland hyperplasia. Thymectomy may improve the myasthenia in a proportion of cases. There is no diagnostic pathology seen by routine light microscopy in muscle biopsy.

Diseases caused by defective ion transport in muscle

Several diseases of muscle have been shown to be due to abnormal ion transport across muscle membranes. The main syndromes are manifest by sudden reversible attacks of paralysis and flaccidity (**periodic paralysis**), abnormal relaxation of muscles (**myotonia**), or **fatiguability**.

Hypokalemic periodic paralysis is most common in adult women. Attacks of paralysis typically occur on waking in the morning and can last for many hours. There is a fall in the serum potassium level to 2–2.5 mmol/L.

Mutations in muscle dihydropyridine (DHP)-sensitive calcium channel alpha-1 sub-unit have been found.

Hyperkalemic periodic paralysis is most common in childhood and adolescence. Attacks are precipitated when the individual is at rest following a period of exercise, but are short-lived (1–2 hours). There is elevation of the serum potassium to 5–7 mmol/L during an attack. Fixed muscle weakness develops in most patients with time. This syndrome is caused by mutations in the gene ▶

for the alpha sub-unit of the skeletal muscle Na⁺ channel located on chromosome 17.

Paramyotonia congenita (PC) is an autosomal dominant non-progressive muscle disorder characterized by cold-induced stiffness followed by muscle weakness. The weakness is also caused by a dysfunction of the sodium channel in muscle fibers, caused by mutation in the sodium channel gene located on chromosome 17. Thus, paramyotonia congenita and hyperkalemic periodic paralysis are caused by allelic mutations at the same locus.

Autosomal recessive generalized myotonia (Becker's disease) and **autosomal dominant myotonia congenita (Thomsen's disease)** are characterized by skeletal muscle stiffness manifest by difficulty in relaxing grip. These diseases are the result of muscle membrane hyperexcitability due to mutation in the gene for a skeletal muscle chloride channel protein on chromosome 7. Defective ion transport causes failure of muscle relaxation.

Lambert–Eaton myasthenic syndrome (LEMS) is characterized by abnormal fatiguability. It is an autoimmune disorder of neuromuscular transmission, often found in patients with lung cancer. Autoantibodies bind to presynaptic voltage-dependent calcium channels at motor nerve terminals to cause functional loss. This in turn causes reduced release of acetylcholine in response to nerve stimulation. Small-cell lung carcinoma cells express calcium channels, suggesting that autoantibody production is triggered by these tumor antigens.

Malignant hyperthermia is an inherited disorder in which exposure to certain drugs, especially those used in anesthesia, leads to sustained muscle contraction, hypermetabolism and pyrexia; this may be fatal. Disease is due to defects in the gene coding for a sarcoplasmic reticulum release-channel called the ryanodine receptor; ryanodine is an artificial ligand which bonds to the channel. Mutation in this gene can also cause central core disease, one of the congenital myopathies. Some patients with muscle weakness and thymoma have autoantibodies to the ryanodine receptor, simulating myasthenia gravis.

Ophthalmic pathology

Clinical Overview

The most common diseases of the eye are the common deteriorations in visual acuity due to short-sightedness or long-sightedness. In the vast majority of cases these are corrected by the use of spectacles or contact lenses, and fall within the province of the optician rather than the ophthalmic surgeon.

The eyelids are specialized skin and, as such, may develop many of the lesions which occur in skin elsewhere, such as seborrheic keratoses, viral warts, various inflammatory diseases, and (particularly important) basal cell carcinoma. The management of malignant tumors in the eyelid is particularly difficult due to the functional and cosmetic implications of achieving wide safe excision.

Trauma to the eye, especially to the cornea, is extremely common in clinical practice. Infective autoimmune and inflammatory processes are common in the conjunctiva, cornea and uvea. Although the most frequently encountered tumors related to the eye are skin tumors in the eyelid, the most common tumor of the globe is malignant melanoma of the choroid. In children, retinoblastoma is an important embryonal tumor.

The retina is affected by systemic disorders which have an impact on small retinal blood vessels (e.g, diabetes and systemic hypertension), and degenerative processes of the retina are also common. Macular degeneration of aging is a very common cause of blindness.

Abnormalities in the fluid drainage pathways of the eye lead to the severe disease glaucoma, which has several different pathological causes.

Introduction

The eye, the anatomy of which is shown in *Fig. 22.1*, is designed to focus light onto the specialized photoreceptors of the retina. Diseases of the eye are common and frequently present to family practitioners, arising from the whole range of pathological causes. Importantly, several systemic diseases have major manifestations as eye disorders.

This chapter will consider diseases affecting the coverings of the eye (eyelids, conjunctiva and cornea), disorders affecting the pigmented uveal tissues, the lens, the retina and vitreous. The pathology of the common problems of glaucoma, eye trauma, and space-occupying lesions of the orbit will then be discussed.

DISEASES OF THE EYELIDS, CONJUNCTIVA AND CORNEA

Inflammatory and neoplastic diseases of the eyelids are common

The structure of the eyelid is shown in *Fig. 22.2*. The tarsal plate is a tough collagenous sheet in which the sebaceous-like meibomian glands are located. Minor skin-appendage glands are associated with the eyelashes. The conjunctiva, which is a two-layered columnar epithelium containing mucin-secreting goblet cells, lines the eyelids (palpebral conjunctiva) and covers the anterior part of the globe (bulbar conjunctiva) up to the corneal epithelium (the limbus).

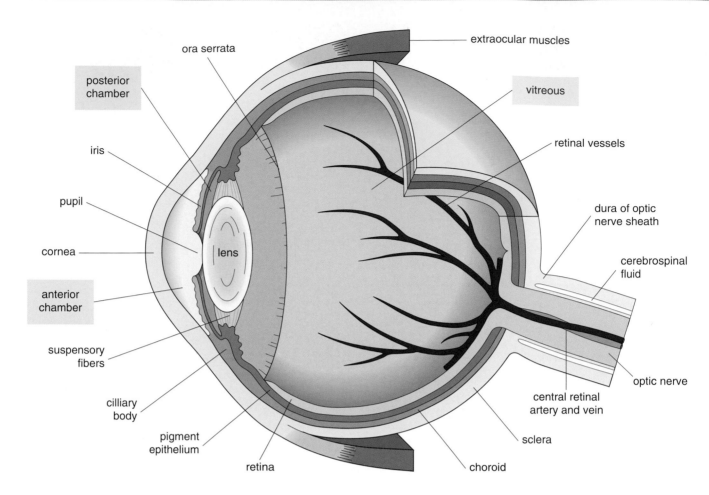

Fig. 22.1 Normal anatomy of the eye. The anterior and posterior chambers are filled with aqueous and are anterior to the lens. The vitreous is a specialized support tissue, not merely a gelatinous fluid.

Diseases of the eyelids and conjunctiva are extremely common, ranging from self-limiting infections to malignant tumors.

Blockage and infection of a meibomian gland causes swelling and acute inflammation of the affected gland. A chalazion is a firm swelling in the eyelid, which bulges under the palpebral conjunctiva (see *Fig. 22.6a*). Caused by rupture of a meibomian gland, it histologically consists of a foreign-body histiocytic chronic inflammatory response to lipid-rich material derived from the destroyed gland (*Fig. 22.3*).

The conjunctiva is frequently the site of infections causing **conjunctivitis**. Adenovirus types 3 and 7 cause follicular conjunctivitis, whereas types 8 and 19 cause epidemic keratoconjunctivitis. Allergic conjunctivitis is common in association with allergy to pollens. Bacterial conjunctivitis may also occur due to *Haemophilus* or, uncommonly, there may be neonatal infection with gonococcus. Granulomatous inflammation of the conjunctiva may be caused by several diseases, particularly sarcoidosis (see page 539) and TB, and may arise with allergies such as hayfever. Involvement of the skin of the eyelid with molluscum contagiosum gives rise to typical umbilicated lesions (see page 491).

Proliferation of sub-epithelial support tissues gives rise to **pingueculas**, which are small areas of yellow thickening of the bulbar conjunctiva. Caused by cumulative exposure to damaging environmental stimuli such as sun, wind and dust, they increase in incidence with age. Similar areas that encroach over the limbus onto the cornea are termed **pterygia**.

The eyelids are the site of several tumors and cysts. The main tumors of the eyelid are derived from skin and skin appendages, and are histologically similar to those arising elsewhere in the skin. Cysts may develop from blockage and dilatation of skin appendages and minor glands in the eyelid.

- **Xanthelasmas**, plaque-like, yellow lesions seen in the skin around the eyelids, are collections of lipid-filled histiocytes in the dermis. They may be associated with hyperlipidemic states.

- **Conjunctival melanocytic nevi** are the most common tumor of the conjunctiva. They are classified in a similar way to those seen in the skin (see page 501).

- **Primary acquired melanosis** is the term used to describe flat, stippled pigmentation of the conjunctiva

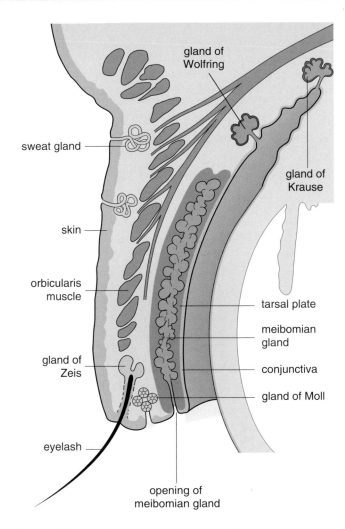

Fig. 22.2 Normal anatomy of the eyelid.
The eyelid contains meibomian glands, which may become
inflamed to form a chalazion. Cysts may develop from any of
the skin appendages or mucus glands.

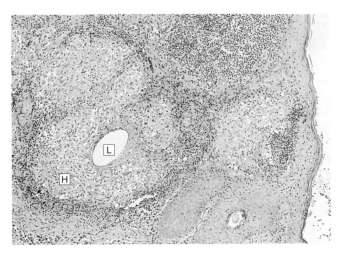

Fig. 22.3 Chalazion.
A chalazion represents a histiocytic inflammatory response (**H**)
to lipid material (**L**) released from damaged meibomian glands.

- **Lymphomas** may develop in the conjunctiva and
these have the characteristics of a lymphoma of
mucosal-associated lymphoid tissue (MALT).

- **Sebaceous gland carcinomas** are uncommon but
highly malignant tumors arising from the meibomian
glands.

Corneal diseases commonly cause scarring and loss of visual acuity

The cornea is covered by a non-keratinized squamous
epithelium and is composed of a stroma with a lining
endothelium. The endothelium is vital to normal corneal
function because it actively pumps fluid out of the corneal
stroma. The stroma is composed of highly organized
parallel layers of collagen. Deposition of abnormal collagen
leads to an opaque scar termed a **leukoma**.

Arcus senilis, seen as a yellow-white line at the corneal
margin, is due to accumulation of lipid in between the
corneal stromal lamella. It is normal with aging, but is
associated with hyperlipidemia when it arises in young
patients.

Squamous metaplasia of the surface corneal epithelium
may occur, causing corneal opacification. This is usually
secondary to lack of normal lubrication by tears, e.g. in dry-
eye syndromes or when diseases prevent eyelids covering
the cornea. It can also be caused by vitamin A deficiency.

The important diseases of the cornea result in structural
changes leading to opacification and impairment of visual
acuity.

Minor trauma to the cornea can cause painful loss of
surface epithelium, termed corneal abrasion. This may be
complicated by secondary infection, but in most cases heals
with regeneration.

Infective or inflammatory disorders of the cornea,
which are collectively termed **keratitis**, can result in scarring leading to opacification. Infection is most commonly

which develops in the elderly. Histologically such
lesions may be entirely benign or may show cytological
atypia when they may be a precursor lesion of
conjunctival malignant melanoma.

- **Conjunctival papillomas** are benign, red polypoid
lesions that arise from the palpebral or bulbar
conjunctiva; some have a viral etiology.

- **Basal-cell carcinomas** are common tumors that
involve the skin of the eyelid up to the lid margin
(see *Fig. 22.6c*). They are locally invasive and identical
to those arising in other sites.

- **Squamous-cell carcinomas** arise from the skin of the
eyelid or, less commonly, from the conjunctiva, where
they may be preceded by intraepithelial carcinoma.

- **Malignant melanomas** can arise in the conjunctiva
or from the skin of the eyelid. Both intraepithelial and
invasive lesions are seen, which are like those described
in the skin (see page 503).

due to viruses (herpes simplex), *Chlamydia trachomatis* (causing trachoma) and bacteria.

Corneal edema is caused by loss of, or damage to, corneal endothelium. As the cornea becomes opaque with accumulation of interstitial fluid from failure of endothelial function, blurring of vision occurs. In severe cases, extremely painful bullas form beneath corneal surface epithelium, with secondary superficial scarring.

Keratoconus is characterized by abnormal thinning of central corneal stroma, leading to conical protrusion of the cornea associated with central scarring causing opacification. This condition is associated with atopy and allergic conjunctivitis.

Corneal dystrophies are uncommon diseases (often inherited) that result in deposition of abnormal material within the cornea, causing opacification. There are many different sub-types, which are categorized according to the site and nature of the abnormal material deposited, e.g. **lattice dystrophy** shows amyloid and **macular dystrophy** shows mucopolysaccharide accumulation.

Corneal transplantation is possible, replacing a damaged cornea by a healthy graft. Failure of grafts is mainly related to loss of endothelial cells in the donor graft causing development of corneal edema.

DISEASES OF THE UVEA

The uvea is an intermediate layer between the sclera and the retina. It contains blood vessels, nerves, support cells and melanocytes. Functionally the uvea is divided into three special areas: the choroid (beneath the retina), the ciliary body, and the iris.

Uveal inflammation is associated with several systemic diseases as well as being caused by local infection

The uvea is the site of several inflammatory processes, collectively known as **uveitis**. Depending on the preferential site of inflammation, these may be manifest as **choroiditis**, **iritis**, **cyclitis** (inflammation of ciliary body), **iridocyclitis** or, when all sites are involved, **generalized uveitis**.

Uveitis is one of the causes of an acutely painful, red, inflamed eye. Histologically, there is lymphocytic and sometimes granulomatous inflammation of the uvea. In **iritis** this causes exudates in the aqueous, which are visible as keratic precipitates. In **choroiditis**, inflammatory exudation can cause detachment of the retina, whereas inflammatory destruction of the pigment epithelial layer causes degeneration of overlying photoreceptors, which normally depend on this layer for support.

Uveitis can be caused by several disease processes, the most common being **immune-mediated** and associated with other systemic diseases such as sarcoidosis, rheumatoid disease, ankylosing spondylitis, Reiter's syndrome, and inflammatory bowel disease. Infection with **cytomegalovirus**

or *Toxoplasma*, often as a complication of immunosuppression, can cause severe choroiditis leading to blindness. The larva of *Toxocara canis* can reach the eye to cause severe inflammation in the choroid, spreading to the retina (**chorioretinitis**) and vitreous, at which stage blindness results.

Melanocytic tumors commonly arise in the uvea and may be benign or malignant

The melanocytes of the uvea are the cells of origin for benign melanocytic nevi as well as ocular malignant melanomas.

Most **benign melanocytic nevi** arise in the iris and are seen as abnormal areas of pigmentation. They often change in appearance with time, bringing them to medical attention. Most lesions are proliferations of spindle-shaped melanocytes.

Ocular malignant melanomas can arise anywhere in the uvea (5% arise in the iris, 10% in the ciliary body, and 85% in the choroid). Depending on the site of origin, tumors cause different types of symptom leading to impaired vision. Macroscopically, tumors are darkly pigmented lesions, typically 1–2 cm in diameter, which cause detachment of overlying retina (*Fig. 22.4*). There are two main histological patterns of ocular melanoma:

- **Spindle-cell melanomas** tend to have little pleomorphism and few mitoses, and are usually localized to the globe. If they are excised completely, 10-year survival is around 90%.

- **Epithelioid melanomas** show large cells with pleomorphism and many mitoses. This type is associated with a 10-year survival of 35%, orbital invasion frequently being encountered at time of diagnosis.

Spread of ocular melanomas occurs directly into the orbit, or hematogenously to cause systemic metastasis. Late manifestation of metastatic disease from excised orbital melanomas is a well-recognized phenomenon.

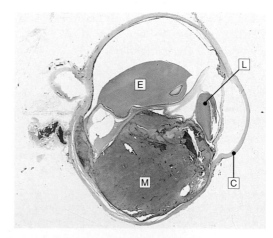

Fig. 22.4 Uveal malignant melanoma.
Histological section of globe (lens (**L**), cornea (**C**)) showing mass of melanoma (**M**). The retina has become detached with a sub-retinal exudate (**E**).

LENS ABNORMALITIES

Dislocation of the lens may be spontaneous or traumatic in origin

The lens is normally suspended by fibers of the ciliary zonule, which are composed of the protein fibrillin, and attached to the ciliary body. When dislocation of the lens occurs, which may be spontaneous or traumatic, the lens becomes detached from its normal position. In anterior dislocation the lens falls forward, obstructs the pupil, and causes acute glaucoma (see page 481). In posterior dislocation the lens falls back towards the vitreous, with loss of visual acuity.

Spontaneous dislocation is predisposed to by Marfan's syndrome, caused by mutation in one of the genes for fibrillin. Traumatic dislocation is seen with both penetrating and non-penetrating injuries (see page 482).

Cataracts, which are areas of opacification in the lens, have a wide range of causes

The normal lens is composed of a capsule, lens epithelial cells, and a central mass of tightly packed cells that have lost their nuclei and contain highly stable transparent proteins termed 'crystallins'. In cataract formation, there is degeneration of lens crystallins, which become opaque. Structural changes in the lens occur with hyaline globules, liquefaction, and focal calcification. Degenerate lens material may gain access to the aqueous, where it is phagocytosed by macrophages and may cause blockage of the trabecular meshwork, leading to secondary open-angle glaucoma (see page 482).

The main cause of cataracts is thought to be metabolic derangement in lens nutrition, which is derived from diffusion from the aqueous. There are several predisposing factors for development. The most common cataracts are those that develop in aging (**senile cataracts**). Predisposing conditions for cataract formation include trauma, diabetes mellitus, corticosteroid therapy, inflammation in the globe (e.g. uveitis), glaucoma, and irradiation of the eye. Congenital cataracts may develop after rubella infection *in utero*.

DISEASES OF THE RETINA AND VITREOUS

Retinal diseases are mainly inflammatory, vascular or degenerative in etiology

The retina is the specialized neural layer of the eye. It contains the photoreceptors (rods and cones), which detect light, and the interneurons, which integrate input into the retinal ganglion cells (which give rise to the axons in the optic nerve). The ends of the retinal photoreceptors are embedded in the pigment epithelium of the uvea, which provides essential metabolic support. At its surface, the retina is separated from the vitreous by a basement membrane, underlining the fact that the vitreous is not merely a ball of fluid, but a complex transparent support tissue that contains cells as well as specialized matrix proteins.

The retina can be secondarily damaged by several disease processes such as disorders of vasculature (discussed below) and inflammatory diseases of the choroid, or there may be secondary damage from the high pressure in the globe caused by glaucoma (see page 481). Primary retinal diseases are degenerative or, uncommonly, infective.

Age-related macular degeneration (ARMD) is one of the most common causes of severe loss of vision in the elderly. The pathogenesis of this condition is not completely understood but appears to involve disturbance in the normal mechanisms for photoreceptor turnover and renewal. Histologically, the affected area shows atrophy of the photoreceptor cell layer with loss of cells from the outer nuclear layer with gliotic scarring. Lipohyaline material may accumulate beneath the pigment epithelium ('drusen'). ARMD may progress to a condition termed **disciform degeneration of the macula** in which there is fibrous and vascular proliferation immediately beneath the pigment epithelium, predisposing to sub-retinal bleeding and blindness.

Pigmentary retinopathy is a term applied to a group of diseases in which there is retinal degeneration associated with melanin pigment migrating from the choroid to be sequestered in macrophages located around retinal vessels. The main type encountered is the hereditary disease **retinitis pigmentosa**. Other causes are secondary to primary neurometabolic storage diseases (see page 458).

Infection by *Toxoplasma*, **cytomegalovirus** and **herpes** is seen in immunosuppressed patients, particularly those with AIDS, and is growing in importance as a cause of blindness.

Loss of retinal ganglion cells due to retinal disease causes optic nerve atrophy, seen as a small pale optic disc on fundoscopy. This indicates severe irreversible retinal damage, as retinal neurons cannot be replaced once lost.

Vascular diseases of the retina are a common cause of blindness

Vascular disorders are a major cause of eye disease, having their main impact on the retina. The main predisposing factors for vascular disease are hypertension and diabetes mellitus. Retinal complications of diabetes mellitus are now one of the most common causes of blindness in western countries.

Among the main vascular diseases is **benign hypertension**, which is associated with development of hyaline thickening in retinal vessels. In accelerated-phase hypertension, flame hemorrhages, exudates, and areas of retinal ischemia develop, causing microinfarcts termed **cotton-wool spots**.

Diabetic retinal disease causes thickening of the basement membrane of capillaries and hyaline arteriolosclerosis.

Microaneurysms occur as dilatations of arterioles and capillaries with abnormally fragile and permeable walls. Exudates develop, with 'blot hemorrhages' from leaking capillary vessels. Areas of ischemia cause **cotton-wool spots**. Retinal ischemia causes secretion of angiogenesis factors, inducing formation of new vessels (**proliferative retinopathy**).

Neovascularization is the term used to describe the formation of new vessels on the inner surface of the retina (leading to hemorrhages) and on the anterior surface of the iris (leading to secondary closed-angle glaucoma).

Retinal artery occlusion occurs with blockage of the central retinal artery as a result of embolism or, less commonly, from vasculitis such as giant-cell arteritis (see page 171). The retina undergoes necrosis and there is loss of retinal ganglion cells, leading to optic atrophy and proliferation of retinal glial cells (**retinal gliosis**).

Retinal vein occlusion is predisposed by polycythemia and chronic glaucoma. Thrombosis leads to suffusion of the retina with blood, resulting in widespread hemorrhage.

Pathology of common fundoscopic abnormalities

Papilledema is swelling of the optic disc, a clinical sign seen on fundoscopy. However, this is not simply edema as seen in other tissues. The swelling is due to pressure on the optic nerve as it enters the CSF-filled optic nerve sheath, usually the result of a focal lesion causing raised intracranial pressure. The increased pressure on the optic nerve leads to impairment of the normal flow of cytoplasm along the axon, causing the axons to become dilated and swollen. More severe pressure on the optic nerve impairs venous return and leads to development of secondary hemorrhages in the retina.

Hard exudates are lipid-rich accumulations of plasma proteins, which leak out of vessels and accumulate in the outer plexiform layer.

Cotton-wool spots are areas of microinfarction in the retina. The spots are the ballooned ends of damaged retinal axons.

Flame hemorrhages are caused by disease affecting arterioles. The flame shape is caused by blood tracking in the superficial nerve-fiber layer.

Blot hemorrhages are caused by capillary rupture deep in the outer plexiform layer of the retina.

Silver wiring of vessels is caused by arteriolosclerosis of retinal vessels, which demonstrate replacement of their walls by hyaline material (see page 167).

If lysis of the thrombus occurs, normal function is regained. However, persistent occlusion causes development of neovascularization and glaucoma.

In retinal detachment the retina is separated from the pigment epithelium, thereby losing metabolic support

Retinal detachment occurs when the neural retinal layer becomes separated from the retinal pigment epithelium. Provided that the photoreceptor layer is brought back into contact, the retina may regain function; however, prolonged detachment leads to loss of metabolic support from the retinal pigment epithelium, with degeneration of photoreceptor cells and permanent loss of function.

There are three main reasons for retinal detachment:

- **Traction on the retina** from abnormalities in the vitreous. This occurs with organization of previous trauma or with development of neovascularization. In diabetic proliferative retinopathy this is termed **vasoproliferative retinopathy** (VPR). Following trauma to the retina, retinal glial cells and cells from the pigment epithelium may grow up to the vitreous, termed **proliferative vitreoretinopathy** (PVR).

- **Shearing of the retina** may cause formation of small retinal tears and development of detachment. These tears are predisposed by degenerative conditions of the retina or vitreous and develop when the vitreous focally loses contact with the retina at the vitreoretinal junction. Instead of transmitting rotational forces uniformly, loss of contact with vitreous causes forces to be focally concentrated, leading to tearing of the retina. This loss of contact is predisposed in patients with severe myopia.

- **Pressure on the retina** from accumulation of fluid in the sub-retinal space, commonly from inflammatory exudate, hemorrhage, or neoplasm.

Retinoblastoma is an uncommon tumor of childhood

Retinoblastoma is a very rare malignant tumor of the retina, occurring in children under the age of 5 years. Its importance lies in the fact that it is inherited in about a third of cases, and molecular genetics have shown it to be predisposed by loss of a specific tumor-suppressor gene termed RB. Patients with the heritable form have a high incidence of bilateral disease, whereas patients with sporadic disease tend to have unilateral tumor.

Composed of primitive neuroblast-like cells, lesions macroscopically appear as a mass of white tissue that arises in the retina and replaces the vitreous. Tumors behave aggressively, with spread to the orbit and along the optic nerve to the CNS. Children present with enlargement of the globe, or with a white pupil due to tumor in the vitreous.

GLAUCOMA

In glaucoma there is an abnormally raised intraocular pressure which can potentially cause damage to the retina and optic nerve

A very common syndrome in which there is increased intraocular pressure, glaucoma affects 2% of the population over the age of 40 years. It is important in that if it remains untreated, blindness develops.

The maintenance of normal intraocular pressure is achieved through the continuous secretion of aqueous by the ciliary body being balanced by its removal from the anterior chamber by filtration from the trabecular mesh-work at the periphery of the iris into the canal of Schlemm. In glaucoma the balance is disturbed, nearly always by an abnormality in the filtration and removal of aqueous.

There are two main clinical syndromes. **Chronic glaucoma** occurs with gradual increase in intraocular pressure, leading to slow, gradual deterioration in visual acuity if untreated. **Acute glaucoma** is associated with rapid increase in intraocular pressure, which causes severe pain and redness in the eye (see *Fig. 22.6b*), and rapid deterioration in visual function (this can be permanent if not urgently treated).

The effects of raised intraocular pressure are **cupping and atrophy of the optic disc**, detected on fundoscopy, and **degeneration of retinal ganglion cells**. Clinically, there is progressive peripheral visual-field loss, leading to blindness in untreated cases. In acute glaucoma there is

breakdown of the endothelium, leading to edema of the cornea and formation of painful corneal bullas. In chronic glaucoma the sclera may stretch to form bulges termed **staphylomas**.

In glaucoma there is interference with filtration of aqueous at the trabecular meshwork

There are several common causes of glaucoma, divisible into primary and secondary groups.

Primary glaucoma is caused by two main abnormalities in drainage of aqueous:

- Closing-up of the trabecular meshwork, which normally leads to the canal of Schlemm, can occur as a degenerative process, the incidence of which increases with age; it is mainly encountered in those over the age of 40 years, often being familial. Because the drainage angle is normal, this is termed **primary open-angle glaucoma** (*Fig. 22.5a*).

- With age, some patients develop narrowing of the angle between the iris and the cornea, causing functional blockage to aqueous drainage. This may be predisposed by the normal reduction of the size of the eye with aging, and the normal increase in the size of the lens with age. An acute attack occurs particularly when the pupil is dilated, as the iris thickens with contraction. Acute attacks may therefore be precipitated by being in the dark. Because the drainage angle is abnormal, this is termed **primary closed-angle glaucoma** (*Fig. 22.5b*).

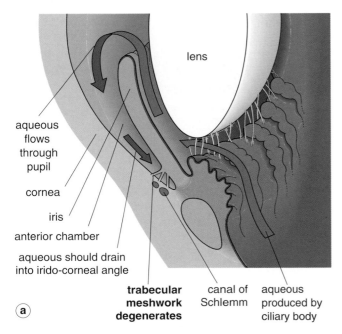

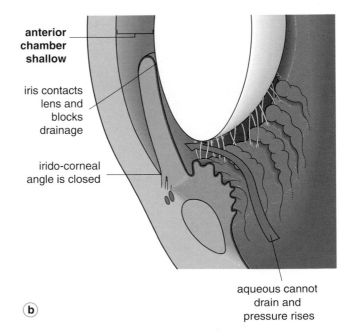

Fig. 22.5 Glaucoma. (a) **Primary open-angle glaucoma**. With age, the channels in the trabecular meshwork degenerate. However, aqueous continues to be produced, so the pressure in the eye increases. As the angle between the cornea and iris root is normal (open), this is termed open-angle glaucoma. (b) **Primary closed-angle glaucoma**. If the anterior chamber becomes shallow, then the drainage angle is functionally closed. If the pupil dilates, this further compromises the drainage of aqueous and may precipitate an acute attack of glaucoma.

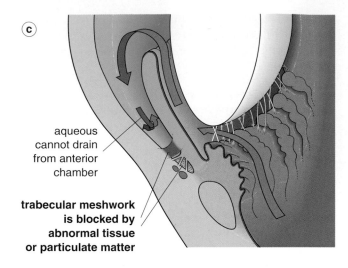

Fig. 22.5 (c) Secondary glaucoma.
If abnormal tissue (e.g. new blood vessels) blocks the trabecular meshwork, then aqueous cannot drain and glaucoma may develop; this is termed secondary closed-angle glaucoma. If particulate matter (such as inflammatory cells) occludes the trabecular meshwork, it is termed secondary open-angle glaucoma, since the irido-corneal angle remains open.

Secondary glaucoma is caused by diseases that obstruct the drainage of aqueous. For example, there may be adhesions between the iris and cornea that are caused by uveitis or are secondary to vascular proliferation due to retinal ischemia (**secondary closed-angle glaucoma**). Alternatively, there may be blockage of the trabecular meshwork by particulate material in the aqueous, especially degenerate lens material, pigment from melanocytic lesions, or macrophages accumulating in response to hemorrhage or inflammation (**secondary open-angle glaucoma**) (*Fig. 22.5c*).

Congenital glaucoma seen in childhood with enlargement of the globe, is very rare. It is mainly due to developmental defects in the drainage of aqueous.

TRAUMA TO THE EYE

Trauma to the eye is a common cause of visual impairment

Mostly preventable by the use of suitable eye protection, trauma is a common cause of eye disease. Damage may be immediately apparent or may develop after the injury as a secondary complication.

- **Contusion of the globe** can cause intraocular hemorrhage or tearing of the retina and uvea.
- **Dislocation of the lens** may occur with severe trauma (see page 141).
- **Penetrating injuries** (those that pass into the cornea) cause permanent scarring if there is damage to Bowman's membrane, whereas **perforating injuries** (those that pass through cornea) can be complicated

by hemorrhage or infection. Healing of a corneal perforation may be complicated by adhesion of the iris to the back of the cornea at the site of injury.

- **Secondary glaucoma** is an important complication of bleeding into the anterior chamber.
- **Siderosis bulbi** is caused by retention of an iron-containing foreign body in the globe. Iron pigment is deposited within the tissues of the eye, causing retinal degeneration.
- **Sympathetic ophthalmitis** is an uncommon T-cell-mediated immune response, causing granulomatous inflammation in a normal eye that has been stimulated by damage to the other eye. The trigger for this immune reaction is exposure of retinal antigens (normally sequestered by a blood–retinal barrier) to the immune system after trauma to the globe. Histologically, there is severe granulomatous inflammation of the eye. The development of this condition can be prevented if the damaged eye is removed.

DISEASES OF THE ORBIT

Diseases of the orbit present with displacement of the eye (**proptosis**) or orbital pain. The main causes for swelling in the orbit are thyroid eye disease, vascular lesions, inflammatory diseases, and tumors. Clinical evaluation includes imaging of the orbit to establish the site and nature of the swelling, followed by biopsy in many cases. Thyroid disease (Graves' disease) may cause orbital swelling and proptosis due to accumulation of extracellular matrix material in the orbital tissues (see page 334).

Orbital inflammatory diseases are of diverse etiology and are usually biopsied only to exclude presence of tumor

Orbital inflammatory diseases present as swelling of the orbit, proptosis, and orbital pain. There are many causes for inflammation in the orbit, and biopsy is sometimes performed to establish a cause and to distinguish lesions from infiltration by tumor. These conditions were once called orbital pseudotumors, a name that should be avoided as a mass (tumor) is not always evident on investigation. Arteritis, connective tissue diseases, fungal infection, and specific inflammatory conditions related to the sclera (e.g. **sclerotenonitis**) can all present in this manner.

Vascular lesions and tumors are the most common cause of orbital swellings in adults

Vascular lesions and tumors are a common cause of orbital mass lesions. Rapid increase in size may be caused by thrombosis within a lesion.

Cavernous hemangiomas are well-circumscribed lesions, 1–2 cm in diameter. The most common orbital tumors seen in adults, they are usually easy to remove surgically.

Capillary hemangiomas are poorly circumscribed lesions, most commonly seen in childhood. Their extensive involvement of orbital tissues makes surgical treatment very difficult.

Lymphangiomas may involve the orbit and, based on the extent of orbital involvement, can be divided into superficial, deep, and combined types.

Hemangiopericytomas are tumors derived from the vascular-related pericytes. They vary in malignant potential, 30% being locally recurrent, even if histologically benign.

In addition to these lesions, less well-defined AVMs and varicose veins are also encountered within the orbit.

Lymphoma is the most common type of primary malignant orbital tumor

The most common primary tumor of the orbit is non-Hodgkin's lymphoma. The majority are low-grade B-cell tumors; less common are high-grade centroblastic/immuno-blastic tumors. Burkitt's lymphoma, a high-grade lympho-blastic B-cell tumor, is the most common orbital tumor in some parts of Africa.

Macroscopically, tumors form masses within the orbit, often involving the extraocular muscles. Many arise from the lacrimal gland. Tumors that are of the low-grade type have a low risk (< 25%) of systemic disease and an excellent prognosis, whereas those that are intermediate- or high-grade have a high risk (> 60%) of developing systemic disease.

Benign reactive lymphoid infiltrates of the orbit are also seen and must be distinguished from lymphomas by immunohistochemistry.

Orbital tumors of mesodermal and neural origin may be benign or malignant

Orbital tumors may arise from neural or mesodermal tissues. Different tumors, both benign and malignant, are encountered in different age groups.

Ocular tumor extension into the orbit is a frequent development, the main ocular tumors being retinoblastoma in childhood (see page 480), and uveal melanoma in adults (see page 478).

Rhabdomyosarcoma of the orbit is a tumor of child-hood, being of the embryonal sub-type. Although highly malignant, treatment with radiotherapy and chemotherapy shows a 3-year survival rate of 93%.

Fibrous histiocytoma is the most common mesenchy-mal tumor of the orbit in adults. It is a spindle-cell tumor composed of fibroblast-like cells and histiocyte-like cells with a collagenous matrix, classified into benign, locally aggressive, and malignant types. As they are poorly circum-scribed, these tumors often recur, with a recurrence rate of 30% for benign lesions, 57% for locally aggressive lesions, and 64% for malignant lesions.

Fibro-osseous lesions from the skull often encroach on the orbit, particularly fibromatoses, primary bone tumors,

fibrous dysplasia of bone, and Langerhan's cell histiocytosis (histiocytosis X) (see page 326).

Benign nerve-sheath tumors account for about 2% of all orbital tumors. They are either well-circumscribed schwannomas (neurilemmomas) or less easily excised plexi-form neurofibromas.

Meningiomas of the orbit arise from the arachnoidal meningothelial cells of the optic nerve sheath and are similar to those that occur in the CNS.

Optic-nerve gliomas are astrocytomas of low-grade malignancy, classed as juvenile pilocytic astrocytomas. Histologically they are spindle-cell tumors with a fine fibrillarity.

Metastatic tumors in the orbit are most commonly from breast, lung, kidney and prostate

Metastatic tumor commonly involves the orbit, tumors of the breast, lung, kidney and prostate being the most commonly reported. The diagnosis of the primary site of a metastatic deposit can be aided by immunocyto-chemistry to determine the presence of marker substances within tumor cells. This is particularly useful with small samples removed from the orbit in cases in which the pathologist is not aided by architectural features of the tumor.

Clinically, diffuse invasion of the orbital tissues produces proptosis, pain from involvement of nerves, and paralysis of eye movements. In severe cases the eye is immobile (a frozen orbit).

Developmental lesions of the orbit are common in childhood

In childhood, developmental lesions account for many orbital swellings. Among the most common types are dermoid cysts lined by squamous epithelium, with skin appendages such as sebaceous glands, hair follicles, and sweat glands in the wall. These account for 46% of all orbital tumors in childhood, and for 24% of all tumors in all age groups.

Brain heterotopias may affect the orbit and are part of the spectrum of neural-tube defects (see page 456). Anterior encephalocele may involve the orbit, with meninges, glial tissue or brain tissue present in the orbit.

Lacrimal gland swellings may be inflammatory or neoplastic

Enlargement of lacrimal gland may be due to specific or non-specific inflammation (including granulomatous diseases), or to primary (benign and malignant) and meta-static neoplasms.

Infection (commonly due to bacteria) of the lacrimal gland or ducts may cause swelling. Blockage of the duct may occur with local overgrowth of *Actinomyces*, forming the basis for a calculus composed of filamentous organisms.

Cysts of the lacrimal gland or associated ducts are common. Some are developmental dermoid cysts, whereas others are retention cysts caused by duct blockage.

Sjögren's disease is associated with autoimmune infiltration and enlargement of the gland by lymphoid cells, with gland loss causing dry eyes.

Sarcoidosis (see page 539) is associated with expansion of the gland by non-caseating granulomas.

Lymphoma of the lacrimal gland is the most common primary tumor (usually low-grade B-cell non-Hodgkin's lymphoma of MALT type).

Common eye disorders in family practice

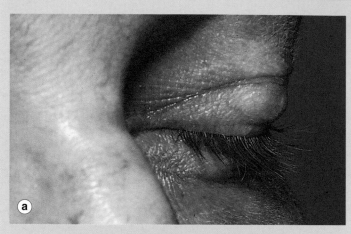

Fig. 22.6 (a) Chalazion.
A chalazion (meibomian cyst) develops from blockage and inflammation of a meibomian gland. At first, lesions are red and tender, but later form firm nodules in the lid. Most resolve with local antibiotic ointment but some require curettage. Lesions that do not resolve should be regarded with suspicion, as uncommon malignant tumors of the lid may present in this manner.

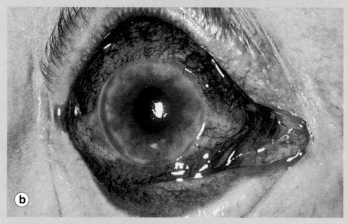

(b) Acute red eye.
A painful red eye can be caused by three main processes: conjunctivitis, uveitis, and acute glaucoma. In this case, the patient has acute closed-angle glaucoma; failure to detect this and treat the condition would lead to permanent damage to the eye and blindness.

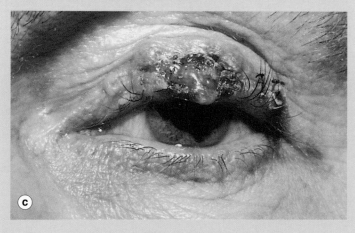

(c) Skin-appendage tumor.
The eyelids may be involved in diseases that affect the skin elsewhere. Dermatological conditions such as allergic dermatitis (usually to eye make-up or shampoo), discoid lupus erythematosus, and sarcoid may affect the lid. Tumors such as syringomas, and sebaceous gland tumors also affect the lid. In this case, this ulcerated lesion on the lid margin was a basal-cell carcinoma.

Dermatopathology

Clinical Overview

Patients are very aware of their skin, and are sensitive to any minor abnormalities in appearance, texture and sensation, changes which, if they occurred in the gastric or colonic mucosa would probably be asymptomatic and therefore ignored. Hence a vast number of medical consultation events at all levels are concerned with abnormalities of skin. The body surface is exposed to the full range of potential external damaging factors such as physical trauma, heat, cold, UV irradiation, toxic chemicals, etc, and it is therefore not surprising that there is a much wider range of skin diseases than in any other tissue or organ system.

The most commonly encountered skin diseases are inflammatory (**dermatitis**) due either to allergic reactions, infections, contact toxins, or an unknown cause. With the expanding repertoire of therapeutic pharmaceutical agents, drug reactions in skin are becoming increasingly common.

Benign hyperplastic lesions of epidermis (e.g. **seborrheic keratoses**, **skin tags**) and benign **epidermal cysts** are extremely common, increasing in incidence from middle age, but rarely require treatment unless they are unsightly (much medical and surgical intervention in skin disease is for cosmetic purposes rather than to manage morbidity or potential fatality). In children and young people the most common non-inflammatory lesions of the skin are pigmented moles (**nevi**) due to proliferation of benign melanocytes in epidermis and dermis. These may require excision because they are unsightly, but a few may eventually transform into malignant tumors of melanocytes (**malignant melanoma**). Like the other two common malignant tumors of skin, **basal-cell carcinoma** and **squamous-cell carcinoma**, this malignant tumor of melanocytes is predisposed to by prolonged exposure to UV rays in sunlight.

The full panoply of skin disease is enormous, but many are rare. The diseases discussed and illustrated in this chapter are those which a student is most likely to encounter in a short attachment to a dermatology specialist or a family practice during training.

INTRODUCTION

Most epithelial surfaces, e.g. those lining the respiratory, alimentary and urinary tracts, show a very limited range of disease processes, rarely more than half a dozen common inflammatory disorders, and a similar number of neoplastic or growth disorders. In contrast, the skin exhibits many hundreds of different inflammatory patterns and probably 30 or 40 tumors or tumor-like lesions, the great majority of

which are common. The breadth of dermatopathology is therefore immense; fortunately, much of the detail lies within the province of the specialist clinical dermatologist and dermatopathologist, and is not essential for medical students and non-specialist doctors.

The study of dermatopathology is further complicated by the fact that the pathogenesis of many of the skin conditions is unknown. In addition, the nomenclature of the various skin lesions, particularly that for inflammatory skin diseases, is an arcane mixture of Latin and Greek that disguises the fact that the nomenclature is purely descriptive of the visual appearance of the rash. Thus, euphonious but uninformative names like 'pityriasis lichenoides et varioliformis acuta' exist.

DERMATITIS

'Dermatitis' is the name given to inflammatory lesions in the skin, irrespective of whether they involve dermis or epidermis; in most cases both components of the skin are involved.

Some patterns of inflammatory skin disease have characteristic features, e.g. lichenoid dermatitis, psoriasiform dermatitis (see below), which enable them to be identified more accurately, both clinically and histologically. Other patterns are caused by microorganisms such as bacteria (e.g. impetigo, folliculitis), fungi (e.g. athlete's foot, ringworm), viruses (e.g. herpes, varicella) or other organisms (e.g. scabies), but many are **non-specific**. The most common pattern of non-specific dermatitis is traditionally called **eczema**, and may have many causes.

Non-specific (eczematous) dermatitis may be acute, subacute or chronic

In acute dermatitis the skin becomes red (erythema), itchy and tender, with tiny blisters called **vesicles** forming in the epidermis (*Fig. 23.1*). The vesicles burst, discharging clear, yellow fluid, and then crust over. The reddening of the skin is due to a chronic inflammatory cell infiltrate around blood vessels in the upper dermis; leakage of fluid from the vessels may produce swelling of the upper dermis, which may cause the lesion to be slightly raised above the level of normal skin.

Vesicles develop because fluid accumulates between the epidermal cells (**spongiosis**), eventually forming small fluid-filled collections. Some of the chronic inflammatory cells around the vessels in the upper dermis may migrate into the epidermis. The vesicles enlarge until they burst onto the surface.

Because the lesion is itchy in the acute stage, it is almost invariably scratched by the patient. As a result, secondary changes occur due to repeated trauma rather than the background skin disease. Repeated trauma to lesions of acute eczema leads to **chronic dermatitis**.

Chronic non-specific dermatitis is usually the result of chronic trauma to acute dermatitis lesions. The skin is thickened, often cracked, and covered by thick, opaque scale (*Fig. 23.2*). This scale is a greatly thickened layer of surface keratin (hyperkeratosis), which overlies an epidermis markedly thickened by increase in the number of cells in the various layers (particularly stratum spinosum and the granular layer). Such thickening, termed **acanthosis**, is a common feature of chronic inflammatory skin diseases of many types.

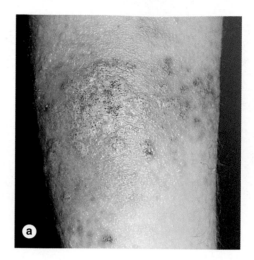

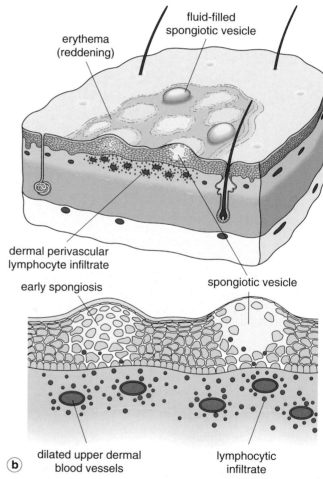

Fig. 23.1 Acute dermatitis.
(a) Typical acute dermatitis with reddening (erythema) of the skin and numerous tiny vesicles, some of which have burst due to scratching because of severe itch. (b) The histological basis of erythema and of vesicle formation.

The epidermis also shows elongation and accentuation of the rete ridge system, an arrangement that, in normal skin, is designed to resist shearing forces. The dermis shows increased fibrosis, with prominent thick-walled vessels.

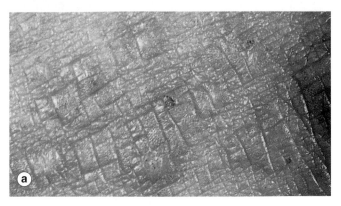

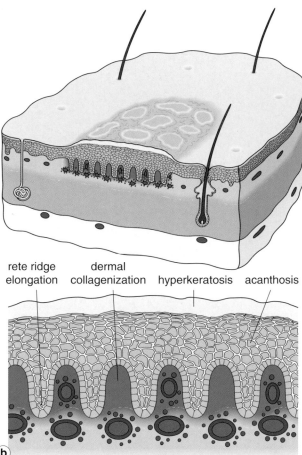

rete ridge
elongation   dermal
collagenization   hyperkeratosis   acanthosis

Fig. 23.2 Chronic dermatitis.
(a) Close-up of chronic dermatitis with raised areas of skin thickening due to chronic scratching of a healing acute dermatitis. (b) The histological basis of chronic dermatitis.

Constant scratching and picking at itchy inflammatory lesions in the skin leads to localized lesions with greatly thickened epidermis and thick horny keratin scale on top, together with localized fibrous thickening of the dermis. Called **prurigo nodularis**, the lesions often continue to be picked and traumatized so that there is surface ulceration, a lesion sometimes called 'picker's nodule'.

The term **subacute dermatitis** is sometimes used to describe skin inflammation in which there are features of

chronic dermatitis (acanthosis, hyperkeratosis, dermal fibrosis, etc.), but with the addition of active spongiosis and vesicle formation.

The cause of non-specific dermatitis usually has to be inferred from the distribution and nature of the rash rather than from histological differences

Among the most common types of non-specific dermatitis seen in community practice is **atopic dermatitis**. Often starting in infancy and childhood but persisting into adult life, this pattern is associated with a strong family history, e.g. the patient and other family members may have asthma, hayfever or a predisposition to urticarial skin rashes. The atopic state, and its mechanisms, are discussed in Chapter 7.

Gravitational dermatitis (*Fig. 23.3a*) affects the ankle and lower leg of patients with varicose veins, and is sometimes called **varicose eczema**. The dermatitis features are superimposed on chronic changes in the skin due to inadequate venous drainage, e.g. thick-walled dermal vessels or extravasation of red blood cells (leading to brown pigmentation by hemosiderin).

Irritant contact dermatitis (*Fig. 23.3b*), which is due to contact of the skin with strong agents such as detergents and alkalis, most commonly affects the hands. The disease is particularly common in housewives who do not wear gloves when handling strong detergents, and in some people who have occupational exposure.

Allergic contact dermatitis is usually a reaction to metals such as nickel, materials in cosmetics, dye mixtures and rubber. It tends to occur in people who have a probable inherited predisposition, and the lesions are localized to the site of contact, e.g. around the wrist in response to nickel in the back or strap of a watch.

In **seborrheic dermatitis** (*Fig. 23.3c*) the reddened and inflamed skin is covered by thick waxy or white scale. In infants this is largely confined to the scalp (**cradle cap**), whereas in adults the face is also involved. Obese elderly people may develop this pattern in skin creases. This condition has recently been linked with *Pityrosporum* yeasts.

Some types of specific dermatitis have characteristic histological and clinical appearances

Lichen planus is a common inflammatory skin disease that often affects the flexor aspects of the forearm, wrist and ankle. It also occurs on the trunk, as well as affecting various mucosal surfaces, particularly in the mouth and vulva; it occasionally arises on the penis. On the skin the lesions are raised, itchy papules, often purplish red in colour, which sometimes form flat and shiny raised plaques (*Fig. 23.4*). The cause is unknown and the lesions often persist for many months or even years. When each lesion resolves, it frequently leaves a pigmented patch of flat skin.

The main histological abnormality in lichen planus is damage to the basal layer of the epidermis, destroying both basal cells and any contained melanocytes. It is this destruction of basal melanocytes that allows melanin to drop down into the dermis, where it accumulates in dermal macrophages, giving a healed lesion a brown discoloration. Associated with the destruction of the basal layer is a characteristic pattern of lymphocytic infiltration, which is closely applied to the dermoepidermal junction in the upper dermis. This pattern of inflammation is called **lichenoid** and can occasionally be seen in other skin conditions.

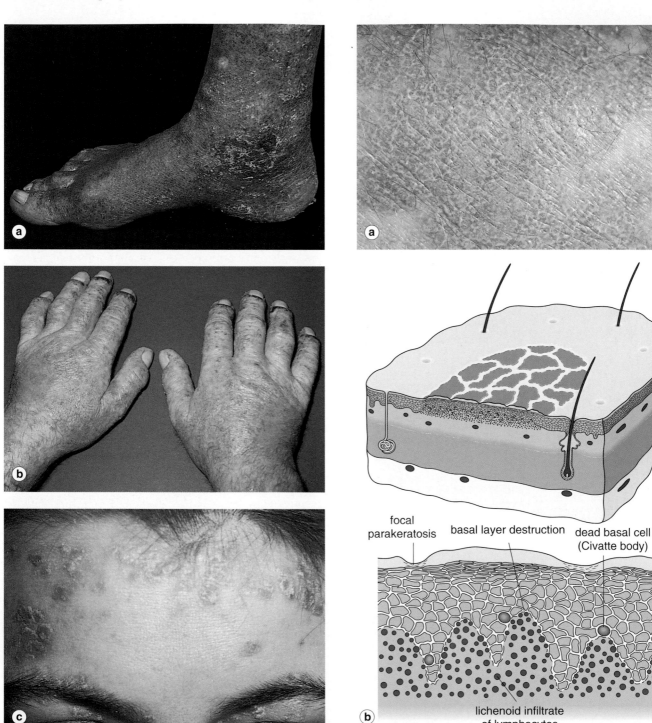

Fig. 23.3 Common clinical patterns of dermatitis.
(a) Gravitational dermatitis. (b) Irritant contact dermatitis due to immersion of hands in strong detergent. (c) Seborrhic dermatitis in a young girl.

Fig. 23.4 Lichen planus.
(a) Clinical appearance of raised, red plaques with thick, opaque, white lines (Wickham's striae). (b) The histopathological basis of lichen planus.

Lichen planus affecting the buccal and genital mucosae has a tendency to lead to separation of the epidermis from the underlying submucosa, as a result of destruction of the basal layer of the epidermis. The ensuing erosion leaves naked areas of inflamed submucosa; this change rarely occurs in skin. Another variant of lichen planus, **follicular lichen planus**, causes destruction of the basal layer of hair follicles, which may result in hair loss; follicular lichen planus is one of the causes of inflammatory **alopecia** (see page 509).

Destruction of the basal layer of the epidermis, sometimes associated with a lichenoid pattern of upper dermal inflammatory cell infiltrate, can be seen in certain other conditions without the clinical features of lichen planus; they are sometimes known as **lichenoid dermatitis**. Some drug reactions may be responsible, and in some cases the inflammation is clinically and histologically indistinguishable from spontaneous lichen planus.

Psoriasis (*Fig. 23.5*) is a chronic intermittent disease in which red, raised plaques covered by thick, white scale appear on knees, elbows, trunk and scalp. They may also occur in skin creases, where the silvery-white surface scale is often less obvious and may even be absent. A characteristic feature is that when the scale is lifted off, it reveals small areas of punctate bleeding.

Histologically, the scale is composed of flakes of thickened surface keratin, which contain remnants of the nuclei from the superficial squames from which they are derived (**parakeratosis**). The epidermis shows a characteristic pattern of abnormality, with long rete ridges separated by markedly edematous papillary dermis in which there are large numbers of dilated capillaries. It is these capillaries which bleed when the scale is lifted, for the epidermis overlying the swollen papillary dermis is often very thin. Another characteristic feature of psoriasis is that the major inflammatory cell involved is the neutrophil polymorph; these cells migrate through the epidermis and may be trapped beneath the thickened horny layer (Monro microabscesses). In some types of psoriasis, very large numbers of neutrophil polymorphs migrate through the epidermis, accumulating beneath the parakeratotic scale to form neutrophil collections visible to the naked eye as yellowish purulent blobs (**pustules**). Known as **pustular psoriasis**, this pattern commonly affects the palms of the hands and the soles of the feet. Psoriasis may also affect the nail bed leading to pitting, thickening and eventual destruction of the nail.

Inflammatory skin disease with some of the clinical and histological features of psoriasis can also be seen in some other conditions (psoriasiform dermatitis), e.g. the skin lesions in Reiter's syndrome.

Pityriasis rosea is a common skin condition in young people, a typical pityriasis lesion being a red patch with a rim of scale. The first lesion is usually a large patch, up to 2 cm in diameter ('herald patch'), but subsequent lesions are usually smaller; all are characterized by an area of scale that begins in the center of the lesion, spreading peripherally as the lesion enlarges. Pityriasis rosea is the most common of the patterns of dermatitis known as 'pityriasiform', all of which are characterized by the presence of white scale that histologically corresponds to an area of parakeratosis. Other types of pityriasiform eruption such as pityriasis lichenoides chronica and pityriasis rubra pilaris are much less common.

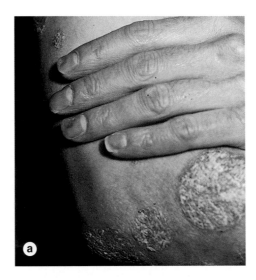
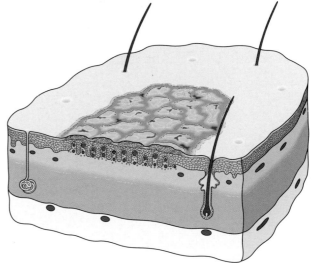
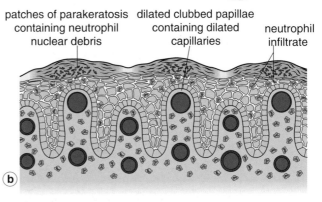

patches of parakeratosis containing neutrophil nuclear debris — dilated clubbed papillae containing dilated capillaries — neutrophil infiltrate

Fig. 23.5 Psoriasis.
(a) Clinical appearance showing typical red patches covered with thick, white scale; note the nail involvement. (b) The histopathological basis of psoriasis.

INFECTIONS OF THE SKIN

Infections of the skin may be due to viruses, fungi or bacteria, viruses being the most common causative organisms.

Viruses can have both direct and indirect effects in skin infections

Three main groups of viruses affect the skin **directly**, producing lesions in which the virus particles are present (often in large numbers), sometimes in the form of intracellular inclusions.

Herpes virus produces blistering lesions of the epidermis, with viral inclusions in the epidermal cells (*Fig. 23.6*). Examples include herpes simplex type 1 (**non-genital herpes**), herpes simplex type 2 (**genital herpes**), and herpes zoster-varicella (**chicken pox** and **shingles**).

Human papillomavirus produces proliferative epidermal lesions (**viral warts**), the nature of which differs from site to site, varying from exophytic filiform fronded lesions (*Fig. 23.7a*) or small flat plaques (e.g. planar warts on the face) to deeply inverted hyperkeratotic lesions (e.g. plantar warts on the sole of the foot) (*Fig. 23.7c*). In the skin of the perineum, human papillomavirus produces florid papillomatous exophytic growths called **condyloma acuminata** (*Fig. 23.7b*); the virus may also infect the genital and anal mucosa in both males and females, and is regarded as an etiological factor in the development of carcinoma at these sites.

Pox virus produces multiple, pale, domed lesions on the trunk and face of children, adolescents and young adults (**molluscum contagiosum**) (*Fig. 23.8*). These are due to localized nodular thickening of the epidermis, the epidermal cells being packed with large viral inclusions.

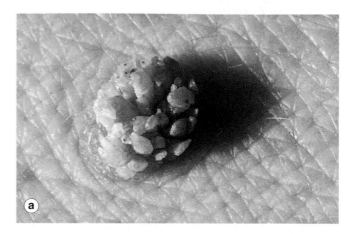

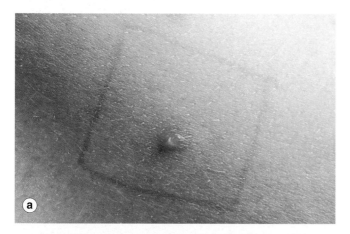

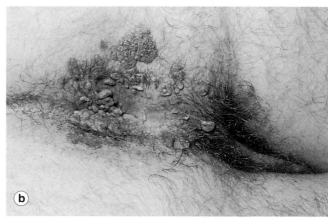

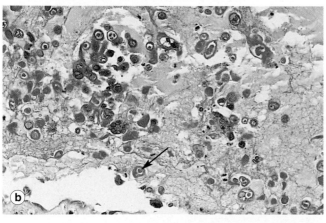

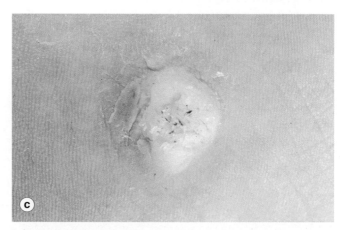

Fig. 23.6 Herpes virus. (a) Typical herpes virus vesicle in chicken pox. (b) Histology of chicken pox, showing destruction of epidermal cells, many of which contain viral inclusions (arrow).

Fig. 23.7 Human papillomavirus. (a) Typical filiform skin wart. (b) Perineal condylomata acuminata. (c) Plantar wart (verruca).

The **indirect effects** of generalized viremia are much more common than the direct effects, and are very variable in pattern, distribution and severity. Many viremias are associated with the development of a transient red (**erythematous**) rash with no specific features, although in the case of parvovirus infection the erythema is most marked and may be confined to the cheeks and buttocks (**slapped cheek syndrome**). Other common viral skin lesions include those of measles and rubellas in which the clinical appearance of the rash, its distribution, and associated systemic symptoms are diagnostic.

Fungi are common commensals on the skin surface and may give rise to skin disease

Superficial fungal infections of the skin are the most common type of pathogenic fungal infection. In the vast majority of cases the fungal hyphae or yeast forms reside in the keratin layer on the skin surface, and are associated with a minimal inflammatory response in the epidermis and upper dermis (*Fig. 23.9*).

These infections are commonly seen in community practice, the nature of the lesion being dependent on the type of causative organism and the particular area of skin involved. Common diseases such as athlete's foot (caused by *Trichophyton* and *Epidermophyton*) and ringworm (caused by *Microsporum* or *Trichophyton rubrum*) are conditions most familiar to the general public (*Fig. 23.10*).

Occasionally the fungi populate the hair follicles, in which case the inflammatory reaction may be more vigorous, resulting in a destructive folliculitis. This is becoming more common, particularly in immunosuppressed patients (e.g. those with AIDS).

Subcutaneous fungal infections usually result from introduction of pathogenic fungi into the subcutaneous tissues following a penetrating injury

Subcutaneous fungal infections are relatively uncommon in the western world. The foot is the most common site, and people who spend much of their day barefoot are particularly prone.

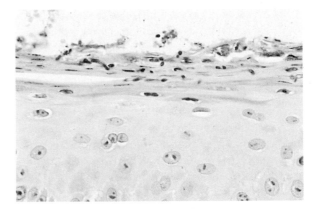

Fig. 23.9 Dermatophytic fungi in horny layer of epidermis. The fungal hyphae, which are stained magenta, are confined to the keratinous horny layer (DPAS stain).

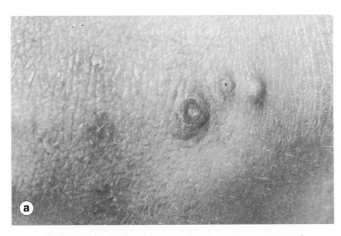

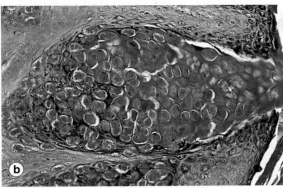

Fig. 23.8 Molluscum contagiosum.
(a) Clinical appearance showing raised nodules with a central keratotic core. (b) Histology showing part of a lesion, the keratotic core being composed of infected epidermal cells containing large red or purple viral inclusions.

Fig. 23.10
Common fungal infections of skin

Disease	Site	Features
Athlete's foot	Toes and feet	Redness, erosion and scaling
Ringworm	Face and trunk	Ring lesion with red scaly edge
Tinea capitis	Scalp	Hair loss and scaling
Tinea cruris	Groin	Red, scaly rash with brown patches
Tinea unguium	Finger/toe nails	Thick, crumbling nails
Pityriasis versicolor	Trunk, mainly upper	Flat patches of increased or decreased pigmentation

Infection usually presents with extensive soft-tissue swelling, and the soft tissues become very hard. In the foot, there may be evidence of underlying bone destruction. In response to the presence of the fungi, deep abscess cavities form, frequently discharging as sinuses onto the surface. In such cases there is usually a very florid acute inflammatory reaction with suppuration, and the material that discharges from the sinuses is pus from the abscess cavities; fungi are often discharged with the pus. The most common type of infection is called 'Madura foot', the causative organism of which is *Madurella*.

Bacterial infections of the skin are usually due to staphylococci or streptococci

Both staphylococci and streptococci can produce a condition called **impetigo**, which is highly contagious and spreads rapidly through populations, e.g. in schools. Large epidermal blisters (**bullae**) develop (*Fig. 23.11*), which may be filled either with clear fluid or with neutrophil polymorphs to form a pus-containing blister (**pustule**). In infants, some staphylococci produce a potent toxin that can lead to extensive disruption of the epidermis, with widespread confluent blistering and separation of the upper layers of the epidermis (**staphylococcal scalded skin syndrome**).

Infection of hair follicles by bacteria, usually *Staphylococcus aureus*, produces tiny pustules located in the necks of the follicles (**superficial folliculitis**) (*Fig. 23.12a*). Deep, severe follicle infection leads to an expanding collection of pus, which destroys the follicle and extends into surrounding dermis to form a **boil**.

Erysipelas is a spreading acute inflammation of the deep dermis and upper subcutis by streptococci, most commonly seen on the face (*Fig. 23.12b*).

Cellulitis is a similar infection but involves the dermis and subcutis. Sometimes the bacteria extend into deep subcutis, fascia and underlying muscle, where they proliferate rapidly and secrete toxins which lead to extensive spreading necrosis of the involved tissues. This is called **necrotizing fasciitis** and is difficult to control even with massive doses of antibiotics. It occurs particularly in the limbs (sometimes following a penetrating injury) and may necessitate amputation to prevent overwhelming septicemia. The most common causative organisms causing both cellulitis and necrotizing fasciitis are streptococci and staphylococci, but anaerobic organisms may also be responsible for necrotizing fasciitis (see *Fig. 23.12c*). A specific form of deep infection of muscle is **gas gangrene**, caused by *Clostridium perfringens* and some other clostridium.

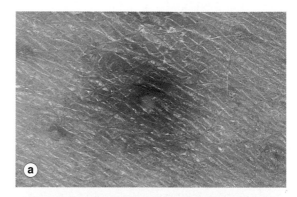
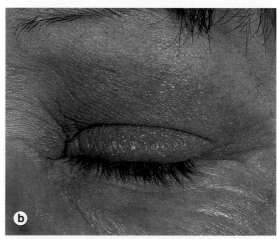
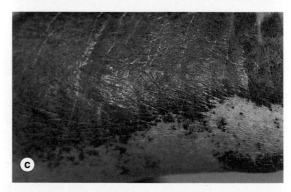

Fig. 23.12 Other common bacterial infections of skin.
(a) Folliculitis. Bacterial infection of a hair follicle. (b) Erysipelas.
(c) Severe spreading cellulitis.

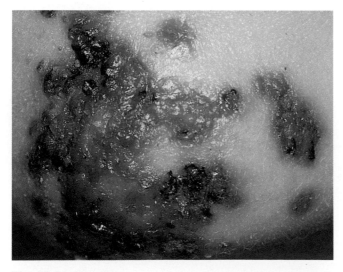

Fig. 23.11 Impetigo.
Clinical appearance showing typical yellow, crusting blisters.

Tuberculous infection of the skin is now rare, but other mycobacteria can cause skin disease

Infection of the skin by *M. tuberculosis* produces the slowly progressive chronic skin lesion called **lupus vulgaris**, in which there is giant-cell granulomatous inflammation in the dermis, leading to destruction of dermal collagen and skin appendages. The lesions are now mainly seen in elderly people, who often claim that they have been present for many years. In such lesions, there may be extensive fibrous scarring, skin appendage destruction, and epidermal atrophy, although the epidermis may occasionally be irregularly thickened and raised, mimicking squamous carcinoma (pseudocarcinomatous hyperplasia).

Other mycobacteria may gain access to the dermis through small cuts, setting up chronic inflammatory granulomatous inflammation, often with ulceration. Examples include mycobacteria contracted through bathing (*M. balnei*) or through contact with infected tropical fish and their aquaria (see also page 121).

Worldwide, the most important and common mycobacterial infection of skin is **leprosy**. The dermis of patients may be extensively infiltrated by swollen macrophages, the cytoplasm of which is packed with the causative *Mycobacterium leprae* (**lepromatous leprosy**), producing numerous raised nodules (papules) and plaques. In another form of cutaneous leprosy known as **tuberculoid leprosy**, small granulomas can be found in all layers of the dermis, but are particularly common around nerves, and may produce nerve damage. The causative organism can rarely be found in this form, the clinical lesions of which are very variable; they may be raised, reddish purple patches or flat areas (macules) in which there is loss of sensation and often loss of skin pigment.

The most important protozoal infection of the skin is caused by leishmania

Infection of the skin by leishmania is usually acquired following a sandfly bite. The organism is introduced into the dermis, where it excites an initially macrophagic reaction; the macrophages phagocytose the organisms, producing a small, raised, red nodule. At a later stage, a very heavy lymphocytic and plasma-cell infiltrate produces a much larger skin nodule (known as an 'oriental sore'), which frequently ulcerates. The causative organism is *L. tropica*. Other forms of leishmania infection occur in the tropics and may involve mucous surfaces such as the mouth and nose. There may be skin nodules in systemic leishmaniasis due to *L. donovani* (see also page 133).

The most common parasitic infection of the skin in the UK, Europe and USA is scabies

Caused by the mite *Sarcoptes scabiei*, scabies presents with a very itchy raised lesion, which is often red and scaling. Lesions sometimes show a linear pattern caused by the mites burrowing a track in the epidermis, with inflammatory changes in the dermis beneath. Occasionally the mite can be found at the head of the track. The presence of the mite excites an inflammatory reaction in which eosinophils are numerous in both the epidermis and the underlying dermis. It is the eosinophils that are responsible for the severe itching of the scabies lesion.

BLISTERING DISEASES OF THE SKIN

Many skin diseases mainly affect the epidermis, causing the formation of a blister either in or immediately beneath the epidermis. If the blisters are small (less than 5 mm in diameter), they are known as **vesicles**; if they are larger (greater than 5 mm in diameter), they are termed **bullae**. Blister formation requires the separation of the keratinocytes in the epidermis from each other, or from the underlying basement membrane.

Depending on where the separation occurs, blisters are classified as **intraepidermal** and **subepidermal** (or **basal**). Intraepidermal and basal blisters are divided according to different criteria, intraepidermal blisters being grouped according to the nature of the process producing the blister, and basal blisters being grouped according to the nature of the inflammatory cell infiltrate associated with the blister formation.

Intraepidermal blisters may form through one of three different mechanisms

Intraepidermal blisters may form as a result of excess fluid accumulation (spongiosis), separation of abnormal keratinocyte attachments (acantholysis), or because of degeneration of keratinocytes (reticular degeneration).

Spongiosis (*Fig. 23.13a*) is by far the most common cause of intraepidermal blister formation, but it tends to produce much smaller blisters (**vesicles**) than the other mechanisms; it is the cause of blistering in many forms of acute dermatitis including atopic dermatitis, seborrheic dermatitis and contact dermatitis (see page 486).

Acantholysis (*Fig. 23.13b*) is the cause of blister formation in pemphigus vulgaris, in which large, flaccid bullae form on reddened skin, affecting the middle-aged and elderly. Blisters arise spontaneously in buccal mucosa and skin, but can be induced by rubbing apparently normal skin (Nikolsky's sign). The disease is thought to be immunologically mediated (see pink box on page 494).

Reticular degeneration blisters (*Fig. 23.13c*) are associated with necrosis of epidermal keratinocytes, often following a phase of marked keratinocyte swelling (ballooning degeneration). It is the pattern responsible for viral blisters such as herpes and varicella, and viral inclusions are present in the degenerating and dying keratinocytes. It may also be seen in some forms of blistering drug reaction, e.g. erythema multiforme (see page 497).

Mechanisms in pemphigus vulgaris

Direct immunofluorescence can demonstrate both IgG and C3 in the intercellular spaces between keratinocytes in all levels of the epidermis (particularly in the stratum spinosum). Pemphigus vulgaris patients have a serum antibody (pemphigus antibody), which can be demonstrated by indirect immunofluorescence on normal squamous epithelium. It is postulated that the pemphigus antibody binds to the intercellular region of the epidermis, and the binding stimulates complement activation and proteolytic enzyme release, damaging the cell attachments and leading to separation and acantholysis.

The severity of the skin lesion appears to be directly proportional to the titer of antibody in the serum.

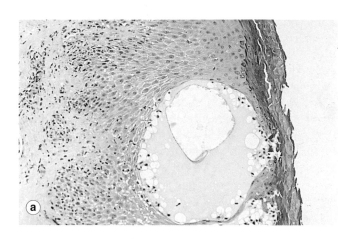

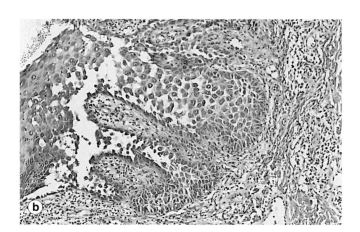

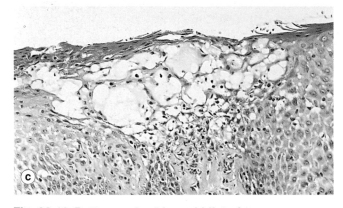

Fig. 23.13 Patterns of epidermal blistering.
(a) Spongiosis, due to fluid accumulation. (b) Acantholysis, due to separation of abnormal epidermal cells. (c) Reticular degeneration, due to rupture of bloated epidermal cells.

Basal blisters arise by separation of the epidermis from the basement membrane, or of epidermis and basement membrane from the underlying dermis

The exact site of separation is often difficult to determine once the blister has formed; electron microscopy of a very early separation is required if identification is to be accurate. In most cases the specific site of separation is not relevant to the diagnosis, but in the important inherited disease **epidermolysis bullosa** the site of separation is vital to classify the type (*Fig. 23.14*). Accurate classification of the type is important in prognosis and genetic counselling. The various types are:

- **Epidermolysis bullosa simplex.** Separation occurs above the basement membrane, through the basal cell cytoplasm. This form has a good prognosis, is inherited as an autosomal dominant condition, and the blisters heal without scarring or deformity.

- **Junctional epidermolysis bullosa.** Separation occurs through the lamina lucida of the basement membrane, separating and damaging the hemidesmosomal attachments of the basal cell to the basement membrane. Also known as the 'lethal' variant, it is present at birth, the child usually dying within the first few weeks of life. The defect also affects other squamous epithelia, e.g. in the esophagus, leading to blistering in sites other than the skin.

- **Dystrophic epidermolysis bullosa.** Separation occurs below the basement membrane, by separation of the anchoring fibrils. Because the separation is below the basement membrane, in the upper dermis, this type leads to dermal scarring and considerable tissue destruction in some of the more severe forms.

Epidermolysis bullosa

495

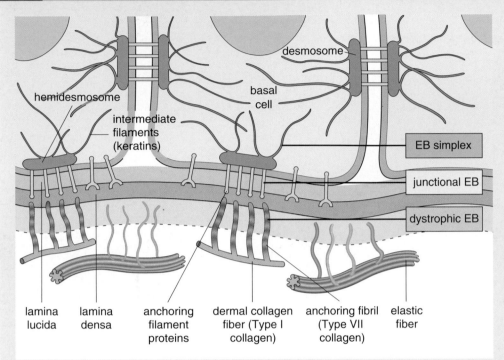

Fig. 23.14 This diagram shows the sites of separation in the various types of epidermolysis bullosa.

Labels in diagram: desmosome, basal cell, hemidesmosome, intermediate filaments (keratins), EB simplex, junctional EB, dystrophic EB, lamina lucida, lamina densa, anchoring filament proteins, dermal collagen fiber (Type I collagen), anchoring fibril (Type VII collagen), elastic fiber

Molecular biology of epidermolysis bullosa

Epidermolysis bullosa simplex shows autosomal dominant inheritance. The separation occurs in the lower part of the basal cell layer, above the basement membrane. The mechanism is believed to be:

```
Mutations in keratin 5, keratin 14 or
intermediate filament-associated proteins
            ↓
Defective keratin intermediate
       filament assembly
            ↓
Defect in cellular cytoskeleton
            ↓
Cellular fragility and disintegration
          of basal cell
            ↓
Blistering above basement membrane
```

Junctional epidermolysis bullosa shows autosomal recessive inheritance. The separation occurs within the membrane. The mechanism is believed to be:

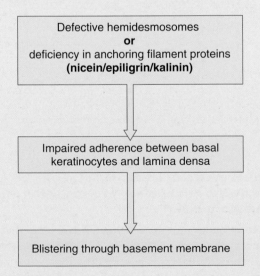

```
Defective hemidesmosomes
           or
deficiency in anchoring filament proteins
      (nicein/epiligrin/kalinin)
            ↓
Impaired adherence between basal
  keratinocytes and lamina densa
            ↓
Blistering through basement membrane
```

▶ **Dystrophic epidermolysis bullosa** may be either autosomal dominant or recessive, different mechanisms operating in each.

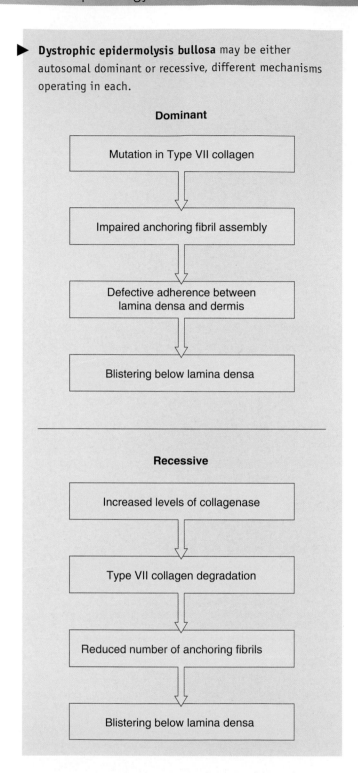

Dominant

Mutation in Type VII collagen

⬇

Impaired anchoring fibril assembly

⬇

Defective adherence between lamina densa and dermis

⬇

Blistering below lamina densa

Recessive

Increased levels of collagenase

⬇

Type VII collagen degradation

⬇

Reduced number of anchoring fibrils

⬇

Blistering below lamina densa

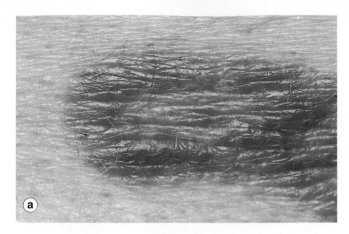

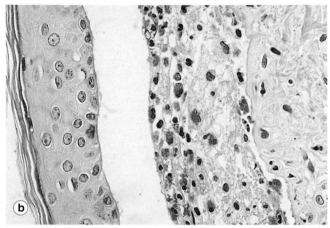

Fig. 23.15 Pemphigoid.
(a) Clinical features showing incipient blister formation in an area of reddening. The epidermis has already begun to separate in the pale central area. (b) Histology showing complete separation of the epidermis from the dermis, and a heavy infiltrate of eosinophils.

The likely cause of a basal blister can be determined by the nature of associated inflammatory cells

Blisters forming around the basement membrane often do so in an area that shows infiltration by inflammatory cells, and the nature of the inflammatory cell gives a clue to the diagnosis. For example, **eosinophils** are characteristic of pemphigoid (*Fig. 23.15*) (a blistering disease of the elderly) and herpes gestationis (a rare but important blistering rash occurring in mid or late pregnancy), and **neutrophil polymorphs** are mainly seen in dermatitis herpetiformis (an itchy, blistering disease in young and middle-aged adults, which is associated with celiac disease). **Lymphocytes** are seen in cases of blistering lichen planus (see page 489) and erythema multiforme.

Some basal blisters form in areas in which there is no inflammatory cell infiltrate; the most common example is the friction blister formed by shearing forces in non-specialized skin, e.g. ankle blisters from badly fitting shoes. Epidermolysis bullosa is another condition in which there are no inflammatory cells.

Increased activity or numbers of mast cells in the skin produces dermal edema and itching known as urticaria

Urticaria has many causes, the most familiar of which is 'hives' or 'nettle rash'. In addition, many patients with an atopic tendency or family history (see page 109) have a predisposition to develop urticaria, although the stimulus that provokes it may be difficult to identify; sometimes certain foods, heat, cold or sunlight are implicated. Degranulation of mast cells releases substances that increase vascular permeability, transudation of fluid into the dermis (leading to edema) and activation of platelets and eosinophils (leading to itch). In atopy the mast-cell degranulation is probably immunologically mediated by interaction of an antigen with IgE, which is bound to the mast-cell membrane (Type I hypersensitivity reaction, see page 109), but many cases are probably non-immunologically mediated.

Localized accumulations of mast cells in the skin can produce multiple brownish raised patches, which urticate on pressure (**urticaria pigmentosa**); less commonly, there may be a solitary tumor-like nodule (**solitary mastocytoma**), usually in young children.

Small vessel vasculitis may be confined to the skin, or the skin can be one of many tissues affected

The most frequently involved vessels are the small capillaries, arterioles and venules in the upper dermis. Vasculitic damage to the walls leads to extravasation of red cells into the upper dermis, producing the lesions known as **petechiae** (when minute) or **purpura** (when larger). Some lesions may be slightly raised and nodular (palpable purpura); the lesions may be widespread, but the lower limb (particularly the area below the knee) is by far the most common site.

The most common causes of a vasculitic rash of this type are drug reaction (*Fig. 23.16*), systemic connective tissue disease (e.g. SLE), and bacteremia or septicemia (particularly acute meningococcal type).

Although the skin lesion is the most obvious manifestation, there may be evidence of other system involvement, e.g. joint and abdominal symptoms in Henoch–Schönlein purpura. When larger blood vessels are involved, the vasculitis occurs in the mid and deep dermis or subcutis. Larger, deeper, ill-defined nodules develop, again commonly on the lower limb. The most common cause is **polyarteritis nodosa**.

Some vasculitic lesions in the lower limb lead to necrosis of epidermis and dermis, producing an ulcer that is characterized by a raised, purplish edge.

Most acute purpuric vasculitic lesions of the skin show destruction of the vessel wall, with an associated neutrophil polymorph infiltrate (**neutrophilic or 'leukocytoclastic' vasculitis**), occasionally with fibrinoid necrosis of the vessel wall. Sometimes the infiltrate in the vessel wall is largely composed of lymphocytes (**lymphocytic vasculitis**) without fibrinoid necrosis. This pattern shows less red-cell extravasation, and purpura is not such an important clinical feature; often the lesion appears to be a localized area of erythema. Lymphocytic vasculitis is particularly seen in association with systemic connective tissue disease (e.g. SLE, rheumatoid arthritis), and as a drug reaction.

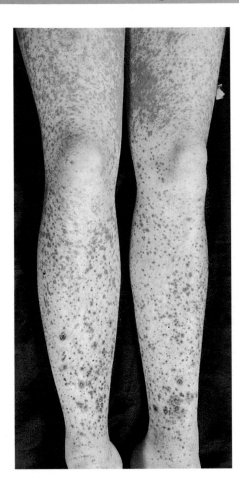

Fig. 23.16 Vasculitic skin rash producing purpura.
In this case the purpura was due to a neutrophilic vasculitis, which occurred as part of an adverse drug reaction.

Many skin lesions are iatrogenic, due to ingested drugs

Skin lesions of this nature are becoming increasingly common and show a wide variation in appearance, pattern and duration. The most common pattern is a **toxic erythema**, clinically and histologically identical to that seen as an indirect effect of virus infection (see page 491).

Skin reactions to drugs can mimic almost any other type of inflammatory skin disease. Common patterns are:

- **Lichenoid drug eruptions**, resembling lichen planus both clinically and histologically.
- **Vasculitic eruptions**, usually a small-vessel neutrophilic vasculitis in the upper dermis, producing purpura.
- **Urticarial eruptions**, producing blotchy, raised, itchy rashes.
- **Blistering and exfoliating eruptions**, particularly erythema multiforme (*Fig. 23.17*) and toxic epidermal necrolysis. The latter is the most severe, and often fatal, drug reaction in the skin, leading to extensive shedding of epidermis, together with severe metabolic disorder.
- **Erythema nodosum**, a characteristic deep dermal and subcutaneous reaction that produces firm, reddish purple nodules, usually on the legs (*Fig. 23.18*).

In general, skin rashes due to drugs develop at least a week after first exposure, improving within 3–4 days of stopping

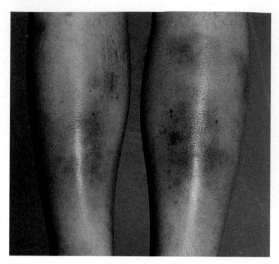

Fig. 23.17 Erythema nodosum. Typical erythema nodosum on the shins (in this case the result of an adverse reaction to sulfonamide therapy).

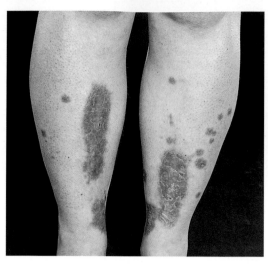

Fig. 23.19 Necrobiosis lipoidica. These advanced lesions had been present for many months on the shins of this diabetic.

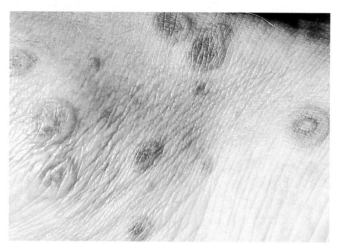

Fig. 23.18 Erythema multiforme.
In this case the erythema multiforme was due to an adverse reaction to antibiotics.

These diseases are dealt with in more detail in Chapter 25, and the skin lesions are discussed there (see pages 534 and 536).

Other systemic diseases in which there are important cutaneous manifestations are **diabetes mellitus** and **sarcoidosis**. In diabetes mellitus some patients develop red or yellowish, shiny, depressed plaques on the leg, due to degeneration of dermal collagen, known as **necrobiosis lipoidica** (*Fig. 23.19*). In **sarcoidosis**, cutaneous sarcoid granulomas are very common and can have many different clinical patterns, although the presence of non-caseating giant-cell granulomas is common to them all. Patients with sarcoidosis may also present with, or develop, erythema nodosum (see page 539).

Internal malignant disease may be associated with the development of a range of skin lesions (such as dermatomyositis), many of which are bizarre both clinically and histologically.

TUMORS OF THE SKIN

Tumors of the skin can be divided into those derived from the cells of the epidermis, those from the skin appendages, and those from the connective tissues in the dermis.

The epidermis contains a number of different cell types, namely, keratinocytes, melanocytes, Langerhans' cells, and Merkel's cells. Tumors in the epidermis most commonly originate from keratinocytes or melanocytes.

Keratinocyte-derived tumors of the epidermis are of two main types: basal-cell carcinoma and squamous-cell carcinoma

Both basal-cell carcinoma and squamous-cell carcinoma are predisposed to by exposure to light and ionizing radiations, and are therefore most commonly seen in exposed areas

the drug; the rash recurs within 20 days of re-exposure. However, certain drug rashes persist for a very long time after the drug is stopped, e.g. the extensive erythematous rash following ingestion of captopril and enalapril.

It is not sufficiently appreciated that drug reactions in skin are frequently due to non-prescription drugs bought over the counter (e.g. aspirin) or to agents included in food items (e.g. some coloring agents). A very detailed clinical history must be taken.

Many systemic diseases have cutaneous manifestations

Many systemic diseases have skin lesions as part of their general picture, and the first manifestation of disease may be the skin lesions. The most important group are the systemic autoimmune diseases such as SLE and systemic sclerosis.

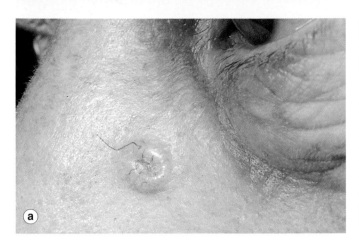

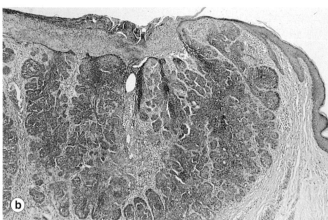

Fig. 23.20 Basal-cell carcinoma: nodular pattern.
(a) A typical raised nodule with a pearly-white edge and central ulceration. (b) Histology showing the typical nodular pattern.

such as the head and neck, and the dorsum of the hands. Both types of tumor arise most frequently in the elderly, and multiple lesions are not uncommon.

Basal-cell carcinoma, which occurs in three main patterns, is a locally invasive tumor that does not metastasize

The three main patterns are nodular basal-cell carcinoma, morpheic basal-cell carcinoma, and superficial basal-cell carcinoma.

Nodular basal-cell carcinoma is the most common pattern, occurring most frequently in those over the age of 50 years. Arising on areas exposed to light, such as the face and forehead, it is relatively rare on the trunk and limbs. It presents as a firm, raised nodule, often showing central ulceration, with a raised, pearly edge, which may show numerous telangiectatic vessels (*Fig. 23.20*). It is composed of clusters of small, dark cells resembling those of the basal layer of the epidermis. The edge of each cluster often shows a regular palisaded pattern. In the larger more protuberant lesions, cystic change is frequently seen.

Morpheic basal-cell carcinoma appears as a flat, thickened, whitish or yellowish plaque, which may be sunken and firm, with focal areas of ulceration. In contrast to nodular basal-cell carcinoma, it has indistinct edges and the tumor may extend in the dermis for some way beyond the visible or palpable borders. Histologically, small clumps and cords of basal cells are separated by a dense fibrous stroma (*Fig. 23.21*).

Superficial basal-cell carcinoma usually appears as a flat, red plaque, often with an irregular edge (*Fig. 23.22*). It is most common on the face, but this variant can occur on the trunk. Sometimes there are raised areas within the tumor, representing the development of a nodular basal-cell carcinoma within the pre-existing superficial lesion. Histologically, there are usually many small buds or nodular downgrowths of basal cells from the overlying epidermis. This superficial pattern may be multifocal, e.g. occurring in

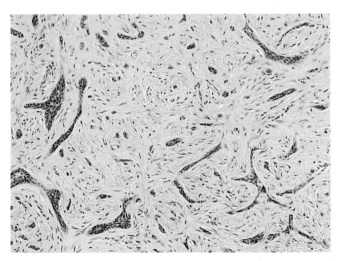

Fig. 23.21 Basal-cell carcinoma: morpheic pattern.
Histology showing narrow, compressed cords of basal cells in a dense fibrous stroma.

the irradiation field over the vertebrae in patients previously given radiotherapy for ankylosing spondylitis.

All basal-cell carcinomas can be cured if completely excised. However, local recurrence is a problem, particularly in the morpheic and superficial types, which are less clearly defined to the naked eye. Neglected basal-cell carcinomas cause considerable local destruction of the soft tissues and, occasionally, the bones of the face (hence their old name of 'rodent ulcer'). Although most seem to originate from the basal cells of the epidermis, some appear to arise from the necks of hair follicles, and can be confused with a tumor of hair follicles known as 'trichoepithelioma'.

Invasive squamous carcinoma of the skin may arise in pre-existing epidermal dysplastic lesions

Two patterns of intraepidermal dysplasia are recognized. One is **actinic keratosis** (also known as **solar keratosis**), which occurs most commonly on the face, scalp and backs of the hands (i.e. light-exposed skin). It arises as irregular plaques or patches (frequently multiple), up to 1 cm in diameter, with a rough, hard hyperkeratotic surface. Histologically, the cells in the lower half of the epidermis show marked dysplasia and atypia.

The other pattern shows epidermal atypia, with pleomorphism and mitoses, throughout all layers of the epidermis to the surface (*Fig. 23.23a*). This is regarded as squamous carcinoma *in situ* (**intraepidermal carcinoma**) and, like actinic keratoses, occurs on light-exposed skin, but may also occur on skin that is normally covered, e.g. on the trunk.

Clinically, lesions appear as flat or raised reddish-brown plaques, sometimes with surface keratinous scale, and occasionally with focal ulceration.

The incidence of malignant invasive change supervening in intraepidermal carcinoma is very much greater than that in actinic keratoses.

Most squamous carcinomas of the skin are locally invasive and well-differentiated, with the formation of keratin nests; occasionally, poorly differentiated non-keratinizing squamous carcinoma can develop in an area of pre-existing intraepidermal carcinoma. Invasive squamous carcinoma (*Fig. 23.23b*), unlike basal-cell carcinoma, has the potential for metastasis, usually metastasizing to regional lymph nodes initially.

One variant of invasive squamous carcinoma, verrucous carcinoma, is particularly common on the vulva in elderly women, presenting as a well-differentiated, exophytic, cauliflower-like lesion. This tumor grows locally, rarely metastasizing.

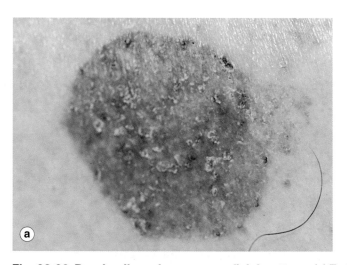
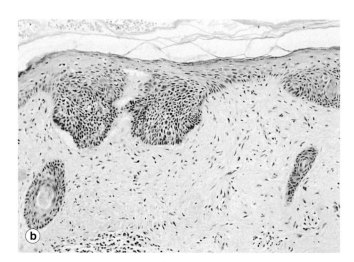

Fig. 23.22 Basal-cell carcinoma: superficial pattern. (a) Typical flat, red plaque with slight scaliness. (b) Histology showing multiple nests of basal-cell carcinoma growing down from the overlying epidermis.

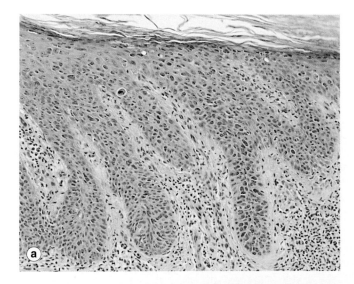
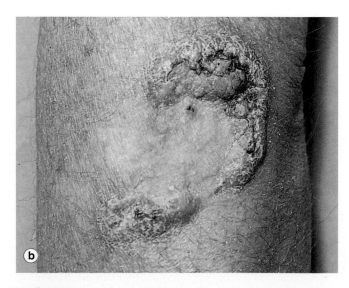

Fig. 23.23 Intraepidermal carcinoma and invasive squamous carcinoma.
(a) Histology of intraepidermal carcinoma showing thickening of the epidermis by pleomorphic dysplastic epidermal cells, without invasion into the dermis. (b) Invasive squamous-cell carcinoma of the skin showing the characteristic raised keratotic edges.

Melanocytes in the basal layer of the epidermis are an important source of tumor-like hamartomas (nevi) and invasive malignant tumors (malignant melanoma)

Melanocytic nevi (commonly known as 'moles') are extremely common and most individuals have a few somewhere on the skin, some people having very large numbers. They are regarded as hamartomatous malformations, and five main patterns are recognized.

In **junctional nevus** (*Fig. 23.24a* and *d*) the abnormal clumps of melanocytes are confined to the epidermis and are located in the basal layer. Clinically the lesions are flat (macular) and uniformly and deeply pigmented. They usually develop in childhood and adolescence.

Compound nevi (*Fig. 23.24b* and *e*) are raised, pale brown, slightly nodular lesions with an irregular surface, but the pigmentation is uniform. They are most common in adolescents and young adults. Histologically, there are clumps of melanocytes in both the epidermis (similar to those seen in junctional nevi) and the upper dermis. Those intradermal nevus cells that are closest to the junctional nests are histologically similar to the intraepidermal nevus cells. However, in the deeper levels they are smaller and more compact, a feature that is said to indicate maturation of the nevus cells. It is believed that the natural history of intraepidermal junctional nevus cells is for them to drop into the dermis and to become smaller and more compact the longer they have been in the dermis. It is not uncommon for coarse hairs to emerge from compound nevi (hairy mole).

Intradermal nevi (*Fig. 23.24c* and *f*) are also raised, but are normally smoothly domed, and may be flesh-coloured or slightly brown. They are usually seen in adults and are rare in adolescents and children. They appear to be entirely composed of nevus cells within the dermis, and there is no nested junctional component, although there may be a slight increase in melanocytes in the basal layer.

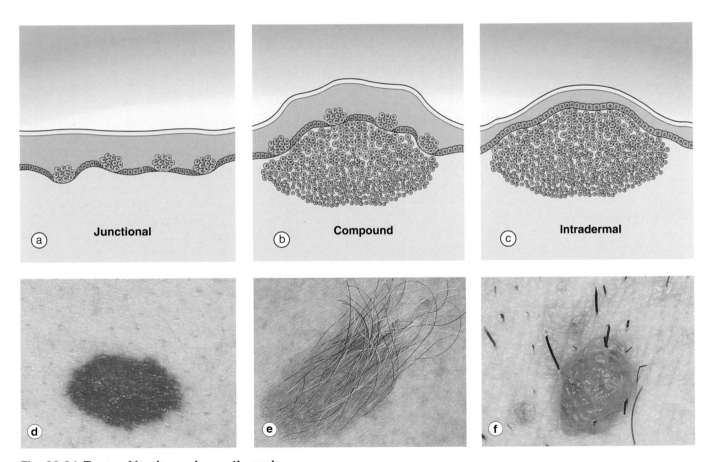

Fig. 23.24 Types of benign melanocytic nevi.
The distribution of melanocytes in junctional, compound and intradermal nevi. (a) In junctional nevus, there are rounded nests of melanocytes, some of which contain melanin granules in the cytoplasm, in the lower epidermis at the dermoepidermal junction.
(b) In compound nevus, there is a junctional nevus component, combined with an intradermal mass of benign melanocytic nevus cells.
(c) An intradermal nevus is entirely composed of melanocytic nevus cells in clusters within the upper dermis; there is no junctional component, and the intradermal melanocytes are usually small and entirely benign. (d) This flat pigmented lesion is regular in outline; it is a junctional nevus in a 17-year-old girl. In someone younger it would probably be more deeply pigmented. (e) This benign nevus is less intensely pigmented than the junctional nevus. It is becoming slightly raised as more of the melanocytes drop down from the epidermis into the upper dermis. The presence of coarse hairs is a frequent finding. (f) The clinical photograph shows a typical raised, slightly brown and wrinkled polypoid benign intradermal nevus. The color is uniform, as is the physical outline.

Blue nevi are entirely intradermal lesions, in which usually very heavily pigmented melanocytes are scattered in an ill-defined nodule separated by coarse bands of collagen. On cut surface these are brown due to the pigment, but they appear blue-black when viewed through the epidermis. They are usually first noted in childhood and can grow slowly, but are rarely more than 1 cm in diameter. Occasional very large blue nevi may be present on the buttocks, whereas the smaller blue nevi are most common on the head and arms. Malignant change is extremely rare.

Spitz nevus or **juvenile nevus**, as its name implies, is seen mainly in children, presenting as a raised, reddish brown, smooth-surfaced nodule. Although clinically they appear innocuous, histologically these melanocytic lesions show frightening degrees of pleomorphism and atypia and can be histologically confused with malignant melanoma.

The vast majority of nevi are entirely benign, but malignant change can occasionally supervene

It is the junctional component of junctional/compound nevi that is most at risk of conversion to malignancy. In the benign nevi the junctional melanocytes are arranged either in nests or in a linear (lentiginous) pattern. The individual melanocytes show no evidence of pleomorphism or mitotic activity and have the cytological characteristics of benign cells. Occasionally, both cytological and architectural atypia develop, the individual cells showing marked nuclear pleomorphism with increased numbers of mitoses; architectural atypia frequently takes the form of loss of roundness of the junctional cell nests, which often become flat and follow the general contour of the epidermal rete ridges.

Clinically, such nevi appear larger than usual (greater than 1 cm in diameter) and have irregularity of edge, surface and pigmentation. This irregularity of surface texture and outline, and the development of variable degrees of brown pigmentation, may develop in a nevus which has formerly been smooth and uniform in surface, outline and colour. These changes in a pre-existing mole should be regarded as an indication of possible early malignant change, and excision biopsy should be performed as a matter of urgency. There is no place for shave, punch or incision biopsies (see page 510). They may be single, but some people have many such atypical nevi, and there is often a family history (**dysplastic nevus syndrome**).

Lentigo maligna is a pattern of junctional melanocyte proliferation affecting the faces of the elderly

Clinically the lesions appear as flat, variegated, brown-black areas of pigmentation on the faces of elderly men and women. They gradually increase in size and have an irregular outline. Histologically, the basal layer of the epidermis is largely replaced by an almost continuous line of large atypical melanocytes, which sometimes partially extend down skin appendages such as hair follicles. Occasionally a solid, raised nodule arises within such an area, often indicating the development of a supervening early nodular malignant melanoma (lentigo maligna melanoma).

Malignant melanoma is increasing in incidence in white-skinned races

Malignant melanoma is predominantly a tumor of adults, but it does occasionally occur in children. It may arise within the junctional component of a pre-existing melanocytic nevus (see 'dysplastic nevus' and 'lentigo maligna'), or may apparently develop of its own accord within otherwise normal skin. The most important predisposing factor is excessive exposure to ultraviolet (UV) light, and the increasing incidence of malignant melanoma has been ascribed to both the reduced filtering power of the thinning ozone layer, and increased social exposure to sunshine. The tumor is uncommon in dark-skinned races, possibly because of the protective effect of increased epidermal melanin against UV irradiation. Women are slightly more likely to develop a tumor than men, the legs being a common site in women, and the trunk (particularly the back) being a common site in men. Malignant melanoma may occur in other mucosal surfaces, e.g. the mouth and nose.

Malignant melanomas of the skin present as irregular pigmented lesions

Compared to benign pigmented melanocytic lesions, malignant melanomas are often larger (with a history of recent increase in size), with an irregular border leading to asymmetry, and variable pigmentation. Ulceration may be present. Some forms are flat, others manifesting as raised nodular lesions. Malignant melanomas can be classified into three main groups:

- **Lentigo malignant melanoma.** A nodular lesion arising in a pre-existing facial lentigo maligna.
- **Superficial spreading malignant melanoma.** Usually a flat lesion with variable pigmentation and irregular edges. This is the most common type, accounting for about 75% of all malignant melanomas; it is in this group that the recent increase in incidence has been most marked.
- **Nodular malignant melanoma.** Presents as a raised brown-black nodule, usually without preceding benign melanocytic lesion. These account for about 5% of all malignant melanomas (see *Fig. 23.25f*).

A further group that is worth recognizing is the so-called **acral lentiginous malignant melanoma.** This is confined to the hands and feet, and some occur beneath the finger nails and toe nails (**sub-ungual melanoma**). Although it is most common in elderly Caucasians, it is particularly common in Orientals. Histologically, it resembles superficial spreading malignant melanoma.

Superficial spreading malignant melanoma may be either *in situ* or invasive

In superficial spreading malignant melanoma *in situ*, the atypical melanocytes are confined to the epidermis (*Fig. 23.26*). In contrast, with invasive superficial spreading malignant melanoma, in addition to the *in situ* change, clusters of malignant melanocytes invade the dermis. In the invasive type, the prognosis largely depends on the depth of dermal invasion (see blue box on page 504). In most cases, at the time of excision biopsy to establish the diagnosis, the invasion is very superficial; the prognosis is good for these tumors if they are adequately excised.

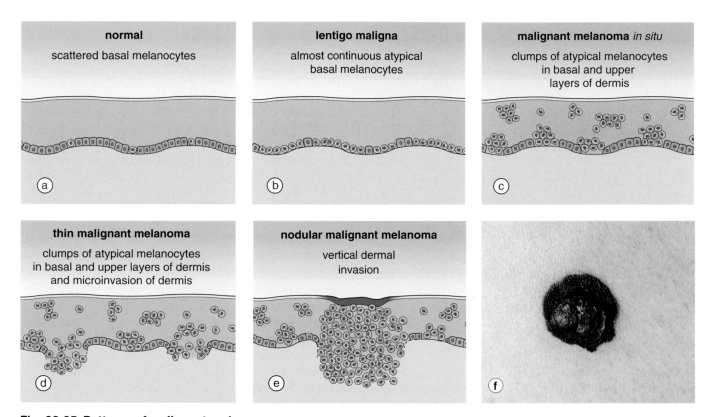

Fig. 23.25 Patterns of malignant melanoma.
(a) Melanocytes in normal skin. (b) Lentigo maligna. (c) Malignant melanoma *in situ* (melanocytic intraepidermal neoplasia).
(d) Thin malignant melanoma with microinvasion of dermis. (e) Nodular malignant melanoma with vertical growth pattern.
(f) Malignant melanoma (note the spreading pigmentation and the raised central nodule).

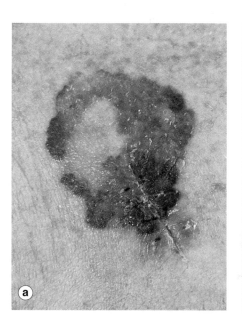

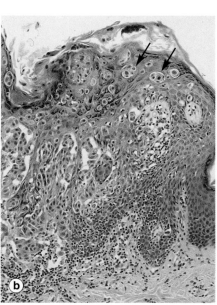

Fig. 23.26 Superficial spreading malignant melanoma.
(a) This pigmented lesion of the skin shows marked irregularity in outline and in degree of pigmentation. This was originally a dysplastic compound nevus, which has transformed into a superficial spreading malignant melanoma. A biopsy has been taken from the most obviously malignant area. (b) There are malignant melanocytes invading upwards into the epidermis (pagetoid change – see arrows). At bottom left of the picture, melanocytes can also be seen beginning to invade downwards into the dermis.

Prognostic factors in invasive malignant melanoma

Patients can be divided into three groups according to the risk of metastasis.

- **Low risk.** The best prognostic criterion is a Breslow thickness of less than 0.76 mm. The Breslow thickness is the measured thickness (on a histological section) from the deepest level of the malignant melanoma to the granular layer of the overlying epidermis.
- **Moderate risk.** Tumors with a Breslow thickness of between 0.76 mm and 1.5 mm.
- **High risk.** Tumors with a Breslow thickness of greater than 1.5 mm.

Clarke's levels express the depth of invasion of the tumor according to structural levels in the skin. For example, level 1 is confined within the epidermis, level 2 shows invasion of papillary dermis only, and later levels express varying degrees of invasion of the reticular dermis and subcutis. However, Clarke's levels are not as consistently reproducible as the Breslow thickness, which is the measurement of choice.

Malignant melanoma in the skin can metastasize via lymphatics and blood vessels

Malignant melanoma can metastasize **by lymphatics** to the lymph nodes draining the area in which the primary lesion occurs, e.g. inguinal nodes in leg lesions. Sometimes clusters of melanoma cells become trapped in lymphatic vessels in the skin on the way to the lymph nodes, setting up metastases within the skin (**satellite deposits**).

Bloodstream spread can also occur, common sites for bloodstream metastasis being the liver, lung and brain. However, melanoma is notorious for producing blood-borne metastases in bizarre sites such as the myocardium.

For malignant melanoma to metastasize, it has to gain access to the lymphatics and blood vessels in the dermis. The more extensive the growth and the deeper it extends into dermis, the more lymphatics and blood vessels it can invade. The risk of metastasis, and therefore the prognosis, are thus largely dependent on the depth of invasion. The two ways of expressing this are Clarke's levels and the Breslow thickness (see blue box).

Proliferation of Langerhans' cells in the skin is rare and largely confined to young children

Langerhans' cells are slightly increased in number in a large range of inflammatory skin diseases, and may be found in their normal location in the epidermis as well as around upper dermal blood vessels. There is a group of conditions called **Langerhans' cell histiocytosis** (also known as **histiocytosis X**), in which there is extensive proliferation of Langerhans' cells, either alone or in conjunction with other cells such as eosinophils, fibroblasts and lymphocytes.

There are three components to the Langerhans' cell histiocytosis group: **Letterer–Siwe disease** (a disease of infants, usually presenting with a skin rash), **Hand–Schüller–Christian disease** (in which there are localized accumulations in bone, producing osteolytic lesions, together with pulmonary infiltration and occasional lymph node involvement), and **eosinophil granuloma** (in which there is usually a solitary osteolytic lesion in bone, composed largely of Langerhans' cells with eosinophils). There is considerable overlap between these three syndromes, but Letterer–Siwe disease is the most clear cut. It is largely confined to infants, presenting with a variable skin rash that often resembles seborrheic dermatitis. It behaves in a malignant fashion, with extensive infiltration of the upper dermis and many other systemic tissues by large abnormal Langerhans' cells.

Tumors of Merkel cells are rare, highly malignant, and usually found in the elderly

Merkel cells are neuroendocrine cells in the basal layer of the epidermis, associated with peripheral nerve endings by synaptic connection. Tumors of Merkel cells usually occur in the elderly, mainly around the head and neck, with the arm being the next most common site. Lesions principally occur in sun-damaged skin as raised painless nodules, which grow progressively. They have a poor prognosis and metastasize widely and early.

TUMORS OF SKIN APPENDAGES

The skin appendages that most frequently give rise to tumors are the pilosebaceous apparatus and the eccrine ducts and glands. Tumors of apocrine glands are rare.

Two common tumors are derived from hair follicles: trichoepithelioma and pilomatrixoma

Trichoepithelioma commonly presents as a skin-covered nodule, less than 1 cm in diameter, on the faces of teenagers and young and middle-aged adults. Both clinically and histologically, these lesions resemble small nodular basal-cell carcinomas. The difference in age incidence is the main distinction between the two.

Pilomatrixomas occur mainly in children, arising on the face, neck and shoulders. They are raised, knobbly, dermal tumors, up to 2 cm in diameter, which are often very pale or white with thin epidermis stretched over them.

Tumors or tumor-like nodules derived from the sebaceous component of the hair follicle most frequently occur on the face. The most common is **sebaceous hyperplasia**, in which there are a number of yellow papules, usually on the forehead, cheeks and the area around the nose. They mainly affect elderly men and, less commonly, women; clinically they may be mistaken for small basal-cell carcinomas.

Tumors derived from eccrine sweat glands and their ducts are not common, but there are many different types

The main types are:

- **Syringoma.** Multiple, small, pale white nodules or papules on the lower eyelids and cheek, usually in women.
- **Eccrine poroma.** A raised, solitary, fleshy tumor, usually situated on the sole but occasionally seen in the palm.
- **Hidroacanthoma simplex.** Usually located on the lower leg in elderly people, often confused clinically with basal-cell carcinoma or seborrheic keratosis.
- **Clear-cell acanthoma.** A flat or slightly raised reddish lesion on the legs.
- **Clear-cell or eccrine hidradenoma.** Usually located on the head or neck of young adults. Arises as a solitary nodular tumor which may appear cystic. Solid lesions are usually flesh-colored or slightly red; cystic lesions may have a bluish tinge.
- **Cylindroma.** One of the most common tumors, the majority occurring on the head, scalp and neck as slow-growing, pink, raised nodules. They are particularly common in women, and multiple cylindromas may occur with an autosomal dominant mode of inheritance. Multiple tumors on the scalp are sometimes called 'turban tumor'.

Most skin cysts are derived from skin appendages

The most common skin cyst derived from a skin appendage is the so-called **pilar cyst**, which occurs on the scalp of the elderly as a well-circumscribed, round tumor. Histologically, lesions are lined by squamous epithelium similar to that of hair follicles and contain thick, white, compacted keratin. They may be multiple.

Epidermal cysts are also believed to be derived from hair follicles and are very similar to pilar cysts. They are mainly seen on the face, neck and upper trunk in young and middle-aged adults, and may occur in an area previously damaged by severe acne. Similar epidermal cysts may be seen at the angle of the eye in children (**external angular dermoid**) and are regarded as congenital malformations. Epidermal cysts may also be seen anywhere on the body following penetrating injury and are believed to be derived from squamous epithelium from the epidermis, implanted during trauma (**inclusion dermoid**). The skin and subcutaneous tissue around some epidermal cysts may show reddening and swelling, and the lesion becomes tender. This is commonly called 'infected epidermoid cyst', but the inflammation is caused by leakage of keratin into surrounding tissues following trauma and is not associated with infection.

TUMORS AND TUMOR-LIKE ENLARGEMENTS OF THE DERMIS

Although many of the lesions originating from the cells in the dermis appear to be tumor-like, they are in fact hamartomatous malformations rather than true neoplastic proliferations. The most common are: **angioma** and angioma-like proliferations (e.g. pyogenic granuloma), **fibrohistiocytic lesions** (e.g. dermatofibroma), **neurofibroma** and **neurilemmoma**, and **leiomyoma**.

Dermal lesions due to abnormal blood vessels are common, most being developmental malformations rather than true neoplasms

The most frequently seen vascular lesions in the dermis are hamartomatous, and the most common examples include capillary hemangioma, cavernous hemangioma and port-wine stain.

Capillary hemangiomas are common in babies (strawberry nevus) and are usually located on the trunk, buttocks or face. They are not present at birth, but manifest in the first few months of life; they spontaneously enlarge and then regress over the first couple of years of life. These firm, dark-pink tumors protrude from the surface of the skin and are usually 2–3 cm in diameter.

Cavernous hemangiomas are clinically similar to capillary hemangiomas, occurring in the same location and in the same group. However, they tend to be larger, less clearly defined, and show no tendency to involution.

Port-wine stain usually presents at birth as a flat, purplish red or pink area on the face and neck. It occasionally arises on the limbs. These lesions show no tendency to regress and may continue to grow; they are sometimes associated with intracerebral vascular malformations (Sturge–Weber syndrome).

Pyogenic granuloma is a common, raised, red, vascular-looking lesion (*Fig. 23.27*). Histologically, it appears to

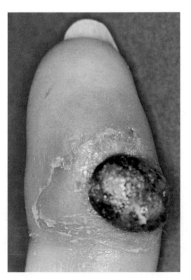

Fig. 23.27 Pyogenic granuloma. Typical site and appearance of pyogenic granuloma, a raised angioma-like lesion, in this case due to trauma from a rose thorn.

be composed of highly vascular granulation tissue with inflammatory cells in the stroma. Often showing surface ulceration, they grow rapidly up to 1–2 cm in a matter of weeks until they are pedunculated red nodules. They are most common on the head and neck, and also involve the buccal and gingival mucosa (see Chapter 12), particularly in young pregnant women. They also occur on the limbs, particularly around the lower arms and hands, and there is sometimes a history of penetrating trauma.

The most important true tumors of vascular origin in the skin are glomus tumor, angiosarcoma and Kaposi's sarcoma

Glomus tumors most commonly occur in the fingers, particularly underneath the fingernails. They are small, reddish nodules (sometimes slightly blue), which are exquisitely tender particularly when pressed, but may also be spontaneously painful. They are derived from special arteriovenous anastomoses called 'glomus bodies', which are most frequently found in the hands.

Angiosarcoma is a highly malignant tumor in the skin. It is usually seen in elderly people, arising mainly in the head and neck region, particularly the scalp and forehead. Lesions appear as slightly raised purplish red patches or plaques, which spread and then undergo ulceration.

Kaposi's sarcoma was formerly uncommon in the western world, being mainly confined to Central Africa. However, occasional cases were seen in elderly Caucasians, usually men, and principally in the hands and feet.

Kaposi's sarcoma has become a much more important tumor because of its high incidence in young adults (mainly males) who have AIDS; in this group the lesions are often multiple and grow rapidly, sometimes involving the oral mucosa, with a tendency to metastasize widely. They usually begin as a small, reddish patch, which enlarges and becomes a raised plaque or nodule (see page 173).

Fibrous histiocytic tumors are the most common true tumors of the dermis

The cell of origin is considered to be the myofibroblast, a connective tissue cell that shows features of smooth muscle and fibroblast, together with some histiocytic characteristics.

Fibrous histiocytic tumors arise most commonly on the limbs in middle-aged adults, and are slightly more common in women. The lesions are solitary raised nodules, usually brownish in colour, and the overlying epidermis may show some thickening and hyperkeratosis.

The most common histological pattern is that of **dermatofibroma** in which the dermal nodule is ill defined and composed of spindle-shaped myofibroblasts which lies between dermal collagen bands, expanding the dermis. Of the two less common variants, one (histiocytoma cutis) contains a much higher proportion of lipid-filled histiocytic cells, giving the lesion a yellow colour on cut surface; this is particularly common around the ankle. The other variant,

the so-called 'sclerosing hemangioma' is more densely sclerotic, with increased numbers of vessels. Often hemosiderin from leaked blood gives the lesion a brownish cut-surface appearance.

Dermal fibrous histiocytic tumors of this type are entirely benign, but there are two tumors with histological similarities, which behave as malignant tumors. **Dermatofibrosarcoma protuberans** is a much larger, slowly growing dermal tumor, which is irregular in outline and has multiple nodules within it. **Malignant fibrous histiocytoma** is one of the most common soft tissue tumors affecting the deep tissues (particularly of the thigh and buttock), but some malignant fibrous histiocytomas appear to arise in subcutaneous fat and may initially present as a deep skin tumor.

Non-neoplastic fibrous lesions of the dermis are common

The most common non-neoplastic fibrous lesions of the dermis are **keloids**. These occur as raised, firm, collagenous lesions, which are often covered by smooth, rather thin epidermis. They grow slowly and become harder with time. They are usually found around the head, neck, upper chest and upper arms of young people (there is a female preponderance), and young women of Afro-Caribbean origin are particularly prone. Lesions follow a history of trauma, e.g. keloids on the earlobe are commonly the result of ear piercing, and keloidal change in surgical scars is an important cosmetic problem in the areas of the body where keloid change tends to occur (*Fig. 23.28*). They probably represent excessive reactive collagen formation by fibroblasts after trauma, with the proliferation of fibroblasts and collagen deposition extending beyond the original site of trauma. In this way they are distinguished from hypertrophic scarring, in which a slowly resolving scar remains localized to the area of trauma.

The **fibromatoses** are diffuse proliferations of fibrous and fibrohistiocytic tissues in the subcutis and adipose tissue. There are many types, most of which are rare. The most frequently seen is **palmar fibromatosis (Dupuytren's contracture)**, in which there is fibrous thickening of the tissues in the palm of the hand, usually in the form of a single long cord. This leads to fixed flexion deformities of the fingers, most commonly the fourth or ring finger, giving rise to puckering of the palmar skin, a palpable rigid bar of firm tissue running to the finger, and a claw-like deformity of one or more fingers. It occurs most commonly in adult Caucasian males and has a particularly high incidence in alcoholics. There may also be plantar fibromatosis, in which a similar thickening occurs on the soles of the feet but rarely, if ever, produces flexion deformity of the toe.

Neurofibromas may be solitary or multiple; neurilemmoma is a solitary tumor

Neurofibromas are characteristically soft, raised, fleshy dermal tumors, which are often pedunculated.

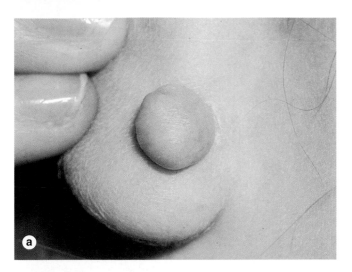

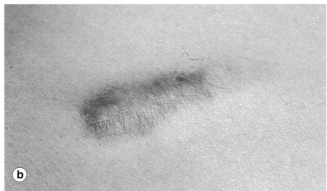

Fig. 23.28 Keloid.
(a) Keloid in earlobe following ear piercing. (b) Keloid in scar, common in the upper trunk in young women.

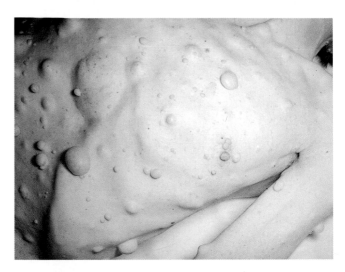

Fig. 23.29 Multiple neurofibromas in von Recklinghausen's disease. Very large numbers of soft, fleshy dermal tumors are present, together with some less protuberant subcutaneous tumors.

In **von Recklinghausen's disease** there are large numbers of such tumors in many areas of the skin (*Fig. 23.29*), and similar lesions are present in the internal organs. They are complex benign tumors containing Schwann cells, but elements of endoneurium and perineurium are also present; they are sometimes considered to be hamartomatous malformations (see also page 467). Malignant change may occasionally supervene in one of the larger skin tumors in von Recklinghausen's disease, but the solitary tumors are benign.

Schwannomas (neurilemmomas) are solitary tumors of the Schwann cells of peripheral nerves, and usually lie in the line of a peripheral nerve. They are usually located in the subcutis rather than the dermis. They occur in middle-aged adults, with equal sex incidence, and are mainly seen on the limbs and head and neck. They are benign, but may undergo degenerative change if long-standing (ancient Schwannoma).

Leiomyomas in the skin are derived either from the walls of dermal vessels or from arrector pili muscles. They present as raised, red lesions, up to 1 cm across, and are both painful and tender. Those derived from arrector pili may be multiple and usually arise on the trunk and limbs in young adults; those derived from blood vessel smooth muscle are usually solitary, and may be larger than 1 cm in diameter.

The most common lymphoma to present in the skin is cutaneous T-cell lymphoma (CTCL)

B-cell lymphoma in the skin usually occurs as part of a systemic lymphoma. It manifests either as a solitary, raised, reddish purple nodule or as a series of coalescing nodules, particularly in the head and neck.

T-cell lymphoma may present in the skin, sometimes remaining in the skin for many years before becoming systematized. The florid lesions of T-cell lymphoma in the skin are known as **mycosis fungoides**, appearing as multiple, raised, red nodules or indurated plaques. However, many patients have a long history of red skin patches with a wrinkled, scaly surface (often for many years), which occasionally become slowly more raised to form reddish confluent plaques (*Fig. 23.30a*).

Histologically, these are manifestations of infiltration of upper dermis and epidermis by increasing numbers of malignant T-lymphocytes (*Fig. 23.30b*), and are known respectively as the 'patch' and 'plaque' stages of CTCL. By the time the patient has developed a nodular lesion of mycosis fungoides, the dermis contains nodular infiltrates of malignant T-lymphocytes.

Some patients with CTCL present with general widespread reddening of the skin (erythroderma), and a few of them have lymphadenopathy and malignant T-lymphocytes in the peripheral blood (**Sézary's syndrome**).

There are many conditions that mimic CTCL both clinically and histologically, and the diagnosis of the disease may be difficult until the late stages, when plaques and nodular tumors are prominent.

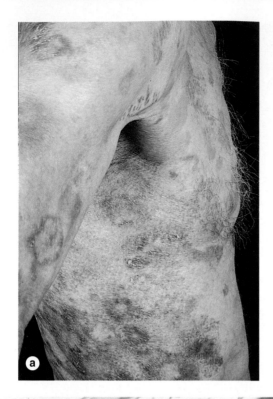

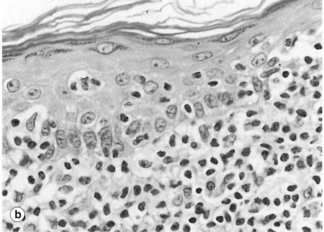

Fig. 23.30 Cutaneous T-cell lymphoma (mycosis fungoides). (a) The skin shows a mixture of red patches and raised plaques due to skin infiltration by malignant T-lymphocytes. (b) Histology shows large numbers of pleomorphic T-lymphocytes in the dermis, and invading the epidermis.

IMPORTANT MISCELLANEOUS SKIN CONDITIONS

There are many common and important lesions of the skin that are very difficult to fit into the categories used above, mainly because their etiology and pathogenesis are not known. They can be divided into: non-neoplastic squamous keratoses, disorders of hair and hair follicles, and chronic skin ulcers.

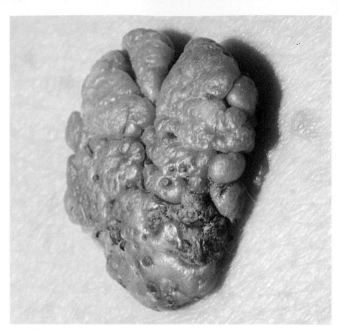

Fig. 23.31 Raised benign seborrheic keratosis (seborrheic wart). These are often covered by a thick layer of warty, grey keratin.

Seborrheic warts, keratoacanthomas and cutaneous horns are benign epidermal proliferations characterized by excess keratin production

Seborrheic keratoses are extremely common, increasing in number with age. They are almost invariably multiple and present as slightly raised, greyish brown keratotic lesions, the larger examples of which may have an obviously warty surface (*Fig. 23.31*). They are due to proliferation of epidermal cells resembling those that occupy the basal layer, and there is excessive production of keratin. They are invariably benign.

Keratoacanthoma most commonly occurs in the elderly, particularly on the face. A characteristic and frightening feature is that they clinically resemble squamous-cell carcinomas and grow extremely rapidly, changing in a matter of weeks from a slightly raised, red papule to a large domed nodule with raised, firm edges and a central mass of keratin (*Fig. 23.32*). At certain stages in their growth, keratoacanthomas also share histological features with squamous-cell carcinoma, and the differential diagnosis can be very difficult. Most keratoacanthomas spontaneously regress within some months, but those that persist should be excised because of the difficulty of distinguishing them from squamous-cell carcinomas.

Cutaneous horns are hard, protruding lumps of keratin that arise from an area of abnormal epidermis. The underlying epidermal abnormality is usually benign, e.g. a viral wart or seborrheic keratosis, but occasionally cutaneous horns can arise on an area of intraepidermal carcinoma.

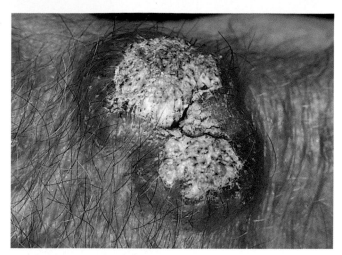

Fig. 23.32 Keratoacanthoma.
Typical lesion with a raised, red edge. It is filled with creamy grey masses of keratin. These can be clinically mistaken for squamous-cell carcinoma of the skin.

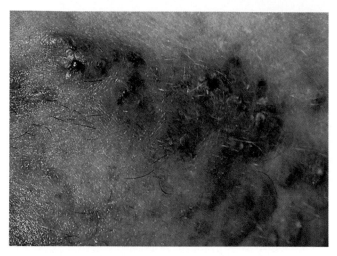

Fig. 23.33 Acne vulgaris. Severe acne, some lesions showing pustule formation and crusting.

Disorders of the hair and hair follicles are very commonly encountered in community practice

Hair follicles are the site of both keratin retention and bacterial and fungal infection (**superficial folliculitis**). Acute superficial folliculitis is usually due to *Staphylococcus aureus*. It is most common in the beard area in adolescent and young adult males, but may also occur elsewhere, e.g. the thighs and buttocks. Clinically it presents as minute, yellowish, rounded pustules, often with a central hair. **Deep folliculitis** occurs when the infection (also usually staphylococcal) occurs deep in the hair follicle. This causes an expanding mass that destroys the follicle, producing a 'boil'.

Acne vulgaris, which most commonly affects adolescents, is a form of chronic folliculitis associated with excess keratin accumulation in the pilosebaceous duct. The infective lesion probably arises in obstructed hair follicles, which produce small, raised, white nodules (whiteheads or blackheads). Rupture of these nodules releases a mixture of keratin, sebaceous-gland secretion and bacteria into the surrounding dermis, where there is a mixed inflammatory reaction, both acute inflammatory and chronic granulomatous (*Fig. 23.33*). Sometimes acne forms large tender keratin-filled cysts (**cystic acne**). The cause is not known, but high circulating androgens are thought to be significant.

Rosacea is a follicle-related disease in which there is marked reddening of the skin of the face, associated with telangiectatic dilatation of upper dermal vessels and a perivascular chronic inflammatory infiltrate which, when heavy, leads to persistent indurated reddening of the skin. Papules or pustules frequently develop, and are based on markedly dilated hair follicles in which fragments, live or dead, of the mite *Demodex folliculorum* are commonly found. The most floridly lumpy forms of rosacea are those

that occur when the follicles rupture, their contents exciting a giant-cell granulomatous reaction (granulomatous rosacea), or when the lesion occurs in an area of marked sebaceous gland hyperplasia, commonly the noses of elderly men (**rhinophyma**).

Abnormal hair loss is called alopecia and there are many types

Hair loss from the scalp is a normal aging change, with exaggerated or early loss in those in whom there is a family predisposition (particularly men). There are many causes of hair loss outside the normal range, the most common being **alopecia areata**. Other types of alopecia include **alopecia totalis and universalis** (loss of all head hair and all body hair, respectively), **trichotillomania** (traumatic hair loss due to avulsion, usually self-inflicted, of the hair from the follicle for esthetic or psychological reasons), and **scarring alopecia** (usually the result of inflammatory destruction of hair follicles due to some other disease, e.g. lupus erythematosus or lichen planus, affecting the hair follicles).

Alopecia areata is the most common type of pathological hair loss

In alopecia areata there is sudden onset of round or oval patches of baldness in the scalp, leaving unusually smooth, almost shiny skin. The patches persist for many months, but in most cases the hair grows back within 12–18 months, although further patches may develop. A few progress to alopecia totalis.

The disease is multifactorial, and there is often a family history; more than half of the patients have a history of atopic eczema, asthma, or an autoimmune disease (particularly of the thyroid). It is common in association with Down's syndrome. There appears to be a sudden loss of anagen (growing) hairs, and the follicles enter the resting catagen/telogen phase, during which time there is a perifollicular infiltrate by lymphocytes.

The most common ulcers of the skin occur on the lower legs and are associated with chronic venous insufficiency

Most common in middle-aged and elderly women with varicose veins, chronic venous insufficiency in the lower legs and gravitational dermatitis, 'varicose' or 'venous' ulcers are a common and persistent problem in community practice.

They are shallow but often spreading ulcers, forming on a background of chronic gravitational dermatitis and pigmentation in the fragile atrophic skin around the ankles and lower shin (*Fig. 23.34*). They show little tendency to heal spontaneously, and secondary infection is common; some of the topical applications used to treat or prevent bacterial infection produce a contact dermatitis, leading to deterioration of the ulcer.

Occasionally, chronic skin ulcers have a slightly raised purplish edge; these ulcers may be the result of vasculitic lesions in dermal vessels.

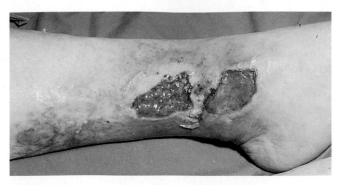

Fig. 23.34 Chronic leg ulcers.
The characteristic location and appearance of chronic leg ulcers, on the medial side of the leg, just above the ankle. In this case the ulcers are due to chronic venous insufficiency (note the brown pigmentation in surrounding skin). This is an important cause of morbidity in the elderly, but may also occur in middle-aged women with varicose veins, and in the obese. Healing is slow, and the skin remains fragile and predisposed to further ulceration even after complete healing.

Skin biopsy

Most dermatological disorders are easily diagnosed by a competent dermatologist on their clinical features alone, but some have an atypical appearance or an unusual distribution, leading to doubt about the diagnosis. In these cases, histological examination of a skin biopsy may be useful. The various biopsy techniques are:

- **Curette biopsy:** in which the skin lesion (usually raised) is scraped off piecemeal with a curette, and the fragments are sent for histological examination. This is not recommended if an accurate histological diagnosis is required.
- **Shave biopsy:** in which a raised skin lesion is 'shaved off' with a sharp blade. This is sometimes carried out as a part diagnostic/part therapeutic maneuver for raised melanocytic lesions such as compound nevi, but is unsafe if there is any clinical doubt about the malignant potential of the lesion, since excision is rarely complete.
- **Punch biopsy:** a 3, 4 or 6 mm punch-biopsy sample is obtained. This method is useful to sample a uniform skin lesion, particularly an inflammatory disease such as psoriasis or discoid lupus erythematosus.
- **Incision biopsy:** in which a biopsy of a large skin lesion is taken by scalpel in the form of a sliver which includes both normal and abnormal skin.
- **Excision biopsy:** in which a small skin lesion is completely excised, usually as an ellipse with normal skin all around, for diagnostic purposes. However, where the lesion is solitary, and particularly when a skin tumor is suspected, an excision biopsy is also curative. This is the method of choice for all solitary skin tumors, particularly melanocytic lesions, basal-cell carcinomas, squamous-cell carcinomas and skin appendage tumors. If there is a clinical doubt about the extent of local spread, the lesion can be excised with a large area of normal skin.

Although histological examination of the biopsy forms the basis of laboratory diagnosis, immunfluorescent examination (e.g. pemphigoid, dermatitis herpetiformis) and electron microscopy (e.g. T-cell lymphoma) may be useful.

24

Orthopedic and rheumatological pathology

Clinical Overview

The most important diseases of the bones, joints and tendons which the medical student will meet during an attachment to an orthopedic and rheumatological unit will be those due either to **acute trauma** (such as fracture of bone, rupture of tendons and sprains of joints) or to **chronic degenerative diseases** due to wear and tear (such as osteoarthrosis and the various wear and tear lesions of tendons, tendon sheaths and ligaments).

Thus in bone pathology it is important that students understand the structure of bone and the processes involved in the healthy healing of bone fracture; a knowledge of the processes involved in healing underpins the various techniques of conservative and surgical management of fracture. An understanding of the normal histology and physiology of mineralized bone is essential if the student is to appreciate the mechanisms involved in the important metabolic disorders of bone.

In the western world infections of bone are now unusual, and are mostly seen as a result of bacterial contamination during penetrating injury, or associated with bacteremia due to a limited number of bacteria. Bone tumors are rare as primary lesions, but the bone is a common site of metastasis for important and common malignant tumors such as carcinomas of the breast, bronchus, prostate, kidney and thyroid.

Diseases of joints are an important cause of morbidity, with pain and loss of mobility the most important and distressing symptoms. Not only are joints prone to wear and tear with age, the ligaments and tendons inserted into bone are also prone to degenerative disease, as well as acute injury. Joint damage is a particularly common and crippling manifestation of rheumatoid disease, and the joints are frequently involved in other systemic connective tissue diseases such as systemic lupus erythematosus and scleroderma.

BONE

Bone is composed of specialized collagen (osteoid), which is mineralized by the deposition of hydroxyapatite

Bone is composed of a collagen-containing extracellular matrix (osteoid) synthesized by **osteoblasts**, which is mineralized by calcium-containing salts. There are two main patterns of bone deposition (*Fig. 24.1*).

In normal **lamellar bone** the osteoid collagen is deposited in a mechanically strong, parallel stratified pattern. The collagen is deposited in a direction dependent upon the maximal stresses to which the bones will be exposed, giving the maximum strength for the minimum bone bulk.

In abnormal **woven bone** the osteoblasts deposit osteoid collagen in a haphazard pattern. With its random arrangement of osteoid collagen fibers, this woven pattern is far less efficient and much weaker than lamellar bone, with a greater tendency to fracture under stress.

Bone is constantly being refashioned by osteoblastic new bone formation and osteoclastic removal of old bone

Osteoclasts are highly specialized cells capable of removing bone; they are multinucleate giant cells derived from the

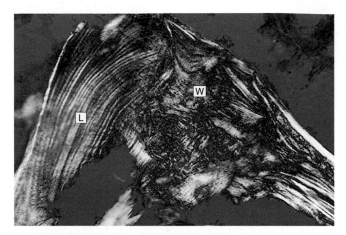

Fig. 24.1 Woven and lamellar bone.
Polarizing light micrograph showing recently formed woven bone (**W**). The haphazard collagen arrangement contrasts with the regular lamellae of lamellar bone (**L**).

Several factors are involved in bone formation and destruction

Parathyroid hormone (PTH) is secreted by the parathyroids in response to a fall in blood calcium, and restores the plasma calcium level by directly or indirectly stimulating osteoclastic bone resorption. PTH also increases both resorption of calcium ions and phosphate ion excretion by the kidney.

Vitamin D acts as a hormone, promoting the mineralization of bone (see page 514). Vitamin D deficiency leads to **osteomalacia**, a disease in which there is failure of mineralization of osteoid collagen (see page 514).

Calcitonin, a hormone produced by the parafollicular cells of the thyroid, is secreted in response to a rise in plasma calcium and has the opposite effects to PTH. It depresses osteoclast activity, thus reducing bone resorption and is used as a therapeutic agent to suppress abnormally increased osteoclast activity in diseases such as Paget's disease (see page 515).

Many other factors exert some influence on bone formation, e.g. growth hormone, corticosteroids, androgens and estrogens, insulin and some vitamins, local growth factors, cytokines and prostaglandins.

monocyte–macrophage series. Combined activity of osteoblasts and osteoclasts can produce reshaping of bone in order to meet new directional stresses. Unbalanced pathological increase in osteoclastic activity leads to destruction of bone, a feature of some metabolic bone diseases (discussed later in this chapter). The control of osteoblast and osteoclast activity, and therefore the balance between bone formation and destruction in normal remodeling, is not completely understood, but many factors play a role.

METABOLIC BONE DISEASE

Metabolic bone disease comprises four fairly common conditions in which there is imbalance between osteoblastic (bone forming) and osteoclastic (bone destroying) activity.

In **osteoporosis**, there is a slowly progressive increase in bone erosion, which is not adequately counteracted by new bone formation. Thus, the cortical bone is thinned, and the bone trabeculae are thinned and reduced in number, leading to general reduction in bone mass, but without distortion of architecture.

In **osteomalacia**, osteoblastic production of bone collagen is normal, but mineralization is inadequate. This leads to trabecular bone that is only partially mineralized and therefore soft and weak.

In **Paget's disease of bone**, there is excessive uncontrolled destruction of bone by abnormally large and active osteoclasts, with concurrent inadequate attempts at haphazard new bone formation by osteoblasts, producing physically weak woven bone.

In **hyperparathyroidism**, excessive secretion of PTH produces increased osteoclastic activity. There is excessive destruction of cortical and trabecular bone, with inadequate compensatory osteoblastic activity.

Patients with chronic renal failure develop the bone disease known as **renal osteodystrophy** as a result of mixed metabolic disturbance (mainly the combined effects of osteomalacia and hyperparathyroidism). The mechanisms are discussed below.

Osteoporosis is characterized by reduced bone mass and is the most common metabolic bone disease

Osteoporosis is characterized by generalized reduction in the mass of bone, the bone being composed of abnormally thin trabeculae. It is widespread in the elderly and is an important cause of morbidity and even mortality, the weakened bone being particularly predisposed to fracture with minimal trauma. In established osteoporosis, thinning of the cortical bone is combined with thinning and reduction in number of bone trabeculae (*Fig. 24.2*). The consequences of osteoporosis are related to the general weakening of both cortical and trabecular bone.

Bone pain, particularly in the back, is a common symptom, and imaging often shows a so-called 'compression fracture' of one or more vertebral bodies. Multiple compressions of vertebrae can lead to an overall loss of height, which may be compounded by uneven compression of vertebrae leading to bending of the spine anteroposteriorly (**kyphosis**).

Fractures of the neck of the femur and of the wrists are common complications of osteoporosis in the elderly; the cause is often relatively trivial (usually a fall). Elderly patients with a fractured neck of femur are an important component of the orthopedic workload, representing a substantial cost to the health services because of the often long and difficult postoperative return to mobility.

There are several different predisposing factors for the development of osteoporosis (see pink box).

It is most commonly encountered in post-menopausal women, when it is termed **senile osteoporosis**. It is believed that a major reduction in bone mass occurs in the 10 years after the onset of menopause, implying a hormonal influence for estrogen in maintaining bone mass.

Osteoporosis localized to one or both lower limbs is a common finding in people with paralysis due to neurological disease, in which case it is considered to be a form of **disuse atrophy**. Reduction in general mobility and activity may be a factor in osteoporosis in the elderly.

Osteoporosis is seen as a common complication of prolonged **corticosteroid therapy**. It is particularly important when the corticosteroids are being administered for diseases such as rheumatoid arthritis, in which there is also an element of disuse atrophy due to reduction in mobility. Osteoporosis can also be seen in some other endocrine disorders such as thyrotoxicosis and panhypopituitarism, and associations have been reported with liver disease and diabetes.

Genetics of osteoporosis

There is mounting evidence that there are genetic predispositions to osteoporosis. Linkage analysis suggests that there are multiple genes involved.

- A G-to-T polymorphism in a regulatory region of the collagen COL1A1 gene is significantly related to bone mass and risk of osteoporotic fracture in post-menopausal osteoporosis.
- Early-onset osteoporosis has been described in families associated with mutations in the COL1A1 gene on 17q and the COL1A2 gene on 7q.
- Polymorphisms in the vitamin D receptor gene and the calcitonin receptor gene (CALCR) have been suggested as genetic risk factors for osteoporosis in some studies.

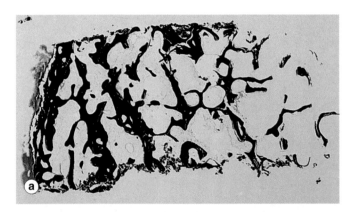

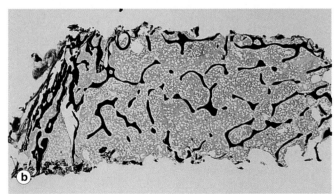

Fig. 24.2 Osteoporosis.
(a) Micrograph of a resin section of a bone biopsy from the iliac crest, showing normal cortical and trabecular bone. It has been stained with a silver method, which stains calcified bone black.
(b) Micrograph of bone from a patient with osteoporosis. When compared with (a), which shows bone mass of a normal patient of the same age, it is obvious that the cortical zone is narrower, and that the trabeculae are thinner and less numerous.

KEY FACTS
Main associations with osteoporosis

- Old age: particularly in post-menopausal women.
- Disuse: particularly in limb paralysis and, temporarily, in an immobilized limb following fracture.
- Peri-menopausal state: osteoporosis in post-menopausal women may be minimized by hormone replacement therapy.
- Prolonged corticosteroid therapy: particularly when given for rheumatoid arthritis and immunosuppression.
- Assorted endocrine disorders: there is a strong association with Cushing's disease and Cushing's syndrome, and a less strong association with thyrotoxicosis, diabetes and hypopituitarism.
- Miscellaneous factors include: liver disease, particularly alcoholic liver disease.

Osteomalacia is due to failure of mineralization of osteoid; 'rickets' is osteomalacia affecting children

In osteomalacia there is normal deposition of bone osteoid by osteoblasts, and bone architecture is normal. However, there is inadequate mineralization so that, for example, only the center of bony trabecula is adequately mineralized, the periphery being composed of soft unmineralized osteoid (*Fig. 24.3*). In adults this results in bone pain, sometimes due to microfractures of cortical plate and trabecular bone; the cortical microfractures can sometimes be seen radiologically (Looser's zone) and are most common in the bones of

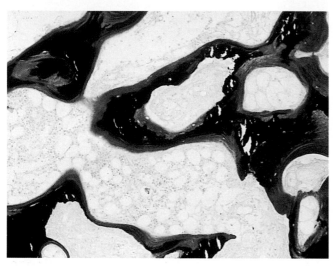

Fig. 24.3 Osteomalacia.
Micrograph of iliac crest bone embedded in acrylic resin without prior decalcification from a patient with osteomalacia. Note the broad zone of unmineralized osteoid (red) and the central zone of mineralized bone (black), in this section stained by the von Kossa silver technique.

the lower limb, which are also the site of major bone pain. In severe long-standing untreated osteomalacia in adults, softening of the long bones may lead to bowing of the legs.

In children, in whom the skeleton is not fully formed, osteomalacia leads to characteristic structural deformities of the long bones of the leg (severe bowing), distortion of the skull bone (leading to bossing), and enlargement of the costochondral junctions of the ribs (producing a characteristic 'rickety rosary').

Osteomalacia is usually the result of abnormalities of vitamin D metabolism

The metabolism of vitamin D and its association with bone mineralization is illustrated in *Fig. 24.4*. Through its effect on calcium metabolism, an inadequate supply of vitamin D, for whatever reason, is the most important cause of osteomalacia. Vitamin D deficiency may be due to:

- **Inadequate dietary intake**. Formerly the most common cause of osteomalacia in children, this is now rare in the western world, except in people who have extreme diets, e.g. pure vegans.

- **Inadequate body synthesis of vitamin D**. As vitamin D is synthesized in the skin under the influence of UV light, extensive covering of the skin for social and cultural reasons may be an important contributory factor in osteomalacia.

The above two factors are responsible for the high incidence of osteomalacia in natives of the Indian subcontinent living in the UK and other European countries. In Caucasians living in the west, the most important causes are:

- **Malabsorption due to intestinal disease**, for example after extensive small-bowel resection, treated and untreated Crohn's disease, and untreated celiac disease.

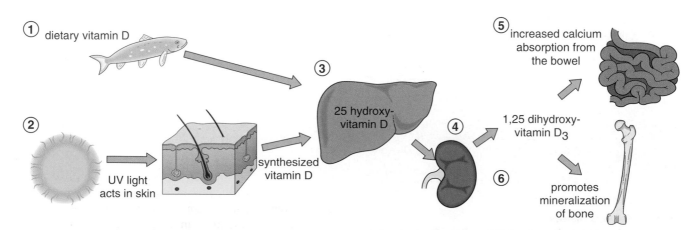

Fig. 24.4 Metabolism of vitamin D.
Some vitamin D is dietary (1) e.g. from fish and fish oil, but most is synthesized in skin (2) by the action of UV light on the precursor 7 hydrocholesterol. Both dietary and synthesized vitamin D undergo hydroxylation in the liver (3) to form 25 hydroxyvitamin D, which is further hydroxylated in the kidney (4) to the major active substance 1,25 dihydroxyvitamin D_3 which increases absorption of calcium by the small bowel (5) and promotes mineralization of bone (6).

• **Renal disease**. In chronic renal failure, conversion of vitamin D to its active metabolite (1,25 dihydroxy-vitamin D_3) by renal tubular epithelial cells is impaired, and osteomalacia is one of the important metabolic bone diseases associated with renal failure.

Rarely, liver disease and some drug therapies may interfere with vitamin D metabolism and have a role in the development of osteomalacia.

Metabolism of vitamin D

Vitamin D_3, from diet or produced in the skin, is metabolized in liver and kidney to produce the active form, which has effects on bone and gut (*Fig. 24.4*).

Paget's disease of bone is a common disease of unknown cause affecting bones in the elderly

In Paget's disease there is excessive uncontrolled resorption of bone by large abnormal multinucleated osteoclasts. Excessive osteoclastic erosion occurs in waves, leading to localized destruction of trabecular and cortical bone; each wave of bone destruction is followed by a vigorous but uncoordinated osteoblastic response, producing new osteoid in an attempt to fill the defects left by the osteoclasts. Both the osteoclastic erosion and the osteoblastic response are random, haphazard and unrelated to the functional stresses on the bone. As a result, the bone architecture is greatly distorted and, although there may be an increase in bone bulk, it is paradoxically weaker than normal. New bone formed as a repair attempt by the osteoblasts often has the characteristic woven, non-lamellar pattern indicative of rapid reparative deposition. Disruption of the bone architecture is followed by progressive fibrosis of the marrow spaces (*Fig. 24.5*).

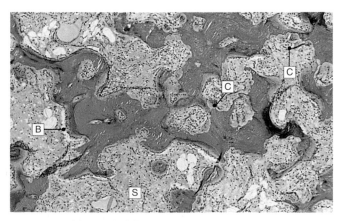

Fig. 24.5 Paget's disease.
Micrograph of a resin-embedded section of bone from a patient with Paget's disease. The bone trabeculae are irregular and abnormally broad. They are composed of woven bone with haphazard deposition of collagen. Osteoclasts (**C**) resorb bone, while osteoblasts (**B**) deposit new bone osteoid. There is associated fibrosis of marrow spaces (**S**).

Paget's disease may be widespread, affecting many bones, or confined to one area in a single bone (monostotic Paget's disease). Its cause is unknown, but a viral infection of osteoclasts has been postulated because of the observation that some abnormal osteoclasts in Paget's disease contain paracrystalline inclusions resembling paramyxovirus. However, no virus has been shown using sophisticated molecular techniques.

There are two common effects of Paget's disease. **Bone pain** is usually localized to the site of most active disease, Paget's disease characteristically waxing and waning. **Bone deformity** is usually seen only where there is extensive involvement of an entire bone or series of bones, e.g. there may be marked enlargement of the skull, or thickening, enlargement and bowing of the tibia. Most patients present with one or both of the above features, but some occasionally present with the complications of Paget's disease. For example, **nerve compression symptoms** are usually seen in association with Paget's disease of the skull, in which enlargement of the Pagetic bone can lead to cranial nerve palsies.

In cases of **pathological fracture**, although the bone is increased in bulk, it is weaker than normal and more likely to fracture with trivial trauma. Imaging illustrates that the fracture has occurred at a site of bone abnormality, and there may be radiological evidence of Paget's disease elsewhere in the same or other bones.

Malignant tumor, usually osteosarcoma, may develop in areas of long-standing active Paget's disease. Osteosarcoma is normally a disease of children (see page 520), and its development as a complication of Paget's disease is one of the very rare instances in which it is seen in the elderly.

Hyperparathyroidism produces bone erosion by stimulation of osteoclast activity

Parathyroid hormone (PTH) stimulates osteoclastic resorption of bone, with the release of calcium from the bone into the plasma. Its activity is normally finely controlled by a feedback mechanism whereby PTH secretion from the parathyroid gland is suppressed by a rise in plasma calcium concentration and stimulated by a fall. Failure of the feedback mechanism leads to excessive parathormone secretion, with continuing PTH output and excessive osteoclastic destruction of bone.

There are two main patterns of hyperparathyroidism. In **primary hyperparathyroidism** an autonomous parathyroid tumor, usually a parathyroid adenoma, secretes excess PTH continuously outside of the control of the feedback mechanism. In **secondary hyperparathyroidism** a persistently low serum calcium level (due to excess calcium loss in the urine in chronic renal disease) leads to continuous stimulation of the parathyroids by the feedback mechanism. This results in hyperplasia of all the parathyroid glands and a constant excessive secretion of PTH.

The effects on bone of constant PTH stimulation are unremitting osteoclastic resorption of bone, followed by compensatory attempts by osteoblasts to deposit new bone. In addition to the diffuse bone resorption affecting all bones, single or multiple focal osteolytic lesions are occasionally present in bone. To the naked eye, these lesions appear to be filled with soft, semi-fluid, brown material. These are the so-called **brown tumors**, which are composed of large masses of giant osteoclast-like cells and spindle cells associated with old and recent hemorrhage. Multiple brown tumors produce numerous osteolytic lesions in many bones, a condition sometimes called 'von Recklinghausen's disease of bone' or **osteitis fibrosa cystica**. Whether single or multiple, brown tumors are most common in primary hyperparathyroidism. In secondary hyperparathyroid bone disease due to renal failure, there is usually associated osteomalacia due to vitamin D₃ abnormalities resulting from renal tubular disease.

In primary hyperparathyroidism the serum calcium level is often greatly increased (**hypercalcemia**) because of the continuous release of calcium from bone in the absence of an effective feedback mechanism. In secondary hyperparathyroidism it is the presence of a pathologically low serum calcium level that stimulates PTH activity and calcium release from bone; the serum calcium level is therefore low (**hypocalcemia**) or normal because any calcium mobilized from the bone is almost immediately lost through the abnormal kidneys.

DATA SET
Renal bone disease

A 31-year-old man with polycystic kidney disease:

Plasma

Calcium	1.83 mmol/L	(2.2–2.6)
Phosphate	2.33 mmol/L	(0.7–1.4)
Albumin	32 g/L	(35–50)
Alkaline phosphatase	391 U/L	(80–280)
Urea	34 mmol/L	(1–6.5)
PTH	123 ng/L	(10–55)

Hypocalcemia is a common complication of chronic renal failure. Contributory causes include the lack of the active form of vitamin D, 1,25 dihydroxycholecalciferol, which is normally formed in the kidney by 1α hydroxylation of 25 hydroxycholecalciferol. Renal phosphate retention may also cause hypocalcemia, by precipitation of calcium phosphate. Hypocalcemia stimulates the release of parathyroid hormone (PTH). Secondary hyperparathyroidism and 1,25 dihydroxycholecalciferol deficiency result in metabolic bone disease, reflected in the raised alkaline phosphatase released from osteoblasts.

Renal osteodystrophy is a metabolic bone disorder associated with chronic renal failure

The term 'renal osteodystrophy' refers to metabolic and structural abnormalities of bone caused by the presence of chronic renal failure. There are two main components to renal osteodystrophy: **osteomalacia of renal origin** (due to failure of conversion of 25 hydroxyvitamin D₃ to the active principle 1,25 dihydroxyvitamin D₃ in the kidney because of tubular damage) and **secondary hyperparathyroid effects** (secondary to low serum calcium because of a combination of vitamin D deficiency, excess calcium loss in urine, and phosphate retention).

The bone in renal osteodystrophy therefore shows a combination of secondary hyperparathyroidism changes, excessive bone erosion by osteoclasts, and failure of mineralization of osteoid collagen.

A further factor occurs in patients who receive long-term hemodialysis for chronic renal failure. Such patients often retain increased quantities of aluminium, which become deposited in the bone in the site in which mineralization by calcium should be taking place, blocking calcification of the osteoid, and thus playing a role in the osteomalacia.

BONE FRACTURE

Bone fractures heal by granulation tissue formation and fibrous repair, followed by new bone formation in the fibrous granulation tissue

Caused by physical trauma, bone fracture is one of the most common abnormalities of bone. The degree of fracture can vary widely from a simple crack in the cortical bone to a complex multiple fracture with fragmentation and displacement of the bone pieces, associated with severe damage to the surrounding soft tissues and, sometimes, exposure of the bone fragments to the exterior through a large gaping wound (open 'compound' fracture).

The sequence of events in healing of a simple undisplaced fracture is illustrated in *Fig. 24.6*. For a fracture to heal efficiently it is important that all conditions are optimal; there are many factors that interfere with the satisfactory healing of fractures.

Delayed or abnormal healing of fractures can lead to non-union, in which the fractured bone ends do not join by bone

For proper fracture healing to take place it is essential that the fractured bone ends be in close apposition, that the fracture is immobilized, and that the patient's healing capacity is adequate.

Among the factors that detrimentally affect healing of bone is **poor blood supply** to the affected area. This is particularly important in certain areas such as the scaphoid bone in the wrist and the neck of the femur, both of which

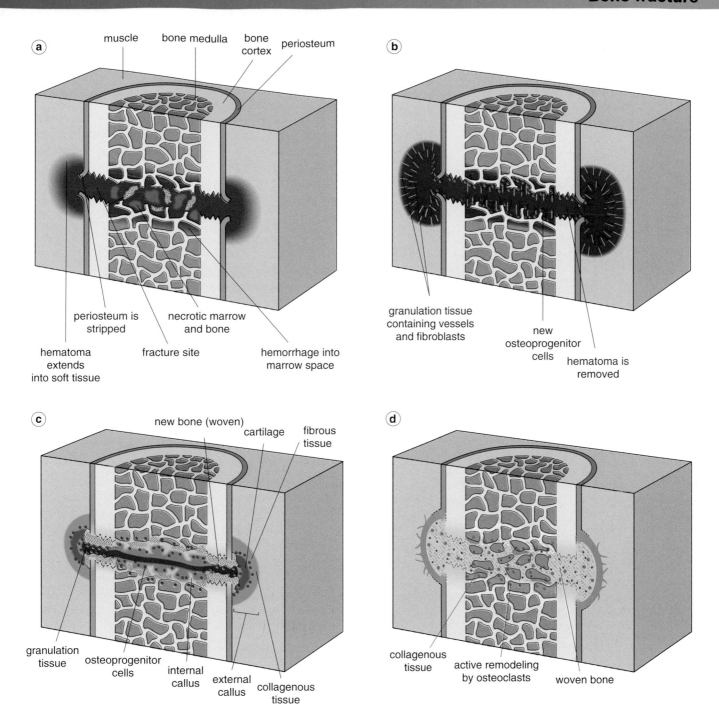

Fig. 24.6 Bone fracture.

(a) Due to tearing of blood vessels in the medullary cavity, cortex and periosteum, hematoma forms at the site of fracture. The periosteum is stripped from the bone surface. (b) Organization of the hematoma is associated with the migration of neutrophils and macrophages into the fracture hematoma; these cells phagocytose the hematoma and necrotic debris. This is followed by in-growth of capillaries and fibroblasts from surrounding tissue, producing fibrovascular granulation tissue. New osteoprogenitor cells develop from mesenchymal precursor cells. (c) Osteoblasts derived from osteoprogenitor cells migrate into the granulation tissue and differentiate into osteoid-synthesizing units, which proceed to deposit large quantities of osteoid collagen in a haphazard way, producing a woven bone pattern. **External callus** bridges the fracture site outside the bone and, if there is a significant gap between the bone ends, it may include cartilage. **Internal callus** bridges the fracture in the medullary cavity and rarely contains cartilage. When bone ends are closely apposed, direct ossification between fractured ends occurs. (d) Callus is usually well-established by the third week after fracture, but initial bony union is by woven bone, which is mechanically weak. Remodeling of callus occurs once the defect between the two bone ends is bridged by bony callus, taking many months. A combination of osteoclastic erosion and organized osteoblastic osteoid synthesis removes surplus calcified callus, replacing the inefficient bulky woven bone with compact organized lamellar bone.

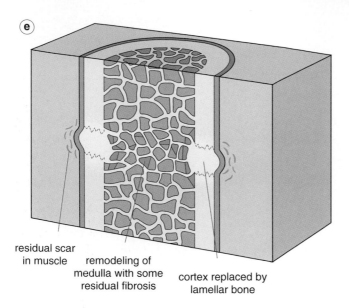

Fig. 24.6 (e) With time, remodeling creates new lamellar trabecular bone, which is orientated in a direction determined by the stresses to which the bone is exposed with mobilization. Even with remodeling, cortical irregularity and minor marrow space fibrosis persist at the site of fracture.

can be associated with avascular necrosis of fracture fragments. **Poor general nutritional status** (particularly where there is protein malnutrition or vitamin deficiencies) and **poor apposition of the fractured bone ends** (e.g. wide displacement, entrapped viable soft tissue between the bone ends, or excessive mobility) can also contribute to delayed or abnormal healing, as can **presence of foreign bodies** or large quantities of necrotic bone, **the presence of infection** (particularly in open fractures) and **corticosteroid therapy**.

The aim of treatment in fractures is to ensure close apposition of the bone ends, followed by firm immobilization so that the fractured bone ends cannot move during the formation of granulation tissue and callus.

When fractured bone ends are not closely apposed, or if any of the above local complicating factors are present, ossification of the callus does not occur, and the two bone ends are joined by fibrous tissue (**fibrous ankylosis**) which is unstable.

Fracture may occur with minimal trauma if the underlying bone is abnormal

For fracture of normal bone to occur, the causative trauma usually has to be severe. In contrast, trivial trauma may cause fracture when the underlying bone is abnormal (**pathological fracture**).

Among the common abnormalities predisposing to pathological fracture are **osteoporosis** (particularly in the femur and vertebral column in the elderly), **osteomalacia** (the fractures are often small microfractures without displacement), **Paget's disease of bone** (the Pagetic bone being structurally weak despite the increase in bulk), and **primary** or **metastatic tumor**. Metastatic carcinoma in bone is an important cause of pathological fracture. Bone metastases from carcinoma of the breast, bronchus, thyroid and kidney produce bone destruction (osteolytic metastases), which predisposes to fracture. Primary tumors of bone or bone marrow, such as giant-cell tumor of bone and myeloma, also play a role, as do some non-neoplastic bone lesions such as bone cysts.

Congenital bone disorders can also predispose to pathological fracture. The most important disorder is osteogenesis imperfecta, in which multiple fractures occur, often *in utero* and in infancy, with minimal trauma.

INFECTION OF BONE

Infection of bone is called 'osteomyelitis' and usually involves the cortex, medulla and periosteum

The main causative organisms include *Staphylococcus aureus*, *Escherichia coli* (particularly in infants and the very elderly), *Salmonella* (particularly in patients with sickle-cell disease), and *Mycobacterium tuberculosis*.

In osteomyelitis the infective organisms gain access to the medullary cavity of the bone by two main routes:

- **Direct access through an open wound.** This is an important cause after trauma, particularly when trauma has been followed by an open fracture, and can lead to failed or delayed fracture repair. It is also an important cause in postoperative patients who have had surgery on bones.

- **Blood-borne spread** following bacteremia from a focus of sepsis elsewhere, e.g. acute pyelonephritis. Tuberculous osteomyelitis is the result of blood-borne spread from a primary tuberculous infective lesion in the lung.

Occasionally, bone infection can be a complication of sepsis in adjacent soft tissues or organs, e.g. mastoiditis complicating bacterial middle-ear infection.

In all forms of osteomyelitis (except for TB) the marrow cavity becomes filled with a purulent acute inflammatory exudate, leading to necrosis of medullary bone trabeculae. Destruction of the cortical bone may lead to the discharge of pus into extraosseus connective tissue, and the infection may track through to the skin surface, producing a chronic discharging sinus.

Because the infection is localized to the confined space of the marrow cavity, the pus has little chance to drain without surgical intervention; inflammation tends to become chronic, with organisms remaining viable within the marrow cavity for many years.

Chronic osteomyelitis results, with extensive bone destruction, marrow fibrosis and recurrent focal suppuration. With chronicity, there is reactive new-bone formation, particularly around the inflamed periosteum, leading to a thickened and abnormally shaped bone.

In **tuberculous osteomyelitis**, the marrow cavity contains rapidly enlarging caseating granulomas which destroy trabecular and cortical bone.

BONE TUMORS

It is important to distinguish between tumors **of** bone and tumors **in** bone, since the most commonly seen tumors in bone are blood-borne metastases from other primary sites, and tumors of hemopoietic cells located within the marrow spaces of bones, particularly myeloma.

Primary tumors derived from the cells involved in bone formation and modeling are comparatively rare, the most common lesions being **osteosarcoma** and **chondrosarcoma**. Less common primary tumors of bone are summarized in *Fig. 24.7*.

Some intraosseous lesions with the appearance of bone tumors are not true neoplasms, but represent hamartomatous malformations, non-neoplastic proliferative disorders, or non-neoplastic cysts.

The most common malignant tumor in bone is metastatic blood-borne malignancy, usually metastatic carcinoma

Five common carcinomas have a particular predilection for metastasizing to bone: adenocarcinoma from the breast, carcinoma of the bronchus (particularly small-celled undifferentiated carcinoma), adenocarcinoma of the kidney, adenocarcinoma of the thyroid, and adenocarcinoma of the prostate (which often produces sclerotic reaction in bone).

Most metastatic tumor cells within bone marrow spaces lead to erosion of trabecular bone, either directly or through osteoclast stimulation, and to erosion of bone cortex (osteolytic metastases). This leads to bone weakness, predisposing to **pathological fracture**, which may be the first presenting feature. Carcinoma of the prostate often produces metastatic deposits in which there is stimulation of new bone formation (osteosclerotic metastases), particularly in the lumbo-sacral vertebrae.

Metastatic carcinoma in bone commonly produces bone pain, usually localized to the site of metastatic deposits. In addition to bone pain and fracture, it may produce symptoms due to three effects: **extensive replacement of**

Fig. 24.7
Important primary tumors of bone

Name	Presumed cell of origin	Age and sex incidence	Common sites	Behavior
Osteoid osteoma	Osteoblast	Adolescents M > F	Lower limb	Benign, osteosclerotic; painful
Non-ossifying fibroma	Uncertain	Child/adol M > F	Long bones of lower limb	Benign, osteolytic; occasionally multiple
Chondromyxoid fibroma	Uncertain	Adol/young adult M > F	Long bones esp. tibia	Benign osteolytic
Enchondroma	Chondrocyte	Young adults M > F	Bones of hands	Usually benign and expansile
Giant-cell tumor	Osteoclast	20–40 yrs M > F	Around knee	Mostly benign, may recur; rarely malignant
Chordoma	Notochord tissue	40+ yrs M > F	Sacrum	Local bone destruction and invasion
Osteosarcoma	Primitive osteoblast	(i) 10–25 yrs (ii) over 65 yrs M > F	(i) Around knee (ii) At site of Paget's disease	Highly malignant; early metastasis to lungs
Chondrosarcoma	Chondrocyte	30–60 yrs M > F	Spine and pelvis	Malignant; local spread and distant metastasis
Ewing's tumor	Uncertain	Child/adol M > F	Midshaft of long bones	Malignant; early and extensive metastasis

bone marrow, leading to leukoerythroblastic anemia; **symptoms due to hypercalcemia**, caused by release of calcium from bone by the destructive osteolytic process; and **nerve and spinal compression**, particularly in vertebral metastases.

Myeloma is a tumor of plasma cells that commonly presents as single or multiple bone tumors

The vast majority of plasma-cell tumors occur in bone (see page 314), arising in one of three patterns: **diffuse plasma-cell infiltration of marrow**, in which there is no discrete tumor formation; **solitary osteolytic bone lesion** (**solitary plasmacytoma**), which is an unusual pattern; and **multiple osteolytic lesions in many bones** (**multiple myelomatosis**).

Bone pain (and occasional pathological fracture) is an important clinical feature of myeloma. However, symptoms are not confined to bone because the neoplastic plasma cells produce abnormal amounts of immunoglobulin (usually IgG); this is of a single clonal type (monoclonal gammopathy) as it is produced by a single clone of neoplastic plasma cells. Many of the clinical features of myeloma are the result of the replacement of normal marrow cells by malignant plasma cells, together with the impact of the abnormal IgG (and its component heavy and light chains) on blood viscosity and renal function. Myeloma is discussed in greater detail in Chapter 15.

The most common malignant primary tumors of bone are osteosarcomas and chondrosarcomas

Osteosarcoma is a malignant tumor of osteoblasts, which occurs in adolescent children, most commonly in boys. The majority arise around the knee, either in the lower end of the femur or in the upper end of the tibia, although a small percentage occur in other long bones such as the humerus, or in the upper end of the femur.

The tumor causes gradually increasing pain around the knee, and is often well-advanced at the time of clinical and radiological diagnosis. The tumor originates in the medullary cavity close to the metaphyseal plate and spreads extensively within the medullary cavity, eventually eroding through cortical plate and extending into soft tissue. The malignant osteoblasts produce varying amounts of osteoid collagen, some of which becomes mineralized (*Fig. 24.8*); this mineralization in the tumor can be demonstrated radiologically and by other imaging methods, and is particularly apparent when the tumor is invading soft tissues.

The tumor grows rapidly and metastasizes early via the bloodstream, usually producing pulmonary metastases. The prognosis has generally been poor (5–10% 5-year survival), but is improving with the adoption of earlier surgical treatment, combined with radiotherapy and chemotherapy. Osteosarcoma in adults is largely confined to elderly patients

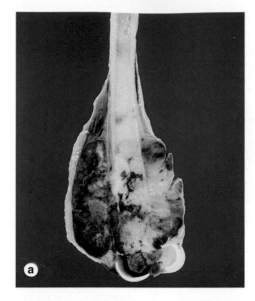

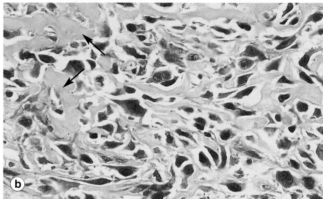

Fig. 24.8 Osteosarcoma. An osteosarcoma is seen at the lower end of the femur. Tumor expands and destroys the bone (a). Histologically (b), neoplastic osteoblasts secrete pink-stained osteoid (arrows) between cells.

with a long history of active Paget's disease of bone, the tumor occasionally developing in an area of Paget's disease.

Chondrosarcoma mainly occurs in adults, usually the middle-aged or elderly, and is particularly common in the bones of the pelvis

Chondrosarcomas are slow-growing tumors that often reach a large size, expanding the bone and eventually breaking through the periosteum into surrounding soft tissue, but usually maintaining a clearly defined border. Although malignant, they metastasize very late in most cases, the majority being low-grade well-differentiated tumors, histologically very similar to benign cartilaginous tumors; a few are high-grade poorly-differentiated tumors with marked pleomorphism and high mitotic activity; they grow rapidly with early blood-borne metastases.

Macroscopically, tumors have a glistening white appearance (*Fig. 24.9*). Radical local surgery may be curative in the low-grade group.

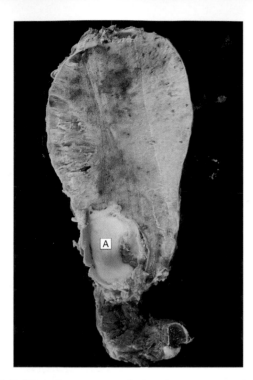

Fig. 24.9 Chondrosarcoma. A chondrosarcoma replaces much of the bone of the pelvis. The acetabulum (**A**) is still visible. Cartilage tumors have a glistening white appearance, similar to that of normal cartilage.

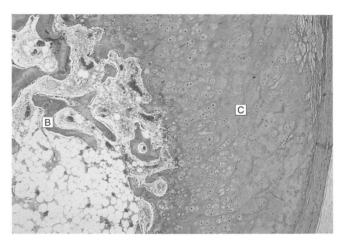

Fig. 24.10 Cartilage-capped exostosis. Histology of an exostosis shows a cartilage cap (**C**) overlying bone (**B**).

The most common benign bone-forming tumor is osteoid osteoma

Osteoid osteomas are mainly found in the long bones of the lower leg, arising in adolescents and young adults. They present with bone pain localized to the area of the lesion. Usually less than 2 cm in diameter, they are radiologically characteristic, with a central dense area surrounded by a halo of bone lucency. Histologically they are composed of active osteoblasts, which deposit large irregular masses of osteoid collagen in a haphazard manner.

So-called **giant osteoid osteoma** or **benign osteoblastoma** is a larger tumor with similar histological features, mainly affecting the bones of the hands and feet and vertebrae; these are often more cellular than small osteoid osteomas, more locally aggressive, and can recur after incomplete excision.

Ivory osteoma is composed of densely compact bone of cortical type with Haversian systems. It arises as small round nodules, usually in the skull bones.

The most common benign tumor of cartilage-forming tissue is the chondroma

Chondromas, most commonly found in the small bones of the hands and feet, may be single (solitary enchondroma) or multiple (enchondromatosis). The tumors arise in the metaphysis and may originate from residual nests of cartilage cells left behind as bone growth proceeds. They are composed of cartilaginous matrix containing scattered benign chondrocytes. A solitary chondroma at the periphery rarely undergoes malignant change, but this occasionally happens in multiple enchondromatosis. The term 'enchondroma' is used to indicate that these tumors arise within the bone, to distinguish them from the benign osteochondroma, which grows as a nodular exophytic lesion.

Benign osteochondroma grows as an exophytic nodule from the metaphysis of a long bone

Benign osteochondromas, also known as **cartilage-capped exostoses**, may be solitary (as a sporadic abnormality in childhood and adolescence) or multiple (as in the autosomal dominant condition **hereditary multiple exostoses**). They are composed of a nodule of protuberant bone covered by a cap of cartilage and an outer layer of perichondrium (*Fig. 24.10*). In children the cartilage layer may be thick, but this thins as the patient ages. Lesions are found most commonly in the humerus, femur and upper end of the tibia. Chondrosarcomatous change is rare in single sporadic lesions, but is more common in hereditary multiple lesions.

Giant-cell tumor of bone, sometimes called 'osteoclastoma', arises in the epiphysis of a long bone

Giant-cell tumors of bone are osteolytic lesions that occur in young and middle-aged adults, generally being more common in women. The bone is replaced by a mass of large multinucleated giant cells resembling large osteoclasts, which are embedded in a supporting spindle-celled stroma. The lesions expand into the metaphysis and, with enlargement, may erode the cortical bone. However, they rarely penetrate the periosteum or articular cartilage. These locally aggressive tumors are difficult to treat because of frequent recurrence at the site of inadequate local excision, particularly if an attempt has been made to eradicate the tumour by curettage. Because of their apparent osteoclast component, and the presence of hemorrhage and cystic change associated with bone destruction, giant-cell tumors of bone can be difficult to distinguish from the **brown tumor of hyperparathyroidism** and also from an unusual lesion called **aneurysmal bone cyst**. The latter can usually be distinguished by the different site, most commonly in the vertebrae or in the shaft of a long bone. Unlike giant-cell tumors, aneurysmal bone cysts can usually be cured by curettage.

BONE DISEASE IN CHILDREN

Children have a general predisposition to fracture for many reasons to do with their levels of physical activity in play and sport, and their limited ability to sense risk and danger. However, they are more likely to be physically abused than any other group, and multiple or repeated fractures in a child should ring alarm bells. The most important malignant tumor of bone, osteosarcoma, is principally limited to children. A rarer malignant tumor in bone, **Ewing's tumor**, is also largely confined to children. Pediatric bone disorders resulting from abnormal skeletal development are an important group of diseases, the most important examples being **achondroplasia** and **osteogenesis imperfecta**.

Achondroplasia is an inherited disorder of growth cartilage that results in dwarfism due to short limbs

Achondroplasia is an autosomal dominant condition, caused by mutations in the fibroblast growth factor-3 (FGF-3) receptor located on chromosome 4. Mutations cause permanent activation of the receptor, causing arrest of bone growth. There is a high incidence of spontaneous mutation, accounting for its sudden appearance in a child with normal parents. The condition is recognizable at birth and is compatible with normal survival and life-span. The trunk develops normally, but the head may be enlarged, with a depressed bridge of the nose and prominent forehead.

Osteogenesis imperfecta may lead to spontaneous fractures with minimal trauma in infancy and childhood and, occasionally, *in utero*

Osteogenesis imperfecta is due to mutations in the gene coding for Type I collagen, resulting in abnormal collagen formation in osteoid. This leads to widespread weakness of bone, with multiple fractures frequently leading to severe deformity. Formation of the teeth is also affected, and the collagen of the sclera of the eye is poorly formed, giving rise to the characteristic physical sign of pale-blue sclerae.

The pattern of inheritance can be either dominant or recessive, and there is marked variation in severity; the most severe cases are usually stillborn because of extensive intrauterine fractures.

In community practice, Osgood–Schlatter's disease is a common cause of bone pain in children

Osgood–Schlatter disease mainly affects children between 10 and 12 years of age. Patients present with pain just below the knee, and have a tender spot at the site of the tibial tubercle at the upper end of the tibia. This is due to the tendon insertion separating from the front of the tibia, pulling away with it a small fragment of bone from the tibial tubercle; the bone fragment may undergo avascular necrosis as a result of this avulsion fracture.

Perthes' disease is an important cause of hip pain in children

Perthes' disease mainly affects boys and usually begins between the ages of 5 and 10 years. It is due to avascular

Molecular genetics of osteogenesis imperfecta

Osteogenesis imperfecta ranges in severity from minor increase in the rate of fractures to the most severe form, which leads to intrauterine or perinatal death. It results from mutations in the genes that encode the chains of Type I collagen, the major structural protein in bone osteoid.

There are over 20 genes coding for collagen, distributed over 10 chromosomes; more than 50 mutations in the COL1A1 and COL1A2 genes (responsible for coding for Type I pro-collagen) are known to produce various types of osteogenesis imperfecta. Some are point mutations in which, for example, glycine is replaced by cystine or arginine. When such point mutations occur near the carboxy-terminus, they seem to produce lethal disease, those near the amino-terminus producing mild disease.

All collagen-gene mutations resulting in osteogenesis imperfecta are associated with decreased production of normal Type I pro-collagen. When abnormal Type I pro-collagen is produced, the phenotype can range from very mild to lethal, depending on the nature of the mutation. However, when minimally abnormal Type I pro-collagen is produced, the phenotype is generally very mild, i.e. with normal stature and little or no bone deformity.

necrosis of the femoral head and epiphysis. As a result, the head of the femur undergoes collapse, fragmentation and flattening, and the femoral neck becomes shorter. The dead bone of the epiphysis becomes revascularized and there is some new bone formation, but the deformity of the femoral head persists, predisposing to osteoarthritis in adulthood. The lesion is usually unilateral, and there may be a family history. The pathogenesis is uncertain.

DISEASES OF JOINTS, TENDONS AND SOFT TISSUES

Bones are joined together by **joints**, which allow varying degrees of movement between the adjacent bone ends; some joints permit considerable movement, others allowing only limited movement. The most important type of joint that permits considerable movement is the synovial joint, illustrated in *Fig. 24.11*. Excessive movement at the joint is limited by a strong joint capsule and an enclosing ligament, assisted by attached muscles and tendons. In joints in which there is only limited movement the bones are joined by fibrous or cartilaginous tissue, e.g. the fibrocollagenous and cartilaginous intervertebral discs between adjacent vertebral bodies.

Patients with diseases in the joints and associated tendons and soft tissues may present to the orthopedic surgeon,

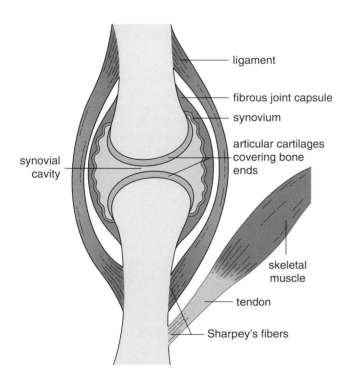

Fig. 24.11 Synovial joint.
Diagram of a simple synovial joint showing the two articulating bone ends separated from each other by synovial fluid and enclosed within a fibrocollagenous capsule. Surrounding ligaments and tendinous muscle attachments prevent excess movement.

rheumatologist or, in the case of acute post-traumatic lesions, in Accident and Emergency Departments. Furthermore, such patients are numerous in general community practice, comprising a significant percentage of the persistent uncured attenders at clinics of all types. Thus, these diseases are an important cause of morbidity in patients of all ages (with the exception of very young children), although the nature of the disorder is different at different ages. For example, osteoarthritis of the hip is the most common disease in the elderly, whereas in adolescents and young adults the consequences of trauma to tendons, ligaments and joints are most common. Constant repetitive actions involving the same series of joints over a long period of time (often in the course of the patient's occupation) can lead to repetitive strain symptoms, with mixed features of joint, tendon and ligament disease (see page 529).

Inflammatory disease of joints (arthritis and synovitis) has four main causes

Inflammatory disease of joints, which is grouped under the terms **arthritis** and **synovitis**, has four main causes: **degenerative**, e.g. osteoarthritis; **autoimmune**, e.g. rheumatoid arthritis, SLE, rheumatic fever (see page 525); **crystal depositions**, e.g. gout and other crystalline arthropathies; and **infective**, e.g. tuberculous arthritis.

Osteoarthritis is a common and important degenerative disease with both destructive and reparative components

Osteoarthritis may arise as a primary disorder, as well as arising secondary to other joint malfunctions (particularly abnormal loading or structural deformities). The pathological changes involve cartilage, bone, synovium and joint capsule, with secondary effects on muscle (*Fig. 24.12*). The main factors in development of osteoarthritis are aging, abnormal load on joints, crystal deposition, and inflammation of joints.

In general, osteoarthritis affects joints that are constantly exposed to wear and tear. It is an important component of occupational joint disease, e.g. osteoarthritis of the fingers in typists, and of the knee in professional footballers.

Previous abnormality of the joint predisposes to the early development of severe osteoarthritis (sometimes called 'secondary osteoarthritis'); causes include:

- Congenital abnormality of joints.
- Trauma to joints (including trauma resulting from lack of sensory innervation).
- Inflammatory joint disease.
- Avascular necrosis of bone.

Clinically, osteoarthritis can be classified according to the main presenting features, namely:

- **Primary generalized osteoarthritis** is usually associated with the development of Heberden's nodes on the fingers and is commonest in post-menopausal women.

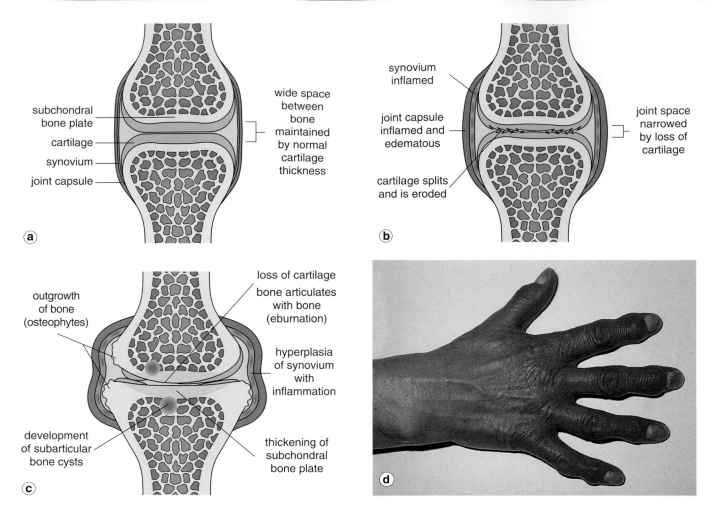

Fig. 24.12 Pathological changes in osteoarthritis.
(a) In a normal synovial joint the distance between the bone ends seen on radiography is maintained by the thickness of articular cartilage. (b) The early change in osteoarthritis is **destruction of articular cartilage**, which splits (fibrillation), becomes eroded and leads to narrowing of the joint space on radiography. There is inflammation and thickening of the joint capsule and synovium. (c) With time, there is **thickening of subarticular bone** caused by constant friction of the two naked bone surfaces, leading to a highly polished bony articular surface (eburnation). **Small cysts** develop in the bone beneath the abnormal articular surface. **Osteophytes** form around the periphery of the joint by irregular outgrowths of bone. There may be **reactive thickening of the synovium** due to inflammation caused by bone and cartilage debris. Inflammatory changes are also often seen. **Atrophy of muscle** is caused by disuse following immobility of the diseased joint. (d) In osteoarthritis of the hands, osteophytes on the interphalangeal joints of the fingers are termed 'Heberden's nodes' and appear as small nodules.

- **Erosive inflammatory osteoarthritis** describes forms of osteoarthritis in which there is severe inflammation and erosion of cartilage, with rapid progression.
- **Hypertrophic osteoarthritis** describes forms with florid osteophyte formation and bone sclerosis, with a slow progression and relatively good prognosis.

Irrespective of the site, osteoarthritis causes pain and limitation of movement at the affected joint, sometimes associated with visible swelling; this is partly due to the presence of bony osteophytes and partly to fluid accumulation in the joint cavity and synovial fibrosis. In osteoarthritis affecting the cervical vertebrae (**cervical spondylosis**), osteophytes compressing emerging spinal nerves are responsible for much of the symptomatology.

Rheumatoid disease is a systemic autoimmune disease that particularly affects the joints, leading to arthritis

Rheumatoid arthritis is a common and important cause of inflammatory joint disease, although it is but one manifestation of a generalized systemic disorder (see Chapter 25). It is characterized by the presence of a circulating autoantibody, 'rheumatoid factor' (**seropositive arthritis**), which distinguishes this form of disease from several other inflammatory joint diseases (**seronegative arthritis**).

Rheumatoid arthritis mainly affects peripheral synovial joints such as the fingers and wrists, but can also affect the knees and more proximal joints. Women are affected two to three times more commonly than men, and the usual

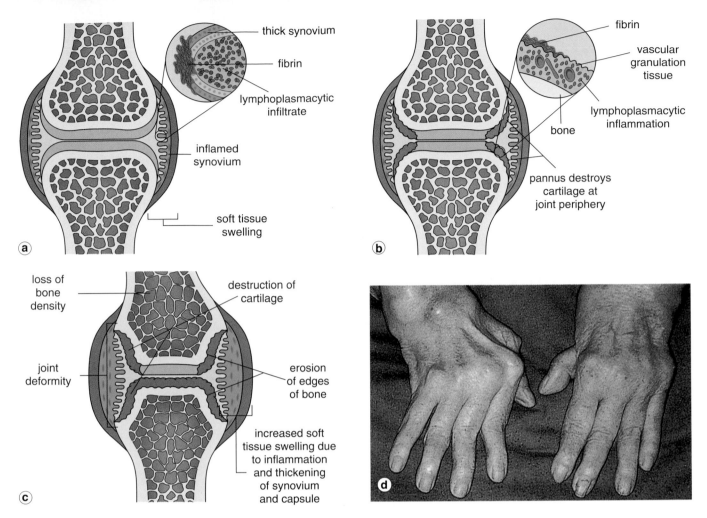

Fig. 24.13 Rheumatoid arthritis.
(a) The early pathological change in rheumatoid arthritis is **rheumatoid synovitis**. The synovium is swollen and shows a villous pattern. There is a great increase in chronic inflammatory cells (mainly lymphocytes and plasma cells) in the synovial stroma, often with an exudate comprising **fluid**, which produces an effusion in the joint space, and **fibrin** which is deposited on the synovial surface. Soft tissue swelling from synovial inflammation can be marked. (b) With time, there is **articular cartilage destruction**; vascular granulation tissue grows across the surface of the cartilage (**pannus**) from the edges of the joint, and the articular surface shows loss of cartilage beneath the extending pannus, most marked at the joint margins. (c) The inflammatory pannus causes **focal destruction of bone**. At the edges of the joint there is osteolytic destruction of bone, responsible for 'erosions' seen on radiographs. This phase is associated with joint deformity. (d) The characteristic deformity and soft tissue swelling associated with long-standing rheumatoid disease of the hands.

age of onset is between 35 and 45 years. The affected joints become swollen, painful and warm, often with redness of the overlying skin. There are three main pathological changes, as illustrated in *Fig. 24.13*.

In long-standing chronic disease the articular cartilage may be largely destroyed and replaced by fibrous pannus; the underlying bone shows osteolytic erosions, and the synovium lining the joint capsule is greatly thickened and chronically inflamed. The loss of articular surface can lead to the development of secondary osteoarthritic changes, particularly in weight-bearing joints such as the knee. Unlike most other autoimmune arthropathies, rheumatoid arthritis is chronic and progressive. It usually leads to eventual joint deformity, with secondary features (e.g. muscle wasting) due to disuse of the disorganized joint.

The joint changes are often associated with the development of subcutaneous **rheumatoid nodules**; these, and other features seen in systemic rheumatoid disease, are discussed in Chapter 25.

Autoimmune arthritis also occurs in patients with SLE, rheumatic fever and systemic sclerosis

Several types of arthritis are associated with systemic autoimmune disease processes.

SLE is a systemic disease in which joint involvement is a frequent but minor feature. The arthropathy is often transient, affecting the same type of joints as rheumatoid disease (i.e. fingers, wrists and knees), but is rarely progressive and does not lead to joint deformity.

Rheumatic fever is described in Chapter 10 because of its severe impact on the heart. A transient flitting arthritis is a characteristic feature of the acute stage, and the larger joints (e.g. elbow, knee and ankle) are most frequently involved. Like the arthritis of SLE, it is transient and does not lead to chronicity and joint deformity. There may occasionally be subcutaneous nodules similar to those seen in rheumatoid arthritis, but they are localized to the region of the affected joint; these nodules are transient and do not persist as in rheumatoid arthritis.

Systemic sclerosis is a systemic connective tissue disease that mainly affects the skin, bowel, lung and kidneys; occasionally there is an associated arthritis, with features similar to those of mild rheumatoid arthritis.

The crystal arthropathies are caused by deposition of crystals in joints causing arthritis

The crystal arthropathies are diseases characterized by deposition of crystals in joints and soft tissues. Affected patients usually present with an episode of acute mono-arthritis or oligoarthritis, inflammation being caused by the deposition of the crystals, sometimes called a 'chemical' arthritis. With time, inflammatory changes lead to development of a chronic arthritis with features of osteoarthritis (secondary osteoarthritis).

The nomenclature of this group of disorders is in a state of change; the term 'gout' is used as a clinical description for joints affected by crystal deposition, which must then be refined by demonstrating the type of crystal involved. There are two main types of crystal arthropathy: **urate gout** (gout) and **calcium pyrophosphate gout** (pseudogout).

Less common forms of crystal arthritis are caused by deposition of hydroxyapatite, which also causes peri-arthritis and tendinitis. Oxalate arthritis may be seen in patients with hyperoxaluria, and in some patients on hemodialysis.

The most important crystal arthropathy is caused by deposition of uric acid, causing true gout

Urate gout is characterized by deposition of urate crystals in joints and soft tissues, which is caused by the presence of hyperuricemia. Uric acid is normally derived from the breakdown of purines and is excreted in the urine. Urate gout is largely confined to men, although some women develop it after the menopause. It can present at any time between the ages of 20 and 60 years, most cases presenting with an acute attack of arthritis, often affecting the big toe.

There are two main reasons for hyperuricemia:

- **Underexcretion of uric acid**. Seen in the majority of patients with urate gout, but of uncertain origin. It is clinically associated with hyperlipidemia, renal failure, alcohol consumption, and some drugs (diuretics).

- **Overproduction of uric acid**. High-cell turnover (leukemia and chemotherapy for tumors).
- Rare congenital enzyme defects of purine metabolism.

In the majority of patients with urate gout, disease is probably the result of polygenic factors leading to under-excretion of uric acid (primary gout). Only a small proportion of patients develop urate gout as a result of overproduction of uric acid.

Urate crystals are deposited in certain joints, particularly the metatarsophalangeal joint of the big toe, stimulating an acute inflammatory reaction leading to a painful acute arthritis (*Fig. 24.14*). Uric acid crystals are also deposited in the soft tissues around joints, where their presence excites a foreign-body giant-cell reaction. These soft tissue masses may enlarge to produce a palpable mass composed of white chalky material (**tophi**) (*Fig. 24.15*).

In the joint, the urate crystals are deposited on the surface of the articular cartilage to form a white powdery deposit, beneath which the cartilage shows degenerative changes. Attacks of acute gouty arthritis are intermittent and may be precipitated by dietary indiscretion. The pain of an acute attack is excruciating, and various inflammatory

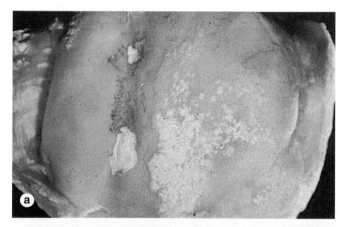

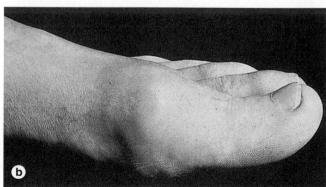

Fig. 24.14 Gouty arthritis.
This is an opened joint showing a white deposit of urate crystals on the articular surface in gout (a). The most commonly affected site is the big toe (b); the metatarsophalangeal joint becomes inflamed, often developing secondary osteoarthritis with deformity.

mediators (particularly interleukin-1) have been implicated in the pain, edema and redness seen in the acutely inflamed joint. The stimulus to inflammatory mediator release is probably the deposition of crystals in the joint cavity, synovium and periarticular soft tissues, and neutrophil polymorphs can be seen to phagocytose urate crystals in the joint fluid. The diagnosis is best made by examining aspirated synovial fluid from the joint for the presence of crystals.

Recurrent attacks of acute gout affecting the same joint eventually lead to articular cartilage destruction, chronic synovial thickening and a secondary osteoarthritis; this is called **chronic gouty arthritis**.

Urate crystals deposited in the kidney may lead to an interstitial nephritis and to renal calculi composed of uric acid. Precipitation of urates in renal tubules may produce acute tubular necrosis and acute renal failure in leukemic patients with massive purine release after chemotherapy.

Hyperuricemic gout has a familial tendency and is believed to be polygenically inherited (see page 76). It is associated with an increased predisposition to hypertension and coronary artery disease.

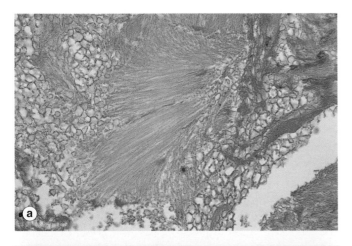

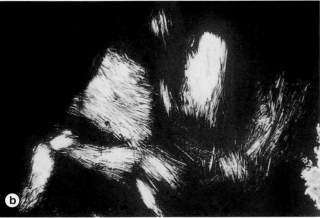

Fig. 24.15 Uric acid crystals forming tophi.
(a) This photomicrograph shows characteristic fine feathery crystals of urate from a gouty tophus. (b) The crystals are particularly obvious and beautiful when viewed under polarized light.

Calcium pyrophosphate crystal arthritis is also known as 'pseudogout'

Crystals of calcium pyrophosphate dihydrate may be deposited in the articular cartilage of joints (**chondrocalcinosis**). The cartilage deposition may be entirely asymptomatic, but if the crystals are shed into the joint space, patients develop an acute arthritis similar to that seen in urate gout. The shedding of crystals may be precipitated by trauma, intercurrent illness, or may be spontaneous. The joint most commonly affected is the knee, followed by the wrist, shoulder and ankle. The diagnosis is made by demonstrating pyrophosphate crystals in aspirated joint fluid; as the disease may closely mimic true urate gout, it is often also called 'pseudogout'.

This type of crystal arthritis is most common in the elderly as a primary degenerative disorder, some cases being due to an autosomal dominant trait. Patients under the age of 60 years with this form of arthritis may have a secondary form associated with hyperparathyroidism, hemochromatosis or less common metabolic or endocrine disorders.

With time, damage to cartilage by pyrophosphate may lead to development of secondary osteoarthritis.

Infective arthritis is mainly due to pyogenic bacteria and mycobacteria

Pyogenic bacteria may gain access to a joint either by bloodstream spread or, more commonly, by local trauma or spread from adjacent infective foci. Infective arthritis is a well-recognized complication of prosthetic surgery at the knee and hip (the most common sites for infective arthritis of all types and causes).

A wide range of bacteria may be responsible, but *Staphylococcus aureus*, streptococci and *Haemophilus* are the most important. Blood-borne infection by the gonococcus is an important cause in teenagers and young adults. Children and young adults are the most likely groups to develop septic arthritis, most cases in older adults being associated with penetrating injury such as open fractures, insertion of surgical prosthesis, and non-sterile intra-articular injections of steroids for established autoimmune arthritis. Intravenous drug users are particularly likely to develop septic arthritis associated with Gram-negative bacteremia.

Almost all cases of infective arthritis affect a single joint only, but some cases of gonococcal arthritis and arthritis in intravenous drug abusers may affect more joints. The diagnosis can be established with certainty only by aspiration of fluid from the joint space, which is examined cytologically for evidence of pus and microorganisms, and then cultured.

Tuberculous arthritis is now rare, and is the result of bloodstream spread from pulmonary TB. In adults the vertebral column is most often affected; tuberculous osteomyelitis leads to collapse of affected vertebrae, particularly in the lumbar and lower thoracic spine (Pott's disease), and paravertebral collection of tuberculous caseous material occasionally tracks down the psoas muscle (psoas abscess) to point in the groin. In children, tuberculous arthritis mainly affects the hip and knee. Synovial biopsy shows caseating tuberculous granulomas.

Infective arthritis in syphilis and brucellosis is now rare. Arthritis due to the spirochete *Borrelia burgdorferi* (Lyme disease) and to some fungal infections such as blastomycosis occurs in outbreaks in the USA and Europe.

The seronegative spondylarthritides are characterized by peripheral joint inflammation without circulating rheumatoid factor

The seronegative spondylarthritides are a set of inflammatory arthritides that involve peripheral joints, as well as the sacroiliac joint and spine; they are distinguished from rheumatoid disease by the absence of circulating rheumatoid factor. The cause and pathogenesis of these diseases are not known, but an autoimmune reaction is suggested by a high incidence of the antigen HLA B27. The most important conditions are **ankylosing spondylitis, psoriatic arthropathy, enteropathic arthropathy** and **reactive arthritis**.

Ankylosing spondylitis is almost as common as rheumatoid disease, but is often not clinically diagnosed. It typically presents in late adolescent and young adult Caucasian males, as an ankylosing arthropathy that begins in the lumbar vertebral spine and sacroiliac joints, extending upwards to involve thoracic and cervical vertebrae. In addition, there is often involvement of peripheral joints, mainly the hips and knees. The disease progresses slowly and unremittingly. In the early stages, there is inflammation (with a heavy lymphocytic infiltrate) of the ligaments around the vertebrae, which subsequently heals by dense fibrosis and ossification of the ligaments to form a rigid shell linking the periphery of the vertebral bodies. Eventually the vertebral column becomes fused, inflexible and rigid (bamboo spine). Systemic manifestations include recurrent iritis and aortic valve incompetence. Over 90% of men with ankylosing spondylitis have the HLA B27 antigen (less than 10% of the normal population have this antigen).

Reactive arthritis follows genital infection with *Chlamydia trachomatis* in some susceptible individuals, or arises after bacterial gastroenteritis due to *Salmonella*, *Yersinia* or *Campylobacter*. The HLA B27 antigen is present in 80% of affected patients.

Reiter's syndrome comprises arthritis, urethritis, and conjunctivitis. The arthritis usually affects the knee or the ankle, and the clinical and histological features of the arthropathy resemble those seen in rheumatoid arthritis, with chronic inflammatory synovitis. There is spontaneous resolution in some affected patients, but symptoms are still present in 80% of patients after 5 years. In a minority of cases, severe spondylitis and features very similar to ankylosing spondylitis develop.

Psoriatic arthropathy occurs in 5–10% of patients with psoriasis. It tends to involve the distal interphalangeal joints

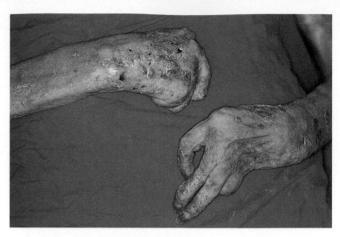

Fig. 24.16 Psoriatic arthropathy.
The arthropathy associated with some cases of psoriasis can be severely destructive leading to marked deformity, pain and loss of function, particularly in the hands. Note that the patient has severe active psoriasis of the skin of the hands and arms.

(a characteristic feature), but there may be a more widespread symmetrical multi-joint involvement, with sacroiliitis and spondylitis. The joint changes are similar to those seen in rheumatoid arthritis, and osteolytic destruction of bone is particularly common in association with the arthritis involving the distal interphalangeal joints (*Fig. 24.16*). Patients who have associated spondylitis usually have the HLA B27 antigen.

Acute trauma to joints and associated tendons, ligaments and soft tissues is responsible for considerable morbidity

Direct trauma to joints may lead to **dislocation**, a condition predisposed to by lax ligaments. Although the trauma required to produce dislocation is usually severe, some patients have a predisposition to dislocation of certain joints, particularly the shoulder joint; in severe cases, dislocation may occur without trauma when the joint is held in a certain position. Most dislocations that occur without associated fracture are the result of sports injuries, and are therefore seen in the young and otherwise healthy. Shoulders and finger joints are particularly commonly affected by sports injuries. When the dislocated bones have been relocated in their proper configuration in the joint, there may be residual inflammation because of direct trauma of the dislocated bone on the joint capsule and surrounding ligaments; this trauma sometimes leads to permanent weakness of the soft tissues surrounding the joint, predisposing to further episodes of dislocation.

Lacerations of the menisci in the knee joint may occur in either normal or degenerate menisci

The **menisci** of the knee joint are principally composed of dense compact collagen in which the fibers are mainly

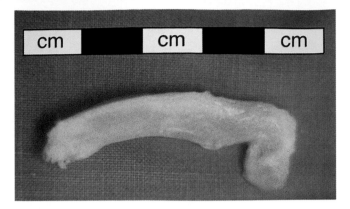

Fig. 24.17 Torn knee meniscus.
The specimen is a severely damaged knee meniscus showing the so-called 'bucket-handle' appearance. The inner part of the meniscus has completely separated away.

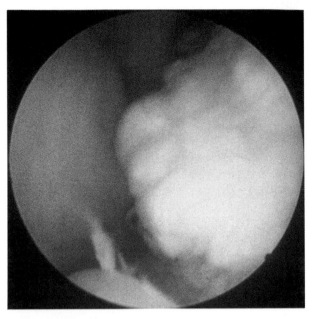

Fig. 24.18 Torn cruciate ligament.
This photograph was taken during arthroscopic exploration of the knee. It shows the completely separated remains of a cruciate ligament, now shrunken and white following its detachment after rupture. It is from the knee of an English soccer player.

arranged in a circumferential pattern, probably to withstand the circumferential stress to which they are exposed. In addition there are some radial fibers which probably hold the circumferential fibers together and resist splitting (which might result from excessive compression).

Lacerations of a structurally normal meniscus in young people are almost invariably the result of sporting injury, usually severe rotational stress in a partly bent knee. They mainly involve the medial meniscus, the laceration commonly initially appearing as a split separating the circumferential fibers. The split tends to extend throughout the meniscus to produce the so-called 'bucket-handle tear' (*Fig. 24.17*). Occasionally there is a partial radial tear which may lead to irregular fragmentation on the medial aspect of the meniscus.

In the elderly, laceration of the meniscus usually occurs with minimal trauma in menisci that are abnormal as a result of myxoid degeneration of the collagen, leading to separation, fraying and occasional cyst formation. Focal calcification of the menisci is a characteristic feature of pseudogout due to pyrophosphate crystal deposition (see page 527).

Torn ligaments are a common consequence of overstretching at a joint

Ligament tears are usually the result of excessive physical exercise, and are therefore a common sporting injury, although the ligaments on the lateral aspect of the ankle are frequently damaged by acute overstretching during trivial stumbles (sprained ankle).

The intra-articular cruciate ligaments within the knee joint are frequently torn in sporting injury (*Fig. 24.18*). Rupture of the cruciate ligaments leads to chronic instability of the knee; because these ligaments are long structures stretched between two bone surfaces, tearing leads to their pulling apart and spontaneous natural healing is usually unsuccessful because of the distance between the separated ends. Current treatment options include replacement by various types of prosthetic ligament.

Acute tendon damage is usually due to either penetrating injuries or spontaneous rupture

Industrial or domestic injuries, particularly to the hand, are an important cause of laceration of one or more **flexor or extensor tendons of the hand**, with consequent loss of the ability to flex or extend the affected fingers. Spontaneous rupture of the Achilles tendon usually occurs as a sporting injury following acute over-stretching. Healing is slow even when the torn ends of the long cylindrical tendons are closely apposed surgically. Tendon is very slow to heal because it is a densely collagenous fibrous tissue with a comparatively poor blood supply and very scanty fibroblasts. For good healing accurate apposition of the torn ends is essential. The gap is filled by vascular granulation tissue, with eventual fibroblast proliferation and deposition of new densely hyaline collagen. A further problem is that these long tendons frequently run in a surrounding synovial-lined tendon sheath, and healing by fibrosis of the damaged tendon sheath leads to fibrous adhesions between sheath and tendon, limiting the sliding movement of the tendon within the sheath. Repeat surgery to separate these adhesions and to mobilize the healed tendon is frequently necessary, as is strenuous physiotherapy.

'Tennis elbow' is due to repeated damage to the tendinous insertion of the extensor muscles of the forearm on the lateral aspect of the elbow

'Tennis elbow' (also called lateral epicondylitis) is pain and tenderness at the lateral epicondyle of the elbow joint where the common tendon of the extensor muscles of the forearm is inserted into bone. Minor tears in this tendon occur with certain strenuous movements (particularly vigorous single-handed backhand strokes in tennis), and repetition of these movements perpetuates the damage. Since tendon tissue is relatively acellular, healing is slow and incomplete. The repeatedly damaged tendon shows areas of myxoid degeneration of collagen, increased vascularity, replacement of dense tendon with looser collagenous scar, and there may be foci of calcification. In some cases there may be reactive thickening of the periosteum of the lateral epicondyle around the site of insertion.

Although tennis elbow is frequently the result of a sporting injury, it also occurs in manual workers whose job involves repeated rotation and gripping movements of the wrist and lower arm with the elbow partially flexed. Because of the different strains involved, 'golfer's elbow' involves the medial epicondyle of the elbow, with tendon damage similar to that seen in tennis elbow.

Carpal tunnel syndrome is a common condition affecting the hand, particularly in women

The flexor tendons of the fingers enter the hand at the wrist through a space called the **carpal tunnel**. This is floored by the carpal bones of the wrist and the roof is formed by a strong dense fibrocollagenous band called the flexor retinaculum. With the flexor tendons in the tunnel is the median nerve (see *Fig. 24.19*), and compression of this nerve is responsible for the symptoms of the syndrome, mainly pain and paresthesia in the distribution of the median nerve (thumb, all of the index and middle fingers, and the radial half of the ring finger). In severe or late cases there may be loss of sensation in this distribution, wasting of the muscles of the thenar eminence, and occasionally pain up to the elbow. The syndrome is due to reduction in the size of the space in the carpal tunnel and may result from degeneration and thickening of the flexor retinaculum, thickening of the synovium on the inner surface of the flexor retinaculum and the outer surfaces of the flexor tendons, a reduction in the fluid in the space, or a combination of all three.

It is about four times more common in women than in men, and can be a transient symptom in the later stages of pregnancy, the symptoms frequently occurring early in the morning and improving during the day. Persistent carpal tunnel syndrome is thought to be related to excessive use of the wrist in sport or the work place, but some cases follow Colles' fracture of the wrist, rheumatoid arthritis and patients with renal failure on hemodialysis with long-standing arteriovenous shunts at the wrist.

de Quervain's tenosynovitis is due to thickening of the tendon sheath of the thumb abductors at the radiostyloid process

The tendons of the thumb abductors (extensor pollicis brevis and abductor pollicis longus) pass through a small

normal carpal tunnel

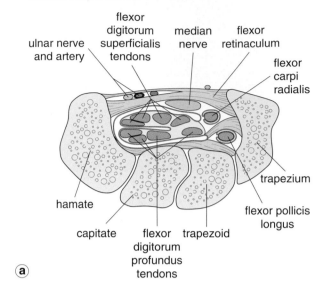

(a)

carpal tunnel syndrome

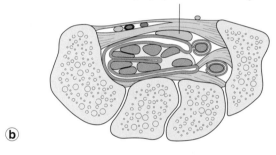

(b)

Fig. 24.19 Diagram showing carpal tunnel syndrome.
(a) The contents of the normal carpal tunnel containing the long flexor tendons of the fingers and thumb, together with the median nerve, enclosed by the bones of the hand and the flexor retinaculum. The outer surface of the long flexor tendons is coated by a synovial sheath (blue) which is normally thin.
(b) The features of carpal tunnel syndrome in which the median nerve is compressed and damaged, usually by thickening of the synovium over the long flexor tendons.

compartment roofed by a tight fibrous bridge just before the styloid process of the radius. This compartment is very variable in size and shape, and is sometimes divided into two compartments by a vertical septum.

Certain repetitive twisting movements at the wrist with the fingers and thumb flexed may produce localized thickening of the tendon sheaths of the two tendons, reducing the space within the compartment. The tendon sheaths show increased vascularity and marked edema, often followed by varying degrees of fibrous thickening. This produces pain and tenderness on the radial side of the wrist at the site of the compartment.

'Trigger finger' is due to thickening of the tendon sheath of a flexor profundus longus tendon

The most commonly affected fingers are the middle and ring fingers, but it may involve the thumb in infants. The mechanism in most cases is thought to be repeated external trauma or chronic friction to the tendon and tendon sheath leading to local thickening of the tendon sheath by fibrosis, edema and hypervascularity, and probably also to the anular ligament which overlies it at the base of the finger. As a result of the thickening the tendon finds it increasingly difficult to slide under the anular ligament, often making a popping noise as it passes through with difficulty. Repeated attempts to pass through lead to a worsening of the thickening of the two components until eventually the tendon will not pass through unless manually assisted by forced extension of the finger. Eventually the tendon and finger become stuck in the flexed position.

Repetitive strain injury (RSI) particularly involves the upper limb

Repeated overuse of muscle, tendons and joints in the upper limb, particularly on a regular basis over a long period of time in an occupational activity, may lead to a combination of degenerative changes of the joints (osteoarthritis – see page 523), and degenerative changes in tendons and ligaments, often leading to laxity of ligaments and fibrous thickening of the tendon sheath (stenosing tenosynovitis – see page 530). Although the individual components may be quite minor, together they can lead to significant morbidity, with joint pain and tenderness, limitation of movement, and swelling if there is a significant degree of osteoarthritis.

The details of all the pathological changes involved are not fully documented, but the symptom complex is known as **repetitive strain injury**. It is not yet clear whether the overuse is causative or merely exacerbates abnormalities already present. The etiological role of repetitive strain injury in such common wrist and hand conditions as carpal tunnel syndrome and de Quervain's tenosynovitis is still in dispute, but the recognition of the entity has led to better ergonomic design of seating, work desk heights and equipment, particularly in occupations involving keyboard work.

Intervertebral disc disease is a common and important cause of back pain and neurological symptoms

The intervertebral discs not only permit a limited degree of movement between adjacent vertebrae, they also act as shock absorbers, and are constantly exposed to vertical compressive forces. Each disc is composed of cartilaginous end-plates, with densely collagenous anulus fibrosus surrounding a central slightly gelatinous nucleus pulposus (*Fig. 24.20*). The narrow cartilaginous end-plate is most prominent in the young.

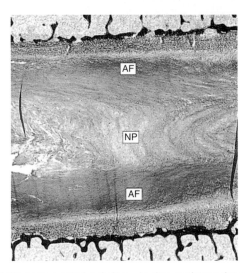

Fig. 24.20 Intervertebral disc. In disc prolapse the soft nucleus pulposus (**NP**) herniates through the tough anulus fibrosus (**AF**) to compress nerve roots.

Abnormalities of the disc occur with increasing age; in the elderly the disc becomes shrunken and has a less gelatinous nucleus pulposus. Most clinically significant episodes of intervertebral disc disease occur in young people, who have a bulky, non-shrunken disc with abundant nucleus pulposus.

The most common disease is that associated with displacement of the nucleus pulposus from its central position, the most clinically significant being posterior displacement, which can produce pressure on the emerging nerve roots or on the contents of the spinal canal. This can lead to nerve-root compression with pain in the distribution of the damaged nerve.

Sometimes the nerve is involved in the acute inflammatory reaction to the displaced disc material, and the symptoms abate when the inflammatory changes settle down. However, symptoms are always likely to recur if there is further disc displacement, further inflammation, or fibrous healing of the inflammation. The displacement of nucleus pulposus material is often called **disc herniation**. It may be mild, with nucleus pulposus causing an intact but thinned anulus fibrosus to bulge (**protrusion** and **prolapse**), or severe, with nucleus pulposus extruding through the ruptured anulus fibrosus (**extrusion**).

DISORDERS OF SOFT TISSUE

The most commonly seen soft-tissue disorders in community practice are those due to trauma. They include **skeletal muscle injury** due to tearing of fibers, which is the result of over-stretching after vigorous or extraordinary exercise. This is most frequently seen in young healthy adults participating in vigorous sports. There may be associated ligament and tendon damage (see page 529). **Blunt trauma** produces hematomas in muscle, subcutaneous fat and fascia,

open trauma producing laceration of skeletal muscle and fascia with bleeding (usually the result of a road traffic accident or a severe fall). There is often an associated fracture of underlying bone.

Skeletal muscle can heal by fibrosis, although some functional fiber loss is experienced, together with disuse atrophy (which follows immobilization during healing).

Tumors of soft tissue are rare except for subcutaneous lipoma

Benign tumors composed of adipose tissue are very common in the subcutaneous fat, but may also occur deep within muscle masses (**intramuscular lipoma**). They are slowly growing, soft, lobulated, well-circumscribed tumors on the trunk or limbs of adults, and are usually solitary but may be multiple. Multiple lipomas are often tender, histologically showing an increased number of blood vessels (**angiolipoma**) or increased amounts of fibrous tissue (**fibrolipoma**). The subcutaneous tumors are entirely benign and usually well circumscribed, although the deep intramuscular lipomas have ill-defined margins, are difficult to remove surgically, and recur frequently, with occasional malignant change to a **liposarcoma** supervening.

The most important group of connective-tissue tumors with malignant potential are those that show fibrohistiocytic differentiation. Believed to be derived from primitive fibroblasts that retain the potential to show histiocytic differentiation, their histogenesis is still uncertain. Benign **fibrous histiocytomas** are very common tumors in the dermis (see page 506), but **malignant fibrous histiocytoma** (**MFH**) is rare (although it is still the most common malignant soft-tissue tumor). They occur in adults, principally the elderly, and usually present as an enlarging painless mass deeply located in the thigh and, occasionally, the lower leg. Some are deeply located in the muscle compartments, but others are more superficial, often being subcutaneous. These tumors are slowly infiltrative, with a high recurrence rate; a proportion show blood-borne metastatic spread. A variant of this tumor can occur in the retroperitoneum, producing a large mass compressing the ureters and distorting the kidneys.

True tumors of skeletal muscle are very rare, although **rhabdomyosarcoma** is probably the most common primary soft-tissue tumor in infants and children.

Tumors derived from nerve sheath are common within soft tissues and in the subcutis

One of the most common tumors of soft tissues is derived from support cells of peripheral nerves and is termed a **peripheral nerve sheath tumor**.

Benign schwannoma (**neurilemmoma**) occurs in adults as a well-circumscribed, slow-growing tumor, usually in the subcutaneous tissue in the head and neck or upper limb. These lesions are completely benign, but surgical removal entails damaging the nerve to which they are attached.

Neurofibroma is a benign tumor that is usually solitary, but multiple in von Recklinghausen's neurofibromatosis. The solitary lesions most commonly occur in the subcutaneous tissue of young adults, whereas the multiple lesions occur in other sites as well, particularly in the cauda equina. Malignant change may occur in the multiple lesions, but is virtually unknown in solitary tumors. These tumors are also discussed in Chapter 21.

Important multisystem diseases

Clinical Overview

Many diseases are specific to one organ or system, but there are a number of important diseases that cause damage in many tissues and organs and that involve a number of systems, being termed **multisystem diseases**. Multisystem disorders can be divided into three main categories:

- **Disorders of immune or autoimmune basis.** In this chapter we discuss in some detail systemic lupus erythematosus (SLE), progressive systemic sclerosis, rheumatoid disease and sarcoidosis, although some aspects of each are also discussed in other chapters relating to other systems which are particularly affected (e.g. see Chapter 24 for the joint manifestation of rheumatoid disease, Chapter 17 for the renal lesions in SLE). Systemic vasculitis could also easily have been included in this chapter, but is mainly dealt with in Chapter 10.

- **Disorders involving the storage or deposition of abnormal substances.** Amyloidosis is still an important disease in this group, though its incidence is falling. The metabolic storage disorders such as the glycogenoses and lipidoses are particularly important in pediatrics since the responsible gene defects are now being identified, offering greater accuracy of prenatal diagnosis early in pregnancy. Also, bone marrow transplant offers hope of a cure in some of the disorders. Hemochromatosis and Wilson's disease are also examples of this type of multisystem disorder.

- **Disorders involving systemic metabolic defects affecting many tissues.** Diabetes mellitus is the most important example. It is dealt with here in recognition of its impact on many organs and tissues, rather than in association with the islets of Langerhans of the pancreas in Chapter 16.

SYSTEMIC LUPUS ERYTHEMATOSUS

This is a very common (though frequently undiagnosed) condition in the general population, particularly common in young and middle-aged women. It is one of the so-called 'connective tissue disorders' in which patients produce antibodies to a very wide range of their own tissues ('auto-antigens'). The cause is unknown, but it has been postulated that the stimulus to the production of the abnormal autoantibodies may be sensitizing drugs or chemicals, or unidentified viral infection. Drugs and chemicals have been implicated because of the known development of SLE following the use of many drugs, particularly hydralazine.

Many tissues and organs are involved in SLE, but synovial joints, skin, kidneys and brain are the major target organs

The diagnosis of SLE is based on a combination of clinical features and the result of laboratory investigation, primarily the identification of the autoantibodies, and particularly those antibodies directed against nuclear DNA (see blue box on page 535). As so many different organs and tissues may be involved, the ways in which the disease can present are many and varied (*Fig. 25.1*). The range of features that can occur in SLE is shown well by the American Rheumatism Association List of Diagnostic Criteria for SLE (in order of specificity):

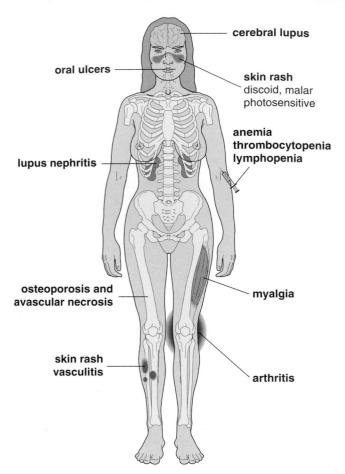

Fig. 25.1 Multisystem manifestations of systemic lupus erythematosus. SLE affects a wide range of tissues and organ systems.

- Discoid skin rash.
- Neurological disorder.
- Malar skin rash.
- Skin photosensitivity.
- Oral ulceration.
- Renal abnormality (lupus nephritis).
- Evidence of immunological disorder.
- Hematological disorder.
- Serosal inflammation.
- Presence of antinuclear antibody.
- Arthritis.

Skin rashes of various types occur in about 80% of all patients with systemic lupus

One of the most common tissues affected in SLE is the skin. The most common patterns of skin rash are:

- **Chronic discoid LE:** round ('discoid'), red scaly telangiectatic plaques, usually on face and scalp, and less commonly on the hands. Follicular plugging with keratin is common, particularly in the scalp and facial lesions. The lesions heal from the center, with the skin

becoming atrophic, often with loss of pigment. Involvement of the scalp may lead to patchy hair loss (see page 509); this is a cause of **scarring alopecia**.

- **Malar skin rash:** a symmetrical, slightly raised red erythematous rash on the cheeks and across the bridge of the nose. The characteristic distribution of broad patches on the cheeks joined by a narrower band across the nose has led to this being called the 'butterfly' rash.
- **Photosensitivity reactions:** rashes in light-exposed areas, worse when there has been increased sun exposure, may be of either of the above malar or discoid patterns, but may also be non-specific. Direct immunofluorescence of sun-exposed but non-lesional skin shows IgG, IgM and complement in the epidermal basement membrane in patients with SLE, irrespective of the clinical pattern of the skin disease. These represent immune complex deposits on the dermal side of the basement membrane, within the intercellular matrix and between collagen fibers.
- **Vasculitic skin lesions:** these occur as either an acute purpuric neutrophilic vasculitis in the upper dermis, or a lymphocytic vasculitis producing slightly raised erythematous patches, and are important features of skin rashes in lupus. Their significance is often missed because the rashes do not conform to the classical discoid or malar types described above.

The SLE variant that is known as **mixed connective tissue disease** (MCTD) has skin lesions less commonly than classic SLE, but many patients have a non-specific lymphocytic vasculitis at some stage in the illness, and eventually develop Raynaud's phenomenon.

Oral mucosal lesions in SLE produce superficial erosions and ulcers

Clinically and histologically, the oral lesions in SLE closely resemble oral lichen planus (see page 225) with red erosions, but they are found rather more commonly on the hard palate than is lichen planus. A characteristic histological feature of oral LE is the presence of extensive basal layer destruction, similar to that seen in lichen planus and in skin lesions. Oral mucosal lesions occur in about 20% of patients with SLE.

Neurological and psychiatric disorders are common in SLE, and may be the presenting symptom

The most common feature of neurological involvement in SLE is a non-organic psychiatric disorder of unknown cause; occasional cases that come to autopsy show either acute neutrophilic or lymphocytic vasculitis in the brain. Patients may also have a wide range of organic brain disorders, such as focal demyelination, microinfarction and neuronal loss, leading to a variety of symptoms. Grand mal epileptic seizures are an important clinical manifestation of cerebral lupus. Vascular occlusion is the result of anti-phospholipid antibodies causing platelet aggregation.

It is important to remember that some of the neurological manifestations in SLE may be the result of the treatment rather than the disease, particularly corticosteroid therapy.

Kidney involvement in SLE is common, and is an important cause of morbidity and mortality

Renal involvement in lupus is common, and the severity can vary from minor abnormalities (such as asymptomatic albuminuria) to severe glomerular disease leading to renal failure. The main abnormalities in renal involvement in SLE are in the glomerulus, where there can be a wide range of structural abnormalities. There may also be extra-glomerular vascular abnormalities and tubular damage, particularly interstitial nephritis.

Lupus nephritis may mimic other forms of glomerular disease by showing the following patterns: focal segmental mesangial glomerulonephritis, focal segmental proliferative glomerulonephritis with tuft damage, membranous nephropathy, and membranoproliferative pattern of lupus nephritis.

These patterns of glomerular structural abnormality are discussed and illustrated in greater detail on page 366. The basis of the glomerular damage in all patterns is the deposition of immune complexes in the glomerulus. The complexes may be deposited in the basement membrane (leading to basement membrane thickening), or in the mesangium (leading to mesangial expansion); immuno-fluorescence methods show that the immune complexes contain three types of immunoglobulin, IgG, IgA and IgM, and two types of complement, C3 and C1q.

The detection of this 'full house' of immunoglobulins and complement factors, together with the particular locations of the immune complexes in relation to the glomerular basement membrane, are important factors in distinguishing lupus glomerulonephritis from non-lupus patterns.

Hematological abnormalities are common in SLE

Patients with SLE frequently have hematological abnormalities, some having an unknown cause, and others having an autoimmune mechanism.

- **Normocytic hypochromic anemia**.
- **Autoimmune hemolytic anemia** (approximately 10% of cases), with red-cell antibodies and positive Coombs test.
- **Reduced peripheral white cell count**, usually due to disproportionate reduction of lymphocytes (lymphopenia).
- **Thrombocytopenia**, sometimes associated with the presence of antiplatelet antibodies.

- **Predisposition to thrombosis**, particularly if there are anticardiolipin/lupus anticoagulant antibodies.

Musculoskeletal symptoms may be the earliest presenting feature of SLE

SLE frequently presents clinically with musculoskeletal symptoms. Joint pain and other symptoms of arthritis occur in about 90% of all patients, and may precede the recognition of SLE by some years. The main rheumatological disorders of SLE are **arthritis**, **bone disease** and **myalgia**.

Arthritis which is misdiagnosed sometimes as rheumatoid arthritis or asymmetrical polyarticular arthritis, usually begins in the fingers, wrists and knees. Avascular bone necrosis may contribute to the arthropathy. The synovial surfaces may show fibrin deposition, and the articular cartilage shows changes similar to those seen in mild rheumatoid arthritis.

Bone disease usually presents as disproportionately severe osteoporosis for the age. It is difficult to separate the osteoporosis due to SLE from that due to the corticosteroids used in treatment. Avascular bone necrosis is common in SLE, appearing to be polyarticular, and usually being associated with the joints showing the most severe arthritis.

Myalgia in the form of pain in skeletal muscles, is a very common feature of SLE, and is frequently neglected clinically since it is difficult to dissociate from the pain due to co-existing arthritis. Muscle biopsy in patients with significant myalgia frequently shows a lymphocytic vasculitis.

Immunological investigation of suspected SLE

There is a cluster of antibodies that are aimed against the nuclei (antinuclear antibodies – ANAs) that can be used for diagnosis. These are not specific to SLE, as they can occur in some of the lupus-overlap syndromes with other connective tissue diseases.

- **Anti-dsDNA** (antibody against double-stranded DNA) is the most frequently detected and specific autoantibody.

- **Anti-ssDNA** (antibody against single-stranded DNA) may be found in SLE, but is also found in other diseases.

- **Anti-DNA histone** is found particularly commonly in drug-induced SLE.

Antibodies are useful in the detection of other types of systemic connective tissue disease.

PROGRESSIVE SYSTEMIC SCLEROSIS (PSS)

Systemic sclerosis is one of the so-called 'connective tissue diseases', and affects many systems and organs. It is three times more common in women than in men, and occurs mainly in middle-aged or elderly women. The main abnormality is an excess formation of fibrous tissue in tissues. The fibrous tissue is particularly collagenous, and leads to rigidity of the affected tissue, often with the destruction of specialized cells. Vessel wall thickening and perivascular fibrosis are characteristic features of systemic sclerosis, and are responsible for slowly progressive ischemic damage in a wide range of tissues. The skin is the most commonly affected organ in systemic sclerosis, but the alimentary tract, lung, kidney and heart may also be involved (*Fig. 25.2*).

Skin involvement in systemic sclerosis is called 'scleroderma'

In systemic sclerosis, the skin involvement consists of dermal thickening through the process of fibrous replacement of normal dermal structures. This thickening often extends into the subcutis, and leads to gradually increasing rigidity of the skin with tightening and atrophy of the overlying epidermis. The lesions affect particularly the fingers and the face: the fingers becoming hard, rigid and shiny (*Fig. 25.3*), and the face showing a characteristic tautness of the skin with overlying epidermal atrophy and indrawn margins of the mouth.

In the fingers there may be associated Raynaud's phenomenon, and, in old long-standing cases, there may be calcification of the soft tissues, particularly around the finger joints (calcinosis cutis). The dermal fibrosis leads to destruction of skin appendages, so the skin becomes hairless and eccrine sweat ducts are damaged.

This pattern of skin involvement is usually associated with involvement of the internal organs, but there are a few cases where the scleroderma remains localized to the skin. **Morphea** is the name given to single (rarely multiple) skin lesions which have the histological and clinical features of localized scleroderma. Morpheic lesions are initially creamy-coloured, thickened plaques on the trunk or limbs, sometimes with a purple edge in the actively growing phase. The lesions eventually become depressed with atrophic epidermis. Multiple areas may coalesce.

Involvement of the alimentary tract in systemic sclerosis particularly affects the esophagus

Proliferating fibrosis with collagenosis in the esophageal muscle wall leads to the destruction of the smooth muscle, and its replacement by collagenous fibrous tissue; nerve fibers in the esophageal wall are also damaged by the fibrosis, and there is often thickening of the blood vessels. These changes result in a thickened, rigid esophageal wall,

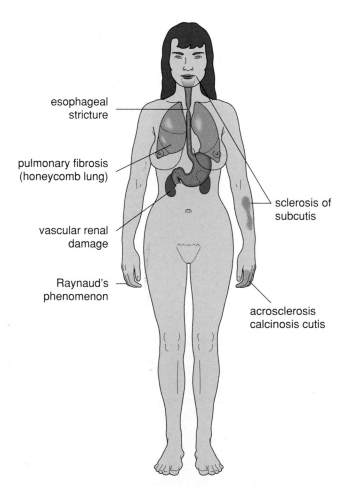

Fig. 25.2 Multisystem manifestations of systemic sclerosis. Systemic sclerosis affects a wide range of tissues and organ systems, often as a result of vascular obliteration.

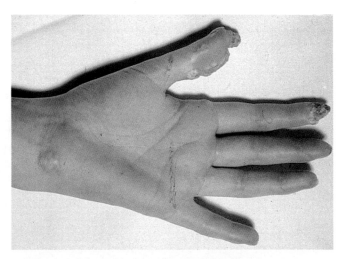

Fig. 25.3 Systemic sclerosis. The fingers in some patterns of systemic sclerosis are narrowed with tight shiny skin. Subcutaneous calcification (**calcinosis cutis**) can also be seen as white spots on the ends of the fingers.

which is often incapable of coordinated contraction and therefore unable to produce efficient peristalsis. As a result, reflux esophagitis with inflammation and even ulceration are common, and these may lead to the presence of fibrous strictures.

Lung involvement in systemic sclerosis leads to extensive interstitial fibrosis and 'honeycomb lung'

Progressive fibrosis of the pulmonary interstitium leads to appearances that are similar to those seen in end-stage interstitial pneumonitis. Respiratory bronchioles, alveolar ducts and alveolar walls are progressively destroyed, until the lung is a fibrous network that contains large cystic spaces; this is termed 'honeycomb lung' (see page 207).

Kidney involvement in systemic sclerosis is largely the result of vessel abnormalities and their effects on the glomeruli

Kidney involvement in systemic sclerosis usually presents acutely with evidence of severe small vessel and glomerular damage. The appearances of the afferent arterioles are very similar to those seen in malignant hypertensive disease of the kidney, with an intimal proliferation of small arteries and arterioles leading to the almost complete occlusion of the lumen; this is also associated with fibrinoid necrosis of some of the afferent arterioles and of portions of the glomerular tuft. These renal changes in progressive systemic sclerosis are called **acute scleroderma kidney**.

RHEUMATOID DISEASE

Rheumatoid disease is a multisystem connective tissue disease in which the dominant effects are on the joints, giving **rheumatoid arthritis**; the changes in the joints are described in Chapter 24.

The disease is more common in women than in men, and there is a genetic predisposition, although the cause or causes remain unknown. Rheumatoid disease also affects the skin, lungs, blood vessels, eyes, and the hemopoietic and lymphoreticular systems (*Fig. 25.4* on page 538). The treatment for rheumatoid disease may itself cause pathology, e.g. steroid-induced osteoporosis, analgesic-related ulceration of stomach, and drug-induced renal disease.

Rheumatoid arthritis is a symmetrical polyarthritis, characterized by the destruction of articular cartilage and its replacement by chronic inflammatory pannus

The histological changes in rheumatoid arthritis have been described on page 525. In most cases, the disease first attacks the finger joints, followed, in order of frequency, by the metatarsophalangeal joints and the joints of the

ankles, wrists, knees, shoulders, elbows and hips (*Fig. 25.4*). However, the disease may also affect joints such as the temporomandibular joint, the synovial joints of the spine (particularly the upper cervical spine), and occasionally the joints of the larynx.

Skin is involved in rheumatoid disease by the formation of rheumatoid nodules or the presence of vasculitis

The most frequent skin lesion in rheumatoid disease is the **rheumatoid nodule** (*Fig. 25.4b*), a subcutaneous firm nodule located usually over the extensor aspect of the forearm but also found occasionally in the skin overlying other bony prominences. The rheumatoid nodules are composed of extensive areas of degenerate collagen that are surrounded by a giant-cell granulomatous reaction (see *Fig. 25.4c*). These nodules are seen in approximately 25% of cases of rheumatoid arthritis, particularly in patients with severe arthritic disease and other visceral involvement such as pulmonary fibrosis. Occasionally, the nodules can antedate the development of arthritis.

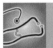

Laboratory diagnosis of rheumatoid disease

The laboratory diagnosis of rheumatoid disease is based on demonstrating the presence of antibodies known as **rheumatoid factors**. These factors react with antigenic sites on the C_H2 domain of the Fc portion of IgG. The most common type of rheumatoid factor is an immunoglobulin IgM molecule, which can form complexes with circulating IgG.

High rheumatoid factor titers are associated with severe progressive disease, particularly when there are systemic complications and rheumatoid nodules in the subcutis of the skin. There are two methods for demonstrating the presence of rheumatoid factors:

- **Rose–Waaler test:** based on the ability of IgM rheumatoid factor to agglutinate sheep red cells which have been coated with rabbit anti-sheep antibody.
- **Latex agglutination test:** in which the rheumatoid factor antibody agglutinates latex particles which have been coated with human IgG. This test is less specific than the Rose–Waaler test.

Radio-immunoassays and enzyme-linked immunosorbent assay (ELISA) can be used to measure rheumatoid factors of all types, including the most common IgM form.

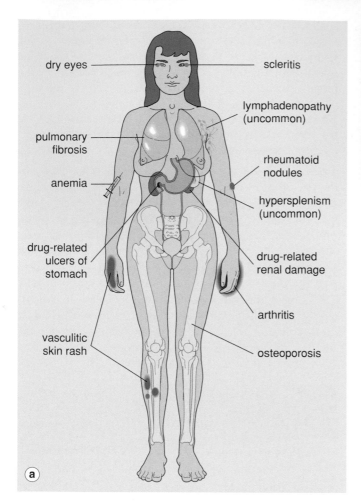

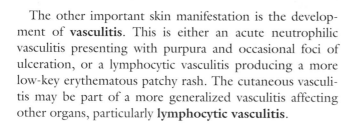

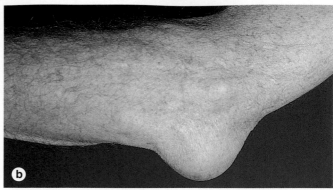

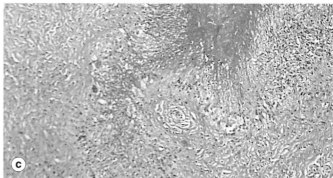

Fig. 25.4 Multisystem manifestations of rheumatoid disease. (a) Rheumatoid disease may cause primary disease, or damage may be caused by drug treatment. (b) Subcutaneous nodule of rheumatoid disease. (c) Histologically, such nodules contain areas of degenerate collagen surrounded by a granulomatous inflammatory response.

The other important skin manifestation is the development of **vasculitis**. This is either an acute neutrophilic vasculitis presenting with purpura and occasional foci of ulceration, or a lymphocytic vasculitis producing a more low-key erythematous patchy rash. The cutaneous vasculitis may be part of a more generalized vasculitis affecting other organs, particularly **lymphocytic vasculitis**.

Rheumatoid disease can cause 'dry-eye syndrome' and degeneration of the sclera

In rheumatoid disease, both the lacrimal and mucous glands may be affected by lymphocytic inflammation, leading to the destruction of the glands and to dry eyes (**keratoconjunctivitis sicca**). The lack of tears leads to secondary inflammation of the cornea. The degeneration of collagenous tissue may occur in the eye, analogous to that which is present in rheumatoid nodules, causing **scleritis**. In severe cases, this progresses to cause perforation of the globe, termed **scleromalacia perforans**.

Pulmonary involvement in rheumatoid disease causes interstitial fibrosis

The most common form of pulmonary involvement in rheumatoid disease is **interstitial pneumonitis and**

fibrosing alveolitis, which leads, eventually, to a pattern of interstitial pulmonary fibrosis that is very similar to that seen in progressive systemic sclerosis, 'honeycomb lung' (see page 207). In addition, patients may develop lesions that are very similar to the subcutaneous rheumatoid nodule, both within the lung and on the pleural surfaces.

Intrapulmonary rheumatoid granulomas are particularly common in patients who already have industrial lung disease due to the inhalation of various types of silica; the association of coalminer's lung with rheumatoid granulomas in sero-positive miners is called **Caplan's syndrome** (see page 209).

Anemia of chronic disorders is common in rheumatoid disease, and a minority of patients develop hypersplenism or lymphadenopathy

Anemia is very common in rheumatoid disease, usually being of the normocytic hypochromic type that is characteristic of chronic disease (see page 319). Despite the hypochromia there is no regular iron deficiency, but there is probably a defect of iron incorporation and utilization. The bone marrow may show follicular lymphocytic aggregates.

Lymph nodes may be enlarged in rheumatoid disease as a result of follicular hyperplasia. Enlargement of the spleen is usual, but it is rarely great enough to be palpable except in cases of **Felty's syndrome**, in which splenomegaly, lymphadenopathy, anemia and leukopenia are present in a patient with sero-positive rheumatoid arthritis; there is an increased susceptibility to infection, and sepsis is an important and common cause of death in these patients.

SARCOIDOSIS

Sarcoidosis is a chronic granulomatous disease of unknown cause, in which many tissues are infiltrated by non-caseating granulomas (see page 59). It is slightly more common in women than in men, and most patients present before the age of 40 years. The organs and systems that are most commonly involved clinically are the lymphoreticular system, the lungs, skin, eyes and the brain, although histological examination in sarcoidosis shows asymptomatic granulomas in many other organs and tissues, such as the heart, skeletal muscle, lacrimal glands and gastrointestinal tract (*Fig. 25.5*).

As so many systems and organs are involved, the clinical presentation patterns are wide and varied; there are also marked differences in the clinical expression of the disease on a geographical and racial basis.

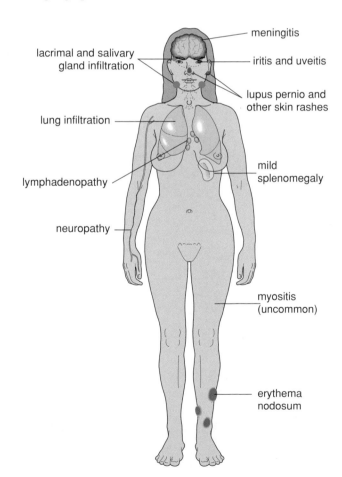

Fig. 25.5 Multisystem manifestations of sarcoidosis.
The granulomatous infiltrate of sarcoidosis may be seen in most tissues.

The etiology and pathogenesis are completely unknown, although numerous immunological abnormalities can be detected in patients with sarcoidosis; however, these may be an effect of the disease rather than the cause. Nevertheless, in lung involvement particularly, it is thought that one important factor is an enhanced cell-mediated immune response.

Lymphoreticular involvement in sarcoidosis is manifest as enlarged lymph nodes

The lymph nodes that are most commonly enlarged in sarcoidosis are the intrathoracic lymph nodes at the hilum of the lung. The enlargement of these nodes is invariably bilateral and almost symmetrical, and can be associated with diffuse pulmonary infiltration. Sarcoid enlargement of peripheral nodes, such as the axillary or cervical nodes, is less common.

The spleen is histologically involved in many patients, but the enlargement of the spleen is clinically manifest only in about 5% of cases in Caucasians; it is more common in Afro-Caribbeans, probably being manifest in about 15% of cases. Massive splenomegaly may be associated with secondary hematological features such as pancytopenia.

Lung involvement in sarcoidosis is common, and is responsible for much of the morbidity

In addition to the bilateral hilar lymphadenopathy, there is frequently a diffuse pulmonary infiltration which leads to a restrictive ventilatory defect and reduced gas transfer. The lung shows interstitial infiltration by typical sarcoid granulomas in the early stages, but these eventually heal by fibrosis. Much of the permanent pulmonary damage, whether structural or functional, is the result of progressive pulmonary interstitial fibrosis.

Skin lesions in association with sarcoidosis are very common

Skin manifestations occur in sarcoidosis in about one-quarter to one-third of all cases. There are two main patterns of involvement:

Erythema nodosum presents as characteristic, tender, red or purple subcutaneous lumps, usually on the shins and thighs, sometimes accompanied by fever and malaise, and frequently by associated arthralgia (see *Fig. 23.17*). It is an inflammatory lesion of the subcutaneous fat, usually associated with inflammation of a large vein. Although occasional giant cells are seen in relation to necrotic fat, true sarcoid granulomas are not seen. This pattern is particularly associated with the bilateral hilar lymphadenopathy pattern in the thorax, and is said to have a good prognosis.

Sarcoid granulomas in the skin may have several clinical manifestations, including brown papules (sometimes associated with hair follicles, leading to hair loss), reddish/brown fixed nodules and plaques, and a characteristic pattern called **lupus pernio**. In this pattern, which is associated with severe systemic involvement (including the nasal passages, lung and eye), there are persistent, rubbery, purple shiny plaques on the face, the tip of the nose and the ends of fingers and ears.

Eye involvement in sarcoidosis is a common presenting symptom, particularly in women

The most common type of ophthalmic involvement in sarcoidosis is an **acute uveitis**. This is often transient and mild, and is particularly associated with erythema nodosum and bilateral hilar lymph node enlargement. It is probable that uveitis occurs in over a quarter of all cases of sarcoidosis, but is sub-clinical in the majority.

More severe eye involvement occurs in **chronic uveitis**, which is persistent and is more likely to lead to permanent impairment of vision. It is usually associated with more severe sarcoidosis, e.g. with extensive pulmonary infiltration and fibrosis, or with cutaneous lupus pernio.

Involvement of the central and peripheral nervous system in sarcoidosis is important and often underdiagnosed

Neurological involvement occurs in at least 10% of patients with sarcoidosis, and is particularly common in patients with diffuse pulmonary infiltration and eye lesions. Sarcoid granulomas that are developing and proliferating in the nervous system can produce a wide range of clinical effects, which are dependent on their location; some of the more common are:

- **Chronic meningitis** with cerebrospinal fluid abnormalities and non-caseating granulomas in the meninges.
- **Cranial nerve lesions**, often as a result of chronic sarcoid meningeal inflammation at the base of the brain.
- **Space-occupying lesions** in the cerebral hemispheres, pituitary or hypothalamus.
- **'Mononeuritis multiplex'**, due to the involvement of many peripheral nerves.

DIABETES MELLITUS

Diabetes mellitus (DM) is a multisystem disease with both biochemical and structural consequences. It is a chronic disease of carbohydrate, fat and protein metabolism, resulting from an inadequate action of the hormone, insulin.

Two main types of **primary diabetes mellitus** are identified, mainly on clinical grounds (*Fig. 25.6*): **Type I diabetes** (insulin dependent diabetes mellitus – IDDM, or juvenile-onset diabetes), and **Type II diabetes** (non-insulin dependent diabetes – NIDDM, or maturity-onset diabetes).

Type III diabetes refers to specific types of diabetes caused by rare genetic defects in islet insulin-secreting cell function and genetic defects in insulin action. **Type IV disease** refers to diabetes related to pregnancy.

Diabetes may also occur **secondarily** to generalized disease of the pancreas, e.g. chronic pancreatitis and hemochromatosis, or may be caused by the secretion of hormones which antagonize the effects of insulin, e.g. in Cushing's syndrome and acromegaly; such diabetes is called **secondary diabetes mellitus**.

Type I diabetes is an organ-specific autoimmune disease

As one of its synonyms implies, Type I diabetes usually presents in childhood or adolescence, mainly as a result of the biochemical disorders leading to hyperglycemia and diabetic ketoacidosis. This type of diabetes is an autoimmune phenomenon; the majority of patients have circulating antibodies to the endocrine-cell population of the islet cells of the pancreas, including antibodies against the insulin-secreting cells. It is therefore an example of an **organ-specific autoimmune disease** (see page 111).

The pancreas in Type I diabetes shows lymphocytic infiltration and destruction of the insulin-secreting cells of the islets of Langerhans. This destruction of insulin-secreting cells leads to an insulin deficiency, which in turn leads to hyperglycemia and other secondary metabolic complications.

Type II diabetes is the result of insulin resistance in peripheral tissues

Type II diabetes is four or five times more common than Type I diabetes. Unlike Type I diabetes, where there is an absolute absence of insulin, in Type II diabetes the blood insulin levels are initially normal, or may even increase in the early stages, before falling eventually to below normal.

Fig. 25.6
Comparison of Type I and Type II diabetes

Type I	Type II
Childhood and adolescence onset	Late middle-age/elderly onset
Thin	Obese
Ketoacidosis common	Ketoacidosis rare
Severe insulin deficiency	Relative deficiency and end-organ resistance
Islet-cell antibodies	No islet-cell antibodies
Autoimmune mechanism	No autoimmune mechanism
Genetic predisposition associated with HLA-DR genotype	Polygenic inheritance

The defect in the Type II pattern is a combination of the effects of the relative deficiency of insulin when compared to the need, and the phenomenon of **insulin resistance**, in which the tissues are unable to respond to insulin. Insulin resistance is thought to be due to an impairment of the function of receptors for insulin on the surfaces of target cells, meaning that glucose does not enter the cell.

A protein called **amylin** is produced in the insulin-secreting cells of the pancreatic islets, and is secreted with the insulin. In Type II diabetics, this protein accumulates in excess around the pancreatic islet cells, producing an amorphous deposit of material with the characteristics of amyloid (see page 543). Its role is not understood, but it may interfere with the subsequent secretion of insulin by the islet cells.

Pathogenesis of Type II diabetes

The precise pathogeneses in Type II diabetes are not known, although etiological factors such as age, obesity and a genetic predisposition are well-recognized. Although Type II diabetics do not have the HLA-DR4 genotype, there is a strong genetic factor: 90–100% of identical twins show concordance. Inheritance is considered to be polygenic (see page 76).

Pathogenesis of Type I diabetes mellitus

Patients with Type I diabetes are usually HLA-DR3 or HLA-DR4 positive, a feature which is shown by other organ-specific autoimmune diseases. It is thought possible that a viral infection may be the trigger for the autoimmune destruction of insulin-secreting cells; viruses implicated include the common childhood viral infections, such as mumps, measles and coxsackie B. One postulated mechanism is that the viruses induce mild structural damage to the islet cells of the pancreas, thereby altering their antigenicity, and that certain individuals with the genetic susceptibility to organ-specific autoimmune disease, e.g. the possession of HLA-DR4, then mount an autoimmune response against the damaged insulin-secreting cells. Another postulate is that an endogenous retrovirus is responsible for eliciting an immune response directed against islet cells.

Laboratory diagnostic criteria for diabetes mellitus

There are currently two widely used sets of diagnostic criteria for diabetes mellitus based on assessment of plasma glucose levels. One is promoted by WHO (1985) while the other more recent criteria are promoted by the American Diabetic Association (1997) (see *Fig. 25.7*).

A condition of **impaired glucose tolerance** is defined as plasma glucose < 7.8 mmol/L fasting and 7.8–11.0 mmol/L 2 hours after a 75 g glucose load (WHO).

The American Diabetic Association recognize the state of **impaired fasting glucose** defined as plasma glucose 6.1–6.9 mmol/L (fasting).

These two states carry the implications of a higher than normal risk for development of diabetes mellitus and cardiovascular disease.

Fig. 25.7
Biochemical criteria in diabetes mellitus

WHO criteria

Fasting plasma glucose	≥ 7.8 mmol/L
AND	
Plasma glucose	≥ 11.1 mmol/L 2 hours after an oral 75 g glucose load

American Diabetic Association

Fasting plasma glucose	> 7.0 mmol/L
OR	
Random plasma glucose	≥ 11.1 mmol/L with appropriate clinical symptoms
OR	
Plasma glucose	≥ 11.1 mmol/L 2 hours after an oral 75 g glucose load

Morbidity and mortality in diabetes mellitus is now mainly the result of its structural complications

Whereas in former years the biochemical disturbances in diabetes mellitus usually led to an early death, the development of insulin treatment for Type I diabetes and of various oral hypoglycemic agents (when combined with diet) for Type II diabetes, have greatly reduced mortality due to hyperglycemia, hypoglycemia and the complications of ketoacidotic coma. Nevertheless, diabetes remains an important cause of morbidity and mortality due to a series of common complications (*Fig. 25.8*). The major complications of diabetes are:

- Predisposition to infection.
- Increased severity of atherosclerosis and its complications.
- Extensive small vessel disease (arteriolosclerosis).
- Renal glomerular disease (see page 368).
- Retinal vascular disease (see page 480).
- Peripheral nerve damage (see page 466).

As a result of these complications, diabetics of both types have a predisposition to develop ischemic heart disease, cerebrovascular disease, peripheral gangrene of lower limbs, chronic renal disease, reduced visual acuity leading to blindness, and peripheral neuropathy.

Diabetics are particularly prone to infection

Patients with diabetes have an increased tendency to develop infections, usually of a bacterial or fungal nature. The main target organs are the skin, the oral and genital mucosae, and the urinary tract.

In the skin, diabetics are particularly vulnerable to follicular infections by staphylococci, and the lesions tend to be more severe than in non-diabetics; boils are particularly frequent in Type II elderly diabetics. Other skin conditions that are more common in diabetics are superficial fungal infections, cellulitis and erysipelas (see Chapter 23).

Diabetics may have particularly severe oral or genital mucosal infections with *Candida*.

In the kidney, in addition to the other abnormalities due to small and large vessel disease, there is an increased predisposition to **acute pyelonephritis**, often associated with recurrent lower urinary tract infections, and sometimes complicated by **papillary necrosis** (see page 369).

Diabetics have very severe atherosclerosis

Although atherosclerosis is widespread and common, diabetics in general suffer much more severe and extensive atherosclerosis than non-diabetics of the same age and gender. Furthermore, in diabetics the atherosclerotic changes extend into much smaller artery branches than in the non-diabetic. The main clinical sequelae of this are seen in:

- The heart, where coronary atherosclerosis is more severe and extensive than in non-diabetics, predisposing to ischemic heart disease.
- The brain, where atherosclerosis of the internal carotid and vertebrobasilar arteries and their branches predisposes to cerebral ischemia.
- The legs and feet, where severe atherosclerosis of the iliofemoral and smaller arteries in the lower leg predisposes to the development of gangrene. Ischemia of a single toe, or ischemic areas on the heel, are characteristic features of diabetic gangrene, which is due to the involvement of smaller, more peripheral arteries than is the case in non-diabetic generalized atherosclerosis.
- The kidney, where extension of atherosclerosis into the main renal arteries and their intrarenal branches makes a major contribution towards chronic nephron ischemia, an important component of the multiple renal lesions in diabetes (see below).

Microvascular disease is an important feature of diabetes, and is responsible for many of the pathological complications

Small arterioles and capillaries in diabetes show a characteristic pattern of wall thickening, which is due to a marked

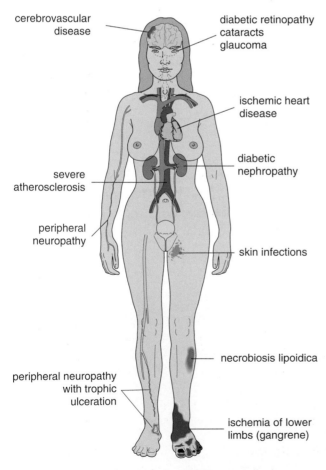

cerebrovascular disease

diabetic retinopathy
cataracts
glaucoma

ischemic heart disease

severe atherosclerosis

diabetic nephropathy

peripheral neuropathy

skin infections

necrobiosis lipoidica

peripheral neuropathy with trophic ulceration

ischemia of lower limbs (gangrene)

Fig. 25.8 Multisystem manifestations of diabetes mellitus. The most important complications are vascular disease, renal disease, and eye disease.

expansion of the basement membrane, termed **hyaline arteriolosclerosis** (see page 167). This small vessel abnormality is widespread, and is responsible for ischemic changes which are symptomatic in the kidney, the retina, the brain and in peripheral nerves.

In the kidney, the capillaries of the glomerular tuft show marked basement membrane thickening associated with increased leakiness of the capillary wall. This permits the leakage of plasma proteins into the glomerular filtrate in amounts greater than can be re-absorbed in the tubular part of the nephron, leading to **proteinuria**, and eventually **glomerular hyalinization with development of chronic renal failure**.

In the retina, the vessel wall changes lead to retinal hemorrhage and vascular proliferation. In the brain, the small vessel lesions lead to lacunar infarction and ischemic white matter degeneration. In peripheral nerves, the capillary wall changes are believed to be a major factor in the development of peripheral neuropathy.

Peripheral neuropathy is an important cause of intractable ulceration of the foot in diabetics

The various patterns of diabetic neuropathy are discussed briefly on page 466. The most common is symmetrical peripheral polyneuropathy, which particularly affects the hands and feet in a 'glove and stocking' distribution. This leads to impairment or loss of sensation, including the loss of pain sensation. The normal pain withdrawal from injury reflex is lost, and areas of the skin become damaged repeatedly by trivial trauma such as friction from tight-fitting footwear (see *Fig. 25.9*). This form of trophic ulceration becomes chronic, healing being impaired by a combination of repeated trauma and the ischemia almost invariably present in the feet of diabetics with severe co-existing vascular disease.

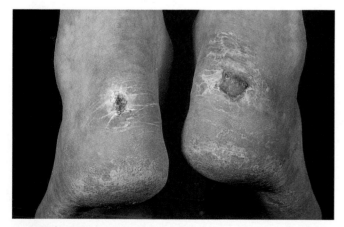

Fig. 25.9 Diabetic trophic ulcers.
The combination of peripheral sensory neuropathy and ischemia, caused by diabetic small vessel disease, makes diabetics particularly prone to develop trophic ulcers at sites of pressure and friction. These are notoriously difficult to heal.

Diabetic nephropathy is an important cause of mortality in diabetics

The kidney is affected in many ways in diabetes. As well as the predisposition to urinary tract infection and the tendency to chronic ischemia associated with severe atherosclerosis, there are certain renal lesions which are particularly associated with diabetes; these are glomerular basement membrane thickening, diabetic glomerulosclerosis (both diffuse and nodular), glomerular exudative lesions, and papillary necrosis. These are considered in more detail in Chapter 17. The end result is development of chronic renal failure.

Diabetes is an important cause of acquired blindness in the western world

Diabetes can affect the eyes in five main ways:

1 **Background retinopathy** is due to small vessel abnormalities in the retina leading to hard exudates, hemorrhages and micro-aneurysms; this does not usually affect acuity.
2 **Proliferative retinopathy** is caused by the extensive proliferation of new small blood vessels in the retina. Sudden deterioration in vision can result from vitreous hemorrhage from the proliferating new vessels or the development of retinal detachment.
3 **Maculopathy** is caused by edema, hard exudates or retinal ischemia, and causes marked reduction in acuity.
4 **Cataract formation** is greatly increased in diabetics.
5 **Glaucoma** shows an increased incidence in diabetics due to neovascularization of the iris, **rubeosis iridis** (see page 482).

AMYLOIDOSIS

Amyloidosis is a condition in which there is a deposition, in many tissues, of an abnormal extracellular fibrillar protein, termed **amyloid**. Amyloid is derived from many different precursor peptides, with the precursors themselves often being fragments derived from larger proteins; it is deposited as a meshwork of rigid, straight fibrils that are 10–15 nm in diameter, being composed of the precursor peptides lined up in an antiparallel β-pleated sheet structure. It is therefore the physical arrangement of the constituent peptides that makes a protein an amyloid, rather than any specific peptide sequence.

Amyloid is detected histologically as a bright-pink hyaline material. It also takes up certain special stains, with the most widely known being Congo red, with electron microscopy showing it to have a fibrillar ultrastructure (*Fig. 25.10*).

Amyloid can be classified according to the nature of the precursor protein

Despite uncertainty about why amyloid is formed, there are well-characterized associations between particular diseases and the deposition of amyloid. In each case, there is an accumulation of a precursor peptide which is processed into an amyloid protein. In some of these diseases there is an identifiable reason for the accumulation of the precursor peptide, and the amyloid is termed **secondary amyloid**. In other cases, the cause of the accumulation of a precursor peptide is not known, and the amyloid is termed **primary amyloid**. In addition, there are several inherited disorders, the **heredofamilial amyloidoses**.

Amyloid is deposited outside cells, and can be classified into localized or systemic patterns

Amyloid is deposited in the extracellular compartment of tissues, and in H&E preparation it is seen as a uniformly eosinophilic (pink-staining) material. It can be highlighted in histological sections by the use of special stains such as Sirius red and Congo red. Congo red staining is commonly used for diagnostic purposes, with amyloid staining orange, and exhibiting a green coloration when viewed with polarized light (*Fig. 25.12*).

Amyloidosis may involve many tissues in the body as it is particularly deposited in the blood vessel walls and basement membranes. The progressive accumulation of amyloid leads to cellular dysfunction, either by preventing the normal processes of diffusion through extracellular tissues, or by the physical compression of functioning parenchymal cells. In some diseases, amyloidosis is a systemic process affecting many organs simultaneously (**systemic amyloid**); there is also a group of conditions in which amyloid only affects one organ or tissue (**localized amyloid**).

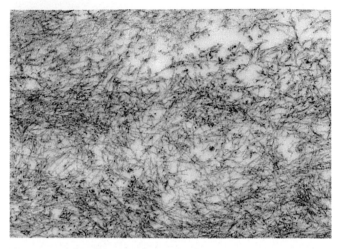

Fig. 25.10 Amyloid ultrastructure. Amyloid is composed of filaments of protein deposited extracellularly.

 Amyloidogenesis

Amyloid is derived in two main ways (*Fig. 25.11*):

- A precursor is produced in abnormally large amounts (examples are given).

- Polymorphisms of normal proteins give rise to peptides which are predisposed to form amyloid, termed amyloidogenic (the two most common examples are given). The nature of the peptide sequences required for this process is still uncertain.

It is thought that cells of the mononuclear-phagocyte system are responsible for processing the precursor peptide to form amyloid fibrils, often by producing fragments of the main precursor peptide.

In addition to the precursor peptide, amyloid contains another serum protein which may assist in nucleation, called serum amyloid P.

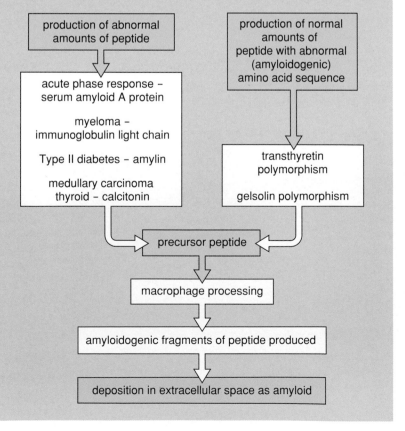

Fig. 25.11 Amyloidogenesis.

Amino-acid sequencing of amyloid proteins in different disease states has enabled a classification of amyloid to be made on biochemical grounds (*Fig. 25.13*).

The commonest example of amyloid deposition is in the nervous system, in both Alzheimer's disease and normal aging (*Fig. 21.34a*). The amyloid is derived from a normal, neuronal membrane protein termed **Alzheimer precursor protein (APP)**, being formed from a peptide fragment termed **Aβ protein** or **A4 protein**.

Amyloid that is associated with an abnormal proliferation of plasma cells is made up of immunoglobulin light chains, with such amyloid deposition occurring in diseases such as myeloma and plasmacytoma (see page 314).

Reactive amyloid may be associated with long-standing chronic inflammatory processes. As in any inflammatory disorder, the associated systemic acute-phase response causes excessive production of serum amyloid A protein (a normal, acute-phase protein) by the liver. With time, and for uncertain reasons, some of this protein is deposited as amyloid. Diseases that lead to this type of secondary amyloid include tuberculosis, rheumatoid arthritis, bronchiectasis and chronic osteomyelitis.

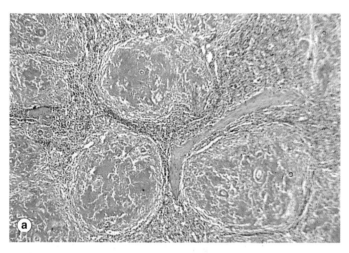
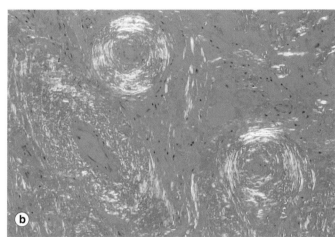

Fig. 25.12 Histology of amyloid.
(a) Amyloid appears as homogeneous bright-pink staining material. In this example, from the spleen, amyloid is deposited as rounded masses. (b) If amyloid is stained with Congo red and viewed under polarized light, it shows apple-green birefringence.

Fig. 25.13
Classification of amyloid

Localization	Clinical association	Precursor protein
Systemic amyloid	Plasma cell tumors	Immunoglobulin light chain
	Chronic inflammation	Serum amyloid A protein
	Familial Mediterranean fever	Serum amyloid A protein
	Familial neuropathy	Transthyretin (prealbumin)
	Dialysis associated	β_2-microglobulin
Localized amyloid	Senile cardiac amyloid	Transthyretin (prealbumin)
	Medullary carcinoma	Calcitonin
	Islet-cell amyloid	Amylin
	Alzheimer's disease	Aβ protein (A4 protein)
	Cerebral angiopathy	Aβ protein (A4 protein)

Diagnosis of amyloidosis

The diagnosis of systemic amyloidosis is usually confirmed by tissue biopsy. The most useful site for biopsy is the rectal mucosa, where amyloid can be detected in the submucosal vessels in 60–70% of cases of generalized amyloidosis. Amyloid may also be detected in renal biopsies or liver biopsies.

More recently, radiolabeled serum amyloid P can be injected into patients and imaged; it localizes to any amyloid deposits.

Tumors of peptide-secreting endocrine cells may form amyloid from the hormone peptide, e.g. in the calcitonin-derived amyloid in medullary carcinoma of the thyroid. In Type II diabetes, the excessive secretion of amylin by the β-cells of the pancreas is associated with its deposition as **islet amyloid**. Uncommon familial types of amyloid are believed to be caused by gene polymorphisms in normal proteins. The amino-acid substitutions are believed to make the proteins, or their peptide fragments, susceptible to amyloid formation.

Amyloid is mainly deposited in the kidney, heart, liver, spleen and nerves

The kidneys are the organs most commonly functionally impaired by systemic amyloidosis, usually presenting with proteinuria or the nephrotic syndrome (see page 351).

Deposition of amyloid in the spleen can occur in either a diffuse pattern or a nodular pattern.

In the liver, amyloid is deposited in the space between the sinusoidal lining cells and the hepatocytes. Clinically, hepatic amyloidosis may be a cause of hepatomegaly. However, there is rarely significant clinical evidence of impaired liver function.

Amyloid involvement of the heart may be a manifestation of senile cardiac amyloid, which is derived from trans-thyretin (prealbumin). The most severe form of cardiac amyloid is seen in systemic amyloidosis, causing cardiomyopathy (see page 180).

INHERITED METABOLIC DISEASES

Several multisystem diseases are the result of inherited metabolic defects, the vast majority of such disorders being inherited as recessive traits. It is possible to categorize such diseases according to the main result of the metabolic defect (*Fig. 25.14*). In some diseases, the metabolic defect results in the accumulation of a metabolic product in cells, giving rise to the term **metabolic storage disease**.

Fig. 25.14
Classification of inherited metabolic diseases according to main result of defect

Decreased formation of a product due to the lack of function of enzyme

Mitochondrial cytopathy (see page 471)

Accumulation of substrate due to the lack of function of enzyme

Phenylketonuria
Glycogenoses
Galactosemia
Lysosomal storage diseases
Peroxisomal diseases
Hemochromatosis (see page 292)
Wilson's disease (see page 292)

Increased formation of metabolites

Steroid 21 hydroxylase deficiency (congenital adrenal hyperplasia)

Failure of membrane transport system

Cystic fibrosis (see page 221)
Muscle ion-channel diseases (see page 472)

Storage diseases result in the accumulation of abnormal metabolic products in cells

Diseases that cause accumulation of metabolic substrates in cells, are termed **storage disorders**. In many cases, the metabolic product accumulates in lysosomal-derived vesicles (**lysosomal storage disease**). In other instances, the abnormal product accumulates free in the cell cytoplasm.

Storage disorders can be sub-classified according to the type of substance that accumulates in cells:

- **Lipidoses:** defects in enzymes that degrade glycolipids, leading to the accumulation of sphingolipids, e.g. Gaucher's disease, Niemann–Pick disease, Tay–Sachs disease.
- **Mucopolysaccharidoses:** the accumulation of mucopolysaccharides (glycosaminoglycans, such as dermatan sulfate and heparin sulfate) in cells, e.g. Hunter's syndrome, Hurler's syndrome.
- **Mucolipidoses:** Types II–IV defects in lysosomal-enzyme transport systems.
- **Glycoproteinoses:** lack of enzymes that degrade glycoproteins, e.g. sialidosis, mannosidosis, fucosidosis.
- **Glycogenoses:** diseases characterized by the accumulation of glycogen in cells (discussed in more detail below).

Fig. 25.15
Main sub-types of glycogenosis

Type	Enzyme deficiency	Features
IA (von Gierke's)	Glucose-6-phosphatase	Hypoglycemia in early life with hepatomegaly
IC	Glucose-6-phosphate translocase	Neutropenia and infections
II (Pompe's)	Lysosomal acid maltase	Cardiac failure in early infancy with cardiomegaly and hepatomegaly
II (Adult onset)	Lysosomal acid maltase	Proximal myopathy or cardiomyopathy
III	Debrancher enzyme	Hypoglycemia, hepatomegaly, cirrhosis
IV	Branching enzyme	Hepatomegaly and cirrhosis
V (McArdle's)	Myophosphorylase	Muscle cramps, rhabdomyolysis, myopathy
VI (Her's)	Hepatic phosphorylase	Hepatomegaly
VII	Phosphofructokinase	Muscle cramps, myopathy

Disease variously affects:

- The lymphoreticular system (spleen, liver, bone marrow, lymph nodes) resulting in splenomegaly and hepatomegaly.
- The nervous system, resulting in mental retardation or progressive failure of intellectual development.
- Endothelium, smooth muscle, skeletal muscle.
- Hepatocytes, resulting in hepatomegaly.

Diagnosis is based upon the clinical recognition of disease complemented by the detection of the abnormal product in cells or, in some cases, the urine. The enzyme defect may be demonstrated in lymphoid cells or in cultured fibroblasts.

The glycogenoses result in abnormal accumulation of glycogen in tissues

The glycogenoses are a group of diseases in which there is an abnormal accumulation of glycogen in tissues; this is caused by diverse enzyme abnormalities in the enzymes involved in the glycogen metabolism. There are over 12 sub-types, the majority of which have defined enzyme deficiencies (*Fig. 25.15*). Diagnosis is often made initially by demonstrating the presence of glycogen in tissue biopsy samples, followed by demonstrating a lack of the appropriate enzyme activity. Increasingly, genetic techniques are being used to refine diagnosis.

Familial defects in lipid metabolism cause hyperlipidemias and are an important cause of atheroma

Hyperlipidemias are a set of conditions in which there is an abnormally high level of one or more lipoproteins in the plasma. In cases where this is the result of a systemic metabolic disturbance, it is termed a **secondary hyperlipidemia** – the main causes being obesity, excess alcohol intake, diabetes mellitus, nephrotic syndrome and hypothyroidism. When hyperlipidemia is caused by a genetic predisposition to an abnormal lipid metabolism, the term **primary hyperlipidemia** is used.

Such primary hyperlipidemias have been shown to be due to a wide range of abnormalities in genes that code for enzymes, apolipoproteins, or receptors involved in the lipid metabolism.

There are several types of hyperlipidemia, which can be characterized by the determination of the lipoprotein profile in plasma. The WHO classification is based on that proposed by Fredrickson, and divides cases into Types I–V. Unfortunately, this does not indicate the cause of a hyperlipidemia (i.e. whether primary or secondary). Recent developments in the biochemistry of these disorders is allowing precise diagnosis to be made, based on metabolic or genetic characterization.

One of the most important consequences of certain types of hyperlipidemia (mainly WHO Type IIa) is a raised serum cholesterol concentration, mainly a reflection of serum LDL, predisposing to atheroma.

The main types of hyperlipidemia and their most important features are listed in *Fig. 25.16*.

In addition to the effects of hyperlipidemia, high levels of one particular lipoprotein termed lipoprotein (a) confers a high risk of the development of both ischemic heart disease and cerebrovascular disease, independent of LDL/cholesterol levels.

Fig. 25.16
Hyperlipidemias

Type	Inheritance	Features	Mechanism
Familial hypercholesterolemia	Autosomal dominant 1:500 population	Increased plasma cholesterol Increased plasma LDL Arcus senilis and tendon xanthomas Increased atheroma risk	Caused by abnormalities in LDL synthesis, transport, receptor binding or internalization. Many different mutations and genes involved
Familial combined hyperlipidemia	Autosomal dominant 1:300 population	Increased plasma cholesterol Increased plasma VLDL Increased plasma LDL Increased atheroma risk	Abnormally high levels of apolipoprotein B produced by liver, thought to be caused by defect in a regulatory gene
Familial hypertriglyceridemia	Autosomal dominant 1:600 population	Increased VLDL in plasma Increased atheroma risk in some cases	Possible polymorphisms in some of the genes coding for apo A and C. Patients with associated low HDL develop premature atheroma
Familial dysbetalipoproteinemia	Autosomal polymorphism Uncommon	Increased chylomicrons Increased IDL Palmar xanthomas Eruptive xanthomas Increased atheroma risk	Apolipoprotein E phenotype E2/2
Familial alphalipoproteinemia	Uncommon	Increased serum cholesterol Increased HDL Reduced atheroma risk	HDL increased
Familial chylomicronemia	Autosomal recessive Rare	Increased chylomicrons Xanthomas in some cases Pancreatitis in some cases	1) Reduced endothelial lipoprotein lipase 2) Reduced apo C-II levels

This table shows the main types of hyperlipidemia and the most important features of each. About 6:1000 of the population have an autosomal dominant predisposition to develop an abnormality of lipid metabolism that increases the risk of developing atheroma. In addition, others have a polygenic increased risk. Some of these cases will come to medical attention because of the trend for the routine screening of blood for cholesterol levels. Other cases will come to light having presented with a complication of atheroma at a young age, e.g. ischemic heart disease or cerebrovascular disease.

Questions

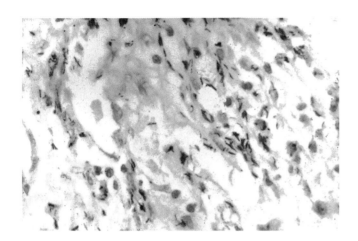

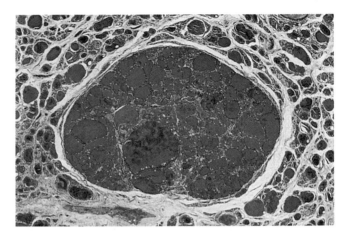

1. This photograph shows a section of lung, specially stained to show the causative organism in a patient with confluent bronchopneumonia. Which of the following statements is **most correct**?

(a) The stain used is demonstrating streptococci.

(b) The stain used is the Ziehl–Neelsen stain for mycobacteria.

(c) The organism can only be demonstrated in tissue sections because it cannot be cultured outside the body.

(d) This organism has excited an acute inflammatory reaction dominated by neutrophils.

(e) The fact that the organisms have stained red means that they are dead, having been killed by antibiotics.

Answer on page 593

2. In this histology picture of a nodule removed from the thyroid gland, which of the following statements is **most correct**?

(a) The well-circumscribed nature of the nodule implies that is benign.

(b) The patient would have low thyroid function (hypothyroidism).

(c) Metastatic spread to regional lymph nodes is likely to be present.

(d) The nodule is due to excess secretion of TSH (thyroid stimulating hormone) by the pituitary gland.

(e) The nodule is an enlarged collection of thyroid C (calcitonin-secreting) cells.

Answer on page 593

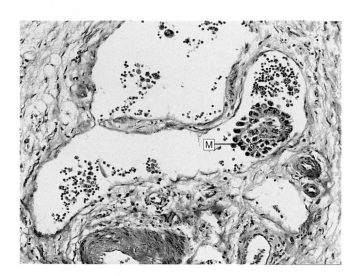

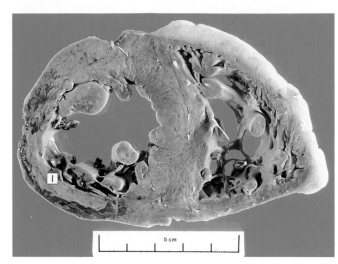

3. These findings were seen in a tissue biopsy from the mediastinal soft tissues. Which statement is **most correct**?

(a) The hyperchromatic, large cell cluster (**M**) is within a lymphatic vessel and indicates spread of a malignant tumor.

(b) The large clump of epithelioid macrophages (**M**) with central necrosis indicates infection by *M. tuberculosis*.

(c) This is a classical whorl from a meningioma (**M**).

(d) There is a clump of atypical lymphoid cells present in a lymphatic vessel indicating a malignant lymphoma (**M**).

(e) Serological testing for Epstein–Barr virus is indicated, as clumps of large atypical lymphoid cells occur in lymphatics in glandular fever (infectious mononucleosis).

Answer on page 593

4. This photograph shows a cross-section through the ventricles of a heart removed at autopsy. Which of the following statements is **most correct**?

(a) The main abnormality is in the wall of the right ventricle.

(b) The lesion labeled (**I**) is less than 24 hours old.

(c) The lesion labeled (**I**) is greater than 8 weeks old.

(d) The lesion labeled (**I**) is 5–7 days old.

(e) The focal involvement of part of the heart wall (**I**) is indicative of a viral myocarditis.

Answer on page 593

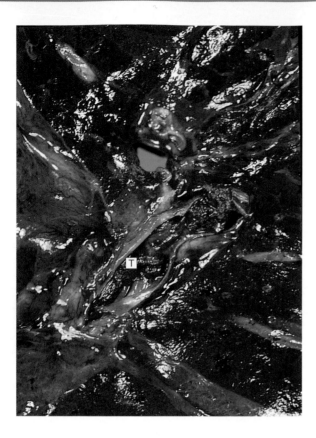

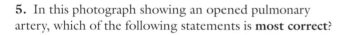

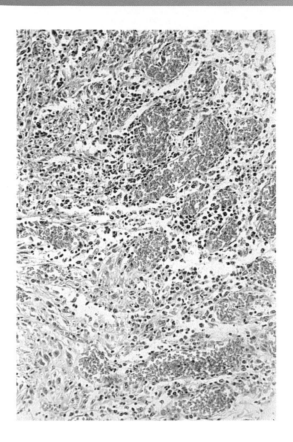

5. In this photograph showing an opened pulmonary artery, which of the following statements is **most correct**?

(a) Invasion of the main pulmonary arteries by malignant tumor (**T**) of the adjacent bronchus has produced occlusion.

(b) The lesion is caused by thrombosis (**T**) superimposed on intimal atheroma within the pulmonary artery.

(c) Thrombotic material (**T**) in the pulmonary arteries has originated in the deep veins of the leg.

(d) Propagation of ventricular thrombus, originating from mural thrombosis in the right ventricle, caused vascular occlusion.

(e) A careful search for systemic arterial thromboemboli is likely to reveal significant lesions.

Answer on page 594

6. This is the histology from the base of an ulcer of the leg of a 60-year-old woman. Which statement is **most correct**?

(a) The dominant presence of thin-walled vessels with a background of lymphoid and macrophagic cells indicates an early phase of wound healing.

(b) The dominant presence of thin-walled vessels in the ulcer base indicates a poor chance of wound healing.

(c) The lack of fibroblast infiltration with dominant vascular and inflammatory cells seen on biopsy suggests that steroid therapy should be implemented to promote healing.

(d) All of the thin-walled vessels will undergo arterialization as wound healing progresses.

(e) The absence of neutrophils, with the dominance of lymphoid cells and monocytic cells suggests a problem with leukocyte function.

Answer on page 594

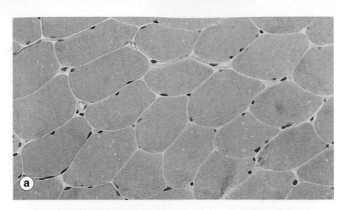

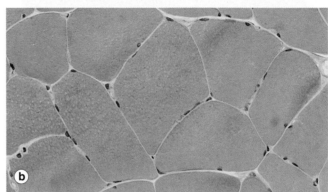

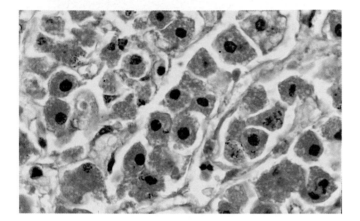

7. This picture shows liver cells which are abnormal, in a tissue biopsy. Which of the following statements is **most correct**?

(a) The nuclear pleomorphism and dense staining of nuclei indicates that the cells are in a state of high proliferative activity.

(b) The dense, hyperchromatic nuclei with cytoplasmic eosinophilia indicates that these cells are undergoing coagulative necrosis.

(c) The homogeneous, glassy cytoplasm is characteristic of liver cells infected by hepatitis B virus.

(d) The absence of visible accumulated fat within hepatocytes suggests starvation.

(e) The dark-staining nuclei indicate that this is from a malignant tumor.

Answer on page 594

8. In these photomicrographs of skeletal muscle cells, the upper picture shows normal fibers. Which of the following statements is **most correct** about the lower picture?

(a) The larger skeletal muscle fiber size in the lower picture is due to hyperplasia.

(b) The larger skeletal muscle fiber size in the lower picture is an example of hypertrophy.

(c) The larger skeletal muscle fiber size in the lower picture is due to metaplasia.

(d) The larger skeletal muscle fiber size in the lower picture is due to denervation.

(e) The larger skeletal muscle fiber size in the lower picture is an indication that it is part of a benign neoplasm.

Answer on page 595

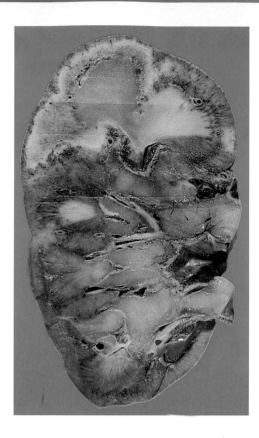

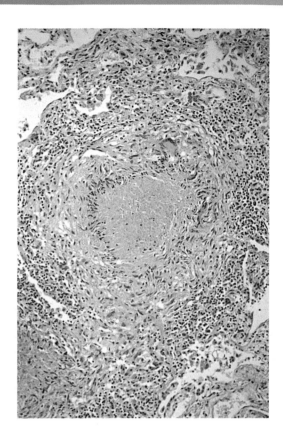

9. This kidney was removed at autopsy in a patient. Which statement is **most correct**?

(a) Segmental pallor of the upper pole indicates a focal glomerulonephritis.

(b) A geographic, non-expansile lesion in the upper pole, replacing the normal architecture, indicates an adenocarcinoma.

(c) This is acute pyelonephritis spreading down the kidney from an origin in the upper pole.

(d) A segmental pale lesion such as this, corresponding to part of the vascular territory within the kidney, indicates a recent renal infarct.

(e) This photograph shows typical acute papillary necrosis of the kidney.

Answer on page 595

10. In this photomicrograph of one of many small lesions in the lung, which of the following statements is **most correct**?

(a) The central homogenous pink material is liquefactive necrosis.

(b) The patient has tuberculosis.

(c) The patient has bronchial carcinoma.

(d) The lesion is the result of viral pneumonia.

(e) The giant cells seen around the margin of the lesion indicate that this is due to an inhaled foreign body.

Answer on page 595

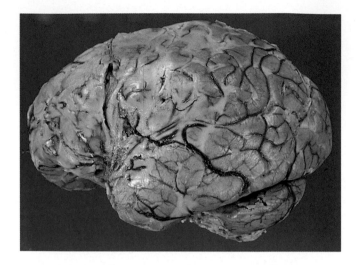

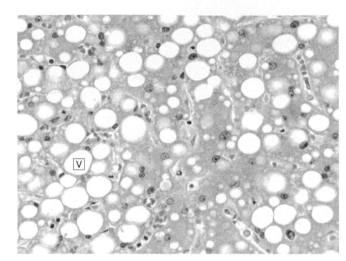

11. In this photograph of the brain from a child who died after an acute febrile illness, which of the following is **most correct?**

(a) The white material under the arachnoid is due to diffuse tumor infiltration.

(b) The white material indicates an underlying cerebral infarct.

(c) The changes are those of a viral encephalitis.

(d) The material is pus, composed mainly of neutrophils and bacteria.

(e) This is meningeal edema due to acute hydrocephalus.

Answer on page 595

12. This illustration shows a liver biopsy stained with hematoxylin and eosin. Which statement is **most correct?**

(a) The abnormal liver cells (**V**) are necrotic.

(b) The pale unstained areas in cells are due to intracytoplasmic water accumulation.

(c) The pale unstained areas in the cells are due to triglyceride accumulation.

(d) The pale areas seen in most cells are characteristic of virus-infected cells.

(e) The change is most commonly due to diabetes mellitus and the accumulation of glycogen.

Answer on page 596

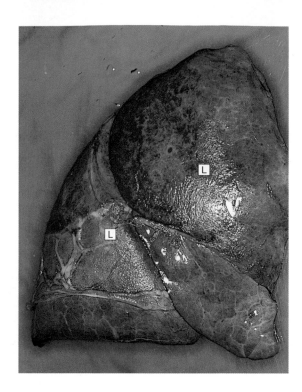

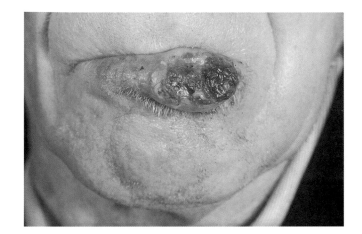

13. In this lung removed at post mortem, which of the following is **most correct**? The surface material (**L**):

(a) Contains fibrin and neutrophils.

(b) Is old fibrous thickening of the pleura.

(c) Is the result of the primary pleural tumor, malignant mesothelioma.

(d) Is the result of diffuse infiltration by metastatic carcinoma.

(e) Produces no clinical symptoms or signs.

Answer on page 596

14. The photograph shows a lesion on the lower lip. Which of the following statements is **most correct**?

(a) It is a large viral lesion ('cold sore').

(b) It is a benign tumor derived from the salivary tissue in the lip.

(c) It is most common in young adult men.

(d) It will resolve with antibiotic therapy.

(e) It is malignant and may metastasize to lymph nodes in the neck.

Answer on page 596

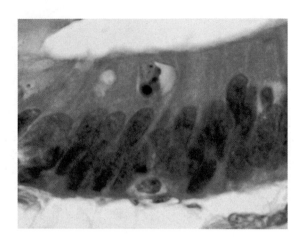

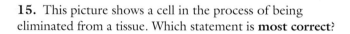

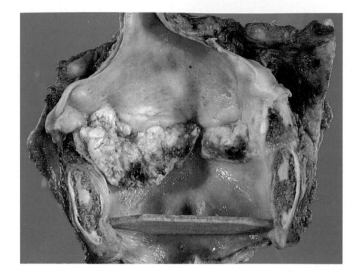

15. This picture shows a cell in the process of being eliminated from a tissue. Which statement is **most correct?**

(a) The morphology of the affected cell is characteristic of coagulative necrosis.

(b) The morphology of the affected cell is characteristic of a cell undergoing autophagy.

(c) The morphology indicates that the affected cell is undergoing cellular atrophy.

(d) The morphology of the affected cell indicates that programmed cell death has taken place.

(e) The morphology is characteristic of an inflammatory destruction of the affected cell.

Answer on page 596

16. This photograph is of the opened larynx. Which of the following statements is **most correct?**

(a) The patient would have presented with difficulty in swallowing.

(b) The patient would have presented with hemoptysis.

(c) The lesion is a non-destructive benign tumor.

(d) The lesion may spread to the lymph nodes in the neck.

(e) Excessive shouting or loud singing is a common and important predisposing factor to this laryngeal lesion.

Answer on page 597

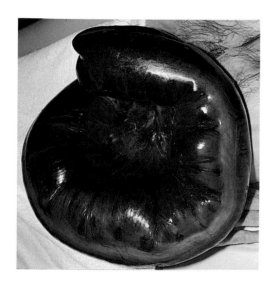

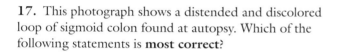

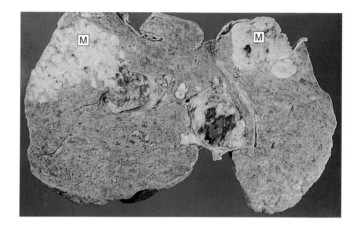

17. This photograph shows a distended and discolored loop of sigmoid colon found at autopsy. Which of the following statements is **most correct**?

(a) The discoloration of the colon is due to melanosis coli.

(b) The discoloration of the colon is due to arterial infarction following a mesenteric thromboembolus.

(c) The discoloration of the colon is due to venous infarction secondary to torsion.

(d) The discoloration is due to severe Crohn's disease of the colon.

(e) This disease is a well-recognized complication of diverticular disease of colon.

Answer on page 597

18. This is a photograph of a liver removed at *post mortem*. Which of the following statements is **most correct**?

(a) The areas marked (**M**) are pale infarcts due to hepatic artery occlusion.

(b) The areas marked (**M**) are abscesses due to ascending cholangitis.

(c) The areas marked (**M**) are metastatic tumor deposits from a primary carcinoma of the ovary.

(d) The areas marked (**M**) are multifocal primary malignant tumors of the liver.

(e) The areas marked (**M**) are nodules of malignant lymphoma.

Answer on page 597

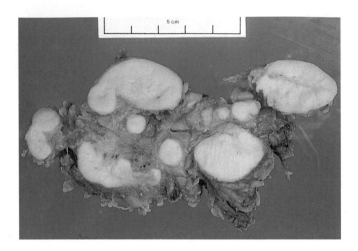

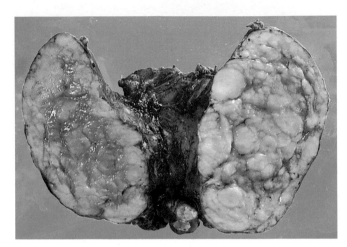

19. This photograph shows part of a mass removed from the neck. Which statement is **most correct**?

(a) The white masses are lymph nodes replaced by malignant lymphoma.

(b) The white masses are lymph nodes showing caseating cervical tuberculosis.

(c) The white masses are parathyroid adenomas.

(d) The white masses are normal lymph nodes.

(e) The white masses are pleomorphic salivary adenomas of the submandibular salivary glands.

Answer on page 597

20. This photograph shows a diffusely enlarged thyroid gland sliced to show the cut-surface of both lateral lobes. Which of the following statements is **most correct**?

(a) The pale fleshy appearance is normal.

(b) The pale fleshy appearance is due to diffuse destruction of follicles by carcinoma.

(c) The pale fleshy appearance is due to diffuse destruction of follicles by lymphocytes.

(d) The patient would have been hyperthyroid.

(e) The patient would have been euthyroid.

Answer on page 598

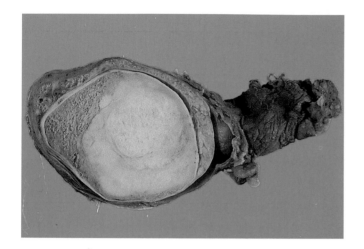

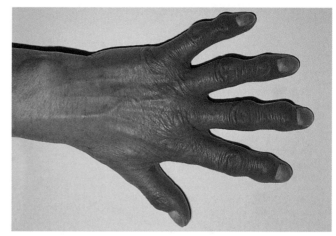

21. This photograph shows a testis removed at operation. Which of the following statements is **most correct**?

(a) Testicular enlargement is due to mumps orchitis.

(b) The pale area in the testis is due to a benign tumor of interstitial (Leydig) cells.

(c) The pale area in the testis is a malignant seminoma.

(d) The pale area in the testis is a malignant mixed teratoma.

(e) The pale area in the testis is a choriocarcinoma.

Answer on page 598

22. This is a photograph of the hand of a 58-year-old woman. Which of the following statements is **most correct**?

The joint changes in the fingers are characteristic of:

(a) Rheumatoid arthritis.

(b) Chronic tophaceous gout.

(c) Osteoarthritis.

(d) Septic arthritis.

(e) Psoriatic arthropathy.

Answer on page 598

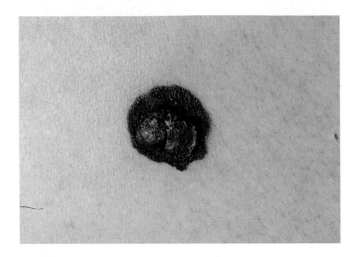

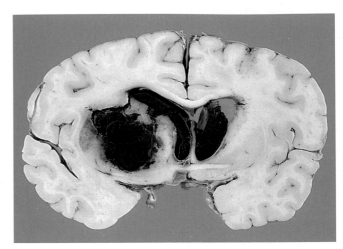

23. This is a photograph of a skin lesion. Which of the following statements is **most correct**?

It is:

(a) A highly pigmented benign compound nevus.

(b) A junctional nevus.

(c) A superficial spreading malignant melanoma *in situ*.

(d) A pigmented hemangioma ('birthmark')

(e) An invasive malignant melanoma.

Answer on page 598

24. This photograph shows a slice through the cerebral hemispheres. Which of the following statements is **most correct**?

The most important predisposing factor in this lesion is:

(a) Cerebral trauma due to head injury.

(b) Systemic hypertension.

(c) Embolism from a mural thrombosis on a myocardial infarct.

(d) Atheroma and thrombosis at the carotid bifurcation.

(e) Severe thrombocytopenia in acute leukemia.

Answer on page 599

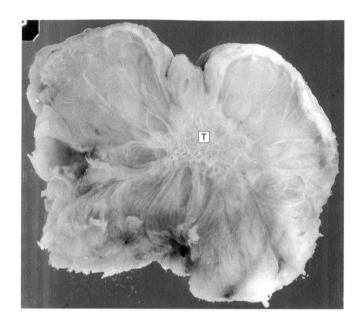

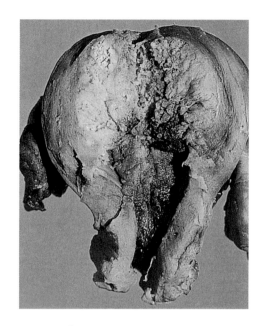

25. This photograph shows breast tissue. Which of the following statements is **most correct**?

(a) The mass (**T**) is a benign nipple adenoma.

(b) Complete local excision effects a cure.

(c) The ill-defined outline of the mass indicates that it is a malignant tumor.

(d) This is sclerosing adenosis.

(e) This is gynecomastia of the male breast.

Answer on page 599

26. This photograph shows a uterus removed at surgery. Which of the following statements is **most correct**?

(a) The patient would have presented with irregular and heavy menstrual bleeding.

(b) The lesion is associated with HPV infection.

(c) This disease is most common in women aged 35–45 years.

(d) The lesion is a degenerating uterine leiomyoma (fibroid).

(e) The lesion is an endometrial adenocarcinoma.

Answer on page 599

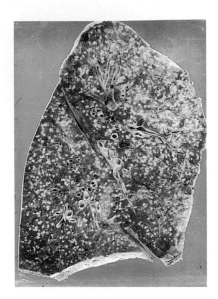

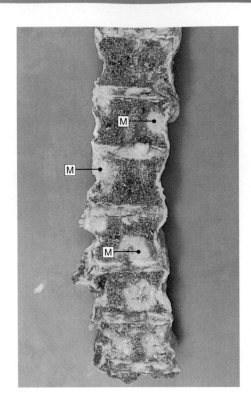

27. This photograph shows a lung affected by miliary tuberculosis. Which of the following statements is **most correct**?

(a) Miliary tuberculosis arises as a result of bloodstream spread of organisms.

(b) The prognosis is good.

(c) This pattern, with tiny areas of infection, occurs in patients with a high patient resistance to the organism.

(d) Miliary tuberculosis is confined to the lungs.

(e) Each small focus eventually enlarges into a large cavitating mass.

Answer on page 599

28. This photograph shows metastatic tumor deposits (**M**) in the vertebral bodies. Of the following statements, which is the **most correct**?

(a) Tumor has spread to the bone by direct local invasion.

(b) Tumor has spread to the bone via lymphatics.

(c) In a man, the most likely primary site of the tumor is the testis.

(d) In a woman, a carcinoma of the breast is the most likely primary site.

(e) Most bone metastases are osteosclerotic and are radio-dense on X-ray.

Answer on page 600

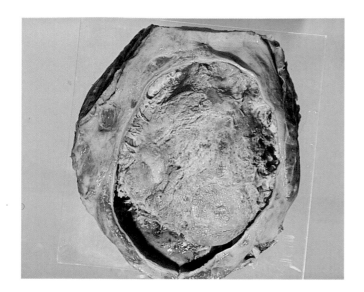

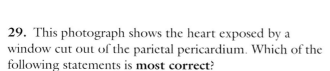

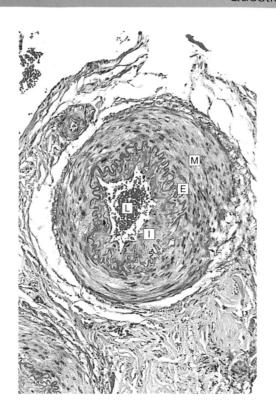

29. This photograph shows the heart exposed by a window cut out of the parietal pericardium. Which of the following statements is **most correct**?

(a) The pericardial cavity and pericardial surfaces are normal.

(b) The pericardial cavity is filled with tuberculous caseous necrosis.

(c) The pericardial cavity is partly obliterated by an acute fibrinous exudate.

(d) The pericardial cavity is partly obliterated by old fibrous adhesions due to an old healed episode of bacterial pericarditis.

(e) The pericardial surfaces are irregular because of malignant tumor deposition from a nearby carcinoma of bronchus.

Answer on page 600

30. This photomicrograph shows an artery in transverse section. Which of the following statements is **most correct**?

(a) The lumen (**L**) of the artery is reduced in size because of atheroma.

(b) The irregular elastic lamina (**E**) means that the artery has been damaged in the past by an episode of necrotizing vasculitis.

(c) The red material in the lumen (**L**) means that the vessel is occluded by thrombosis.

(d) The hypertrophy of the muscular media (**M**) combined with intimal thickening (**I**) means that the patient suffers from 'benign' essential hypertension.

(e) The hypertrophy of the muscular media (**M**) combined with intimal thickening (**I**) means that the patient suffers from 'malignant' accelerated hypertension.

Answer on page 600

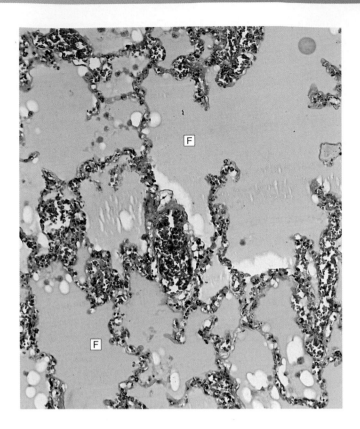

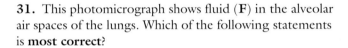

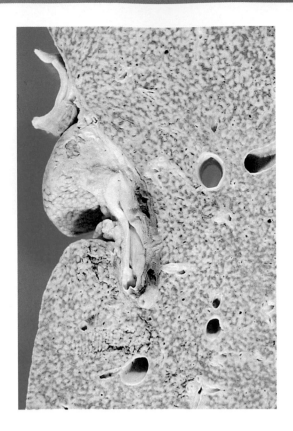

31. This photomicrograph shows fluid (**F**) in the alveolar air spaces of the lungs. Which of the following statements is **most correct**?

(a) The fluid is part of an acute inflammatory exudate due to infection.

(b) The fluid is a transudate which has been pushed into the air sacs from the alveolar capillaries because of a high pressure in the capillary system.

(c) The fluid is a mucoid secretion because the patient suffers from asthma.

(d) The fluid is a transudate which is the result of extensive microthrombosis in pulmonary capillaries and arterioles.

(e) The pink-staining of the fluid is due to seepage of hemoglobin from pulmonary capillaries.

Answer on page 600

32. This picture shows the cut surface of a liver removed at post mortem from a patient with long-standing mitral valve stenosis. The liver slice has been fixed in formalin before photography. Which of the following statements is **most correct**?

(a) The pale areas in the liver are due to acute hepatic necrosis.

(b) The dark areas in the liver are due to excessive iron pigmentation (hemosiderosis) following repeated blood transfusions.

(c) This pattern of the liver is characteristic of chronic ischemia due to hepatic artery atheroma.

(d) This pattern is usually the result of acute left ventricular failure.

(e) This pattern is usually due to chronic right heart failure.

Answer on page 601

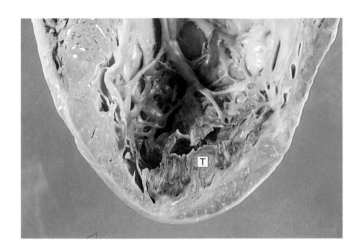

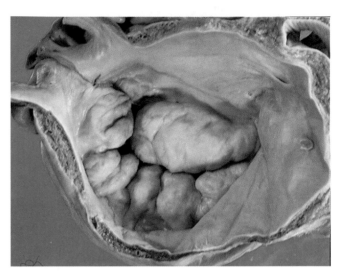

33. This photograph shows mural thrombus (**T**) forming on an area of endocardium damaged by disease. Which of the following statements is **most correct**?

(a) The underlying endocardial abnormality is bacterial endocarditis.

(b) Thrombus has formed because the patient has anti-cardiolipin antibodies.

(c) Thrombus has formed because the patient has atrial fibrillation.

(d) Embolization from this thrombus may occlude a pulmonary artery branch and lead to pulmonary embolism and infarction.

(e) Embolization from this thrombus may lead to a cerebral infarct.

Answer on page 601

34. This photograph looks down on the mitral valve affected by mitral valve prolapse ('floppy valve syndrome'). Which of the following statements is **most correct**?

(a) The irregular thickening of the valve is due to calcification.

(b) The valve is usually functionally stenosed due to narrowing of the valve lumen.

(c) The anterior valve leaflet is usually most severely involved.

(d) Acute rupture of one of the chordae tendinae is an important potentially fatal complication.

(e) The disease is most common in the elderly as a manifestation of senile degeneration of the valve.

Answer on page 601

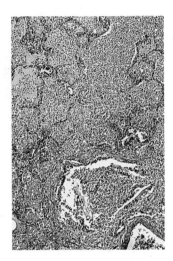

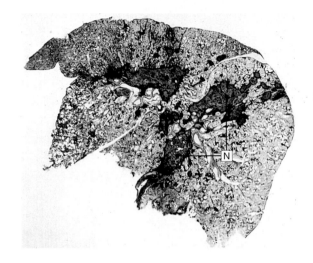

35. This photomicrograph shows the histology of the lung in bronchopneumonia. Which of the following statements is **most correct**?

(a) Bacteria are inhaled into the alveolar air sacs and infection then spreads into the bronchioles.

(b) The most common causative organism is *Klebsiella pneumoniae*.

(c) Bronchopneumonia is often preceded by an upper respiratory infection such as acute tracheobronchitis.

(d) It is a disease of sudden onset in young and middle-aged adults.

(e) It particularly affects the apical segments of the upper lobes.

Answer on page 601

36. This preserved thin slice through a diseased lung shows areas of consolidation (**N**). Which of the following statements is **most correct**?

(a) The areas marked (**N**) are areas of old healed tuberculosis.

(b) The areas marked (**N**) are metastatic deposits of malignant tumor.

(c) The areas marked (**N**) are the consequences of an industrial lung disease.

(d) The areas marked (**N**) are enormously enlarged peribronchial lymph nodes containing carbon inhaled over a long period (anthracosis).

(e) The areas marked (**N**) will contain numerous asbestos bodies.

Answer on page 602

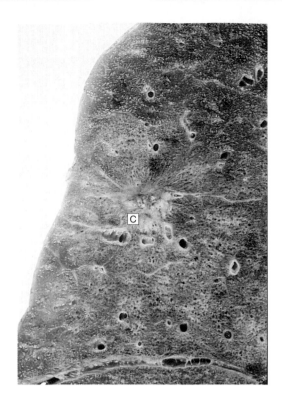

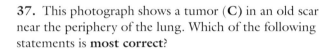

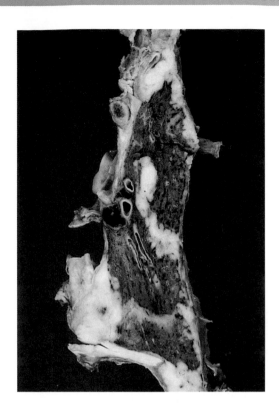

37. This photograph shows a tumor (**C**) in an old scar near the periphery of the lung. Which of the following statements is **most correct?**

(a) Because of its small size, the tumor is most likely to be benign.

(b) Smoking is an important etiological factor in the development of this type of tumor.

(c) Extra-pulmonary metastatic tumor spread is very unlikely.

(d) This is most likely an adenocarcinoma.

(e) Fibrosis within the tumor has led to the scarred appearance.

Answer on page 602

38. This photograph shows a compressed and collapsed lung encased in a shell of white tumor which is a pleural mesothelioma. Which of the following statements is **most correct?**

(a) Mesothelioma of the pleura metastasizes to peribronchial lymph nodes.

(b) Mesothelioma of the pleura is associated with the recent inhalation of substantial amounts of asbestos fibers in a long occupational setting.

(c) Persistent pleural effusion is an early common clinical feature.

(d) Pleural biopsy is of no value in establishing the diagnosis.

(e) There is a 60% 5-year survival rate.

Answer on page 602

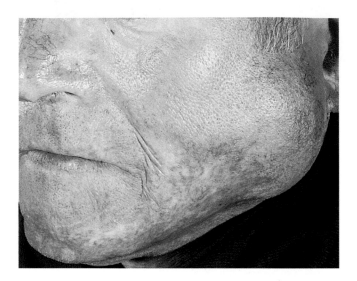

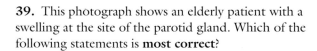

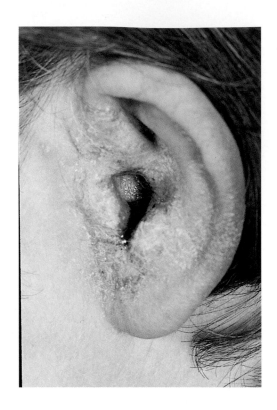

39. This photograph shows an elderly patient with a swelling at the site of the parotid gland. Which of the following statements is **most correct**?

(a) The majority of tumors in the parotid gland are malignant adenoid-cystic carcinomas.

(b) Mumps parotitis is high in the differential diagnosis in this case.

(c) This is most likely a pleomorphic salivary adenoma.

(d) Salivary gland tumors are confined to the parotid, submandibular and sublingual salivary glands.

(e) Benign tumors of the parotid gland are well-circumscribed and encapsulated, so can be easily shelled out without complication.

Answer on page 602

40. This photomicrograph shows acute inflammation of the external ear. Which of the following is **most correct**?

(a) The inflammation is always due to bacterial infection.

(b) This condition may be complicated by a perforated eardrum.

(c) This condition may be complicated by acute mastoiditis.

(d) This condition may be complicted by 'glue ear' in a child.

(e) This condition may be complicated by an allergic reaction to ear drops.

Answer on page 603

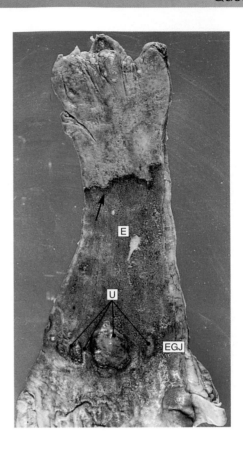

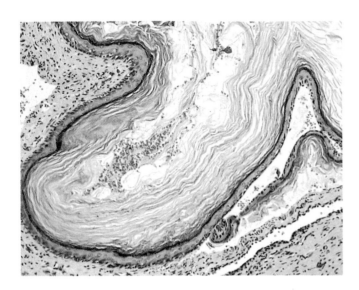

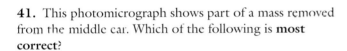

41. This photomicrograph shows part of a mass removed from the middle ear. Which of the following is **most correct?**

(a) It is a benign cholesteatoma.

(b) It is a well-differentiated keratinizing squamous carcinoma.

(c) It remains confined to the middle ear cavity.

(d) Surgical removal is easy and curative.

(e) The lesion is usually asymptomatic except for symptoms of earache.

Answer on page 603

42. This photomicrograph shows the lower end of the esophagus, with the esophago-gastric junction indicated by the label (**EGJ**). Which of the following is **most correct?**

(a) The lower esophageal mucosa (**E**) in this picture is lined by non-keratinizing squamous epithelium.

(b) This is Barrett's esophagus, with columnar epithelium at (**E**).

(c) The ulcerated areas (**U**) at the esophago-gastric junction are due to early carcinoma.

(d) The darker red mucosa at (**E**) is the result of inflammation due to severe Candida infection in this immunosuppressed patient.

(e) The changes seen are the consequences of long-standing esophageal achalasia.

Answer on page 603

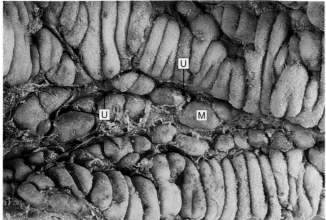

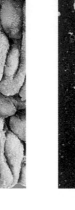

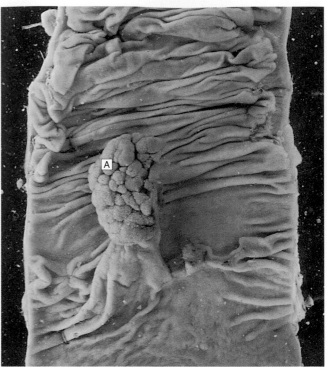

43. This photograph shows the mucosa of the small intestine. Which of the following statements is **most correct**?

(a) The structures labeled (**U**) are linear deep fissured ulcers.

(b) The raised areas labeled (**M**) represent malignant infiltration of mucosa and submucosa by small intestinal malignant lymphoma.

(c) The abnormalities are most likely confined to the mucosal and submucosal layers of the small bowel.

(d) The abnormalities are most likely to involve the entire small intestine.

(e) The abnormalities are cured by antibiotic treatment.

Answer on page 603

44. This photograph shows a mass protruding into the colon in a patient who passed blood per rectum on a number of occasions. Which of the following is **most correct**?

(a) The lesion (**A**) is a metaplastic (hyperplastic) polyp.

(b) The lesion (**A**) is a tubular adenoma.

(c) The lesion (**A**) is a villous adenoma.

(d) The lesion (**A**) is a colonic adenocarcinoma Dukes' Stage B.

(e) The lesion (**A**) is a post-inflammatory polyp following chronic ulcerative colitis.

Answer on page 604

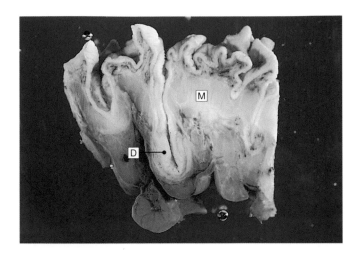

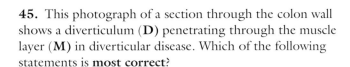

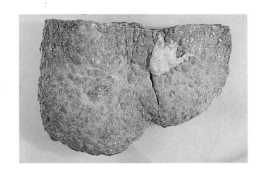

45. This photograph of a section through the colon wall shows a diverticulum (**D**) penetrating through the muscle layer (**M**) in diverticular disease. Which of the following statements is **most correct**?

(a) The muscle layer (**M**) is normal thickness.

(b) The diverticulum (**D**) is infected.

(c) Diverticular disease occurs in young people.

(d) Diverticular disease can be complicated by development of a paracolic abscess.

(e) Diverticular disease is most common in cecum and ascending colon.

Answer on page 604

46. This photograph shows a liver affected by cirrhosis. Which of the following is **most correct**?

(a) The irregular surface is indicative that hepatocellular carcinoma has supervened.

(b) The irregular surface is due to regenerative nodules and fibrosis.

(c) Cirrhosis presents as acute hepatic failure.

(d) Cirrhosis is usually secondary to long-standing extra-hepatic biliary obstruction.

(e) Cirrhosis can be complicated by systemic venous hypertension.

Answer on page 604

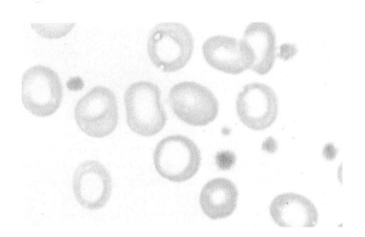

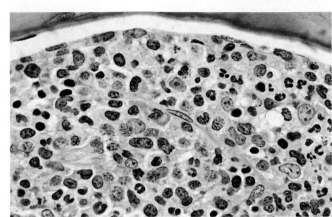

47. This photomicrograph shows red cells and platelets in a blood film from a patient with anemia. Which of the following statements is **most correct**?

(a) The red cells are macrocytic and suggest a diagnosis of B_{12}/folate deficiency.

(b) The red cells are microcytic and hypochromic, suggesting a diagnosis of iron deficiency.

(c) Platelet numbers are increased, suggesting a hemolytic anemia due to hereditary spherocytosis.

(d) Absence of white cells in this field suggests an aplastic anemia due to failure of hemopoietic stem cells.

(e) Examination of a bone marrow aspirate is essential to establish the cause of anemia in this case.

Answer on page 604

48. This photomicrograph shows the bone marrow appearances in a patient with leukemia. Which of the following statements is **most correct**?

(a) The predominant cell is a primitive lymphoblast, and the diagnosis is acute lymphoblastic leukemia.

(b) The predominant cell is the mature lymphocyte, and the diagnosis is chronic lymphocytic leukemia.

(c) The predominant cell is the primitive myeloblast, and the diagnosis is acute myeloblastic leukemia.

(d) The predominant cell is the monocyte, and the diagnosis is acute monocytic leukemia.

(e) The predominant cells are a mixture of early, middle and late cells of the myeloid series, and the diagnosis is chronic myeloid (granulocytic) leukemia.

Answer on page 605

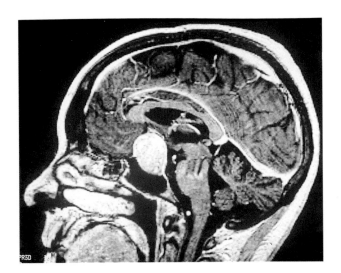

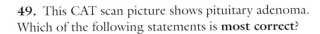

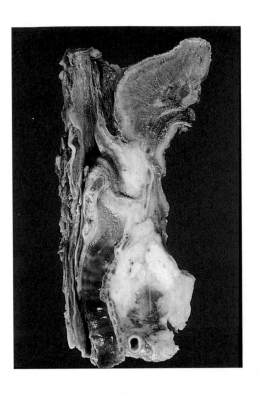

49. This CAT scan picture shows pituitary adenoma. Which of the following statements is **most correct**?

(a) All pituitary adenomas cause illness by excessive secretion of pituitary hormones.

(b) An important presenting symptom of pituitary adenoma is bitemporal hemianopia.

(c) The commonest hormone disturbance syndrome produced by a pituitary adenoma is Cushing's disease due to ACTH excess.

(d) Pituitary adenoma often produces diabetes insipidus.

(e) Sheehan's syndrome is a complication of pituitary adenoma.

Answer on page 605

50. This photograph shows a carcinoma of the thyroid compressing and infiltrating the trachea. Which of the following statements is **most correct**?

(a) This example is most likely to be a papillary carcinoma of the thyroid.

(b) This example is most likely to be a follicular carcinoma of the thyroid.

(c) This example is most likely to be anaplastic carcinoma of the thyroid.

(d) Papillary carcinoma mainly occurs in the elderly and has a bad prognosis.

(e) Anaplastic carcinoma sometimes presents with metastases in bone.

Answer on page 605

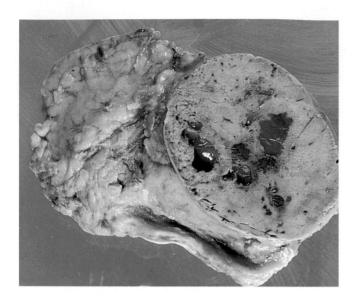

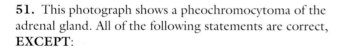

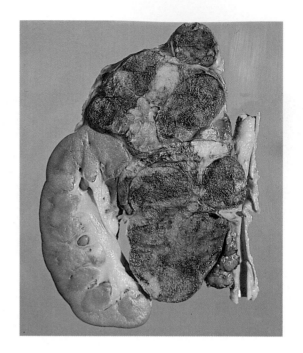

51. This photograph shows a pheochromocytoma of the adrenal gland. All of the following statements are correct, **EXCEPT**:

(a) Pheochromocytomas are derived from the adrenal medulla.

(b) Pheochromocytoma is one of the endocrine tumor seen in the MEN 1 syndrome.

(c) Pheochromocytoma can be diagnosed by measuring urinary VMA levels which are greatly increased.

(d) Pheochromocytoma may be bilateral.

(e) Pheochromocytoma is a cause of surgically-treatable systemic hypertension.

Answer on page 605

52. This photograph shows a large tumor in a young child. Which of the following is **most correct**?

(a) The most likely diagnosis is nephroblastoma.

(b) The most likely diagnosis is a malignant pheochromocytoma.

(c) The most likely diagnosis is malignant lymphoma affecting the para-aortic lymph nodes.

(d) The most likely diagnosis is neuroblastoma of the adrenal medulla.

(e) The most likely diagnosis is a carcinoma of the adrenal cortex.

Answer on page 605

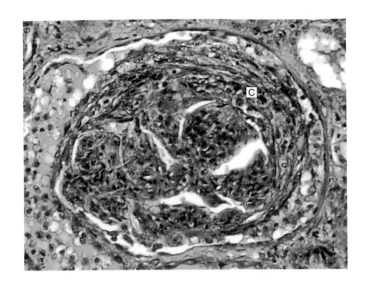
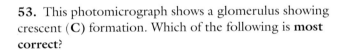

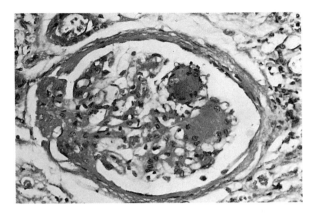

53. This photomicrograph shows a glomerulus showing crescent (**C**) formation. Which of the following is **most correct?**

(a) Crescent formation has a good prognosis.

(b) Crescent formation is frequent in membranous nephropathy.

(c) Crescent formation is due to proliferation of epithelial cells lining Bowman's capsule.

(d) Crescent formation is a component of diabetic nephropathy.

(e) Crescent formation only affects the elderly.

Answer on page 606

54. This photomicrograph shows spherical 'Kimmelstiel–Wilson nodules' forming in the glomerular mesangium in a patient with diabetic renal disease. The following are other features of diabetic renal disease, **EXCEPT:**

(a) Diffuse glomerular basement-membrane thickening.

(b) Diffuse diabetic glomerulosclerosis.

(c) Increased susceptibility to chronic ischemic glomerular damage.

(d) Increased susceptibility to bacterial infection (acute pyelonephritis).

(e) Acute cortical necrosis.

Answer on page 606

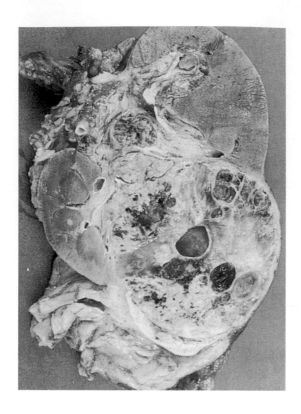

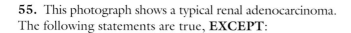

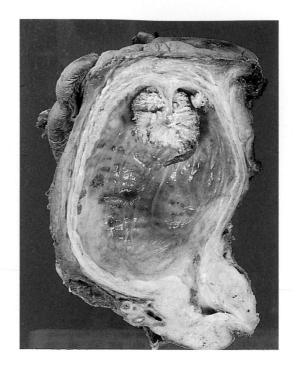

55. This photograph shows a typical renal adenocarcinoma. The following statements are true, **EXCEPT**:

(a) The variegated yellow cut-surface appearance with foci of necrosis and hemorrhage is typical.

(b) A clear cell pattern, with the tumor composed of vacuolated cells, is common.

(c) It is most common in women over the age of 50 years.

(d) Blood-borne metastases to lung and bone are common.

(e) Common presenting symptoms include hematuria, loin pain and a loin mass.

Answer on page 606

56. This photograph shows a tumor (**T**) at the fundus of the bladder. Which of the following statements is **most correct**?

(a) The fact that it has an identifiable stalk means that the tumor is benign.

(b) The fact that it has a well-formed papillary surface pattern means that it is benign.

(c) Papillary transitional cell carcinomas are only found in the bladder.

(d) Sessile tumors which develop in an area of carcinoma *in situ* of transitional cell epithelium have a poor prognosis.

(e) A bladder carcinoma situated (as here) in the dome of the bladder is most likely to be an adenocarcinoma derived from the urachal remnant.

Answer on page 606

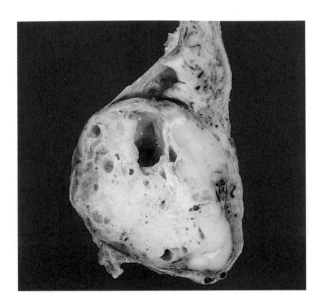

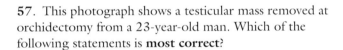

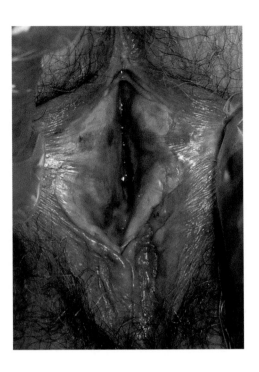

57. This photograph shows a testicular mass removed at orchidectomy from a 23-year-old man. Which of the following statements is **most correct**?

(a) The slightly yellow color means that it is most likely to be a Leydig cell tumor.

(b) The foci of necrosis suggest that this is due to tuberculous infection.

(c) If a tumor, the patient's age would suggest that seminoma is the most likely diagnosis.

(d) Preoperative investigations should include measurement of the tumor markers alpha fetoprotein (AFP) and human chorionic gonadotrophin (HCG).

(e) Most painless testicular swellings are due to benign tumor.

Answer on page 606

58. This photograph shows lichen sclerosus of the vulva. The following statements are true, **EXCEPT**:

(a) Lichen sclerosus can lead to severe narrowing of the introitus.

(b) Lichen sclerosus is a general skin disease with a predilection for the vulva.

(c) Long-standing lichen sclerosus can predispose to squamous carcinoma of the vulva.

(d) Lichen sclerosus is a disease confined to post-menopausal women.

(e) Epidermal atrophy is a characteristic histological feature.

Answer on page 606

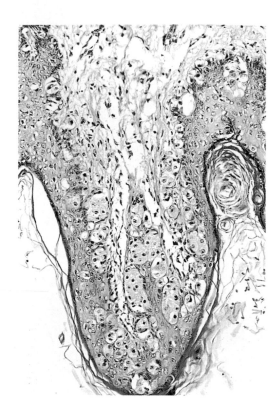

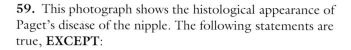

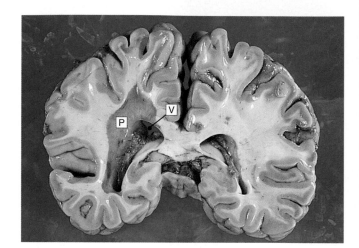

59. This photograph shows the histological appearance of Paget's disease of the nipple. The following statements are true, **EXCEPT**:

(a) The large pale cells in the epidermis are breast carcinoma cells.

(b) Clinically the disease can be confused with eczema (acute dermatitis) of the nipple.

(c) Paget's disease is associated with ductal carcinoma of the breast.

(d) Paget's disease is associated with lobular carcinoma of the breast.

(e) Clinically the disease presents as reddening and thickening of the skin of the nipple and surrounding areola.

Answer on page 606

60. This slice of brain shows an abnormal dark area (**P**) alongside the lateral ventricle (**V**). Which of the following is **most correct**?

(a) It represents an area of recent infarction due to occlusion of the middle cerebral artery.

(b) It is an area of old hemorrhage with hemosiderin staining.

(c) It is a well-differentiated primary astrocytoma.

(d) It is an area of brain necrosis due to herpes simplex encephalitis.

(e) It is an area of demyelination in multiple sclerosis.

Answer on page 606

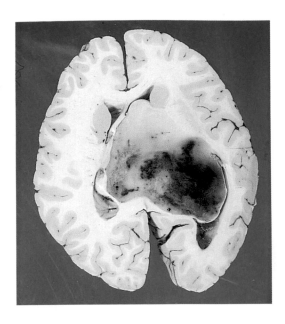

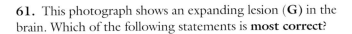

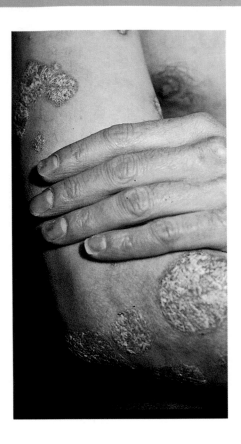

61. This photograph shows an expanding lesion (**G**) in the brain. Which of the following statements is **most correct**?

(a) The lesion is mainly well-circumscribed and is benign.

(b) Because of its brown color, it is most likely a metastasis from malignant melanoma.

(c) It is an organizing hematoma following a non-fatal cerebral hemorrhage in the basal ganglia region.

(d) It is a low-grade, well-differentiated primary glial tumor.

(e) It is a high-grade, poorly differentiated primary glial tumor.

Answer on page 607

62. This photograph shows a typical lesion of active psoriasis on the forearm. All of the following statements are true, **EXCEPT**:

(a) Epidermal pustules sometimes form in psoriasis.

(b) Psoriasis can lead to damage to finger-nails.

(c) Psoriasis may lead to a specific joint disease.

(d) The white material on the surface of the psoriasis plaque is an acute inflammatory exudate.

(e) Elbows and knees are characteristic sites for psoriasis lesions.

Answer on page 607

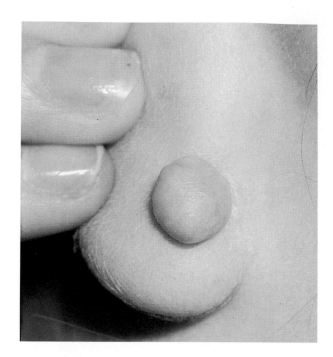

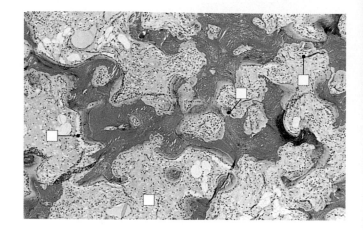

63. This photograph shows a keloid in the earlobe. Which of the following statements is **most correct**?

(a) Keloids are most common on the lower limbs.

(b) Keloids are most common in post-menopausal women.

(c) Keloids only form at sites of trauma to the skin.

(d) Keloids may proliferate and become an autonomous tumor called dermatofibrosarcoma protruberans.

(e) Keloids quickly regress leaving a depressed scar.

Answer on page 607

64. This photomicrograph shows the histology of bone with active Paget's disease. The following are true, **EXCEPT**:

(a) The distortion of bone architecture is the result of haphazard osteoclastic resorption and osteoblastic new bone formation.

(b) The red-staining material covering some of the bone (green) surfaces is unmineralized osteoid recently produced by active osteoblasts.

(c) Replacement of marrow spaces by fibrous tissue is a feature of severe Paget's disease.

(d) Failure of mineralization of the red-staining osteoid is due to Vitamin D deficiency.

(e) Long-standing active Paget's disease of bone may be complicated by the development of the highly malignant tumor, osteosarcoma.

Answer on page 607

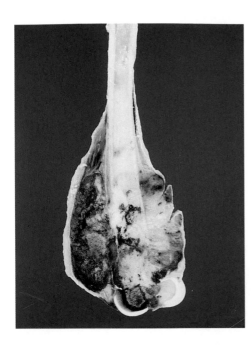

65. This photograph shows the highly malignant tumor of bone, osteosarcoma. The following are correct, **EXCEPT**:

(a) Osteosarcoma is a disease mainly seen in children.

(b) Osteosarcoma is a malignant tumor derived from osteoclasts.

(c) This site (lower end of femur) is a characteristic location for the tumor.

(d) Blood-borne metastases to lungs are common.

(e) Calcification within the tumor is a useful diagnostic sign on imaging.

Answer on page 607

66. Nomenclature of tumors

(a) Adenoma

(b) Adenocarcinoma

(c) Hepatoma

(d) Hamartoma

(e) Papilloma

(f) Sarcoma

(g) Lymphoma

(h) Granuloma

(i) Teratoma

(j) Embryonal tumor

For each description of a neoplasm, select the **most likely** name from the list above.

1. Diffuse infiltration of the liver by large, pleomorphic lymphocytes which are all B-cell in type expressing a single light chain.

2. A mass in the sacrum in any infant containing cartilage, squamous epithelium, neural tissue, thyroid epithelium and bone.

3. A mass in the adrenal gland of a child containing small, mitotically active cells identified as neuroblasts.

4. A mass in the thigh containing pleomorphic spindle-shaped cells with abundant mitoses and necrosis, associated with vascular invasion and metastatic spread to the lung.

5. A mass in the lung composed of smooth muscle and cartilage.

Answer on page 608

67. A patient with a known large anterior myocardial infarct, sustained 2 days previously, suddenly develops a left hemiplegia and dies shortly afterwards. Which of the following is the **most likely** cause?

(a) Thrombosis in the right internal carotid artery, superimposed on vascular atheroma.

(b) Embolization of thrombus from the endocardial surface of the infarcted left ventricle into the right carotid artery.

(c) Rupture of the infarcted myocardium leading to cardiac tamponade.

(d) Development of a leg vein thrombosis with embolization to the brain.

(e) Development of a cerebral abscess following embolization of infected material from endocarditis affecting the aortic valve.

Answer on page 608

68. The process of apoptosis is associated with the following features, **EXCEPT**:

(a) Cleavage of chromatin by endonucleases to form nucleosome-sized fragments.

(b) Stimulation of a local tissue inflammatory response.

(c) Activation of caspases.

(d) Phagocytosis of apoptotic fragments by local macrophages.

(e) Condensation of chromatin beneath the nuclear membrane in the early stage.

Answer on page 608

69. Potentially reversible cell injury caused by hypoxia includes the following, **EXCEPT**:

(a) Reduction in cellular ATP concentration.

(b) Fall in cell pH.

(c) Accumulation of cell glycogen.

(d) Retention of Na^+ and water within the cell.

(e) Low amplitude swelling of mitochondria.

Answer on page 608

70. The following are true, **EXCEPT**:

(a) Fatty change is a form of sublethal metabolic derangement.

(b) Fatty change leads to accumulation of apoproteins within affected cells.

(c) Fatty change can be caused by agents that increase the esterification of free fatty acids to triglycerides.

(d) Fatty change can be stimulated by factors that decrease the oxidation of free fatty acids.

(e) Fatty change in the liver can be caused by ethanol, halogenated hydrocarbons as well as chronic hypoxia.

Answer on page 608

71. The following definitions are true, **EXCEPT**:

(a) Failure of formation of an embryonic cell mass leads to agenesis of an organ.

(b) Failure of differentiation of an embryonic cell mass to organ-specific tissues leads to aplasia of an organ or tissue.

(c) Failure of the structural organization of tissues to form an anatomically correct organ is termed dysgenesis.

(d) Failure of a developing organ to reach full size is termed atrophy.

(e) Differentiation of a mature tissue to a very mature stable type of cell is termed metaplasia.

Answer on page 608

72. The following statements are correct, **EXCEPT**:

(a) Hyperplasia is an increase in the number of cells in a tissue caused by increase in cell division.

(b) Hypertrophy is an increase in the size of existing cells in a tissue, brought about through increased protein synthesis.

(c) Hyperplasia persists once the stimulus causing it has been removed.

(d) Reduction in the functional mass of a tissue can occur through apoptosis or decrease in the size of individual cells.

(e) Cellular atrophy is associated with accumulation of lipofuscin.

Answer on page 608

73. The cell stress response is associated with the following features, **EXCEPT**:

(a) Upregulation of housekeeping genes.

(b) Production of heat shock proteins.

(c) Activation by hypoxia and irradiation.

(d) Resistance of the cell to denaturation of proteins.

(e) Upregulation of proteolytic pathways responsible for eliminating damaged proteins.

Answer on page 609

74. Which of these statements is **least correct**?

(a) Neoplastic cells show nuclear hyperchromatism compared to normal counterparts.

(b) Neoplastic cells show a disproportionately large increase in the size of nuclei relative to the size of the cell cytoplasm compared to normal counterparts.

(c) Benign neoplasms can spread via the bloodstream and cause metastases.

(d) Cells in a benign neoplasm are generally uniform in appearance throughout the tumor.

(e) Cells in a malignant neoplasm vary in shape and size throughout the tumor.

Answer on page 609

75. Which of the following statements is **least correct?**

(a) In acute inflammation the affected area is occupied by a transient material called an exudate.

(b) In acute inflammation small blood vessels adjacent to the affected area initially dilate followed by slowing of blood flow in them.

(c) In acute inflammation circulating neutrophil polymorphs adhere to endothelial cells prior to migration through the vessel wall into tissues.

(d) In acute inflammation resolution is usually followed by scarring.

(e) In acute inflammation fibrinogen is polymerized to fibrin when plasma proteins leak from vessels into tissues.

Answer on page 609

76. Which of the following statements is **least correct?**

(a) Histamine is a pre-formed mediator of acute inflammation found in mast cells and platelets.

(b) Histamine is an important cause of increased vascular permeability.

(c) Both prostaglandins and leukotrienes are derived from local synthesis from arachidonic acid.

(d) Interleukin-1 (IL-1) and Interleukin-8 (IL-8) directly cause endothelial necrosis in the early phase of acute inflammation.

(e) C5a increases vascular permeability by liberating histamine from mast cells and platelets.

Answer on page 609

77. The following situations would all be associated with impaired wound healing, **EXCEPT:**

(a) Healing of an abdominal surgical incision in a patient taking corticosteroids.

(b) Healing of an abrasion on the ankle of a 68-year-old man with diabetes mellitus.

(c) Healing of a bone fracture in the paralysed limb of a person with a dense hemiplegia.

(d) Healing of a surgical incision in the axilla of a woman who had irradiation of the area 2 years previously to treat breast cancer.

(e) Healing of an abdominal surgical incision in a patient taking prophylactic antibiotics for chronic rheumatic mitral valve disease.

Answer on page 609

78. Which of the following statements is **least correct?**

(a) In chronic inflammation the processes of tissue damage, organization and repair occur concurrently.

(b) Chronic inflammation is characterized by a dominant infiltration of tissues by neutrophil polymorphs.

(c) Chronic inflammation always heals by organization and never heals by resolution.

(d) Chronic inflammation is predisposed by an inadequate host response to infection.

(e) Chronic inflammation is a feature of persistent autoimmune diseases.

Answer on page 610

79. Which of the following statements is **least correct**?

(a) Granulomatous inflammation is characterized by a Type IV hypersensitivity response.

(b) The main histological feature seen in granulomatous inflammation is aggregates of plasma cells.

(c) Granulomatous inflammation is seen in diseases caused by mycobacteria.

(d) Foreign material which gains entry to tissues, such as an inorganic dust, can cause a granulomatous response.

(e) Sarcoid is an example of a disease dominated by granulomatous inflammation.

Answer on page 610

80. Which of the following statements is **least correct**?

(a) Mosaicism is caused by a chromosomal abnormality that develops during mitotic division after fertilization.

(b) Genomic imprinting causes the differential expression of a gene depending on whether it is inherited from the mother or father.

(c) Uniparental disomy is an uncommon cause of non-Mendelian inheritance.

(d) A maternal translocation can cause Down's syndrome and this is associated with a low recurrence in subsequent pregancies.

(e) The most important abnormalities of sex chromosome number arise from non-disjunction during meiotic division of gametes.

Answer on page 610

81. Which of the following statements is **least correct**?

(a) In autosomal recessive inheritance, affected individuals are homozygous for the causative gene.

(b) In autosomal recessive inheritance there is 25% chance of heterozygous carrier parents producing an affected homozygous child.

(c) In X-linked recessive inheritance, unaffected males do not carry the causative gene.

(d) In mitochondrial inheritance the progeny of unaffected males may be affected by disease.

(e) In penetrant autosomal dominant inheritance, clinically unaffected individuals cannot pass on the disease.

Answer on page 610

82. Which of the following statements is **least correct**?

(a) In grading a tumor the degree of differentiation of tumor cells is assessed.

(b) In grading a tumor the proportion of cells in cycle, as assessed by the mitotic index, is commonly used.

(c) In staging a tumor it is important to consider the degree of necrosis in the lesion.

(d) In most systems of tumor staging, spread to lymph nodes denotes an advanced stage.

(e) An *in situ* neoplasm is a stage of tumor prior to the development of invasion.

Answer on page 610

83. Which of the following statements about breast disease is **least correct**?

(a) Fibrocystic disease would be the appropriate diagnosis in a lesion from the breast of a 40-year-old woman showing proliferation of ducts and lobular tissue with cyst formation, apocrine metaplasia and surrounding collagenous fibrosis.

(b) Atypical hyperplasia in fibrocystic disease is a risk factor for the subsequent development of carcinoma.

(c) Duct papillomas of the breast are most commonly seen in the large ducts near the nipple.

(d) Paget's disease of the nipple is caused by spread of adenocarcinoma cells from underlying breast into the epidermis of the skin of the nipple.

(e) A mobile discrete breast lump in a female aged 48 is most likely to be a fibroadenoma.

Answer on page 610

84. Which of the following situations is **least likely** to predispose to renal papillary necrosis?

(a) Urinary tract infection in a patient with diabetes mellitus.

(b) A patient with sickle cell disease who develops a lobar pneumonia.

(c) A patient with bilateral hydronephrosis due to bladder outflow obstruction, complicated by urinary tract infection.

(d) A patient who develops severe hypotension as a complication of bleeding from a stab wound to the chest.

(e) A patient with acute pyelonephritis in pregnancy.

Answer on page 611

85. Which of the following statements about disease of the hemopoietic system is **least correct**?

(a) An anemia in which there is borderline microcytosis with a normal serum ferritin level is likely to be due to iron deficiency.

(b) Myelodysplasia is characterized by an increased risk of the development of leukemia.

(c) Hemolysis is an important feature of sickle cell anemia.

(d) Eosinophils are a feature of a response to parasitic infections.

(e) In myeloma, Bence–Jones protein is composed of free light chains or their fragments.

Answer on page 611

86. Which of these statements about disease of the lymphoid system is **least correct**?

(a) Hodgkin's disease is the most common form of primary neoplasm of the lymphoid system.

(b) A person with Hodgkin's disease shown to have disease confined to cervical and mediastinal nodal groups has stage II disease.

(c) A lymphoma affecting the stomach is most likely to be a tumor of mucosal-associated lymphoid tissue.

(d) T-cell lymphoma is associated with HTLV-1 infection in a proportion of cases.

(e) Bone marrow involvement by a neoplasm of lymphoid cells excludes the possibility that it is a lymphoma and proves it is a leukemia.

Answer on page 611

87. Which of these statements about portal hypertension is **least correct?**

(a) In portal hypertension back pressure in the portal vascular bed leads to splenomegaly, ascites and venous varices.

(b) The least common sinusoidal cause of portal hypertension is cirrhosis.

(c) Portal vein thrombosis is a cause of pre-sinusoidal portal hypertension.

(d) Disorders that cause destruction and obliteration of central veins in the liver lead to post-sinusoidal portal hypertension.

(e) Severe, acute portal hypertension is precipitated by hepatic vein thrombosis.

Answer on page 611

88. A 32-year-old man is seen because of severe abdominal pain, pyrexia, and abdominal swelling. He has a mass in the right iliac fossa and a laparotomy is performed. This reveals a thickened, red terminal ileum, enlarged lymph nodes in the adjacent small bowel mesentery and some thickening in the cecum. Which of these statements is **least correct?**

(a) Ileocecal tuberculosis should be considered as a possible diagnosis.

(b) Crohn's disease is a strong possibility.

(c) *Yersinia enterocolitica* infection is a diagnostic possibility.

(d) Localized ulcerative colitis is a probable diagnosis.

(e) A small bowel lymphoma may be the cause of these findings.

Answer on page 611

89. Which of these statements is **least correct?**

(a) Carcinoid tumors of the small bowel are derived from neuroendocrine cells and may secrete endocrine hormones.

(b) Lymphoma of the small bowel may be a complication of celiac disease.

(c) Hyperplastic polyps of the large bowel are a precursor lesion of carcinomas.

(d) In Peutz–Jegher's syndrome multiple hamartomatous polyps develop in the bowel.

(e) Adenocarcinoma of the colon is predisposed by long-standing ulcerative colitis.

Answer on page 611

90. Which of the following statements is **least correct?**

(a) In celiac disease, the small bowel mucosa shows crypt hyperplasia with villous atrophy.

(b) In celiac disease serum antibodies to gliadin are found.

(c) Deficiency of vitamins D and A may occur as a complication of pancreatic atrophy in cystic fibrosis.

(d) In celiac disease, biopsy assessment of mucosal architecture is not helpful in diagnosis.

(e) Disaccharidase enzymes are located on the brush border of small bowel enterocytes.

Answer on page 611

91. The following statements about myeloma are true, **EXCEPT**:

(a) Myeloma is a tumor of a clone of plasma cells.

(b) It is most common over the age of 50.

(c) Bence–Jones protein in the urine consists of whole molecules of abnormal immunoglobulin produced by the tumor cells.

(d) Myeloma may lead to amyloid deposition in tissues.

(e) Myeloma may lead to a leuko-erythroblastic anemia.

Answer on page 612

92. The following statements about Cushing's syndrome are true, **EXCEPT**:

(a) The commonest cause is an adrenal cortical adenoma.

(b) Severe osteoporosis is a complication.

(c) Wound healing is poor in Cushing's syndrome.

(d) Diagnosis is confirmed by raised plasma cortisol levels.

(e) It can occur as a non-metastatic effect of small-cell undifferentiated carcinoma of the bronchus due to ectopic ACTH secretion by the tumor cells.

Answer on page 612

93. Which of the following statements about minimal change nephropathy is **most correct**?

(a) It is a common cause of nephritic syndrome in children.

(b) It is a focal and segmental glomerular disease.

(c) Loss of podocyte foot processes is associated with immune complex deposits in glomerular basement membrane.

(d) Progressive mesangial sclerosis supervenes over many years, leading to chronic renal failure.

(e) Loss of podocyte foot processes is associated with loss of the high polyanionic charge on the outer aspect of the glomerular basement membrane and inner surface of the podocytes.

Answer on page 612

94. The following statements about salpingitis are all true, **EXCEPT**:

(a) Salpingitis may be complicated by tubo-ovarian abscess or pyosalpinx.

(b) Healed salpingitis may lead to hydrosalpinx.

(c) Chronic salpingitis may lead to primary adenocarcinoma of the Fallopian tube.

(d) Chronic or healed scarred salpingitis is a common cause of tubal obstruction leading to infertility.

(e) Chronic or healed scarred salpingitis predisposes to tubal ectopic pregnancy.

Answer on page 612

95. The following are all virus infections of the skin, **EXCEPT**:

(a) *Molluscum contagiosum.*

(b) Condyloma acuminatum.

(c) Condyloma latum.

(d) Shingles.

(e) Plantar wart.

Answer on page 612

96. The following statements about basal cell carcinoma of the skin are true, **EXCEPT**:

(a) Basal cell carcinoma is commonest on sun-exposed areas, particularly the face.

(b) Basal cell carcinoma of the head and neck metastasizes via lymphatics to the cervical lymph nodes.

(c) Basal cell carcinoma may show nodular, morpheic and superficial growth patterns.

(d) Basal cell carcinoma may arise in areas of the skin which have previously been exposed to radiotherapy.

(e) Basal cell carcinoma is the commonest malignant tumor of the skin.

Answer on page 612

97. The following statements about osteomalacia are true, **EXCEPT**:

(a) Osteomalacia is a condition in which there is failure of mineralization of osteoid.

(b) Osteomalacia is due to Vitamin D deficiency.

(c) Osteomalacia can be induced by prolonged corticosteroid therapy.

(d) Osteomalacia can result from malabsorption due to extensive intestinal disease.

(e) Osteomalacia can occur as a complication of chronic renal failure.

Answer on page 612

98. Which of the following statements about parathyroid adenoma is **most correct**?

(a) Parathyroid adenoma is usually multiple, affecting more than one of the four parathyroid glands.

(b) Excessive secretion of parathyroid hormone leads to osteomalacia by stimulating osteoblastic synthesis of excess osteoid.

(c) Chronic renal failure is an important factor in the development of most parathyroid adenomas.

(d) Hypercalcemia is an important feature of parathyroid adenoma.

(e) Malignant change is a risk in long-standing parathyroid adenomas.

Answer on page 612

99. The following are true statements about progressive systemic sclerosis, **EXCEPT**:

(a) The skin is the most commonly affected organ.

(b) Lung involvement may lead to 'honeycomb lung' due to chronic interstitial fibrosis.

(c) Scleroderma is more common in men than women.

(d) Scleroderma can produce acute renal failure via small vessel damage.

(e) Submucosal fibrosis affecting the esophagus may interfere with peristalsis.

Answer on page 612

100. The following are true statements about sarcoidosis, **EXCEPT**:

(a) Lung involvement may lead to pulmonary interstitial fibrosis.

(b) Skin involvement is common.

(c) Uveitis is an important component of eye involvement.

(d) Renal involvement may lead to renal failure.

(e) Lymphadenopathy commonly involves intrathoracic nodes.

Answer on page 612

101. Which of the following statements about cerebrovascular disease is **least correct?**

(a) Lacunar infarcts are predisposed by hyaline arteriolosclerosis and are common in the basal ganglia.

(b) Cortical laminar necrosis is caused by generalized failure of cerebral perfusion or severe hypoxia.

(c) Thrombosis of the sagittal sinus is a cause of cerebral infarction.

(d) If an occlusive thrombus in a large cerebral artery undergoes lysis after it has caused infarction of brain tissue then a hemorrhagic infarct develops.

(e) The commonest site for primary intracerebral hemorrhage caused by hypertension is the subarachnoid space.

Answer on page 612

102. Which of these statements is **least correct?**

(a) Normal intraocular pressure is determined by continuous secretion of aqueous by the ciliary body and the filtration rate of the trabecular meshwork at the periphery of the iris.

(b) In one form of primary glaucoma there is closing up of the trabecular meshwork and this has a familial basis.

(c) Adhesions between iris and the cornea can cause secondary glaucoma.

(d) Papilledema is a sign of increased intraocular pressure in glaucoma.

(e) Untreated glaucoma leads to permanent loss of retinal ganglion cells.

Answer on page 613

103. Which of these statements is **least correct?**

(a) A chalazion represents a histiocytic inflammatory response to lipid material released from damaged meibomian glands.

(b) Damage to the corneal endothelium leads to corneal edema.

(c) Epithelioid-pattern uveal malignant melanoma carries an excellent prognosis and orbital involvement is prevented in most cases by the thick sclera.

(d) Cotton wool spots have a pathological correlate with areas of microinfarction in the retina.

(e) Hard exudates have a pathological correlate with the accumulation of lipid-rich material in the retina.

Answer on page 613

104. Which of the following statements is **least correct?**

(a) If the surface of an atheromatous plaque breaks down, collagen and other tissue components exposed to blood stimulate local thrombus formation.

(b) Severe atheroma of the aorta can be associated with loss of elastic in the vessel wall, leading to development of an aneurysm.

(c) The initial lesion of atheroma is in the intima of the vessel.

(d) Atheroma of the left ventricular wall is an important cause of mural thrombus in the heart.

(e) Angina on exertion is a clinical feature associated with high-grade stenosis of coronary arteries affected by atheroma.

Answer on page 613

105. Which of the following statements is **least correct?**

(a) Ethylene glycol ingestion is seldom harmful and produces effects similar to ethanol ingestion.

(b) Carbon tetrachloride exposure at toxic levels causes fatty change and centrilobular necrosis of liver.

(c) Exposure to lead produces a motor neuropathy in adults.

(d) Chronic effects of excessive ethanol ingestion include cardiomyopathy, peripheral neuropathy and ataxia due to cerebellar degeneration.

(e) Methanol poisoning is associated with development of metabolic acidosis.

Answer on page 613

106. Which of the following statements about malaria is **least correct?**

(a) The female Anopheles mosquito ingests red blood cells from an infected human containing male and female gametocytes.

(b) Sporozoites enter the salivary gland of the mosquito from where they can leave in saliva to infect another host.

(c) Hepatocytes containing merozoites rupture allowing parasites to enter the bloodstream.

(d) Phases of infection of red cells, red cell rupture, and re-invasion of other red cells by merozoites occurs cyclically.

(e) Merozoites released into standing water provide a reservoir of infection amenable to control by insecticide spraying.

Answer on page 613

107. Which of the following infective organisms **do not** characteristically produce a granulomatous inflammatory response?

(a) *Mycobacterium tuberculosis.*

(b) *Yersinia enterocolitica.*

(c) *Mycobacterium leprae.*

(d) *Mycoplasma pneumoniae.*

(e) *Brucella abortus.*

Answer on page 613

Answers

1. Answer (b) is **most correct**.

(a) Streptococci are round coccal organisms, not bacilli as shown here. Although streptococci are an important cause of pneumonia, they can be demonstrated in tissues by the Gram stain, which stains them blue-black.

(b) This is a Ziehl–Neelsen stain for mycobacteria, including *Mycobacterium tuberculosis* which is the cause of this patient's confluent pneumonia. The stain is based on the acid- and alcohol-fast nature of the organism.

(c) *Mycobacterium tuberculosis* can be cultured outside the body using a special medium (Lowenstein–Jensen) but can take up to 6 weeks to produce identifiable colonies. The mycobacterium which cannot be cultured outside the body is *Mycobacterium leprae*, which is responsible for leprosy.

(d) There are no pus cells (viable and necrotic neutrophils) here; neutrophils are unable to handle mycobacteria and the reaction is macrophagic/granulomatous.

(e) The red staining with the ZN stain depends on the organisms being alive with an intact capsule.

2. Answer (a) is **most correct**.

(a) This is a well-circumscribed spherical benign tumor of the thyroid (thyroid adenoma).

(b) The patient's thyroid function would almost certainly have been normal. Occasionally one of these nodules produces excess thyroid hormone, leading to hyperthyroidism.

(c) This is a benign tumor. Malignant tumors of the thyroid may spread to regional lymph nodes, particularly papillary carcinoma and follicular carcinoma.

(d) Excess secretion of thyroid stimulating hormone by the pituitary affects all parts of the thyroid and does not produce focal solitary lesions like this.

(e) The tumor is composed of thyroid follicle cells, as can be seen from the content of thyroid colloid within it. Abnormalities of thyroid C (calcitonin-secreting) cells are rare.

3. Answer (a) is **most correct**.

(a) This is a clump of malignant epithelial (carcinoma) cells within a lymphatic. It is on its way from the primary tumor to a regional lymph node where it will settle down and continue to grow to produce a lymph node metastasis.

(b) These are not macrophages, but are epithelial cells.

(c) These are not cells from a meningioma. Although meningioma can grow into local vessels, they are very unlikely to get to the mediastinum.

(d) These are epithelial cells, not lymphocytes. The neoplastic cells which form lymphoma do not clump.

(e) Although it is true that large atypical lymphoid cells are characteristic of infectious mononucleosis, they never appear as clumps within lymphatic vessels.

4. Answer (d) is **most correct**.

(a) The main abnormality is in the lateral wall of the left ventricle.

(b) This is a myocardial infarct with a pale area of complete muscle necrosis surrounded by a zone of hyperemia. At less than 24 hours old a myocardial infarct may be invisible to the naked eye or just show slight reddish discoloration.

(c) After 8 weeks of healing a myocardial infarct is entirely composed of collagenous white scar tissue.

(d) 5–7 days is the approximate age of this infarct. By 5 days the necrotic area is clearly identifiable and defined, surrounded by a variable red hyperemic zone but organization of the infarcted area is not yet advanced.

(e) Viral myocarditis affects the myocardium diffusely and does not produce focal areas of necrosis.

5. Answer (c) is **most correct**.

(a) This material is not tumor. Carcinoma of the bronchus, though highly locally invasive, almost never infiltrates the wall of one of the main pulmonary arteries.

(b) Although the material labeled (**T**) is indeed thrombus, it has not arisen *in situ* on intimal atheroma within the pulmonary artery. The pulmonary artery is a low pressure system and does not develop atheroma unless there is pulmonary hypertension. Even so, thrombosis occurring on atheroma in the pulmonary artery in pulmonary hypertension is exceedingly rare.

(c) This thrombus has arisen in the deep veins of the leg, and has broken off to pass in the femoral and iliac veins, through the inferior vena cava, into the right atrium, then right ventricle and finally out through the pulmonary valve into the main pulmonary trunk. The thrombus has impacted in a pulmonary artery branch which is too small to permit its passage. This is an example of pulmonary embolism.

(d) This is not thrombus which has propagated from the right ventricle. Thrombosis in the right ventricle is very rare. It is the left ventricle where mural thrombus may develop on top of a myocardial infarct.

(e) The pulmonary arterial tree terminates in minute pulmonary capillaries and thrombotic masses of this size will not pass through the pulmonary capillary bed to enter the left side of the heart and the systemic circulation.

6. Answer (a) is **most correct**.

(a) This is vascular granulation tissue, the earliest stage of wound healing which will eventually culminate in a fibrous scar.

(b) A good vascular supply is essential for good wound healing.

(c) Fibroblasts will come along at a later stage to convert this tissue into fibrous granulation tissue. Steroid therapy is very detrimental to wound healing and should be avoided at all costs.

(d) Many of the new thin-walled vessels will disappear, leaving only a few which will acquire muscle layers and become a permanent feature of the scar.

(e) This stage of the process occurs without the intervention of neutrophils. Neutrophils would have been the dominant cell in the earlier stages of tissue reaction to damage, and some may be present on the ulcer surface as part of the inflammatory slough.

7. Answer (b) is **most correct**.

(a) These nuclei are becoming small and dense-staining, a feature called pyknosis. A large nucleus in a proliferating cell has a prominent nucleolus.

(b) These cells show the first signs of cell death.

(c) The appearance of the cytoplasm is indicative of the early stage of cytoplasmic necrosis. The cytoplasm is dense and eosinophilic.

(d) Fatty accumulation is not seen here. When it does occur it appears as pale vacuoles in the cytoplasm.

(e) Hyperchromatic nuclei in a tumor have coarse clumped chromatin with prominent nucleoli. These are solid, uniformly dense, pyknotic nuclei.

8. Answer (b) is **most correct**.

(a) Hyperplasia is a response to an altered environment by an increase in cell numbers. Skeletal muscle does not undergo hyperplasia.

(b) This is an example of work hypertrophy. The increase in muscle fiber size is due to assiduous sports training.

(c) Metaplasia is a change of one mature cell form to another which is better able to handle the altered environment.

(d) Denervation of skeletal muscle fibers leads to atrophy, a reduction in cell size and number.

(e) This is not a neoplasm but an adaptive response. Benign tumors of skeletal muscle are extremely rare.

9. Answer (d) is **most correct**.

(a) Focal glomerulonephritis is a microscropic disease affecting some glomeruli. The damage cannot be seen naked eye.

(b) Adenocarcinoma in the kidney presents as a creamy yellow nodule, often spherical.

(c) Acute pyelonephritis is an infective disease of the kidney involving the presence of small microabscesses in the cortex, linear abscesses in the medulla, and acute inflammatory changes with pus in the pelvicalyceal system.

(d) The extensive wedge-shaped area of pallor is characteristic of a recent renal infarct due to occlusion of (in this case) the renal artery branch to the upper pole. The infarcted area is extremely pale.

(e) Acute papillary necrosis of the kidney affects only the papillae at the tips of the medulla. The cortex is not involved.

10. Answer (b) is **most correct**.

(a) In liquefactive necrosis the dead material is liquid and cannot usually be seen on a histological section.

(b) This is a typical tubercle, a granuloma with central caseous necrosis surrounded by histiocytes, giant cells, and lymphocytes. The infecting tubercle bacilli mainly lie within the area of caseous necrosis.

(c) The cells here are not neoplastic, but part of a chronic granulomatous inflammatory reaction.

(d) Viral pneumonia does not form caseating granulomas, although multinucleate giant cells are a feature of some types of viral pneumonia, e.g. measles pneumonia.

(e) Foreign bodies are only one of the causative factors of a giant cell reaction. Here, the necrosis is the most important feature, and necrosis is rarely seen in response to foreign bodies.

11. Answer (d) is **most correct**.

(a) CSF spread of tumors in childhood is very rare compared to the correct answer below.

(b) Cerebral infarction is rare in childhood and would not produce thickening of the meninges.

(c) A viral encephalitis affects the brain substance and does not produce meningeal thickening.

(d) There is an acute purulent exudate composed of fluid, the causative bacteria, living and dead neutrophils, and some fibrin in the subarachnoid space. This is characteristic of the naked eye appearance of the brain in acute bacterial meningitis.

(e) Acute hydrocephalus produces enlargment of the brain with flattening of the surface gyri, not meningeal thickening.

12. Answer (c) is **most correct**.

(a) The abnormal liver cells are degenerate but not dead.

(b) Intracytoplasmic water accumulation produces the change known as hydropic or cloudy degeneration.

(c) The spherical pale areas of varying size within the liver cells contain triglycerides. This is fatty degeneration, which is a sublethal metabolic degeneration often seen in liver cells in response to exposure to toxins, most frequently alcohol.

(d) Virus-infected liver cells can have a pale glassy cytoplasm but do not develop spherical vacuoles.

(e) Diabetics may accumulate glycogen in their liver cells but it does not accumulate in the form of spherical vacuoles.

13. Answer (a) is **most correct**.

(a) This is an acute inflammatory exudate over the surface of the visceral pleura from a patient with lobar pneumonia (acute fibrinous pleurisy).

(b) Old fibrous thickening of the pleura produces dense white hyaline thickening.

(c) The primary pleural tumor, malignant mesothelioma, produces dense white thickening which eventually compresses the lung.

(d) In infiltration of the pleura by metastatic carcinoma, discrete small white tumors can usually be seen.

(e) Acute fibrinous pleurisy is associated with severe chest pain on breathing, and on auscultation of the lungs on the affected side, a loud pericardial friction rub should be audible with every inhalation and exhalation.

14. Answer (e) is **most correct**.

(a) This is much too large and protruberant to be a large cold sore.

(b) Although the lip contains salivary tissue, and benign tumors of salivary tissue are common, the lip is not a frequent site for true salivary tumors which, in any case, usually appear as smooth spherical non-ulcerated masses.

(c) The disease is most common in elderly men (as seen here).

(d) This is an invasive malignant tumor and will not resolve with antibiotic therapy.

(e) This is an invasive squamous carcinoma of the lower lip. In addition to progressive local invasion, this tumor spreads via lymphatics to the regional lymph nodes in the neck.

15. Answer (d) is **most correct**.

(a) The cell morphology, of a single cell fragmented into particles, is characteristic of apoptosis.

(b) Autophagy produces cellular atrophy leaving residual lipofuscin in the cell as a brown pigment.

(c) The affected cell has fragmented into small bodies, not undergone atrophy.

(d) This is a later stage of apoptosis and the small particles of cell are apoptotic bodies.

(e) There are no inflammatory cells present. This is one of the hallmarks of apoptotic cell death, that it does not result in recruitment of inflammatory cells.

16. Answer (d) is **most correct**.

(a) Difficulty in swallowing is a symptom of a tumor in the esophagus.

(b) Hemoptysis is an uncommon presentation of this lesion, although it may occur. It is much more common as a presenting feature of carcinoma of the bronchus. This patient would have presented with a hoarse voice.

(c) This lesion is obviously destroying both vocal cords and is therefore invasive and malignant.

(d) This is a squamous carcinoma of the larynx. In the early stages when it is confined to the true vocal cords it has little potential for lymphatic spread because the true cords have few lymphatics. When it has invaded extensively it reaches and invades lymphatics which drain into the lymph nodes in the neck and cervical lymph node metastases are common.

(e) So-called 'singer's nodule' is a small benign thickening, often nodular, on the free edge of the true cord. Smoking is the most important predisposing factor to carcinoma of the larynx.

17. Answer (c) is **most correct**.

(a) Discoloration due to melanosis coli is confined to the mucosal surface.

(b) Although the color is right for arterial infarction, it rarely occurs as an acute event confined to the sigmoid colon. It is much more common in the small intestine.

(c) The loop of sigmoid colon has twisted on itself leading to occlusion of the venous drainage. This has led to venous infarction of the twisted loop (sigmoid volvulus).

(d) This loop of bowel is obviously ischemic. Ischemia of the colon does not occur in Crohn's disease.

(e) Although diverticular disease is common in the colon of the elderly, it plays no part in the development of sigmoid volvulus.

18. Answer (d) is **most correct**.

(a) True infarcts of the liver due to hepatic artery occlusion are extremely rare, and largely confined to hepatic artery damage due to surgical trauma.

(b) Liver abscesses, from whatever cause, are not solid but have a liquid center containing necrotic liver tissue and pus.

(c) Although metastatic tumors are the most frequent tumors in the liver, the outline and distribution of the tumors in this case are not those of secondary tumors.

(d) These are primary hepatocellular carcinomas arising multifocally within a liver already damaged by hepatic cirrhosis.

(e) Although malignant lymphoma does occur in the liver, the most common pattern is diffuse infiltration or multiple small nodules. Also, there is no association between lymphoma in the liver and hepatic cirrhosis.

19. Answer (a) is **most correct**.

(a) All lymph nodes are enlarged to varying degrees and show homogeneous replacement by white tumor tissue, which completely obliterates the architecture of the lymph nodes. This is characteristic of nodal involvement in malignant lymphoma.

(b) Although tuberculosis can involve the lymph nodes of the neck, it rarely involves multiple nodes and there is always necrosis within the node.

(c) Parathyroid adenomas are brown and almost always solitary and closely related to the thyroid gland.

(d) These lymph nodes are variably enlarged and the wrong color, normally being pinkish-brown.

(e) Pleomorphic salivary adenomas are usually solitary and embedded within salivary gland tissue.

pathology

20. Answer (c) is **most correct**.

(a) The normal thyroid gland is brownish due to the iodine in the stored thyroid colloid.

(b) Although carcinoma of the thyroid produces a pale fleshy lesion, it is never uniformly infiltrative as here.

(c) This is Hashimoto's autoimmune thyroiditis. The thyroid follicular structure has been infiltrated and destroyed by a heavy lymphocytic infiltrate, with eradication of the stored brown thyroid colloid. The characteristic pale appearance is due to a combination of destruction of brown thyroid colloid and extensive lymphocytic infiltrate (lymphocytes in bulk are white).

(d) The patient would have been hypothyroid due to destruction of thyroid follicle cells and depletion of thyroid colloid stores. In the early stages there may be a transient phase of hyperthyroidism, but this photograph shows a late stage of Hashimoto's disease.

(e) The patient would have been hypothyroid (see answer (d) above).

21. Answer (c) is **most correct**.

(a) Mumps orchitis leads to diffuse enlargement of the entire testis, not a localized lesion within normal testis as shown in this photograph. Orchidectomy is also unnecessarily aggressive and inappropriate treatment for mumps orchitis!

(b) Although benign tumors of interstitial (Leydig) cells do occur in the testis, their color is usually brownish. They are very rare, most tumors being derived from the germ cells.

(c) Seminoma of the testis is the most common germ cell tumor, and the homogeneous pale cut-surface appearance of this tumor is characteristic of seminoma.

(d) Teratoma of the testis has a characteristically variably cystic cut-surface appearance.

(e) Choriocarcinoma (malignant trophoblastic tumor) has a characteristically hemorrhagic reddish/brown cut-surface appearance.

22. Answer (c) is **most correct**.

(a) In rheumatoid arthritis there is much more deformity of the knuckles with marked deviation of the fingers.

(b) In chronic tophaceous gout there is rarely involvement of as many of the finger joints as seen here. Often the lumps are pale due to the fact that they contain large aggregations of urate crystals, and may even ulcerate discharging white pasty material.

(c) These are the typical appearances of osteoarthritis affecting the fingers; the nodules at the interphalangeal joints are called 'Heberden's nodes', and represent osteophytic outgrowths of new bone material at the bone ends.

(d) Septic arthritis usually involves a single joint, is very red shiny and swollen, and rarely affects the fingers.

(e) The joint changes in psoriatic arthropathy commonly involve the hands but closely resemble rheumatoid arthritis.

23. Answer (e) is **most correct**.

(a) This lesion is irregular in outline and pigmentation, is partly flat with a central raised nodule. Benign compound nevi are raised but regular in outline and pigmentation.

(b) A junctional nevus is flat and uniform in outline without any raised element. It may be almost as dark as this, but the pigmentation is usually even.

(c) A superficial spreading malignant melanoma in situ shows irregularity in outline and pigmentation as seen in this lesion, but does not have any raised areas.

(d) Pigmented hemangiomas are usually golden-brown and regular.

(e) The central raised black nodule indicates a malignant melanoma which is invading the dermis. It may originally have been a superficial spreading malignant melanoma *in situ* (see answer (c) above) before invasion took place.

24. Answer (b) is **most correct**.

(a) Head injury usually produces either an extradural or subdural hemorrhage. When the injury is severe, the cerebral hemispheres may also show contusional hemorrhage, but it is not localized in the basal ganglia region like this, being located in the cerebral cortex immediately beneath the site of impact and on the opposite side ('*contre coup* hemorrhage').

(b) Hypertension is the commonest cause of intracerebral hemorrhage, and the basal ganglia region is the most common site.

(c) Embolism from a mural thrombus on a myocardial infarct causes a cerebral infarct.

(d) Atheroma and thrombosis at the carotid bifurcation causes cerebral infarcts, often small and multiple.

(e) Bleeding in the brain due to very low platelet counts usually produces large numbers of small petechial hemorrhages throughout the brain, not a large localized lesion.

25. Answer (c) is **most correct**.

(a) Although the lesion is attached to the nipple, it has infiltrated the nipple from below and drawn it in. Nipple adenoma is benign and very rare; this lesion is malignant and common.

(b) This is a malignant tumor, and complete local excision is supplemented by radiotherapy to the site and removal of regional lymph nodes to assess lymphatic spread.

(c) This is the typical irregular outline of a malignant invasive tumor of the breast, adenocarcinoma. Invasion of the overlying nipple and adjacent fatty breast tissue can be seen.

(d) Sclerosing adenosis is one of the components of the common benign proliferative breast disease called fibroadenosis or fibrocystic disease.

(e) Gynecomastia of the male breast does not invade the nipple, nor surrounding fat.

26. Answer (e) is **most correct**.

(a) The majority of women with highly invasive extensively infiltrating endometrial adenocarcinomas are post-menopausal.

(b) HPV infection is strongly associated with carcinoma of the uterine cervix, but not with carcinoma of the endometrium.

(c) Women with this pattern of endometrial adenocarcinoma are usually elderly and well post-menopausal. There is a less aggressive form of endometrial carcinoma which can occur about the menopause.

(d) Uterine leiomyomas are well-circumscribed even if they undergo central degeneration.

(e) It is a highly aggressive infiltrating endometrial adenocarcinoma which has invaded the full-thickness of the myometrium almost to the serosal surface, particularly at the fundus.

27. Answer (a) is **most correct**.

(a) Tubercle bacilli from either an apical cavitating tuberculous mass or from a cavitating hilar lymph node enter blood vessels and are widely spread through the pulmonary and systemic circulations.

(b) The prognosis is poor, even with vigorous anti-tuberculous therapy.

(c) It occurs in patients with low resistance, e.g. malnourished, immune-suppressed, etc.

(d) Liver, spleen and kidneys are frequently involved.

(e) The patient usually dies before this can happen. Confluence of expanding tubercles occurs in tuberculous bronchopneumonia.

28. Answer (d) is **most correct**.

(a) Metastatic tumor in bone usually spreads via the bloodstream.

(b) See answer (a).

(c) In men, bronchus and prostate are the most common primary sites of tumor which metastasize to bone, followed by kidney.

(d) Breast and bronchus are the most common primary sites of malignant tumors which metastasize to bone in women.

(e) Most metastatic tumor deposits lead to osteolytic destruction of bone and are therefore radio-lucent on X-ray. Only bone metastases from carcinoma of the prostate are regularly osteosclerotic.

29. Answer (c) is **most correct**.

(a) The pericardial surfaces are normally smooth, not rough and shaggy, as here.

(b) Tuberculous pericarditis is now very rare, and the reaction is not so florid.

(c) This is a classical acute fibrinous pericarditis with the pericardial surfaces covered by a fibrinous acute inflammatory exudate.

(d) These are very recent loose adhesions between visceral and parietal pericardium. Old fibrous adhesions are more compact, and with a more complete obliteration of the pericardial cavity.

(e) Although local spread of cancer from the bronchus to the pericardium can occur, it appears as white patches and nodules on the pericardial surfaces.

30. Answer (d) is **most correct**.

(a) Although the lumen is reduced, it is because of the thickening of the intimal (**I**) and tunica media (**M**) layers. There is no atheroma deposition in the intima.

(b) The elastic lamina, though thickened and reduplicated, is intact. Had there been a previous episode of vasculitis, there would have been breaks in the elastic lamina.

(c) These are normal red cells.

(d) The features shown and described (together with elastic lamina reduplication), are the characteristic small- and medium-sized artery changes in 'benign' essential hypertension.

(e) The changes in a small or medium artery 'malignant' accelerated hypertension are largely confined to the intima. The media is rarely hypertrophied unless there has been pre-existing 'benign' essential hypertension.

31. Answer (b) is **most correct**.

(a) An exudate should contain fibrin and neutrophils.

(b) The fluid is water which contains protein (pulmonary edema), usually due to a high pulmonary capillary and venous pressure. It is most commonly due to acute left ventricular failure.

(c) The mucoid secretions in asthma are in bronchi and bronchioles, not alveolar air sacs.

(d) Although the fluid is a transudate, there is no microthrombosis in alveolar blood vessels.

(e) Hemoglobin only gets into the alveolar air sacs when there is bleeding into them.

32. Answer (e) is **most correct**.

(a) The pale areas are due to fatty change in hepatocytes at the periphery of the lobules.

(b) The dark areas are due to blood suffusing into the sinusoids from the central veins of each lobule, because of high pressure in the central veins.

(c) Chronic ischemia of the liver due to arterial disease is very rare. The hepatic artery is a sturdy little chap and laughs in the face of atheroma.

(d) Acute left ventricular failure leads first to acute pulmonary edema.

(e) These appearances ('nutmeg liver') are due to chronic passive venous congestion resulting from high pressure in central hepatic veins and inferior vena cava. This is usually a consequence of long-standing right heart failure.

33. Answer (e) is **most correct**.

(a) Bacterial endocarditis is almost always located on heart valves, not at the ventricular apex, as here.

(b) Thrombi may form on heart valves in patients with SLE who have anti-cardiolipin antibodies, not at the ventricular apex as here.

(c) In patients who develop thrombosis due to atrial fibrillation, the thrombus is almost always located in the left atrial appendage.

(d) This thrombus has formed in the left ventricle, on an area of endocardium damaged by myocardial infarction. If an embolus breaks off, it passes in the systemic arterial system to organs such as the brain, kidneys, spleen and bowel, NOT to the lungs. Pulmonary emboli and infarcts arise from thrombosis formed in the systemic venous system, usually in the legs.

(e) Emboli may break off and pass into the cerebral arteries, leading to infarction of the brain, often fatal.

34. Answer (d) is **most correct**.

(a) The valve is thickened by myxoid degeneration of the central zona fibrosa.

(b) The valve is functionally incompetent because of hypermobility of the affected leaflets.

(c) The posterior leaflet is usually most severely affected.

(d) This is an important complication, acute valve incompetence usually leading to uncontrollable acute left ventricular failure.

(e) It is most common in young and middle-aged adults, particularly women.

35. Answer (c) is **most correct**.

(a) The other way round.

(b) *Klebsiella pneumoniae* usually causes a lobar pattern of pneumonia, and is rare.

(c) Almost all cases are preceded by a viral or bacterial infection of the upper respiratory tract, with infected secretions passing down into the distal bronchioles under the influence of gravity.

(d) It is most common in infants and the weak and debilitated elderly.

(e) It most frequently affects the basal parts of the lower lobes (see answer to (c) above). If the patient is unconscious and nursed flat on the back or on the right side, gravity may take infected secretions from the trachea into the right upper lobe.

pathology

Answers

36. Answer (c) is **most correct**.

(a) Old healed tuberculosis is usually located at the lung apex.

(b) Metastatic tumor deposits in lung are usually white and spherical.

(c) This is an example of the progressive massive fibrosis pattern of coalminer's pneumoconiosis.

(d) Although the areas contain carbon (hence their grey-black color), they also contain abundant silica particles which have induced lung fibrosis. These masses are in the lung, not in lymph nodes.

(e) Asbestos fibers are usually deposited at the periphery of the lung, leading mainly to sub-pleural fibrosis.

37. Answer (d) is **most correct**.

(a) The tumor is ill-defined and irregular, not well-circumscribed and encapsulated. Benign tumors in the lung periphery are very rare.

(b) Smoking is an important etiological factor in malignant squamous and undifferentiated bronchial carcinomas at the lung hilum, not in peripheral tumors.

(c) In so-called peripheral 'scar cancers' (adenocarcinomas) there is often very extensive blood-borne metastasis to other organs, e.g. brain, liver or adrenals, despite the small size of the primary tumor.

(d) Most primary carcinomas in the lung periphery are adenocarcinomas, including 'scar cancers'.

(e) The cancer has arisen in an old long-standing lung scar.

38. Answer (c) is **most correct**.

(a) Mesothelioma spreads and infiltrates locally but rarely spreads to distant sites by lymphatic or bloodstream spread.

(b) The exposure is often in the distant past (often 20–40 years) and may be a minor exposure of quite brief duration.

(c) After radiological confirmation of pleural effusion, cytological examination of the aspirated pleural fluid can point to the diagnosis of mesothelioma.

(d) Pleural biopsy and histological examination are the cornerstones of diagnosis.

(e) Death usually occurs within 10 months of clinical presentation.

39. Answer (c) is **most correct**.

(a) Most parotid tumors are benign, either salivary adenomas or adenolymphoma (Warthin's tumor).

(b) Although mumps parotitis can produce swelling of this size it is always bilateral and affects younger people.

(c) Pleomorphic salivary adenoma is the commonest tumor in all salivary glands.

(d) Tumors, both benign and malignant, can also occur in minor salivary gland tissue in the lips, buccal region, palate or tongue.

(e) The appearance of circumscription is false, and shelling out leaves behind fragments which may regrow. A significant hazard of surgery for parotid tumors is surgical trauma to the facial nerve which runs through the parotid gland.

40. Answer (e) is **most correct**.

(a) This is acute otitis externa, and may be caused by a bacterium or fungus.

(b) Perforated eardrum is a complication of otitis media (acute inflammation of the middle ear).

(c) Acute mastoiditis is a complication of acute otitis media.

(d) 'Glue ear' is a form of otitis media with effusion of mucoid fluid which accumulates in the middle ear.

(e) Acute otitis externa may be either initiated by an allergic reaction to ear drops, or more commonly perpetuated and worsened by an allergic reaction to ear drops given for the original bacterial or fungal infection.

41. Answer (a) is **most correct**.

(a) A cholesteatoma is a form of epidermoid cyst in the middle ear.

(b) Squamous cell carcinoma occurs in the external ear (particularly on the pinna in the elderly), but is exceptionally rare in the middle ear.

(c) It slowly enlarges and may erode the labyrinth and mastoid air cells, as well as destroying the ossicles. Large cholesteatomas may even erode the bone of the skull which forms the base of the middle cranial fossa.

(d) Complete surgical removal is very difficult, and regrowth is common.

(e) Cholesteatomas cause deafness by destroying the fine structures in the middle ear.

42. Answer (b) is **most correct**.

(a) The darker red mucosa is lined by gastric-type columnar epithelium.

(b) Barrett's esophagus is characterized by the replacement of the normal squamous mucosa of the lower esophagus by gastric-type columnar epithelium. The demarcation of the two types of mucosa is indicated by the arrow.

(c) The ulcers are flat, without the hard raised edges which would suggest carcinoma. However, very early malignancy can only be excluded by histological examination of a biopsy from the ulcer edge.

(d) Although Candidal infection causes inflammation of the esophageal mucosa, the surface usually shows white patches due to fungal hyphal colonies.

(e) Achalasia of the esophagus leads to esophageal dilatation, but no mucosal changes or ulceration.

43. Answer (a) is **most correct**.

(a) The deep fissured ulcers produce the 'cobblestone' mucosal pattern characteristic of Crohn's disease.

(b) The areas labeled (**M**) are raised areas of mucosa swollen by submucosal edema and inflammation, contributing (with the intervening fissured ulcers) to the 'cobblestone' appearance of the mucosa.

(c) The pathological changes of inflammation affect the full thickness of the bowel wall (i.e. are transmural).

(d) In the small intestine, the affected areas are patchy and discontinuous ('skip lesions'), with normal bowel wall in between.

(e) Although the cause of Crohn's disease is unknown, it does not respond to antibiotic therapy.

44. Answer (b) is **most correct**.

(a) Metaplastic polyps are smaller and sessile. This has a stalk (**S**).

(b) The lobulated appearance is characteristic.

(c) Villous adenomas have a frond-like surface.

(d) Although tubular adenomas can convert into carcinoma, this has not done so to the naked eye, and is certainly not a Dukes' B (with invasion of muscle wall). Early Dukes' A carcinoma can only be excluded by histological examination of the stalk (**S**) to rule out early stalk invasion.

(e) Inflammatory polyps in chronic ulcerative colitis are small and multiple. In any case, the surrounding colonic mucosa shows no evidence of old or active colitis.

45. Answer (d) is **most correct**.

(a) The muscle layer (**M**) is hypertrophied, a characteristic of diverticular disease.

(b) If this diverticulum were infected, it would be distended and possibly contain pus.

(c) Diverticular disease occurs in the elderly.

(d) If a diverticulum becomes obstructed, then inflamed, pus accumulates in the obstructed diverticulum. Rupture leads to formation of a paracolic abscess, and often perforation leading to fecal peritonitis.

(e) It is most common in sigmoid and descending colon.

46. Answer (b) is **most correct**.

(a) Hepatocellular carcinoma can supervene in long-standing cirrhosis, but is usually a distinct large mass.

(b) The characteristic features of cirrhosis are liver cell necrosis, followed by progressive fibrosis, with regenerative nodules of hepatocytes between the fibrous bands.

(c) Although acute hepatic failure can supervene in cirrhosis, most patients present with symptoms due to chronic hepatic failure or portal hypertension.

(d) It is a rare cause.

(e) An important complication of the architectural distortion of the intra-hepatic vessels in cirrhosis is high pressure in the hepatic portal venous system ('portal hypertension'), not in the systemic venous system.

47. Answer (b) is **most correct**.

(a) Although there is no scale, these red cells are smaller than normal by comparison with the platelets also present. Also, in B_{12}/folate deficiency, platelets are greatly reduced in number, not increased as here.

(b) A hypochromic microcytic anemia is typical of iron deficiency. The increased numbers of platelets in this film suggest that the iron deficiency is due to blood loss, with a recent episode.

(c) In hereditary spherocytosis the red cells are spherical and lack the central pallor, being packed with hemoglobin.

(d) In aplastic anemia, all blood cells are reduced in number (including platelets, which are increased here). Also the red cells are scanty but adequately hemoglobinized, with immature and nucleated forms present.

(e) In this case, the diagnosis can be established on the blood film appearances alone, supported by estimations of serum iron and iron-binding capacity. Marrow examination is unnecessary.

48. Answer (e) is **most correct**.

(a) In acute lymphoblastic leukemia, immature lymphoblasts wipe out almost all other cells, giving the marrow a uniform cellular content, not the mixture as shown here.

(b) There are no mature lymphocytes here. The cells with dark round nuclei are red cell precursors.

(c) As in answer (a), but substitute immature myeloblasts for immature lymphoblasts.

(d) There are no monocytes, immature or mature, in this marrow.

(e) **The marrow is almost overwhelmed by proliferation of myeloid series cells, some of which are maturing into myelocytes, metamyelocytes and neutrophils.**

49. Answer (b) is **most correct**.

(a) Most pituitary adenomas are non-functioning and do not produce hormonal syndromes.

(b) **This is a common presentation in both functioning and non-functioning adenomas. It is due to pressure on the optic chiasma by the enlarging pituitary gland.**

(c) Cushing's disease is quite rare. The most common functioning adenomas are those which produce prolactin, leading to menstrual disturbances and infertility in women.

(d) Diabetes insipidus is due to failure of ADH secretion by the hypothalamus and posterior pituitary. It may complicate surgery for pituitary adenoma when the posterior pituitary and its stalk connection to the hypothalamus are removed.

(e) Sheehan's syndrome is due to destruction of the anterior pituitary by acute ischemic necrosis as a result of hypovolemia following intrapartum or postpartum hemorrhage. It leads to hypopituitarism.

50. Answer (c) is **most correct**.

(a) Papillary carcinoma rarely extends outside the thyroid capsule by local invasion.

(b) Thyroid carcinoma rarely infiltrates local structures.

(c) **Rapid local growth, with extension out of the thyroid capsule and invasion of adjacent structures is typical of anaplastic carcinoma.**

(d) Papillary carcinoma occurs particularly in young adults and in early middle-age. Anaplastic carcinoma is the type which mainly occurs in elderly people.

(e) Anaplastic carcinoma is so rapid in its growth that it usually kills by local invasion of vital structures such as trachea and jugular vein. Follicular carcinoma sometimes first presents with pathological fracture due to bone metastasis.

51. Answer (b) is the **EXCEPTION**.

Pheochromocytoma is one of the endocrine tumors seen in MEN 2 syndrome (the others are medullary carcinoma of the thyroid and sometimes parathyroid hyperplasia). The other statements are correct.

52. Answer (d) is **most correct**.

(a) Nephroblastoma is a fleshy white tumor originating in the kidney. Here the tumor is brown, and the kidney is intact.

(b) Pheochromocytoma is a well-circumscribed tumor, almost always benign, and very rare in young children.

(c) Lymphoma is white and fleshy.

(d) **The brown color with focal hemorrhagic necrosis, large size, extensive local spread, and patient's age are characteristic.**

(e) Tumors of the adrenal cortex are almost always yellow.

53. Answer (c) is **most correct**.

(a) Crescent formation is an indication of poor prognosis because each affected glomerulus is crushed out of existence by the crescent. If more than 75% of glomeruli are affected, irreversible renal failure occurs.

(b) It does not occur in membranous nephropathy.

(c) Absolutely true.

(d) Crescents are not a feature of diabetic nephropathy.

(e) Crescents can form in association with glomerular disease at any age, but is rare in infants.

54. Answer (e) is the **EXCEPTION**.

Diabetics are susceptible to acute papillary necrosis in which the papillary tips of the medullary pyramids undergo necrosis and are shed. Acute cortical necrosis is a rare disease in which there is extensive necrosis of the peripheral cortex of both kidneys due to microthrombotic occlusion of small arteries.

55. Answer (c) is the **EXCEPTION**.

It is most common in MEN over the age of 50 (male:female rate is about 3:1).

56. Answer (d) is **most correct**.

(a) There may be micro-invasion of the stalk.

(b) This is not a reliable sign. Histological examination is essential.

(c) They may be found anywhere in the urothelial tract, e.g. in ureter, renal pelvis and calyces.

(d) They are usually high-grade, solid carcinomas which invade the bladder wall deeply and extensively, and are often advanced on first presentation.

(e) Although adenocarcinoma can occur at that site it is rare. Transitional cell carcinoma is much more common.

57. Answer (d) is **most correct**.

(a) Leydig cell tumors are rare, usually well-circumscribed and small, without cystic spaces.

(b) Tuberculosis mainly affects the epididymis.

(c) Seminoma usually occurs in men over the age of 35. The patient's age would suggest that this is an embryonal carcinoma or immature teratoma. Choriocarcinoma is unlikely because of the lack of hemorrhage in the tumor.

(d) Preoperative measurement and postoperative monitoring of these tumor markers is a vital component of management, particularly in arriving at a decision about chemotherapy treatment.

(e) All painless testicular swellings should be regarded as due to malignant tumors, with urgent investigation and treatment.

58. Answer (d) is the **EXCEPTION**.

Lichen sclerosus of the vulva can occur at any age, even in young girls. The other statements are true.

59. Answer (d) is the **EXCEPTION**.

Paget's disease is due to spread of a **ductal** carcinoma of the breast along the nipple ducts and out into the epidermis of the nipple.

60. Answer (e) is **most correct**.

(a) Cerebral infarcts due to middle cerebral artery occlusion are peripheral and involve white and grey matter of the cerebral cortex.

(b) Looks nothing like it.

(c) Primary astrocytomas look like white matter when they are well-differentiated.

(d) Herpes simplex encephalitis mainly affects the temporal lobes.

(e) The color and location are characteristic. There are usually multiple small foci scattered in the white matter, not seen in this single slice.

61. Answer (e) is **most correct**.

(a) It is not particularly well-circumscribed, has an irregular shape, and a variegated cut-surface appearance. It is unlikely to be benign.

(b) Although melanoma metastases in the brain are often brown, they are usually small, multiple and spherical.

(c) Only part of it is hemorrhagic. A hemorrhage of this size would have been fatal.

(d) Low-grade, well-differentiated primary glial tumors are usually white and homogeneous, closely resembling normal white matter.

(e) The large size, irregular outline and variegated appearance with areas of hemorrhage suggest that this is a high-grade, poorly differentiated primary glial tumor, a glioblastoma.

62. Answer (d) is the **EXCEPTION**.

(a) One form of psoriasis which particularly affects palms and soles is characterized by small epidermal pustules ('pustular psoriasis').

(b) Damage to the nail bed can lead to nail damage.

(c) Some patients with psoriasis develop a severe arthropathy (psoriatic arthropathy) which resembles rheumatoid arthritis.

(d) The white material on the surface of psoriatic patches is made up to parakeratotic keratin forming a silvery scale. Removal of the scale often leads to punctate areas of bleeding.

(e) Elbows, knees, trunk, scalp and forehead are common sites for psoriasis.

63. Answer (c) is **most correct**.

(a) Keloids are most common on head and neck, upper trunk and upper arms.

(b) Although more common in women, the great majority occur in young women under the age of 30.

(c) Previous penetrating trauma is a prerequisite, e.g. operation scars. The illustrated example occurred following ear piercing.

(d) They are completely benign.

(e) They are unusually persistent and regress very slowly and never to the extent of leaving a depressed scar.

64. Answer (d) is the untrue **EXCEPTION**.

(a) This is the basis of Paget's disease of bone.

(b) Active osteoblasts deposit new osteoid in an attempt to repair the damage caused by excessive osteoclastic bone resorption.

(c) Marrow fibrosis occurs in long-standing disease.

(d) The osteoid is unmineralized because it is being deposited so quickly and extensively that mineralization cannot keep pace in all the sites.

(e) Osteosarcoma is usually a disease of children. It only occurs in the elderly in the context of pre-existing Paget's disease.

65. Answer (b) is the untrue **EXCEPTION**.

Osteosarcoma is a malignant tumor of **osteoblasts**. All other statements are correct.

66. The matching pairs are:

1. (g) Lymphoma is correct. A monotypic proliferation of B-cells suggests a non-Hodgkin's lymphoma.

2. (i) This is most likely to be a teratoma – a form of neoplasm containing elements from different germ cell elements and representing a form of germ cell tumor. Common sites are testis, ovary, sacrum, mediastinum and pineal region.

3. (j) This is a neuroblastoma, a form of embryonal tumor. Others include medulloblastoma, nephroblastoma, hepatoblastoma.

4. (f) This is a sarcoma. At this site it might be a fibrosarcoma or a rhabdomyosarcoma. If arising in bone it might be an osteosarcoma.

5. (d) This is a hamartoma, a local overgrowth of tissue indigenous to the part affected.

67. Answer (b) is the **most likely cause.**

(a) This is entirely possible, however it is not the most likely.

(b) This is the most likely cause. Mural thrombus develops over the area of infarction.

(c) This is a complication of recent myocardial infarction but will not cause a hemiplegia.

(d) While leg vein thrombosis can develop after a myocardial infarct, embolization would cause pulmonary embolism, not embolization to the systemic arterial system.

(e) A cerebral abscess can cause a hemiplegia but is not likely to have developed in the setting of endocarditis complicating a myocardial infarct.

68. Answer (b) is the **EXCEPTION**.

In apoptosis, caspase activation leads to controlled elimination of the cell. The action of endonucleases cleaves chromatin in between nucleosomes and this is reflected in chromatin condensation early in the process. Apoptotic fragments are phagocytosed by local cells including tissue macrophages. Apoptosis does *not* stimulate a local inflammatory response.

69. Answer (c) is the **EXCEPTION**.

Following hypoxia there is reduction of ATP production in the cell. Glycogen is broken down anaerobically to form lactate, which reduces cell pH. Loss of ATP causes failure of membrane iron pumps with retention of sodium and water within the cell. Morphologically, mitochondria undergo low amplitude swelling.

70. Answer (b) is the **EXCEPTION**.

Reduced apoprotein availability leading to impaired export of triglyceride from cells is a factor in the development of fatty change.

71. Answer (d) is the untrue **EXCEPTION**.

Failure of a developing organ to reach full size is termed hypoplasia.

72. Answer (c) is the untrue **EXCEPTION**.

Once the stimulus which has caused hyperplasia is removed a tissue returns to normal. This contrasts with abnormal cell proliferation in neoplasia where cell division takes place in the absence of the initiating stimulus.

73. Answer (a) is the **EXCEPTION**.

The cell stress response is activated by many deleterious stimuli including hypoxia and irradiation. Housekeeping genes are downregulated and cell stress genes are upregulated to produce heat shock proteins (also called cell stress proteins). These proteins give the cell resistance to protein denaturation. Any proteins that are damaged can be eliminated by proteolytic pathways, notably the ubiquitin system.

74. Answer (c) is **least correct**.

(a) This is a feature used in diagnostic cytology to spot malignant cells.

(b) This is also a useful cytological feature for recognizing an atypical cell.

(c) By definition a benign neoplasm does *not* metastasize.

(d) This is true for most benign tumors.

(e) This is true for most malignant tumors.

75. Answer (d) is **least correct**.

(a) The acute inflammatory exudate is the key player in the acute inflammatory response.

(b) Vascular dilatation is responsible for the redness seen in acutely inflamed tissues.

(c) Neutrophil adhesion is first transient (rolling) then firmer (adhesion). Rolling is mediated by selectin binding. Adhesion is mainly mediated by integrin binding.

(d) Resolution implies that the exudate is removed and tissue architecture restored without damage or scarring. This happens for example after some pneumonias.

(e) Fibrinogen deposition in the tissues is believed to form a scaffold to help cell migration. It may also limit the spread of some bacteria.

76. Answer (d) is **least correct**.

(a) Histamine is also seen in basophils.

(b) Histamine is especially important in the early phase of acute inflammation.

(c) The cyclo-oxygenase pathway produces prostaglandins while the lipoxygenase pathway produces leukotrienes.

(d) The leukotrienes are produced from activated lymphoid cells and monocytes. They have a variety of actions including induction of cell adhesion molecules, neutrophil chemotaxis, cell activation, and stimulation of fever. They do *not* cause endothelial necrosis.

(e) The complement system is important in acute inflammation.

77. Answer (e) is the **EXCEPTION**.

(a) Steroids impair wound healing.

(b) Diabetes mellitus impairs wound healing – it may also predispose to wound infection.

(c) Denervation and impaired sensation cause poor healing in the affected part.

(d) Previous irradiation impairs wound healing – even if many years ago.

(e) Antibiotic administration should not cause impaired wound healing.

78. Answer (b) is **least correct**.

(a) This is a defining characteristic of chronic inflammation.

(b) The dominant cells in chronic inflammation are lymphocytes and macrophages.

(c) The end result is usually scarring in the affected tissues.

(d) An example would be the development of chronic inflammation in response to an infection in a patient with diabetes mellitus.

(e) For example in rheumatoid disease.

79. Answer (b) is **least correct**.

(a) This is a T-cell mediated cytotoxic response.

(b) The dominant cells are T-cells and recruited macrophages.

(c) For example in tuberculosis.

(d) A granulomatous reaction with numerous giant cells is a characteristic reaction to the presence of insoluble foreign bodies in tissues.

(e) Sarcoid is a granulomatous disease affecting lungs, lymphoreticular system, and less commonly other tissues.

80. Answer (d) is **least correct**.

(a) This causes an embryo to develop with several cell lines.

(b) For example in Prader–Willi syndrome and Angelman syndrome due to loss of a region in chromosome 15.

(c) This is a rare but important genetic mechanism.

(d) While this is a cause of Down's syndrome (approximately 4% of cases) it has a *high risk* for occurring in subsequent pregnancies.

(e) This is the most important mechanism for development of sex chromosome abnormalities.

81. Answer (d) is **least correct**.

(a) They carry two copies of the gene.

(b) There is a 1:4 chance of carriers transmitting the disease to an affected offspring.

(c) As they carry only one X-chromosome, being unaffected must mean the chromosome is normal.

(d) An unaffected male will not be carrying the gene.

(e) As only one copy is needed for disease, an unaffected person cannot carry the causative gene.

82. Answer (c) is **least correct**.

(a) Grading involves assessment of differentiation – low-grade tumors resemble the tissue of origin.

(b) High-grade tumors tend to have a high proliferation rate and mitotic index is used in several grading schemes.

(c) Tumor necrosis is *not* used to stage a tumor. Staging assesses how far a tumor has spread. Necrosis is a feature of the grading of some tumors, when it links with high-grade lesions.

(d) Nodal spread goes with advanced disease.

(e) *In situ* neoplasia is a potentially treatable and curable non-invasive condition.

83. Answer (e) is **least correct**.

(a) This would be a good description for the histological findings in fibrocystic disease.

(b) This would increase the risk of a person developing a subsequent carcinoma.

(c) They may present with blood-stained nipple discharge.

(d) This is a pattern of spread of breast cancer.

(e) Fibroadenomas are commonest in the 25–35 years age group. It is never safe to assume the nature of a breast lump in a woman of any age.

84. Answer (d) is **least likely**.

There are several predisposing factors to renal papillary necrosis, most of which are listed, with the exception of (d). Hypotension is more likely to cause acute tubular necrosis.

85. Answer (a) is **least correct**.

(a) This is most suggestive of an anemia of chronic disorders.

(b) There are several sub-types of myelodysplasia.

(c) Hemolysis of deformed red cells is important in sickle cell disease.

(d) There may be tissue or blood eosinophilia.

(e) This is detected in the urine of affected patients.

86. Answer (e) is **least correct**.

(a) This is the commonest form of lymphoma.

(b) Involvement of groups on one side of the diaphragm.

(c) A so-called MALT tumor.

(d) This is an oncogenic retrovirus.

(e) Nodal or extranodal lymphomas may spread to bone marrow.

87. Answer (b) is **least correct**.

(a) The commonest varices are in the lower esophagus.

(b) Cirrhosis is the *commonest* reason for esophageal varices due to portal hypertension.

(c) Predisposing factors include polycythemia, local sepsis.

(d) For example after some cytotoxic drug therapies.

(e) This is called Budd–Chiari syndrome.

88. Answer (d) is **least correct**.

(a) Diagnosis could be made on biopsy and culture of affected tissues.

(b) This would be a classical type of presentation.

(c) Ileocecal infection with nodal involvement occurs.

(d) Ulcerative colitis is a distal process, which would *not* be expected to affect the ileum with nodal involvement.

(e) A tumor such as a lymphoma should be considered.

89. Answer (c) is **least correct**.

(a) Secretion of 5 Hydroxy tryptamine causes the carcinoid syndrome.

(b) Lymphoma is believed to develop in the setting of massive lymphoid infiltration seen in gluten-induced enteropathy.

(c) Hyperplastic polyps are flat, dome-shaped mucosal lesions that are not pre-neoplastic. Adenomatous polyps carry a high risk of development of carcinoma.

(d) These can occur in any part of the bowel.

(e) Extensive long-standing disease carries the highest risk.

90. Answer (d) is **least correct**.

(a) Crypts increase in depth with increased epithelial turnover, however villi do not form.

(b) This is a help in diagnosis along with detection of anti-endomysial antibodies.

(c) This is due to failure of absorption of fat soluble vitamins as a result of lack of lipase activity.

(d) Biopsy detection of mucosal changes is very useful in diagnosis.

(e) Loss of these enzymes in mucosal disease leads to failure of absorption of disaccharides.

91. Answer (c) is the **EXCEPTION**.

Bence–Jones protein consists only of the light chain component of immunoglobulin molecules.

92. Answer (a) is the **EXCEPTION**.

The commonest cause of Cushing's syndrome is therapeutic administration of corticosteroids.

93. Answer (e) is **most correct**.

(a) It is a common cause of the NEPHROTIC syndrome in children, *not* nephritic syndrome.

(b) It affects all parts of all glomeruli, i.e. it is global and diffuse.

(c) No immune complexes have been seen in minimal change nephropathy.

(d) The glomerular abnormalities resolve spontaneously and never progress to renal failure.

(e) The loss of the polyanionic charge is thought to cause collapse of the podocyte foot processes and to permit leakage of protein across the glomerular filtration barrier.

94. Answer (c) is the **EXCEPTION**.

Primary adenocarcinoma of the Fallopian tube is extremely rare, and there is no link with acute or chronic salpingitis.

95. Answer (c) is the **EXCEPTION**.

Condyloma latum is the name given to the wart-like thickening of the skin in the genital region which occurs in secondary syphilis. These lesions contain the causative bacterium, *Treponema pallidum*.

96. Answer (b) is the **EXCEPTION**.

Basal cell carcinoma, though it may show extensive local invasion and destruction of invaded tissues, never metastasizes to distant sites.

97. Answer (c) is the **EXCEPTION**.

Osteoporosis can be induced by prolonged corticosteroid therapy, but not osteomalacia.

98. Answer (d) is **most correct**.

(a) Parathyroid adenoma usually only affects one gland; the others often undergo atrophy.

(b) Excessive secretion of parathyroid hormone stimulates osteoclasts to erode bone, leading to parathyroid bone disease.

(c) Chronic renal failure may stimulate hyperplasia of all parathyroid glands (secondary hyperparathyroidism) but does not stimulate the growth of an adenoma.

(d) Patients often present with symptoms due to a high serum calcium or to the associated bone disease.

(e) Parathyroid carcinoma is extremely rare.

99. Answer (c) is the **EXCEPTION**.

Scleroderma is three times more common in women than men.

100. Answer (d) is the **EXCEPTION**.

Renal involvement is extremely rare. The other statements are true.

101. Answer (e) is **least correct**.

(a) These are small, slit-shaped infarcts mainly seen in the deep grey matter and internal capsule region.

(b) For example after an anesthetic disaster.

(c) This causes venous infarction, typically hemorrhagic.

(d) Reperfusion of a cerebral infarct causes it to become hemorrhagic.

(e) The commonest site is in the internal capsule, basal ganglia region, *not* the subarachnoid space.

102. Answer (d) is **least correct**.

(a) Aqueous eventually drains via the canal of Schlemm.

(b) This is usually seen after 40 years-of-age.

(c) This may happen after inflammatory disease of the eye.

(d) Papilledema is seen with raised intracranial pressure, *not* glaucoma.

(e) The fundoscopic correlate is a pale optic disk which is cupped due to the raised intraocular pressure.

103. Answer (c) is **least correct**.

(a) A chalazion is a common cause of a localized swelling in an eyelid.

(b) This is often painful due to development of small corneal epithelial bullae.

(c) Such tumors have often spread down vessels or along nerves penetrating the sclera and have only a 35% 10-year survival.

(d) The spots are the ballooned ends of damaged retinal axons.

(e) These leak from vessels and accumulate in the outer plexiform layer.

104. Answer (d) is **least correct**.

(a) This an important cause of arterial thrombosis, for example in the coronary arteries.

(b) Most atheromatous aneurysms are seen in the abdominal aorta below the origin of the renal arteries.

(c) Infiltration of the intima by macrophages containing lipid is believed to be the earliest lesion in atheroma.

(d) Mural thrombus in the heart is most often caused by a previous myocardial infarct. For all practical purposes you do not see atheroma in the ventricular wall.

(e) A very common clinical consequence of atheroma.

105. Answer (a) is **least correct**.

(a) Ethylene glycol is highly toxic causing oxalate deposition in kidneys, renal failure due to acute tubular necrosis, and metabolic acidosis.

(b) This is an important hepatotoxin.

(c) Estimation of blood lead levels is useful in differential diagnosis of denervating disorders.

(d) These may occur independently of other effects such as hepatic damage or development of pancreatitis.

(e) It also causes neurological damage.

106. Answer (e) is **least correct**.

(a) After ingestion the gametocytes reproduce sexually to produce infective sporozoites.

(b) This is how malaria is transmitted.

(c) This is an asexual reproductive phase. Some organisms may lie dormant in liver to produce late relapses of disease.

(d) While most cycles of reproduction are asexual there is also sexual reproduction to produce gametocytes that can infect a mosquito.

(e) Malaria parasites have no reservoir in standing water. Mosquito larvae can be controlled in this way.

107. Answer (d) is **correct**.

(a) *M. tuberculosis* produces granulomas with characteristic central caseous necrosis.

(b) *Yersinia enterocolitica* can cause a terminal ileitis with granulomas in local lymph nodes.

(c) *M. leprae* can produce granulomas in so-called tuberculoid leprosy.

(d) *Mycoplasma pneumoniae* does not cause a granulomatous response.

(e) Brucellosis is characterized by granulomatous inflammation in tissues

Laboratory methods and terminology

acidophilic

Staining with acidic dyes, for example eosin (see 'hematoxylin and eosin').

autopsy

see '*post-mortem* examination'

basophilic

Staining with basic dyes, for example hematoxylin (see 'hematoxylin and eosin').

biopsy methods

There are many ways in which samples can be taken for histological examination to establish an accurate tissue diagnosis:

- Excision biopsy. The entire abnormal area is excised and submitted for microscopical examination; this is usually both diagnostic and curative, for example, the complete excision of a neoplastic polyp in the colon.

- Incision biopsy is undertaken where it is impossible or inappropriate to excise the whole of the diseased area; a sample is removed by incising the lesion with a scalpel to provide a substantial amount of tissue for microscopical examination.

- Needle biopsy is undertaken for both superficial and deep lesions; a hollow needle is introduced into the lesion, upon which a small core of tissue occupies the needle lumen from where it is removed gently and sent for microscopical examination. This technique is widely used in the examination of liver disease and kidney disease. Where the lesion to be sampled is fairly superficial, for example an abnormal enlarged lymph node in the neck, accurate guiding of the needle is simple; for deeper lesions the needle may need to be introduced under imaging control.

- Trephine biopsies are usually confined to the removal of samples of bone, such as to investigate either disease of the bone itself or, in hematological disorders, the bone marrow. The trephine is like a hollow drill which is inserted by hand, the biopsy sample occupies the hollow centre of the trephine from which it can be extracted after removal.

- Endoscopic biopsy is performed by using fine biopsy forceps that are passed down the channel of an endoscope. The lesion to be sampled is viewed directly, and samples 1–2 mm in diameter are removed for histological examination. This is mainly used in the upper and lower gastrointestinal tracts, upper and lower airways, and the lower urinary tract.

- Stereotactic biopsy is a special technique in which imaging is used to locate precisely a deep-seated lesion with reference to surface landmarks or an attached frame. A needle can then be guided to biopsy an area with accuracy to within 1 mm. This is particularly used in biopsy of brain lesions.

bone marrow aspiration

A trephine or needle is inserted into a bone marrow cavity, usually the sternum, iliac crest or tibia (in infants), and hemopoietic marrow is aspirated; smears are prepared and stained, and are then examined microscopically to determine the cell types present. This process is undertaken in the diagnosis of severe intractable anemia of unknown cause, leukemias (both proven and suspected), myelodysplastic syndromes, and many other conditions. As well as being used for initial diagnosis, marrow aspiration is used to assess the effectiveness of treatment in leukemia and lymphoma, and to diagnose early relapse.

cervical cytology

This branch of cytology concentrates on the analysis of exfoliative cytology of the cervix as a means of detecting cervical neoplasia. Infective and inflammatory conditions of the female genital tract may also be detected by this technique. A special spatula is used to scrape cells from the endocervical junction and these are smeared on a slide, fixed, and sent to the laboratory. Papanicolaou technique is used to stain smears, resulting in blue nuclei, pink superficial cells, and blue-green parabasal cells.

clinical chemistry

Investigations are now largely carried out in automated systems, and many can be carried out on small samples of blood or other body fluids. In the majority of cases, estimations can be made on 5 ml of clotted blood; these include frequent investigations such as urea and electrolytes, serum calcium, proteins, enzymes, hormone assays, and most drug level estimations. Occasionally it is necessary to place the blood in a container with an anticoagulant so that it does not clot; lithium–heparin and fluoride–oxalate are the most frequently used anticoagulants. For most estimations on body fluids, such as urine, all that is required is an untreated sample of the fresh fluid, but occasionally 24-hour samples of urine are required. Each laboratory has its own set of normal standards, according to the technique used in the estimations; similarly, some laboratories vary in the way in which they prefer their samples presented. Every student and practising doctor should pay great attention to the instructions of their particular laboratory if samples, time and money are not to be wasted.

cytogenetics

Culture of cells is performed and chromosome spreads made for analysis. Alterations in chromosome number or fine structure can be detected, and may be useful in analysis of congenital abnormalities, mental retardation, and certain tumours. Tissue must be rapidly transported in specialized tissue culture medium to the laboratory.

cytological examination

In this technique, a diagnosis is based on the appearances of isolated cells taken, or shed, from an abnormal area. The technique is mainly used in the diagnosis of malignant disease, using the cytological criteria which indicate that a cell is both neoplastic and malignant (e.g. nuclear atypia, high mitotic rate, high nucleus to cytoplasm ratio). Cells can be obtained from an abnormal area by:

- Exfoliation methods, in which cells are scraped from the surface of an abnormal area. This method is limited to disorders in which the abnormality is in an accessible epithelial surface, for example the cervix of the uterus, or the mucosal lining of the esophagus, stomach or proximal tracheobronchial tree. The specimen may be obtained either by using a specially designed spatula which scrapes the cells from the surface, or by a brush which is passed over the abnormal surface – superficial cells becoming adherent to the brush bristles. Cells are transferred to a microscope slide, fixed, and then stained with various stains to show the nuclear and cytoplasmic characteristics.

- Fluid aspiration is a method in which fluid is aspirated from hollow viscera such as the pleural and peritoneal cavities, and the cell content of the fluid is examined microscopically. The cell population is frequently small, and various methods are used to provide a concentrated sample of cells. Similar methods can be used to examine cerebrospinal fluid in the diagnosis of malignancy involving the brain and meninges, and sometimes clues about the nature of inflammatory diseases in the CNS can be obtained by nothing the type of inflammatory cells present, for example, neutrophils in bacterial meningitis, lymphocytes in tuberculous meningitis and viral meningoencephalitis. Naturally voided fluids, such as urine and sputum, can also be examined for cell content to detect atypical or reactive cells.

- Aspiration of cells from solid lesions – 'fine needle aspiration' – is an important and clinically convenient method of diagnosing suspected malignancy without the necessity for a surgical maneuver involving excision or incision biopsy. A needle is inserted into a solid lump (usually in an organ or tissue close to the surface such as breast, thyroid, or superficial lymph node) and suction applied so that some of the cells in the lump pass into the needle. These are then expressed onto a microscope slide, fixed and stained for microscopical examination. As with most diagnostic cytological techniques, it is mainly used in the diagnosis of malignant tumours, looking for the cytological criteria of malignancy.

Fixation and staining of cytological preparations is discussed under 'fixation and fixatives' and 'special stains'.

electron microscopy (EM)

This is used to supplement analysis performed by light microscopy. It is particularly valuable in the assessment of renal biopsies for glomerulonephritis when location of immune complexes can be determined. It is used in the diagnosis of tumours by looking for fine detail of cell differentiation. Muscle biopsy relies on electron microscopy for the diagnosis of several important myopathies. Viral disorders can also be diagnosed by the analysis of characteristic viral particles. Tissue samples for **EM** should be fixed in a specially prepared, buffered, glutaraldehyde fixative. Samples should be 1–2 mm in diameter to ensure that adequate fixation occurs.

enzyme histochemistry

This is a technique for demonstrating the location of specific enzymes in tissue sections. It is particularly used for the analysis of skeletal muscle biopsies, allowing delineation of different fiber types. Fresh, unfixed tissue is essential (see also 'frozen section').

erythrocyte sedimentation rate (ESR)

This is a test performed in hematology departments. Blood is allowed to stand in special tubes and the rate of sedimentation is measured and expressed in mm/hr. If red blood cells are induced to form aggregates then the sedimentation time is rapid. Conditions in which there are acute phase proteins in the blood, or when there are high concentrations of immunoglobulin, are particularly associated with a high ESR.

fixation and fixatives

The histological diagnosis of disease processes is still largely based on the microscopical examination of a thin (3–5 μm) section of the tissue, which has been embedded in paraffin wax after the tissue has been fixed. The most common and widely used protein-linking substances that are used as fixatives are aldehydes, particularly formaldehyde and glutaraldehyde. Formaldehyde is used as a 10% aqueous solution (formalin), which is often buffered to prevent the fixative solution becoming acidic (since the formaldehyde spontaneously converts to formic acid).

Why does the tissue have to be fixed? Fixation achieves a number of objectives:

- First of all it prevents the tissue undergoing autolysis (i.e. self-breakdown by the release of tissue enzymes when cells die). Autolysed tissues lose all their architectural and cytological characteristics, rendering accurate microscopical diagnosis impossible. Fixation inactivates the enzymes responsible for autolysis, as well as killing microorganisms which may be present in the sample.

- Secondly, fixation hardens the tissues by cross-linking the structural-protein component of the cells and stromal components, so that the architectural and cytological relationships are retained in a state which pretty-much resembles the true living state.

- Thirdly, fixation protects the tissues from the possible untoward effects of the various processes that it has to go through during the embedding of the tissue sample in paraffin or other supporting medium. When the tissues may need to be examined by special laboratory techniques (for example, electron microscopy or immunocytochemistry), special fixatives may be required.

frozen section

A frozen section is performed by freezing a sample of fresh tissue rapidly in a special mounting medium, and then making histological sections in a machine called a cryostat (basically a freezer containing a microtome). The tissue is held at about −20°C, at which temperature it becomes hard enough to cut sections at about 8 μm thick. These sections can be stained, and a rapid diagnosis can be made, for example, while a patient is under anaesthetic. Frozen sections are also used for some special examinations, particularly enzyme histochemistry and immunohistochemistry. A disadvantage of this technique is that sections lack the resolution obtainable with wax-embedded material.

full blood count

These are the basis of initial hematological investigation, and are carried out mainly by machinery that provides figures for hemoglobin levels, red-cell numbers, size (diameter and volume), white-cell numbers and platelet numbers. Microscopical examination of the blood smear gives valuable information about the nature of red cells and white cells – particularly in the presence of abnormal forms of any of the cells. The cytological appearance of these cells may give a strong clue to the diagnosis, but not all films are examined microscopically because it is very time-consuming, costly and labour intensive. In most cases, the staff of the Hematology Laboratory will make a decision on whether to examine a smear, which is based on the information given on the request form and on the figures obtained from the full blood count; they will always examine a film if requested to do so. To get the maximum information from a basic hematology request, it is vital that full clinical information is supplied on the request form.

hematoxylin and eosin

This is the standard histological stain in use in histology laboratories. Hematoxylin stains nuclei deep-purple; eosin stains cytoplasm shades of pink. Structures that stain with eosin are termed eosinophilic or, because eosin is an acidic dye, acidophilic. Structures that stain with hematoxylin are termed basophilic as this is a basic dye.

immunofluorescence

This is a technique for staining histological sections in order to detect the presence of a specific protein or antigen in the tissue. An antibody that is directed at the antigen is applied to the section, and detected by a fluorescent dye. Sections need to be viewed with a special fluorescence microscope. This is useful in the diagnosis of renal disease and skin disease that are caused by autoimmune or immune-complex reactions.

immunohistochemistry

This is a staining technique that allows the detection of specific proteins or antigens in tissue sections. Antibodies to specific proteins or antigens are applied to tissue sections and are detected by a coloured reaction product. In most cases, there is a brown reaction product generated by the detection of a marker enzyme, peroxidase – hence the term 'immunoperoxidase reaction'. This technique is routinely performed in most laboratories and allows very specific identification of cell types as well as tumor markers.

necropsy

see 'post-mortem examination'

neuropathology

Examination of the tissues of the nervous system is traditionally carried out in specialized laboratories. Examination of the post-mortem brain takes many weeks, as fixation, tissue processing, and staining of large sections of brain is much more prolonged than for small tissue samples.

post-mortem examination

The investigation of disease should not end with the death of the patient. *Post-mortem* examination should be carried out to confirm or establish the structural diseases present, to note the effect or failure of any treatment given during life and, most importantly, to establish a cause of death and list of conditions present at the time of death for accurate registration. Considerable weight is placed on the officially registered cause of death when devising statistics on which to base distribution of health care resources, and it is vital that the national figures are accurate. Unfortunately, many studies in western countries have shown that cause of death registration is frequently very inaccurate unless a *post-mortem* examination has been performed. (Comparative studies in which practitioners were invited to list the cause of death before autopsy, and the pathologist asked to provide a cause of death afterwards, shows a very high level of inaccuracy without adequate *post-mortem* examination.) A *post-mortem* is therefore a vital component of clinical audit, but is sadly neglected in most countries, resulting in spurious and highly inaccurate figures for disease incidence and causes of death. There are important implications, as inappropriate allocation of healthcare resources is inevitable because of diagnostic inaccuracies. It should be the intention of clinical practitioners to request a *post-mortem* examination on any death occurring in hospital, and it should be possible for practitioners in the community to request *post-mortem* on any of their patients of whom they are not absolutely certain of the cause or mechanism of death.

Some deaths require a *post-mortem* examination by law, for example, those of medico-legal significance, where there is a possibility that death was not due to natural disease, or where death may be attributable to an accident or industrial disease. There are many such categories where *post-mortem* examination is compulsory by law, and these cases come under the aegis of the Coroner in England and Wales, the Medical Examiner in the United States, and the Procurator Fiscal in Scotland.

Post-mortem examination

A *post-mortem* examination is carried out by the dissection of the internal organs, which are usually removed through a single longitudinal incision extending from the neck to the suprapubic region in the anterior mid-line. The brain is examined after the lifting of the calvarium through an incision passing over the back of the head. In most cases, a provisional diagnosis is established by naked-eye examination of the organs after dissection. Histological and microbiological examination of tissue samples removed at *post mortem* are performed to establish an accurate diagnosis.

Unless the case has been referred by one of the medicolegal authorities, the written permission of the next of kin is required before a *post-mortem* examination can be carried out. If it is the wish of the next of kin, it may be possible to carry out a 'limited post mortem' in which, for example, only the heart or brain is examined if the disease is believed to be localized to that area.

After the removal and dissection of the organs, they are replaced in the body cavities which are cleaned, and then the skin incisions are sewn together. Reconstitution of the body is an important part of examination. When the deceased is dressed in a shroud, it is possible to view the body without visible signs of the examination having been performed.

preservation of operative and biopsy specimens

Fixatives can provide their beneficial effects only if they penetrate the tissues. Most fixatives penetrate fairly slowly. Small tissue fragments, such as needle-biopsy samples, fix very quickly, and the architecture and cytology are usually very well preserved. However, large tissue samples fix more slowly since the immersed specimen can only be fixed by diffusion of fixative from the outer surface; furthermore, large specimens require large volumes of fixative. A compact organ such as the spleen, even if immersed in a large volume of fixative in a large container, will reach the laboratory a few hours after removal with only the outer 2–5 mm fixed; the remainder of the splenic tissue will have already undergone some degree of autolysis and subsequent architectural and cytological distortion. Therefore, the only part of the spleen that will show good preservation for microscopical analysis will be the splenic capsule and the underlying couple of millimetres of splenic parenchyma. The same applies to any solid organ; this is particularly important in the case of enlarged lymph nodes, where accurate diagnosis is dependent upon the high quality preservation of cytology and architecture. There are four main rules for handling tissue samples and for presenting them to the histopathology laboratory (see following blue box).

Rules for handling tissues for the laboratory

Rule 1

If a pathological lesion is unusual, or is likely to be one that may require special techniques such as electron microscopy, ring the laboratory to check whether the specimen should be fixed or sent down fresh and, if fixed, which fixative should be used. This is becoming increasingly important with the wider use of immunocytochemical techniques and electron microscopy in the accurate diagnosis of lymphoma and certain tumor types. Some tissues, for example skeletal muscle, can be diagnosed only if unfixed and received promptly. Some tissue samples may need to undergo enzyme histochemistry or have frozen sections made to reach a diagnosis. If the laboratory requires the specimen fresh, arrange for *immediate transfer* of the specimen to a named person in the laboratory. Do not rely on a hospital portering system. Many biopsy specimens are ruined by the amount of autolysis and drying out that occurs when small specimens such as Tru-cut needle biopsies are delayed either in theatre, in the porter's pocket, or because they are hanging around in the laboratory because no member of laboratory staff has been notified of its arrival. If a fresh specimen is to be sent, always warn the laboratory that it is on its way. All fresh tissue should be handled as if it potentially infective. Samples should be placed in sealed containers and labeled with the nature of the specimen, the name and details of the patient, and appropriate clinical details.

Rule 2

If a specimen is to be fixed, always ensure that the specimen is placed in sufficient fixative and in a large enough container to take the specimen and fixative solution (preferably 4–5 times the volume of the specimen) without distortion to the specimen. Remember that soft, unfixed tissues are pliable and can be squashed into quite a small container, but that the space left for fixative solution will be so small that insufficient fixative will be used and the specimen will remain largely unfixed. Also, if the specimen has been squashed, when the specimen is hardened by the fixative it will retain the shape of the container into which it has been forced.

Rule 3

If the pathological lesion is at the centre of the excised specimen, it will not be fixed properly unless one

surface of the lesion is exposed to the fixative; it is therefore advisable to transect the excised specimen through the lesion so that the fixative will hit the main pathology immediately upon immersion. For example, a carcinoma in the centre of a mastectomy specimen will show severe autolysis unless the specimen is transected through the pathological lesion. A word of caution here – although a simple transection through a lesion will facilitate fixation, repeated slicing or the use of a random hacking technique, applied to the specimen by the surgeon before insertion into fixative, will render accurate reconstruction impossible after fixation. Although this will not interefere with the histological diagnosis, it may mean that the pathologist is unable to offer any valid comment on the extent of spread or completeness of excision of a neoplastic lesion. In many large laboratories, pathologists encourage receipt of fresh material within minutes of removal so that tissue can be fixed properly or, alternatively, preserved by other techniques.

A small tissue sample such as a needle biopsy will be completely fixed within a couple of hours, and embedding into paraffin wax can begin on the same day that the biopsy is taken, with a good chance that a histology report may be available by the following day (within 24 hours of the biopsy being taken). Larger specimens may take 12–24 hours to fix, even if every precaution to ensure good fixation has been taken. Since processing into paraffin cannot take place until the sample has been fully fixed, a histopathology report from a large specimen may take 3–4 days. This time can be shortened if the main pathological lesion in a large specimen is transected so that it is exposed to the formalin; the pathologist can then take a sample from the fixed part of the lesion, and a report on the nature of the lesion can be issued within 24 hours, even though the report on the remainder of the specimen may need to follow in 2–3 days time.

Rule 4

All specimens must be fully labeled with patient details and the nature of sample. A request card which is also labeled with the patient details, nature of sample, and full clinical details of the case must accompany the samples.

resin sections

Resin rather than paraffin wax (see 'tissue processing') can be used to embed tissue samples; it allows much thinner sections and greater resolution of fine structure. This is particularly done for the histology of bone, as it allows sectioning of the densely calcified matrix.

special stains

Certain structures can be highlighted by use of special staining techniques. Common methods used in histopathology laboratories are:

- PAS stain (periodic-acid Schiff) detects mucin and mucopolysaccharides. It will also detect many fungi.

- Reticulin stain detects reticulin and basement membranes.

- Methenamine-silver stain detects basement membranes.

- Trichrome stains distinguish collagen, cells, and elastic tissues.

- Masson-Fontana stain detects melanin.

- Perls' stain detects iron pigment

- Ziehl-Nielsen stain detects acid-fast bacilli such as *M. tuberculosis.*

- Gram stain detects bacteria.

tissue processing

Once received by the laboratory, fixed tissues must be processed into paraffin wax. A pathologist examines specimens, and portions of tissue are taken for examination by histology. For small samples, such as needle biopsies, the whole specimen is processed. For large, resected specimens, small samples are dissected using a scalpel. In most laboratories, automated machines expose tissues to increasing concentrations of alcohol, xylene and finally paraffin wax at 60°C. Specimens are then embedded in wax in moulds and allowed to harden. Sections are cut on a microtome at 3–5 μm thickness, mounted on glass slides, and stained for histological examination. The whole process from specimen to section (including adequate fixation) takes about 24 hours.

viral diagnosis

Virus diseases can be diagnosed by microbiological, histological and immunological means. Histological examination of tissue samples is not used frequently, but can be useful in the diagnosis of viral disorders of the skin (e.g. herpes, and HPV infection producing warts). The diagnosis is based upon the characteristic histological and cytological features of virus-infected cells, or the presence of characteristic viral inclusions. Electron microscopy can be used to visualize the viral particles. Immunocytochemical methods can also be used on tissue sections to identify certain types of virus, such as some strains of human papillomavirus.

Using microbiological and immunological methods, viral diagnosis can be established early in the course of the illness by fluorescence of viral antigen in smears of infected cells, by isolation in cell culture, and by the detection of virus-specific IgM in the serum.

The detection of antibodies during the period of convalescence enables the virus infection to be diagnosed retrospectively by the demonstration of changing titers of antibody during the illness and subsequent convalescence. For this reason, at least two serum samples need to be taken, one during the illness, and at least one during the convalescence period; the presence of detectable antibody on a single occasion indicates only that the patient has been exposed to the virus in the past. Changing antibody levels are necessary to establish current or recent infection.

Index

anatomy 475–476
diabetes 479, 543
dry-eye syndromes *see* Dry-eye
   syndromes
sarcoidosis 540
sickle-cell disease 322
trauma 482

Fabry's disease 467
Factor V 154, 155, 156
Factor VII 155
Factor VIII 154, 155, 156
Factor IX 155
Factor X 155
Factor XI 155
Factor XII (Hageman factor) 44
   coagulation cascade 155
   endotoxic shock syndrome 114
Fallopian tubes 410–411
   tuberculosis 58
Fallot's tetralogy 61, 187, 188
Familial adenomatous polyposis coli
      71, 95, 102, 260, 261
Familial amyloidosis syndromes 467, 544
Familial hypercholesterolemia 71, 548
Familial juvenile nephronophthisis 382
Familial Mediterranean fever 545
Familial retinoblastoma 102
Fanconi's syndrome 373
Farmer's lung 208
Fasciitis, necrotizing 117, 492
Fas-Fas ligand-mediated apoptosis 18
Fat
   dietary 100
   embolism 159, 441
   metabolism 274
   necrosis 30, 301, 421–422
Fatiguability 472
Fatty streak 162, 163
Felty's syndrome 539
Feminization 346
Fetal alcohol syndrome 146, 456
Fetus
   congenital syphilis 116
   developmental disorders 61–64
Fiber, dietary 100
Fibrillin 166, 479
Fibrin
   acute inflammatory exudate 36, 37, 44
   coagulation cascade 154, 155
   degradation products (FDPs) 155
   thrombus formation 152, 153
Fibrinogen
   acute inflammatory exudate 36, 37, 44
   coagulation cascade 154, 155
Fibrinolysis 152, 155
Fibrinolytic drugs (thrombolytic therapy)
      157, 177
Fibrinopeptides 44
Fibroadenomas 421, 424
Fibroblast growth factor 53, 94
Fibroblasts
   adaptability to environmental change
      9, 32
   hypoxia 32
   surgical wound healing 49
   tissue repair 47–49
   tuberculosis 54
Fibrocytes 49
Fibroelastosis, endocardial 183
Fibrogenesis 50
Fibrohistiocytic lesions 505, 506
Fibroids, uterine 409–410

Fibrolipomas 532
Fibromas 90
   ameloblastic 233
   chondromyxoid 519
   non-ossifying 519
   ovaries 414
   renal 374
   testes 384
Fibromatoses 506
   palmar (Dupuytren's contracture) 506
   plantar 506
Fibronectin 50
Fibro-osseous lesions, orbital 483
Fibrosarcomas 90
Fibrosis
   cirrhosis 279, 293
   endomyocardial 183
   interstitial *see* Interstitial fibrosis
   liver 274, 279, 288
   mammary 423
   muscle 468
   myocardial 176
   parasitic infections 131
   progressive massive 209
   pulmonary *see* Pulmonary fibrosis
   schistosomiasis 136
Fibrothecomas 414
Filiariasis 138
Fine needle aspiration cytology 103, 430
Fish tank granuloma 58
Fissures, anal 268
Fistulas
   anal 268
   tracheo-esophageal 269
Flatworms (cestodes) 130, 136–138
Floppy baby syndrome 469, 472
Flow cytometry 21
Flukes 130, 135–136
Fluorescent *in situ* hybridization (FISH)
      96, 129
Folate deficiency 150
   marrow hypoplasia 323
   megaloblastic anemia 318–319
   post-infective 256
Follicle-stimulating hormone (FSH) 346
   Klinefelter's syndrome 390
   polycystic ovaries 412
Follicular hyperplasia 305, 306
Follicular lymphoma 96, 312
Folliculitis 116
   deep 509
   fungal 491
   superficial 492, 509
Food allergies 109
Food poisoning 118, 248, 255
Foreign bodies
   ears 238, 241
   granulomas 53, 58, 211
Formaldehyde solution 104
Formalin 33
Fournier's gangrene 393
Fractures 141–142, 516–518
   bone cancer 518
   compound 516
   compression 512–513
   healing 516–518
   nasal 234
   osteomalacia 518
   osteoporosis 513
   pathological 215, 515, 518, 519
Fragile-X syndrome 71
Free radicals
   apoptosis 18, 22
   cell damage 23

scavengers 24–25
Fresh-frozen biopsies 104
Friedreich's ataxia 454
Frontal dementias 454
Frontal sinuses, absent 221
Frostbite 142, 143
Fucosidosis 546
Fungal infections 124–126
   acute tubular necrosis 372
   central nervous system 449
   colon 254
   dermatophytic 124–125
   drug addiction 146
   endocarditis 183
   granulomatous inflammation 53
   HIV infection 108
   lungs 198, 199
   lymphadenopathy 307
   myocarditis 182
   nervous system 449
   oral 224
   pneumonia 199
   skin 491–492
   subcutaneous 491–492
   type IV hypersensitivity reactions 110
   vulva 397
Fusobacterium 197, 225

ß-Galactocerebroside deficiency 458
Gallbladder
   calcification (porcelain gallbladder) 299
   carcinoma 300
   cholesterolosis 298
   disease 298–300
   empyema 299
   mucocele 299
Gallstones 298–300
Gamma-glutamyl transpeptidase 291
Gamma-interferon 53
Gammopathy, benign monoclonal 314
Gangliocytomas 463
GanglMAgliogliomas 463
Ganglioneuroblastomas 347
Gangliosidoses 458
Gangrene 151, 166
   acute appendicitis 266
   diabetes mellitus 542
   Fournier's 393
   gas 119, 492
GAP proteins 459
Gardner's syndrome 261
Gardnerella vaginalis 399, 400
Gargoylism 458, 546
Gas gangrene 119, 492
Gastric acid 197
Gastric cancer 252–254
   5-year survival rate 104
   chronic gastritis 100
   dietary factors 101
   early 253–254
   Japan 101
   nitrates/nitrites 100
   nitrosamines 97
Gastrin 346
Gastritis 250–252
   acute 251
   autoimmune (type A) 111
   autoimmune atrophic 319
   autoimmune chronic 251
   chronic 100, 251–252
   erosive 251
   necrotizing ulcerative 251
   reactive (reflux) 251

Teratogens 61
Teratomas 91, 316, 386–388
  nervous system 464
  ovaries 415
  testes 386–388
Terminal transferase (TdT) 313
Terminology 3
Testes 383–390
  atrophy 14
  cancer, 5-year survival rate 104
  choriocarcinoma 389
  development 383
  germ-cell tumors 385–389
  hemorrhagic necrosis 31
  hormone secretion 346–347
  infection 384
  lymphomas 390
  maldescent 383–384, 385
  syphilis 116
  teratomas 386–388
  torsion 160, 383, 384
  tumors 383, 385–390
Testosterone
  depletion 346
  excess 347
  secretion 346
Tetanus (lockjaw) 119
Tetraplegia 443
Thalassemia 73, 320–321
Thalidomide
  anti-angiogenic effects 83
  brain abnormalities 456
  teratogenicity 61, 62
Thecomas 414
Thiamine 150
Thiols 25
Thomsen's disease (autosomal dominant
    myotonia congenita) 473
Thorns 58
Thorotrast 296
Threadworms 139, 267
Thrombasthenia, Glanzmann's 153
Thrombin 154, 155, 161
Thrombocythemia, primary 326, 327
Thrombocytopenia
  autoimmune 112
  idiopathic (ITP) 327
  pernicious anemia 319
  systemic lupus erythematosus 535
Thrombocytosis, reactive 327
Thromboembolism 151, 157–159
  pulmonary 157–158, 191, 193
Thrombolytic pathway 44
Thrombolytic therapy 157, 177
Thrombomodulin 155, 156
Thrombosis 1, 151, 152–157
  acute ischemic heart disease 176–177
  atheroma 164
  bowel 264
  carotid artery 438
  cerebral venous sinus 156
  deep vein 157–158, 178
  fibrinolytic drugs 177
  heart valves 183
  hemorrhoids 268
  hepatic vein 269
  mural 156, 178, 180
  occlusive 156
  oral contraception 156
  organization 157
  pancreatic carcinoma 303
  pathological 153
  portal vein 269, 281
  predisposing factors 156

propagation 157
pulmonary infarction 193, 194
recanalization 157
renal infarcts 355
sagittal sinus 440
systemic lupus erythematosus 535
vegetations 156, 183, 186
venous 151, 156
venous sinus occlusion 160, 439
Thrombospondin (platelet factor 4) 18, 21,
    83
Thromboxane A$_2$ (TXA$_2$)
  acute inflammation 43, 45
  asthma 202
  endothelial secretion 39
  thrombus formation 153
Thrush see Candida albicans
Thymectomy 472
Thymomas 316–317
  myasthenia gravis 472
  ryanodine 473
Thymus gland 316–317
  B-cell lymphomas 316
  diffuse large B-cell lymphoma 313
  hormone secretion 346
  hyperplasia 317
  hypoplasia 106
  involution 14
  lymphomas 316
  myasthenia gravis 111, 316–317, 472
  nodular sclerosing Hodgkin's disease
    316
  precursor T-cell lymphoblastic lymphoma
    315, 316
  severe combined immune deficiency 106
  tumors 316–317
Thyroglobulin (thyroid colloid) 332
Thyroid carcinoma 244, 329, 337–338
  5-year survival rate 104
  adenoma 329, 334, 336–337
  anaplastic 337–338
  follicular 337
  irradiation-related 99
  lymphoma 100, 338
  medullary 91, 338, 347, 545, 546
  papillary 337
Thyroid disease
  cardiomyopathy 181
  orbital swelling 482
  type 2 fiber atrophy myopathy 471
Thyroid gland 329, 332–338
  amyloid 545, 546
  autoimmune disease 111
  benign neoplasm 82
  carcinoma see Thyroid carcinoma
  cysts 246
  disease see Thyroid disease
  enlargement see Goiter
  follicle cells 332
  goiter see Goiter
  hyperplasia 9, 333
  lymphoma 100, 338
  nodular hyperplasia 12
  parafollicular (C) cells 332, 338
  solitary nodules 244, 336–337
Thyroid stimulating hormone (TSH) 330,
    332, 333
Thyroiditis
  autoimmune 333–334, 342
    chronic hepatitis 289
    preneoplastic 100
  de Quervain's (giant-cell; granulomatous)
    333–334
  focal lymphocytic 334

Hashimoto's 106, 111, 112, 329,
    332–336
  lymphomas 316
  primary atrophic 335
  viral 333–334
Thyrotoxicosis 332, 334, 513
Thyroxine (T$_4$) 332–333
Tinea capitis 491
Tinea cruris 491
Tinea unguium 491
Tinnitus 240
Tissue factor 155
Tissue-plasminogen activator (TPA) 155, 177
Tissues
  acute inflammation see Acute
    inflammation
  basic pathological responses 3
  chronic inflammation see Chronic
    inflammation
  collagenous scar 35, 47–49
  healing 46–50
  regeneration 35
  response to environmental change 17
  responses to damage 35–59
  restitution 35
Togaviruses 129, 286
Tonsillitis 117, 233–234
Tonsils, palatine/lingual 232–234
Tophi 526
TORCH 297
Total body irradiation 144
Toxic epidermal necrolysis 497
Toxic shock syndrome 113, 114, 117, 399
Toxins
  central nervous system 455–456
  myocarditis 182
  respiratory tract 191
Toxocara canis 138, 139, 478
Toxocara catis 138, 139
Toxocariasis (larva migrans) 138, 139, 478
Toxoplasma gondii (toxoplasmosis)
    134–135
  acute lymphadenopathic 134
  brain 449, 456
  cerebral abscesses 446
  cervical lymph nodes 245
  choroiditis 478
  congenital 135
  cysts 134
  deafness 241
  encephalitis 134
  HIV infection 108, 134
  lymphadenopathy 134, 306
  ocular (choroidoretinitis) 135
  retinal infection 479
  spontaneous abortion 417
  teratogenicity 61
Tracheobronchitis 121, 191, 194, 197
Tracheo-esophageal fistula 269
Transcription regulatory systems 16
Transferrin 277
Transforming growth factor 50
Transglutaminase 21, 155
Transient ischemic attacks (TIAs) 437
Transitional cell carcinomas 236, 350
Transitional cell papillomas 236
Transitional-cell tumors 378–380
Transplantation
  antigens 111–112
  bone marrow 327
  cornea 478
  heart 186
  hypersensitivity reactions 110
  immune responses 111–112

649

oral 223, 225
peptic 51–52, 247, 252
skin 138, 510
snail track 115, 225
solitary ulcer syndrome 265
stomach 247, 252
varicose 510
venous 510
Ulegyria 457, 458
Ultrasound scanning 4
Ultraviolet radiation 7
skin cancers 99, 143, 485
malignant melanoma 101, 143, 502
Upper respiratory tract 192
infection (URTI) 191, 242
Upper urinary tract see Kidneys
Urachus, persistent 382
Urate crystals
granulomatous inflammation 53, 58
nephropathy 373
Ureaplasma urealyticum 393
Uremia 351, 352, 353
Ureteritis 376
Ureterocele 382
Ureters
colic 378
developmental defects 382
obstruction 377
Urethra, obstruction 377
Urethral valves, posterior 382
Urethritis 376
Chlamydia trachomatis 123, 393
gonococcal 393
non-gonococcal 391, 393
Proteus 119
trichomonas 135
Ureaplasma urealyticum 393
Uric acid
gout 526–527
stones 378
Urinary tract 349–382
calculi 349, 378
carcinoma in situ 379
development 350
developmental diseases 380–382
infection 376
E. coli 119, 376
Enterobacter 119
Klebsiella 119
obstruction 377–378
pregnancy 416
Proteus 119
pyelonephritis 376
Serratia 119
Staphylococcus saprophyticus 117
tumors 378–380
Urinary-type plasminogen activator (uPA) 155
Urolithiasis 378
Urticaria 109, 496–497
Uterus
adenomyosis 405
fibroids 409–410
Uvea 478
Uveitis 478
acute 540
chronic 540
immune-mediated 478
sarcoidosis 540
Uvula, bifid 223

Vagina 399
cancer 99
tumors 399
Vaginitis 135, 399, 400
Valve disease 183–187
endocardial thickening 183
incompetence 183
infection 185–187
mitral see Mitral valve disease
rheumatic fever 183, 184
scarring 184
stenosis 183
structural abnormalities 185
thrombosis 156
tricuspid 185
vegetations see Vegetations
Valvulitis, infective 183
Vanillylmandelic acid (VMA) 343, 348
Varicella see Chickenpox
Varicella-zoster virus (HHV3) 113, 127
Varices
esophageal 172, 250, 280
saphenous veins 172
Varicoceles 172, 383, 384
Varicose ulcers 510
Varicose veins 172
gravitational dermatitis 487, 488, 510
portal hypertension 280
pregnancy 172
Vascular cell adhesion molecule 1 (VCAM-1) 39
Vascular disease
colon 264–265
diabetes mellitus 466
liver 280–281
peripheral 164, 166
peripheral nerve damage 466–467
renal function 354–356
retina 479–480
small intestine 264–265
Vascular endothelial growth factor (VEGF) 83
Vascular tumors/malformations 172–173
Vasculitis 169–171
cerebral 447
connective tissue disease 169, 171, 497
drug-induced 169, 170, 497
Henoch-Schönlein purpura 169, 170
hypersensitivity 169, 170
lymphocytic 170–171, 497, 538
mononeuropathies 467
necrotizing 170–171, 193
neutrophilic (leukocytoclastic) 170, 497
peripheral nerve damage 467
polyarteritis nodosa 467
pulmonary (pulmonary angiitis) 193
rheumatoid arthritis 169, 467, 538
skin 497
systemic 169
systemic lupus erythematosus 169, 171, 467, 497, 534
type III hypersensitivity reactions 110
Vasoactive factors 39
Vasoactive intestinal peptide (VIP) 346
Vasopressin see Antidiuretic hormone
Vasostatin 83
Vegetations 183–184, 186
infective endocarditis 186
marantic 183–184
thrombosis 156, 183, 186
Veins
infarction (hemorrhagic necrosis) 29–30, 31, 160
structural abnormalities 172
thrombosis see Thrombosis
varicose see Varicose veins

Venezuelan encephalitis 448
Venous sinus thrombosis 160, 439
Ventricles
aneurysms 133, 180
thrombosis 156
Ventricular septal defects (VSDs) 61, 187
Verrucas 127, 490
Verrucous carcinoma 244, 398
Vertebrobasilar territory occlusions 439
Vertigo, paroxysmal 240
Vesicles 486, 493
Vesicoureteric reflux 382
Vestibular membrane of Reissner 240
Vestibulocochlear nerve 241
Vibrio cholerae 120, 255
Vinca alkaloids 466
Vinyl chloride 173, 296
Viral infections 126–130
asthma 200
bronchitis 194
cell necrosis 126
cell proliferation 126
central nervous system 447–449
drug addiction 146
encephalitis 433
genetic abnormalities 66
hepatitis 281–286
histological diagnosis 129
inclusion bodies 129
latent 126
liver disease 273
lungs 197
meningitis 447
myocarditis 181
nervous system 447–449
neurons 126
oral 223
pericarditis 182
persistent 126–127
pleura 220
skin 490–491
thyroiditis 333–334
vulva 397
warts 126, 127, 393, 490
Viral oncogenes (v-oncs) 94
Virchow's node 254
Viremia 113
Virilization 347
Viruses
acute-transforming 99
carcinogenesis 99
colon 254
pneumonia 197
slow-transforming 99
type IV hypersensitivity reactions 110
Vitamin A deficiency 150
corneal squamous metaplasia 477
malabsorption 256
squamous metaplasia 16
Vitamin B$_1$ (thiamine) deficiency 150, 455
peripheral neuropathies 466
Vitamin B$_2$ (riboflavine) deficiency 150
Vitamin B$_6$ (pyridoxine) deficiency 150
Vitamin B$_{12}$ (cobalamin) deficiency 150, 455
malabsorption 256
marrow hypoplasia 323
megaloblastic anemia 318
peripheral neuropathies 466
pernicious anemia 251
post-infective 256
tapeworms 137
Vitamin C
deficiency 150
wound healing 50